Pharmacotherapy Handbook

Eleventh Edition

Pharmacotherapy Handbook

Eleventh Edition

Terry L. Schwinghammer, PharmD, FCCP, FASHP, FAPhA
Professor Emeritus, Department of Clinical Pharmacy
School of Pharmacy
West Virginia University
Morgantown, West Virginia

Joseph T. DiPiro, PharmD, FCCP
Professor and Dean
Archie O. McCalley Chair
School of Pharmacy
Virginia Commonwealth University
Richmond, Virginia

Vicki L. Ellingrod, PharmD, FCCP
John Gideon Searle Professor of Pharmacy
Associate Dean for Research and Graduate Education, College of Pharmacy
Professor of Psychiatry, Medical School
University of Michigan
Ann Arbor, Michigan

Cecily V. DiPiro, PharmD
Consultant Pharmacist
Richmond, Virginia

New York   Chicago   San Francisco   Athens   London   Madrid   Mexico City
Milan   New Delhi   Singapore   Sydney   Toronto

Pharmacotherapy Handbook, Eleventh Edition

1 2 3 4 5 6 7 8 9   LCR   25 24 23 22 21

ISBN 978-1-260-11669-4
MHID 1-260-11669-7

This book was set in Minion Pro by MPS Limited.
The editors were Michael Weitz and Peter J. Boyle.
The production supervisor was Catherine H. Saggese.
Project management was provided by Touseen Qadri, MPS Limited.

Cataloging-in-publication data for this book is on file at the Library of Congress.

Contents

Contents

SECTION 6: GYNECOLOGIC AND OBSTETRIC DISORDERS

Edited by Vicki L. Ellingrod

SECTION 7: HEMATOLOGIC DISORDERS

Edited by Cecily V. DiPiro

SECTION 8: INFECTIOUS DISEASES

Edited by Joseph T. DiPiro

SECTION 9: NEUROLOGIC DISORDERS

Edited by Vicki L. Ellingrod

Contents

SECTION 16: UROLOGIC DISORDERS

Edited by Cecily V. DiPiro

APPENDICES

Edited by Terry L. Schwinghammer

Preface

The 11th edition of this companion to *Pharmacotherapy: A Pathophysiologic Approach* is designed to provide practitioners and students with critical information that can be used to guide medication decision-making in collaborative, interprofessional health-care settings. To ensure brevity, clarity, and portability, the bulleted format provides essential textual information, key tables and figures, and treatment algorithms.

Corresponding to the major sections in the *Pharmacotherapy* textbook, medical conditions are alphabetized within the following sections: Bone and Joint Disorders; Cardiovascular Disorders; Dermatologic Disorders; Endocrinologic Disorders; Gastrointestinal Disorders; Gynecologic and Obstetric Disorders; Hematologic Disorders; Infectious Diseases; Neurologic Disorders; Nutrition Support; Oncologic Disorders; Ophthalmic Disorders; Psychiatric Disorders; Renal Disorders; Respiratory Disorders; and Urologic Disorders. The *Handbook* includes nine tabular appendices (four more than the 10th edition) involving pediatric pharmacotherapy, nutrition, and neonatal critical care; geriatric assessment and pharmacotherapy; critical care patient assessment and pharmacotherapy; drug allergy; drug-induced hematologic disorders; drug-induced liver disease; drug-induced pulmonary disease; drug-induced kidney disease; and drug-induced ophthalmic disorders. This edition also includes new chapters on the pharmacists' patient care process, opioid use disorder, and superficial fungal infections.

Each chapter is organized in a consistent format:

- Disease State Definition
- Pathophysiology
- Clinical Presentation
- Diagnosis
- Treatment
- Evaluation of Therapeutic Outcomes

The Treatment section may include goals of treatment, general approach to treatment, nonpharmacologic therapy, drug selection guidelines, dosing recommendations, adverse effects, pharmacokinetic considerations, and important drug-drug interactions. When more in-depth information is required, the reader is encouraged to refer to the corresponding chapter in the primary textbook, *Pharmacotherapy: A Pathophysiologic Approach*, 11th edition. These chapters now provide guidance on application of the pharmacists' patient care process for specific conditions.

The authors gratefully acknowledge Barbara G. Wells, PharmD, FASHP, FCCP, retired Dean Emeritus and Professor Emeritus, School of Pharmacy, The University of Mississippi, for her substantial contributions to the creation, design, and production of all previous editions of this work. Her vision, insight, and passion for the provision of patient-centered medication therapy are evident throughout the pages of the *Handbook*. In addition, this edition of the *Handbook* is dedicated to the memory of her late husband, Richard M. Wells: pharmacist, colleague, and friend.

It is our hope that students and practitioners find this book to be helpful on their daily journey to provide the highest quality individualized, patient-centered care. We invite your comments on how we may improve subsequent editions of this work.

Terry L. Schwinghammer
Joseph T. DiPiro
Vicki L. Ellingrod
Cecily V. DiPiro

Please provide your comments about this book, Schwinghammer et al., *Pharmacotherapy Handbook*, 11th edition, to its authors and publisher by writing to userservices@mheducation.com. Please indicate the author and title of this handbook in the subject line of your e-mail.

The Patient Care Process

INTRODUCTION

Health professionals who provide direct patient care are often called *practitioners*. Health professionals *practice* when they use their unique knowledge and skills to serve patients. A healthcare practice is not a physical location or simply a list of activities. Rather, a professional practice requires three essential elements: (1) a philosophy of practice, (2) a process of care, and (3) a practice management system.

A *practice philosophy* is the moral purpose and commonly held set of values that guides the profession. It is the critical foundation on which the practices of pharmacy, medicine, nursing, and dentistry are built. Although the concept of pharmaceutical care is not formally included in the code of ethics for the pharmacy profession or the oath of a pharmacist, pharmacists understand that they have a unique responsibility for addressing the drug-related needs of patients and should be held accountable for preventing, identifying, and resolving drug therapy problems.

The *patient care process* is a fundamental series of actions that guide the activities of health professionals. In 2014, the Joint Commission for Pharmacy Practitioners (JCPP)—representing 11 national pharmacy organizations—endorsed a framework for providing clinically oriented patient care services called the Pharmacists' Patient Care Process. This process includes five essential steps: (1) collecting subjective and objective information about the patient; (2) assessing the collected data to identify problems, determine the adequacy of current treatments, and set priorities; (3) creating an individualized care plan that is evidence-based and cost-effective; (4) implementing the care plan; and (5) monitoring the patient over time during follow-up encounters to evaluate the effectiveness of the plan and modify it as needed (**Fig. 1**). In addition to the five fundamental steps, a patient-centered approach to decision making is essential.

A *practice management system* is necessary to support the efficient and effective delivery of services, including physical, financial, and human resources with policies and procedures to carry out the work of patient care.

This chapter provides a brief summary of the patient care process applied to drug therapy management and the practice management issues influencing adoption and application of this process by pharmacists.

IMPORTANCE OF A STANDARD CARE PROCESS

The stimulus for developing the patient care process for pharmacy was the wide variation observed as pharmacists provided direct patient care, often using the same terminology to describe diverse services or, conversely, using different terminology to describe the same service. Without a consistent patient care process, it has been challenging for the pharmacy profession to communicate the pharmacist's role to external groups and establish the distinct value pharmacists bring to an interprofessional care team. Moreover, the patient must know and understand what is to be delivered to determine how best to receive the care provided. Likewise, other members of the healthcare team must determine how best to integrate the pharmacist's work into their efforts caring for the patient. A process of care must be built on a set of fundamental steps that can address the wide range of complexity that exists among patients. The process needs to be adaptable to varied settings, diverse populations, and different acuity levels.

FIGURE 1. **The pharmacists' patient care process.** *Joint Commission of Pharmacy Practitioners. Pharmacists' Patient Care Process. May 29, 2014.* Available at: https://jcpp.net/wp-content/uploads/2016/03/PatientCareProcess-with-supporting-organizations.pdf. Reprinted with permission.

THE PATIENT CARE PROCESS TO OPTIMIZE PHARMACOTHERAPY

The application or focus of a profession-specific process of care depends upon the profession's knowledge and expertise. For pharmacy, the patient care process is focused on patient medication-related needs and experience with medication therapy. Each health profession then addresses patient needs by assessing patient-specific information in a unique manner. For pharmacists providing comprehensive medication management (CMM), the assessment step involves a systematic examination of the *indication, effectiveness, safety,* and *adherence* for each of the patient's medications. This is a unique way of approaching a patient's health needs; no other discipline applies a systematic assessment process to medications and the medication experience in this manner.

The pharmacists' patient care process is standardized and is not specific to a care setting—it can be applied wherever CMM is performed. However, the type of information collected, its sources, and the duration of time to complete the process may vary depending on the practice setting and acuity of care. The subsequent sections in this chapter briefly describe the steps in the patient care process for pharmacists.

COLLECT PATIENT-SPECIFIC INFORMATION

Collect relevant subjective and objective information about the patient and analyze the data to understand the medical/medication history and clinical status of the patient. Information from the health record may include patient demographics, active medical problem list, admission and discharge notes, office visit notes, laboratory values, diagnostic tests, and medication lists. Conduct a comprehensive medication review with the patient that also includes alcohol, tobacco and caffeine use; immunization status; allergies; and adverse drug effects. Ask whether the patient has questions or concerns for the visit. Document a complete medication list that includes all prescription and nonprescription medications as well as dietary supplements the patient is taking (ie, name, indication, strength and formulation, dose, frequency, duration, and response to medication). Gather past medication history, if pertinent. Collect information about the patient's medication experience (eg, beliefs, expectations, and cultural considerations related to medications) and personal goals of therapy. Ask about the patient's ability to access medications, manage medications at home, adhere to the therapy, and use medications appropriately. Gather additional important information (eg, physical assessment findings, review of systems, home-monitored blood glucose, blood pressure readings).

ASSESS INFORMATION AND FORMULATE A MEDICATION THERAPY PROBLEM LIST

Analyze the information collected to formulate a problem list consisting of the patient's active medical problems and medication therapy problems in order to prioritize medication therapy recommendations that achieve the patient's health goals. Assess the *indication* of each medication the patient is taking, including the presence of an appropriate indication; consider also whether the patient has an untreated medical condition that requires therapy. Assess the *effectiveness* of each medication, including progress toward achieving therapeutic goals; optimal selection of drug product, dose, and duration of therapy; and need for additional laboratory data to monitor medication response. Assess the *safety* of each medication by identifying adverse events; excessive doses; availability of safer alternatives; pertinent drug-disease, drug-drug, or drug-food interactions; and need for additional laboratory data to monitor medication safety. Assess *adherence* and the patient's ability to take each medication (eg, administration, access, affordability). Ensure that medication administration times are appropriate and convenient for the patient. From all of this information, formulate and prioritize a medication therapy problem list, classifying the patient's medication therapy problems based on indication, effectiveness, safety, and adherence (Table 1).

TABLE 1	Medication Therapy Problem Categories Framework
Medication-Related Needs	**Medication Therapy Problem Category**
Indication	Unnecessary medication therapy
	Needs additional medication therapy
Effectiveness	Ineffective medication
	Dosage too low
	Needs additional monitoring
Safety	Adverse medication event
	Dosage too high
	Needs additional monitoring
Adherence	Adherence
	Cost

Pharmacy Quality Alliance. PQA Medication Therapy Problem Categories Framework. August 2017. Available at: https://www.pqaalliance.org/assets/Measures/PQA%20MTP%20Categories%20 Framework.pdf.

DEVELOP THE CARE PLAN

Working in collaboration with other healthcare professionals and the patient or caregiver, develop an individualized, patient-centered care plan that is evidence based and affordable for the patient. Design the plan to manage the patient's active medical conditions and resolve the identified medication therapy problems. Coordinate care with the primary care provider and other healthcare team members to reach consensus on the proposed care plan, when needed. Identify the monitoring parameters necessary to assess effectiveness, safety, and adherence, including frequency of follow-up monitoring. Design personalized education and interventions for the patient, and reconcile all medication lists (eg, from the medical record, patient, pharmacy) to arrive at an accurate and updated medication list. Determine who will implement components of the care plan (ie, patient, clinical pharmacist, other providers). Decide on the appropriate time frame and mode for patient follow-up (eg, phone, face-to-face).

IMPLEMENT THE CARE PLAN

Implement the care plan in collaboration with other healthcare professionals and the patient or caregiver. Discuss the care plan with the patient, educate the patient about the medications and goals of therapy, make sure the patient understands and agrees with the plan, and implement recommendations that are within your scope of practice. For recommendations that cannot be independently implemented, communicate the care plan to the rest of the team, indicating where input is required by other team members. Document the encounter in the health record (eg, assessment, medication therapy care plan, rationale, monitoring, and follow-up). Arrange patient follow-up based on the determined time frame and communicate follow-up instructions with the patient.

FOLLOW-UP WITH THE PATIENT

Provide targeted follow-up and monitoring (whether in person, electronically, or via phone) to assess the effectiveness and safety of the care plan. Modify the plan when needed in collaboration with other team members and the patient or caregiver to achieve patient and clinical goals of therapy. Plan for a CMM follow-up visit at least once within a year of the initial visit, and repeat all steps of the patient care process at that time to ensure continuity of care and ongoing medication optimization. Refer the patient back to the provider (and document accordingly) if all medication therapy problems have been resolved, no new problems are identified, and it is determined that the patient no longer needs CMM services.

PRACTICE MANAGEMENT ISSUES

A practice management system is essential to the care process and includes the metrics to ensure patient health outcomes are being achieved; efficient workflow; communication and documentation using the power of information technology (IT); and data that accurately reflect the attribution and value the practitioner brings to patient care.

QUALITY METRICS

The patient care process sets a standard of achievable performance by defining the parameters of the process that can be measured. With the movement toward outcome-based healthcare models and value-based payment systems, it is critical to objectively measure the impact a patient care service has on a patient's health and well-being. For the process to be measurable, each element must be clearly defined and performed in a similar manner during each patient encounter. The lack of clarity and consistency has hindered collection of robust evidence to support the value of pharmacists' patient care services. The standard patient care process gives pharmacists an opportunity to show value on a large scale because the services are comparable and clearly understood across practice settings.

WORKFLOW, DOCUMENTATION, AND INFORMATION SYSTEMS

Healthcare systems are rapidly embracing the power of technology to analyze information and gain important insights about the health outcomes being achieved. The uniform patient care process sets a standard for the practice workflow that allows IT systems to capture and extract data for analysis and sharing. The ability to capture clinical data is currently available through a number of coding systems, such as the International Classification of Diseases 10th edition (ICD-10) and the Systematized Nomenclature of Medicine—Clinical Terms (SNOMED-CT). Practitioners need to understand how coding systems operate behind the scenes when performing and documenting their clinical activities. This will enable practitioners to assist information technologists to effectively design systems to accurately document the elements of the process that can produce the data on medication-related outcomes.

DOCUMENTATION, ATTRIBUTION, AND PAYMENT

Payment to healthcare providers for patient care services in the United States has traditionally been based on the documentation and reporting of standard processes of care. Rules and guidance from Medicare and the Centers for Medicare and Medicaid Services (CMS) are considered the billing and payment standard for healthcare providers both for governmental and commercial payers. Reporting the complexity of care provided is built on top of the documentation requirements; complexity is determined by the number of required elements in each documentation domain. A billing code is then assigned to the patient encounter that equates to a payment commensurate with the level of care provided. This process is the basis for the current fee-for-service payment structure, and it is likely that this general format will remain in any future payment model. The traditional SOAP (Subjective, Objective, Assessment, Plan) note format is often used by pharmacists when documenting patient care and is particularly appropriate when providing services incident to an eligible Medicare Part B provider. However, some elements of the SOAP note that are required when using certain billing codes are not routinely performed by pharmacists (eg, comprehensive physical examination). The pharmacists' patient care process establishes a standard framework that reflects the pharmacist's work. Using a standard care process accompanied with a standard documentation framework will result in efficiencies of practice, enable appropriate and accurate billing, and facilitate the attribution of care to desired patient outcomes needed in value-based payment models.

See Chapter 1, The Patient Care Process, authored by Stuart T. Haines, Mary Ann Kliethermes, and Todd D. Sorensen for a more detailed discussion of this topic.

1

Gout and Hyperuricemia

- *Gout* involves hyperuricemia, recurrent attacks of acute arthritis with monosodium urate (MSU) crystals in synovial fluid leukocytes, deposits of MSU crystals in tissues in and around joints (tophi), interstitial kidney disease, and uric acid nephrolithiasis.

Acute Gouty Arthritis

PATHOPHYSIOLOGY

- Uric acid is the end product of purine degradation. An increased urate pool in individuals with gout may result from overproduction or underexcretion.
- Purines originate from dietary purine, conversion of tissue nucleic acid to purine nucleotides, and de novo synthesis of purine bases.
- Overproduction of uric acid may result from abnormalities in enzyme systems that regulate purine metabolism (eg, increased activity of phosphoribosyl pyrophosphate [PRPP] synthetase or deficiency of hypoxanthine-guanine phosphoribosyl transferase [HGPRT]).
- Uric acid may also be overproduced because of increased breakdown of tissue nucleic acids, as with myeloproliferative and lymphoproliferative disorders. Cytotoxic drugs can result in overproduction of uric acid due to lysis and the breakdown of cellular matter.
- Dietary purines are insignificant in generating hyperuricemia without some derangement in purine metabolism or elimination.
- Two-thirds of uric acid produced daily is excreted in urine. The remainder is eliminated through gastrointestinal (GI) tract after degradation by colonic bacteria. Decline in urinary excretion to a concentration below the rate of production leads to hyperuricemia and an increased pool of sodium urate.
- Drugs that decrease renal uric acid clearance include diuretics, nicotinic acid, salicylates (<2 g/day), ethanol, pyrazinamide, levodopa, ethambutol, cyclosporine, and cytotoxic drugs.
- Deposition of urate crystals in synovial fluid results in inflammation, vasodilation, increased vascular permeability, complement activation, and chemotactic activity for polymorphonuclear leukocytes. Phagocytosis of urate crystals by leukocytes results in rapid lysis of cells and discharge of proteolytic enzymes into cytoplasm. The ensuing inflammatory reaction causes intense joint pain, erythema, warmth, and swelling.
- Uric acid nephrolithiasis occurs in ~10% of patients with gout. Predisposing factors include excessive urinary excretion of uric acid, acidic urine (pH <6), and highly concentrated urine.
- In acute uric acid nephropathy, acute kidney injury occurs because of blockage of urine flow from massive precipitation of uric acid crystals in collecting ducts and ureters. Chronic urate nephropathy is caused by long-term deposition of urate crystals in the renal parenchyma.
- Tophi (urate deposits) are uncommon and are a late complication of hyperuricemia. The most common sites are the base of the fingers, olecranon bursae, ulnar aspect of forearm, Achilles tendon, knees, wrists, and hands.

CLINICAL PRESENTATION

- Acute gout attacks are characterized by rapid onset of excruciating pain, swelling, and inflammation. The attack is typically monoarticular, most often affecting the first metatarsophalangeal joint (podagra), and then, in order of frequency, the insteps, ankles, heels, knees, wrists, fingers, and elbows. Attacks commonly begin at night, with the patient awakening with excruciating pain. Affected joints are erythematous, warm, and swollen. Fever and leukocytosis are common. Untreated attacks last from 3 to 14 days before spontaneous recovery.

- Acute attacks may occur without provocation or be precipitated by stress, trauma, alcohol ingestion, infection, surgery, rapid lowering of serum uric acid by uric acid-lowering agents, and ingestion of drugs known to elevate serum uric acid concentrations.

DIAGNOSIS

- Definitive diagnosis requires aspiration of synovial fluid from the affected joint and identification of intracellular crystals of MSU monohydrate in synovial fluid leukocytes.
- When joint aspiration is not feasible, a presumptive diagnosis is based on presence of characteristic signs and symptoms as well as the response to treatment.

TREATMENT

- <u>Goals of Treatment</u>: Terminate the acute attack, prevent recurrent attacks, and prevent complications associated with chronic deposition of urate crystals in tissues.

NONPHARMACOLOGIC THERAPY

- Local ice application is the most effective adjunctive treatment.
- Dietary supplements (eg, flaxseed, cherry, celery root) are not recommended.

PHARMACOLOGIC THERAPY (FIG. 1-1)

- Most patients are treated successfully with nonsteroidal anti-inflammatory drugs (NSAIDs), corticosteroids, or colchicine. Treatment should begin as soon as possible after the onset of an attack.

NSAIDS

- NSAIDs have excellent efficacy and minimal toxicity with short-term use. Indomethacin, naproxen, and sulindac have Food and Drug Administration (FDA) approval for gout, but others are likely to be effective (Table 1-1).
- Start therapy within 24 hours of attack onset and continue until complete resolution (usually 5–8 days). Tapering may be considered after resolution, especially if comorbidities such as impaired hepatic or kidney function make prolonged therapy undesirable.
- The most common adverse effects involve the GI tract (gastritis, bleeding, and perforation), kidneys (renal papillary necrosis, reduced glomerular filtration rate), cardiovascular system (increased blood pressure, sodium and fluid retention), and central nervous system (impaired cognitive function, headache, and dizziness).
- Selective cyclooxygenase-2 inhibitors (eg, celecoxib) may be an option for patients unable to take nonselective NSAIDs, but the risk-to-benefit ratio in acute gout is unclear, and cardiovascular risk must be considered.

Corticosteroids

- Corticosteroid efficacy is equivalent to NSAIDs; they can be used systemically or by intra-articular (IA) injection. If only one or two joints are involved, either IA or oral corticosteroids are recommended. Systemic therapy is necessary for polyarticular attacks.
- **Prednisone** or **prednisolone** oral dosing strategies include (1) 0.5 mg/kg daily for 5–10 days followed by abrupt discontinuation, or (2) 0.5 mg/kg daily for 2–5 days followed by tapering for 7–10 days. Tapering is often used to reduce the hypothetical risk of a rebound attack upon steroid withdrawal.
- **Methylprednisolone dose pack** is a 6-day regimen starting with 24 mg on day 1 and decreasing by 4 mg each day that may be considered.
- **Triamcinolone acetonide** 20–40 mg given by IA injection may be used if gout is limited to one or two joints; give 10–40 mg IA (large joints) or 5–20 mg IA (small joints). IA corticosteroids should be used with an oral NSAID, colchicine, or corticosteroid therapy.

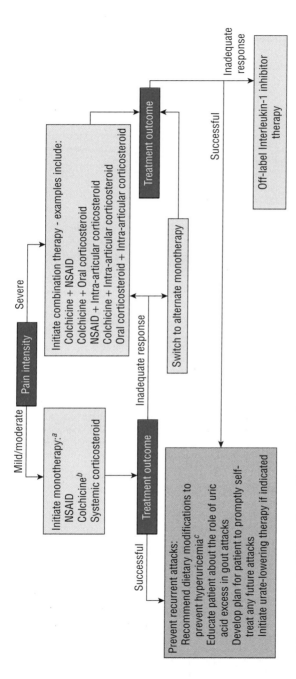

a) Recommendation for initial monotherapy with one of these medication groups supported unanimously by guidelines of the American College of Rheumatology (ACR), European League Against Rheumatism (EULAR), and American College of Physicians (ACP)

b) Colchicine should be started as soon as possible, ideally within 12-36 hours of pain onset

c) Noted as an area of inconclusive evidence by 2017 ACP guidelines

(Algorithm derived from 2017 ACP, 2016 EULAR, and 2012 ACR gout guidelines.)

FIGURE 1-1. Algorithm for management of an acute gout attack.

TABLE 1-1	Dosage Regimens of Oral Nonsteroidal Anti-inflammatory Drugs for Treatment of Acute Gout	
Generic Name	**Initial Dose**	**Usual Range**
Etodolac	300 mg twice daily	300–500 mg twice daily
Fenoprofen	400 mg three times daily	400–600 mg three to four times daily
Ibuprofen	400 mg three times daily	400–800 mg three to four times daily
Indomethacin	50 mg three times daily	50 mg three times daily initially until pain is tolerable then rapidly reduce to complete cessation
Ketoprofen	75 mg three times daily or 50 mg four times daily	50–75 mg three to four times daily
Naproxen	750 mg followed by 250 mg every 8 hours until the attack has subsided	—
Piroxicam	20 mg once daily or 10 mg twice daily	—
Sulindac	200 mg twice daily	150–200 mg twice daily for 7–10 days
Meloxicam	5 mg once daily	7.5–15 mg once daily
Celecoxib	800 mg followed by 400 mg on day one, then 400 mg twice daily for 1 week	—

- **Methylprednisolone** (a long-acting corticosteroid) given by a single intramuscular (IM) injection followed by a short course of oral corticosteroid therapy is another reasonable approach. Alternatively, IM corticosteroid monotherapy may be considered in patients with multiple affected joints who cannot take oral therapy.
- Short-term corticosteroid use is generally well tolerated. Use with caution in patients with diabetes, GI problems, bleeding disorders, cardiovascular disease, and psychiatric disorders. Avoid long-term use because of risk for osteoporosis, hypothalamic–pituitary–adrenal axis suppression, cataracts, and muscle deconditioning.
- **Adrenocorticotropic hormone (ACTH) gel:** 40–80 USP units IM every 6–8 hours for 2 or 3 days and then discontinued. Limit use to patients with contraindications to first-line therapies (eg, heart failure, chronic kidney disease, and history of GI bleeding) or patients unable to take oral medications. However, the high drug price excludes ACTH as a viable treatment option.

Colchicine

- **Colchicine** is highly effective in relieving acute gout attacks; when it is started within the first 24 hours of onset, about two-thirds of patients respond within hours. Use only within 36 hours of attack onset because the likelihood of success decreases substantially if treatment is delayed.
- Colchicine causes dose-dependent GI adverse effects (nausea, vomiting, and diarrhea). Non-GI effects include neutropenia and axonal neuromyopathy, which may be worsened in patients taking other myopathic drugs (eg, statins) or with impaired kidney function. Use colchicine with caution in patients taking P-glycoprotein or strong CYP450 3A4 inhibitors (eg, clarithromycin) due to increased plasma colchicine levels and potential toxicity; colchicine dose reductions may be required. Also use colchicine with caution in patients with impaired kidney or hepatic function.
- **Colcrys** is an FDA-approved colchicine product available in 0.6 mg oral tablets. The recommended dose is 1.2 mg (two tablets) initially, followed by 0.6 mg (one tablet) 1 hour later. Although not an FDA-approved regimen, the American College of Rheumatology (ACR) gout treatment guidelines suggest that colchicine 0.6 mg once or

twice daily can be started 12 hours after the initial 1.2-mg dose and continued until the attack resolves. Colchicine is also available generically.

Hyperuricemia In Gout

- Recurrent gout attacks can be prevented by maintaining low uric acid levels, but adherence with nonpharmacologic and pharmacologic therapies is poor.

NONPHARMACOLOGIC THERAPY

- Patient education should address the recurrent nature of gout and the objective of each lifestyle/dietary modification and medication.
- Promote weight loss through caloric restriction and exercise in all patients to enhance renal urate excretion.
- Alcohol restriction is important because consumption correlates with gout attacks. ACR guidelines recommend limiting alcohol use in all gout patients and avoidance of any alcohol during periods of frequent gout attacks and in patients with advanced gout under poor control.
- Dietary recommendations include limiting consumption of high-fructose corn syrup and purine-rich foods (organ meats and some seafood) and encouraging consumption of vegetables and low-fat dairy products. The DASH diet (Dietary Approaches to Stop Hypertension) may lower serum uric acid by ~1.0 mg/dL in hyperuricemic patients who are adherent. However, no studies have demonstrated that dietary intervention improves clinical outcomes such as reduction in gout flares.
- Evaluate the medication list for potentially unnecessary drugs that may elevate uric acid levels. The ACR guidelines recommend elimination of nonessential uric acid-elevating medications in patients with hyperuricemia when feasible (eg, thiazide and loop diuretics, calcineurin inhibitors, niacin). Low-dose aspirin for cardiovascular prevention should be continued because aspirin has a negligible effect on elevating serum uric acid.

PHARMACOLOGIC THERAPY (FIG. 1-2)

- After the first attack of acute gout, prophylactic pharmacotherapy is recommended if patients have two or more attacks per year, even if serum uric acid is normal or only minimally elevated. Other indications include presence of tophi, kidney disease, or history of uric acid urolithiasis.
- Urate-lowering therapy can be started during an acute attack if anti-inflammatory prophylaxis has been initiated.
- Apply a stepwise approach to hyperuricemia (**Fig.** 1-2). Xanthine oxidase inhibitors are recommended first-line therapy, with uricosurics reserved for patients with a contraindication or intolerance to xanthine oxidase inhibitors. In refractory cases, combination therapy with a xanthine oxidase inhibitor plus a drug with uricosuric properties (probenecid, losartan, or fenofibrate) is suggested. Pegloticase may be used in severe cases in which the patient cannot tolerate or is not responding to other therapies.
- The ACR guideline goal of urate-lowering therapy is to achieve and maintain serum uric acid <6 mg/dL (357 μmol/L), and preferably <5 mg/dL (297 μmol/L) if gout is severe or signs and symptoms of gout persist. Urate lowering should be prescribed for long-term use.

Xanthine Oxidase Inhibitors

- Xanthine oxidase inhibitors reduce uric acid by impairing conversion of hypoxanthine to xanthine and xanthine to uric acid. Because they are effective in both overproducers and underexcretors of uric acid, they are the most widely prescribed agents for long-term prevention of recurrent gout attacks.
- **Allopurinol** lowers uric acid levels in a dose-dependent manner. ACR guidelines recommend a starting dose no greater than 100 mg daily in patients with normal kidney function and no more than 50 mg/day in patients with chronic kidney disease (stage 4 or worse) to avoid allopurinol hypersensitivity syndrome and prevent acute gout attacks common during initiation of urate-lowering therapy. The dose should be titrated gradually every 2–5 weeks up to a maximum of 800 mg/day until the serum urate target is achieved.

a) Indications for urate-lowering therapy include: 1) presence of tophus 2) ≥ 2 gout attacks per year 3) kidney disease 4) past urolithiasis. EULAR, but not ACR or ACP Guidelines, also recognize the following indications for ULT: 1) first diagnosis of gout at age < 40 years 2) uric acid > 8.0 mg/dL 3) high-risk comorbidities (hypertension, ischemic heart disease, hear failure)

b) Recognized as first line by ACR Guidelines but cardiovascular safety concerns have been reported since guideline publication

c) EULAR Guidelines also recognize calcium channel blockers and statins as add-on therapy for uric acid lowering when indicated for treatment of comorbidities

d) The effectiveness of dietary intervention in improving clinical outcomes is noted as an area of inconclusive evidence by 2017 ACP guidelines

e) Targeting and maintaining a specific urate level is noted as an area of inconclusive evidence by 2017 ACP guidelines

NSAID, nonsteroidal anti-inflammatory drug; ULT, urate-lowering therapy; XOI, xanthine oxidase inhibitor. (Algorithm derived from 2017 ACP, 2016 EULAR, and 2012 ACR gout guidelines.)

FIGURE 1-2. Algorithm for management of hyperuricemia in gout.

- Mild adverse effects of allopurinol include skin rash, leukopenia, GI problems, headache, and urticaria. A more severe adverse reaction known as allopurinol hypersensitivity syndrome, which includes severe rash (toxic epidermal necrolysis, erythema multiforme, or exfoliative dermatitis), hepatitis, interstitial nephritis, and eosinophilia, occurs rarely but is associated with a 20%–25% mortality rate.
- **Febuxostat** (Uloric) also lowers serum uric acid in a dose-dependent manner. The recommended starting dose is 40 mg once daily. Increase the dose to 80 mg once daily for patients who do not achieve target serum uric acid concentrations after 2 weeks of therapy. Adverse events include nausea, arthralgias, and minor hepatic transaminase elevations. Febuxostat does not require dose adjustment in hepatic or kidney dysfunction. Recent clinical trial evidence demonstrated an increase in all-cause and cardiovascular mortality compared to allopurinol, resulting in addition of a warning in the FDA-approved labeling. Because of these safety concerns, lack of evidence of superior efficacy compared to equivalent-dosed allopurinol, and increased cost, febuxostat is considered a second-line option. Due to rapid mobilization of urate deposits during initiation, give concomitant therapy with colchicine or an NSAID for at least the first 8 weeks of therapy to prevent acute gout flares.

Uricosurics

- Uricosuric drugs increase renal clearance of uric acid by inhibiting the postsecretory renal proximal tubular reabsorption of uric acid. Patients with a history of urolithiasis should not receive uricosurics. Start uricosuric therapy at a low dose to avoid marked uricosuria and possible stone formation. Maintaining adequate urine flow and urine alkalinization during the first several days of therapy may also decrease likelihood of uric acid stone formation. Uricosuric treatment is limited to patients with creatinine clearance (CrCl) >45–50 mL/min.
- **Probenecid:** The initial dose is 250 mg twice daily for 1–2 weeks, then 500 mg twice daily for 2 weeks. Increase the daily dose thereafter by 500-mg increments every 1–2 weeks until satisfactory control is achieved or a maximum dose of 2 g/day is reached. Major side effects include GI irritation, rash and hypersensitivity, precipitation of acute gouty arthritis, and urolithiasis.
- **Lesinurad** (Zurampic) inhibits urate transporter 1 in proximal renal tubules, thereby increasing uric acid excretion. It is approved as combination therapy with a xanthine oxidase inhibitor for treatment of hyperuricemia associated with gout in patients who have not achieved target serum uric acid concentrations with xanthine oxidase inhibitor monotherapy. The approved lesinurad dose is 200 mg once daily in the morning with food and water in combination with a xanthine oxidase inhibitor. Lesinurad should not be used in patients with CrCl <45 mL/min. Adverse effects include urticaria and elevated levels of serum creatinine, lipase, and creatine kinase. It carries a black box warning about increased risk of acute renal failure when used in the absence of xanthine oxidase inhibitor therapy. A combination product (Duzallo) is available that contains two different allopurinol strengths: lesinurad 200 mg/allopurinol 200 mg (for patients with CrCl 45–59 mL/min) and lesinurad 200 mg/allopurinol 300 mg (for patients with CrCl >59 mL/min).

Pegloticase

- **Pegloticase** (Krystexxa) is a pegylated recombinant uricase that reduces serum uric acid by converting uric acid to allantoin, which is water soluble. Pegloticase is indicated for antihyperuricemic therapy in adults refractory to conventional therapy.
- The dose is 8 mg by IV infusion over at least 2 hours every 2 weeks. Because of potential infusion-related allergic reactions, patients must be pretreated with antihistamines and corticosteroids. Pegloticase is substantially more expensive than first-line urate-lowering therapies.
- The ideal duration of pegloticase therapy is unknown. Development of pegloticase antibodies resulting in loss of efficacy may limit the duration of effective therapy.
- Because of its limitations, reserve pegloticase for patients with refractory gout who are unable to take or have failed all other urate-lowering therapies.

Miscellaneous Urate-Lowering Agents

- **Fenofibrate** is thought to increase clearance of hypoxanthine and xanthine, leading to a sustained reduction in serum urate concentrations of 20%–30%.
- **Atorvastatin** and **rosuvastatin** have also been associated with serum uric acid lowering, although the effect is less than with fenofibrate. The mechanism is unclear but is thought to be due to decreased renal reabsorption of uric acid.
- **Losartan** inhibits renal tubular reabsorption of uric acid and increases urinary excretion, properties that are not shared with other angiotensin II receptor blockers. It also alkalinizes the urine, which helps reduce the risk for stone formation.
- **Amlodipine**, **nifedipine**, and **diltiazem** (calcium channel blockers) have been associated with a lower risk of gout, which has been attributed to increased renal elimination of uric acid.

ANTI-INFLAMMATORY PROPHYLAXIS DURING INITIATION OF URATE-LOWERING THERAPY

- Initiation of urate-lowering therapy can precipitate an acute gout attack due to remodeling of urate crystal deposits in joints after rapid lowering of urate concentrations. Prophylactic anti-inflammatory therapy is often used to prevent such gout attacks.
- The ACR guidelines recommend low-dose oral colchicine (0.6 mg twice daily) or low-dose NSAIDs (eg, naproxen 250 mg twice daily) as first-line prophylactic therapies, with stronger evidence supporting use of colchicine. For patients on long-term NSAID prophylaxis, a proton pump inhibitor or other acid-suppressing therapy is indicated to protect from NSAID-induced gastric problems.
- Low-dose corticosteroid therapy (eg, prednisone $\leq$10 mg/day) is an alternative for patients with intolerance, contraindication, or lack of response to first-line therapy. The potential severe adverse effects of prolonged corticosteroid therapy preclude their use as first-line therapy.
- Continue prophylaxis for at least 6 months or 3 months after achieving target serum uric acid, whichever is longer. For patients with one or more tophi, continue prophylactic therapy for 6 months after achieving the serum urate target (**Fig. 1-2**).

EVALUATION OF THERAPEUTIC OUTCOMES

- Check the serum uric acid level in patients suspected of having an acute gout attack, particularly if it is not the first attack, and a decision is to be made about starting prophylaxis. However, acute gout can occur with normal serum uric acid concentrations.
- Monitor patients with acute gout for symptomatic relief of joint pain as well as potential adverse effects and drug interactions related to drug therapy. Acute pain of an initial gout attack should begin to ease within about 8 hours of treatment initiation. Complete resolution of pain, erythema, and inflammation usually occurs within 48–72 hours.
- For patients receiving urate-lowering therapy, obtain baseline assessment of kidney function, hepatic enzymes, complete blood count, and electrolytes. Recheck the tests every 6–12 months in patients receiving long-term treatment.
- During titration of urate-lowering therapy, monitor serum uric acid every 2–5 weeks; after the urate target is achieved, monitor uric acid every 6 months.
- Because of the high rates of comorbidities associated with gout (diabetes, chronic kidney disease, hypertension, obesity, myocardial infarction, heart failure, and stroke), elevated serum uric acid concentrations or gout should prompt evaluation for cardiovascular disease and the need for appropriate risk reduction measures. Clinicians should also look for possible correctable causes of hyperuricemia (eg, medications, obesity, malignancy, and alcohol abuse).

See Chapter 109, Gout and Hyperuricemia, authored by Michelle A. Fravel and Michael E. Ernst, for a more detailed discussion of this topic.

CHAPTER 2

Osteoarthritis

- *Osteoarthritis* (OA) is a common, progressive disorder affecting primarily weight-bearing diarthrodial joints, characterized by progressive destruction of articular cartilage, osteophyte formation, pain, limitation of motion, deformity, and disability.

PATHOPHYSIOLOGY

- *Primary (idiopathic) OA*, the more common type, has no known cause.
- *Secondary OA* is associated with a known cause such as inflammation, trauma, metabolic or endocrine disorders, and congenital factors.
- OA usually begins with damage to articular cartilage through injury, excessive joint loading from obesity or other reasons, or joint instability. Damage to cartilage increases activity of chondrocytes in attempt to repair damage, leading to increased synthesis of matrix constituents with cartilage swelling. Normal balance between cartilage breakdown and resynthesis is lost, with increasing destruction and cartilage loss.
- Subchondral bone adjacent to articular cartilage undergoes pathologic changes and releases vasoactive peptides and matrix metalloproteinases. Neovascularization and increased permeability of adjacent cartilage occur, which contribute to cartilage loss and chondrocyte apoptosis.
- Cartilage loss causes joint space narrowing and painful, deformed joints. Remaining cartilage softens and develops fibrillations, followed by further cartilage loss and exposure of underlying bone. New bone formations (osteophytes) at joint margins distant from cartilage destruction are thought to help stabilize affected joints.
- Inflammatory changes can occur in the joint capsule and synovium. Crystals or cartilage shards in synovial fluid may contribute to inflammation. Interleukin-1, prostaglandin E_2, tumor necrosis factor-α, and nitric oxide in synovial fluid may also play a role. Inflammatory changes result in synovial effusions and thickening.
- Pain may result from distention of the synovial capsule by increased joint fluid; microfracture; periosteal irritation; or damage to ligaments, synovium, or the meniscus.

CLINICAL PRESENTATION

- Risk factors include increasing age, obesity, sex, certain occupations and sports activities, history of joint injury or surgery, and genetic predisposition.
- The predominant symptom is deep, aching pain in affected joints. Pain accompanies joint activity and decreases with rest.
- Joints most commonly affected are the distal interphalangeal (DIP) and proximal interphalangeal (PIP) joints of the hand, first carpometacarpal joint, knees, hips, cervical and lumbar spine, and first metatarsophalangeal (MTP) joint of the toe.
- Limitation of motion, stiffness, crepitus, and deformities may occur. Patients with lower extremity involvement may report weakness or instability.
- Upon arising, joint stiffness typically lasts less than 30 minutes and resolves with motion.
- Presence of warm, red, and tender joints suggests inflammatory synovitis.
- Physical examination of affected joints reveals tenderness, crepitus, and possibly enlargement. Heberden and Bouchard nodes are bony enlargements (osteophytes) of the DIP and PIP joints, respectively.

DIAGNOSIS

- Diagnosis is made through patient history, physician examination, radiologic findings, and laboratory testing.
- American College of Rheumatology criteria for classification of OA of the hips, knees, and hands include presence of pain, bony changes on examination, normal erythrocyte sedimentation rate (ESR), and radiographs showing osteophytes or joint space narrowing.
- For hip OA, patients must have hip pain and two of the following: (1) ESR <20 mm/hr (5.6 μm/sec), (2) radiographic femoral or acetabular osteophytes, and/or (3) radiographic joint space narrowing.
- For knee OA, patients must have knee pain and radiographic osteophytes in addition to one or more of the following: (1) age >50 years, (2) morning stiffness lasting ≤30 minutes, (3) crepitus on motion, (4) bony enlargement, (5) bony tenderness, and/or (6) palpable joint warmth.
- ESR may be slightly elevated if inflammation is present. Rheumatoid factor is negative. Analysis of synovial fluid reveals high viscosity and mild leukocytosis (<2000 white blood cells/mm³ [2×10^9/L]) with predominantly mononuclear cells.

TREATMENT

- <u>Goals of Treatment</u>: (1) Educate the patient, family members, and caregivers; (2) relieve pain and stiffness; (3) maintain or improve joint mobility; (4) limit functional impairment; and (5) maintain or improve quality of life.

NONPHARMACOLOGIC THERAPY

- Educate the patient about the disease process and extent, prognosis, and treatment options. Promote dietary counseling, exercise, and a weight loss program for overweight patients.
- Physical therapy—with heat or cold treatments and an exercise program—helps maintain range of motion and reduce pain and need for analgesics.
- Assistive and orthotic devices (canes, walkers, braces, heel cups, and insoles) can be used during exercise or daily activities.
- Surgical procedures (eg, osteotomy, arthroplasty, joint fusion) are indicated for functional disability and/or severe pain unresponsive to conservative therapy.

PHARMACOLOGIC THERAPY (TABLE 2-1)

General Approach

- Drug therapy is targeted at relief of pain. A conservative approach is warranted because OA often occurs in older individuals with other medical conditions.
- Apply an individualized approach (Figs. 2-1 and 2-2). Continue appropriate nondrug therapies when initiating drug therapy.

Knee and Hip OA

- **Acetaminophen** is a preferred first-line treatment; it may be less effective than oral nonsteroidal anti-inflammatory drugs (NSAIDs) but has a lower risk of serious gastrointestinal (GI) and cardiovascular (CV) events. Acetaminophen is usually well tolerated, but potentially fatal hepatotoxicity with overdose is well documented. It should be avoided in chronic alcohol users or patients with liver disease.
- **Nonselective NSAIDs** or **cyclooxygenase-2 (COX-2) selective inhibitors** (eg, **celecoxib**) are recommended if a patient fails acetaminophen. Nonselective NSAIDs may cause minor GI complaints such as nausea, dyspepsia, anorexia, abdominal pain, and diarrhea. They may cause gastric and duodenal ulcers and bleeding through direct (topical) or indirect (systemic) mechanisms. Risk factors for NSAID-associated ulcers and ulcer complications (perforation, gastric outlet obstruction, and GI bleeding) include longer duration of NSAID use, higher dosage, age older than

TABLE 2-1 Medications for the Treatment of Osteoarthritis		
Drug	**Starting Dose**	**Usual Range**
Oral analgesics		
Acetaminophen	325–500 mg three times a day	325–650 mg every 4–6 hours or 1 g three to four times/day
Tramadol	25 mg in the morning	Titrate dose in 25-mg increments to reach a maintenance dose of 50–100 mg three times a day
Tramadol ER	100 mg daily	Titrate to 200–300 mg daily
Hydrocodone/ acetaminophen	5 mg/325 mg three times daily	2.5–10 mg/325–650 mg three to five times daily
Oxycodone/acetaminophen	5 mg/325 mg three times daily	2.5–10 mg/325–650 mg three to five times daily
Topical analgesics		
Capsaicin 0.025%–0.15%		Apply to affected joint three to four times per day
Diclofenac 1% gel		Apply 2 or 4 g per site as prescribed, four times daily
Diclofenac 1.3% patch		Apply one patch twice daily to the site to be treated, as directed
Diclofenac 1.5% solution		Apply 40 drops to the affected knee, applying and rubbing in 10 drops at a time. Repeat for a total of four times daily.
Intra-articular corticosteroids		
Triamcinolone	5–15 mg per joint	10–40 mg per large joint (knee, hip, shoulder)
Methylprednisolone acetate	10–20 mg per joint	20–80 mg per large joint (knee, hip, shoulder)
NSAIDs		
Aspirin (plain, buffered, or enteric-coated)	325 mg three times a day	325–650 mg four times a day
Celecoxib	100 mg daily	100 mg twice daily or 200 mg daily
Diclofenac IR	50 mg twice a day	50–75 mg twice a day
Diclofenac XR	100 mg daily	100–200 mg daily
Diflunisal	250 mg twice a day	500–750 mg twice a day
Etodolac	300 mg twice a day	400–500 mg twice a day
Fenoprofen	400 mg three times a day	400–600 mg three to four times a day
Flurbiprofen	100 mg twice a day	200–300 mg/day in two to four divided doses

(Continued)

TABLE 2-1	Medications for the Treatment of Osteoarthritis *(Continued)*	
Drug	**Starting Dose**	**Usual Range**
Ibuprofen	200 mg three times a day	1200–3200 mg/day in three to four divided doses
Indomethacin	25 mg twice a day	Titrate dose by 25–50 mg/day until pain controlled or maximum dose of 50 mg three times a day
Indomethacin SR	75 mg SR once daily	Can titrate to 75 mg SR twice daily if needed
Ketoprofen	50 mg three times a day	50–75 mg three to four times a day
Meclofenamate	50 mg three times a day	50–100 mg three to four times a day
Mefenamic acid	250 mg three times a day	250 mg four times a day
Meloxicam	7.5 mg daily	15 mg daily
Nabumetone	500 mg daily	500–1000 mg one to two times a day
Naproxen	250 mg twice a day	500 mg twice a day
Naproxen sodium	220 mg twice a day	220–550 mg twice a day
Naproxen sodium CR	750–1000 mg once daily	500–1500 mg once daily
Oxaprozin	600 mg daily	600–1200 mg daily
Piroxicam	10 mg daily	20 mg daily
Salsalate	500 mg twice a day	500–1000 mg two to three times a day

CR, controlled-release; ER, extended-release; IR, immediate-release; SR, sustained-release; XR, extended-release.

60 years, past history of peptic ulcer disease of any cause, history of alcohol use, and concomitant use of glucocorticoids or anticoagulants. Options for reducing the GI risk of nonselective NSAIDs include using (1) the lowest dose possible and only when needed, (2) misoprostol four times daily with the NSAID, and (3) a PPI or full-dose H_2-receptor antagonist daily with the NSAID.

• COX-2 inhibitors pose less risk for adverse GI events than nonselective NSAIDs, but this advantage is substantially reduced for patients taking aspirin. Both nonselective and selective NSAIDs are associated with an increased risk for CV events (hypertension, stroke, myocardial infarction, and death).

• NSAIDs may also cause kidney diseases, hepatitis, hypersensitivity reactions, rash, and CNS complaints of drowsiness, dizziness, headaches, depression, confusion, and tinnitus. NSAIDs inhibit COX-1–dependent thromboxane production in platelets, thereby increasing bleeding risk. Unlike aspirin, celecoxib and nonspecific NSAIDs inhibit thromboxane formation reversibly, with normalization of platelet function 1–3 days after drug discontinuation. Avoid NSAIDs in late pregnancy because of risk of premature closure of the ductus arteriosus. The most potentially serious drug interactions include use of NSAIDs with lithium, warfarin, oral hypoglycemics, methotrexate, antihypertensives, angiotensin-converting enzyme inhibitors, β-blockers, and diuretics.

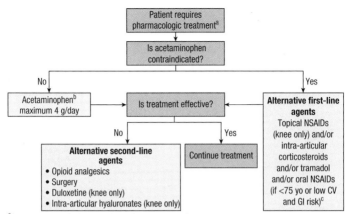

aSelection of a medication should consider patient-specific characteristics.
bThe patient must be counseled regarding all acetaminophen-containing products.
cWhen used for chronic management of OA, consider addition of a proton-pump inhibitor.

(CV, cardiovascular; GI, gastrointestinal; NSAID, nonsteroidal anti-inflammatory drug.)

FIGURE 2-1. Treatment recommendations for hip and knee osteoarthritis.

- **Topical NSAIDs** are recommended for knee OA if acetaminophen fails, and they are preferred over oral NSAIDs in patients older than 75 years. Topical NSAIDs provide similar pain relief with fewer adverse GI events than oral NSAIDs but may be associated with adverse events at the application site (eg, dry skin, pruritus, and rash). Patients using topical products should avoid oral NSAIDs to minimize the potential for additive side effects. Use of topical NSAIDs has not been linked with increased risk of CV events.
- **Intra-articular (IA) corticosteroid injections** are recommended for both hip and knee OA when analgesia with acetaminophen or NSAIDs is suboptimal. They can provide excellent pain relief, particularly when joint effusion is present. Local anesthetics such as lidocaine or bupivacaine are commonly combined with corticosteroids to provide rapid pain relief. Injections may also be given with concomitant oral analgesics for additional pain control. After aseptic aspiration of the effusion and corticosteroid injection, initial pain relief may occur within 24–72 hours, with peak relief occurring after 7–10 days and lasting for 4–8 weeks. Local adverse effects can include infection, osteonecrosis, tendon rupture, and skin atrophy at the injection site. Do not administer injections more frequently than once every 3 months to minimize systemic adverse effects. Systemic corticosteroid therapy is not recommended in OA, given lack of proven benefit and well-known adverse effects with long-term use.
- **Tramadol** is recommended for hip and knee OA in patients who have failed scheduled full-dose acetaminophen and topical NSAIDs, who are not appropriate candidates for oral NSAIDs, and who are not able to receive IA corticosteroids. Tramadol can be added to partially effective acetaminophen or oral NSAID therapy. Tramadol is associated with opioid-like adverse effects such as nausea, vomiting, dizziness, constipation, headache, and somnolence. However, tramadol is not associated with life-threatening GI bleeding, CV events, or renal failure. The most serious adverse event is seizures. Tramadol is classified as a Schedule IV controlled substance due to its potential for dependence, addiction, and diversion. There is increased risk of serotonin syndrome when tramadol is used with other serotonergic medications, including duloxetine.
- **Opioids** should be considered in patients not responding adequately to nonpharmacologic and first-line pharmacologic therapies. Patients who are at high surgical risk and cannot undergo joint arthroplasty are also candidates for opioid therapy. Use opioid analgesics in the lowest effective dose and the smallest quantity needed. Avoid combinations of opioids and sedating medications whenever possible.

^aSelection of a medication should consider patient-specific characteristics.
^bWhen used for chronic management of OA, consider addition of a proton-pump inhibitor.
^cShould not combine topical NSAIDs and oral NSAIDs.

(CV, cardiovascular; GI, gastrointestinal; NSAID, nonsteroidal anti-inflammatory drug.)

FIGURE 2-2. Treatment recommendations for hand osteoarthritis.

Inform patients on how to use, store, and dispose of opioid medications. Sustained-release compounds usually offer better pain control throughout the day. Common adverse effects include nausea, somnolence, constipation, dry mouth, and dizziness. Opioid dependence, addiction, tolerance, hyperalgesia, and issues surrounding drug diversion may be associated with long-term treatment. Assess opioid use at least every 3 months, evaluating patient progression toward functional treatment goals, risks of harm, and adverse effects.

- **Duloxetine** can be used as adjunctive treatment of knee (not hip) OA in patients with partial response to first-line analgesics (acetaminophen, oral NSAIDs). It may be a preferred second-line medication in patients with both neuropathic and musculoskeletal OA pain. Pain reduction occurs after about 4 weeks of therapy. Duloxetine may cause nausea, dry mouth, constipation, anorexia, fatigue, somnolence, and dizziness. Serious rare events include Stevens-Johnson syndrome and liver failure. Concomitant use with other medications that increase serotonin concentration (including tramadol) increases risk of serotonin syndrome.

- **IA hyaluronic acid** (sodium hyaluronate) is not routinely recommended because injections have shown limited benefit for knee OA and have not been shown to benefit hip OA. Injections are usually well tolerated, but acute joint swelling, effusion, stiffness, and local skin reactions (eg, rash, ecchymoses, or pruritus) have been reported. IA preparations and regimens for OA knee pain include:
  ✓ **Cross-linked hyaluronate 30 mg/3 mL** (Gel-One) single injection
  ✓ **Hyaluronan 30 mg/2 mL** (Orthovisc) once weekly for three injections
  ✓ **Hyaluronan 88 mg/4 mL** (Monovisc) single injection

✓ **Hylan polymers 16 mg/2 mL** (Synvisc) once weekly for three injections
✓ **Hylan polymers 48 mg/6 mL** (Synvisc-One) single injection
✓ **Sodium hyaluronate 20 mg/2 mL** (Hyalgan) once weekly for five injections
✓ **Sodium hyaluronate 20 mg/2 mL** (Euflexxa) once weekly for three injections
✓ **Sodium hyaluronate 25 mg/2.5 mL** (Supartz FX) once weekly for five injections
✓ **Sodium hyaluronate 25 mg/2.5 mL** (GenVisc 850) once weekly for five injections

- **Glucosamine and/or chondroitin** and **topical rubefacients** (eg, **methyl salicylate, trolamine salicylate**) lack uniform improvement in pain control or functional status for hip and knee pain and are not preferred treatment options. Glucosamine adverse effects are mild and include flatulence, bloating, and abdominal cramps. The most common adverse effect of chondroitin is nausea.

Hand OA

- **Topical NSAIDs** are a first-line option for hand OA. Topical diclofenac has efficacy similar to oral NSAIDs with fewer adverse GI events, albeit with some local application site events. Efficacy with topical NSAIDs typically occurs with 1–2 weeks.
- **Oral NSAIDs** are an alternative first-line treatment for patients who cannot tolerate the local skin reactions or who received inadequate relief from topical NSAIDs.
- **Capsaicin cream** is an alternative first-line treatment; small clinical trials have demonstrated about 50% reduction in pain scores. It is a reasonable option for patients unable to take oral NSAIDs. Capsaicin must be used regularly to be effective, and it may require up to 2 weeks to take effect. Adverse effects are primarily local and include burning, stinging, and/or erythema that usually subsides with repeated application. Warn patients not to get cream in their eyes or mouth and to wash hands after application. Application of the cream, gel, solution, or lotion is recommended four times daily.
- **Tramadol** is an alternative first-line treatment and is a reasonable option for patients who do not respond to topical therapy and are not candidates for oral NSAIDs because of high GI, CV, or renal risks. Tramadol may also be used in combination with partially effective acetaminophen, topical therapy, or oral NSAIDs.

EVALUATION OF THERAPEUTIC OUTCOMES

- To monitor efficacy, assess baseline pain with a visual analog scale, and assess range of motion for affected joints with flexion, extension, abduction, or adduction.
- Depending on the joint(s) affected, measurement of grip strength and 50-ft walking time can help assess hand and hip/knee OA, respectively.
- Baseline radiographs can document extent of joint involvement and follow disease progression with therapy.
- Other measures include the clinician's global assessment based on patient's history of activities and limitations caused by OA, the Western Ontario and McMaster Universities Arthrosis Index, Stanford Health Assessment Questionnaire, and documentation of analgesic or NSAID use.
- Ask patients about adverse effects from medications. Monitor for signs of drug-related effects, such as skin rash, headaches, drowsiness, weight gain, or hypertension from NSAIDs.
- Obtain baseline serum creatinine, hematology profile, and serum transaminases with repeat levels at 6- to 12-month intervals to identify specific toxicities to the kidney, liver, GI tract, or bone marrow.

See Chapter 106, Osteoarthritis, authored by Lucinda M. Buys and Sara A. Wiedenfeld, for a more detailed discussion of this topic.

Osteoporosis

CHAPTER 3

- *Osteoporosis* is a bone disorder characterized by low bone density, impaired bone architecture, and compromised bone strength predisposing to fracture.

PATHOPHYSIOLOGY

- Bone loss occurs when resorption exceeds formation, usually from high bone turnover when the number or depth of bone resorption sites greatly exceeds the ability of osteoblasts to form new bone. Accelerated bone turnover can increase the amount of immature bone that is not adequately mineralized.
- Men and women begin to lose bone mass starting in the third or fourth decade because of reduced bone formation. Estrogen deficiency during menopause increases osteoclast activity, increasing bone resorption more than formation. Men are at a lower risk for developing osteoporosis and osteoporotic fractures because of larger bone size, greater peak bone mass, increase in bone width with aging, fewer falls, and shorter life expectancy. Male osteoporosis results from aging or secondary causes.
- Age-related osteoporosis results from hormone, calcium, and vitamin D deficiencies; decreased production or function of cytokines; decreased body water; less exercise; and other factors that result in accelerated bone turnover and reduced osteoblast formation.
- Drug-induced osteoporosis may result from systemic corticosteroids, excessive thyroid hormone replacement, antiepileptic drugs (eg, phenytoin, phenobarbital), depot medroxyprogesterone acetate, and other agents.

CLINICAL PRESENTATION

- Many patients are unaware that they have osteoporosis and only present after fracture. Fractures can occur after bending, lifting, or falling or independent of any activity.
- The most common fractures involve vertebrae, proximal femur, and distal radius (wrist or Colles fracture). Vertebral fractures may be asymptomatic or present with moderate to severe back pain that radiates down a leg. Pain usually subsides after 2–4 weeks, but residual back pain may persist. Multiple vertebral fractures decrease height and sometimes curve the spine (kyphosis or lordosis).
- Patients with a nonvertebral fracture frequently present with severe pain, swelling, and reduced function and mobility at the fracture site.

DIAGNOSIS

- The FRAX tool uses the following risk factors to predict the percent probability of fracture in the next 10 years: age, race/ethnicity, sex, previous fragility fracture, parent history of hip fracture, body mass index, glucocorticoid use, current smoking, alcohol ($\geq$3 drinks per day), rheumatoid arthritis, and select secondary causes with femoral neck or total hip bone mineral density (BMD) data optional.
- The Garvan calculator uses four risk factors (age, sex, low-trauma fracture, and falls) with the option to also use BMD. It calculates 5- and 10-year risk estimates of any osteoporotic/fragility fracture and hip fracture. This tool corrects some disadvantages of FRAX because it includes falls and number of previous fractures, but it does not use as many other risk factors.
- Physical examination findings may include bone pain, postural changes (ie, kyphosis), and loss of height (>1.5 in [3.8 cm]).

- Laboratory testing: complete blood count, serum creatinine, calcium, phosphorus, electrolytes, alkaline phosphatase, albumin, thyroid-stimulating hormone, total testosterone (for men), 25-hydroxyvitamin D, and 24-hour urine concentrations of calcium and phosphorus.
- Measurement of central (hip and spine) BMD with dual-energy x-ray absorptiometry (DXA) is the diagnostic standard. Measurement at peripheral sites (forearm, heel, and finger) with DXA or quantitative ultrasonography is used only for screening and for determining need for further testing.
- A T-score compares the patient's BMD to the mean BMD of a healthy, young (20- to 29-year-old), sex-matched, white reference population. The T-score is the number of standard deviations from the mean of the reference population.
- Diagnosis of osteoporosis is based on low-trauma fracture or femoral neck, total hip, and/or spine DXA using World Health Organization (WHO) T-score thresholds. Normal bone mass is T-score above −1, low bone mass (osteopenia) is T-score between −1 and −2.4, and osteoporosis is T-score at or below −2.5.

TREATMENT

- <u>Goals of Treatment</u>: The primary goal of osteoporosis care is prevention. Optimizing peak bone mass when young reduces the future incidence of osteoporosis. After low bone mass or osteoporosis develops, the objective is to stabilize or improve bone mass and strength and prevent fractures. Goals in patients with osteoporotic fractures include reducing pain and deformity, improving function, reducing falls and fractures, and improving quality of life.
- **Figure 3-1** provides an osteoporosis management algorithm for postmenopausal women and men ages 50 and older.

NONPHARMACOLOGIC THERAPY

- All individuals should have a balanced diet with adequate intake of **calcium** and **vitamin D** (**Table 3-1**). Achieving daily calcium requirements from calcium-containing foods is preferred.
  - ✓ Consumers can calculate the amount of calcium in a food serving by adding a zero to the percentage of the daily value on food labels. One serving of milk (8 oz or 240 mL) has 30% of the daily value of calcium; this converts to 300 mg of calcium per serving.
  - ✓ To calculate the amount of vitamin D in a food serving, multiply the percent daily value of vitamin D listed on the food label by 4. For example, 20% vitamin D = 80 units.
- Protein is required for bone formation; the recommended dietary allowance (RDA) is 0.8 g/kg body weight per day for adults, increasing to 1–1.2 g/kg body weight in older adults.
- Alcohol consumption should not exceed 1–2 drinks per day for women and 2–3 drinks per day for men.
- Ideally, caffeine intake should be limited to 2 or fewer servings per day.
- Smoking cessation helps optimize peak bone mass, minimize bone loss, and ultimately reduce fracture risk.
- Weight-bearing aerobic and strengthening exercises can decrease risk of falls and fractures by improving muscle strength, coordination, balance, and mobility.
- Fall prevention programs that are multifactorial can decrease falls, fractures, other injuries, and nursing home and hospital admissions.
- Vertebroplasty and kyphoplasty involve injection of cement into fractured vertebra(e) for patients with debilitating pain from compression fractures. Although intended to stabilize damaged vertebrae, reduce pain, and decrease opioid intake, recent research demonstrated only short-term benefit with no major pain relief and the potential for post-procedure complications.

Presence of a low-trauma fracture (vertebrae or hip) → **No** →
- Woman ≥65 years of age
- Man ≥70 years of age
- Postmenopausal woman <65 years of age with a FRAX 10-year major osteoporotic fracture score >8.4%
- Man 50 to 69 years old with clinical risk factors for fracture[a]
- Abnormal peripheral BMD test
- Radiographic evidence of low bone mass
- Medical conditions or medications known to increase the risk for bone loss and fracture (eg, rheumatoid arthritis, glucocorticoids ≥3 months, certain chemotherapies)

Yes (from fracture box, down)

Yes (from clinical risk factors box, down) → Send for central DXA testing

Presence of a low-trauma fracture — Yes branch:
- Evaluate for secondary causes
- Bone healthy lifestyle[b]
- Dietary calcium 1,000 to 1,200 mg daily[c]
- Vitamin D at least 800 to 1,000 units daily
- Medication therapy[d] – treatment dosed
  - First line: alendronate, risedronate, zoledronic acid or denosumab
  - Alternate therapy: abaloparatide,[e] ibandronate, raloxifene,[f] romosozumab,[e] or teriparatide[g]
  - Last line: intranasal calcitonin

  Obtain baseline central BMD testing for monitoring response to therapy.

  Re-evaluate BMD using central DXA in 2 to 5 years

Normal BMD
T-score ≥ –1.0
- Bone healthy lifestyle[b]
- Dietary calcium 1,000 to 1,200 mg daily[c]
- Vitamin D 800 to 1,000 units daily

  Re-evaluate BMD using central DXA in 5 years or as appropriate

Low bone mass
T-score –1.1 to –2.4 at femoral neck or spine AND a FRAX 10-year probability of hip fracture ≤3% or all major osteoporosis-related fracture ≤20%[h]
- Bone healthy lifestyle[b]
- Dietary calcium 1,000 to 1,200 mg daily[c]
- Vitamin D 800 to 1,000 units daily
- Medication therapy – prevention doses
  - Considered if risk factors exist
  - Generally not for women who are or are considering pregnancy

  Re-evaluate BMD using central DXA in ≥2 years or as appropriate

Osteoporosis or high fracture risk
T-score ≤–2.5 at femoral neck or spine OR T-score –1.1 to –2.4 at femoral neck or spine AND a FRAX 10-year probability of hip fracture ≥3% or all major osteoporosis-related fracture ≥20%[h]
- Evaluate for secondary causes
- Bone healthy lifestyle[b]
- Dietary calcium 1,000 to 1,200 mg daily[c]
- Vitamin D at least 800 to 1,000 units daily
- Medication therapy[d] – treatment doses
  - First line: alendronate, risedronate, zoledronic acid or denosumab
  - Alternate therapy: abaloparatide,[e] ibandronate, raloxifene,[f] romosozumab,[e] or teriparatide[g]
  - Last line: intranasal calcitonin

  Re-evaluate BMD using central DXA in 2 to 5 years or as appropriate

[a]Major clinical risk factors for fracture: current smoker, low body weight or body mass index, personal history of fracture as an adult (after age 50 years), history of osteoporosis/low trauma fracture in a first-degree relative, excessive alcohol intake.

[b]Bone-healthy lifestyle includes well-balanced diet with adequate calcium, vitamin D, and protein intakes; smoking cessation; limited alcohol intake; weight-bearing/resistance exercises; and fall prevention.

[c]Dietary calcium preferred. If diet is inadequate, supplement as necessary.

[d]Sometimes men with hypogonadism also receive testosterone replacement; sometimes women with menopausal symptoms receive low-dose hormone therapy for a short time.

[e]Newer agents marketed after osteoporosis guidelines published; similar uses as teriparatide.

[f]Raloxifene can be a good option in women at high risk for breast cancer.

[g]Teriparatide can be considered a first-line option in patients with a very high risk of fracture (e.g, multiple low trauma fractures) or intolerant to other medications.

[h]Some providers use age-adjusted FRAX thresholds versus set thresholds for all age groups.

(BMD, bone mineral density; DXA, dual-energy x-ray absorptiometry; FRAX, World Health Organization Fracture Risk Assessment Tool.)

FIGURE 3-1. **Algorithm for the management of osteoporosis in postmenopausal women and men aged 50 and older.**

TABLE 3-1	Calcium and Vitamin D Recommended Dietary Allowances (RDAs) and Tolerable Upper Intake Levels (ULs)				
Group and Ages	**Elemental Calcium RDA (mg)**	**Calcium Tolerable Upper Intake Level (mg)**	**Vitamin D RDA (Units)[a]**	**Vitamin D Tolerable Upper Intake Level (Units)**
Infants				
Birth–6 months	200[b]	1000	400[b]	1000
7–12 months	260[b]	1500	400[b]	1500
Children				
1–3 years	700	2500	600	2500
4–8 years	1000	2500	600	3000
9–18 years	1300	3000	600	4000
Adults				
19–50 years	1000	2500	600[b,c]	4000
51–70 years (men)	1000	2000	600[b,c]	4000
51–70 years (women)	1200	2000	600[b,c]	4000
>70 years	1200	2000	800[b,c]	4000

[a]Some guidelines recommend intake to achieve a 25(OH) vitamin D concentration >30 ng/mL (mcg/L; 75 nmol/L), which is higher than the Institute of Medicine goal of >20 ng/mL (mcg/L; 50 nmol/L).
[b]Adequate intake (evidence insufficient to determine an RDA).
[c]Guidelines recommend 800–1000 units or 1000–2000 units for adults with osteoporosis.

PHARMACOLOGIC THERAPY

GENERAL APPROACH

- Combined with adequate calcium and vitamin D intakes, alendronate, risedronate, zoledronic acid, and denosumab are the prescription medications of choice because they reduce both hip and vertebral fracture risks.
- Abaloparatide, bazedoxifene/conjugated equine estrogens, ibandronate, raloxifene, romosozumab, and teriparatide are second-line alternatives because they decrease vertebral but not hip fracture risks.
- Calcitonin is last-line therapy.
- Estrogen and testosterone are not used for osteoporosis treatment but can have a positive bone effect when prescribed for other conditions.

ANTIRESORPTIVE THERAPY

Calcium Supplementation

- Calcium generally maintains or increases BMD slightly, but its effects are less than those of other therapies. There are insufficient data to support using calcium and vitamin D supplementation to reduce fracture incidence. Because the fraction of calcium absorbed decreases with increasing dose, maximum single doses of 600 mg or less of elemental calcium are recommended.
- **Calcium carbonate** is the salt of choice because it contains the highest concentration of elemental calcium (40%) and is typically least expensive. It should be ingested with meals to enhance absorption in an acidic environment.

- **Calcium citrate** (21% calcium) has acid-independent absorption and need not be taken with meals. It may have fewer GI side effects than calcium carbonate.
- **Tricalcium phosphate** contains 38% calcium, but calcium-phosphate complexes could limit overall calcium absorption. It may be useful in patients with hypophosphatemia that cannot be resolved with increased dietary intake.
- Constipation is the most common calcium-related adverse reaction; treat with increased water intake, dietary fiber (given separately from calcium), and exercise. Calcium carbonate can sometimes cause flatulence or upset stomach. Calcium causes kidney stones rarely.
- Calcium can decrease the oral absorption of some drugs including iron, tetracyclines, quinolones, bisphosphonates, and thyroid supplements.

Vitamin D Supplementation

- **Vitamin D** supplementation using 700–800 units per day has been shown to significantly reduce the incidence of both hip and nonvertebral fractures with small increases in BMD.
- Supplementation is usually provided with daily nonprescription cholecalciferol (vitamin D_3) products. Higher-dose prescription ergocalciferol (vitamin D_2) regimens given weekly, monthly, or quarterly may be used for replacement and maintenance therapy. The RDAs in Table 3-1 should be achieved through food and supplementation.
- Current guidelines recommend treating patients with osteoporosis to a 25-hydroxyvitamin D concentration of at least 30 ng/mL (mcg/L; 75 nmol/L) or 30–50 ng/mL.
- Because the half-life of vitamin D is about 1 month, recheck the vitamin D concentration after about 3 months of therapy.
- Medications that can induce vitamin D metabolism include rifampin, phenytoin, barbiturates, valproic acid, and carbamazepine. Vitamin D absorption can be decreased by cholestyramine, colestipol, orlistat, and mineral oil. Vitamin D can enhance the absorption of aluminum; therefore, aluminum-containing products should be avoided to prevent aluminum toxicity.

Bisphosphonates

- Bisphosphonates (Table 3-2) mimic pyrophosphate, an endogenous bone resorption inhibitor. Therapy leads to decreased osteoclast maturation, number, recruitment, bone adhesion, and life span. Incorporation into bone gives bisphosphonates long biologic half-lives of up to 10 years.
- Bisphosphonates consistently increase BMD and reduce fracture risk, with differences in sites of fracture reduction among agents. Ibandronate is not a first-line therapy because of the lack of hip fracture reduction data.
- BMD increases are dose dependent and greatest in the first 12 months of therapy. After discontinuation, the increased BMD is sustained for a prolonged period that varies per bisphosphonate.
- **Alendronate, risedronate,** and **IV zoledronic acid** are Food and Drug Administration (FDA) indicated for postmenopausal, male, and glucocorticoid-induced osteoporosis. **IV and oral ibandronate** are indicated only for postmenopausal osteoporosis. Weekly alendronate, weekly and monthly risedronate, and monthly oral and quarterly IV ibandronate therapy produce equivalent BMD changes to their respective daily regimens.
- Oral bisphosphonates must be administered correctly to optimize clinical benefit and minimize adverse GI effects. Each oral tablet should be taken in the morning with at least 6 oz (180 mL) of plain water (not coffee, juice, mineral water, or milk) at least 30 minutes (60 minutes for oral ibandronate) before consuming any food, supplements, or medications. An exception is delayed-release risedronate, which is administered immediately after breakfast with at least 4 oz (120 mL) of plain water. The patient should remain upright (sitting or standing) for at least 30 minutes after alendronate and risedronate and 1 hour after ibandronate to prevent esophageal irritation and ulceration.

TABLE 3-2 Medications Used to Prevent and Treat Osteoporosis

Drug	Brand Name	Dose	Comments
Antiresorptive Medications—Nutritional Supplements			
Calcium	Various	*Adequate daily intake:* IOM: 200–1200 mg/day, varies per age); supplement dose is difference between required adequate intake and dietary intake. Immediate-release doses should be <500–600 mg.	Recommend food first to achieve goal intake. Available in different salts including carbonate and citrate, absorption of other salts not fully quantified. Different formulations including chewable, liquid, gummy, softgel, drink, and wafer; different combination products. Review package to determine number of units to create a serving size and desired amount of elemental calcium. Give calcium carbonate with meals to improve absorption.
Vitamin D D₃ (cholecalciferol) D₂ (ergocalciferol)	Over the counter: Tablets, 400, 1000, and 2000 units Capsule, 400, 1000, 2000, 5000, and 10,000 units Gummies, 300, 500, 1000 units Drops 300, 400, 1000, and 2000 units/mL or drop Solution, 400 and 5000 units/mL Spray 1000 and 5000 units/spray Creams and lotions 500 and 1000 units per ¼ teaspoonful Prescription: Capsule, 50,000 units Solution, 8000 units/mL	Adequate daily intake: IOM: 400–800 units/day to achieve adequate intake; NOF: 800–1000 units orally daily; if low 25(OH) vitamin D concentrations, malabsorption, or altered metabolism higher doses (>2000 units daily) might be required. *Vitamin D deficiency:* 50,000 units orally once to twice weekly for 8–12 weeks; repeat as needed until therapeutic concentrations.	Vegetarians and vegans need to read label to determine if a plant-based product. Slight advantage of D₃ over D₂ for increasing serum 25(OH) vitamin D concentrations. For drops, make sure measurement is correct for desired dose. Ability of sprays, lotions, and creams to resolve deficiencies or maintain adequate intakes is unknown.

(continued)

TABLE 3-2 Medications Used to Prevent and Treat Osteoporosis *(Continued)*

Drug	Brand Name	Dose	Comments
Antiresorptive Prescription Medications			
Bisphosphonates			
Alendronate	Fosamax Fosamax Plus D Binosto (effervescent tab)	Treatment: 10 mg orally daily or 70 mg orally weekly Prevention: 5 mg orally daily or 35 mg orally weekly	Generic available for weekly tablet product. 70 mg dose is available as a tablet, effervescent tablet, oral liquid or combination tablet with 2800 or 5600 units of vitamin D_3. Administered in the morning on an empty stomach with 6–8 ounces of plain water. Do not eat and remain upright for at least 30 minutes following administration. Do not coadminister with any other medication or supplements, including calcium and vitamin D.
Ibandronate	Boniva	Treatment: 150 mg orally monthly, 3 mg IV quarterly Prevention: 150 mg orally monthly	Generic available for oral product. Administration instructions same as for alendronate, except must delay eating and remain upright for at least 60 minutes.
Risedronate	Actonel Atelvia (delayed-release)	Treatment and prevention: 5 mg orally daily, 35 mg orally weekly, 150 mg orally monthly	Generic available for immediate-release product. 35 mg dose is also available as a delayed-release product. Administration instructions same as for alendronate, except delayed-release product is taken immediately following breakfast.

Zoledronic acid	Reclast	Treatment: 5 mg IV infusion yearly Prevention: 5 mg IV infusion every 2 years	Can premedicate with acetaminophen to decrease infusion reactions. Contraindicated if CrCl <35 mL/min Also marketed under the brand name Zometa (4 mg) for treatment of hypercalcemia and prevention of skeletal-related events from bone metastases from solid tumors with different dosing.

RANK Ligand Inhibitor

Denosumab	Prolia	Treatment: 60 mg SC every 6 months	Administered by a healthcare practitioner. Correct hypocalcemia before administration. Also marketed under the brand name Xgeva (70 mg/mL) for treatment of hypercalcemia and prevention of skeletal-related events from bone metastases from solid tumors with different dosing.

Estrogen Agonist/Antagonist and Tissue Selective Estrogen Complex

Raloxifene	Evista	60 mg orally daily	Generic available
Bazedoxifene with conjugated equine estrogens (CEE)	Duavee	20 mg plus 0.45 mg CEE orally daily	For postmenopausal women with a uterus; no progestogen needed. Bazedoxifene monotherapy available in some countries.
Calcitonin (salmon)	Fortical	200 units (1 spray) intranasally daily, alternating nares every other day.	Generic available. Also available as an SC injection. Refrigerate nasal spray until opened for daily use, then room temperature. Prime with first use.

(continued)

TABLE 3-2	Medications Used to Prevent and Treat Osteoporosis (Continued)		
Drug	Brand Name	Dose	Comments
Formation Medications			
Recombinant human parathyroid hormone (PTH 1–34 units)			
Teriparatide	Forteo	20 mcg SC daily for up to 2 years	First dose sitting or lying. Refrigerate before and after each use. Use new needle with each dose. Inject thigh or stomach. Discard after 28 days or if cloudy.
	PF708 approved biosimilar; under investigation to determine therapeutic equivalence		
Human parathyroid hormone–related peptide (PTHrP[1–34]) analog			
Abaloparatide	Tymlos	80 mcg SC daily for up to 2 years	First dose sitting or lying. Refrigerate before use then keep at room temperature. Use new needle with each dose. Inject in abdomen. Discard after 30 days.
Formation and Antiresorptive Medication			
Sclerostin inhibitor			
Romosozumab	Evenity	210 mg SC monthly for 1 year; administered as two single-use 105-mg/1.17-mL prefilled syringes	Correct hypocalcemia before administration. Refrigerate. Leave at room temperature for at least 30 minutes before use. Inject in abdomen, thigh, or upper arm; preferably each injection at a different site.

IOM, Institute of Medicine; IV, intravenously; NOF, National Osteoporosis Foundation; NSAID, nonsteroidal anti-inflammatory drug; SC, subcutaneously.
Data from product prescribing information.

- If a patient misses a weekly dose, it can be taken the next day. If more than 1 day has elapsed, that dose is skipped. If a patient misses a monthly dose, it can be taken up to 7 days before the next scheduled dose.
- The most common bisphosphonate adverse effects include nausea, abdominal pain, and dyspepsia. Esophageal, gastric, or duodenal irritation, perforation, ulceration, or bleeding may occur. The most common adverse effects of IV bisphosphonates include fever, flu-like symptoms, and local injection-site reactions.
- Rare adverse effects include osteonecrosis of the jaw (ONJ) and subtrochanteric femoral (atypical) fractures. ONJ occurs more commonly in patients with cancer receiving higher-dose IV bisphosphonate therapy and other risk factors including glucocorticoid therapy and diabetes mellitus.
- The optimal duration of bisphosphonate therapy is unknown. Some experts recommend considering a bisphosphonate holiday (defined as disruption of therapy during which medication effects exist with a plan for medication reinstitution) in postmenopausal women after 5 years of oral bisphosphonates or 3 years of IV bisphosphonates if no significant fracture history, hip BMD T-score is above −2.5, and fracture risk is not high. In women with a high fracture risk or lower hip BMD T-scores, continuing oral bisphosphonates for 10 years or IV bisphosphonates for 6 years should be considered. A bisphosphonate holiday should last for ≤5 years with BMD and patient assessment done every 2–4 years.

Denosumab

- **Denosumab** (Prolia) is a RANK ligand inhibitor that inhibits osteoclast formation and increases osteoclast apoptosis. It is indicated for treatment of osteoporosis in women and men at high risk for fracture, for glucocorticoid-induced osteoporosis, to increase bone mass in men receiving androgen-deprivation therapy for nonmetastatic prostate cancer, and in women receiving adjuvant aromatase inhibitor therapy for breast cancer who are at high risk for fracture.
- Over 3 years, denosumab significantly decreased vertebral fractures, nonvertebral fractures, and hip fractures in postmenopausal women with low bone density. Continued increases in BMD occur with long-term treatment with no plateau in BMD effects over 10 years.
- Denosumab is administered as a 60-mg subcutaneous (SC) injection in the upper arm, upper thigh, or abdomen once every 6 months.
- Adverse reactions not associated with the injection site include back pain, arthralgia, and infection. ONJ and atypical femoral shaft fracture occur rarely. Denosumab is contraindicated in patients with hypocalcemia until the condition is corrected.
- After 5–10 years of therapy, patients should be reevaluated for medication continuation, discontinuation, or switching to a different medication.

Mixed Estrogen Agonists/Antagonists and Tissue-Selective Estrogen Complexes

- **Raloxifene** (Evista) is an estrogen agonist/antagonist that is an estrogen agonist on bone receptors but an antagonist at breast receptors, with minimal effects on the uterus. It is approved for prevention and treatment of postmenopausal osteoporosis and for reducing the risk of invasive breast cancer in postmenopausal women with and without osteoporosis.
- **Bazedoxifene** is an estrogen agonist/antagonist that is an agonist at bone and antagonist at the uterus and breast; however, it has no breast cancer prevention effects. The proprietary product Duavee is combined with **conjugated equine estrogens** (CEE), making it a tissue-selective estrogen complex. It is approved for prevention of postmenopausal osteoporosis and vasomotor menstrual symptoms.
- Raloxifene and bazedoxifene decrease vertebral but not hip fractures. The drugs increase spine and hip BMD, but to a lesser extent than bisphosphonates. Data for both drugs support beneficial effects for up to 7–8 years of use. However, the benefit is lost after discontinuation, and bone loss returns to age- or disease-related rates.

- Hot flushes are common with raloxifene but decreased with bazedoxifene/CEE. Raloxifene rarely causes endometrial thickening and bleeding; bazedoxifene decreases these events making progestogen therapy unnecessary when combined with CEE. Leg cramps and muscle spasms are common with these agents. Thromboembolic events are uncommon (<1.5%) but can be fatal. Bazedoxifene/CEE has all of the contraindications and precautions for estrogens as a class.

Calcitonin

- **Calcitonin** is an endogenous hormone released from the thyroid gland when serum calcium is elevated. Salmon calcitonin is used clinically because it is more potent and longer lasting than the mammalian form.
- Calcitonin is indicated for osteoporosis treatment for women at least 5 years past menopause. An FDA Advisory Committee Panel voted against continued use for postmenopausal osteoporosis, but it can be used if alternative therapies are not appropriate.
- Only vertebral fractures have been documented to decrease with intranasal calcitonin therapy. Calcitonin does not consistently affect hip BMD. No calcitonin data exist for men. Intranasal calcitonin may provide some pain relief in patients with acute vertebral fractures, but such use should be short-term (4 weeks) and not in place of other more appropriate analgesic or osteoporosis therapy.

Hormone Therapies

- Hormone therapies (**estrogen** and **testosterone**) are not recommended solely for osteoporosis but have positive bone effects when used for other indications. Estrogen therapy can be a good choice for women going through early menopause when protection against bone loss is needed in addition to reduction of vasomotor symptoms, reserving other osteoporosis therapy until treatment is reassessed closer to the average age of menopause.
- Estrogen with or without a progestogen significantly decreases fracture risk and bone loss in women. Oral and transdermal estrogens at equivalent doses and continuous or cyclic regimens have similar BMD effects. Effect on BMD is dose dependent, with some benefit seen with lower estrogen doses. When estrogen therapy is discontinued, bone loss accelerates and fracture protection is lost.
- Testosterone is used to treat hypogonadism in men, but an osteoporosis medication should be added when risk for osteoporotic fracture is high. No fracture data are available, but some data support minor bone loss prevention for testosterone use in men and women.

FORMATION MEDICATIONS

Parathyroid Hormone Analogs

- **Abaloparatide** (Tymlos) is an analog of parathyroid hormone-related peptide (PTHrP), and **teriparatide** (Forteo) and **PF708** (approved with Forteo [teriparatide injection] as the reference drug) are analogs of parathyroid hormone (PTH); these agents are indicated for the treatment of postmenopausal women with osteoporosis at high risk for fracture, defined as multiple risk factors for fracture, history of osteoporotic fracture, or failure or intolerance to other therapies. Teriparatide is also FDA approved for men with idiopathic or hypogonadal osteoporosis who are at high risk for fracture, men intolerant to other osteoporosis medications, and patients with glucocorticoid-induced osteoporosis.
- Teriparatide increases bone formation with a minor increase in bone resorption for a net anabolic effect when administered intermittently (ie, subcutaneously once daily). Abaloparatide has a greater anabolic effect with less activation of bone resorption and remodeling than teriparatide. Both medications improve bone mass.
- Two years of teriparatide or abaloparatide reduces vertebral and nonvertebral fracture risk in postmenopausal women. Observational teriparatide data suggest a similar fracture benefit in men, whereas no data are available regarding abaloparatide use in men. Discontinuation of PTH analog therapy results in decreased BMD, which can be alleviated with subsequent antiresorptive therapy.

- Transient hypercalcemia can occur and is less common with abaloparatide than teriparatide (3.4% vs 6.4%, respectively). Because of an increased incidence of osteosarcoma in rats, both medications contain a box warning against use in patients at increased risk for osteosarcoma; this adverse effect has not occurred in people. PTH analogs should not be used in patients with hypercalcemia, metabolic bone diseases other than osteoporosis, metastatic or skeletal cancers, or premenopausal women of childbearing potential.

FORMATION AND ANTIRESORPTIVE MEDICATION

Romosozumab

- **Romosozumab** (Evenity) is a humanized monoclonal antibody that binds to sclerostin to prevent inhibition of bone formation and decrease bone resorption, an activity that differentiates this medication from other anabolic therapies. It indicated for postmenopausal women at high risk for fracture defined as multiple risk factors for fracture, a history of osteoporotic fracture, or failure or intolerance to other therapies.
- After 1 year of therapy in postmenopausal women, vertebral fractures decreased by 73%, with a nonsignificant decrease in nonvertebral fractures of 25%; lumbar spine and hip BMD statistically increase after 1 year of treatment. To prevent BMD loss after discontinuation, 1 year of denosumab or alendronate after romosozumab resulted in BMD continuing to increase at both sites.
- The most common adverse effects are headache and arthralgia; hypercalcemia occurs in <1% of patients. Mild injection site irritation occurs in 6%–8% of patients. Romosozumab antibodies may occur in 10%–20% of patients but are generally not neutralizing and do not reduce efficacy. Serious cardiovascular events have been reported, and the labeling contains a boxed warning of an increased risk of myocardial infarction (MI), stroke, and cardiovascular death. Romosozumab should not be used within 1 year of an MI or stroke, and benefit–risk evaluation should be conducted in patients with or at risk for these conditions. Rare cases of ONJ and atypical femoral fractures have been reported.
- Therapy should be limited to 12 monthly doses. If osteoporosis therapy remains warranted, continued therapy with an antiresorptive agent should be considered.

SEQUENTIAL AND COMBINATION THERAPY

- In sequential therapy, an anabolic agent is given first to increase bone remodeling units and bone mass, followed by an antiresorptive agent to continue with bone formation. This regimen is generally reserved for patients with severe osteoporosis because of the cost of anabolic agents.
  - ✓ Starting with an antiresorptive first and then switching to teriparatide results in lower BMD increases but may be especially useful for patients who have fractured or continue to lose bone mass while on antiresorptive therapy.
  - ✓ Small increases in BMD can occur after switching from an oral bisphosphonate to denosumab. This sequential therapy can be used during a bisphosphonate drug holiday or for bisphosphonate treatment failures (ie, no BMD changes or fracture).
- Combination therapy is rarely used because of no documented fracture benefit, increased cost, concern for dual suppression of bone turnover, and potential for more adverse effects. When raloxifene is used for breast cancer prevention, another antiresorptive agent is sometimes prescribed, especially if hip fracture risk is high.

GLUCOCORTICOID-INDUCED OSTEOPOROSIS

- Glucocorticoids decrease bone formation through decreased proliferation and differentiation as well as enhanced apoptosis of osteoblasts. They also increase the number of osteoclasts, increase bone resorption, decrease calcium absorption, and increase renal calcium excretion.
- All glucocorticoid doses and formulations have been associated with increased bone loss and fractures; however, risk is much greater with oral prednisone doses ≥5 mg daily (or equivalent) and oral therapy vs inhaler or intranasal therapy.

- Bone losses are rapid, with up to 12%–15% loss over the first year; the greatest decrease occurs in the first 6 months of therapy. Bone loss is about 2%–3% per year after the first year.
- Perform an initial BMD assessment prior to or within 6 months of glucocorticoid initiation for adults ≥40 years of age and for adults <40 years of age with a history of fragility fracture or other risk factors. Repeat BMD testing is recommended every 2–3 years during osteoporosis therapy for those taking very high glucocorticoid doses (≥30 mg prednisone per day or a cumulative dose >5 g in the past year), a fracture 18 months or more after starting osteoporosis therapy, medication adherence or absorption concerns, or other risk factors for osteoporosis.
- All patients starting or receiving systemic glucocorticoid therapy (any dose or duration) should practice a bone-healthy lifestyle and ingest 1000–1200 mg elemental calcium and 600–800 units of vitamin D daily to achieve therapeutic 25-hydroxyvitamin D concentrations. Use the lowest possible corticosteroid dose and duration.
- Treatment guidelines divide recommendations for prescription medication use by fracture risk and age. Alendronate, risedronate, zoledronic acid, denosumab, and teriparatide are FDA approved for glucocorticoid-induced osteoporosis.
- Standard osteoporosis therapy doses are used. Oral bisphosphonates are recommended first-line, although IV bisphosphonates can be used in nonadherent patients or those unable to take the oral preparations. Teriparatide is recommended for patients who cannot use a bisphosphonate, and denosumab is recommended if neither a bisphosphonate nor teriparatide can be used. Denosumab is not recommended as first-line therapy due to limited safety data in this population. Raloxifene does not have an FDA indication for this use, but there are clinical data documenting improved BMD at the lumbar spine in patients taking glucocorticoids.

EVALUATION OF THERAPEUTIC OUTCOMES

- Assess medication adherence and tolerability at each visit.
- Ask patients about possible fracture symptoms (eg, bone pain, disability) at each visit. Assessment of fracture, back pain, and height loss can help identify worsening osteoporosis.
- Obtain a central DXA BMD measurement after 1–2 years or 3–5 years after initiating a medication therapy to monitor response. Repeat a central DXA every 2 years until BMD is stable, at which time the reassessment interval can be lengthened. More frequent monitoring may be warranted in patients with conditions associated with high rates of bone loss (eg, glucocorticoid use).

See Chapter 108, Osteoporosis, authored by Mary Beth O'Connell, Jill S. Borchert, Erin M. Slazak, and Joseph P. Fava for a more detailed discussion of this topic.

Rheumatoid Arthritis

- *Rheumatoid arthritis* (RA) is a chronic, progressive autoimmune condition that primarily affects joints and the synovium but can also have systemic manifestations.

PATHOPHYSIOLOGY

- RA results from a combination of genetic susceptibility, nongenetic factors, and a triggering event. An unknown infectious process is thought to be the primary trigger.
- Antigen-presenting cells process and present antigens to T cells; activated T cells stimulate B cells to produce autoantibodies that form large complexes that deposit throughout the body. Antibodies to immunoglobulin G (IgG) are known as rheumatoid factor (RF) and have a strong correlation to the pathogenesis and poor prognosis of RA. B cells also produce proinflammatory cytokines, including tumor necrosis factor (TNF) and the interleukin (IL) system, which induce expression of adhesion molecules on the endothelium, further enhancing T-cell proliferation and differentiation, encouraging cell migration, and regulating matrix modeling.
- Overexpression of tumor suppressor gene p53 prevents normal DNA repair and interferes with appropriate cell apoptosis and increased anti-citrullinated protein antibodies (ACPA). ACPA positivity is associated with a worse prognosis in patients with RA.
- Migration of lymphocytes, macrophages, and mononuclear cells into the synovium and synovial cavity increases synovial mass, causing hypertrophy and angiogenesis. Angiogenesis is driven by IL-8, prostaglandins, vascular endothelial growth factor, and macrophage angiogenic factor. As the vessels develop, cytokines stimulate further migration of cells into the synovium, causing inflammation. The inflamed, fibrotic synovium (*pannus*) invades cartilage and bone around it, promoting further destruction and dysregulation.
- Cytokines within cartilage cause generation of reactive nitrogen and oxygen species and increase chondrocyte catabolism, inhibit chondrocyte anabolism, and increase extracellular matrix destruction. Proinflammatory cytokines travel to bone, provide the source for receptor activator of NFkB ligand (RANKL), and enhance osteoclast activity, leading to bone matrix destruction.
- Chronic inflammation in vascular endothelial and visceral, cutaneous, and pleural tissues leads to complications including vasculitis, fibrosis, anemia, and renal amyloidosis.

CLINICAL PRESENTATION

- Nonspecific prodromal symptoms developing over weeks to months include fatigue, weakness, low-grade fever, anorexia, and joint pain. Stiffness and myalgias may precede development of synovitis.
- Joint involvement tends to be symmetric and affects small joints of the hands, feet, wrists, and ankles; elbows, knees, shoulders, hips, cervical spine, and temporomandibular joints may also be affected.
- Joint stiffness is typically worse in the morning, usually exceeds 30 minutes, and may persist all day.
- On examination, joint swelling may be visible or apparent only by palpation. Tissue is soft, spongy, warm, and may be erythematous. If left untreated, long-term joint inflammation may lead to bony erosions and subluxations of wrists, metacarpophalangeal joints, and proximal interphalangeal joints (swan neck deformity, boutonnière deformity, and ulnar deviation).
- Extra-articular involvement may include rheumatoid nodules, interstitial lung disease, pleural effusions, vasculitis, ocular manifestations, pericarditis, cardiac conduction abnormalities, bone marrow suppression, and lymphadenopathy.

- RF is detected in 70%–80% of patients; higher titers generally reflect a more severe disease course. ACPA antibodies are more specific for RA and may be detectable very early in the disease; they generally predict a more aggressive disease course. Antinuclear antibodies (ANAs) are detected in 25% of patients with RA. Elevated erythrocyte sedimentation rate (ESR) and C-reactive protein (CRP) indicate the presence of a nonspecific inflammatory process. Normocytic anemia, thrombocytosis or thrombocytopenia, and leukopenia may also be present. Analysis of aspirated synovial fluid typically demonstrates a high white blood cell count without crystals or infection.
- Early radiologic findings include soft tissue swelling and periarticular osteoporosis. With disease progression, joint space narrowing, bony erosions, and joint subluxations and deviations may occur.

DIAGNOSIS

- The American College of Rheumatology (ACR) and the European League Against Rheumatism (EULAR) revised criteria for diagnosis of RA in 2010. These criteria are intended for patients early in their disease to allow for earlier treatment targeted toward preventing structural joint damage. Patients with synovitis at least one joint and no other explanation for the finding are candidates for assessment. The criteria use a scoring system with a combined score of 6 or more out of 10 indicating that the patient has definite RA.

TREATMENT

- <u>Goals of Treatment</u>: The ultimate goal is to induce complete remission or low disease activity (referred to as "treat to target"). Additional goals are to reduce inflammation and symptoms, maintain ability to function in daily activities, slow destructive joint changes, and delay disability.

NONPHARMACOLOGIC THERAPY

- Patient education about the disease and medications (eg, potential adverse effects, self-administration of injectable agents) is important.
- Physical therapy can reduce pain and inflammation while preserving joint function. Exercise and physical activity (including aerobic activity and muscle-strengthening exercises) can improve disease outcomes.
- Assistive devices and orthoses such as braces and supports are useful to improve pain and function. Occupational therapy can provide benefits such as appropriate footwear and splinting.
- Weight loss can help decrease stress on joints.
- Surgical options (eg, joint replacements) are reserved for patients with more severe disease with significant cartilage loss.

PHARMACOLOGIC THERAPY

General Approach

- Therapies to treat RA and slow disease progression include conventional and biologic disease-modifying antirheumatic drugs (DMARDs) and the small-molecule oral Janus-kinase (JAK) inhibitors.
  - ✓ Conventional DMARDs include **methotrexate, leflunomide, sulfasalazine**, and **hydroxychloroquine.**
  - ✓ Biologic DMARDs include TNF inhibitors (**adalimumab, certolizumab, etanercept, golimumab**, and **infliximab**) and non-TNF biologics (**abatacept, sarilumab, tocilizumab, rituximab**, and **anakinra**).
  - ✓ JAK inhibitors include **baricitinib, tofacitinib**, and **upadacitinib.**
- Current RA treatment guidelines recommend initiating conventional DMARDs irrespective of disease activity in treatment-naive patients once a diagnosis is established (Fig. 4-1).

(DMARD, disease-modifying antirheumatic drug; MTX, methotrexate; TNFi, tumor necrosis factor inhibitor.)

FIGURE 4-1. **Algorithm for treatment of rheumatoid arthritis (RA) in early (<6 months) or established (≥6 months) RA with low to high disease activity.**

- The preferred conventional DMARD is methotrexate unless a contraindication exists. However, choice of therapy may depend on the level of disease activity, comorbid conditions, patient preference, and insurance coverage.
- For patients with early RA (<6 months duration) and low disease activity, DMARD monotherapy is recommended. Double or triple DMARD therapy is recommended for moderate or high disease activity. A biologic agent can be used as monotherapy or with conventional DMARD(s) in patients with moderate or high disease activity. A JAK inhibitor is an alternate option if disease activity remains moderate or high with combination conventional DMARDs.
- If disease activity remains moderate or high despite conventional DMARDs or biologics, a low-dose glucocorticoid (prednisone ≤10 mg/day or equivalent) can be added for the shortest duration necessary. If patients achieve remission, DMARDs and biologic agents can be tapered, but patients should remain on DMARD therapy at some dosage level.
- For patients with established RA (duration ≥6 months), DMARD monotherapy is recommended despite disease activity in DMARD-naive patients. Combination conventional DMARDs, a biologic DMARD, or a JAK inhibitor can be used if disease activity remains moderate or high after an adequate trial with DMARD monotherapy.

In patients taking TNF inhibitor monotherapy with moderate or high disease activity, one or two conventional DMARDs can be added to the TNF inhibitor. A non-TNF biologic can be used in place of a TNF inhibitor if disease activity remains moderate or high on a TNF inhibitor and is recommended over a JAK inhibitor. Therapy can be switched to another non-TNF biologic if the first non-TNF agent cannot adequately control disease activity. A non-TNF biologic can also be started if separate courses of two different TNF inhibitors have not adequately controlled disease activity. A JAK inhibitor can be initiated if disease activity persists despite multiple TNF inhibitors in patients for whom non-TNF biologics are not an option. Dual biologic therapy should be avoided due to the risk of infection associated with immunosuppression. A glucocorticoid can be added if disease flares occur or disease activity is inadequately controlled despite DMARD, TNF inhibitor, or non-TNF biologic therapy.

- Because DMARDs can take weeks to months to take effect, nonsteroidal anti-inflammatory drugs (NSAIDs), glucocorticoids, and other analgesics (eg, acetaminophen) can be used to provide more rapid symptomatic relief ("bridge therapy"). NSAIDs do not slow disease progression, and glucocorticoids can have serious side effects, making both drug classes less desirable for long-term use.
- See Tables 4-1 and 4-2 for usual dosages and monitoring parameters for NSAIDs, glucocorticoids, and conventional and biologic DMARDs.

Conventional DMARDs

- **Methotrexate** inhibits dihydrofolate reductase, thereby inhibiting DNA synthesis and repair and cellular replication. Injectable (subcutaneous [SC], intramuscular [IM]) methotrexate has higher bioavailability than oral methotrexate and thus provides superior clinical efficacy; it is typically better tolerated with less potential to cause gastrointestinal (GI) side effects as well. Oral methotrexate doses >15 mg weekly may not have significant added clinical benefit; changing to SC methotrexate may increase bioavailability and clinical benefit in this situation. Clinical benefit can be seen 3–6 weeks after starting therapy. Methotrexate has numerous adverse effects (Table 4-2); concomitant folic acid 1–5 mg/day may reduce some adverse effects without loss of efficacy. Methotrexate is teratogenic, and patients should use contraception and discontinue the drug if conception is planned. Methotrexate is contraindicated in pregnant and nursing women, chronic liver disease, immunodeficiency, and preexisting hematologic disorders (eg, leukopenia, thrombocytopenia). Methotrexate excretion is reduced in renal impairment and may require dose reduction or discontinuation in some cases.
- **Leflunomide** inhibits pyrimidine synthesis, which reduces lymphocyte proliferation and modulation of inflammation. It can be used as monotherapy or in combination with other DMARDs. Efficacy for RA is similar to that of methotrexate. A loading dose of 100 mg/day for 3 days may achieve steady state more rapidly but may increase the risk for toxicities. The usual maintenance dose of 20 mg/day may be lowered to 10 mg/day in cases of GI intolerance, alopecia, or other dose-related toxicity. Adverse effects are listed in Table 4-2. Leflunomide is teratogenic and should not be used in pregnant or nursing mothers or in patients with severe hepatic impairment.
- **Sulfasalazine** can be used as monotherapy or in combination with other DMARDs. Clinical benefit usually occurs in 4 weeks, but some patients may require 12 weeks. Sulfasalazine use is limited by GI adverse effects (Table 4-2). Sulfasalazine crosses the placenta and is present in breast milk but can be used in pregnant and nursing mothers with caution.
- **Hydroxychloroquine** is typically used in combination with other DMARDs, but it can be used as monotherapy in mild cases. Clinical benefit is delayed and may take several weeks. Its main advantage is that it does not require frequent, routine laboratory monitoring because it is not generally associated with infection risk or hepatic, renal, or blood cell abnormalities. GI side effects can sometimes be mitigated by taking the medication with food or splitting the dose into two doses. Hydroxychloroquine can be continued during pregnancy because no studies have

TABLE 4-1 Usual Doses for Disease-Modifying Antirheumatic Drugs

Drugs	Brand Names	Routes of Administration	Starting Dose	Usual Ranges or Maintenance Dose	Comments
Conventional DMARDs					
Methotrexate	Rasuvo Trexall Otrexup (SC)	Oral, SC, IM	Oral: 7.5 mg once weekly or 2.5 mg every 12 hours for 3 doses once weekly SC/IM: 7.5 mg once weekly	7.5–20 mg every week	May be given with folic acid 1–5 mg/day to reduce adverse effects
Leflunomide	Arava	Oral	Loading dose: 100 mg daily for 3 days, then 20 mg daily or 10–20 mg daily without loading dose	10–20 mg daily	Not recommended in liver disease (ALT >3 times ULN)
Hydroxychloroquine	Plaquenil	Oral	200 mg twice daily or 400 mg daily	200 mg twice daily or 400 mg daily	Take with food or milk; use with caution in renal or hepatic impairment
Sulfasalazine	Azulfidine	Oral	500 mg once or twice daily	1000 mg twice daily (maximum dose 3000 mg/day if inadequate response after 12 weeks of 2000 mg/day)	Not recommended in renal or hepatic impairment
Tumor Necrosis Factor (TNF) Inhibitors					
Adalimumab	Humira	SC	40 mg every 2 weeks	40 mg every 2 weeks (may increase to 40 mg once weekly if not taking methotrexate)	

(Continued)

TABLE 4-1 Usual Doses for Disease-Modifying Antirheumatic Drugs (Continued)

Drugs	Brand Names	Routes of Administration	Starting Dose	Usual Ranges or Maintenance Dose	Comments
Certolizumab	Cimzia	SC	400 mg at 0, 2, 4 weeks	200 mg every other week or 400 mg every 4 weeks	
Etanercept	Enbrel	SC	50 mg once weekly or 25 mg twice weekly	Same as starting dose	
Golimumab	Simponi	SC	50 mg once monthly	Same as starting dose	
Infliximab	Remicade	IV	3 mg/kg at 0, 2, 6 weeks, and then every 8 weeks	3–10 mg/kg every 4–8 weeks	Given in combination with methotrexate; pretreat with methylprednisolone, acetaminophen, and antihistamine
Costimulation Modulator					
Abatacept	Orencia	IV, SC	IV: <60 kg: 500 mg, 60–100 kg: 750 mg, >100 kg: 1000 mg at 0, 2, and 4 weeks or initial IV dose followed by 125 mg SC within 24 hours SC: 125 mg weekly	IV: dose based on weight every 4 weeks SC: 125 mg weekly	

IL-6 Receptor Antagonists

Sarilumab	Kevzara	SC	200 mg every 2 weeks	Same as starting dose
Tocilizumab	Actemra	IV, SC	IV: 4 mg/kg every 4 weeks, SC: <100 kg: 162 mg every other week, >100 kg: 162 mg weekly	IV: 4–8 mg/kg every 4 weeks (maximum 800 mg per infusion) SC: <100 kg: 162 mg every other week, followed by an increase to weekly injections if needed; >100 kg: 162 mg weekly	Can increase metabolism of CYP3A4 substrates

Janus Kinase (JAK) Inhibitors

Baricitinib	Olumiant	Oral IR	2 mg once daily	Same as starting dose	1 mg once daily in patients taking strong organic anion transporter 3 (OAT3) inhibitors (eg, probenecid)
Tofacitinib	Xeljanz	Oral	IR: 5 mg twice daily ER: 11 mg daily	Same as starting dose	5 mg once daily in moderate-to-severe renal insufficiency, moderate hepatic impairment, or concomitant CYP3A4 or CYP2C19 inhibitors
Upadacitinib	Rinvoq	Oral ER	15 mg once daily	Same as starting dose	Use with caution with strong CYP3A4 inhibitors; coadministration with strong CYP3A4 inducers is not recommended.

(Continued)

TABLE 4-1 Usual Doses for Disease-Modifying Antirheumatic Drugs *(Continued)*

Drugs	Brand Names	Routes of Administration	Starting Dose	Usual Ranges or Maintenance Dose	Comments
Anti-CD20 Monoclonal Antibody					
Rituximab	Rituxan	IV	1000 mg in 2 doses given 2 weeks apart	Initial dose may be repeated every 16–24 weeks based on response	Pretreat with methylprednisolone, acetaminophen, and antihistamine
IL-1 Receptor Antagonist					
Anakinra	Kineret	SC	100 mg once daily	Same as starting dose	

ALT, alanine transaminase; CYP, cytochrome P; ER, extended release; IM, intramuscular; IR, immediate release; IV, intravenous; SC, subcutaneous; ULN, upper limit of normal.

shown an increased risk of birth defects or ocular toxicities. Hydroxychloroquine is excreted into breast milk, and caution should be used in nursing mothers. Periodic ophthalmologic examinations are necessary for early detection of irreversible retinal toxicity (Table 4-2).

Biologic DMARDs

- Biologic agents are genetically engineered proteins that decrease inflammation by various mechanisms. They are categorized as either TNF inhibitors or non-TNF biologics. They may be effective when conventional DMARDs fail to achieve adequate disease control but are considerably more expensive.
- Biologic DMARDs are associated with an increased risk of infection due to immunosuppressive effects. A tuberculin skin test or interferon gamma release assay (IGRA) blood test should be obtained before starting a biologic to detect and treat latent or active tuberculosis. Patients should also be screened for hepatitis B before starting biologic therapy because of the risk for reactivation.
- Biologics can be used in combination with conventional DMARDs, but multiple biologics should not be used concomitantly due to additive immunosuppressive effects. In general, if patients are switched from one biologic to another, the new agent should be initiated when the patient is due for a dose of the previous biologic. Because of immunosuppressive effects, patients taking biologics should notify their providers if they are being treated for an infection or plan to undergo major surgery. Treatment may need to be held until appropriate postsurgical healing and/or resolution of infection can be confirmed. Live vaccines should not be given to patients taking biologic agents.
- *Biosimilars* are biologic products that have been verified to have no clinically meaningful differences compared to an FDA-approved reference biologic product. These agents can increase access to RA treatment because their costs are lower than the originator products. However, concerns that limit their use include lack of regulatory guidelines about switching from the original biologic product to the biosimilar and uncertainty about extrapolation of indications for biosimilars from the original biologic product.

TNF-α Inhibitors

- TNF inhibitors block the proinflammatory cytokine TNF-α. It may take several weeks for clinical benefit to be noted and up to 3 months to achieve full clinical benefit. These agents are typically used when disease activity remains moderate or high despite conventional DMARD therapy. TNF inhibitors are more expensive than conventional DMARDs.
- Selection of a particular TNF inhibitor depends on cost and patient preference for route and frequency of administration. They should not be used in patients with moderate-to-severe heart failure (New York Heart Association [NYHA] class III/IV) because new-onset and worsening heart failure have been reported. These agents increase the risk of serious infection and malignancies (eg, lymphoma, skin cancers), and new-onset or exacerbation of demyelinating disorders such as multiple sclerosis has been observed.
- See Tables 4-1 and 4-2 for dosing and monitoring information.

  ✓ **Adalimumab** (Humira) binds to TNF-α and blocks its interaction with the p55 and p75 cell surface TNF receptors. It is available as a prefilled syringe or pen for SC injection.

  ✓ **Certolizumab** (Cimzia) is a pegylated humanized antibody Fab fragment of TNF-α monoclonal antibody. Because it lacks the Fc region, it does not induce complement activation, antibody-dependent cell-mediated cytotoxicity, or apoptosis. Pegylation allows for delayed elimination and extended half-life. It is available as a prefilled syringe for SC injection.

  ✓ **Etanercept** (Enbrel) is a recombinant DNA-derived protein composed of TNF receptor linked to the Fc fragment of human IgG1. It is available as a prefilled syringe or pen for SC injection.

TABLE 4-2	Clinical Monitoring of Drug Therapy in Rheumatoid Arthritis		
Drugs	Adverse Drug Reactions	Initial Monitoring	Maintenance Monitoring
NSAIDs	GI ulceration, bleeding, perforation; renal damage	SCr, CBC every 2–4 weeks after starting therapy	Same as initial plus stool guaiac every 6–12 months
Corticosteroids	Fluid retention, hyperglycemia, hypertension, behavioral and mood changes, increased appetite, weight gain, electrolyte imbalances, impaired healing, hirsutism, Cushing syndrome, HPA axis suppression, osteonecrosis of femoral and humeral heads, osteoporosis and fractures, myopathy, glaucoma, cataracts	Glucose, CBC periodically, BP every 3–6 months	Same as initial
Methotrexate	Infection, hepatic fibrosis, cirrhosis, interstitial pneumonitis, stomatitis, rash, GI perforation, diarrhea, thrombocytopenia, leukopenia	SCr, CBC with differential, AST, ALT, hepatitis B and C screening, tuberculosis screening	SCr, CBC with differential, AST, ALT, every 2–4 weeks for 3 months after starting or following a dose increase, then every 8–12 weeks during 3–6 months of therapy, and every 12 weeks after 6 months of therapy; signs of infection
Leflunomide	Hepatitis, diarrhea/nausea, alopecia, elevated BP	CBC with differential, SCr, ALT, AST, BP	CBC with differential, SCr, ALT, AST every 2–4 weeks for 3 months after starting or following a dose increase, then every 8–12 weeks during 3–6 months of therapy, and every 12 weeks after 6 months of therapy; BP periodically
Sulfasalazine	Rash, nausea, vomiting, diarrhea, photosensitivity, alopecia	CBC with differential, SCr, ALT, AST	CBC with differential, SCr, ALT, AST every 2–4 weeks for 3 months after starting or following a dose increase, then every 8–12 weeks during 3–6 months of therapy, and every 12 weeks after 6 months of therapy

Drug	Adverse Effects	Baseline Monitoring	Ongoing Monitoring
Hydroxychloroquine	Retinal damage, rash, diarrhea	Ophthalmologic exam within 5 years of starting therapy	Ophthalmologic exam annually if risk factors for retinal damage present or annually beginning after 5 years of use if no risk factors
Etanercept, adalimumab, golimumab, certolizumab	Local injection-site reactions, infection, malignancy	Tuberculosis screening, hepatitis B screening, CBC with differential	Periodic skin examination, signs/symptoms of infection and malignancy, CBC with differential periodically
Infliximab	Immune reactions, infection, malignancy	Tuberculosis screening, hepatitis B screening, CBC with differential, LFTs	CBC with differential, LFTs, signs/symptoms of infection and malignancy
Abatacept	Immune reactions, infection, malignancy	Tuberculosis screening, hepatitis B screening	Signs/symptoms of infection and malignancy
Sarilumab	Local injection-site reactions, infection, malignancy	Tuberculosis screening, hepatitis B screening, CBC with differential, LFTs, lipid panel	CBC with differential and LFTs 4–8 weeks after starting and then every 3 months, FLP 4–8 weeks after starting and every 6 months during therapy; signs/symptoms of infection and malignancy
Tocilizumab	Local injection-site reactions, infection, malignancy, GI perforation, neutropenia, thrombocytopenia	Tuberculosis screening, hepatitis B screening, CBC with differential, AST, ALT, FLP	AST, ALT, CBC with differential every 4–8 weeks after starting then every 3 months; FLP after 4–8 weeks of starting then every 6 months; signs/symptoms of infection and malignancy
Baricitinib, tofacitinib, upadacitinib	Infection, malignancy, GI perforations, upper respiratory tract infections, headache, diarrhea, nasopharyngitis	Tuberculosis screening, hepatitis B screening, CBC with differential, Hgb, LFTs, FLP, HR, and BP	CBC with differential and Hgb after 4–8 weeks and every 3 months, FLP after 4–8 weeks and periodically, LFTs periodically, periodic skin examinations, HR and BP, signs/symptoms of infection and malignancy

(Continued)

45

TABLE 4-2	Clinical Monitoring of Drug Therapy in Rheumatoid Arthritis *(Continued)*		
Drugs	**Adverse Drug Reactions**	**Initial Monitoring**	**Maintenance Monitoring**
Rituximab	Immune reactions, infection, malignancy	Tuberculosis screening, hepatitis B screening, CBC with differential	CBC with differential prior to each treatment course and at 2- to 4-month intervals, signs/symptoms of infection
Anakinra	Local injection site reactions, infection, malignancy	CBC with differential, tuberculosis screening, SCr, hepatitis B screening	CBC with differential every 3 months up to 1 year, SCr periodically, signs/symptoms of infection and malignancy

ALT, alanine transaminase; AST, aspartate transaminase; BP, blood pressure; CBC, complete blood count; FLP, fasting lipid panel; GI, gastrointestinal; Hgb, hemoglobin; HPA, hypothalamic–pituitary–adrenal; HR, heart rate; LFTs, liver function tests; NSAIDs, nonsteroidal anti-inflammatory drugs; SCr, serum creatinine.

✓ **Golimumab** (Simponi) is a human monoclonal antibody that binds to human TNF-α. It is available as a prefilled syringe or pen for SC injection. It is also available as an intravenous (IV) product.

✓ **Infliximab** (Remicade) is a chimeric monoclonal antibody that binds to human TNF-α. It is administered as an IV infusion. To prevent formation of an antibody response to this foreign protein, methotrexate must be given orally in doses used to treat RA for as long as the patient continues infliximab. Premedication with an antihistamine, acetaminophen, and/or a glucocorticoid can decrease development of infusion-related reactions. Patients on infliximab plus methotrexate have been shown to have a better clinical response than patients treated with methotrexate alone.

Costimulation Modulator

- **Abatacept** (Orencia) inhibits T-cell activation by binding to CD80 and CD86, which blocks the interaction between T cells CD28, thus inhibiting the activation of T cells. Abatacept is indicated for moderate-to-severe RA and can be used as monotherapy or in conjunction with conventional DMARDs. Abatacept is typically initiated if disease activity persists after conventional DMARD monotherapy and can be an alternative to TNF inhibitors with or without methotrexate. It can also be initiated in patients who have failed or have had an inadequate response to TNF inhibitors. Abatacept plus methotrexate has similar efficacy and incidence of adverse events as adalimumab plus methotrexate in biologic-naive patients who had an incomplete response to methotrexate. Abatacept is available in a prefilled syringe or auto-injector for SC injection and as an IV infusion.

IL-6 Receptor Antagonists

- **Sarilumab** (Kevzara) is indicated for treatment of patients with moderate-to-severe RA who have had an incomplete response or intolerance to one or more DMARDs. It can be used as monotherapy or with conventional DMARDs. It is available as prefilled syringes for SC injection.
- **Tocilizumab** (Actemra) can be used for patients with moderate-to-severe RA who have had an incomplete response to one or more DMARDs. It can be used alone or in combination with conventional DMARDs. It is available as prefilled syringes for SC injection and as an IV infusion.

Anti-CD20 Monoclonal Antibody

- **Rituximab** (Rituxan) is a monoclonal antibody that binds the CD20 antigen on the surface of B cells. Binding of rituximab to B cells results in nearly complete depletion of peripheral B cells, with a gradual recovery over several months. Rituximab can be initiated in patients with moderate-to-severe RA who have had an incomplete response to one or more TNF inhibitors. Methotrexate should be given concurrently in the usual doses for RA to achieve optimal outcomes. An observational cohort study showed that patients who failed one TNF inhibitor had greater reductions in disease activity scores when treated with rituximab than with a second TNF inhibitor. Rituximab is given as two 1000-mg infusions separated by 2 weeks. Because recovery of B-cells can take several months, rituximab can be given every 24 weeks. The decision to re-dose should be based on the return of RA symptoms. Methylprednisolone 100 mg IV is recommended 30 minutes before each infusion as well as acetaminophen and an antihistamine to reduce the incidence and severity of infusion reactions.

IL-1 Receptor Antagonist

- **Anakinra** (Kineret) is an IL-1 receptor antagonist; it is less effective than other biologics, is used infrequently, and is not included in the current ACR treatment recommendations. However, it can be used in patients with moderate-to-severe RA who have failed one or more DMARDs. Anakinra can be used alone or in combination with DMARDs other than TNF-α inhibitors.

Janus-Kinase Inhibitors
- **Baricitinib** (Olumiant), **tofacitinib** (Xeljanz), and **upadacitinib** (Rinvoq) are oral, small-molecule, nonbiologic JAK inhibitors. Baricitinib is FDA approved for adults with moderately to severely active RA who have had an inadequate response to one or more TNF inhibitors; it may be used alone or in combination with methotrexate or other conventional DMARDs. Tofacitinib and upadacitinib have FDA approval for treatment of adults with moderately to severely active RA who have had an inadequate response or intolerance to methotrexate; these drugs may be used as monotherapy or in combination with methotrexate or other nonbiologic DMARDs. JAK inhibitors should not be given concomitantly with biologic agents.
- Labeling for all JAK inhibitors includes black-box warnings about serious infections, lymphomas, and other malignancies. Live vaccinations should not be given during treatment. Patients should be tested and treated for latent tuberculosis before starting therapy.

Nonsteroidal Anti-inflammatory Drugs
- NSAIDs inhibit prostaglandin synthesis, which is a small portion of the inflammatory cascade. They possess both analgesic and anti-inflammatory properties and reduce stiffness, but they do not slow disease progression or prevent bony erosions or joint deformity and should not be used as monotherapy for RA treatment. They have a more rapid onset of action than DMARDs and may be beneficial to "bridge" patients while DMARDs take effect. Common NSAID dosage regimens are shown in Table 4-3.

TABLE 4-3	Dosage Regimens for Nonsteroidal Anti-inflammatory Drugs		
	Recommended Total Daily Anti-inflammatory Dosage		
Drug	**Adult**	**Children**	**Dosing Schedule**
Aspirin	2.6–5.2 g	60–100 mg/kg	4 times daily
Celecoxib	200–400 mg	–	Once or twice daily
Diclofenac	150–200 mg	–	3 or 4 times daily; extended release: twice daily
Diflunisal	0.5–1.5 g	–	Twice daily
Etodolac	0.2–1.2 g (max. 20 mg/kg)	–	2–4 times daily
Fenoprofen	0.9–3 g	–	4 times daily
Flurbiprofen	200–300 mg	–	2–4 times daily
Ibuprofen	1.2–3.2 g	20–40 mg/kg	3 or 4 times daily
Indomethacin	50–200 mg	2–4 mg/kg (max. 200 mg)	2–4 times daily; extended release: once daily
Meclofenamate	200–400 mg	–	3–4 times daily
Meloxicam	7.5–15 mg	–	Once daily
Nabumetone	1–2 g	–	Once or twice daily
Naproxen	0.5–1 g	10 mg/kg	Twice daily; extended release: once daily
Naproxen sodium	0.55–1.1 g	–	Twice daily
Nonacetylated salicylates	1.2–4.8 g	–	2–6 times daily
Oxaprozin	0.6–1.8 g (max. 26 mg/kg)	–	1–3 times daily
Piroxicam	10–20 mg	–	Once daily
Sulindac	300–400 mg	–	Twice daily
Tolmetin	0.6–1.8 g	15–30 mg/kg	2–4 times daily

Glucocorticoids

- Glucocorticoids have anti-inflammatory and immunosuppressive properties; although they have been shown to slow RA progression, glucocorticoids should not be used as monotherapy for RA due to the potential for serious, long-term adverse effects (Table 4-2). They should be used at the lowest effective dose for the shortest period of time. According to the ACR, short-term glucocorticoid therapy is defined as <3 months, and low-dose glucocorticoid is defined as prednisone ≤10 mg/day (or equivalent).

- Similar to NSAIDs, oral glucocorticoids (eg, **prednisone**, **methylprednisolone**) can be used to "bridge" patients while DMARDs take effect. They can also be used as adjuncts to DMARDs at the lowest dose possible in patients with refractory disease. High-dose, short-term bursts can be used as needed for acute flares of RA symptoms, followed by tapering to the lowest effective dose to control symptoms or until discontinued over several days.

- The IM route may be useful in nonadherent patients. Depot forms (**triamcinolone acetonide**, **triamcinolone hexacetonide**, and **methylprednisolone acetate**) provide 2–6 weeks of symptom control. Onset of effect may be delayed for several days. The depot effect provides a physiologic taper, avoiding hypothalamic–pituitary axis suppression.

- Intra-articular injections may be useful when only a few joints are involved. Injections should not be repeated more often than every 3 months because of the potential for accelerated loss of joint cartilage.

EVALUATION OF THERAPEUTIC OUTCOMES

- Assess disease activity at baseline and at each follow-up visit to evaluate therapeutic response. Clinical signs of improvement include reduction in joint pain, swelling, and tenderness; less morning stiffness; reduced fatigue; and improved ability to perform activities of daily living.

- Perform a physical examination at each visit to objectively evaluate the number of swollen and tender joints, joint mobility, and presence of deformity.

- Several assessment tools are available to measure RA disease activity, such as the Clinical Disease Activity Index (CDAI), Disease Activity Score (DAS28), Patient Activity Scale (PAS), Routine Assessment of Patient Index Data 3 (RAPID-3), and Simplified Disease Activity Index (SDAI).

- Laboratory monitoring of acute phase reactants such as CRP and ESR can be useful in assessing inflammation.

- Obtain plain radiographs of the hands, wrists, and forefeet at baseline and every 2 years in patients with low disease activity or in remission. Little to no evidence of RA disease progression should be evident if drug therapy is effective. Imaging may be needed more frequently in patients with moderate or high disease activity. Drug therapy should be modified if patients have radiographic changes suggestive of disease progression (eg, periarticular osteopenia, bone erosions, joint space narrowing).

- It is important to monitor and assess for clinical and laboratory adverse effects of the medications used to treat RA (Table 4-2).

See Chapter 107, Rheumatoid Arthritis, authored by Stephanie Gruber, Bianca Lezcano, and Susan Hylland, for a detailed discussion of this topic.

CHAPTER 5 Acute Coronary Syndromes

- *Acute coronary syndrome* (ACS) involves acute myocardial ischemia resulting from imbalance between myocardial oxygen demand and supply. Classification based on electrocardiographic (ECG) changes includes: (1) ST-segment-elevation myocardial infarction (STEMI) or (2) non–ST-segment-elevation ACS (NSTE-ACS), which includes non–ST-segment-elevation MI (NSTEMI) and unstable angina (UA).

PATHOPHYSIOLOGY

- Endothelial dysfunction, inflammation, and formation of fatty streaks contribute to development of atherosclerotic coronary artery plaques. Eventual plaque rupture and subsequent thrombus formation abruptly decreases myocardial blood flow and oxygen supply, leading to ischemia and potentially infarction.
- Atherosclerotic plaques that rupture typically have thin fibrous caps and tend to be nonobstructive, occluding <70% of the luminal diameter; thus, patients may not experience angina prior to plaque rupture due to adequate autoregulation that maintains blood flow and oxygen supply during increased myocardial oxygen demand. Increased catecholamine release during physical or emotional stress may enhance the likelihood of rupture of a thinning fibrous cap.
- Plaque rupture breaches the barrier between the necrotic plaque core and blood components; circulating platelets are attracted and adhere to the area of injury. Platelet adhesion occurs via platelet glycoprotein (GP) VI receptors binding to collagen within the damaged fibrotic cap, as well as platelet GP Ib-IX receptors and von Willebrand factor. Platelets are then activated by collagen, thrombin, thromboxane A_2, adenosine diphosphate (ADP), epinephrine, and serotonin. Binding of these activators to their specific receptors on the platelet surface (eg, $P2Y_{12}$ receptor for ADP, protease-activated receptor [PAR]-1 for thrombin) results in increased platelet surface area and release of further platelet activators from granules within platelets. Assembly of tenase and prothrombinase complexes within activated platelets produces most of the activated factor Xa and IIa (thrombin) in the coagulation cascade. A change in the conformation of the GP IIb/IIIa surface receptors of platelets cross-links platelets to each other through fibrinogen bridges, resulting in platelet aggregation and formation of a platelet plug in the area of plaque rupture.
- Activation of the clotting cascade forms a fibrin meshwork (thrombus) around the platelet plug that traps cellular components such as red blood cells and causes abrupt reduction in myocardial blood flow and oxygen supply. If ischemia is left untreated, myocyte necrosis and cell death may ensue.
- Subtypes of MI are based on etiology: (1) rupture, fissure, or erosion of an atherosclerotic plaque (90% of cases); (2) reduced myocardial oxygen supply or increased demand in the absence of a coronary artery process; (3) MI resulting in death without the possibility of measuring biomarkers; (4) MI associated with percutaneous coronary intervention (PCI; Type 4a) or stent thrombosis (Type 4b); and (5) MI associated with coronary artery bypass graft (CABG) surgery.
- After MI, acute and chronic adaptations occur to prevent hemodynamic collapse but may also lead to ventricular remodeling and post-MI complications. Stimulation of the sympathetic nervous system (SNS) and renin–angiotensin–aldosterone system (RAAS) compensates for decreased cardiac output. However, chronic hyperactivation of these systems can lead to ventricular hypertrophy and further impairment

51

of contractility and cardiac output. Release of inflammatory mediators and collagen deposition contribute to myocardial fibrosis or scarring, which can lead to thinning of the left ventricular (LV) wall and eventual development of dilated cardiomyopathy.

- Complications of MI include ventricular arrhythmias, bradyarrhythmias, heart block, heart failure (HF), cardiogenic shock, LV free-wall or septal rupture, thromboembolism (including stroke secondary to LV thrombus embolization), aneurysm formation, and pericarditis. Many patients with ACS develop depression during the convalescent period.

CLINICAL PRESENTATION

- The patient is typically in acute distress and may present with or develop hypertensive crisis, acute HF, cardiogenic shock, or cardiac arrest.
- The classic symptom of ACS is abrupt-onset substernal chest pain or discomfort often described as a squeezing, heaviness, or tightness that persists for 10 minutes or longer. Symptoms may radiate to the arms and shoulders (especially on the left side), back, abdomen, or jaw. Nausea, vomiting, diaphoresis, or shortness of breath may also be present.
- Many patients have atypical symptoms without chest pain, such as epigastric pain, indigestion, pleuritic chest pain, and increasing exertional dyspnea. Older adults, women, and patients with diabetes mellitus (DM), impaired renal function, and dementia are more likely to present with atypical features.
- No physical examination findings are specific for ACS. Nonspecific findings include S_4 or paradoxical splitting of S_2 heart sounds on auscultation. Signs of acute decompensated HF include jugular venous distention, pulmonary edema, and an S_3 on auscultation. Patients may also present with arrhythmias, heart block, hypertension (HTN), hypotension, or shock.

DIAGNOSIS

- Obtain 12-lead ECG within 10 minutes of presentation. Changes suggestive of acute ischemia include STE, ST-segment depression, and T-wave inversion. Presence of a new left bundle-branch block (LBBB) in patients with suspected ACS is strongly suggestive of acute MI. Some patients with ACS have no ECG changes, so appropriate evaluation and risk stratification must carefully assess medical history, presenting symptoms, and cardiac biomarkers.
- Cardiac troponin (either T or I) is measured at the time of presentation and repeated 3–6 hours later to detect myocardial injury; elevated blood levels (exceeding the 99th percentile of the upper reference limit) occur within 2–4 hours of myocyte injury or necrosis and may remain elevated as long as 2 weeks. Myocardial injury is considered acute if there is a dynamic rise and/or fall by 20% or more in serial troponin values. Elevated levels in a patient with ACS symptoms, ischemic changes on ECG, or other evidence of ischemia confirm the diagnosis of MI. Additional troponin levels should be obtained beyond 6 hours after symptom onset in patients with intermediate- to high-risk features of ACS but normal troponin levels during serial measurements.
- Elevated dynamic cardiac troponin levels with ST-segment elevation of at least 1 mm in two contiguous leads or new LBBB on the presenting ECG confirms the diagnosis of STEMI. In contrast, the diagnosis of NSTEMI is appropriate for patients with symptoms of ACS and elevated troponin levels without at least 1 mm ST-segment elevation on the ECG at presentation. Patients with symptoms consistent with ACS but in whom troponin is not elevated may have UA or an alternative diagnosis.

TREATMENT

- <u>Goals of Treatment</u>: Short-term goals includes: (1) early restoration of blood flow to the affected artery to prevent infarct expansion (in the case of MI) or prevent complete occlusion and MI (in UA), (2) prevention of death and other complications, (3) prevention of coronary artery reocclusion, and (4) relief of ischemic chest discomfort. Long-term goals include control of cardiovascular (CV) risk factors, prevention of additional CV events, and improvement in quality of life.

GENERAL APPROACH TO TREATMENT OF ACS

- The clinical presentation, past medical history, ECG, and biomarkers are used to stratify patients as low, medium, or high risk and determine which patients may benefit from reperfusion therapy, an early invasive approach, or medical management. Treatment decisions are based on the initial and ongoing risk stratification (Fig. 5-1).
- Because STEMI has the highest short-term risk of death, these patients should be emergently referred for primary PCI; confirmation of elevated troponin should not delay treatment.
- General measures include hospital admission, oxygen administration if saturation is <90% (0.90) bed rest with continuous multilead ST-segment monitoring for arrhythmias and ischemia, frequent measurement of vital signs, ischemic pain relief, and prompt initiation of antithrombotic therapy.
- Assess kidney function (serum creatinine, creatinine clearance) to identify patients who may need dosing adjustments and those at high risk of morbidity and mortality.
- Measure serum potassium and magnesium levels, which may affect heart rhythm. Obtain complete blood cell count (CBC), fasting lipid panel, and coagulation tests (aPTT or anti-Xa levels, INR) because most patients will receive antithrombotic therapy.

ACUTE SUPPORTIVE CARE FOR ACS

- **Aspirin** is recommended for all ACS patients without contraindications, regardless of the type of ACS or management strategy. The initial dose is 162–325 mg (non-enteric coated) given as soon as possible and chewed and swallowed to speed dissolution and onset of platelet inhibition (<30 minutes). After the initial dose, aspirin 81 mg daily is continued indefinitely. Contraindications to aspirin include hypersensitivity and major GI intolerance. In these cases, clopidogrel with a loading dose followed by a maintenance dose should be used as an alternative.
- **Nitroglycerin** (NTG) is indicated for relief of anginal symptoms, uncontrolled HTN, and acute HF. The sublingual (SL) dose is 0.3–0.4 mg every 5 minutes for up to 3 doses as needed for angina. Consider intravenous (IV) NTG for persistent angina despite SL NTG at an initial dose of 10 mcg/min titrated to symptom relief and desired blood pressure (BP). Continue IV NTG until symptoms have resolved, BP is controlled, and HF symptoms have subsided. Gradually taper the infusion upon discontinuation. Nitrate administration is contraindicated in patients who have recently taken oral phosphodiesterase-5 (PDE-5) inhibitors (eg, sildenafil).
- **Oxygen** administration (2–4 L/min) should be reserved for select patients, particularly those with oxygen saturation <90% (0.90), because data suggest that routine use may adversely affect patients with ACS by increasing coronary vascular resistance and reducing coronary blood flow.
- **Morphine** is an analgesic, anxiolytic, and venodilator that reduces oxygen demand, but its role in ACS is uncertain because some studies have shown adverse outcomes. Current guidelines recommend IV morphine for pain relief in patients with STEMI. Recommended doses are 4–8 mg IV × 1 (lower dose in elderly), then 2–8 mg IV every 5–15 minutes as needed. In NSTE-ACS, IV morphine use is recommended only in patients refractory to treatment with other anti-ischemic medications; doses between 1 and 5 mg every 5–30 minutes are recommended.
- **β-Blockers** should be administered to all patients without contraindications because they reduce angina and the risk of MI and arrhythmias, even though their mortality benefit in the reperfusion era is uncertain. Current guidelines recommend initiation of an oral β-blocker within the first 24 hours of ACS presentation and continuation for at least 3 years in patients with normal LV ejection fraction (LVEF). For ACS patients with LV dysfunction (LVEF <40% [0.40]), β-blocker therapy is often lifelong. Recommended doses include:
  - ✓ **Carvedilol:** 6.25 mg orally twice daily; target dose is 25 mg twice daily as tolerated.
  - ✓ **Metoprolol:** 25–50 mg orally every 6–12 hours for 2–3 days, then once daily (metoprolol succinate) or twice daily (metoprolol tartrate); target dose is 200 mg daily. The IV dose is 5 mg every 5 minutes as tolerated up to 3 doses, titrated to

FIGURE 5-1. Evaluation and initial management of patients with suspected ACS.

BP and heart rate (HR); the IV route should be reserved for STEMI patients with acute uncontrolled HTN or refractory symptoms.

- **Calcium channel blockers** (CCBs) have anti-ischemic effects but may not have beneficial effects on mortality, MI, or recurrent MI. Guidelines recommend nondihydropyridine CCBs (diltiazem, verapamil) for angina symptoms in patients with ACS who have a contraindication, have intolerance, or are refractory to β-blockers in the absence of LV dysfunction, risk factors for cardiogenic shock, and atrioventricular conduction defects. Long-acting CCBs are recommended for patients with ACS with known or suspected vasospasm. Recommended doses include:
  - ✓ **Diltiazem:** 120–360 mg/day orally
  - ✓ **Verapamil:** 240–480 mg/day orally
  - ✓ **Amlodipine:** 5–10 mg orally once daily
  - ✓ **Nicardipine:** 60–120 mg/day orally
  - ✓ **Nifedipine extended-release** (ER): 30–120 mg orally once daily

TREATMENT STRATEGIES IN STEMI

Primary PCI

- Mechanical reperfusion with PCI using intracoronary balloons, stents, or other devices within 90 minutes of first medical contact is the reperfusion treatment of choice. Patients presenting to hospitals unable to perform PCI should be transferred to a PCI-capable hospital to achieve reperfusion within 120 minutes of the first medical contact. Compared to reperfusion with fibrinolysis, primary PCI improves survival, establishes consistent revascularization to the infarct-related artery, reduces the risk of stroke and intracranial hemorrhage (ICH), and reduces reinfarction and recurrent ischemia.

Fibrinolysis

- Administer fibrinolysis to patients with STEMI when PCI cannot be performed within 120 minutes of first medical contact, provided no contraindications exist. Limit use of fibrinolytics between 12 and 24 hours after symptom onset to patients with clinical and/or ECG evidence of ongoing ischemia.
- Absolute contraindications to fibrinolytic therapy include any prior hemorrhagic stroke, ischemic stroke within 3 months, intracranial neoplasm or AV malformation, active internal bleeding, aortic dissection, considerable facial or closed head trauma in the past 3 months, intracranial or intraspinal surgery within 2 months, severe uncontrolled HTN, and for streptokinase, treatment within previous 6 months (if considering streptokinase again). Primary PCI is preferred in these situations.
- A fibrin-specific agent (alteplase, reteplase, or tenecteplase) is preferred over the non–fibrin-specific agent streptokinase because of greater reperfusion success and less systemic bleeding.
- Treat eligible patients within 30 minutes of hospital arrival with one of the following:
  - ✓ **Alteplase:** 15-mg IV bolus over 1–2 minutes, then 0.75 mg/kg (maximum 50 mg) IV over 30 minutes, then 0.5 mg/kg (maximum 35 mg) IV over 60 minutes; maximum total dose 100 mg
  - ✓ **Reteplase:** 10 units IV over 2 minutes, followed 30 minutes later with another 10 units IV over 2 minutes
  - ✓ **Tenecteplase:** Single IV bolus given over 5 seconds based on patient weight: 30 mg if <60 kg; 35 mg if 60–69.9 kg; 40 mg if 70–79.9 kg; 45 mg if 80–89.9 kg; and 50 mg if ≥90 kg
- Fibrinolytic therapy is associated with a slight but statistically significant risk for stroke, largely attributed to ICH (0.9%–1.0% of patients). Predictors for ICH include advanced age, lower total body weight, female sex, preexisting cerebrovascular disease, and systolic and diastolic HTN at time of presentation.

Antithrombotic Therapy

- Administer antithrombotic therapy with antiplatelet agents and parenteral anticoagulation concomitantly with both primary PCI and fibrinolysis to improve vessel patency and prevent reocclusion (see Antithrombotic Therapy section below).

TREATMENT STRATEGIES IN NSTE-ACS

Early Invasive Approach

- Patients presenting with NSTE-ACS typically have a partially occluded coronary artery with some residual perfusion; therefore, the need for and urgency to perform PCI is not as critical. With an early invasive approach, diagnostic angiography is typically performed within the first 24 hours with the intent to perform revascularization if appropriate. Guidelines recommend this strategy in patients with intermediate to high risk for death, MI, refractory angina, acute HF, cardiogenic shock, or arrhythmias.

Ischemia-Guided Approach (Medical Management)

- If an early invasive strategy using PCI is not considered appropriate, select low-risk patients may receive more conservative ischemia-guided medical management, where antiplatelet and anticoagulants are administered and PCI is not initially planned. Patients are evaluated for signs and symptoms of recurrent ischemia or hemodynamic instability (eg, with noninvasive stress testing) and taken for coronary angiography and possible PCI only if symptoms recur.

ANTITHROMBOTIC THERAPY FOR ACS

- Both antiplatelet and anticoagulant therapy are necessary in the acute treatment phase of ACS because platelets dominate the pathophysiologic processes in arterial thrombosis, and thrombin is involved in both platelet activation and coagulation. After hospital discharge, most patients are continued on long-term antiplatelet therapy only, although long-term anticoagulant therapy may benefit some high-risk individuals.

Antiplatelet Therapy

- **Aspirin:** A dose of 81 mg daily is continued indefinitely (after the initial 162–325 mg dose) in patients with either STEMI or NSTE-ACS, regardless of the management strategy employed. Patients undergoing PCI for STEMI or NSTE-ACS already receiving chronic aspirin 81 mg daily should be given an additional dose of 81–325 mg before the procedure.
- **P2Y$_{12}$ Inhibitors:** An oral agent (clopidogrel, prasugrel, ticagrelor) is typically given with aspirin as dual antiplatelet therapy (DAPT) to prevent stent thrombosis and thrombotic CV events. Cangrelor is an IV drug indicated as an adjunct to PCI to reduce periprocedural MI, repeat revascularization, and stent thrombosis in patients not receiving oral P2Y$_{12}$ inhibitors or planned GP IIb/IIIa inhibitors. Any of the four agents may be given with primary PCI, but only clopidogrel has been evaluated in large clinical trials in patients with STEMI receiving reperfusion with fibrinolysis. Recommended doses are as follows:
  - ✓ **Clopidogrel:** 600-mg oral loading dose before primary PCI for STEMI or NSTE-ACS. Give a 300-mg oral loading dose to patients receiving a fibrinolytic or who do not receive reperfusion therapy. Avoid a loading dose in patients age ≥75 years. The maintenance dose is 75 mg daily.
  - ✓ **Prasugrel:** 60-mg oral loading dose in patients undergoing PCI, followed by 10 mg orally once daily for patients weighing ≥60 kg; use 5 mg once daily for patients weighing <60 kg.
  - ✓ **Ticagrelor:** 180-mg oral loading dose in patients undergoing PCI, followed by 90 mg orally twice daily.
  - ✓ **Cangrelor:** 30 mcg/kg IV bolus prior to PCI followed by 4 mcg/kg/min infusion for duration of PCI or 2 hours, whichever is longer.
- Withhold clopidogrel and ticagrelor for at least 5 days and prasugrel for 7 days before elective surgery (eg, CABG surgery). Cangrelor can be continued until just a few hours before surgery because of its short duration of action.

Glycoprotein IIb/IIIa Inhibitors (GPIs)

- GPIs inhibit GP IIb/IIIa receptors on platelets, blocking the binding of fibrinogen to activated GP IIb/IIIa receptors, which is the final step in platelet aggregation.

- These agents must be given with unfractionated heparin (UFH) or a low-molecular-weight heparin (LMWH) that should be discontinued immediately after PCI to reduce the risk of major bleeding.
- Use of GPIs has been declining in recent years; patients likely to benefit most are those receiving PCI for NSTE-ACS with elevated troponin levels and patients with STEMI who have not been preloaded with a $P2Y_{12}$ inhibitor and are not being treated with bivalirudin. Recommended doses are as follows:
  - ✓ **Abciximab:** 0.25 mg/kg IV bolus given 10–60 minutes before the start of PCI, followed by 0.125 mcg/kg/min (maximum 10 mcg/min) for 12 hours; alternatively, 0.25 mg/kg intracoronary bolus only.
  - ✓ **Eptifibatide:** 180 mcg/kg IV bolus, repeated in 10 minutes, followed by IV infusion of 2 mcg/kg/min for 18–24 hours after PCI; reduce infusion dose by 50% if creatinine clearance (CrCl) is <50 mL/min (0.83 mL/sec).
  - ✓ **Tirofiban:** 25 mcg/kg IV bolus, then 0.15 mcg/kg/min for up to 18–24 hours after PCI; reduce infusion dose by 50% if CrCl is ≤60 mL/min (1.0 mL/sec).
- GPIs are not beneficial and should not be used in patients with NSTE-ACS undergoing an ischemia-driven approach. GPIs should also be avoided in patients with STEMI receiving reperfusion with fibrinolytics because of significant increases in major bleeding and ICH.
- Besides bleeding, GPIs cause significant thrombocytopenia in about 1% of patients receiving abciximab and 0.5% with eptifibatide and tirofiban. Because GPIs are given with heparin, it is important to differentiate GPI-induced thrombocytopenia from heparin-induced thrombocytopenia (HIT).

Anticoagulants

- Although patients with ACS are typically on at least two antiplatelet agents for a year or more, a single anticoagulant is usually given for a short time (the initial few days of hospitalization).
- Current evidence in the acute management of ACS is with injectable anticoagulants. See Table 5-1 for anticoagulant indications and drug doses in ACS.
- **Unfractionated heparin (UFH)** has been widely used in ACS management for several decades. Based on experience, UFH can be used across the spectrum of ACS and regardless of the management strategy. Because of significant interpatient variability in anticoagulant response, therapy must be monitored with the activated partial thromboplastin time (aPTT) every 6 hours until two consecutive readings are within the institution's therapeutic range (1.5–2 times the control value), then every 24 hours for the duration of UFH therapy. The activated clotting time (ACT) is monitored during PCI because it can be measured at the bedside with rapid results. Platelet counts should also be monitored daily or every other day to detect HIT. If HIT is suspected, discontinue UFH and provide anticoagulation with an IV direct thrombin inhibitor.
- **Low-molecular-weight heparins (LMWHs)** provide a predicable anticoagulant dose response with no need for routine therapeutic monitoring. Anti-Xa level monitoring may be helpful in obese patients (>190 kg) and patients with severe renal insufficiency (eg, CrCl <30 mL/min [0.5 mL/sec]). The target peak anti-Xa level is 0.3–0.7 IU/mL (kIU/L) drawn 4 hours after the third dose. The utility of anti-Xa monitoring is limited because patients with ACS typically receive anticoagulant therapy for only a few days. Although the incidence of HIT is lower with LMWHs (<2%) than with UFH (2%–5%), monitoring of platelet counts is still warranted. Due to 90% crossreactivity between HIT antibodies from LMWH and UFH, LMWH is not a safe alternative in patients who develop HIT from UFH and vice versa.
  - ✓ **Enoxaparin** is the most widely studied agent in ACS and is the only LMWH recommended in current guidelines. Data support its efficacy in patients with STEMI and NSTE-ACS, regardless of the perfusion or management strategy used. However, enoxaparin dosing varies across these different situations (Table 5-1). In patients with STEMI receiving reperfusion with fibrinolytics,

TABLE 5-1	Anticoagulant Drug Use and Dosing for Treatment of Acute Coronary Syndrome			
	STEMI		NSTE-ACS	
Drug	Primary PCI	Fibrinolytic Perfusion	Early Invasive Strategy	Ischemia-Driven Strategy
Bivalirudin	0.75 mg/kg IV bolus, followed by 1.75 mg/kg/hr IV infusion until completion of PCI; CrCl <30 mL/min (0.5 mL/sec): reduce infusion to 1 mg/kg/hr	No recommendation	0.10 mg/kg IV bolus, followed by 0.25 mg/kg/hr IV infusion until completion of PCI	No recommendation
Enoxaparin	0.5 mg/kg one-time IV bolus	30 mg IV bolus, followed within 15 min by 1 mg/kg SC every 12 hours for up to 8 days or hospital discharge; cap first two SC doses at 100 mg; CrCl <30 mL/min (0.5 mL/sec): 30 mg IV bolus, followed by 1 mg/kg SC every 24 hours; cap first dose at 100 mg; Age ≥75 years: omit IV bolus and initiate 0.75 mg/kg SC every 12 hours; cap first two doses at 75 mg; CrCl <30 mL/min (0.5 mL/sec) and age ≥75: omit IV bolus and initiate at 1 mg/kg every 24 hours	1 mg/kg SC every 12 hours until PCI; may give an initial 30 mg IV bolus; Give 0.3 mg/kg IV bolus if PCI occurs before two SC doses have been given, or if the last dose was given 8 hours or more prior to PCI; CrCl <30 mL/min (0.5 mL/s): 1 mg/kg SC every 24 hours	1 mg/kg SC every 12 hours for duration of hospitalization; may give an initial 30 mg IV bolus; CrCl <30 mL/min (0.5 mL/ sec): 1 mg/kg SC every 24 hours

Fondaparinux	No recommendation	2.5 mg IV first dose, followed by 2.5 mg SC daily for up to 8 days or hospital discharge	2.5 mg SC daily until PCI; At time of PCI, if no GPI give 85 units/kg IV UFH[a], if with GPI give 60 units/kg IV UFH[a]	2.5 mg SC daily for up to 8 days or duration of hospitalization.
Unfractionated heparin (UFH)	If no GPI, 70–100 units/kg IV bolus to achieve therapeutic ACT[a]; If taking GPI, 50–70 units/kg IV bolus to achieve therapeutic ACT[a]	60 units/kg (max. 4000 units) IV bolus, followed by 12 units/kg/hr (max. initial infusion rate 1000 units/hr)	60 units/kg (max. 4000 units) IV bolus, followed by 12 units/kg/hr (max. initial infusion rate 1000 units/hr)[a]	60 units/kg (max. 4000 units) IV bolus, followed by 12 units/kg/hr (max. initial infusion rate 1000 units/hr)

[a]Additional IV UFH boluses may be needed to maintain a therapeutic ACT.

ACT, activated clotting time; CrCl, creatinine clearance; GPI, glycoprotein IIb/IIIa inhibitor; IV, intravenous; NSTE-ACS, non-ST-segment elevation acute coronary syndrome; PCI, percutaneous coronary intervention; SC, subcutaneous; STEMI, ST-segment elevation myocardial infarction; UFH, unfractionated heparin.

enoxaparin demonstrated a significant 17% reduction in death and MI compared to UFH. Based on clinical trial data, either UFH or enoxaparin is recommended in patients with NSTE-ACS.

- **Fondaparinux** provides a predicable anticoagulant dose response with no need for therapeutic monitoring (similar to LMWH). A clinical trial in NSTE-ACS patients receiving either an ischemia-driven or invasive management strategy demonstrated similar efficacy between fondaparinux and enoxaparin, with significantly less major bleeding in patients receiving fondaparinux. Although confounding factors may account for the bleeding difference, fondaparinux can be considered in patients undergoing an ischemia-driven approach who are at high risk of bleeding. Fondaparinux is not recommended in patients receiving primary PCI for STEMI because of clinical trial results demonstrating higher rates of catheter-related thrombosis compared to UFH. In patients with STEMI receiving fibrinolytics, fondaparinux had efficacy and safety similar to UFH. However, fondaparinux is rarely used in patients with STEMI based on the lack of superiority to UFH and the benefit shown with enoxaparin over UFH in this population.
- **Bivalirudin** is a direct thrombin inhibitor that is used only in patients with ACS who receive PCI and can be monitored with the ACT in the catheterization laboratory. Although current guidelines recommend bivalirudin use, UFH is often used instead because recent trials suggested that bivalirudin does not offer efficacy or safety benefits over UFH alone in the setting of primary PCI for STEMI. Bivalirudin has not been evaluated in patients with STEMI receiving reperfusion with fibrinolytics or in patients with NSTE-ACS undergoing an ischemia-driven approach.

SECONDARY PREVENTION OF ISCHEMIC EVENTS

- After a diagnosis of ACS, patients are considered to have atherosclerotic cardiovascular disease (ASCVD) and should be treated aggressively because they are at the highest risk of recurrent major adverse cardiovascular events (MACE).
- Aggressive risk factor modification strategies should be initiated and continued indefinitely (eg, increased physical activity, dietary modification, weight loss, BP modification, and smoking cessation).
- Pharmacotherapy proven to decrease mortality, HF, reinfarction, stroke, and stent thrombosis should be initiated prior to hospital discharge in all patients without contraindications. This includes anti-ischemic, antiplatelet, lipid-lowering, and antihypertensive therapies.
- Medication reconciliation at discharge should include assessment for the medication classes listed below as appropriate unless a contraindication exists; drug regimen examples within medication classes listed here are not intended to be exhaustive.
- **Aspirin:** Treat with aspirin 81 mg once daily indefinitely.
- **$P2Y_{12}$ inhibitor:** Because the ischemic risk following ACS is high, DAPT with aspirin plus a $P2Y_{12}$ receptor inhibitor is indicated for most patients for at least 12 months regardless of the management strategy employed. Continuation of DAPT beyond 12 months may be reasonable for patients at higher ischemic risk if they also have a low bleeding risk. For patients with STEMI treated with fibrinolysis, the minimum recommended duration of DAPT is 14 days.
  - ✓ Clopidogrel: 75 mg once daily
  - ✓ Prasugrel: 10 mg once daily (5 mg daily if body weight <60 kg)
  - ✓ Ticagrelor: 90 mg twice daily
- **β-Blocker:**
  - ✓ Carvedilol: 6.25 mg twice daily; target dose (in patients with HF with reduced ejection fraction [HFrEF]) 25 mg twice daily as tolerated
  - ✓ Metoprolol: 25–50 mg every 6–12 hours for 2–3 days, then once daily (metoprolol succinate) or twice daily (metoprolol tartrate); target dose (in patients with HFrEF) 200 mg daily

    Other β-blockers may be considered; in patients with HFrEF, use either metoprolol succinate, carvedilol, or bisoprolol, Continue therapy for at least 3 years and indefinitely in patients with concomitant HFrEF.

- **Statin:** Initiate high-intensity statin therapy during the index hospitalization once the patient has been stabilized and continue treatment indefinitely. All patients should receive the highest dose of maximally tolerated statin:
  - ✓ Atorvastatin: 80 mg daily
  - ✓ Rosuvastatin: 20–40 mg daily

  Moderate-intensity statins or lower doses of high-intensity statins may be considered for ACS patients with a history of statin intolerance or those at high risk for statin-related adverse effects. Patients over age 75 may be prescribed a moderate-intensity statin as initial therapy. Reassess a lipid panel 4–6 weeks after initiation of therapy with the goal of a 50% reduction in LDL-C from baseline.

- **Non-statin cholesterol-lowering medications:** For patients with very high risk ASCVD (eg, post-ACS) and LDL-C >70 mg/dL (1.81 mmol/L) on maximally tolerated statin therapy.
  - ✓ Ezetimibe: 10 mg daily
  - ✓ Simvastatin: 40 mg/ezetimibe 10 mg daily
  - ✓ Alirocumab: 75 mg SC every 2 weeks

- **Angiotensin-converting enzyme (ACE) inhibitor:** Early administration (within 48 hours of presentation) is associated with lower mortality within the first month of therapy with additional benefit observed during over longer treatment durations.
  - ✓ Lisinopril: 2.5–5 mg daily; target dose 10–40 mg daily
  - ✓ Captopril: 6.25–12.5 mg three times daily; target dose 25–50 mg three times daily
  - ✓ Ramipril: 2.5 mg twice daily; target dose 5 mg twice daily
  - ✓ Trandolapril: 0.5–1 mg daily; target dose 4 mg daily

- **Angiotensin receptor blocker (ARB):** Patients intolerant to ACE inhibitors:
  - ✓ Valsartan: 20 mg twice daily; target dose 160 mg twice daily

- **Aldosterone antagonist:** To reduce mortality, consider administration within the first 14 days after MI in patients treated with both an ACE inhibitor (or ARB) and β-blocker with LV dysfunction (LVEF ≤40% [0.40]) and either HF symptoms or DM.
  - ✓ Eplerenone: 25 mg daily; target dose 50 mg daily
  - ✓ Spironolactone: 12.5–25 mg daily; target dose 25–50 mg daily

- **Nitroglycerin:** All patients not taking PDE-5 inhibitors should be prescribed and instructed on appropriate use of short-acting NTG, either SL tablets (0.3–0.4 mg SL every 5 minutes, up to 3 doses) or lingual spray to relieve acute anginal symptoms on an as-needed basis.

EVALUATION OF THERAPEUTIC OUTCOMES

- Evaluation of short-term efficacy focuses on restoration or preservation of coronary blood flow, symptom relief, and prevention of MACE.
- Determine restoration of blood flow and relief of ischemia by resolution of ischemic ECG changes on presentation, which should occur soon after revascularization.
- Although troponin levels may remain elevated for several days, levels in patients with MI should peak within 12–24 hours and then decline steadily once ischemia is relieved.
- Monitor for development of ACS complications (eg, HF, arrhythmias) frequently.
- Prior to hospital discharge, perform echocardiogram or equivalent modality to identify patients with LV dysfunction (LVEF <40% [0.40]) who are at high risk of death and candidates for guideline-directed medical therapy and device therapy.
- Assure that evidence-based therapies shown to reduce the risk of MACE following ACS have been initiated.
- Long-term outcome evaluation is directed at maintaining functional capacity, quality of life, and continued focus on risk reduction.
- Monitor patients at every healthcare encounter for development of adverse effects from ACS pharmacotherapy (Table 5-2).

See Chapter 33, Acute Coronary Syndrome, authored by Robert J. DiDomenico, Paul P. Dobesh, and Shannon W. Finks, for a more detailed discussion of this topic.

TABLE 5-2	Adverse Drug Effect Monitoring for Acute Coronary Syndrome	
Drug	**Adverse Effects**	**Monitoring Parameters**
Fibrinolytics	Bleeding (ICH)	Clinical signs of bleeding[a]; baseline aPTT, INR; Hgb, Hct, platelet count at baseline then daily; mental status every 2 hours for signs of ICH
Aspirin	Dyspepsia, GI bleeding	Clinical signs of bleeding[a]; GI upset; Hgb, Hct, and platelet count at baseline and every 6 months
P2Y$_{12}$ inhibitors	Bleeding, rash	Clinical signs of bleeding[a]; evidence of rash; Hgb, Hct, platelet count at baseline and every 6 months
	Ticagrelor: dyspnea, ventricular pauses, bradycardia	Ticagrelor: dyspnea, HR, telemetry during hospitalization
Glycoprotein IIb/ IIIa inhibitors	Bleeding, thrombocytopenia (can be profound with abciximab)	Clinical signs of bleeding[a]; Hgb, Hct, and platelet count at baseline, 2 hours, then daily
		Eptifibatide and tirofiban: SCr at baseline then daily
Anticoagulants	Bleeding	Clinical signs of bleeding[a]; baseline aPTT, INR; Hgb, Hct, platelet count at baseline then daily
	UFH and LMWH: heparin-induced thrombocytopenia	UFH: aPTT every 6 hours until two consecutive aPTT values are at goal, then every 24 hours; monitor the ACT during PCI
		Enoxaparin, bivalirudin, and fondaparinux: SCr at baseline then daily
		Enoxaparin: may consider steady-state anti-Xa levels in select populations
β-Blockers	Hypotension, HF, bradycardia, cardiogenic shock, AV block, exacerbation of asthma or reactive airway disease	Continuous telemetry (while hospitalized); BP, HR, signs and symptoms of HF; monitor every 5 min before each IV bolus dose; monitor every shift while hospitalized then at each healthcare encounter after discharge
Nitroglycerin	Flushing, headache, hypotension, tachycardia	BP and HR; monitor every 5–15 min following dosage adjustment of IV NTG then every 1–2 hours; monitor every 5 min following administration of short-acting NTG

Morphine	Hypotension, respiratory depression, sedation, hypersensitivity	BP, HR, respiratory rate, sedation level 5 min after administration then every 1–2 hours for 4 hours after the last dose
Calcium channel blockers	Hypotension Verapamil and diltiazem: HF, cardiogenic shock, bradycardia, AV block	BP and HR every shift while hospitalized then at each healthcare encounter after discharge Verapamil and diltiazem: continuous telemetry (while hospitalized); signs and symptoms of HF every shift while hospitalized then at each healthcare encounter after discharge
Statins	GI discomfort, arthralgia, myalgia, musculoskeletal pain, hepatotoxicity	Liver function tests at baseline (prior to discharge) and if signs or symptoms of hepatotoxicity develop; creatine kinase if severe myalgia or musculoskeletal symptoms occur; LDL-C at baseline, 4–12 weeks after initiation or dose adjustment, then every 3–12 months
Nonstatin therapies for cholesterol management	Ezetimibe and combination: GI discomfort, arthralgia, myalgia, musculoskeletal pain Alirocumab: injection site pain, hypersensitivity	Simvastatin/ezetimibe: liver function tests at baseline (prior to discharge) and if signs or symptoms of hepatotoxicity develop; creatinine kinase if severe myalgia or musculoskeletal symptoms occur; LDL-C at baseline, 4–12 weeks after initiation or dose adjustment, then every 3–12 months Alirocumab: LDL-C at baseline and 4–8 weeks after initiation or dose adjustment; evaluation of injection site if injection site pain develops, signs and symptoms of hypersensitivity with each healthcare encounter
ACE inhibitors	Hypotension, hyperuricemia, hyperkalemia, worsening renal function, chronic cough, angioedema	BP every shift while hospitalized, 1–2 weeks after initiation or dose adjustment, then with each healthcare encounter; SCr and potassium at baseline, 1–2 weeks after initiation, then every 6–12 months; signs and symptoms of angioedema or cough with each healthcare encounter
ARBs	Hypotension, hyperuricemia, hyperkalemia, worsening renal function	BP every shift while hospitalized, 1–2 weeks after initiation or dose adjustment, then with each healthcare encounter; SCr and potassium at baseline, 1–2 weeks after initiation, then every 6–12 months
Aldosterone antagonist	Hyperkalemia, worsening renal function	BP every shift while hospitalized, 1–2 weeks after initiation or dose adjustment, then with each healthcare encounter; SCr and potassium at baseline, after initiation or dose adjustment: at 3 days, 1 week, monthly for 3 months, then every 3 months

[a] Clinical signs of bleeding include bloody stools, melena, hematuria, hematemesis, bruising, and oozing from arterial or venous puncture sites.
ACE, angiotensin-converting enzyme; ACT, activated clotting time; aPTT, activated partial thromboplastin time; ARB, angiotensin receptor blocker; AV, atrioventricular; BP, blood pressure; GI, gastrointestinal; Hct, hematocrit; HF, heart failure; Hgb, hemoglobin; HR, heart rate; ICH, intracranial hemorrhage; INR, international normalized ratio; LDL-C, low-density lipoprotein cholesterol; NTG, nitroglycerin; PCI, percutaneous coronary intervention; SCr, serum creatinine; UFH, unfractionated heparin.

CHAPTER 6

Arrhythmias

- *Cardiac arrhythmia* involves a group of conditions in which the heartbeat is irregular, too slow, or too fast. *Supraventricular arrhythmias* occur above the ventricles, and *ventricular arrhythmias* occur within the ventricles.

PATHOPHYSIOLOGY

SUPRAVENTRICULAR ARRHYTHMIAS

Atrial Fibrillation and Atrial Flutter

- Atrial fibrillation (AF) has extremely rapid (400–600 atrial beats/min) and disorganized atrial activation. There is loss of atrial contraction (atrial kick), and supraventricular impulses penetrate the atrioventricular (AV) conduction system to variable degrees, resulting in irregular ventricular activation and an irregularly irregular pulse. The AV junction will not conduct most of the supraventricular impulses, causing the ventricular response to be considerably slower than the atrial rate.
- Atrial flutter has rapid (270–330 atrial beats/min) but regular atrial activation. Ventricular response usually has a regular pattern and a pulse of 300 beats/min. This arrhythmia is less common than AF but has similar precipitating factors, consequences, and drug therapy approach.
- The predominant mechanism of AF and atrial flutter is reentry, which is usually associated with organic heart disease that causes left atrial distention (eg, ischemia or infarction, hypertensive heart disease, and valvular disorders). Additional associated disorders include acute pulmonary embolism and chronic lung disease, resulting in pulmonary hypertension and cor pulmonale, and states of high adrenergic tone such as thyrotoxicosis, alcohol withdrawal, sepsis, and excessive physical exertion.

Paroxysmal Supraventricular Tachycardia

- PSVT arising by reentrant mechanisms includes arrhythmias caused by AV nodal reentry (AVNRT), AV reentrant tachycardia (AVRT) due to an accessory pathway, sinoatrial (SA) nodal reentry, and intraatrial reentry.

VENTRICULAR ARRHYTHMIAS

Premature Ventricular Complexes

- Premature ventricular complexes (PVCs) can occur in patients with or without structural heart disease (SHD). PVCs may be elicited by abnormal automaticity, triggered activity, or reentrant mechanisms. PVCs often occur in healthy individuals and have little, if any, prognostic significance in this situation. PVCs occur more frequently and in more complex forms in patients with SHD than in healthy individuals, and patients with some PVC forms (multifocal or couplets) are at higher risk of sudden cardiac death.

Ventricular Tachycardia

- Ventricular tachycardia (VT) is defined by three or more repetitive PVCs occurring at a rate of >100 beats/min. It is a wide QRS tachycardia that may result acutely from severe electrolyte abnormalities (hypokalemia, hypomagnesemia), hypoxia, drug toxicity (eg, digoxin), or (most commonly) in patients presenting with acute myocardial infarction (MI) or myocardial ischemia complicated by heart failure (HF). The chronic recurrent form is almost always associated with SHD (eg, idiopathic dilated cardiomyopathy or remote MI with left ventricular [LV] aneurysm).
- Sustained VT requires intervention to restore a stable rhythm or persists for a relatively long time (usually >30 seconds). Nonsustained VT self-terminates after a brief duration (usually <30 seconds). Incessant VT refers to VT occurring more

frequently than sinus rhythm, so that VT becomes the dominant rhythm. Monomorphic VT has a consistent QRS configuration, whereas polymorphic VT has varying QRS complexes. Torsade de pointes (TdP) is a polymorphic VT in which the QRS complexes appear to undulate around a central axis.

Ventricular Proarrhythmia

- Proarrhythmia is the development of a significant new arrhythmia, such as VT, ventricular fibrillation (VF), or TdP, or worsening of an existing arrhythmia. Proarrhythmia results from the same mechanisms that cause other arrhythmias or from an alteration in the underlying substrate due to an antiarrhythmic drug (AAD).
  - ✓ Class Ic AADs can cause a rapid, sustained, monomorphic VT with a characteristic sinusoidal QRS pattern resulting from excessive sodium channel blockade and slowed conduction. The proarrhythmia risk continues as long as the AAD is continued. Predisposing factors include the presence of underlying ventricular arrhythmias, coronary artery disease (CAD), and LV dysfunction.
  - ✓ TdP is a rapid form of polymorphic VT associated with evidence of delayed ventricular repolarization due to blockade of potassium conductance. TdP may be hereditary or acquired. Acquired forms are associated with many clinical conditions and drugs, especially class Ia and class III I_{Kr} blockers. Development of clinically significant QTc interval prolongation (ie, QTc interval >500 msec or an increase in QTc interval of >60–70 msec from baseline) after starting a drug is an indication to discontinue the agent or reduce its dose with careful monitoring.

Ventricular Fibrillation

- VF is electrical anarchy of the ventricle resulting in no cardiac output and cardiovascular (CV) collapse. Sudden cardiac death occurs most commonly in patients with CAD or LV dysfunction.

BRADYARRHYTHMIAS

- Sinus bradyarrhythmias (heart rate <60 beats/min) are common, especially in young, athletically active individuals, and are usually asymptomatic and do not require intervention. However, some patients have sinus node dysfunction (sick sinus syndrome) because of underlying SHD and the normal aging process, which attenuates SA nodal function. Sinus node dysfunction is usually representative of diffuse conduction disease, which may be accompanied by AV block and by paroxysmal tachycardias such as AF. Alternating bradyarrhythmias and tachyarrhythmias are referred to as the tachy–brady syndrome.
- AV block or conduction delay may occur in any area of the AV conduction system. AV block may be found in patients without underlying heart disease (eg, trained athletes) or during sleep when vagal tone is high. It may be transient when the underlying etiology is reversible (eg, myocarditis, myocardial ischemia, after CV surgery, or during drug therapy). β-Blockers, digoxin, or nondihydropyridine (non-DHP) calcium channel blockers (CCBs) may cause AV block, primarily in the AV nodal area. Class I AADs may exacerbate conduction delays below the level of the AV node. AV block may be irreversible if the cause is acute MI, rare degenerative diseases, primary myocardial disease, or congenital heart disease.

CLINICAL PRESENTATION

- Patients with AF or atrial flutter may complain of rapid heart rate, palpitations, chest pain, dyspnea, dizziness, and fatigue. Medical emergencies are severe HF (ie, pulmonary edema, hypotension) or AF occurring in the setting of acute MI. These arrhythmias are usually not directly life-threatening and do not generally cause hemodynamic collapse or syncope.
- PSVT caused by reentry can be transient, resulting in few, if any, symptoms. Patients may complain of intermittent episodes of rapid heart rate/palpitations that abruptly

start and stop, usually without provocation (but sometimes with exercise). Patients may also complain of chest pressure or a neck sensation. Life-threatening symptoms (syncope, hemodynamic collapse) are associated with an extremely rapid heart rate (eg, >200 beats/min) and AF associated with an accessory pathway.

- PVCs are non–life-threatening and usually asymptomatic. Patients occasionally complain of palpitations or uncomfortable heartbeats. Because the PVC occurs early and the ventricle contracts when incompletely filled, patients do not feel the PVC itself; rather, the sinus beat following the PVC and a compensatory pause is responsible for the symptoms.
- The symptoms of sustained VT (monomorphic VT or TdP) can range from nearly asymptomatic to pulseless hemodynamic collapse. Fast heart rates and underlying poor LV function result in more severe symptoms. Symptoms of nonsustained, self-terminating VT correlate with duration of episodes (eg, patients with 15-second episodes will be more symptomatic than those with three-beat episodes).
- VF results in hemodynamic collapse, syncope, and cardiac arrest. Cardiac output and blood pressure are not recordable.
- Some patients who develop proarrhythmia may be asymptomatic, others may notice worsening symptoms, and some may die suddenly.
- Symptoms of bradyarrhythmias generally result from decreased cardiac output and may be associated with hypotension (eg, dizziness, syncope, fatigue, confusion). If LV dysfunction exists, patients may experience worsening HF symptoms. Except for recurrent syncope, symptoms associated with bradyarrhythmias are often subtle and nonspecific.

DIAGNOSIS

- On ECG, AF is an irregularly irregular rhythm with no discernible, consistent atrial activity (P waves). Ventricular rate is usually 90–170 beats/min and the pulse is irregular. Atrial flutter is usually a regular supraventricular rhythm with characteristic flutter waves reflecting more organized atrial activity; the ventricular rate is often in factors of 300 beats/min (eg, 150, 100, or 75 beats/min).
- The ECG in patients with PSVT commonly shows a rapid, narrow QRS tachycardia (regular in rhythm) that starts and stops abruptly. Atrial activity, although present, is difficult to ascertain on ECG because P waves are "buried" in the QRS complex or T wave.
- Proarrhythmia can be difficult to diagnose because of the variable nature of underlying arrhythmias.
- TdP is characterized by long QT intervals or prominent U waves on the ECG.
- First-degree AV block is 1:1 AV conduction with a prolonged PR interval. Second-degree AV block is divided into two forms: Mobitz I AV block (Wenckebach periodicity) is <1:1 AV conduction with progressively lengthening PR intervals until a ventricular complex is dropped; Mobitz II AV block is intermittently dropped ventricular beats in a random fashion without progressive PR lengthening. Third-degree AV block is complete heart block where AV conduction is totally absent (AV dissociation).

TREATMENT

- <u>Goals of Treatment</u>: The desired outcome depends on the underlying arrhythmia. For example, the goals of treating AF or atrial flutter are restoring sinus rhythm, preventing thromboembolic complications, and preventing further recurrences.

GENERAL APPROACH

- Use of AADs has declined because clinical trials showed increased mortality with their use due to proarrhythmic side effects. AADs have been increasingly replaced by nonpharmacologic approaches such as ablation and the implantable cardioverter-defibrillator (ICD).

ANTIARRHYTHMIC DRUGS

- Drugs may depress the automatic properties of abnormal pacemaker cells by decreasing the slope of phase 4 depolarization and/or by elevating threshold potential. Drugs may alter conduction characteristics of the pathways of a reentrant loop.
- The Vaughan Williams classification system of AADs is most frequently used for categorizing their electrophysiologic actions (Table 6-1).
    - ✓ Class I drugs are sodium channel blockers. Class Ia drugs slow conduction velocity, prolong refractoriness, and decrease the automatic properties of sodium-dependent (normal and diseased) conduction tissue. Class Ia drugs are effective for both supraventricular and ventricular arrhythmias, but they are infrequently used because of limited efficacy and significant toxicities.
    - ✓ Class Ib drugs probably act similarly to class Ia drugs, except that class Ib agents are considerably more effective in ventricular than supraventricular arrhythmias.
    - ✓ Class Ic drugs slow conduction velocity while leaving refractoriness relatively unaltered. Although effective for both ventricular and supraventricular arrhythmias, their use for ventricular arrhythmias has been limited by the risk of proarrhythmia.
    - ✓ Class II drugs include β-blockers; their antiarrhythmic effects result from antiadrenergic actions. β-Blockers are most useful in tachycardias in which nodal tissues are abnormally automatic or are a portion of a reentrant loop. These agents are also helpful in slowing ventricular response in atrial tachycardias (eg, AF) by effects on the AV node.
    - ✓ Class III drugs prolong refractoriness in atrial and ventricular tissue and include very different drugs that share the common effect of delaying repolarization by

TABLE 6-1	Classification of Antiarrhythmic Drugs				
Class	Drug	Conduction Velocity[a]	Refractory Period	Automaticity	Ion Block
Ia	Quinidine	↓	↑	↓	Sodium (intermediate)
	Procainamide				
	Disopyramide				Potassium
Ib	Lidocaine	0/↓	↓	↓	Sodium (fast on–off)
	Mexiletine				
Ic	Flecainide	↓↓	0	↓	Sodium (slow on–off)
	Propafenone[b]				
II[c]	β-Blockers	↓	↑	↓	Calcium (indirect)
III	Amiodarone[d]	0	↑↑	0	Potassium
	Dofetilide				
	Dronedarone[d]				
	Sotalol[b]				
	Ibutilide				
IV[c]	Verapamil	↓	↑	↓	Calcium
	Diltiazem				

[a]Variables for normal tissue models in ventricular tissue.
[b]Also has β-blocking actions.
[c]Variables for sinoatrial (SA) and atrioventricular (AV) nodal tissue only.
[d]Also has sodium, calcium, and β-blocking actions.
0, no change; ↑, increased; ↓, decreased.

blocking potassium channels. **Amiodarone** and **sotalol** are effective in most supraventricular and VTs. Amiodarone displays electrophysiologic characteristics of all four Vaughan Williams classes. It is a sodium channel blocker with relatively fast on–off kinetics, has nonselective β-blocking actions, blocks potassium channels, and has slight calcium-blocking activity. Sotalol inhibits outward potassium movement during repolarization and also possesses nonselective β-blocking actions. **Dronedarone**, **ibutilide**, and **dofetilide** are indicated only for treatment of supraventricular arrhythmias.

✓ Class IV drugs include the non-DHP CCBs (**verapamil**, **diltiazem**), which inhibit calcium entry into cells, thereby slowing conduction, prolonging refractoriness, and decreasing SA and AV nodal automaticity. They are effective for automatic or reentrant tachycardias that arise from or use the SA or AV nodes.

• See Table 6-2 for recommended doses of oral AADs, Table 6-3 for usual IV antiarrhythmic doses, and Table 6-4 for common side effects.

ATRIAL FIBRILLATION OR ATRIAL FLUTTER

• Treatment of AF involves several sequential goals. First, evaluate need for acute treatment (usually with drugs that slow ventricular rate). Second, determine whether an attempt should be made to restore the patient to SR, taking into consideration the risks (eg, thromboembolism). Lastly, consider ways to prevent long-term complications, such as recurrent arrhythmia and thromboembolism (Fig. 6-1).

Hemodynamically Unstable AF

• In patients with new-onset AF or atrial flutter with signs and/or symptoms of hemodynamic instability (eg, severe hypotension, angina, and/or pulmonary edema), direct-current cardioversion (DCC) is indicated to restore sinus rhythm immediately (without regard to the risk of thromboembolism).

TABLE 6-2	Typical Maintenance Doses of Oral Antiarrhythmic Drugs	
Drug	**Dose**	**Dose Adjusted**
Disopyramide	100–150 mg every 6 hours	HEP, REN
	200–300 mg every 12 hours (SR form)	
Quinidine	200–300 mg sulfate salt every 6 hours	HEP
	324–648 gluconate salt every 8–12 hours	
Mexiletine	200–300 mg every 8 hours	HEP
Flecainide	50–200 mg every 12 hours	HEP, REN
Propafenone	150–300 mg every 8 hours	HEP
	225–425 mg every 12 hours (SR form)	
Amiodarone	400 mg 2 or 3 times daily until 10 g total, and then 200–400 mg daily[a]	
Dofetilide	500 mcg every 12 hours	REN[b]
Dronedarone	400 mg twice daily (with meals)[c]	
Sotalol	80–160 mg every 12 hours	REN[d]

[a]Usual maintenance dose for atrial fibrillation is 200 mg/day (may further decrease dose to 100 mg/day with long-term use if patient clinically stable in order to decrease risk of toxicity); usual maintenance dose for ventricular arrhythmias is 300–400 mg/day.
[b]Dose should be based on creatinine clearance; should not be used when creatinine clearance <20 mL/min.
[c]Should not be used in severe hepatic impairment.
[d]Should not be used for atrial fibrillation when creatinine clearance <40 mL/min.
HEP, hepatic disease; REN, renal impairment; SR, sustained release.

TABLE 6-3	Intravenous Antiarrhythmic Dosing	
Drug	**Clinical Situation**	**Dose**
Amiodarone	Pulseless VT/VF	300 mg IV/IO push (can give additional 150 mg IV/IO push if persistent VT/VF or if VT/VF recurs), followed by infusion of 1 mg/min for 6 hours, and then 0.5 mg/min × 18 hours
	Stable VT (with a pulse)	150 mg IV over 10 min, followed by infusion of 1 mg/min for 6 hours, and then 0.5 mg/min × 18 hours
	AF (termination)	150 mg IV over 10 min, followed by infusion of 1 mg/min for 6 hours, and then 0.5 mg/min × 18 hours
Diltiazem	PSVT; AF (rate control)	0.25 mg/kg IV over 2 min (may repeat with 0.35 mg/kg IV over 2 min), followed by infusion of 5–15 mg/hr
Ibutilide	AF (termination)	1 mg IV over 10 min (may repeat if needed)
Lidocaine	Pulseless VT/VF	1–1.5 mg/kg IV/IO push (can give additional 0.5–0.75 mg/kg IV/IO push every 5–10 min if persistent VT/VF [maximum cumulative dose = 3 mg/kg]), followed by infusion of 1–4 mg/min (1–2 mg/min if liver disease or HF)
	Stable VT (with a pulse)	1–1.5 mg/kg IV push (can give additional 0.5–0.75 mg/kg IV push every 5–10 min if persistent VT [maximum cumulative dose = 3 mg/kg]), followed by infusion of 1–4 mg/min (1–2 mg/min if liver disease or HF)
Procainamide	AF (termination); stable VT (with a pulse)	15–18 mg/kg IV over 60 min, followed by infusion of 1–4 mg/min
Verapamil	PSVT; AF (rate control)	2.5–5 mg IV over 2 min (may repeat up to maximum cumulative dose of 20 mg); can follow with infusion of 2.5–10 mg/hr

AF, atrial fibrillation; HF, heart failure; IO, intraosseous; IV, intravenous; PSVT, paroxysmal supraventricular tachycardia; VF, ventricular fibrillation; VT, ventricular tachycardia.

Ventricular Rate Control

- If patients are hemodynamically stable, the focus should be directed toward controlling ventricular rate. Use drugs that slow conduction and increase refractoriness in the AV node as initial therapy. In patients with normal LV function (left ventricular ejection fraction [LVEF] >40% [0.40]), an IV β-blocker (**propranolol**, **metoprolol**, **esmolol**) or non-DHP CCB (**diltiazem**, **verapamil**) is recommended as first-line therapy. If a high adrenergic state is the precipitating factor, IV β-blockers should be considered first. In patients with LVEF ≤40% (0.40), avoid IV diltiazem and verapamil and use IV β-blockers with caution. In patients having an exacerbation of HF symptoms, use IV **digoxin** or **amiodarone** as first-line therapy for ventricular rate control. IV amiodarone can also be used in patients who are refractory or have contraindications to β-blockers, non-DHP CCBs, and digoxin.
- After treatment with AV nodal blocking agents and a subsequent decrease in ventricular rate, evaluate the patient for the possibility of restoring sinus rhythm if AF persists.

TABLE 6-4	Side Effects of Antiarrhythmic Drugs
Disopyramide	Anticholinergic symptoms (dry mouth, urinary retention, constipation, blurred vision), nausea, anorexia, TdP, HF, conduction disturbances, ventricular arrhythmias
Procainamide[a]	Hypotension, TdP, worsening HF, conduction disturbances, ventricular arrhythmias
Quinidine	Cinchonism, diarrhea, abdominal cramps, nausea, vomiting, hypotension, TdP, worsening HF, conduction disturbances, ventricular arrhythmias, fever
Lidocaine	Dizziness, sedation, slurred speech, blurred vision, paresthesia, muscle twitching, confusion, nausea, vomiting, seizures, psychosis, sinus arrest, conduction disturbances
Mexiletine	Dizziness, sedation, anxiety, confusion, paresthesia, tremor, ataxia, blurred vision, nausea, vomiting, anorexia, conduction disturbances, ventricular arrhythmias
Flecainide	Blurred vision, dizziness, dyspnea, headache, tremor, nausea, worsening HF, conduction disturbances, ventricular arrhythmias
Propafenone	Dizziness, fatigue, blurred vision, bronchospasm, headache, taste disturbances, nausea, vomiting, bradycardia or AV block, worsening HF, ventricular arrhythmias
Amiodarone	Tremor, ataxia, paresthesia, insomnia, corneal microdeposits, optic neuropathy/neuritis, nausea, vomiting, anorexia, constipation, TdP (<1%), bradycardia or AV block (IV and oral use), pulmonary fibrosis, liver function test abnormalities, hypothyroidism, hyperthyroidism, photosensitivity, blue-gray skin discoloration, hypotension (IV use), phlebitis (IV use)
Dofetilide	Headache, dizziness, TdP
Dronedarone	Nausea, vomiting, diarrhea, serum creatinine elevations, bradycardia, worsening HF, hepatotoxicity, pulmonary fibrosis, acute renal failure, TdP (<1%)
Ibutilide	Headache, TdP, bradycardia or AV block, hypotension
Sotalol	Dizziness, weakness, fatigue, nausea, vomiting, diarrhea, bradycardia or AV block, TdP, bronchospasm, worsening HF

[a]Side effects listed are for the IV formulation only; oral formulations are no longer available.
AV, atrioventricular; HF, heart failure; IV, intravenous; TdP, torsade de pointes.

Anticoagulation Prior to Cardioversion

- If sinus rhythm is to be restored, initiate anticoagulation prior to cardioversion because return of atrial contraction may dislodge poorly adherent thrombi and increase the risk of thromboembolism. Initiating anticoagulation prior to cardioversion prevents clot growth and formation of new thrombi and allows existing thrombi to become organized and well adherent to the atrial wall. Patients become at increased risk of thrombus formation and a subsequent embolic event if the duration of AF exceeds 48 hours.
- Patients undergoing elective cardioversion for AF lasting longer than 48 hours or an unknown duration should receive **warfarin** (target international normalized ratio [INR] 2–3) or a direct oral anticoagulant (DOAC; **apixaban**, **dabigatran**, **edoxaban**,

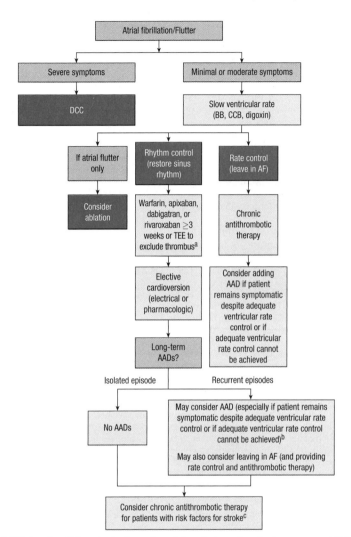

aIf AF is less than 48 hours in duration, anticoagulation prior to cardioversion is unnecessary; initiate anticoagulation with unfractionated heparin, a low-molecular-weight heparin, apixaban, dabigatran, or rivaroxaban as soon as possible either before or after cardioversion for patients at high risk for stroke (this anticoagulant regimen or no antithrombotic therapy may be considered in low-risk patients).
bAblation may be considered for patients who fail or do not tolerate at least 1 AAD or as first-line therapy (before AAD therapy) for select patients with recurrent symptomatic paroxysmal AF or any classification of AF and heart failure with reduced left ventricular ejection fraction.
cChronic antithrombotic therapy should be considered in all patients with AF and risk factors for stroke regardless of whether or not they remain in sinus rhythm.

(AAD, antiarrhythmic drug; AF, atrial fibrillation; AFl, atrial flutter; BB, β-blocker; CCB, calcium channel blocker [ie, verapamil or diltiazem]; DCC, direct current cardioversion; TEE, transesophageal echocardiogram.)

FIGURE 6-1. Algorithm for the treatment of AF and atrial flutter.

or **rivaroxaban**) for at least 3 weeks prior to cardioversion. If cardioversion is success-ful, continue anticoagulation for at least 4 weeks.

- Patients with AF less than 48 hours in duration do not require a prolonged period of anticoagulation prior to cardioversion because there has not been sufficient time to form atrial thrombi. Recommendations regarding short-term anticoagulation therapy given immediately prior to cardioversion differ. The CHEST guidelines recommend anticoagulation with either IV **unfractionated heparin** (UFH) or sub-cutaneous **low-molecular-weight heparin** (LMWH) (with doses used for treating venous thromboembolism) at the time the patient presents with AF that is known to be less than 48 hours in duration. If the patient is successfully cardioverted to sinus rhythm, continue therapeutic anticoagulation with warfarin (INR target range 2–3) or a DOAC for at least 4 weeks. Decisions about long-term antithrombotic therapy beyond 4 weeks should be based on the patient's risk for stroke and not whether the patient is in sinus rhythm. According to the 2019 AHA/ACC/HRS Focused Update, the anticoagulant regimen selected depends on the patient's risk of stroke (refer to the textbook chapter for more information).

Conversion to Sinus Rhythm

- After anticoagulation needs have been addressed (or after transesophageal echocar-diography [TEE] demonstrated absence of a thrombus, obviating need for anticoagula-tion), methods for restoring sinus rhythm are pharmacologic cardioversion and DCC. Disadvantages of pharmacologic cardioversion are the risk of significant side effects (eg, drug-induced TdP, drug–drug interactions) and lower cardioversion rate for AADs compared with DCC. DCC is quick and more often successful (80%–90% success rate), but it requires prior sedation or anesthesia and has a small risk of serious complications, such as sinus arrest or ventricular arrhythmias. Clinicians often elect to use AADs first, and then resort to DCC if these drugs fail. Pharmacologic cardioversion is most effective when initiated within 7 days after the onset of AF. There is good evidence for cardioversion efficacy of class III pure Ik blockers (**ibutilide, dofetilide**), class Ic drugs (eg, **flecainide, propafenone**), and **amiodarone** (oral or IV).

- Single oral loading doses of propafenone (body weight >70 kg: 600 mg; <70 kg: 450 mg) and flecainide (body weight >70 kg: 300 mg; <70 kg: 200 mg) are effective for cardioversion of recent-onset AF. These regimens have been incorporated into the "pill in the pocket" approach, whereby outpatient, patient-controlled self-adminis-tration of a single oral dose of either flecainide or propafenone is used to terminate recent-onset AF in select patients without sinus or AV node dysfunction, bundle-branch block, or SHD. This method should only be considered for patients who have been successfully cardioverted with these drugs on an inpatient basis.

Chronic Anticoagulation for Stroke Prevention

- When initiating chronic antithrombotic therapy to prevent stroke in patients with AF, selection of the appropriate regimen is based on the patient's stroke risk as determined by the CHA_2DS_2-Vasc risk scoring system. Patients are given 2 points each if they have a history of a previous stroke, transient ischemic attack, or throm-boembolism, or if they are at least 75 years old. Patients are given 1 point each for age 65–74 years; having hypertension, diabetes, HF, or vascular disease; and being female.
  - ✓ *Low risk*: No antithrombotic therapy is recommended for males with a CHA_2DS_2-VASc score of 0 and females with a score of 1 because they are at low risk for stroke.
  - ✓ *Intermediate risk*: For patients with one nonsex stroke risk factor (ie, CHA_2DS_2-VASc score of 1 in males or 2 in females), oral anticoagulation is recommended over aspirin monotherapy, aspirin plus clopidogrel, or no antithrombotic therapy.
  - ✓ *High risk*: For patients with more than one nonsex stroke risk factor (ie, CHA_2DS_2-VASc score of ≥2 in males or ≥3 in females), oral anticoagulation is also recommended.

- For stroke prevention in AF, the CHEST guidelines recommend a DOAC (apixaban, dabigatran, edoxaban, or rivaroxaban) over warfarin. However, anticoagulant therapy must be individualized for each patient. If warfarin is used, the target INR is 2–3, and the goal time in therapeutic range (TTR) should ideally be >70%. If a therapeutic INR cannot be maintained on warfarin, a DOAC is recommended. If treatment with oral anticoagulation must be temporarily interrupted, coverage with parenteral UFH or LMWH should be considered.

- In patients with mechanical heart valves, warfarin is the anticoagulant of choice; the target INR is based on the type and location of the valve placed. Dabigatran, edoxaban, and rivaroxaban should be avoided in patients with creatinine clearance <15 mL/min (0.25 mL/sec).

- Decisions regarding the duration of chronic antithrombotic therapy should be based on a patient's risk for stroke using the CHA_2DS_2-VASc scoring system.

Chronic Antiarrhythmic Therapy

- Use of AADs to prevent AF recurrences is controversial; AADs may be reasonable in patients who remain symptomatic despite having adequate ventricular rate control or for patients in whom adequate ventricular rate control cannot be achieved.

- In patients with no SHD, **dofetilide**, **dronedarone**, **flecainide**, **propafenone**, or **sotalol** should be considered initially. **Amiodarone** is second-line if the patient fails or does not tolerate one of these drugs. In patients with HF, amiodarone or dofetilide is first-line therapy, with catheter ablation as second-line. In patients with CAD dofetilide, dronedarone, or sotalol are first-line, with amiodarone as second-line therapy. Flecainide and propafenone should be avoided in the presence of SHD because of the risk of proarrhythmia.

PAROXYSMAL SUPRAVENTRICULAR TACHYCARDIA

- Both pharmacologic and nonpharmacologic methods have been used to treat PSVT. Drugs can be divided into three broad categories: (1) those that directly or indirectly increase vagal tone to the AV node (eg, digoxin), (2) those that depress conduction through slow, calcium-dependent tissue (eg, adenosine, β-blockers, and non-DHP CCBs), and (3) those that depress conduction through fast, sodium-dependent tissue (eg, quinidine, procainamide, disopyramide, and flecainide). Drugs within these categories alter the electrophysiologic characteristics of the reentrant substrate so that PSVT cannot be sustained.

- Acute management for patients with AVNRT or orthodromic AVRT includes vagal maneuvers and/or adenosine. If these options are ineffective or unfeasible in a hemodynamically unstable patient, synchronized DCC is the next step. If vagal techniques and adenosine are ineffective or unfeasible in a hemodynamically stable patient, the next step is administration of an IV β-blocker or non-DHP CCB. If AVNRT cannot be corrected with these measures, IV amiodarone can be used. For patients with AVRT, the next step is synchronized cardioversion.

- After an acute episode of AVNRT or AVRT is terminated, long-term prophylaxis is indicated if frequent episodes necessitate therapeutic intervention or if episodes are infrequent but severely symptomatic. AADs are no longer the treatment of choice to prevent recurrences of reentrant PSVT but may be necessary occasionally, particularly in patients with mild symptoms and infrequent recurrences. Drugs effective in preventing recurrences are the AV nodal blocking drugs (digoxin, β-blockers, non-DHP CCBs, and combinations of these agents) and the class Ic AADs (flecainide, propafenone). Sotalol, dofetilide, and amiodarone can be considered alternatives.

- Catheter ablation using radiofrequency current on the PSVT substrate is the preferred treatment strategy (over AADs) for patients with symptomatic PSVT. It is highly effective and curative, rarely results in complications, obviates need for chronic AAD therapy, and is cost effective.

PREMATURE VENTRICULAR COMPLEXES

- In apparently healthy individuals without SHD, drug therapy is unnecessary because PVCs carry little or no risk. In addition, AADs should not be used to suppress asymptomatic PVCs. In patients with symptomatic PVCs who have risk factors for arrhythmic death (recent MI, LV dysfunction, or complex PVCs), limit chronic therapy to β-blockers. β-Blockers can also be used to suppress symptomatic PVCs in patients without underlying heart disease.

VENTRICULAR TACHYCARDIA

Acute Ventricular Tachycardia

- If severe symptoms are present, institute synchronized DCC immediately to restore sinus rhythm and correct precipitating factors if possible. If VT is an isolated electrical event associated with a transient initiating factor (eg, acute myocardial ischemia or digitalis toxicity), there is no need for long-term antiarrhythmic therapy after precipitating factors are corrected.
- Patients with mild or no symptoms can be treated initially with AADs. IV procainamide, amiodarone, or sotalol may be considered in this situation; lidocaine is an alternative agent. Deliver synchronized DCC if the patient's status deteriorates, VT degenerates to VF, or drug therapy fails.

Sustained Ventricular Tachycardia

- Patients with chronic recurrent sustained VT are at high risk for death; trial-and-error attempts to find effective therapy are unwarranted. Use of invasive electrophysiologic studies and serial Holter monitoring with drug testing have been largely abandoned. These findings and the side-effect profiles of antiarrhythmic agents have led to nondrug approaches.
- The automatic ICD is a highly effective method for preventing sudden death due to recurrent VT or VF.

Ventricular Proarrhythmia

- The proarrhythmia caused by the class Ic AADs is often resistant to resuscitation with cardioversion or overdrive pacing. IV **lidocaine** (which competes for the sodium channel receptor) or **sodium bicarbonate** (which reverses the excessive sodium channel blockade) has been used successfully by some clinicians.

Torsade de Pointes

- For an acute episode of TdP, most patients require and respond to DCC. However, TdP tends to be paroxysmal and often recurs rapidly after DCC.
- IV **magnesium sulfate** is the drug of choice for preventing recurrences of TdP. If ineffective, institute strategies to increase heart rate and shorten ventricular repolarization (ie, temporary transvenous pacing at 105–120 beats/min or pharmacologic pacing with **isoproterenol**). Discontinue agents that prolong the QT interval and correct exacerbating factors (eg, hypokalemia and hypomagnesemia). Lidocaine is usually ineffective, and AADs that further prolong repolarization (eg, IV procainamide) are absolutely contraindicated.

Ventricular Fibrillation

- Manage patients with pulseless VT or VF (with or without associated myocardial ischemia) according to American Heart Association guidelines for cardiopulmonary resuscitation and emergency cardiovascular care (see Chapter 7).

BRADYARRHYTHMIAS

- Asymptomatic sinus bradyarrhythmias usually do not require treatment.
- Treatment of sinus node dysfunction involves eliminating symptomatic bradycardia and potentially managing alternating tachycardias such as AF. In general, permanent pacemaker implantation is the long-term therapy of choice. Drugs commonly used to treat supraventricular tachycardias should be used with caution, if at all, in the absence of a functioning pacemaker.

- Symptomatic carotid sinus hypersensitivity also should be treated with permanent pacemaker therapy. Patients who remain symptomatic may benefit from adding an α-adrenergic stimulant such as **midodrine**.
- Vasovagal syncope has traditionally been treated successfully with oral β-blockers (eg, **metoprolol**) to inhibit the sympathetic surge that causes forceful ventricular contraction and precedes the onset of hypotension and bradycardia. Other drugs that have been used successfully (with or without β-blockers) include **fludrocortisone**, anticholinergics (**scopolamine patches** and **disopyramide**), α-adrenergic agonists (**midodrine**), adenosine analogues (**theophylline, dipyridamole**), and selective serotonin reuptake inhibitors (**sertraline, paroxetine**).

Atrioventricular Block

- If patients with second- or third-degree AV block develop signs or symptoms of poor perfusion (eg, altered mental status, chest pain, hypotension, shock) administer **atropine** (0.5 mg IV given every 3–5 minutes, up to 3 mg total dose). Transcutaneous pacing can be initiated in patients unresponsive to atropine. Infusions of **epinephrine** (2–10 mcg/min) or **dopamine** (2–10 mcg/kg/min) can also be used in the event of atropine failure. These agents usually do not help if the site of the AV block is below the AV node (Mobitz II or trifascicular AV block).
- Chronic symptomatic AV block warrants insertion of a permanent pacemaker. Patients without symptoms can sometimes be followed closely without the need for a pacemaker.

EVALUATION OF THERAPEUTIC OUTCOMES

- The most important monitoring parameters include: (1) mortality (total and sudden cardiac death), (2) arrhythmia recurrence (duration, frequency, and symptoms), (3) hemodynamic consequences (rate, blood pressure, and symptoms), and (4) treatment complications (side effects or need for alternative or additional drugs, devices, or surgery).

See Chapter 39, The Arrhythmias, authored by Jessica J. Tilton, Cynthia A. Sanoski, and Jerry L. Bauman, for a more detailed discussion of this topic.

- *Cardiac arrest* is defined as cessation of cardiac mechanical activity as confirmed by absence of signs of circulation (eg, detectable pulse, unresponsiveness, apnea).

PATHOPHYSIOLOGY

- Coronary artery disease is the most common finding in adults with cardiac arrest and causes ~75% of sudden cardiac deaths. In pediatric patients, cardiac arrest typically results from respiratory failure, asphyxiation, or progressive shock.
- Noncardiac causes include drowning, choking, asphyxia, electrocution, trauma, poisoning, severe asthma, pneumonia, drug overdose, and sudden infant death syndrome.
- Two different pathophysiologic conditions are associated with cardiac arrest:
  - ✓ Primary: arterial blood is fully oxygenated at the time of arrest.
  - ✓ Secondary: respiratory failure with lack of ventilation leads to severe hypoxemia, hypotension, and cardiac arrest.
- Cardiac arrest in adults usually results from arrhythmias. Historically, ventricular fibrillation (VF) and pulseless ventricular tachycardia (PVT) were most common. Recent data indicate that nonshockable rhythms (ie, asystole, pulseless electrical activity [PEA]) are now more prevalent. This change is of concern because survival rates to hospital discharge are higher after shockable rhythms like VF and PVT than with nonshockable rhythms like asystole and PEA.

CLINICAL PRESENTATION

- Cardiac arrest may be preceded by anxiety, shortness of breath, crushing chest pain, nausea, vomiting, and diaphoresis.
- Signs include apnea; hypotension; no detectable pulse; cyanosis; cold, clammy extremities; and unresponsiveness.

DIAGNOSIS

- Rapid diagnosis is vital to success and is made by observing clinical manifestations consistent with cardiac arrest.
- Electrocardiography (ECG) identifies the cardiac rhythm, which in turn determines drug therapy.
  - ✓ VF is electrical anarchy of the ventricle resulting in no cardiac output and cardiovascular collapse.
  - ✓ PEA is absence of a detectable pulse and presence of some type of electrical activity other than VF or PVT.
  - ✓ Asystole occurs when there is no electrical activity in the heart, indicated by a flat line on the ECG.

TREATMENT

- <u>Goals of Treatment</u>: Resuscitation goals are to preserve life; restore health; relieve suffering; limit disability; and respect the individual's decisions, rights, and privacy. This can be accomplished via cardiopulmonary resuscitation (CPR) by return of spontaneous circulation (ROSC) with effective ventilation and perfusion quickly to minimize hypoxic damage to vital organs. After successful resuscitation, the primary outcome is survival to hospital discharge with good neurologic function.

GENERAL APPROACH

- The American Heart Association (AHA) guidelines for CPR and emergency cardio-vascular care (ECC) are now updated annually (published online) and emphasize timely implementation of the "chain of survival":
  - ✓ For out-of-hospital arrests: (1) immediate recognition of cardiac arrest and acti-vation of the emergency response system, (2) immediate high-quality CPR, (3) rapid defibrillation, (4) effective advanced cardiac life support (ACLS), and (5) integrated post-arrest care.
  - ✓ For in-hospital arrests: (1) surveillance and prevention of cardiac arrest, (2) prompt notification and response by a multidisciplinary team of healthcare providers, (3) high-quality CPR, (4) prompt defibrillation and ACLS when appropriate, and (5) integrated post-arrest care.

Basic Life Support Given by Healthcare Providers

- The mnemonic for the CPR sequence is "CAB" (circulation, airway, breathing). Basic life support *given by healthcare providers trained in CPR* includes the following actions performed in this order:
  - ✓ First, determine patient responsiveness. If unresponsive with no breathing or no normal breathing (ie, only gasping), activate the emergency medical response team and obtain an automated external defibrillator (AED).
  - ✓ Check for a pulse, but if not definitely felt within 10 seconds, begin CPR with chest compressions and use the AED when available.
  - ✓ Begin CPR with 30 chest compressions at a rate of 100–120/min and a compres-sion depth of at least 2 in (5 cm) in adults and at least one third of the anteropos-terior chest diameter in infants and children (~1.5 in [4 cm] in infants and 2 in [5 cm] in children).
  - ✓ Open the airway and deliver 2 rescue breaths, then repeat chest compressions. Follow each cycle of 30 chest compressions by 2 rescue breaths.
  - ✓ Continue CPR until an AED is ready for use or ACLS providers take over care.
  - ✓ If/when an AED is available, check rhythm to determine if defibrillation is advised. If so, deliver one shock with immediate resumption of chest compressions/rescue breaths for 2 minutes or until prompted by the AED to allow for another rhythm check.
  - ✓ If the rhythm is not shockable, resume CPR immediately for 2 minutes or until prompted by the AED. Continue this cycle until ACLS providers take over or the victim starts to move.

Advanced Cardiac Life Support

- Once ACLS providers arrive, further definitive therapy is given following the ACLS algorithm shown in **Figure 7-1**.
- A bag-mask device or an advanced airway (eg, endotracheal tube, supraglottic device) may be used to provide ventilation. One provider can deliver 1 breath every 6 seconds while a second provider performs continuous chest compressions.
- Central venous catheter access results in faster and higher peak drug concentrations than peripheral venous administration, but central line access is not needed in most resuscitation attempts. However, if a central line is already present, it is the access site of choice. If IV access (either central or peripheral) has not been established, insert a large peripheral venous catheter. If this is unsuccessful, insert an intraosseous (IO) device.
- If neither IV nor IO access can be established, **lidocaine**, **epinephrine**, **naloxone**, and **vasopressin** may be administered endotracheally. The endotracheal dose should gen-erally be 2–2.5 times larger than the IV/IO dose. Dilute the medications in 5–10 mL of either sterile water (preferred) or normal saline.

FIGURE 7-1. Treatment algorithm for adult cardiac arrest: Advanced cardiac life support (ACLS).

TREATMENT OF VENTRICULAR FIBRILLATION AND PULSELESS VENTRICULAR TACHYCARDIA

Nonpharmacologic Therapy

- Electrical defibrillation is the only effective method of restoring a cardiac rhythm for VF and PVT. For a witnessed adult cardiac arrest, use an AED immediately when available. When the arrest is not witnessed or when an AED is not immediately available, initiate CPR while the AED is being retrieved, and attempt defibrillation as soon as the device is available. For in-hospital cardiac arrest with an AED available, begin CPR while the AED is being placed.

- After 2 minutes of chest compressions, recheck the rhythm; if there is still evidence of VF or PVT, give pharmacologic therapy with repeat attempts at single-discharge defibrillation.
- Obtain IV access and an advanced airway when feasible, but not at the expense of stopping chest compressions. Once an airway is obtained, use caution to avoid providing excessive ventilations.

Pharmacologic Therapy

Epinephrine

- **Epinephrine** is a drug of first choice for treating VF, PVT, asystole, and PEA. It is an α- and β-receptor agonist, causing vasoconstriction and increased rate and forcefulness of heart contractions, thereby augmenting low coronary and cerebral perfusion pressures.
- The recommended adult dose of epinephrine is 1 mg administered by IV or IO injection every 3–5 minutes. Although higher doses have been studied, they are not recommended for routine use in cardiac arrest.

Vasopressin

- **Vasopressin** is a potent nonadrenergic vasoconstrictor that increases blood pressure (BP) and systemic vascular resistance. Despite some theoretical advantages, clinical outcomes are not superior to use of standard-dose epinephrine alone or to the combination of vasopressin and epinephrine. For in-hospital cardiac arrest, the combination of vasopressin, epinephrine, and methylprednisolone with post-arrest hydrocortisone may be considered, but further studies are needed before this can be routinely recommended.

Antiarrhythmics

- The purpose of antiarrhythmic drug therapy after unsuccessful defibrillation and vasopressor administration is to prevent development or recurrence of VF and PVT. However, clinical evidence demonstrating improved survival to hospital discharge is lacking.
- **Amiodarone** may be considered in patients with VF/VT unresponsive to CPR, defibrillation, and vasopressors. The dose is 300 mg IV/IO followed by a second dose of 150 mg.
- **Lidocaine** may be considered as an alternative to amiodarone for VF or PVT unresponsive to CPR, defibrillation, and a vasopressor, but it has not been shown to improve rates of ROSC, admission to the hospital, or survival to discharge. The initial dose is 1–1.5 mg/kg IV. Additional doses of 0.5–0.75 mg/kg can be administered at 5- to 10-minute intervals to a maximum total dose of 3 mg/kg if VF/PVT persists.

Magnesium

- Severe hypomagnesemia has been associated with VF/PVT, but routine administration of magnesium during cardiac arrest has not improved clinical outcomes. Two trials showed improved ROSC in cardiac arrests associated with torsades de pointes; therefore, limit magnesium administration to these patients. The dose is 1–2 g diluted in 10 mL of 5% dextrose in water administered IV/IO push over 15 minutes.

Thrombolytics

- Thrombolytic use during CPR has been investigated because most adult cardiac arrests are related to either myocardial infarction (MI) or pulmonary embolism (PE). Although early small studies demonstrated some benefit, larger randomized trials showed no improvement in ROSC or survival to hospital discharge, and the incidence of intracranial hemorrhage was greater than with placebo. Therefore, fibrinolytic therapy should not be used routinely in cardiac arrest but may be considered when PE is suspected.

TREATMENT OF PULSELESS ELECTRICAL ACTIVITY AND ASYSTOLE

Nonpharmacologic Therapy

- Successful treatment of PEA and asystole depends on diagnosis of the underlying cause. Potentially reversible causes include: (1) hypovolemia, (2) hypoxia, (3) acidosis, (4) hyper- or hypokalemia, (5) hypothermia, (6) hypoglycemia, (7) drug overdose, (8) cardiac tamponade, (9) tension pneumothorax, (10) coronary thrombosis, (11) pulmonary thrombosis, and (12) trauma.
- PEA and asystole are treated the same way. Both conditions require CPR, airway control, and IV access. Avoid defibrillation in asystole because the resulting parasympathetic discharge can reduce the chance of ROSC and decrease the likelihood of survival. If available, transcutaneous pacing can be attempted.

Pharmacologic Therapy

- **Epinephrine** (1 mg by IV or IO injection every 3–5 minutes) is the primary pharmacologic agent used; vasopressin is no longer recommended.
- Atropine is no longer recommended for treatment of asystole or PEA because there are no prospective controlled trials showing benefit and the evidence from observational reports is inconsistent.

ACID–BASE MANAGEMENT

- Acidosis occurs during cardiac arrest because of decreased blood flow or inadequate ventilation. Chest compressions generate only about 25% of normal cardiac output, leading to inadequate organ perfusion, tissue hypoxia, and metabolic acidosis. Lack of ventilation causes CO_2 retention, leading to respiratory acidosis. The combined acidosis reduces myocardial contractility and lowers the fibrillation threshold.
- Routine use of sodium bicarbonate in cardiac arrest is not recommended because there are insufficient data to support its use, and it may have detrimental effects. It can be used in special circumstances (eg, hyperkalemia, tricyclic antidepressant overdose, salicylate toxicity).

POSTRESUSCITATIVE CARE

- ROSC from a cardiac arrest may be followed by a post-cardiac arrest syndrome characterized by hypoxic brain injury, myocardial dysfunction, systemic ischemia/reperfusion response, and the underlying persistent precipitating pathology.
- It is imperative to ensure adequate airway and oxygenation. After use of 100% oxygen during the resuscitation effort, titrate the oxygen fraction down as tolerated to maintain an oxyhemoglobin saturation of at least 94% (0.94). Overventilation can be avoided by using end-tidal (ET) CO_2 measurements.
- Evaluate for ECG changes consistent with acute MI immediately and perform revascularization if present.
- Because cerebral hypoperfusion may persist for several hours after resuscitation, augmenting BP to achieve a goal of mean arterial pressure (MAP) >80 mm Hg has been recommended.
- Therapeutic hypothermia or targeted temperature management is an integral component of postresuscitative care. Hypothermia can protect against cerebral injury by suppressing chemical reactions that occur after restoration of blood flow. All comatose adult patients should have targeted temperature management after ROSC, with a constant temperature maintained between 32° and 36°C for at least 24 hours. A rewarming phase should consist of slow and controlled warming at a rate of 0.2–0.5°C per hour. It is also reasonable to actively prevent fever after targeted temperature management. Potential complications of hypothermia include coagulopathy, dysrhythmias, bradycardia, diuresis, electrolyte disorders, hyperglycemia, infection risks, and effects on drug distribution and clearance.

EVALUATION OF THERAPEUTIC OUTCOMES

- The optimal outcome following CPR is an awake, responsive, spontaneously breathing patient. Patients must remain neurologically intact with minimal morbidity after resuscitation if it is to be considered successful.
- In many cases, rhythm assessment via ECG and pulse checks are the only physiologic parameters available to guide therapy. However, palpating a pulse to determine efficacy of blood flow during CPR has not been shown to be useful.
- Invasive hemodynamic monitoring (eg, coronary perfusion pressure, central venous oxygenation) can provide useful information during CPR but is seldom available. Arterial diastolic pressure may be a reasonable surrogate for coronary perfusion pressure with a suggested goal of >25 mm Hg. An arterial central venous oxygen saturation <30% (0.30) indicates poor CPR quality.
- $ETCO_2$ monitoring is a useful method to assess cardiac output during CPR and has been associated with ROSC. Persistently low $ETCO_2$ values (<10 mm Hg [1.3 kPa]) during CPR in intubated patients suggest that ROSC is unlikely.
- In the postresuscitative phase, monitoring should be directed toward the components of the post-cardiac arrest syndrome. Identify and treat the precipitating cause of the arrest (eg, coronary angiography with prompt recanalization if indicated). Optimize hemodynamics with avoidance of hypotension (MAP <65 mm Hg or SBP <90 mm Hg). Monitor oxygenation closely and maintain arterial blood oxygen saturation >94% (0.94). Because seizures can occur after cardiac arrest, EEG monitoring is indicated. Avoid hyperthermia and maintain normoglycemia. A complete review of systems is recommended because the post-cardiac arrest syndrome can affect most organ systems.

See Chapter 40, Cardiac Arrest, authored by Jeffrey F. Barletta, for a more detailed discussion of this topic.

Dyslipidemia

- *Dyslipidemia* is defined as elevated total cholesterol (TC), low-density lipoprotein cholesterol (LDL-C), or triglycerides (TG); low high-density lipoprotein cholesterol (HDL-C); or a combination of these abnormalities.

PATHOPHYSIOLOGY

- Cholesterol, triglycerides, and phospholipids are transported in blood as complexes of lipids and proteins (lipoproteins). Lipid abnormalities increase the risk of coronary, cerebrovascular, and peripheral arterial disease, collectively known as atherosclerotic cardiovascular disease (ASCVD).
- Atherogenesis is a progressive process initiated by migration of LDL-C and remnant lipoprotein particles into vessel walls. These particles undergo oxidation and are taken up by macrophages, which induces endothelial cell dysfunction that reduces the ability of the endothelium to dilate the artery and causes a prothrombotic state. Unregulated uptake of cholesterol by macrophages leads to foam cell formation and the development of atherosclerotic plaques. Macrophages eventually produce and secrete matrix metalloproteinases, which degrade the collagen matrix of the plaques and cause them to be unstable.
- Repeated injury and repair within an atherosclerotic plaque eventually lead to a fibrous cap protecting the underlying core of lipids, collagen, calcium, and inflammatory cells. Maintenance of the fibrous plaque is critical to prevent plaque rupture and coronary thrombosis. Potential clinical outcomes include angina, myocardial infarction (MI), arrhythmias, stroke, peripheral arterial disease, abdominal aortic aneurysm, and sudden death.
- Primary dyslipidemias include genetic defects resulting in hypercholesterolemia, hypertriglyceridemia, combined hyperlipidemia, and disorders of HDL-C metabolism and an excess of lipoproteins. These disorders have an increased risk of premature ASCVD due to significant elevations in cholesterol levels. In homozygous and heterozygous familial hypercholesterolemia (FH), the primary defect is the inability to bind LDL-C to LDL-C receptors. This leads to lack of LDL-C degradation by cells and unregulated biosynthesis of cholesterol.
- Secondary or acquired dyslipidemias can accompany genetic disorders and may be associated with diet (excessive alcohol use, anorexia, weight gain, excessive intake of carbohydrates or saturated fat), medications (eg, progestins, thiazide diuretics, glucocorticoids, β-blockers, isotretinoin, protease inhibitors, cyclosporine, mirtazapine, sirolimus), and comorbid conditions (eg, nephrotic syndrome, renal failure, hypothyroidism, obesity, diabetes).

CLINICAL PRESENTATION AND DIAGNOSIS

- Most patients are asymptomatic for years before they develop ASCVD, which may produce symptoms including chest pain, palpitations, sweating, anxiety, shortness of breath, loss of consciousness, difficulty with speech or movement, or abdominal pain.
- Perform a thorough medical history in patients presenting with dyslipidemia, including individual characteristics (age, race, gender, pregnancy), history of high-risk comorbid conditions (eg, hypertension, diabetes, peripheral arterial disease, coronary heart disease [CHD], chronic kidney disease [CKD], carotid artery stenosis), family history (eg, early-onset CHD), current medication and prior lipid-lowering medication use, lifestyle assessment (smoking status, exercise, diet, alcohol use), and ischemic symptoms.

- Measure height, weight, BMI, and blood pressure. Physical signs may include eruptive xanthomas, peripheral polyneuropathy, increased blood pressure, and abdominal obesity.
- Laboratory tests may show elevated TC, LDL-C, TG, apolipoprotein B, and high-sensitivity C-reactive protein (hsCRP); HDL-C may be low. Perform other baseline testing (eg, AST/ALT, TSH, glucose, serum creatinine, BUN, and urinalysis). Calculate 10-year ASCVD risk in primary prevention situations.
- Screening may be conducted for manifestations of vascular disease, including carotid ultrasound, coronary calcium score, ankle-brachial index, and heart catheterization.

TREATMENT

- Goals of Treatment: Prevent ASCVD-related morbidity and mortality, including revascularization procedures, MI, and ischemic stroke. Surrogate markers include achieving desired levels of TC, LDL-C, HDL-C, and TG (Table 8-1).

GENERAL APPROACH

- A comprehensive approach to treating dyslipidemia and modifiable major ASCVD risk factors is required to reduce the risk of first and recurrent ASCVD events. Therapeutic lifestyle changes (TLC) are first-line therapy for any lipoprotein disorder, including reducing the percent of calories from saturated and trans fats, increased intake of soluble fiber, weight reduction if overweight or obese, increased physical activity, and avoiding or quitting tobacco use. Hypertensive patients should achieve optimal blood pressure control, and persons with diabetes mellitus should receive glucose-lowering therapies known to reduce ASCVD risk.
- If TLC is insufficient, lipid-lowering agents should be chosen based on which lipid is at an undesirable level and the degree to which it is expected to increase the risk of ASCVD. The decision to initiate lipid-lowering therapy should be based on an individual's ASCVD risk and not merely plasma levels of atherogenic lipoproteins

TABLE 8-1	Classification of Total-, LDL-, HDL-Cholesterol, and Triglycerides in Adults
Total Cholesterol	
<200 mg/dL (5.17 mmol/L)	Desirable
200–239 mg/dL (5.17–6.20 mmol/L)	Borderline high
≥240 mg/dL (6.21 mmol/L)	High
Low-Density Lipoprotein Cholesterol	
<100 mg/dL (2.59 mmol/L)	Optimal
100–129 mg/dL (2.59–3.35 mmol/L)	Near or above optimal
130–159 mg/dL (3.36–4.13 mmol/L)	Borderline high
160–189 mg/dL (4.14–4.90 mmol/L)	High
≥190 mg/dL (4.91 mmol/L)	Very high
High-Density Lipoprotein Cholesterol	
<40 mg/dL (1.03 mmol/L)	Low (Men)
<50 mg/dL (1.3 mmol/L)	Low (Women)
Triglycerides	
<150 mg/dL (1.70 mmol/L)	Normal
150–199 mg/dL (1.70–2.25 mmol/L)	Borderline high
200–499 mg/dL (2.26–5.64 mmol/L)	High
≥500 mg/dL (5.65 mmol/L)	Very high

(eg, LDL-C) alone. Patients with established ASCVD are at highest risk and most likely to benefit from lipid-lowering therapy. Risk assessment in patients without established ASCVD requires careful consideration of risk factors, the risks of lipid-lowering therapy, and patient preference. For patients between 40 and 79 years of age and no history of ASCVD, the ASCVD Risk Estimator Plus (www.tools.acc.org/ascvd-risk-estimator-plus) should be used to facilitate a clinician–patient discussion regarding the benefits and risks of lipid-lowering therapy, especially in patients whose 10-year risk is ≥7.5%. An estimated lifetime risk for ASCVD can also be performed for patients between ages 20 and 39, but the results should only be used to justify the need for lifestyle changes and not initiation of lipid-lowering therapy.

- HMG-CoA reductase inhibitors (statins) are the drugs of choice for most patients with dyslipidemia based on demonstrated effectiveness in reducing first and recurrent cardiovascular (CV) events, CV mortality, and all-cause mortality. The 2018 American College of Cardiology/American Heart Association (ACC/AHA) Blood Cholesterol Guideline identified patient groups for whom clinical trial data demonstrate clear evidence that the benefits of statin therapy outweigh the potential risks (**Table 8-2**).

- Nonstatin therapies (eg, ezetimibe, PCSK9 inhibitors) may be added when adequate LDL-C lowering cannot be achieved with statins alone or in patients unable to tolerate the recommended dose of a statin.

NONPHARMACOLOGIC THERAPY

- Employ TLC in all patients, including those receiving lipid-lowering therapy. Lifestyle modification alone is inappropriate for patients with established ASCVD given the benefit of statins in these high-risk patients.

- Determine weight and BMI at each visit and discuss lifestyle changes to induce a 5%–10% weight loss in overweight or obese persons.

- Recommend moderate-to-vigorous intensity physical activity three to four times per week with each session lasting 40 minutes on average.

- Counsel all patients to stop smoking and avoid tobacco products altogether.

- Advise patients to reduce the percent of daily calories from saturated and trans fats by following a diet that emphasizes vegetables, fruits, whole grains, low-fat dairy, poultry, fish, legumes, and nuts while limiting intake of sweets, sugary beverages, and red meat. Adapt the dietary pattern to a patient's caloric requirements, cultural food preferences, and other medical conditions (eg, diabetes mellitus). It is important to involve all family members, especially if the patient is not the primary person preparing food.

- Increased intake of soluble fiber (oat bran, pectins, certain gums, and psyllium) can reduce total and LDL cholesterol but has little effect on HDL-C or TG. Total daily fiber intake should be about 25 g/day. Fiber products may also help manage constipation associated with bile acid sequestrants (BAS).

- Ingestion of modest to large amounts of oily, cold-water fish (eg, salmon, tuna) may provide CV benefits; however, there are concerns about environmental contaminants and long-term sustainability. Alternatively, fish oil supplementation provides a consistent daily intake of omega-3 polyunsaturated fatty acids (PUFA) such as eicosapentaenoic acid (EPA) and docosahexaenoic acid (DHA) (see Pharmacologic Therapy section below).

- Ingestion of 2–3 g daily of plant sterols and stanols isolated from vegetable oils reduces LDL-C by 5%–15%. They are usually available in butter-like spreads (eg, Benecol). Phytosterols should be administered 2–4 hours before or after BAS to avoid binding of phytosterols in the gut.

- Red yeast rice contains monacolin K, which is chemically identical to lovastatin. However, the amount of monacolin K in OTC products varies by over 120-fold, with some products containing negligible amounts and others likely having higher levels than described on the label, resulting in cases of rhabdomyolysis, liver toxicity, and renal failure. Red yeast rice is not a suitable alternative to statins, but if patients

TABLE 8-2   Key Recommendations to Reduce the Risk of ASCVD in Adults[a]

Heart-healthy lifestyle for everyone

Patient Groups Likely to Benefit from Statin Therapy

Clinical ASCVD[b]	
Very high risk[c]	High-intensity or maximally tolerated statin therapy (Class I)
Not at very high risk	
Age <75 years	High-intensity statin therapy (Class I)
	If high-intensity not tolerated, use moderate-intensity statin therapy (Class I)
Age >75 years	Initiation of moderate- or high-intensity statin is reasonable (Class IIa)
1. Primary prevention: Severe hypercholesterolemia (LDL-C ≥190 mg/dL [4.91 mmol/L])	Rule out secondary causes of dyslipidemia
	Age 20–75 years: Maximally tolerated statin therapy (Class I)
2. Primary prevention: Diabetes 40–75 years and LDL-C 70–189 mg/dL (1.81–4.89 mmol/L)	Moderate-intensity statin therapy regardless of 10-year ASCVD risk (Class I)
	High-intensity statin therapy is reasonable in patients with diabetes and multiple ASCVD risk factors (Class IIa)
	It is reasonable to continue statin therapy in adults ≥75 years of age with diabetes previously taking statin therapy (Class IIa)
	It is reasonable to initiate statin therapy in adults ≥75 years of age with diabetes after a discussion of risks and benefits (Class IIb)
	It is reasonable to initiate statin therapy in adults 20–30 years of age with diabetes if any of the following apply (Class IIb):
	• Long duration of diabetes (≥10 years for type 2 diabetes; ≥20 years for type 1 diabetes)
	• Albuminuria (≥30 mg/g albumin/mg creatinine [3.4 mg/mmol creatinine])
	• Estimated glomerular filtration rate <60 mL/min/1.73 m^2
	• Retinopathy
	• Neuropathy
	• Ankle–brachial index <0.9

3. Primary prevention: No diabetes, 40–75 years, and LDL-C 70–189 mg/dL (1.81–4.89 mmol/L)

Emphasize heart-healthy lifestyle and address other risk factors

Estimate 10-year ASCVD-risk score based on Pooled Cohort Equation:

- High Risk (≥20%): Initiate high-intensity statin therapy (Class I)
- Intermediate Risk (≥7.5% to <20%): If risk enhancers[c] present, consider moderate-intensity statin therapy (Class I)
- If risk decision is uncertain, consider measuring CAC in select adults:
  - ✓ Consider no statin if CAC = 0 unless patient has diabetes or significant family history of ASCVD
  - ✓ Consider initiating statin therapy if CAC 1–99, especially if age >55 years
  - ✓ Initiate statin therapy if CAC ≥100
- Borderline risk (5%–<7.5%): If risk enhancers[d] present, risk discussion regarding moderate-intensity statin therapy (Class IIb)
- Low risk (<5%): Emphasize heart-healthy lifestyle

4. Primary prevention: No diabetes, 20–39 years, and LDL-C 70–189 mg/dL (1.81–4.89 mmol/L)

Estimate lifetime ASCVD-risk based on Pooled Cohort Equation to encourage lifestyle to reduce ASCVD risk

Consider statin therapy if family history of premature ASCVD and LDL-C ≥160 mg/dL (4.14 mmol/L)

[a]American College of Cardiology/American Heart Association (ACC/AHA) Level of Evidence and Class of Recommendation.

[b]Clinical ASCVD includes nonfatal MI, CHD death, and nonfatal and fatal stroke, TIA or peripheral arterial disease presumed to be of atherosclerotic origin.

[c]Very high risk includes history of >1 major ASCVD events including recent acute coronary syndrome (past 12 months), history of MI, ischemic stroke, or peripheral arterial disease; OR one major ASCVD event PLUS multiple high-risk conditions: >65 years, familial hypercholesterolemia, history of coronary bypass graft surgery, diabetes mellitus, hypertension, CKD, current smoking, LDL-C >100 mg/dL (2.59 mmol/L) despite maximally tolerated statin and ezetimibe, or history of heart failure.

[d]Risk enhancers include LDL-C 160–189 mg/dL (4.14–4.89 mmol/L), family history of premature ASCVD, metabolic syndrome, CKD, chronic inflammatory conditions (eg, rheumatoid arthritis), premature menopause (before age 40), preeclampsia, high-risk race/ethnicities (eg, South Asian), TG ≥175 mg/dL (1.98 mmol/L), hsCRP ≥2 mg/L, lipoprotein(a) ≥50 mg/dL (0.5 g/L), apoB ≥130 mg/dL (1.3 g/L), or ankle-brachial index <0.9.

ASCVD, atherosclerotic cardiovascular disease; CAC, coronary artery calcium; CKD, chronic kidney disease; hsCRP, high-sensitivity C-reactive protein; LDL-C, low-density lipoprotein cholesterol; NYHA, New York Heart Association.

choose to take it, recommend that they purchase a reputable product and avoid concurrent use with prescription statins.

PHARMACOLOGIC THERAPY

- Evidence from controlled clinical trials demonstrates that reducing LDL-C lowers ASCVD event rates in the setting of primary and secondary prevention. Epidemiological studies suggest that every 38 mg/dL (0.98 mmol/L) reduction in LDL-C produces a 21% reduction in ASCVD event rates over 5 years. There is a dose-dependent, log-linear association between LDL-C and ASCVD risk, and evidence suggests that lower levels of LDL-C achieve greater risk reductions.
- Lipid-lowering drugs can be broadly divided into agents that primarily decrease atherogenic cholesterol-containing lipoprotein particles (eg, statins) and those that primarily decrease TG levels (eg, fibrates).

Statins

- Statins inhibit 3-hydroxy-3-methylglutaryl coenzyme A (HMG-CoA) reductase, interrupting conversion of HMG-CoA to mevalonate, the rate-limiting step in cholesterol biosynthesis. Reduced LDL synthesis and enhanced LDL catabolism mediated through LDL receptors appear to be the principal mechanisms for lipid-lowering effects.
- Statins significantly reduce LDL-C (20%–60%), modestly increase HDL-C (6%–12%), and decrease TG (10%–29%).
- Statins are first-line lipid-lowering therapy for dyslipidemia due to strong evidence from many controlled trials demonstrating significant reduction in the risk of first (primary prevention) and recurrent (secondary prevention) CV events.
- Statin selection is primarily based on the indicated intensity (Table 8-3). Products in order of decreasing LDL-C lowering potency include **rosuvastatin**, **atorvastatin**, **pitavastatin**, **simvastatin**, **lovastatin**, **pravastatin**, and **fluvastatin**.
- Statins are generally well tolerated. Statin-associated muscle symptoms (SAMS) are reported by 10%–25% of users and are often a reason for discontinuation. Myalgia is the most common SAMS and involves bilateral muscle achiness, weakness, or cramps affecting larger muscle groups (such as thighs and back). The most concerning SAMS

TABLE 8-3 Intensity of Statin Therapy by Drug and Dose		
High-Intensity Therapy	**Moderate-Intensity Therapy**	**Low-Intensity Therapy**
Daily dose lowers LDL on average by ≥50%	Daily dose lowers LDL on average by 30% to <50%	Daily dose lowers LDL on average by <30%
Atorvastatin 40–80 mg	**Atorvastatin 10–20 mg**	Simvastatin 10 mg
Rosuvastatin 20–40 mg	**Rosuvastatin 5–20 mg**	**Pravastatin 10–20 mg**
	Simvastatin 20–40 mg[a]	**Lovastatin 20 mg**
	Pravastatin 40–80 mg	Fluvastatin 20–40 mg
	Lovastatin 40 mg	Pitavastatin 1 mg
	Fluvastatin XL 80 mg	
	Fluvastatin 40 mg BID	
	Pitavastatin 2–4 mg	

[a]Simvastatin is not recommended by the U.S. Food and Drug Administration (FDA) to be started at 80 mg/day due to increased risk of myopathy and rarely rhabdomyolysis.
Boldface type indicates medications that have cardiovascular outcome data from randomized controlled trials when given in the specified dose.

is rhabdomyolysis, which is rapid breakdown of skeletal muscle resulting in creatine kinase (CK) elevations >10 times the upper limit of normal and potentially acute kidney injury. Rhabdomyolysis may be associated with dark ("tea-colored") urine, nausea, vomiting, confusion, coma, cardiac arrhythmias, electrolyte disturbances, and even death. Fortunately, rhabdomyolysis is quite rare (0.1% of statin-treated patients vs 0.04% of patients receiving placebo in controlled clinical trials). Risk factors for developing SAMS include advanced age, female gender, low body mass index, frequent heavy exercisers, comorbidities (eg, kidney disease, hypothyroidism), and increased serum statin concentrations due to drug–drug interactions. Lower starting doses may be advisable for patients with multiple risk factors, with dose titration to the desired potency after the initial dose is tolerated.

- Statins (except pravastatin) are metabolized to some degree by CYP isoenzymes. Lovastatin, simvastatin, and atorvastatin have more significant drug–drug interactions because they are predominantly metabolized by CYP3A4, whereas fluvastatin, pitavastatin, and rosuvastatin are metabolized by other CYP isoenzymes (eg, CYP2C9, CYP2C8, CYP2C19). Concurrent medications that compete with or inhibit the same CYP isoenzyme can increase serum statin concentrations and the risk for SAMS. Concurrent use of medications such as gemfibrozil that interfere with statin glucuronidation, which is responsible for statin clearance, also increase the risk of SAMS.

- A Statin Intolerance App (http://www.acc.org/statinintoleranceapp) can be used to determine the possibility of SAMS and provide guidance on managing patients with possible SAMS. Statin therapy should generally be discontinued in patients with intolerable symptoms. If symptoms resolve, start a different statin at a lower dose. Additionally, hydrophilic statins (eg, atorvastatin, rosuvastatin) may be better tolerated than lipophilic statins (eg, simvastatin). If symptoms do not improve, investigate other potential causes of muscle pain (eg, hypothyroidism, severe vitamin D deficiency) before a statin rechallenge. Every-other-day dosing using statins with long half-lives (eg, atorvastatin, rosuvastatin) may also be considered. Nonstatin therapies may be considered in patients who fail multiple statins. Routine CK monitoring is not recommended, but testing in a patient with symptoms can be used to exclude rhabdomyolysis and help confirm myalgia.

- Mild elevations in serum transaminase levels (primarily alanine aminotransferase [ALT]) may occur, but routine monitoring of liver enzymes is not recommended. Obtain hepatic enzymes before starting statin therapy as a baseline value for comparison if enzymes are later found to be elevated. Statins may be initiated in patients with chronic liver disease, compensated cirrhosis, and nonalcoholic fatty liver disease but are contraindicated in decompensated cirrhosis or acute liver failure.

- Statin use is also associated with a small (<1%) increased risk of new-onset diabetes. Common attributes of statin users who develop new-onset diabetes include higher statin doses and presence of other risk factors for diabetes, including obesity, impaired fasting glucose, A1C >6% (0.06; 42 mmol/mol Hb), or metabolic syndrome.

- Statin products and usual adult starting doses are provided in Table 8-4.

Cholesterol Absorption Inhibitors

- **Ezetimibe** (Table 8-4) is a preferred adjunct therapy because it modestly reduces the risk of recurrent CV events when used in combination with statin therapy. Its primary effect is modest reduction in LDL-C (15%–24%) with higher reductions achievable in combination with statin therapy. Ezetimibe reduces LDL-C by inhibiting the NPC1L1 protein, an important transporter of cholesterol absorption in the small intestine and hepatocytes. Ezetimibe is generally well tolerated and is associated with mild gastrointestinal (GI) complaints (eg, diarrhea), myalgia, and ALT elevations when used with statins. Ezetimibe has no effects on the CYP450 enzyme system; however, concomitant use with cyclosporine can lead to increased exposure to both ezetimibe and cyclosporine.

- **Colesevelam, colestipol,** and **cholestyramine** are BAS that modestly reduce LDL-C (13%–20%) and reduce CV events when used as monotherapy (Table 8-4). They are

TABLE 8-4	Select Drugs Used for Treatment of Dyslipidemia		
Generic (Brand) Name	Dosage Forms	Recommended Adult Starting Dose	Maximum Total Daily Dose
Statins			
Rosuvastatin (Crestor)	5, 10, 20, 40 mg tablets	5 mg once daily	40 mg
Atorvastatin (Lipitor)	10, 20, 40, 80 mg tablets	10–20 mg once daily	80 mg
Pitavastatin (Livalo)	1, 2, 4 mg tablets	2 mg once daily	4 mg
Simvastatin (Zocor)	5, 10, 20, 40, 80 mg tablets	10–20 mg once daily	80 mg
Lovastatin (Mevacor)	20, 40 mg tablets	20 mg once daily with the evening meal	80 mg
Pravastatin (Pravachol)	20, 40, 80 mg tablets	40 mg once daily	80 mg
Fluvastatin (Lescol)	20, 40 mg capsules; 80 mg XL tablets	40–80 mg once daily	80 mg
Cholesterol Absorption Inhibitors			
Ezetimibe (Zetia)	10 mg tablets	10 mg once daily	10 mg
Colesevelam (Welchol)	625 mg tablets; 3.75 and 1.875 g oral suspension packets	6 tablets once daily or 3 tablets twice daily; suspension: 3.75 g packet once daily or one 1.875 g packet twice daily	3750 mg
Colestipol hydrochloride (Colestid)	1 g tablets; 5 g granule packets, bulk powder	Tablets: 2 g once or twice daily; granules: 5 g once or twice daily	16 g tablets; 30 g packets
Cholestyramine (Questran)	4 g packets, bulk powder	4 g once or twice daily	24 g
Proprotein Convertase Subtilisin/Kexin Type 9 (PCSK9) Inhibitors			
Alirocumab (Praluent)	75 mg, 150 mg SC injection	75 mg SC every 2 weeks	150 mg
Evolocumab (Repatha)	140 mg, 420 mg SC injection	140 mg SC every 2 weeks or 420 mg SC once monthly	420 mg
Fibric Acid Derivatives (Fibrates)			
Gemfibrozil (Lopid)	600 mg capsules	600 mg twice daily	1200 mg
Fenofibrate (Tricor, others)	(product dependent)	(product dependent)	(product dependent)
Omega-3 Polyunsaturated Fatty Acids (PUFA)			
Omega-3-acid ethyl esters (Lovaza)	1 g capsules	4 capsules once daily or 2 capsules twice daily	4 g
Omega-3-carboxylic acids (Epanova)	1 g capsules	2 or 4 capsules once daily	4 g
Icosapent ethyl (Vascepa)	0.5, 1 g capsules	Four 0.5 g capsules or two 1 g capsules twice daily	2 g

(Continued)

TABLE 8-4	Select Drugs Used for Treatment of Dyslipidemia (Continued)		
Generic (Brand) Name	Dosage Forms	Recommended Adult Starting Dose	Maximum Total Daily Dose
Niacin			
Niacin (generic)	50, 100, 250, 500 mg tablets; others	250 mg once daily	6 g
Extended-release niacin (Niaspan)	500, 750, 1000 mg tablets	500 mg once daily	2 g
Mipomersen (Kynamro)	200 mg SC injection	200 mg SC once weekly	200 mg
Lomitapide (Juxtapid)	5, 10, 20 mg capsules	5 mg once daily	60 mg
Select Combination Products			
Extended-release niacin + lovastatin tablets (Advicor)	Niacin/lovastatin 500 mg/20 mg, 750 mg/20 mg, 1000 mg/20 mg, 1000 mg/40 mg	500 mg/20 mg once daily at bedtime	1000 mg/ 40 mg
Ezetimibe + simvastatin tablets (Vytorin)	Ezetimibe/ simvastatin 10 mg/10 mg, 10 mg/20 mg, 10 mg/40 mg, 10 mg/80 mg	10 mg/10 mg or 10 mg/20 mg once daily	10 mg/80 mg

SC, subcutaneously.

generally combined with statins when desired LDL-C levels are not achieved with statins alone. BAS are considered first line during pregnancy because they are not systemically absorbed and pose no risk to the fetus.

✓ BAS bind bile acids in the intestinal lumen, interrupting enterohepatic circulation of bile acids, which decreases the bile acid pool size and stimulates hepatic synthesis of bile acids from cholesterol. Depletion of the hepatic cholesterol pool increases cholesterol biosynthesis and the number of LDL receptors on hepatocyte membranes, which enhances the rate of catabolism from plasma and lowers LDL levels. Increased hepatic cholesterol biosynthesis may be paralleled by increased hepatic VLDL production; consequently, BAS may aggravate hypertriglyceridemia and should be avoided in patients with TG levels >300 mg/dL (3.39 mmol/L).

✓ Cholestyramine powders that require mixing with water or juice to create a slurry for oral administration are associated with GI complaints of constipation, bloating, epigastric fullness, nausea, and flatulence. These effects can be minimized by increasing fluid intake, increasing dietary bulk, and using stool softeners. Tablet forms of colesevelam are generally better tolerated than resin powders. Other potential adverse effects include impaired absorption of fat-soluble vitamins A, D, E, and K; GI obstruction; and reduced bioavailability of other drugs such as warfarin, levothyroxine, and phenytoin. Drug–drug interactions may be avoided by taking other medications 1 hour before or 4 hours after the BAS.

✓ Given the better safety and tolerability profile of ezetimibe, BAS should be reserved for patients unable to tolerate ezetimibe who need additional LDL-C lowering despite maximally tolerated statin therapy.

Proprotein Convertase Subtilisin/Kexin Type 9 (PCSK9) Inhibitors

- **Alirocumab** and **evolocumab** are fully human monoclonal antibodies to PCSK9; inhibiting PCSK9 promotes intracellular degradation of hepatic LDL-C, prevents LDL receptor recycling to the cell surface, and reduces LDL-C clearance from the circulation. They reduce LDL-C by as much as 60% when added to statin therapy. Clinical trials have shown that these agents reduce recurrent CV events when added to statin therapy. The drugs are administered by subcutaneous injection either biweekly or once monthly.

- The most common adverse effect is injection site reactions, which can be minimized by allowing the injection to come to room temperature before use and icing the site before injecting. Some patients report flu-like symptoms after the injection. Patients who reach very low LDL-C levels (<20 mg/dL [0.53 mmol/L]) do not appear to be at increased risk of adverse events. Nevertheless, the long-term effects of achieving very low LDL-C levels remain unknown.

- Despite their favorable clinical benefits, PCSK9 inhibitor use has been limited because of high cost. Although these agents should primarily be used in combination with maximally tolerated statins in high-risk patients unable to achieve desired LDL-C levels with a statin alone, evolocumab is FDA-approved for use as monotherapy in patients with primary hyperlipidemia (such as heterozygous FH).

Fibric Acid Derivatives (Fibrates)

- **Gemfibrozil** and **fenofibrate** are potent TG-lowering therapies (20%–50%) but may cause a modest reciprocal rise in LDL-C in patients with severely elevated TG levels. Plasma HDL concentrations may rise 10%–15% or more with fibrates. Gemfibrozil increases the activity of lipoprotein lipase (LPL) and reduces secretion of VLDL from the liver into the plasma. Fenofibrate increases LPL activity and reduces apoprotein C-III (an inhibitor of LPL) by activating peroxisome-proliferator-activated receptor α (PPARα), which regulates the expression of genes involved in the regulation of lipids and other metabolic processes.

- Fibrates have been shown to reduce CV events when used as monotherapy, but there is less evidence to support combination therapy with statins. Fibrates are primarily used in patients with TG levels >500 mg/dL (5.65 mmol/L) to reduce the risk of acute pancreatitis.

- Fibrates are generally well tolerated, but GI complaints and transient hepatic transaminase elevations have been reported. Both agents require dose adjustments for significant renal impairment, and fenofibrate has been reported to transiently worsen renal function.

- SAMS can occur when fibrates are used alone but are more common when used in combination with statins. Gemfibrozil and its glucuronide metabolite have potent effects on CYP450 enzymes (such as CYP3A4) and intestinal, hepatic, and renal transporters making it highly prone to significantly increase serum statin concentrations and the risk of SAMS. Consequently, current guidelines do not recommend gemfibrozil in patients receiving statin therapy; fenofibrate should be used instead.

- Fenofibrate and gemfibrozil may rarely enhance gallstone formation. Fibrates may potentiate the effects of warfarin; the international normalized ratio (INR) should be monitored closely with this combination.

Omega-3 Polyunsaturated Fatty Acids (PUFA)

- High doses of omega-3 PUFA (2–4 g/day of EPA/DHA) significantly reduce TG and VLDL cholesterol levels (20%–50%), but PUFA supplementation has either no effect on TC and LDL-C or may cause slight elevations. Omega-3 PUFA reduce TG levels by increasing hepatic oxidation of free fatty acids, increasing LDL hydrolysis by activating PPARα, and inhibiting apoprotein C-III.

- The omega-3 PUFA formulations approved by the FDA for treating TG levels ≥500 mg/dL (5.65 mmol/L) include **omega-3-acid ethyl esters of EPA/DHA** (Lovaza), **omega-3-carboxylic acids of EPA/DHA** (Epanova), and **ethyl ester of EPA only** (icosapent ethyl; Vascepa). Prescription omega-3 PUFA products contain approximately 1 g of EPA/DHA per capsule, whereas the EPA/DHA content of non–FDA-regulated OTC fish oil supplements is often <300 mg per capsule. Unless patient affordability is an issue, prescription omega-3 PUFA are preferred to minimize pill burden and ensure product quality.
- Randomized clinical trials of omega-3 PUFA have shown mixed results due to variability in study designs and products used. Current recommendations suggest that low-dose omega-3 PUFA supplementation is reasonable in secondary prevention patients with heart failure or at high risk of sudden cardiac death. Low-dose omega-3 PUFA supplementation is not recommended for primary prevention, especially in patients with diabetes. In late 2019, icosapent ethyl received U.S. FDA approval for reducing the risk of CV events in adults with triglyceride levels ≥150 mg/dL and with established CV disease or diabetes plus at least two other CV risk factors and who are already taking maximally tolerated doses of statins.
- GI complaints (eg, abdominal pain, "fishy burps") are common with OTC omega-3 PUFA products but may be minimized by refrigerating the capsules. These products should be used with caution in patients with known sensitivities or allergies to fish or shellfish. Drug–drug interactions are minimal with omega-3 PUFA, although caution is advised when used concomitantly with antiplatelet agents or anticoagulants because omega-3 PUFA may prolong bleeding time.

Niacin

- **Niacin (nicotinic acid)** lowers TG levels (20%–50%) by inhibiting lipolysis with a decrease in free fatty acids in plasma and decreased hepatic esterification of TG. It also significantly raises HDL-C (5%–30%) by reducing its catabolism and decreasing hepatic removal. Niacin reduces hepatic synthesis of VLDL, leading to a modest dose-dependent decrease in LDL-C (5%–20%). Despite these favorable changes, niacin has not been shown to improve CV outcomes in patients already receiving statin therapy with relatively well-controlled lipids at baseline.
- Adverse events frequently limit niacin use. Cutaneous flushing and itching appear to be prostaglandin mediated and can be reduced by taking aspirin 325 mg shortly before niacin ingestion. Flushing seems to be related to rising plasma niacin concentrations and use of immediate-release formulations; taking the dose with meals and slowly titrating the dose upward may also minimize these effects. Concomitant alcohol and hot drinks may magnify flushing and pruritus with niacin and should be avoided at the time of ingestion.
- Niaspan, the only prescription form, is an extended-release product with pharmacokinetics intermediate between immediate- and sustained-release products that are sold as OTC dietary supplements. In controlled trials, Niaspan had fewer dermatologic reactions and a lower risk for hepatotoxicity.
- Niacin therapy may be associated with elevated hepatic enzymes, hyperuricemia, and hyperglycemia. It is contraindicated in patients with active liver disease and active peptic ulcer disease. Nicotinamide should not be used as an alternative to niacin because it does not effectively lower cholesterol or triglyceride levels.

Mipomersen

- **Mipomersen** is indicated as an adjunct to diet and lipid-lowering treatments to reduce LDL-C, TC, apolipoprotein B, and non-HDL-C in patients with homozygous FH. It is an oligonucleotide inhibitor of apolipoprotein B-100 synthesis. When given in combination with maximum tolerated doses of lipid-lowering therapy, mipomersen can produce an additional 25% reduction in LDL-C. Adverse reactions include injection site reactions, flu-like symptoms, nausea, headache, and elevations in serum transaminases. The labeling contains a black box warning for severe hepatotoxicity, and mipomersen is only available through a restricted Risk Evaluation and Mitigation Strategy (REMS) program.

Lomitapide

- **Lomitapide** has the same indication for FH as mipomersen. Lomitapide is a microsomal triglyceride transfer protein (MTP) inhibitor that reduces the amount of cholesterol that the liver and intestines assemble and secrete into the circulation. It may reduce LDL cholesterol by about 40% in patients on maximum tolerated lipid-lowering therapy and LDL apheresis. Like mipomersen, lomitapide contains a black box warning for severe hepatotoxicity and is only available through a restricted REMS program.

TREATMENT RECOMMENDATIONS

Familial Hypercholesterolemia

- Persons with FH have a very high lifetime risk of developing ASCVD. FH should be suspected in adults with untreated LDL-C levels ≥190 mg/dL (4.91 mmol/L) or non-HDL-C levels ≥220 mg/dL (5.69 mmol/L) who have a family history of high cholesterol or ASCVD in first-degree relatives.
- Mipomersen and lomitapide are indicated for patients with FH and reduce LDL-C levels by ~25% and ~40%, respectively, when added to maximum tolerated doses of lipid-lowering therapy.
- Other treatment options for FH patients include LDL apheresis (a process that removes LDL from the blood) and liver transplantation.

Hypertriglyceridemia

- Elevated TG levels are strongly associated with increased ASCVD risk, but the direct role of TG in ASCVD development is debatable.
- Advise all patients with elevated TG to implement lifestyle interventions shown to reduce TG levels, including 5%–10% reduction in body weight, reduced consumption of sugar and refined carbohydrates, increased physical activity, smoking cessation, and restricted alcohol intake.
- Identify and address secondary causes of hypertriglyceridemia (eg, uncontrolled diabetes and CKD, medications such as protease inhibitors and atypical antipsychotics).
- Statins are generally considered first-line therapy after optimizing lifestyle interventions and addressing secondary causes; they can reduce TG levels by up to 30% at higher doses and help achieve desired levels of LDL-C.
- The role of TG-lowering therapies such as fibrates and omega-3 PUFA in patients with TG of 200–499 mg/dL (2.26–5.64 mmol/L) is unclear.
- Fasting TG levels >500 mg/dL (5.65 mmol/L) are associated with pancreatitis and other complications. Dietary fat restriction is essential because it reduces synthesis and entry of additional chylomicrons into the circulation. Lipid-lowering therapies that primarily lower TG (eg, fibrates, omega-3 PUFA, niacin) are recommended as first-line agents. Statins may be reasonable first-line options in patients with an ASCVD risk of ≥7.5%. Treatment success is defined as reducing TG below 500 mg/dL (5.65 mmol/L) and preventing pancreatitis.

Low HDL Cholesterol

- Low HDL-C is a strong independent risk predictor of CHD and is defined as <40 mg/dL (1.03 mmol/L) for men and <50 mg/dL (1.29 mmol/L) for women. There is no specified goal for HDL-C raising, and the primary target in these patients remains lowering LDL-C.
- Lifestyle modifications (eg, smoking cessation, increasing physical activity) are the preferred treatment approach.

- Niacin can produce the greatest increase in HDL-C compared to other lipid-lowering therapies, but no randomized clinical trial data have shown reduction in ASCVD risk by raising HDL-C.

Patients with Diabetes

- Diabetic dyslipidemia is often characterized by hypertriglyceridemia, low HDL-C, and modestly elevated but dense LDL-C forms that are highly atherogenic. Statins are the first-line therapy based on evidence from randomized clinical trials that statins reduce ASCVD events and mortality in persons with diabetes. However, individual risk among patients with no history of ASCVD varies, so the 10-year ASCVD risk score is used to determine the appropriate statin intensity (Table 8-2). High-intensity statin therapy is preferred in patients with a history of ASCVD (secondary prevention) because these patients are at very high risk of recurrent ASCVD events.
- The role of nonstatin therapies in patients with diabetes is complex. Both ezetimibe and evolocumab have shown improved outcomes when added to statin therapy. Although diabetes is associated with a mixed dyslipidemia, the combination of fenofibrate and a statin did not reduce the rate of CV events compared to simvastatin alone in patients with type 2 diabetes. Fenofibrate may offer potential benefit with TG levels >204 mg/dL (2.31 mmol/L) and HDL-C <34 mg/dL (0.88 mmol/L), but this has not been evaluated in a prospective clinical trial. Additionally, fenofibrate appears to reduce the progression of diabetic retinopathy and the need for laser treatment. Colesevelam is FDA-approved to improve both glycemic and lipid control, but it can exacerbate hypertriglyceridemia, which is common in diabetes. Niacin modestly increases fasting plasma glucose (4%–5%) and A1C levels (~0.25%); consequently, niacin should not be routinely used in persons with diabetes.

EVALUATION OF THERAPEUTIC OUTCOMES

- For short-term evaluation, obtain a complete lipid panel 4–12 weeks after initiation or following a dose adjustment of lipid-lowering therapy to assess therapeutic response.
- For long-term evaluation, obtain a repeat lipid panel every 3–12 months to ensure adherence to lipid-lowering therapy and maintenance of desired levels of LDL-C.
  - ✓ Although TC, HDL-C, and TG levels are directly measured, LDL-C is typically estimated using the Friedewald equation: LDL-C = TC − HDL-C − (TG/5) [or LDL-C = TC − HDL-C − (TG/2.2) when lipid levels are all expressed in mmol/L]. However, the equation does not provide an accurate estimate of VLDL-C and can underestimate LDL-C in patients with high TG or very low LDL-C. Useful alternatives in these patients include non-HDL-C (TC − HDL-C) and direct LDL-C measurements, which are more accurate than estimated LDL-C using the Friedewald equation.
  - ✓ A nonfasting lipid panel is generally acceptable except in patients with hypertriglyceridemia, where a fasting lipid panel is preferred to minimize interference from chylomicrons.
- Routine safety monitoring of hepatic function and CK levels is not recommended in statin-treated patients, but these may be obtained if the patient has signs or symptoms suggestive of liver or muscle injury. Perform hepatic function tests in patients taking niacin at baseline, after each dosage increase, and every 6 months thereafter while taking a stable dose.
- Monitor A1C periodically in persons with diabetes receiving niacin and patients treated with statins who are at high risk for developing diabetes.
- In patients treated with lipid-lowering therapy for secondary prevention, symptoms such as angina or intermittent claudication may improve over months to years. Xanthomas or other external manifestations of dyslipidemia should regress with therapy.

• Evaluate modifiable risk factors such as hypertension, smoking, exercise, weight control, and glycemic control in persons with diabetes. Use of food diaries and recall surveys enable collection of information about diet in a systematic manner and may improve patient adherence to dietary recommendations.

See Chapter 31, Dyslipidemia, authored by Dave L. Dixon and Daniel M. Riche, for a more detailed discussion of this topic.

Heart Failure

- *Heart failure* (HF) is a progressive syndrome that can result from any changes in cardiac structure or function that impair the ability of the ventricle to fill with or eject blood. HF may be caused by an abnormality in systolic function, diastolic function, or both. HF with reduced systolic function (ie, reduced left ventricular ejection fraction, LVEF) is referred to as HF with reduced ejection fraction (HFrEF). Preserved LV systolic function (ie, normal LVEF) with presumed diastolic dysfunction is termed HF with preserved ejection fraction (HFpEF).

PATHOPHYSIOLOGY

- Causes of systolic dysfunction (decreased contractility) include reduced muscle mass (eg, myocardial infarction [MI]), dilated cardiomyopathies, and ventricular hypertrophy. Ventricular hypertrophy can be caused by pressure overload (eg, systemic or pulmonary hypertension and aortic or pulmonic valve stenosis) or volume overload (eg, valvular regurgitation, shunts, high-output states).
- Causes of diastolic dysfunction (restriction in ventricular filling) include increased ventricular stiffness, ventricular hypertrophy, infiltrative myocardial diseases, myocardial ischemia and MI, mitral or tricuspid valve stenosis, and pericardial disease (eg, pericarditis and pericardial tamponade).
- The leading causes of HF are coronary artery disease and hypertension.
- Regardless of the index event, decreased cardiac output (CO) results in activation of compensatory responses to maintain circulation: (1) tachycardia and increased contractility through sympathetic nervous system activation, (2) the Frank–Starling mechanism, whereby increased preload (through sodium and water retention) increases stroke volume, (3) vasoconstriction, and (4) ventricular hypertrophy and remodeling. Although these compensatory mechanisms initially maintain cardiac function, they are responsible for the symptoms of HF and contribute to disease progression.
- In the *neurohormonal model* of HF, an initiating event (eg, acute MI) leads to decreased CO; the HF state then becomes a systemic disease whose progression is mediated largely by neurohormones and autocrine/paracrine factors that drive myocyte injury, oxidative stress, inflammation, and extracellular matrix remodeling. These substances include angiotensin II, norepinephrine, aldosterone, natriuretic peptides, and arginine vasopressin (AVP).
- Chronic activation of the neurohormonal systems results in a cascade of events that affect the myocardium at the molecular and cellular levels. These events lead to changes in ventricular size (left ventricular hypertrophy), shape, structure, and function known as *ventricular remodeling*. The alterations in ventricular function result in further deterioration in cardiac systolic and diastolic functions that further promotes the remodeling process.
- Common precipitating factors that may cause a previously compensated HF patient to decompensate include myocardial ischemia and MI, pulmonary infections, nonadherence with diet or drug therapy, and inappropriate medication use. Drugs may precipitate or exacerbate HF through negative inotropic effects, direct cardiotoxicity, or increased sodium and water retention.

CLINICAL PRESENTATION

- Patient presentation may range from asymptomatic to cardiogenic shock.
- Primary symptoms are dyspnea (especially on exertion) and fatigue, which lead to exercise intolerance. Other pulmonary symptoms include orthopnea, paroxysmal nocturnal dyspnea (PND), tachypnea, and cough.

- Fluid overload can result in pulmonary congestion and peripheral edema.
- Nonspecific symptoms may include fatigue, nocturia, hemoptysis, abdominal pain, anorexia, nausea, bloating, ascites, poor appetite or early satiety, and weight gain or loss.
- Physical examination may reveal pulmonary crackles, S_3 gallop, cool extremities, Cheyne–Stokes respiration, tachycardia, narrow pulse pressure, cardiomegaly, symptoms of pulmonary edema (extreme breathlessness and anxiety, sometimes with coughing and pink, frothy sputum), peripheral edema, jugular venous distention (JVD), hepatojugular reflux (HJR), hepatomegaly, and mental status changes.

DIAGNOSIS

- Consider the diagnosis of HF in patients with characteristic signs and symptoms. A complete history and physical examination with appropriate laboratory testing are essential in evaluating patients with suspected HF.
- Laboratory tests for identifying disorders that may cause or worsen HF include complete blood cell count; serum electrolytes (including calcium and magnesium); renal, hepatic, thyroid function tests, and iron studies; urinalysis; lipid profile; and A1C. Hyponatremia (serum sodium <130 mEq/L [mmol/L]) may indicate worsening volume overload and/or disease progression and is associated with reduced survival. Serum creatinine may be increased due to hypoperfusion; preexisting renal dysfunction can contribute to volume overload. B-type natriuretic peptide (BNP) is usually >100 pg/mL (29 pmol/L) and NT-proBNP >300 pg/mL (35 pmol/L).
- Ventricular hypertrophy can be demonstrated on chest radiograph or electrocardiogram (ECG). Chest radiograph may also show pleural effusions or pulmonary edema.
- Echocardiogram can identify abnormalities of the pericardium, myocardium, or heart valves and quantify LVEF to determine if systolic or diastolic dysfunction is present.
- The New York Heart Association Functional Classification System is intended primarily to classify symptoms according to the physician's subjective evaluation. Functional class (FC)-I patients have no limitation of physical activity, FC-II patients have slight limitation, FC-III patients have marked limitation, and FC-IV patients are unable to carry on physical activity without discomfort.
- The American College of Cardiology/American Heart Association (ACC/AHA) staging system provides a more comprehensive framework for evaluating, preventing, and treating HF (see further discussion below).

TREATMENT OF CHRONIC HEART FAILURE

- Goals of Treatment: Improve quality of life, relieve or reduce symptoms, prevent or minimize hospitalizations, slow disease progression, and prolong survival.

GENERAL APPROACH

- The first step is to determine the etiology or precipitating factors. Treatment of underlying disorders (eg, hyperthyroidism) may obviate the need for treating HF.
- *ACC/AHA Stage A:* These are patients at high risk for developing HF. Identify and modify risk factors to prevent development of structural heart disease and subsequent HF. Strategies include smoking cessation and control of hypertension, diabetes mellitus, and dyslipidemia. Although treatment must be individualized, angiotensin-converting enzyme (ACE) inhibitors or angiotensin receptor blockers (ARBs) are recommended for HF prevention in patients with multiple vascular risk factors.
- *ACC/AHA Stage B:* These patients have structural heart disease but no HF signs or symptoms. Treatment is targeted at minimizing additional injury and preventing or slowing the remodeling process. In addition to treatment measures outlined for stage A, patients with reduced LVEF (<40%) should receive an ACE inhibitor

(or ARB) and an evidence-based β-blocker to prevent development of HF, regardless of whether they have had an MI. Patients with a previous MI and reduced LVEF should also receive an ACE inhibitor or ARB, evidence-based β-blockers, and a statin.

- *ACC/AHA Stage C:* These patients have structural heart disease and previous or current HF symptoms and include both HFrEF and HFpEF. In addition to treatments for stages A and B, patients with HFrEF in stage C should receive guideline-directed medical therapy (GDMT) that includes an ACE inhibitor, ARB, or angiotensin receptor–neprilysin inhibitor (ARNI; valsartan–sacubitril) together with an evidence-based β-blocker, and an aldosterone antagonist in eligible patients to reduce morbidity and mortality (**Fig. 9-1**). Loop diuretics, hydralazine–isosorbide dinitrate (ISDN), digoxin, and ivabradine are also used in select patients.
- *ACC/AHA Stage D HFrEF:* These patients have persistent HF symptoms despite maximally tolerated GDMT. They should be considered for specialized interventions, including mechanical circulatory support, continuous IV positive inotropic therapy, cardiac transplantation, or hospice care (when no additional treatments are appropriate).

NONPHARMACOLOGIC THERAPY OF CHRONIC HEART FAILURE

- Interventions include cardiac rehabilitation and restriction of fluid intake and dietary sodium intake (<2–3 g of sodium/day) with daily weight measurements.
- In patients with hyponatremia (serum sodium <130 mEq/L [mmol/L]) or persistent volume retention despite high diuretic doses and sodium restriction, limit daily fluid intake to 2 L/day from all sources.
- Revascularization or anti-ischemic therapy in patients with coronary disease may reduce HF symptoms.
- Drugs that can aggravate HF should be discontinued if possible.

PHARMACOLOGIC THERAPY FOR STAGE C HFrEF

- In general, patients with stage C HFrEF should receive an ACE inhibitor, ARB, or ARNI along with an evidence-based β-blocker, plus an aldosterone antagonist in select patients (**Fig. 9-1**). Administer a diuretic if there is evidence of fluid retention. A hydralazine–nitrate combination, ivabradine, or digoxin may be considered in select patients. Drug dosing recommendations are provided in **Table 9-1**.

Diuretics

- Compensatory mechanisms in HF stimulate excessive sodium and water retention, often leading to systemic and pulmonary congestion. Consequently, diuretic therapy (in addition to sodium restriction) is recommended for all patients with clinical evidence of fluid retention. However, because they do not alter disease progression or prolong survival, diuretics are not required for patients without fluid retention.
- Thiazide diuretics (eg, **hydrochlorothiazide**) are relatively weak and are infrequently used alone in HF. However, thiazides or the thiazide-like diuretic **metolazone** can be used in combination with a loop diuretic to promote very effective diuresis. Thiazides may be preferred over loop diuretics in patients with only mild fluid retention and elevated BP because of their more persistent antihypertensive effects.
- Loop diuretics (**furosemide**, **bumetanide**, and **torsemide**) are usually necessary to restore and maintain euvolemia in HF. In addition to acting in the thick ascending limb of the loop of Henle, they induce a prostaglandin-mediated increase in renal blood flow that contributes to their natriuretic effect. Unlike thiazides, loop diuretics maintain their effectiveness in the presence of impaired renal function, although higher doses may be necessary.
- Adverse effects of diuretics include hypovolemia, hypotension, hyponatremia, hypokalemia, hypomagnesemia, hyperuricemia, and renal dysfunction.

GDMT for HFrEF Stage C

ACEI or ARB (Class I Evidence A)
AND
GDMT β-blocker (Class I Evidence A)

Loop diuretic if needed for volume overload (Class I Evidence C)

Aldosterone antagonist[a] (Class I Evidence A)

ARNI[b] (sacubitril/valsartan) (Class I Evidence B-R)

Isosorbide dinitrate/hydralazine (Class I Evidence A if African-American and
persistently symptomatic on GDMT)
(Class IIa Evidence B if ACEI/ARB intolerant)

Ivabradine[c] (Class II Evidence B-R)

Digoxin[d] (Class IIa Evidence B if persistently symptomatic on GDMT)

[a]NYHA class II-IV symptoms, estimated creatinine clearance >30 mL/min
and K$^+$ <5.0 mEq/L
[b]NYHA class II-III symptoms tolerating an ACEI or ARB – switching to ARNI can
further reduce morbidity/mortality
[c]NYHA class II-III symptoms in normal sinus rhythm and HR ≥70 bpm on
maximally tolerated β-blocker dose
[d]Indication is to reduce hospitalizations

(ACEI, angiotensin-converting enzyme inhibitor; ARB, angiotensin receptor blocker; ARNI, angiotensin receptor–neprilysin inhibitor; bpm, beats per minute; GDMT, guideline-directed medical therapy; HFrEF, heart failure with reduced ejection fraction; K$^+$, serum potassium.)

FIGURE 9-1. Guideline-directed treatment algorithm for patients with ACC/AHA stage C heart failure with reduced ejection fraction. (Adapted from Yancy CW, Jessup M, Bozkurt B, et al. 2013 ACCF/AHA guideline for the management of heart failure: A report of the American College of Cardiology Foundation/American Heart Association Task Force on Practice Guidelines. J Am Coll Cardiol. 2013;62:e147–e239.)

Angiotensin-Converting Enzyme Inhibitors

- ACE inhibitors decrease angiotensin II and aldosterone, attenuating many of their deleterious effects that drive HF initiation and progression. ACE inhibitors also inhibit the breakdown of bradykinin, which increases vasodilation and also leads to cough. ACE inhibitors improve symptoms, slow disease progression, and decrease mortality in patients with HFrEF. Current guidelines recommend that all patients with HFrEF, regardless of whether or not symptoms are present, should receive an ACE inhibitor to reduce morbidity and mortality, unless there are contraindications.
- Clinical trials have documented favorable effects of ACE inhibitors on symptoms, HF progression, hospitalizations, and quality of life. ACE inhibitors improve survival

TABLE 9-1	Drug Dosing Recommendations for Stage C Heart Failure with Reduced Ejection Fraction (HFrEF)	
Generic (Brand) Name	**Initial Dose**	**Usual Range with Normal Renal Function**
Loop Diuretics		
Furosemide (Lasix)	20–40 mg once or twice daily	20–160 mg once or twice daily
Bumetanide (Bumex)	0.5–1 mg once or twice daily	1–2 mg once or twice daily
Torsemide (Demadex)	10–20 mg once daily	10–80 mg once daily
ACE Inhibitors		
Captopril (Capoten)	6.25 mg three times daily	50 mg three times daily[a]
Enalapril (Vasotec)	2.5 mg twice daily	10–20 mg twice daily[a]
Lisinopril (Prinivil, Zestril)	2.5–5 mg once daily	20–40 mg once daily[a]
Quinapril (Accupril)	5 mg twice daily	20–40 mg twice daily
Ramipril (Altace)	1.25–2.5 mg once daily	10 mg once daily[a]
Fosinopril (Monopril)	5–10 mg once daily	40 mg once daily
Trandolapril (Mavik)	1 mg once daily	4 mg once daily[a]
Perindopril (Aceon)	2 mg once daily	8–16 mg once daily
Angiotensin Receptor Blockers		
Candesartan (Atacand)	4–8 mg once daily	32 mg once daily[a]
Valsartan (Diovan)	20–40 mg twice daily	160 mg twice daily[a]
Losartan (Cozaar)	25–50 mg once daily	150 mg once daily[a]
Angiotensin Receptor Blocker–Neprilysin Inhibitor		
Sacubitril/Valsartan (Entresto)	49/51 sacubitril–valsartan twice daily	97/103 mg sacubitril–valsartan twice daily[a]
β-Blockers		
Bisoprolol (Zebeta)	1.25 mg once daily	10 mg once daily[a]
Carvedilol (Coreg)	3.125 mg twice daily	25 mg twice daily[a]
Carvedilol phosphate (Coreg CR)	10 mg once daily	80 mg once daily
Metoprolol succinate CR/XL (Toprol-XL)	12.5–25 mg once daily	200 mg once daily[a]
Aldosterone Antagonists		
Spironolactone (Aldactone)	12.5–25 mg once daily	25–50 mg once daily[a]
Eplerenone (Inspra)	25 mg once daily	50 mg once daily[a]
Other		
Hydralazine–Isosorbide Dinitrate (Bidil)	Hydralazine 37.5 mg 3 times daily	Hydralazine 75 mg 3 times daily[a]
	Isosorbide dinitrate 20 mg 3 times daily	Isosorbide dinitrate 40 mg 3 times daily[a]
Digoxin (Lanoxin)	0.125–0.25 mg once daily	0.125–0.25 mg once daily
Ivabradine (Corlanor)	5 mg twice daily	5–7.5 mg twice daily

[a]Regimens proven in large clinical trials to reduce mortality.
ACEI, angiotensin-converting enzyme inhibitor; ARB, angiotensin receptor blocker.
Data from Brater DC. Pharmacology of diuretics. Am J Med Sci. 2000;319:38-50; Yancy CW, Jessup M, Bozkurt B, et al. 2013 ACCF/AHA guideline for the management of heart failure: A report of the American College of Cardiology Foundation/American Heart Association Task Force on Practice Guidelines. J Am Coll Cardiol. 2013;62:e147–e239.

by 20%–30% compared with placebo. The benefits are independent of HF etiology (ischemic vs nonischemic) and are greatest in patients with the most severe symptoms.

- Start therapy with low doses followed by gradual titration as tolerated to the target or maximally tolerated doses (Table 9-1). Dose titration is usually accomplished by doubling the dose every 2 weeks. Evaluate blood pressure (BP), renal function, and serum potassium at baseline and within 1–2 weeks after the start of therapy and after each dose increase. Although symptoms may improve within a few days of starting therapy, it may take weeks to months before the full benefits are apparent. Even if symptoms do not improve, continue long-term therapy to reduce mortality and hospitalizations.

- The most common adverse effects include hypotension, renal dysfunction, and hyperkalemia. A dry, nonproductive cough (occurring in 15%–20% of patients) is the most common reason for discontinuation. Because cough is a bradykinin-mediated effect, replacement with an ARB is reasonable; however, caution is required because crossreactivity has been reported. Angioedema occurs in approximately 1% of patients and is potentially life threatening; ACE inhibitors are contraindicated in patients with a history of angioedema. ACE inhibitors are contraindicated in pregnancy due to various congenital defects.

Angiotensin Receptor Blockers

- The ARBs block the angiotensin II receptor subtype AT_1, preventing the deleterious effects of angiotensin II on ventricular remodeling. Because they do not affect the ACE enzyme, ARBs do not affect bradykinin, which is linked to ACE inhibitor cough and angioedema.

- ARBs are now a guideline-recommended alternative in patients who are unable to tolerate an ACE inhibitor due to cough or angioedema. Although numerous ARBs are available, only **candesartan**, **valsartan**, and **losartan** are recommended in the guidelines because efficacy has been demonstrated in clinical trials. As with ACE inhibitors, initiate therapy with low doses and then titrate to target doses. Evaluate BP, renal function, and serum potassium within 1–2 weeks after starting therapy and after dosage increases, with these parameters used to guide subsequent dose changes.

- ARBs are not suitable alternatives in patients with hypotension, hyperkalemia, or renal insufficiency due to ACE inhibitors because they are just as likely to cause these adverse effects. Careful monitoring is required when an ARB is used with another inhibitor of the renin-angiotensin-aldosterone system (RAAS) (eg, ACE inhibitor or aldosterone antagonist) because this combination increases the risk of these adverse effects. Because ARBs do not affect bradykinin, they are not associated with cough and have a lower risk of angioedema than ACE inhibitors. Caution should be exercised when ARBs are used in patients with angioedema from ACE inhibitors because crossreactivity has been reported. Similar to ACE inhibitors, ARBs are contraindicated in pregnancy.

Angiotensin Receptor–Neprilysin Inhibitor

- **Valsartan/Sacubitril** is an ARNI approved to reduce the risk of cardiovascular death and hospitalization for HF in patients with NYHA class II–IV HF and reduced LVEF. Neprilysin is an enzyme that degrades bradykinin and other endogenous vasodilator and natriuretic peptides. By reducing neprilysin-mediated breakdown of these compounds, vasodilation, diuresis, and natriuresis are enhanced, and renin and aldosterone secretion is inhibited.

- In patients with HFrEF and NYHA class II–III symptoms tolerating an ACE inhibitor or ARB, current guidelines recommend replacing those drugs with the ARNI to further reduce morbidity and mortality. Discontinue ACE inhibitors 36 hours prior to initiating the ARNI; no waiting period is needed in patients receiving an ARB.

Titrate the initial starting dose to the target dose after 2–4 weeks (see Table 9-1). Closely monitor BP, serum potassium, and renal function after the start of therapy and after each titration step.

- The most common adverse effects include hypotension, dizziness, hyperkalemia, worsening renal function, and cough. Angioedema is most common with sacubitril/valsartan than with enalapril (0.5% vs 0.2%, respectively). Sacubitril/valsartan is contraindicated in patients with a history of angioedema associated with an ACE inhibitor or ARB. It is also contraindicated in pregnancy and should not be used concurrently with ACE inhibitors or other ARBs.

β-Blockers

- β-Blockers antagonize the detrimental effects of the sympathetic nervous systems in HF and slow disease progression. Clinical trial evidence demonstrated that certain β-blockers reduce HF mortality, all-cause hospitalizations, and hospitalizations for worsening HF, among other endpoints.
- The ACC/AHA guidelines recommend use of β-blockers in all stable patients with HFrEF in the absence of contraindications or a clear history of β-blocker intolerance. Patients should receive a β-blocker even if symptoms are mild or well controlled with ACE inhibitor and diuretic therapy. It is not essential that ACE inhibitor doses be optimized before a β-blocker is started because the addition of a β-blocker is likely to be of greater benefit than an increase in ACE inhibitor dose.
- β-Blockers are also recommended for asymptomatic persons with a reduced LVEF (stage B) to decrease the risk of progression to HF.
- **Carvedilol, metoprolol succinate (CR/XL)**, and **bisoprolol** are the only β-blockers shown to reduce mortality in large HF trials. Because bisoprolol is not available in the necessary starting dose of 1.25 mg, the choice is typically limited to either carvedilol or metoprolol succinate. Target doses are those associated with reductions in mortality in placebo-controlled clinical trials (Table 9-1).
- Initiate β-blockers in stable patients who have no or minimal evidence of fluid overload. Because of their negative inotropic effects, start β-blockers in very low doses with slow upward dose titration to avoid symptomatic worsening or acute decompensation. Doses should be doubled no more often than every 2 weeks, as tolerated, until the target or maximally tolerated dose is reached.
- Inform patients that β-blocker therapy is expected to positively influence disease progression and survival even if there is little symptomatic improvement. In addition, dose titration is a long, gradual process; response to therapy may be delayed; and HF symptoms may actually worsen during the initiation period.
- Adverse effects include bradycardia or heart block, hypotension, fatigue, impaired glycemic control in diabetic patients, bronchospasm in patients with asthma, and worsening HF. Absolute contraindications include uncontrolled bronchospastic disease, symptomatic bradycardia, advanced heart block without a pacemaker, and acute decompensated HF. However, β-blockers may be tried with caution in patients with asymptomatic bradycardia, COPD, or well-controlled asthma.

Aldosterone Antagonists

- **Spironolactone** and **eplerenone** block mineralocorticoid receptors, the target for aldosterone. In the kidney, aldosterone antagonists inhibit sodium reabsorption and potassium excretion. However, diuretic effects with low doses are minimal, suggesting that their therapeutic benefits result from other actions. In the heart, aldosterone antagonists inhibit cardiac extracellular matrix and collagen deposition, thereby attenuating cardiac fibrosis and ventricular remodeling. Aldosterone antagonists also attenuate the systemic proinflammatory state, atherogenesis, and oxidative stress caused by aldosterone.
- Current guidelines recommend adding a low-dose aldosterone antagonist to standard therapy to improve symptoms, reduce the risk of HF hospitalization, and increase survival in select patients provided that serum potassium and renal function can be carefully monitored. Based on clinical trial data in HFrEF, low-dose aldosterone

antagonists may be appropriate for: (1) patients with mild to moderately severe HFrEF (NYHA class II–IV) who are receiving standard therapy, and (2) those with LV dysfunction and either acute HF or diabetes early after MI.

- Start with low doses (spironolactone 12.5 mg/day or eplerenone 25 mg/day) especially in older persons and those with diabetes or a creatinine clearance <50 mL/min/1.73m^2 (0.48 mL/sec/m^2 (Table 9-1).

- Avoid aldosterone antagonists in patients with renal impairment, elevated serum potassium (>5 mEq/L [mmol/L]), or history of severe hyperkalemia. Spironolactone also interacts with androgen and progesterone receptors, which may lead to gynecomastia, impotence, and menstrual irregularities in some patients.

Nitrates and Hydralazine

- **Isosorbide dinitrate (ISDN)** is a venodilator that reduces preload, whereas **hydralazine** is a direct arterial vasodilator that reduces systemic vascular resistance (SVR) and increases stroke volume and CO. The beneficial effects of combining a nitrate with hydralazine extend beyond their complementary hemodynamic actions and are likely related to attenuating the biochemical processes driving HF progression.

- Guidelines recommend addition of hydralazine/ISDN to self-described African Americans with HFrEF and NYHA class III–IV symptoms treated with ACE inhibitors (or ARBs) and β-blockers. The combination can also be useful in patients unable to tolerate either an ACE inhibitor or ARB because of renal insufficiency, hyperkalemia, or hypotension.

- Obstacles to successful therapy with the combination include the need for frequent dosing (ie, three times daily with the fixed-dose combination product), high frequency of adverse effects (eg, headache, dizziness, and GI distress), and increased cost for the fixed-dose combination product.

Ivabradine

- Ivabradine inhibits the I_f current in the sinoatrial node that is responsible for controlling HR, thereby slowing spontaneous depolarization of the sinus node and resulting in a dose-dependent slowing of the HR. It does not affect AV conduction, BP, or myocardial contractility. Elevated resting heart rate (HR) (>70–80 bpm) is an independent risk factor for adverse HFrEF outcomes, and β-blockers are frequently underdosed in clinical practice for a variety of reasons. Because of the clear benefits of β-blockers on mortality, clinicians should titrate to the maximum tolerated doses before considering use of ivabradine.

- Ivabradine is indicated to reduce the risk of hospitalization for worsening HF in patients with LVEF ≤35% who are in sinus rhythm with resting HR ≥70 bpm and are either on a maximally tolerated dose of a β-blocker or have a contraindication to β-blocker use.

- The usual starting dose is 5 mg twice daily with meals (Table 9-1). After 2 weeks of treatment, if the resting HR is between 50 and 60 bpm, the dose should be continued. If the HR is >60 bpm, the dose can be increased to the maximum of 7.5 mg twice daily. If at any point the HR is <50 bpm or the patient has symptomatic bradycardia, the dose should be reduced by 2.5 mg twice daily; if the patient is only receiving 2.5 mg twice daily, ivabradine should be discontinued.

- The most common adverse effects are bradycardia, atrial fibrillation, and visual disturbances.

Digoxin

- Although digoxin has positive inotropic effects, its benefits in HF are related to its neurohormonal effects. It attenuates the excessive sympathetic nervous system activation in HF and increases parasympathetic activity, thereby decreasing HR and enhancing diastolic filling. Observational studies of digoxin conducted in the context of contemporary HF therapy showed either neutral effects or reductions in hospitalizations and either neutral or detrimental effects of digoxin on mortality.

- Based on available data, digoxin is not considered a first-line agent in HF, but a trial may be considered in conjunction with GDMT including ACE inhibitors (or ARBs), β-blockers, and diuretics in patients with symptomatic HFrEF to improve symptoms and reduce hospitalizations. Digoxin may also be considered to help control ventricular rate in patients with HFrEF and supraventricular arrhythmias, although β-blockers are generally more effective rate control agents, especially during exercise.
- In the absence of digoxin toxicity or serious adverse effects, digoxin should be continued in most patients. Digoxin withdrawal may be considered for asymptomatic patients who have significant improvement in systolic function with optimal ACE inhibitor and β-blocker treatment.
- The target serum digoxin concentration for most patients is 0.5–0.9 ng/mL (0.6–1.2 nmol/L). Most patients with normal renal function can achieve this level with a dose of 0.125 mg/day. Patients with decreased renal function, low body weight, advanced age, or interacting drugs (eg, amiodarone) should receive 0.125 mg every other day.

PHARMACOLOGIC THERAPY FOR HFpEF

- Treatment includes controlling HR and BP, alleviating causes of myocardial ischemia, reducing volume, and restoring and maintaining sinus rhythm in patients with atrial fibrillation. Many of the drugs are the same as those used to treat HFrEF (eg, diuretics, β-blockers), but the rationale and dosing may be different.
- A loop or a thiazide diuretic should be considered for patients with volume overload. Use a loop diuretic for more severe volume overload or inadequate response to a thiazide. Avoid lowering preload excessively, which may reduce stroke volume and CO. Start diuretics at low doses to avoid hypotension and fatigue.
- ACE inhibitors may be considered in all patients, especially patients with symptomatic atherosclerotic cardiovascular disease or diabetes and one additional risk factor.
- ARBs may be considered in all patients, especially those who are intolerant of ACE inhibitors.
- Aldosterone antagonists can reduce the risk of hospitalization in patients who do not have contraindications and are not at risk for hyperkalemia. They may be beneficial for patients with elevated BNP or NT-proBNP.
- β-Blockers should be considered in patients with one or more of the following conditions: (1) MI, (2) hypertension, and (3) atrial fibrillation requiring ventricular rate control.
- Nondihydropyridine calcium channel blockers (CCB; **diltiazem** or **verapamil**) should be considered for patients with atrial fibrillation warranting ventricular rate control who either are intolerant to or have not responded to a β-blocker. A nondihydropyridine or dihydropyridine (eg, **amlodipine**) CCB can be considered for symptom-limiting angina or hypertension.

TREATMENT OF ACUTE DECOMPENSATED HEART FAILURE (ADHF)

GENERAL APPROACH

- *Acute decompensated heart failure* involves patients with new or worsening signs or symptoms (often resulting from volume overload and/or low CO) requiring medical intervention, such as emergency department visit or hospitalization.
- Goals of Treatment: The overall goals are to relieve symptoms, improve hemodynamic stability, and reduce short-term mortality so the patient can be discharged in a stable compensated state on oral drug therapy.
- Consider hospitalization based on clinical findings. Admission to an intensive care unit (ICU) may be required if the patient experiences hemodynamic instability requiring frequent monitoring of vital signs, invasive hemodynamic monitoring, or rapid titration of IV medications with close monitoring.
- Focus the history and physical exam on potential etiologies of ADHF; presence of precipitating factors (eg, arrhythmias, hypertension, myocardial ischemia or infarction, anemia, and thyroid disorders); onset, duration, and severity of symptoms; and a careful medication history.

- Symptoms of volume overload include dyspnea, orthopnea, PND, ascites, GI symptoms (poor appetite, nausea, early satiety), peripheral edema, and weight gain. Low output symptoms include altered mental status, fatigue, GI symptoms (similar to volume overload), and decreased urine output.
- Signs of volume overload include pulmonary crackles, elevated jugular venous pressure, HJR, S_3 gallop, and peripheral edema. Low output signs include tachycardia, hypotension (more commonly) or hypertension, narrow pulse pressure, cool extremities, pallor, and cachexia.
- Laboratory testing may include BNP or NT-proBNP, thyroid function tests, complete blood count, cardiac enzymes, and routine serum chemistries (eg, serum creatinine, liver function tests).
- Ascertain hemodynamic status to guide initial therapy. Patients may be categorized into one of four hemodynamic subsets based on volume status (euvolemic or "dry" vs volume overloaded or "wet") and CO (adequate CO or "warm" vs hypoperfusion or "cold") (**Fig. 9-2**).
- Reserve invasive hemodynamic monitoring for patients refractory to initial therapy, whose volume status is unclear, or who have significant hypotension or worsening renal function despite appropriate initial therapy.
- Address and correct reversible or treatable causes of decompensation.
- Assess medications being taken prior to admission and determine whether adjustment or discontinuation is required.
- If fluid retention is evident on physical exam, pursue aggressive diuresis, preferably with IV diuretics.
- In the absence of cardiogenic shock or symptomatic hypotension, strive to continue all GDMT for HF. β-blockers may be temporarily held or dose-reduced if recent changes are responsible for acute decompensation. Other GDMT (ACE inhibitors, ARBs, ARNI, and aldosterone antagonists) may also need to be temporarily withheld in the presence of renal dysfunction, with close monitoring of serum potassium. Most patients may continue to receive digoxin at doses targeting a trough serum concentration of 0.5–0.9 ng/mL (mcg/L; 0.6–1.2 nmol/L).

NONPHARMACOLOGIC THERAPY FOR ADHF

- Place all patients with congestive symptoms on sodium restriction (<2 g daily) and consider fluid restriction for refractory symptoms.
- Consider noninvasive ventilation for patients in respiratory distress due to acute pulmonary edema, particularly those at risk for intubation.
- Provide pharmacologic thromboprophylaxis with unfractionated heparin or low-molecular-weight heparin for most patients with limited mobility; consider mechanical thromboprophylaxis with intermittent pneumatic compression devices in patients at high risk for bleeding.
- Most nonpharmacologic therapies for ADHF are reserved for patients failing pharmacologic therapy. Ultrafiltration and wireless invasive hemodynamic monitoring (W-IHM) may be used to manage congestive symptoms. Temporary mechanical circulatory support (MCS) with an intra-aortic balloon pump (IABP), ventricular assist device (VAD), or extracorporeal membrane oxygenation (ECMO) may be considered for hemodynamic stabilization until the underlying etiology of cardiac dysfunction resolves or has been corrected ("bridge to recovery") or until evaluation for definitive therapy (eg, durable MCS or cardiac transplantation) can be completed ("bridge to decision"). IV vasodilators and inotropes may be used with temporary MCS to maximize hemodynamic and clinical benefits or facilitate device removal. Systemic anticoagulant therapy is generally required to prevent device thrombosis, regardless of the method selected.
- Durable MCS with temporary device implantation is used for patients awaiting heart transplantation who are unlikely to survive until a suitable donor is identified ("bridge to transplantation"). Permanent device implantation is used in patients ineligible for heart transplantation due to advanced age or comorbid conditions ("destination therapy").

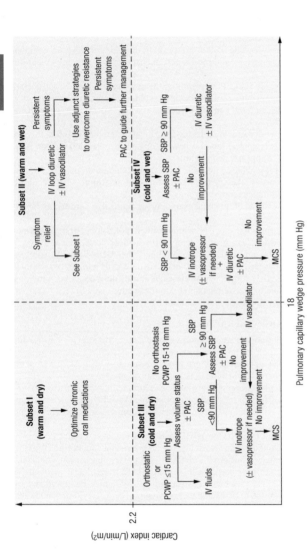

(IV, intravenous; MCS, mechanical circulatory support; PAC, pulmonary artery catheter; PCWP, pulmonary capillary wedge pressure; SBP, systolic BP.)

FIGURE 9-2. General management algorithm for acute decompensated heart failure based on clinical presentation. Patients may be categorized into a hemodynamic subset based on signs and symptoms or invasive hemodynamic monitoring. Adjunct strategies for overcoming diuretic resistance include increasing the dose of loop diuretic; switching to a continuous infusion; adding a diuretic with an alternative mechanism of action, an IV vasodilator, or an IV inotrope; and in select patients, adding mechanical circulatory support.

- Cardiac transplantation is the best option for patients with irreversible advanced HF. New surgical strategies such as ventricular aneurysm resection and myocardial cell transplantation offer additional options for patients ineligible for VAD implantation or heart transplantation.

PHARMACOLOGIC THERAPY FOR ADHF

Loop Diuretics

- Current guidelines recommend IV loop diuretics (**furosemide**, **bumetanide**) as first-line therapy for ADHF patients with volume overload.
- Bolus administration reduces preload by functional venodilation within 5–15 minutes and later (>20 minutes) via sodium and water excretion, thereby improving pulmonary congestion. Although patients with HFrEF can tolerate significant reductions in preload without compromising stroke volume, excessive diuresis can decrease CO. Excessive reductions in venous return may also compromise CO in diastolic dysfunction, intravascular volume depletion, or patients in whom CO is significantly dependent on adequate filling pressure (ie, preload-dependent). Reflex increases in neurohormonal activation (ie, elevated renin, norepinephrine, and AVP) may result in arteriolar and coronary vasoconstriction, tachycardia, and increased myocardial oxygen consumption.
- Use low doses (equivalent to IV furosemide 20–40 mg) initially in ADHF patients who are naïve to loop diuretics. For patients taking loop diuretics prior to admission, a total daily dose of 1- to 2.5-times their home dose is recommended. Higher doses are associated with more rapid relief of congestive symptoms but may also increase the risk of transient worsening of renal function. Doses may be administered as either an IV bolus (ie, divided every 12 hours) or continuous IV infusion. Use diuretic therapy judiciously to obtain the desired improvement in congestive symptoms while avoiding a reduction in CO, symptomatic hypotension, or worsening renal function.
- Diuretic resistance may be improved by administering larger IV bolus doses, transitioning from IV bolus to continuous IV infusions, or adding a second diuretic with a different mechanism of action, such as a distal tubule blocker (eg, oral **metolazone**, oral **hydrochlorothiazide**, or IV **chlorothiazide**). Sequential nephron blockade with a loop and thiazide-type diuretic should generally be reserved for inpatients who can be monitored closely for development of severe electrolyte and intravascular volume depletion. In the outpatient setting, a very low dose of the thiazide-type diuretic or infrequent administration (eg, 1–3 times weekly) is recommended.

Vasopressin Antagonists

- Vasopressin receptor antagonists affect one or two AVP (antidiuretic hormone) receptors, V_{1A} or V_2. Stimulation of V_{1A} receptors (located in vascular smooth muscle cells and myocardium) results in vasoconstriction, myocyte hypertrophy, coronary vasoconstriction, and positive inotropic effects. V_2 receptors are located in renal tubules, where they regulate water reabsorption.
  - ✓ **Tolvaptan** selectively binds to and inhibits the V_2 receptor. It is an oral agent indicated for hypervolemic and euvolemic hyponatremia in patients with syndrome of inappropriate antidiuretic hormone (SIADH), cirrhosis, or HF. Tolvaptan is typically initiated at 15 mg orally daily and then titrated to 30 or 60 mg daily as needed to resolve hyponatremia. It is a substrate of cytochrome P450-3A4 and is contraindicated with potent inhibitors of this enzyme. The most common side effects are dry mouth, thirst, urinary frequency, constipation, and hyperglycemia.
  - ✓ **Conivaptan** nonselectively inhibits both the V_{1A} and V_2 receptors. It is an IV agent indicated for hypervolemic and euvolemic hyponatremia due to a variety of causes but is not indicated for patients with HF.
- Monitor patients closely to avoid an excessively rapid rise in serum sodium that could cause hypotension or hypovolemia requiring drug discontinuation. Therapy may be restarted at a lower dose if hyponatremia recurs or persists and adverse effects resolve.

- The role of vasopressin receptor antagonists in the long-term management of HF is unclear. In a clinical trial of hospitalized patients with HF, tolvaptan improved hyponatremia, diuresis, and signs/symptoms of congestion. However, the study failed to demonstrate improved long-term outcomes, including morbidity and mortality. Another randomized trial in patients with ADHF found worsening renal function in significantly more patients receiving tolvaptan than placebo. Overall, these two trials do not support routine use of tolvaptan in ADHF, and it should be reserved for managing severe hyponatremia.

Vasodilators

- Venodilators reduce preload by increasing venous capacitance, improving symptoms of pulmonary congestion in patients with high ventricular filling pressures. Arterial vasodilators counteract the peripheral vasoconstriction and impaired CO that can result from activation of the sympathetic nervous system, RAAS, and other neurohormonal mediators in HF. Arterial vasodilators reduce impedance, decreasing afterload and causing reflex improvement in LV performance and increased CO. Mixed vasodilators act on both arterial resistance and venous capacitance vessels, reducing congestive symptoms while increasing CO.

- IV vasodilators should be considered before positive inotropic therapy in patients with low CO and elevated SVR (or elevated BP in those without a pulmonary artery catheter). However, hypotension may preclude their use in patients with preexisting low BP or SVR.

- **IV nitroglycerin** is often preferred for preload reduction in ADHF, especially in patients with pulmonary congestion. It reduces preload and pulmonary capillary wedge pressure (PCWP) via functional venodilation and mild arterial vasodilation. In higher doses, nitroglycerin displays potent coronary vasodilating properties and beneficial effects on myocardial oxygen demand and supply, making it the vasodilator of choice for patients with severe HF and ischemic heart disease.
  - ✓ Initiate nitroglycerin at 5–10 mcg/min (0.1 mcg/kg/min) and increase every 5–10 minutes as necessary and tolerated. Maintenance doses usually range from 35 to 200 mcg/min (0.5–3 mcg/kg/min). Hypotension and excessive decrease in PCWP are important dose-limiting side effects. Tolerance to the hemodynamic effects may develop over 12–72 hours of continuous administration.

- **Sodium nitroprusside** is a mixed arteriovenous vasodilator that increases cardiac index (CI) to a similar degree as dobutamine and milrinone despite having no direct inotropic activity. However, nitroprusside generally produces greater decreases in PCWP, SVR, and BP.
  - ✓ Hypotension is an important dose-limiting adverse effect of nitroprusside, and its use should be primarily reserved for patients with elevated SVR. Close monitoring is required because even modest HR increases can have adverse consequences in patients with underlying ischemic heart disease or resting tachycardia.
  - ✓ Nitroprusside is effective in the short-term management of severe HF in a variety of settings (eg, acute MI, valvular regurgitation, after coronary bypass surgery, and ADHF). It does not usually worsen, and may improve, the balance between myocardial oxygen demand and supply. However, an excessive decrease in systemic arterial pressure can decrease coronary perfusion and worsen ischemia.
  - ✓ Nitroprusside has a rapid onset and a duration of action <10 minutes, necessitating continuous IV infusions. Initiate therapy with a low dose (0.1–0.2 mcg/kg/min) to avoid excessive hypotension, and increase by small increments (0.1–0.2 mcg/kg/min) every 5–10 minutes as tolerated. Usual effective doses range from 0.5 to 3 mcg/kg/min. Taper nitroprusside slowly when transitioning to oral medications to avoid the rebound phenomenon of reflex neurohormonal activation after abrupt withdrawal. Nitroprusside-induced cyanide and thiocyanate toxicity are unlikely when doses <3 mcg/kg/min are administered for less than 3 days, except in patients with significant renal impairment (ie, serum creatinine >3 mg/dL [265 μmol/L]).

Inotropes

- Prompt correction of low CO in patients with "cold" subsets (III and IV) is required to restore peripheral tissue perfusion and preserve end-organ function. Although IV inotropes can improve hypoperfusion by enhancing cardiac contractility, potential adverse outcomes limit their use to select patients with refractory ADHF. Inotropes should be considered only as a temporizing measure to maintain end-organ perfusion in patients with cardiogenic shock or severely depressed CO and low systolic BP (ie, ineligible for IV vasodilators) until definitive therapy can be initiated, as a "bridge" for patients with advanced HF who are eligible for MCS or cardiac transplantation, or for palliation of symptoms in patients with advanced HF who are ineligible for MCS or cardiac transplantation.
- Dobutamine and milrinone produce similar hemodynamic effects, but dobutamine usually causes more pronounced increases in HR, and milrinone is associated with greater relaxation in arterial smooth muscle.
- **Dobutamine** is a β_1- and β_2-receptor agonist with some α_1-agonist effects; its positive inotropic effects are due to effects on β_1-receptors. Stimulation of cardiac β_1-receptors does not generally produce a significant increase in HR. Modest peripheral β_2-receptor-mediated vasodilation tends to offset minor α_1-receptor-mediated vasoconstriction; the net vascular effect is usually vasodilation.
  - ✓ CI is increased because of inotropic stimulation, arterial vasodilation, and a variable increase in HR. It causes relatively little change in mean arterial pressure (MAP) compared with the more consistent increases observed with dopamine. Dobutamine should be considered over milrinone when a significant decrease in MAP might further compromise hemodynamic function.
  - ✓ Vasodilation usually reduces PCWP, making dobutamine particularly useful in the presence of low CI and an elevated LV filling pressure; however, these effects may be detrimental in the presence of reduced filling pressure.
  - ✓ Initial doses of 2.5–5 mcg/kg/min may be increased progressively to 20 mcg/kg/min based on clinical and hemodynamic responses. The dose should be tapered rather than abruptly discontinued.
  - ✓ Dobutamine's major adverse effects are tachycardia and ventricular arrhythmias. Potentially detrimental increases in oxygen consumption have also been observed.
- **Milrinone** inhibits phosphodiesterase III and produces positive inotropic and arterial and venous vasodilating effects (an inodilator). It has supplanted use of amrinone, which has a higher rate of thrombocytopenia.
  - ✓ During IV administration, milrinone increases stroke volume and CO with minimal change in HR. However, the vasodilating effects may predominate, leading to decreased BP and a reflex tachycardia. Milrinone also lowers pulmonary PCWP by venodilation and is particularly useful in patients with a low CI and elevated LV filling pressure. However, this decrease in preload can be hazardous for patients without excessive filling pressure, thus blunting the improvement in CO. Use milrinone cautiously in severely hypotensive HF patients because it does not increase, and may even decrease, arterial BP.
  - ✓ Most patients are started on a continuous IV infusion of 0.1–0.3 mcg/kg/min, titrated to a maximum of 0.75 mcg/kg/min. A loading dose of 50 mcg/kg over 10 minutes can be given if rapid hemodynamic changes are required, but its use is uncommon due to an increased risk of hypotension.
  - ✓ The most notable adverse events are arrhythmia, hypotension, and thrombocytopenia. Measure the platelet count before and during therapy.
- **Norepinephrine** and **dopamine** have combined inotropic and vasopressor activity. Although therapies that increase SVR are generally avoided in ADHF, they may be required in select patients where marked hypotension precludes use of traditional inotropes (eg, septic shock, refractory cardiogenic shock). These agents are sometimes combined with traditional inotropes so each drug can be adjusted

independently to achieve the desired hemodynamic response, although little data exist to support that practice.

✓ Norepinephrine stimulates α_1- and β_1-adrenergic receptors. Stimulation of β_1-receptors in myocardial tissue increases HR, contractility, and therefore CO, but peripheral α_1-receptor-induced vasoconstriction is the predominant clinical hemodynamic effect. Lack of affinity for β_2-receptors may be responsible for the limited impact of norepinephrine on CO.

✓ Dopamine is an endogenous precursor of norepinephrine that stimulates α_1, β_1, β_2, and D_1 (vascular dopaminergic) receptors. Positive inotropic effects mediated primarily by β_1-receptors are prominent with doses of 2–5 mcg/kg/min. The CI is increased with minimal changes in SVR. At doses between 5 and 10 mcg/kg/min, chronotropic and α_1-mediated vasoconstriction become more prominent and MAP usually increases as a result of increases in both CI and SVR.

✓ Studies of low-dose dopamine (2–5 mcg/kg/min) given with IV loop diuretics to enhance diuresis demonstrated no improvements in urine output, renal protection, or symptom relief, but increased rates of tachycardia. Thus, low-dose dopamine may not provide any advantages over traditional inotropes in this setting.

EVALUATION OF THERAPEUTIC OUTCOMES

CHRONIC HEART FAILURE

- Ask patients about the presence and severity of symptoms and how symptoms affect daily activities.
- Evaluate efficacy of diuretic treatment by disappearance of the signs and symptoms of excess fluid retention. Focus the physical examination on body weight, extent of JVD, presence of HJR, and presence and severity of pulmonary congestion (crackles, dyspnea on exertion, orthopnea, and PND) and peripheral edema.
- Other outcomes are improvement in exercise tolerance and fatigue, decreased nocturia, and decreased HR.
- Monitor BP to ensure that symptomatic hypotension does not develop as a result of drug therapy.
- Body weight is a sensitive marker of fluid loss or retention, and patients should weigh themselves daily and report changes of 3–5 lb (1.4–2.3 kg) to their healthcare provider so adjustments can be made in diuretic doses.
- Symptoms may worsen initially on β-blocker therapy, and it may take weeks to months before patients notice symptomatic improvement.
- Routine monitoring of serum electrolytes (especially potassium and magnesium) and renal function (BUN, serum creatinine, eGFR) is mandatory in patients with HF.

ACUTE DECOMPENSATED HEART FAILURE

- Assess the efficacy of drug therapy with daily monitoring of weight, strict fluid intake and output measurements, and HF signs/symptoms. Monitor frequently for electrolyte depletion, symptomatic hypotension, and renal dysfunction. Assess vital signs frequently throughout the day.
- Patients should not be discharged until optimal volume status is achieved, they have been successfully transitioned from IV to oral diuretics, and IV inotropes and vasodilators have been discontinued for at least 24 hours.
- Optimize GDMT in hemodynamically stable patients without contraindications, including reinitiation of therapies withheld earlier in the admission. Low-dose β-blockers may be safely initiated at discharge without increasing the risk of readmission. Transitioning eligible patients to the ARNI sacubitril/valsartan may also be considered.

- Schedule a follow-up appointment at 7–10 days postdischarge and a nurse visit or phone call at 3 days for select patients. Also schedule pertinent follow-up labs (eg, potassium, serum creatinine, INR, serum digoxin concentration).
- All patients should be considered for referral to a formal disease management program.

See Chapter 35, Chronic Heart Failure, authored by Robert B. Parker, Jean M. Nappi, and Larisa H. Cavallari, and Chapter 36, Acute Decompensated Heart Failure, authored by Brent N. Reed and Jo E. Rodgers, for more detailed discussions of these topics.

Hypertension 10

- *Hypertension* is defined as persistently elevated arterial blood pressure (BP). See Table 10-1 for the classification of BP in adults.
- Isolated systolic hypertension is diastolic blood pressure (DBP) <80 mm Hg and systolic blood pressure (SBP) ≥130 mm Hg.
- Hypertensive crisis (BP >180/120 mm Hg) is categorized as hypertensive emergency (extreme BP elevation with acute or progressing end-organ damage) or hypertensive urgency (extreme BP elevation without acute or progressing end-organ injury).
- This chapter incorporates elements of the 2017 American College of Cardiology/American Heart Association (ACC/AHA) Guideline for the Prevention, Detection, Evaluation, and Management of High Blood Pressure in Adults, the most recent evidence-based U.S. guideline for hypertension management.

PATHOPHYSIOLOGY

- Hypertension may result from an unknown etiology (primary or essential hypertension) or from a specific cause (secondary hypertension). Secondary hypertension (<10% of cases) is usually caused by chronic kidney disease (CKD) or renovascular disease. Other conditions are Cushing syndrome, coarctation of the aorta, obstructive sleep apnea, hyperparathyroidism, pheochromocytoma, primary aldosteronism, and hyperthyroidism. Examples of drugs that may increase BP include corticosteroids, estrogens, nonsteroidal anti-inflammatory drugs (NSAIDs), amphetamines, cyclosporine, tacrolimus, erythropoietin, and venlafaxine.
- Factors contributing to development of primary hypertension include:
  ✓ Humoral abnormalities involving the renin–angiotensin–aldosterone system (RAAS), natriuretic hormone, and hyperinsulinemia;
  ✓ Disturbances in the CNS, autonomic nerve fibers, adrenergic receptors, or baroreceptors;
  ✓ Abnormalities in renal or tissue autoregulatory processes for sodium excretion, plasma volume, and arteriolar constriction;
  ✓ Deficiency in synthesis of vasodilating substances in vascular endothelium (prostacyclin, bradykinin, nitric oxide) or excess vasoconstricting substances (angiotensin II, endothelin I);
  ✓ High sodium intake or lack of dietary calcium.
- Major causes of death include cerebrovascular events, cardiovascular (CV) events, and renal failure. Probability of premature death correlates with the severity of BP elevation.

TABLE 10-1	Classification of Blood Pressure in Adults		
Classification	**Systolic (mm Hg)**		**Diastolic (mm Hg)**
Normal	<120	and	<80
Prehypertension	120–139	or	80–89
Stage 1 hypertension	140–159	or	90–99
Stage 2 hypertension	≥160	or	≥100

CLINICAL PRESENTATION

- Patients with uncomplicated primary hypertension are usually asymptomatic initially.
- Patients with secondary hypertension may have symptoms of the underlying disorder:
  - ✓ Pheochromocytoma—headaches, sweating, tachycardia, palpitations, orthostatic hypotension;
  - ✓ Primary aldosteronism—hypokalemic symptoms of muscle cramps and weakness;
  - ✓ Cushing syndrome—moon face, buffalo hump, hirsutism, weight gain, polyuria, edema, menstrual irregularities, acne, muscle weakness.

DIAGNOSIS

- Elevated BP may be the only sign of primary hypertension on physical examination. Diagnosis should be based on the average of two or more readings taken at each of two or more clinical encounters. Refer to the textbook chapter for the correct procedure for BP measurement.
- Signs of end-organ damage occur primarily in the eyes, brain, heart, kidneys, and peripheral vasculature.
- Funduscopic examination may reveal arteriolar narrowing, focal arteriolar constriction, arteriovenous nicking, retinal hemorrhages and exudates, and disk edema. Presence of papilledema usually indicates a hypertensive emergency requiring rapid treatment.
- Cardiopulmonary examination may reveal abnormal heart rate or rhythm, left ventricular (LV) hypertrophy, coronary artery disease, or heart failure (HF).
- Peripheral vascular examination may reveal aortic or abdominal bruits, distended veins, diminished or absent peripheral pulses, or lower extremity edema.
- Patients with renal artery stenosis may have an abdominal systolic-diastolic bruit.
- Baseline hypokalemia may suggest mineralocorticoid-induced hypertension. Protein, blood cells, and casts in the urine may indicate renovascular disease.
- *Laboratory tests*: Blood urea nitrogen (BUN), serum creatinine with estimated glomerular filtration rate (eGFR, using the Modification of Diet in Renal Disease [MDRD] equation), fasting lipid panel, fasting blood glucose, serum electrolytes (sodium, potassium, calcium), uric acid, hemoglobin and hematocrit, and spot urine albumin-to-creatinine ratio. A 12-lead electrocardiogram (ECG) should also be obtained.
- *Laboratory tests to diagnose secondary hypertension*: Baseline hypokalemia may suggest mineralocorticoid-induced hypertension. Protein, red blood cells, and casts in the urine may indicate renovascular disease. Obtain plasma norepinephrine and urinary metanephrine levels for pheochromocytoma; plasma and urinary aldosterone concentrations for primary aldosteronism; and plasma renin activity, captopril stimulation test, renal vein renin, and renal artery angiography for renovascular disease.

TREATMENT

- <u>Goals of Treatment</u>: The overall goal is to reduce morbidity and mortality from CV events. The 2017 ACC/AHA guideline recommends a goal BP of <130/80 mm Hg for most patients, including those with clinical arteriosclerotic cardiovascular disease (ASCVD), diabetes, or CKD. For older ambulatory, community-dwelling patients, the goal is SBP <130 mm Hg. For institutionalized older patients and those with a high disease burden or limited life expectancy, consider a relaxed SBP goal of <150 mm Hg (or <140 mm Hg if tolerated).

NONPHARMACOLOGIC THERAPY

- Implement lifestyle modifications in all patients with elevated BP or stage 1 or 2 hypertension. These measures alone are appropriate initial treatment for patients with elevated BP or stage 1 hypertension who are at low risk of ASCVD (ie, primary prevention with a 10-year ASCVD risk <10%). Start drug therapy for these patients when BP is ≥140/90 mm Hg. For patients with stage 1 or 2 hypertension who already have ASCVD (secondary prevention) or an elevated 10-year ASCVD risk ≥10%, the threshold for starting drug therapy is ≥130/80 mm Hg with a goal BP of <130/80 mm Hg.
- Lifestyle modifications shown to lower BP include (1) weight loss if overweight or obese, (2) the Dietary Approaches to Stop Hypertension (DASH) eating plan, (3) reduced salt intake, ideally to 1.5 g/day sodium (3.8 g/day sodium chloride), (4) physical activity (90–150 min/week of aerobic or dynamic resistance training), and (5) moderation of alcohol intake (≤2 drinks/day in men and ≤1 drink/day in women). Although smoking cessation does not control BP, it reduces CV disease risk and should be encouraged.

PHARMACOLOGIC THERAPY

General Approach to Treatment

- Initial drug selection depends on the degree of BP elevation and presence of compelling indications for certain drugs.
- Use a single first-line drug as initial therapy in most patients with newly diagnosed stage 1 hypertension. Start combination drug therapy (preferably with two first-line drugs) as the initial regimen in patients with newly diagnosed stage 2 hypertension (**Fig. 10-1**).
- The four first-line options are **angiotensin-converting enzyme (ACE) inhibitors**, **angiotensin II receptor blockers (ARBs)**, **calcium channel blockers (CCBs)**, and **thiazide diuretics**.
- β-**Blockers** should be reserved to treat a specific compelling indication or in combination with a first-line antihypertensive agent for patients without a compelling indication.
- Other antihypertensive drug classes (α_1-**blockers**, **direct renin inhibitors**, **central** α_2-**agonists**, and **direct arterial vasodilators**) may be used for select patients after implementing first-line agents. They are generally reserved for resistant hypertension or as add-on therapy with multiple other first-line agents. However, they either lack convincing evidence showing reduced morbidity and mortality in hypertension or have a high incidence of adverse effects that hinders tolerability.

COMPELLING INDICATIONS

- Compelling indications are specific comorbid conditions for which clinical trial data support using specific antihypertensive drug classes to treat both hypertension and the compelling indication (**Fig. 10-2**). Selection of drug therapy should follow an evidence-based order.

Heart Failure with Reduced Ejection Fraction (HFrEF)

- Guideline-directed medical therapy consists of three to four drugs: ACE inhibitor or ARB plus diuretic, followed by addition of an evidence-based β-blocker and possibly a mineralocorticoid receptor antagonist.
- Start an ACE inhibitor or ARB in low doses to avoid orthostatic hypotension because of the high renin state in HF.
- Diuretics reduce edema, and loop diuretics are often needed, especially in patients with advanced HF and/or CKD.
- β-Blockers modify disease in HFrEF and are part of standard treatment; adding a β-blocker to a diuretic with an ACE inhibitor or ARB reduces CV morbidity and mortality. Because of the risk of exacerbating HF, β-blockers must be started in very low doses and titrated slowly to high doses based on tolerability. **Bisoprolol,**

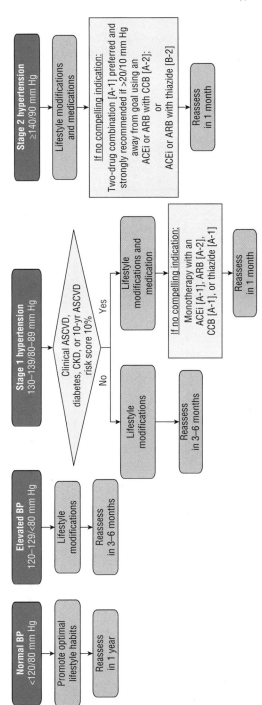

FIGURE 10-1. Algorithm for treatment of elevated BP and hypertension based on BP category at initial diagnosis. Drug therapy recommendations are graded with strength of recommendation and quality of evidence in brackets. Strength of recommendations: A, B, and C are good, moderate, and poor evidence to support recommendation, respectively. Quality of evidence: (1) evidence from more than one properly randomized controlled trial; (2) evidence from at least one well-designed clinical trial with randomization, from cohort or case-controlled studies, or dramatic results from uncontrolled experiments or subgroup analyses; (3) evidence from opinions of respected authorities, based on clinical experience, descriptive studies, or reports of expert communities. *Most patients with diabetes or CKD have a 10-year ASCVD risk score ≥10%.

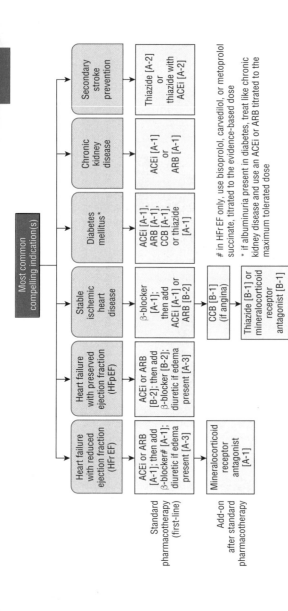

FIGURE 10-2. **Compelling indications for individual drug classes.** Recommendations are evidence-based from outcome studies or clinical guidelines. The order of drug therapies is a general guidance that should be balanced with clinical judgment and patient response. Add-on recommendations are used when additional agents are needed to lower BP to goal values. BP control should be managed concurrently with the compelling indication. Drug therapy recommendations are graded with strength of recommendation and quality of evidence in brackets. Strength of recommendations: A, B, and C are good, moderate, and poor evidence to support recommendation, respectively. Quality of evidence: (1) evidence from more than one randomized controlled trial; (2) evidence from at least one well-designed clinical trial with randomization, from cohort or case-controlled analytic studies or multiple time series, or dramatic results from uncontrolled experiments or subgroup analyses; (3) evidence from opinions of respected authorities, based on clinical experience, descriptive studies, or reports of expert communities.

carvedilol, and **metoprolol succinate** are the only β-blockers proven to be beneficial in HFrEF.

- After implementation of a standard three-drug regimen, other agents may be added to further reduce CV morbidity and mortality, and reduce BP if needed. A mineralocorticoid receptor antagonist (**spironolactone** or **eplerenone**) may be considered at this point. For African Americans, addition of a fixed-dose combination of **isosorbide dinitrate** and **hydralazine** to the standard three-drug regimen is an option to improve CV outcomes.

Heart Failure with Preserved Ejection Fraction (HFpEF)

- Unlike interventions in HFrEF that decrease morbidity and mortality, trials using the same medications in HFpEF have not shown similar benefits. Therefore, treatment should be targeted at signs and symptoms (eg, dyspnea, fatigue, edema), appropriate management of underlying coronary artery disease, and attainment of goal BP to prevent HF progression.
- Patients should use a β-blocker or an ACE inhibitor (or ARB) for treatment of hypertension, and they should receive a diuretic if signs and symptoms of edema are present.

Stable Ischemic Heart Disease (SIHD)

- β-Blockers (without ISA) are first-line therapy in SIHD; they reduce BP and improve angina symptoms by decreasing myocardial oxygen consumption and demand. β-Blockers should be used for hypertension treatment in patients with SIHD. An ACE inhibitor or ARB has been shown to reduce CV events as an add-on to a β-blocker.
- A long-acting nondihydropyridine CCB is an alternative to a β-blocker in SIHD, but β-blockers are the therapy of choice.
- A dihydropyridine CCB may be considered as add-on therapy in SIHD patients who have ongoing ischemic symptoms, but cardiac stimulation makes these agents less desirable.
- For acute coronary syndromes, first-line therapy includes a β-blocker and ACE inhibitor (or ARB); the combination lowers BP, controls acute ischemia, and reduces CV risk.

Diabetes Mellitus

- All four first-line antihypertensive classes (ACE inhibitors, ARBs, CCBs, thiazides) reduce CV events in patients with diabetes, with no evidence of difference in all-cause mortality, CV mortality, HF, or stroke. The risk of kidney disease progression is low in the absence of albuminuria (urine albumin-to-creatinine ratio ≥30 mg/g [3.4 mg/mmol creatinine]). Therefore, any first-line agent can be used to control hypertension in patients with diabetes in the absence of albuminuria. Regardless of the initial agent selected, most patients require combination therapy, which typically includes an ACE inhibitor (or ARB) with a CCB or thiazide.
- After first-line agents, a β-blocker is a useful add-on therapy for BP control in patients with diabetes. However, they may mask symptoms of hypoglycemia (tremor, tachycardia, and palpitations but not sweating) in tightly controlled patients, delay recovery from hypoglycemia, and elevate BP due to vasoconstriction caused by unopposed β-receptor stimulation during the hypoglycemic recovery phase. Despite these potential problems, β-blockers can be used safely in patients with diabetes.

Chronic Kidney Disease

- In addition to lowering BP, ACE inhibitors and ARBs reduce intraglomerular pressure, which may further slow CKD progression.
- Start with low doses and evaluate the serum creatinine soon after starting therapy to minimize the risk of rapid and profound BP drops that could precipitate acute kidney injury (AKI).

Secondary Stroke Prevention

- A thiazide diuretic, either alone or combined with an ACE inhibitor, is recommended for patients with history of stroke or transient ischemic attack. Implement antihypertensive drug therapy only after patients have stabilized after an acute cerebrovascular event.
- The threshold for starting antihypertensive drug therapy in patients with a history of stroke is when BP is >140/90 mm Hg. Once therapy is initiated, patients should be treated to a goal of <130/80 mm Hg.

FIRST-LINE ANTIHYPERTENSIVE AGENTS (TABLE 10-2)

Angiotensin-Converting Enzyme Inhibitors

- ACE inhibitors block conversion of angiotensin I to angiotensin II, a potent vasoconstrictor and stimulator of aldosterone secretion. ACE inhibitors also block degradation of bradykinin and stimulate synthesis of other vasodilating substances (prostaglandin E_2 and prostacyclin).
- Starting doses should be low with slow dose titration. Acute hypotension may occur at the onset of therapy, especially in patients who are sodium or volume depleted, in HF exacerbation, very elderly, or on concurrent vasodilators or diuretics. Starting doses in such patients should be half the normal dose followed by slow dose titration.
- ACE inhibitors decrease aldosterone and can increase serum potassium concentrations. Hyperkalemia occurs primarily in patients with CKD or those also taking potassium supplements, potassium-sparing diuretics, mineralocorticoid receptor antagonists, ARBs, or direct renin inhibitors.
- AKI is an uncommon but serious side effect; preexisting kidney disease increases risk. Bilateral renal artery stenosis or unilateral stenosis of a solitary functioning kidney renders patients dependent on the vasoconstrictive effect of angiotensin II on efferent arterioles, making them particularly susceptible to AKI.
- GFR decreases somewhat when ACE inhibitors are started because of inhibition of angiotensin II vasoconstriction on efferent arterioles. Serum creatinine concentrations often increase, but modest elevations (eg, absolute increases <1 mg/dL [88 μmol/L]) do not warrant treatment changes. Discontinue therapy or reduce dose if larger increases occur.
- Angioedema occurs in <1% of patients. Drug withdrawal is necessary, and some patients may require drug treatment and/or emergent intubation to support respiration. An ARB can generally be used in patients with a history of ACE inhibitor-induced angioedema, with careful monitoring.
- A persistent dry cough occurs in up to 20% of patients and is thought to be due to inhibition of bradykinin breakdown.
- ACE inhibitors (as well as ARBs and direct renin inhibitors) are contraindicated in pregnancy.

Angiotensin II Receptor Blockers

- Angiotensin II is generated by the renin–angiotensin pathway (which involves ACE) and an alternative pathway that uses other enzymes such as chymases. ACE inhibitors block only the renin–angiotensin pathway, whereas ARBs inhibit angiotensin II generated by either pathway. The ARBs directly block the angiotensin II type 1 receptor that mediates the effects of angiotensin II.
- Unlike ACE inhibitors, ARBs do not block bradykinin breakdown. Although this accounts for the lack of cough as a side effect, some of the antihypertensive effect of ACE inhibitors may be due to bradykinin.
- The combination of an ACE inhibitor and ARB has no additional CV event lowering but is associated with a higher risk of side effects (renal dysfunction, hypotension) and should be avoided.
- All ARBs have similar antihypertensive efficacy and fairly flat dose-response curves. Addition of a CCB or thiazide diuretic significantly increases antihypertensive efficacy.

TABLE 10-2	Most Common First-Line and Other Antihypertensive Agents			
Class	**Subclass**	**Medication (Brand Name)**	**Usual Dose Range (mg/day)**	**Daily Frequency**
ACEi		Benazepril (Lotensin)	10–40	1 or 2
		Captopril (Capoten)	12.5–150	2 or 3
		Enalapril (Vasotec)	5–40	1 or 2
		Fosinopril (Monopril)	10–40	1
		Lisinopril (Prinivil, Zestril)	10–40	1
		Moexipril (Univasc)	7.5–30	1 or 2
		Perindopril (Aceon)	4–16	1
		Quinapril (Accupril)	10–80	1 or 2
		Ramipril (Altace)	2.5–10	1 or 2
		Trandolapril (Mavik)	1–4	1
ARB		Azilsartan (Edarbi)	40–80	1
		Candesartan (Atacand)	8–32	1 or 2
		Eprosartan (Teveten)	600–800	1 or 2
		Irbesartan (Avapro)	150–300	1
		Losartan (Cozaar)	50–100	1 or 2
		Telmisartan (Micardis)	20–40	1
		Olmesartan (Benicar)	20–80	1
		Valsartan (Diovan)	80–320	1
Calcium channel blocker	Dihydropyridine	Amlodipine (Norvasc)	2.5–10	1
		Felodipine (Plendil)	5–20	1
		Nifedipine long-acting (Afeditab CR Adalat CC, Nifediac CC, Nifedical XL, Procardia XL)	30–90	1
		Nisoldipine (Sular)	10–40	1
	Nondihydropyridine	Diltiazem sustained release (Cardizem CD, Cartia XT, Dilacor XR, Diltia XT, Tiazac, Taztia XT)	120–480	1
		Diltiazem extended release (Cardizem LA, Matzim LA)	180–480	1 (morning or evening)
		Verapamil sustained release (Calan SR, Isoptin SR, Verelan)	180–420	1 or 2
		Verapamil chronotherapeutic oral drug absorption system (Verelan PM)	100–400	1 (in the evening)

(Continued)

TABLE 10-2 Most Common First-Line and Other Antihypertensive Agents *(Continued)*

Class	Subclass	Medication (Brand Name)	Usual Dose Range (mg/day)	Daily Frequency
Diuretic	Thiazide	Chlorthalidone (Thalitone)	12.5–25	1
		Hydrochlorothiazide (Microzide)	12.5–50	1
		Indapamide (Lozol)	1.25–2.5	1
		Metolazone (Zaroxolyn)	2.5–10	1
	Loop	Bumetanide (Bumex)	0.5–4	2
		Furosemide (Lasix)	20–80	2
		Torsemide (Demadex)	5–10	1
	Potassium sparing	Amiloride (Midamor)	5–10	1 or 2
		Amiloride/ Hydrochlorothiazide (Moduretic)	5–50	1
		Triamterene (Dyrenium)	50–100	1 or 2
		Triamterene/ Hydrochlorothiazide (Dyazide, Maxide)	37.5–75/ 25–50	1
	Mineralocorticoid receptor antagonist	Eplerenone (Inspra)	50–100	1 or 2
		Spironolactone (Aldactone, CaroSpir)	25–50	1 or 2
β-Blocker	Cardioselective	Atenolol (Tenormin)	25–100	1 or 2
		Betaxolol (Kerlone)	5–20	1
		Bisoprolol (Zebeta)	2.5–10	1
		Metoprolol tartrate (Lopressor)	100–200	2
		Metoprolol succinate extended release (Toprol XL)	50–200	1
		Nebivolol (Bystolic)	5–20	1
	Nonselective	Nadolol (Corgard)	40–120	1
		Propranolol (Inderal)	160–480	2
		Propranolol long acting (Inderal LA, Inderal XL, InnoPran XL)	80–320	1
		Timolol (Blocadren)	10–40	1
	Mixed α- and β-blockers	Carvedilol (Coreg)	12.5–50	2
		Carvedilol phosphate (Coreg CR)	20–80	1
		Labetalol (Normodyne, Trandate)	200–800	2

- ARBs have a low incidence of side effects. Like ACE inhibitors, they may cause renal insufficiency, hyperkalemia, and orthostatic hypotension. ARBs are contraindicated in pregnancy.

Calcium Channel Blockers

- Dihydropyridine and nondihydropyridine CCBs are first-line antihypertensive therapies and are also used in addition to or instead of other first-line agents for the compelling indication of ischemic heart disease.
- CCBs cause relaxation of cardiac and smooth muscle by blocking voltage-sensitive calcium channels, thereby reducing entry of extracellular calcium into cells. This leads to vasodilation and a corresponding reduction in BP. Dihydropyridine CCBs may cause reflex sympathetic activation, and all agents (except **amlodipine** and **felodipine**) may have negative inotropic effects.
- **Verapamil** decreases heart rate, slows atrioventricular (AV) nodal conduction, and produces a negative inotropic effect that may precipitate HF in patients with borderline cardiac reserve. **Diltiazem** decreases AV conduction and heart rate to a lesser extent than verapamil.
- Diltiazem and verapamil can cause cardiac conduction abnormalities such as bradycardia, AV block, and HF. Both can cause peripheral edema and hypotension. Verapamil causes constipation in about 7% of patients.
- Dihydropyridines cause a baroreceptor-mediated reflex increase in heart rate because of potent peripheral vasodilating effects. Dihydropyridines do not decrease AV node conduction and are not effective for treating supraventricular tachyarrhythmias.
- Short-acting nifedipine may rarely increase frequency, intensity, and duration of angina in association with acute hypotension. This effect may be obviated by using sustained-release formulations of nifedipine or other dihydropyridines. Other side effects of dihydropyridines are dizziness, flushing, headache, gingival hyperplasia, and peripheral edema.

Diuretics

- Thiazides are the preferred type of diuretic and are a first-line option for most patients with hypertension. **Chlorthalidone** (thiazide-like) is preferred over **hydrochlorothiazide**, especially in resistant hypertension, because it is more potent on a milligram-per-milligram basis.
- Loop diuretics are more potent for inducing diuresis but are not ideal antihypertensives unless edema treatment is also needed. Loop diuretics are sometimes required over thiazides in patients with severe CKD when eGFR is <30 mL/min/1.73 m^2, especially when edema is present.
- Potassium-sparing diuretics are weak antihypertensives when used alone and provide minimal additive effect when combined with a thiazide or loop diuretic. Their primary use is in combination with another diuretic to counteract potassium-wasting properties.
- Mineralocorticoid receptor antagonists (**spironolactone** and **eplerenone**) are also potassium-sparing diuretics that are usually used to treat resistant hypertension because elevated aldosterone concentrations are prevalent in this setting. They are also used as add-on agents in patients with HFrEF with or without concomitant hypertension.
- Acutely, diuretics lower BP by causing diuresis. The reduction in plasma volume and stroke volume associated with diuresis decreases cardiac output and BP. The initial drop in cardiac output causes a compensatory increase in peripheral vascular resistance. With chronic therapy, extracellular fluid volume and plasma volume return to near pretreatment levels, and peripheral vascular resistance falls below baseline. Reduced peripheral vascular resistance is responsible for persistent hypotensive effects. Thiazides also mobilize sodium and water from arteriolar walls, which may contribute to decreased peripheral vascular resistance and lowered BP.
- Combining diuretics with other antihypertensive agents usually results in an additive hypotensive effect because of independent mechanisms of action. Furthermore,

121

many nondiuretic antihypertensive agents induce sodium and water retention, which is counteracted by concurrent diuretic use.

- Side effects of thiazides include hypokalemia, hypomagnesemia, hypercalcemia, hyperuricemia, hyperglycemia, dyslipidemia, and sexual dysfunction. Loop diuretics have less effect on serum lipids and glucose, but hypokalemia is more pronounced, and hypocalcemia may occur.
- Hypokalemia and hypomagnesemia may cause muscle fatigue or cramps, and severe electrolyte abnormalities may result in serious cardiac arrhythmias. Low-dose therapy (eg, 25 mg hydrochlorothiazide or 12.5 mg chlorthalidone daily) causes less electrolyte disturbances than higher doses.
- Potassium-sparing diuretics may cause hyperkalemia, especially in patients with CKD or diabetes and in patients receiving concurrent treatment with a mineralocorticoid receptor antagonist, ACE inhibitor, ARB, direct renin inhibitor, or potassium supplement. Eplerenone has an increased risk for hyperkalemia and is contraindicated in patients with impaired renal function or type 2 diabetes with proteinuria. Spironolactone may cause gynecomastia in up to 10% of patients; this effect occurs rarely with eplerenone.

ALTERNATIVE ANTIHYPERTENSIVE AGENTS (TABLES 10-2 AND 10-3)

β-Blockers

- Evidence suggests that β-blockers may not reduce CV events as well as ACE inhibitors, ARBs, CCBs, or thiazides when used as the initial drug in patients who do not have a compelling indication for a β-blocker.
- β-Blockers are appropriate first-line agents when used to treat specific compelling indications (Fig. 10-2) or when an ACE inhibitor, ARB, CCB, or thiazide cannot be used. β-Blockers also have an important role as add-on therapy to first-line agents in patients with hypertension but no compelling indications.
- Their hypotensive mechanism may involve decreased cardiac output through negative chronotropic and inotropic cardiac effects and inhibition of renin release from the kidney.
- **Atenolol**, **betaxolol**, **bisoprolol**, **metoprolol**, and **nebivolol** are cardioselective at low doses and bind more avidly to β_1-receptors than to β_2-receptors. As a result,

TABLE 10-3	Alternative Antihypertensive Agents	
Class Drug (Brand Name)	**Usual Dose Range (mg/day)**	**Daily Frequency**
α_1-Blockers		
Doxazosin (Cardura)	1–8	1
Prazosin (Minipress)	2–20	2 or 3
Terazosin (Hytrin)	1–20	1 or 2
Direct renin inhibitor		
Aliskiren (Tekturna)	150–300	1
Central α_2-agonists		
Clonidine (Catapres)	0.1–0.8	2
Clonidine patch (Catapres-TTS)	0.1–0.3	1 weekly
Methyldopa (Aldomet)	250–1000	2
Direct arterial vasodilators		
Minoxidil (Loniten)	10–40	1 or 2
Hydralazine (Apresoline)	20–100	2 to 4

they are less likely to provoke bronchospasm and vasoconstriction and are safer than nonselective β-blockers in patients with asthma or diabetes who have a compelling indication for a β-blocker. Cardioselectivity is a dose-dependent phenomenon, and the effect is lost at higher doses.

- **Acebutolol, carteolol**, and **pindolol** possess intrinsic sympathomimetic activity (ISA) or partial β-receptor agonist activity. When sympathetic tone is low, as in resting states, β-receptors are partially stimulated, so resting heart rate, cardiac output, and peripheral blood flow are not reduced when receptors are blocked. Theoretically, these drugs may have advantages in select patients with HF or sinus bradycardia. Unfortunately, they do not reduce CV events as well as other β-blockers and may increase CV risk in patients with SIHD. Thus, agents with ISA are rarely needed and have no role in hypertension management.

- **Atenolol** and **nadolol** have relatively long half-lives and are excreted renally; the dosage may need to be reduced in patients with renal insufficiency. Even though the half-lives of other β-blockers are shorter, once-daily administration still may be effective.

- Cardiac side effects include bradycardia, AV conduction abnormalities, and acute HF. Blocking β_2-receptors in arteriolar smooth muscle may cause cold extremities and aggravate intermittent claudication or Raynaud phenomenon because of decreased peripheral blood flow. Increases in serum lipids and glucose appear to be transient and of little clinical significance.

- Abrupt cessation of β-blocker therapy can produce cardiac ischemia (angina, chest pain), a CV event, or even death in patients with coronary artery disease. In patients without heart disease, abrupt discontinuation of β-blockers may be associated with tachycardia, sweating, and generalized malaise in addition to increased BP. For these reasons, the dose should always be tapered gradually over 1–2 weeks before discontinuation.

α_1-Receptor Blockers

- **Prazosin, terazosin**, and **doxazosin** are selective α_1-receptor blockers that inhibit catecholamine uptake in smooth muscle cells of peripheral vasculature, resulting in vasodilation and BP lowering.

- A first-dose phenomenon characterized by orthostatic hypotension accompanied by transient dizziness or faintness, palpitations, and even syncope may occur within 1–3 hours of the first dose or after later dosage increases. The patient should take the first dose (and subsequent first increased doses) at bedtime. Occasionally, orthostatic hypotension and dizziness persist with chronic administration.

- Sodium and water retention can occur; these agents are most effective when given with a thiazide to maintain antihypertensive efficacy and minimize edema.

- These agents block postsynaptic α_1-adrenergic receptors on the prostate capsule, causing relaxation and decreased resistance to urinary outflow. Although they can provide symptomatic benefit in men with benign prostatic hyperplasia, they should be used to lower BP only in combination with first-line antihypertensive agents.

Direct Renin Inhibitor

- **Aliskiren** blocks the RAAS at its point of activation, resulting in reduced plasma renin activity and BP. It is approved for monotherapy or in combination therapy. It should not be used with an ACE inhibitor or an ARB because of a higher risk of adverse effects without additional reduction in CV events. Its role in the management of hypertension is limited.

- Many of the cautions and adverse effects seen with ACE inhibitors and ARBs apply to aliskiren. It is contraindicated in pregnancy due to known teratogenic effects.

Central α_2-Agonists

- **Clonidine, guanfacine**, and **methyldopa** lower BP primarily by stimulating α_2-adrenergic receptors in the brain, which reduces sympathetic outflow from the vasomotor center and increases vagal tone. Stimulation of presynaptic α_2-receptors peripherally may contribute to reduced sympathetic tone. Consequently, there may be decreases in heart rate, cardiac output, total peripheral resistance, plasma renin activity, and baroreceptor reflexes.

- Clonidine is often used in resistant hypertension, and methyldopa is frequently used for pregnancy-induced hypertension.
- Chronic use results in sodium and fluid retention. Other side effects include depression, orthostatic hypotension, dizziness, and anticholinergic effects (eg, dry mouth, sedation).
- Abrupt cessation may lead to rebound hypertension, perhaps from a compensatory increase in norepinephrine release that follows discontinuation of presynaptic α-receptor stimulation.
- Methyldopa rarely causes hepatitis or hemolytic anemia. A transient elevation in hepatic transaminases occasionally occurs. Discontinue therapy if persistent increases in liver function tests occur, because this may herald onset of fulminant, life-threatening hepatitis. Coombs-positive hemolytic anemia occurs rarely, and 20% of patients exhibit a positive direct Coombs test without anemia. For these reasons, methyldopa has limited usefulness except in pregnancy.

Direct Arterial Vasodilators

- **Hydralazine** and **minoxidil** directly relax arteriolar smooth muscle, resulting in vasodilation and BP lowering. Compensatory activation of baroreceptor reflexes increases sympathetic outflow, thereby increasing heart rate, cardiac output, and renin release. Consequently, hypotensive effectiveness of direct vasodilators diminishes over time unless the patient is also taking a diuretic and a β-blocker. The diuretic minimizes the side effect of sodium and water retention. Direct vasodilators can precipitate angina in patients with underlying SIHD unless the baroreceptor reflex mechanism is blocked with a β-blocker. Nondihydropyridine CCBs can be used as an alternative to β-blockers in patients with contraindications to β-blockers.
- Hydralazine may cause a dose-related, reversible lupus-like syndrome, which is more common in slow acetylators. Lupus-like reactions can usually be avoided by limiting the maximum total daily dose to 200 mg. Because of side effects, hydralazine has limited usefulness for chronic hypertension management.
- Minoxidil is a more potent vasodilator than hydralazine, and compensatory increases in heart rate, cardiac output, renin release, and sodium retention are more dramatic. Due to significant water retention, a loop diuretic is often more effective than a thiazide. Reversible hypertrichosis on the face, arms, back, and chest may be troublesome. Minoxidil is reserved for resistant hypertension and for patients requiring hydralazine who experience drug-induced lupus.

SPECIAL POPULATIONS

Older Persons

- Older patients may present with either isolated systolic hypertension or elevation in both SBP and DBP. CV morbidity and mortality are more directly correlated to SBP than to DBP in patients aged 50 and older.
- First-line antihypertensives provide significant benefits and can be used safely in older patients, but smaller-than-usual initial doses must be used for initial therapy.
- Although the most appropriate BP goal for older patients has been debated, the totality of evidence indicates that older ambulatory patients should be treated to an SBP goal of <130 mm Hg, with careful monitoring. In patients with multiple comorbidities, a relaxed SBP goal of at least <150 mm Hg (or <140 mm Hg if tolerated) may be considered.

Children and Adolescents

- In children, hypertension is defined as SBP or DBP that is >95th percentile for sex, age, and height on at least three occasions. For adolescents, BP values between the 90th and 95th percentile, or >120/80 mm Hg, is considered elevated BP.
- Because secondary hypertension is more common in children and adolescents than in adults, an appropriate workup is required if elevated BP is identified.

- Nonpharmacologic treatment (eg, weight loss if overweight or obese, healthy diet, physical activity) is the cornerstone of therapy for primary hypertension.
- The goal is to reduce the BP to <90th percentile for sex, age, and height and <130/80 mm Hg in adolescents age 13 years and older.
- ACE inhibitors, ARBs, β-blockers, CCBs, and thiazide diuretics are all acceptable drug therapy choices.
- ACE inhibitors, ARBs, and direct renin inhibitors are contraindicated in sexually active girls because of potential teratogenic effects.

Pregnancy

- *Preeclampsia* is defined as hypertension (elevated BP ≥140/90 mm Hg on more than 2 occasions at least 4 hours apart after 20 weeks' gestation or ≥160/110 mm Hg confirmed within a short interval) in association with thrombocytopenia, impaired liver function, new-onset renal insufficiency, pulmonary edema, or new-onset cerebral or visual disturbances. It can lead to life-threatening complications for both mother and fetus.
- *Eclampsia* is the onset of convulsions in preeclampsia and is a medical emergency.
- Definitive treatment of preeclampsia is delivery, and labor induction is indicated if eclampsia is imminent or present. Otherwise, management consists of restricting activity, bed rest, and close monitoring. Salt restriction or other measures that contract blood volume should be avoided. Antihypertensives are used before induction of labor if DBP is >105 mm Hg, with a target DBP of 95–105 mm Hg. Intravenous (IV) hydralazine is most commonly used; IV labetalol is also effective.
- *Chronic hypertension* is hypertension that predates pregnancy. Labetalol, long-acting nifedipine, or methyldopa is recommended as first-line therapy due to favorable safety profiles. β-Blockers (except atenolol) and CCBs are also reasonable alternatives. ACE inhibitors, ARBs, and the direct renin inhibitor aliskiren are known teratogens and contraindicated in pregnancy.

African Americans

- Hypertension is more common and more difficult to control in African Americans than in those of other races; treatment usually requires two or more antihypertensives to reach a BP goal of <130/80 mm Hg.
- CCBs and thiazides are most effective in African Americans and should be first-line in the absence of a compelling indication. Antihypertensive response is significantly increased when either class is combined with a β-blocker, ACE inhibitor, or ARB, perhaps due to the low-renin pattern of hypertension in African Americans.
- Medications recommended for specific compelling indications should be used, even if the antihypertensive effect may not be as great as with another drug class (eg, use a β-blocker first-line for hypertension in African Americans with SIHD).

Pulmonary Disease and Peripheral Arterial Disease

- Although β-blockers (especially nonselective agents) have generally been avoided in hypertensive patients with asthma and COPD because of fear of inducing bronchospasm, cardioselective β-blockers can be used safely. Consequently, cardioselective agents should be used to treat a compelling indication (ie, SIHD or HF) in patients with reactive airway disease.
- Because PAD is a noncoronary form of ASCVD, patients with PAD are at increased risk of stroke and CV events. β-Blockers can theoretically be problematic because of possible decreased peripheral blood flow secondary to unopposed stimulation of α_1-receptors that results in vasoconstriction. However, available data indicate that β-blockers do not worsen claudication symptoms or cause functional impairment. Therefore, antihypertensive treatment for patients with PAD should follow the same general principles as patients without PAD.

HYPERTENSIVE URGENCIES AND EMERGENCIES

- *Hypertensive urgencies* are ideally managed by adjusting maintenance therapy, adding a new antihypertensive, increasing the dose of a current medication, or treating anxiety as applicable. Acute administration of a short-acting oral drug (**captopril**, **clonidine**, or **labetalol**) followed by careful observation for several hours to ensure a gradual BP reduction is an option.
  - ✓ Captopril 25–50 mg orally may be given at 1- to 2-hour intervals. The onset of action is 15–30 minutes.
  - ✓ For treatment of hypertensive rebound after withdrawal of clonidine, 0.2 mg orally is given initially, followed by 0.2 mg hourly until the DBP falls below 110 mm Hg or a total of 0.7 mg has been administered; a single dose may be sufficient.
  - ✓ Labetalol 200–400 mg orally can be given, followed by additional doses every 2–3 hours.
- *Hypertensive emergencies* require immediate BP reduction with a parenteral agent to limit new or progressing end-organ damage. The rate of BP reduction depends on whether the patient has aortic dissection, severe preeclampsia or eclampsia, or pheochromocytoma with hypertensive crisis. In these life-threatening situations, patients should be managed in an intensive care unit, and SBP should be reduced immediately to <140 mm Hg in the first hour, with additional SBP lowering to <120 mm Hg for patients with aortic dissection. For patients with a hypertensive emergency without aortic dissection, severe preeclampsia or eclampsia, or pheochromocytoma with hypertensive crisis, the initial target is reduction in mean arterial pressure of up to 25% over the first hour. If the patient is then stable, BP can be reduced to 160/100–110 mm Hg within the next 2–6 hours. Precipitous drops in BP may cause end-organ ischemia or infarction. If BP reduction is well tolerated, additional gradual decreases toward the goal BP can be attempted after 24–48 hours.
  - ✓ Nitroprusside is the agent of choice for minute-to-minute control in most cases. In aortic dissection, propranolol should be given first to prevent reflex sympathetic activation. When the nitroprusside infusion must be continued longer than 72 hours, measure serum thiocyanate levels, and discontinue the infusion if the level exceeds 12 mg/dL (~2.0 mmol/L). The risk of thiocyanate toxicity is increased in patients with impaired kidney function. Other adverse effects are nausea, vomiting, muscle twitching, and sweating.
  - ✓ Dosing guidelines and adverse effects of parenteral agents for treating hypertensive emergency are listed in **Table 10-4**.

EVALUATION OF THERAPEUTIC OUTCOMES

- Both clinic-based and self-measurement home BP monitoring are important for monitoring and managing hypertension. Encourage patients to obtain a home BP monitor, record the results, and bring them to follow-up clinic visits.
- Evaluate BP response in the clinic 4 weeks after initiating or making changes in therapy and compare the results to home BP readings. Once goal BP is obtained, monitor BP every 3–6 months, assuming no signs or symptoms of acute end-organ damage. Evaluate more frequently in patients with a history of poor control, nonadherence, progressive end-organ damage, or symptoms of adverse drug effects.
- Automated BP monitoring can be useful to establish effective 24-hour control and confirm white coat or masked uncontrolled hypertension.
- Monitor patients routinely for adverse drug events, which may require dosage reduction or substitution with an alternative antihypertensive agent. Perform laboratory monitoring 4 weeks after starting a new agent or dose increase, and then every 6–12 months in stable patients. For patients treated with a mineralocorticoid receptor antagonist (eplerenone or spironolactone) monitor potassium concentrations and kidney function within 3 days of initiation and again at 1 week to detect potential hyperkalemia.
- Monitor patients for signs and symptoms of hypertension-associated complications. Take a careful history for ischemic chest pain (or pressure), palpitations, dizziness,

TABLE 10-4 Parenteral Antihypertensive Agents for Hypertensive Emergency

Drug	Dose	Onset (Minutes)	Duration (Minutes)	Adverse Effects
Clevidipine	1–2 mg/hr (32 mg/hr max)	2–4	5–15	Headache, nausea, tachycardia, hypertriglyceridemia
Enalaprilat	1.25–5 mg IV every 6 hours	15–30	360–720	Precipitous fall in BP in high-renin states; variable response
Esmolol hydrochloride	250–500 mcg/kg/min IV bolus, then 50–100 mcg/kg/min IV infusion; may repeat bolus after 5 min or increase infusion to 300 mcg/min	1–2	10–20	Hypotension, nausea, asthma, first-degree heart block, heart failure
Fenoldopam mesylate	0.1–0.3 mcg/kg/min IV infusion	<5	30	Tachycardia, headache, nausea, flushing
Hydralazine hydrochloride	12–20 mg IV 10–50 mg IM	10–20 20–30	60–240 240–360	Tachycardia, flushing, headache, vomiting, aggravation of angina
Labetalol hydrochloride	20–80 mg IV bolus every 10 min; 0.5–2 mg/min IV infusion	5–10	180–360	Vomiting, scalp tingling, bronchoconstriction, dizziness, nausea, heart block, orthostatic hypotension
Nicardipine hydrochloride	5–15 mg/hr IV	5–10	15–30; may exceed 240	Tachycardia, headache, flushing, local phlebitis
Nitroglycerin	5–100 mcg/min IV infusion	2–5	5–10	Headache, vomiting, methemoglobinemia, tolerance with prolonged use
Sodium nitroprusside	0.25–10 mcg/kg/min IV infusion (requires special delivery system)	Immediate	1–2	Nausea, vomiting, muscle twitching, sweating, thiocyanate and cyanide intoxication

BP, blood pressure; IM, intramuscular; IV, intravenous.

dyspnea, orthopnea, headache, sudden change in vision, one-sided weakness, slurred speech, and loss of balance.
• Monitor funduscopic changes on eye examination, LV hypertrophy on ECG, albuminuria, and changes in kidney function periodically.
• Assess patient adherence with the regimen regularly. Ask patients about changes in their general health perception, physical functioning, and overall satisfaction with treatment.

See Chapter 30, Hypertension, authored by Eric J. MacLaughlin and Joseph J. Saseen, for a more detailed discussion of this topic.

Ischemic Heart Disease

- *Ischemic heart disease* (IHD) is defined as lack of oxygen and decreased or no blood flow to the myocardium resulting from coronary artery narrowing or obstruction. It may present as acute coronary syndrome (ACS), which includes unstable angina and non–ST-segment elevation (NSTE) or ST-segment elevation (STE) myocardial infarction (MI), chronic stable exertional angina, ischemia without symptoms, microvascular angina, or ischemia due to coronary artery vasospasm (variant or Prinzmetal angina). The focus of this chapter is stable IHD.

PATHOPHYSIOLOGY

- Angina pectoris usually results from increased myocardial oxygen demand (MVo_2) in the setting of a fixed decrease in myocardial oxygen supply because of atherosclerotic plaque.
- Major determinants of MVo_2 are heart rate (HR), myocardial contractility, and intramyocardial wall tension during systole. A doubling in any of these individual parameters requires a 50% increase in coronary flow to maintain myocardial supply.
- Coronary atherosclerotic plaques typically develop in larger epicardial (R_1 or conductance) vessels, which normally offer little resistance to myocardial flow. As plaques grow and narrow the lumen, the affected vessel begins to provide considerable resistance to blood flow. Smaller endocardial (R_2 or resistance) vessels provide most resistance to flow in normal coronary arteries and can contract and dilate to maintain blood flow based on metabolic demands of the myocardium (referred to as autoregulation). As a result, coronary plaques that occupy less than 50%–70% of the vessel luminal diameter rarely produce ischemia or angina. However, smaller plaques have a lipid-rich core and thin fibrous cap and are more prone to rupture and cause acute thrombosis. When the luminal diameter of epicardial vessels is reduced by 70% or more, endocardial vessels are maximally dilated, and much of the coronary flow reserve has been used, and minimal physical exertion may result in a flow deficit with myocardial ischemia and often angina. When epicardial stenosis exceeds 90%, endocardial flow reserve is exhausted (referred to as critical stenosis).
- When coronary stenosis exceeds 70%, ischemic episodes lead to production of vascular endothelial growth factor and basic fibroblast growth factor which, combined with endogenous vasodilators (eg, nitrous oxide, prostacyclin), cause native collateral vessels to increase in diameter (arteriogenesis) to maintain perfusion. New collateral vessels can also develop (angiogenesis).
- Inflammation also plays a role in IHD; macrophages and T-lymphocytes produce cytokines, chemokines, and growth factors that activate endothelial cells, increase vasoreactivity, and cause proliferation of vascular smooth muscle cells. C-reactive protein may be elevated and correlates with adverse cardiovascular events.
- Some patients have plaque that causes a fixed decrease in supply but also have reduced myocardial oxygen supply transiently due to vasospasm at the site of the plaque. Vasospasm is typically caused by endothelial damage induced by the plaque. Patient symptoms depend on the extent of the fixed obstruction and the degree of dynamic change in coronary arterial tone. The pattern of ischemic symptoms can change due to a variable amount of vasospasm under certain conditions (referred to as *variable threshold angina*). Ischemic episodes may be more common in the morning hours (due to circadian release of vasoconstrictors) and be precipitated by cold exposure and emotional or mental stress.
- Patients with *variant (Prinzmetal) angina* usually do not have a coronary flow-obstructing plaque but instead have significant reduction in myocardial oxygen supply due to vasospasm in epicardial vessels.

CLINICAL PRESENTATION

- Patients typically complain of chest pain precipitated by exertion or activities of daily living that is described as squeezing, crushing, heaviness, or chest tightness. It can also be more vague and described as a numbness or burning in the chest. The location is often substernal and may radiate to the right or left shoulder or arm (left more commonly), neck, back, or abdomen. Ischemic symptoms may be associated with diaphoresis, nausea, vomiting, and dyspnea. Chest pain generally lasts from 5 to 20 minutes and is usually relieved by rest or sublingual nitroglycerin (SL NTG).
- Some patients (especially women and older individuals) present with atypical chest pain, characterized by midepigastric discomfort, effort intolerance, dyspnea, and excessive fatigue. Patients with diabetes mellitus may have decreased pain sensation due to neuropathy.
- Patients with variant (Prinzmetal) angina are typically younger and may present with chest pain at rest, often early in the morning, and may have transient ST-segment elevation on the ECG.

DIAGNOSIS

- Obtain the medical history to identify the quality and severity of chest pain, precipitating factors, location, duration, pain radiation, and response to nitroglycerin or rest. Ischemic chest pain may resemble pain from noncardiac sources, and diagnosis of anginal pain may be difficult based on history alone.
- Assess nonmodifiable risk factors for coronary artery disease (CAD): age, sex, and family history of premature atherosclerotic disease in first-degree relatives (male onset before age 55 or female before age 65). Identify the presence of modifiable CAD risk factors: hypertension, diabetes mellitus, dyslipidemia, and cigarette smoking.
- Physical exam findings are usually nonspecific, but patients having an ischemic episode may present with tachycardia, diaphoresis, shortness of breath, nausea, vomiting, and lightheadedness. Other findings related to CAD risk factors may include increased blood pressure (BP) and a fourth heart sound reflecting longstanding hypertension. Other positive findings may include pulmonary crackles, displaced point of maximal impulse, and a third heart sound in patients with heart failure with reduced ejection fraction (HFrEF).
- Markers of inflammation, such as high-sensitivity C-reactive protein (hs-CRP), may be elevated.
- Cardiac troponin concentrations are not typically elevated in stable IHD.
- Resting ECG is normal in at least half of patients with angina who are not experiencing acute ischemia. About 50% of patients develop ischemic ST-T wave changes during an episode of angina, which can be observed on the ECG during an exercise stress test. Patients who cannot endure stress testing can have the myocardium stressed pharmacologically with adenosine, regadenoson, dipyridamole, or dobutamine.
- Coronary angiography is the most accurate test for confirming CAD but is invasive and requires arterial access. Myocardial perfusion imaging, cardiac magnetic resonance, coronary artery calcium scoring, and CT angiography can also be used to detect CAD.

TREATMENT

- <u>Goals of Treatment</u>: A primary goal of therapy is complete (or nearly complete) elimination of anginal chest pain and return to normal activities. Long-term goals are to slow progression of atherosclerosis and prevent complications such as MI, heart failure, stroke, and death.

NONPHARMACOLOGIC THERAPY

- Risk factor modification is the primary nondrug approach for primary and secondary prevention of CAD events. Lifestyle modifications include daily physical activity,

- weight management, dietary therapy (reduced intake of saturated fats, trans-fatty acids, and cholesterol), smoking cessation, psychological interventions (eg, screening and treatment for depression if appropriate), limitation of alcohol intake, and avoiding exposure to air pollution.
- Surgical revascularization options for select patients include coronary artery bypass grafting (CABG) or percutaneous coronary intervention (PCI) with or without stent placement.

PHARMACOLOGIC THERAPY

- Guideline-directed medical therapy (GDMT) reduces the rates of death and MI similar to revascularization therapy. See **Figure 11-1** for a treatment algorithm based on the American College of Cardiology/American Heart Association (ACC/AHA) guidelines.
- Approaches to risk factor modification include the following recommendations:
  - ✓ <u>Dyslipidemia</u>: Use moderate- or high-dose statin therapy in the absence of contraindications or adverse effects, in addition to lifestyle changes. Addition of ezetimibe (first) or a PCSK9 inhibitor (second) is reasonable for patients who do not tolerate statins or do not attain a 50% decrease in LDL cholesterol (or LDL remains above 70–100 mg/dL).
  - ✓ <u>Blood pressure</u>: If BP is $\geq$130/80 mm Hg, institute drug therapy in addition to or after a trial of lifestyle modifications.
  - ✓ <u>Diabetes mellitus</u>: Pharmacotherapy to achieve a target A1C of $\leq$7% (53 mmol/mol Hb) is reasonable for select patients (eg, short duration of diabetes and long life expectancy). An A1C goal of <8% is reasonable for other patients, such as those with micro- or macrovascular complications or coexisting medical conditions.
  - ✓ Annual influenza vaccinations are recommended.

Antiplatelet Therapy

- Aspirin irreversibly blocks cyclooxygenase-1 (COX-1) activity and subsequent thromboxane A_2 production, leading to reduced platelet activation and aggregation. A small percentage of patients are nonresponsive to aspirin's antiplatelet effects. Anti-inflammatory drugs (NSAIDs) may interfere with aspirin's antiplatelet effect when coadministered by competing for the site of action in the COX-1 enzyme. The ACC/AHA guidelines contain the following recommendations for stable IHD:
  - ✓ **Aspirin:** 75–162 mg daily should be continued indefinitely in the absence of contraindications.
  - ✓ **Clopidogrel:** 75 mg daily is an appropriate alternative when aspirin is contraindicated. Patient responsiveness to clopidogrel is highly variable, with estimates of nonresponsiveness ranging from 5% to 44% of patients. The most common cause of nonresponsiveness is nonadherence, but genetic polymorphisms to CYP2C19 may contribute in some patients. Some studies have suggested that patients receiving a proton pump inhibitor (most often omeprazole) together with clopidogrel have reduced antiplatelet activity and more ischemic events due to inhibition of cytochrome P450 enzymes involved in converting clopidogrel to its active metabolite. However, the only prospective randomized clinical trial conducted to date found no increased rate of clinical events in patients given clopidogrel plus omeprazole.
  - ✓ **Dual antiplatelet therapy (DAPT)** with aspirin plus a $P2Y_{12}$ inhibitor (clopidogrel, prasugrel, ticagrelor) is beneficial after PCI with coronary stent placement and after treatment for ACS. Its benefits in other situations are less clear. The combination of aspirin (75–162 mg daily) and clopidogrel 75 mg daily may be reasonable in certain high-risk patients.

Angiotensin-Converting Enzyme (ACE) Inhibitors and Angiotensin Receptor Blockers (ARBs)

- In the setting of IHD, ACE inhibitors stabilize coronary plaque, restore or improve endothelial function, inhibit vascular smooth muscle cell growth, decrease

(ACE, angiotensin-converting enzyme; ARB, angiotensin receptor blocker; BP, blood pressure; CABG, coronary artery bypass graft; CCB, calcium channel blocker; CKD, chronic kidney disease; DAPT, dual antiplatelet therapy; DHP, dihydropyridine; DM, diabetes mellitus; Hb, hemoglobin; HTN, hypertension; LA, long-acting; LVEF, left ventricular ejection fraction; PCI, percutaneous coronary intervention; SL NTG, sublingual nitroglycerin.)

FIGURE 11-1. Algorithm for treatment of stable ischemic heart disease (guideline-directed medical therapy).

macrophage migration, and possibly prevent oxidative stress. However, ACE inhibitors have not been shown to improve symptomatic ischemia or reduce chest pain episodes. Clinical trials of the role of ACE inhibitors or ARBs in reducing cardiovascular events (eg, cardiovascular death, MI, stroke) in high-risk patients have produced conflicting results. The ACC/AHA guidelines for stable IHD recommend the following strategies:

✓ Use ACE inhibitors in patients who also have hypertension, diabetes, HFrEF, or chronic kidney disease, unless contraindicated.

✓ ARBs are recommended for the same populations if patients are intolerant to ACE inhibitors.
✓ Combination ACE inhibitor/ARB therapy should be avoided due to the lack of additional benefit and a higher risk of adverse events (eg, hypotension, syncope, renal dysfunction).
✓ Table 11-1 provides the usual dosage ranges for ACE inhibitors and ARBs in stable IHD.

TABLE 11-1	Drugs and Regimens for Stable Ischemic Heart Disease
Drug Class and Generic Names	**Usual Dosage Range[a]**
Angiotensin-Converting Enzyme Inhibitors	
Captopril	6.25–50 mg 3 times daily
Enalapril	2.5–40 mg daily in 1–2 divided doses
Fosinopril	10–80 mg daily in 1–2 divided doses
Lisinopril	2.5–40 mg once daily
Perindopril	4–8 mg once daily
Quinapril	5–20 mg twice daily
Ramipril	2.5–10 mg daily in 1–2 divided doses
Trandolapril	1–4 mg once daily
Angiotensin Receptor Blockers	
Candesartan	4–32 mg once daily
Valsartan	80–320 mg daily in 1–2 divided doses
Telmisartan	20–80 mg once daily
β-Adrenergic Blockers	
Atenolol[b]	25–200 mg once daily
Betaxolol[b]	5–20 mg once daily
Bisoprolol[b]	2.5–10 mg once daily
Carvedilol[c]	3.125–25 mg twice daily
Carvedilol phosphate[c]	10-80 mg once daily
Labetalol[c]	100–400 mg twice daily
Metoprolol[b]	50–200 mg twice daily (once daily for extended release)
Nadolol[d]	40–120 mg once daily
Nebivolol	5–10 mg once daily
Propranolol[d]	20–120 mg twice daily (60–240 mg once daily for long-acting formulation)
Timolol[d]	10–20 mg twice daily
Calcium Channel Blockers: Nondihydropyridine Type	
Diltiazem, extended release	120–360 mg once daily
Verapamil, extended release	180–480 mg once daily

(Continued)

TABLE 11-1	Drugs and Regimens for Stable Ischemic Heart Disease (*Continued*)
Drug Class and Generic Names	**Usual Dosage Range**[a]
Calcium Channel Blockers: Dihydropyridine Type	
Amlodipine	5–10 mg once daily
Felodipine	5–10 mg once daily
Nifedipine, extended release	30–90 mg once daily
Nicardipine	20–40 mg three times daily
Nitrates	
Nitroglycerin extended-release capsules	2.5 mg three times daily initially, with up-titration according to symptoms and tolerance; allow a 10- to 12-hour nitrate-free interval
Isosorbide dinitrate tablets	5–20 mg two to three times daily, with a daily nitrate-free interval of at least 14 hours (eg, dose at 7 AM, noon, and 5 PM)
Isosorbide dinitrate slow-release capsules	40 mg one to two times daily, with a daily nitrate-free interval of at least 18 hours (eg, dose at 8 AM and 2 PM)
Isosorbide mononitrate tablets	5–20 mg two times daily initially, with up-titration according to symptoms and tolerance; doses should be taken 7 hours apart (eg, 8 AM and 3 PM)
Isosorbide mononitrate extended-release tablets	30–120 mg once daily
Nitroglycerin transdermal extended-release film	0.2–0.8 mg/hr, on for 12–14 hours, off for 10–12 hours

[a]Consult official prescribing information. In patients with renal and hepatic dysfunction, adjust initial and maintenance doses for all agents as appropriate based on FDA-approved labeling.
[b]Relatively β_1-selective (selectively is lost at higher doses).
[c]Blocks α_1, β_1, and β_2 receptors.
[d]Nonselective (blocks both β_1 and β_2 receptors).
Data from Landup D, DiDomenico RJ. Stable ischemic heart disease. In: Chisholm-Burns MA, et al., eds. Pharmacotherapy Principles & Practice. 5th ed. New York: McGraw-Hill Education; 2019.

β-Adrenergic Blockers

- β-Blockers competitively inhibit the effects of neuronally released and circulating catecholamines on β-adrenoceptors. Blockade of β_1-receptors in the heart and kidney reduces HR, contractility, and BP, thereby decreasing MVo_2.
- β-Blockers are recommended over calcium channel blockers (CCBs) for initial control of angina episodes in patients with stable IHD. The target is to lower the resting HR to 50–60 beats/min and the exercise HR to <100 beats/min. For patients (eg, elderly) who cannot tolerate these ranges, the target HR should be as low as can be tolerated above 50 beats/min. β-Blockers may be combined with CCBs or long-acting nitrates when initial treatment with β-blockers alone is unsuccessful.
- Only the β-blockers **carvedilol**, **metoprolol succinate**, and **bisoprolol** should be used in patients with HFrEF, starting with low doses and titrating upward slowly.
- Selection of a particular agent depends on the presence of comorbid states, preferred dosing frequency, and cost. β_1-Selective agents are preferred in patients with chronic obstructive pulmonary disease, peripheral arterial disease (PAD), diabetes, dyslipidemia, and sexual dysfunction. Drugs with combined α_1- and β-blockade are effective for IHD, but agents with intrinsic sympathomimetic activity provide little

to no reduction in resting HR and are not preferred except perhaps in patients with PAD or dyslipidemia.

- Common adverse effects include bradycardia, hypotension, heart block, impaired glucose metabolism, altered serum lipids (transiently increased triglycerides, decreased HDL-C, and no change in LDL-C), fatigue, depression, insomnia, and malaise. β-Blockers are contraindicated in patients with preexisting bradycardia, hypotension, 2nd- or 3rd-degree atrioventricular (AV) block, uncontrolled asthma, severe PAD, hypotension, HFrEF with unstable fluid status, and diabetes associated with frequent episodes of hypoglycemia.
- If β-blocker therapy must be discontinued, doses should be tapered over 2–3 weeks to prevent abrupt withdrawal, which can significantly increase in MVo_2 and induce ischemia and even MI because of up-regulation of β-receptors in the myocardium.
- See Table 11-1 for the usual dosage ranges of β-blockers in stable IHD.

Calcium Channel Blockers

- CCBs modulate calcium entry into the myocardium, vascular smooth muscle, and other tissues, which reduces the cytosolic concentration of calcium responsible for activation of the actin–myosin complex and contraction of vascular smooth muscle and myocardium. All CCBs reduce MVo_2 by reducing wall tension via lowering arterial BP and (to a minor extent) depressing contractility. CCBs also provide some increase in supply by inducing coronary vasodilation and preventing vasospasm.
- CCBs or long-acting nitrates should be prescribed for relief of symptoms when β-blockers are contraindicated or cause unacceptable side effects.
- Dihydropyridine CCBs (eg, **nifedipine**, **amlodipine**, **isradipine**, and **felodipine**) primarily affect vascular smooth muscle with little effect on the myocardium. These drugs produce minimal reduction in contractility and either no change or increased HR due to reflex tachycardia from direct arterial dilation. Nifedipine produces more impairment of LV function than amlodipine and felodipine. Short-acting agents should not be used because of their greater propensity to cause reflex tachycardia. Other side effects of these CCBs include hypotension, headache, gingival hyperplasia, and peripheral edema. Although most CCBs are contraindicated in patients with HFrEF, amlodipine and felodipine are considered safe options in these patients.
- Nondihydropyridine CCBs (**verapamil** and **diltiazem**) mostly affect the myocardium with minimal effects on vascular smooth muscle; they reduce HR, contractility, and MVo_2. Initial therapy for relief of symptoms with a long-acting nondihydropyridine CCB instead of a β-blocker is a reasonable approach. Common side effects of these CCBs include bradycardia, hypotension, AV block, and symptoms of LV depression. These agents should be avoided in patients with concomitant HFrEF due to negative inotropic effects. Verapamil may cause constipation in ~8% of patients. Verapamil and diltiazem inhibit clearance of drugs that utilize the cytochrome P450 3A4 isoenzyme such as carbamazepine, cyclosporine, lovastatin, simvastatin, and benzodiazepines. Verapamil, and to a lesser extent diltiazem, also inhibit P-glycoprotein–mediated drug transport, which can increase concentrations of digoxin and cyclosporine. Verapamil also decreases digoxin clearance. Agents that induce the 3A4 isoenzyme can reduce the effectiveness of all CCBs.
- See Table 11-1 for the usual dosage ranges of CCBs in stable IHD.

Nitrates

- Nitrates increase concentrations of cyclic guanosine monophosphate in vascular endothelium, leading to reduced cytoplasmic calcium and vasodilation. Most vasodilation occurs on the venous side, leading to reduced preload, myocardial wall tension, and MVo_2. Arterial vasodilation increases as doses are escalated, which can produce reflex tachycardia that can negate some of the antianginal benefits. This effect can be mitigated with concomitant β-blocker therapy. Nitrates also produce vasodilation of stenotic epicardial vessels and intracoronary collateral vessels, increasing oxygen supply to the ischemic myocardium.

- All patients should have access to sublingual (SL) NTG 0.3 or 0.4 mg tablets or spray to treat acute angina episodes. Relief typically occurs within 5 minutes of administration.
- SL nitrates can also be used to prevent acute episodes if given 2–5 minutes before activities known to produce angina; protection can last for up to 30 minutes with SL NTG and up to 1 hour with SL isosorbide dinitrate (ISDN).
- Long-acting nitrates (or CCBs) should be prescribed for relief of symptoms when β-blockers are contraindicated or cause unacceptable side effects. Various nitrate formulations are available for acute and chronic use (**Table 11-1**).
- Transdermal patches and isosorbide mononitrate (ISMN) are most commonly prescribed for long-term prevention of angina episodes. ISDN is also effective, but the three times daily regimen requires dosing every 4–5 hours during the day to provide a nitrate-free interval. Chronic nitrate use should incorporate a 10- to 14-hour nitrate-free interval each day to reduce nitrate tolerance. Because this approach places the patient at risk for angina episodes, the nitrate-free interval is usually provided during the nighttime hours when the patient has a reduced MVo_2 while sleeping. The extended-release ISMN products that are dosed twice daily should be given 7 hours apart (eg, 7:00 AM and 2:00 PM). An extended-release, once-daily ISMN product is available that provides 12 hours of nitrate exposure followed by a 12-hour nitrate-free interval. Transdermal NTG patches are typically prescribed as "on in the AM and off in the PM" but patients should be given specific application and removal times (eg, apply at 8:00 AM and remove at 8:00 PM).
- Nitrates should not be used routinely as monotherapy for stable IHD because of the lack of angina coverage during the nitrate-free interval, lack of protection against circadian rhythm (nocturnal) ischemic events, and potential for reflex tachycardia. Concomitant β-blocker or diltiazem therapy can prevent rebound ischemia during the nitrate-free interval.
- Common nitrate side effects include headache, flushing, nausea, postural hypotension, and syncope. Headache can be treated with acetaminophen and usually resolves after about 2 weeks of continued therapy. Transdermal NTG may cause skin erythema and inflammation. Initiating therapy with smaller doses and/or rotating the application site can minimize transdermal nitroglycerin side effects.

Ranolazine

- Ranolazine reduces ischemic episodes by selective inhibition of late sodium current (I_{Na}), which reduces intracellular sodium concentration and improves myocardial function and perfusion. It does not impact HR, BP, the inotropic state, or increase coronary blood flow.
- Ranolazine is effective as monotherapy for relief of angina symptoms but should only be used if patients cannot tolerate traditional agents due to hemodynamic or other adverse effects. Because it does not substantially affect HR and BP, it is recommended as add-on therapy to traditional antianginal agents for patients who achieve goal HR and BP and still have exertional angina symptoms, patients who cannot achieve these hemodynamic goals due to adverse effects, and patients who reach maximum doses of traditional agents but still have angina symptoms.
- The initial ranolazine dose is 500 mg twice daily, increased to 1000 mg twice daily within the next 1–2 weeks if tolerated. It can be combined with a β-blocker when initial treatment with β-blockers alone is unsuccessful.
- Adverse effects include constipation, nausea, dizziness, and headache. Ranolazine can prolong the QTc interval and should be used with caution in patients receiving concomitant QTc-prolonging agents.
- Potent inhibitors of CYP3A4 and P-glycoprotein (ketoconazole, itraconazole, protease inhibitors, clarithromycin, and nefazodone) or potent inducers of CYP3A4 and P-glycoprotein (phenytoin, phenobarbital, carbamazepine, rifampin, rifabutin, rifapentine, St. John's wort) are contraindicated with ranolazine due to significant increases and decreases in ranolazine drug concentrations, respectively. Moderate

CYP3A4 inhibitors (eg, diltiazem, verapamil, erythromycin, and fluconazole) can be used with ranolazine, but the maximum dose should not exceed 500 mg twice daily.

TREATMENT OF VARIABLE THRESHOLD ANGINA AND PRINZMETAL ANGINA

- Patients with variable threshold angina require pharmacotherapy for vasospasm. Most patients respond well to SL NTG for acute attacks.
- Both CCBs and nitrates are effective for chronic therapy. CCBs may be preferred because they are dosed less frequently. Nifedipine, verapamil, and diltiazem are equally effective as single agents for initial management of coronary vasospasm; dose titration is important to maximize the response. Patients unresponsive to CCBs alone may have nitrates added.
- β-Blockers are not useful for vasospasm because they may induce coronary vasoconstriction and prolong ischemia.

EVALUATION OF THERAPEUTIC OUTCOMES

- Assess for symptom improvement by number of angina episodes, weekly SL NTG use, and increased exercise capacity or duration of exertion needed to induce angina.
- Use statins for dyslipidemia, strive to achieve BP and A1C goals, and implement the lifestyle modifications of dietary modification, smoking cessation, weight loss, and regular exercise.
- Once patients have been optimized on medical therapy, symptoms should improve over 2–4 weeks and remain stable until the disease progresses. Patients may require evaluation every 1–2 months until target endpoints are achieved; follow-up every 6–12 months thereafter is appropriate.
- The Seattle Angina Questionnaire, Specific Activity Scale, and Canadian Cardiovascular Society classification system can be used to improve reproducibility of symptom assessment.
- If the patient is doing well, no other assessment may be necessary. Although follow-up exercise tolerance testing with or without cardiac imaging can be performed to objectively assess control of ischemic episodes, this is rarely done if patients are doing well because of the expense involved.
- Monitor for adverse drug effects such as headache and dizziness with nitrates; fatigue and lassitude with β-blockers; and peripheral edema, constipation, and dizziness with CCBs.

See Chapter 32, Stable Ischemic Heart Disease, authored by Paul P. Dobesh, Robert J. DiDomenico, and Kelly C. Rogers, for a more detailed discussion of this topic.

Shock Syndromes

- *Shock* involves a group of syndromes that cause acute, generalized circulatory failure associated with inadequate tissue and organ perfusion. Shock is characterized by systolic blood pressure (SBP) <90 mm Hg (or reduction of at least 40 mm Hg from baseline) or mean arterial blood pressure (MAP) <70 mm Hg with tachycardia and organ perfusion abnormalities.
- Classes of shock based on etiologic mechanisms include (1) hypovolemic, (2) cardiogenic, (3) obstructive, and (4) vasodilatory/distributive. Patients may have components of more than one shock syndrome upon presentation.

PATHOPHYSIOLOGY

- Circulatory shock develops when the cardiovascular system is unable to deliver an adequate oxygen supply to meet tissue demands, resulting in cellular dysfunction, a shift in cellular metabolism to anaerobic pathways, and elevated blood lactate concentrations.
- *Hypovolemic shock* is caused by inadequate venous return because of internal or external loss of intravascular fluids (eg, trauma, surgery, hemorrhage), resulting in insufficient cardiac preload and decreased stroke volume.
- *Cardiogenic shock* results from loss of pump function because of decreased cardiac contractility (eg, acute myocardial infarction [AMI]), acute valvular abnormality, or arrhythmia (eg, ventricular tachycardia).
- *Obstructive shock* results from extracardiac obstruction to blood flow into or out of the heart, such as tension pneumothorax, cardiac tamponade, or pulmonary embolism.
- *Vasodilatory/distributive shock* is characterized by loss of vascular tone; this involves tissue hypoperfusion due to decreased systemic vascular resistance (or hypoperfusion despite normal or elevated cardiac output). Distributive shock is a subset of vasodilatory shock characterized by maldistribution of blood flow in organ microcirculation. Most cases of vasodilatory shock result in distributive shock. Almost all cases of septic shock result in vasodilatory/distributive shock.
- The body responds to an abrupt decrease in tissue perfusion with subsequent restoration of perfusion, leading to a systemic inflammatory response syndrome (SIRS) with release of numerous mediators that interact to cause further injury. This "ischemia-reperfusion injury" results in edematous obstruction of capillaries, oxygen free-radical damage of cell membranes, activation of cellular (eg, white blood cells, platelets) and humoral (eg, procoagulants, anticoagulants, complement, kinins) components, release of other inflammatory mediators, and formation of microthrombi.
- As part of the stress response, anti-inflammatory pathways are also activated to counterbalance the proinflammatory effects on tissues. Vagal nerve-mediated release of acetylcholine leads to suppression of proinflammatory cytokines by macrophages. The renin–angiotensin–aldosterone and hypothalamic–pituitary–adrenocortical systems are activated, with release of angiotensin II, vasopressin, and cortisol to maintain blood pressure (BP) via vasoconstriction and renal sodium and water retention. Cortisol and catecholamine release from the adrenal glands also inhibits proinflammatory cytokine production.

CLINICAL PRESENTATION

- Patients may report dizziness, lightheadedness, confusion, and low urine production.
- Symptoms related to the underlying shock etiology will be present (eg, cough, fever, malaise with pneumonia; chest pain with AMI).

- Vital signs may reveal tachycardia (eg, >120 bpm), tachypnea (eg, >30 breaths/min), hypotension (eg, SBP <90 mm Hg), and low or normal body temperature (eg, 36°C–37°C [96.8°F–98.6°F]) in the absence of infection. Temperature may be elevated if infection is present (eg, >38.3°C [101°F]).
- Physical exam findings of tissue hypoperfusion may include neurologic (eg, confusion, obtundation), cutaneous (eg, warm skin with vasodilation and cool, clammy skin with vasoconstriction), and renal (eg, low urine production) system abnormalities. Capillary refill is usually impaired.
- Laboratory test abnormalities may include elevated blood lactate concentration (>2 mmol/L), increased blood urea nitrogen (BUN) and serum creatinine and decreased urine output (<0.5 to 1 mL/kg/hour) with renal dysfunction, elevated transaminase levels with hepatic dysfunction, decreased hemoglobin/hematocrit with hemorrhage, and elevated cardiac troponin concentration with AMI. In septic shock, the white blood cell (WBC) count is usually >12,000 cells/mm³ (12×10^9/L), and thrombocytopenia may occur. In hemorrhagic and septic shock, the prothrombin time (PT) and international normalized ratio (INR) may increase over time.

DIAGNOSIS AND MONITORING

- Rapid assessment by cardiac echocardiography is indicated when the shock etiology is unclear. Transthoracic echocardiograms can lead to rapid (within 5 minutes) diagnosis of the shock type.
- Initial monitoring in suspected circulatory shock should include vital signs, blood lactate concentration, urine production, and physical examination, including mental status.
- Advanced hemodynamic monitoring (eg, central venous catheterization) may be needed to measure central venous pressure (CVP), obtain venous samples for laboratory testing (including central venous oxygen saturation or $ScvO_2$), and administer drugs (including vasopressors) or fluids directly into the central circulation.
- Tissue metabolic requirements are met by both adequate MAP and adequate oxygen delivery (Do_2). MAP is the driving pressure for peripheral blood flow and end-organ perfusion and is a surrogate estimate of tissue blood flow. Because the components of BP are cardiac output (CO) and systemic vascular resistance (SVR) and CO is a determinant of Do_2, BP is integrally related to Do_2. However, compensatory mechanisms such as vasoconstriction may preserve BP while tissue perfusion is inadequate. Therefore, while low BP is commonly present in patients with shock, it is not required to define shock.
- Inadequate Do_2 leads to organ damage in critical illness. In normal individuals, oxygen consumption (Vo_2) depends on Do_2 up to a certain critical level (Vo_2 flow dependency). At this point, tissue oxygen requirements are satisfied and further increases in Do_2 will not alter Vo_2 (Vo_2 flow independency). The point that Vo_2 becomes dependent on Do_2 represents a pathologic transition from aerobic to anaerobic cellular metabolism and lactate production. However, studies in critically ill patients show a continuous, pathologic dependence relationship of Vo_2 with Do_2. The parameters are calculated as follows:

$$Do_2 = CO \times Cao_2 \text{ and } Vo_2 = CO \times (Cao_2 - CVo_2)$$

where CO = cardiac output, Cao_2 = arterial oxygen content determined by hemoglobin concentration and arterial oxygen saturation (Sao_2), and Cvo_2 = mixed venous oxygen content determined by hemoglobin concentration and venous oxygen saturation (Svo_2).

- Venous oximetry (ie, venous oxygen saturations) reflects the adequacy of tissue oxygenation. Svo_2 and central venous oxygen saturation ($Scvo_2$) are the oxyhemoglobin saturation of venous blood obtained from the pulmonary artery and a central vein in the thorax, respectively, and are expressed as a percentage. When tissue oxygen demand exceeds supply, the oxygen extraction ratio (O_2ER) increases and values of

Svo_2 and $Scvo_2$ are low. When hemoglobin, Sao_2, and Vo_2 are stable, Svo_2 or $Scvo_2$ values reflect CO. Thus, venous oximetry may be used as a surrogate for CO and can be useful in shock state differentiation.

- Generally, Svo_2 values >70% (0.70) are considered adequate and normal. However, Svo_2 values <50% (0.50) are low and may approach the critical O_2ER where anaerobic metabolism occurs and lactate concentrations increase. High Svo_2 (>80% [0.80]) can represent a high CO but may also be a poor prognostic sign indicating adequate Do_2 but poor capacity of tissues to extract oxygen.

TREATMENT

- <u>Goals of Treatment</u>: The desired outcome is to reduce morbidity and mortality by preventing organ damage and, to the extent possible, halt or reverse existing organ dysfunction. Treatment of circulatory shock can be divided into four phases, each with different (but sometimes overlapping) treatment goals and strategies: (1) *Salvage*, with goals of obtaining a minimum perfusion pressure and CO to ensure survival and treating the underlying shock etiology (eg, hemostasis, antimicrobials, coronary revascularization); (2) *optimization*, ensuring adequate organ perfusion and Do_2; (3) *stabilization*, to prevent further end-organ dysfunction; and (4) *de-escalation*, which targets patient recovery with goals of weaning (or stopping) vasoactive medications and fluids. This chapter focuses on salvage and optimization, but recognizing the phase of a patient's circulatory shock is necessary to establish treatment goals and therapeutic approaches.

GENERAL APPROACH

- **Figure 12-1** presents an algorithm for managing patients with shock using a stepwise approach to optimize MAP, first with crystalloid fluid resuscitation followed by the vasopressor norepinephrine if appropriate.
- Hospitalization is indicated for patients with circulatory insufficiency that does not respond readily to fluid resuscitation.
- Venous access is generally obtained during the initial examination process. Large-bore peripheral IV lines are preferred over central lines for initial fluid resuscitation, but vasopressors should preferentially be administered via a central venous catheter.
- The stabilization phase should include general supportive care measures such as assessment and management of pain, anxiety/agitation, delirium, immobility, sleep disturbances, nutrition, glycemic control, and thromboembolism prophylaxis.
- A goal MAP >65 mm Hg is often targeted to maintain adequate perfusion to critical organs.
- Consider patient-specific characteristics when establishing a BP goal and determining an adequate perfusion response to resuscitation.
- If MAP or SBP remains below goal, then initiate vasopressors to ensure tissue perfusion.
- Determine adequacy of Do_2 by assessing markers of end-organ perfusion (eg, urine production) and lactate concentrations. Obtain serial lactate concentrations in the early treatment phases because lactate clearance and normalization correspond with improved global tissue perfusion.
- After the salvage treatment phase, give fluids only to patients with ineffective tissue perfusion who are predicted or known to be fluid responsive. The benefits of continued fluid administration (improved CO and tissue perfusion) must be balanced against the risks of fluid overload (eg, pulmonary edema).

NONPHARMACOLOGIC THERAPY

- Give all patients the basic life support measures of a secure airway with appropriate oxygenation.
- For hypovolemic shock, additional measures may include surgery, control of blood loss, blood component transfusion, and prevention of heat loss with hypothermia or cooling measures with heat exposure (eg, heat stroke).

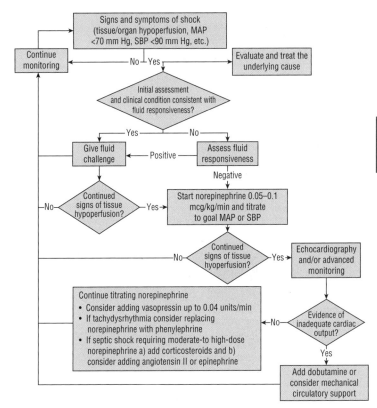

FIGURE 12-1. Algorithm for the management of patients with shock.

- For patients with thermal injuries, cover wound sites with cool, moist sterile dressings until more definitive care can be provided.
- Patients with cardiogenic shock secondary to AMI should undergo emergent coronary revascularization and be considered for CO augmentation via mechanical device (eg, intra-aortic balloon pump or extracorporeal life support).
- Measures for obstructive shock may include pericardiocentesis or surgical evacuation of fluid for cardiac tamponade, needle decompression and/or chest tube thoracostomy for tension pneumothorax, and surgical or catheter thrombectomy for pulmonary embolism.
- Patients with vasodilatory/distributive shock secondary to septic shock should have infectious source control with consideration given to fever control via external cooling.

PHARMACOLOGIC THERAPY

Intravenous Fluids and Blood Products

- The goal of administering IV fluids is to increase venous return in order to increase stroke volume, cardiac output, Do_2, and BP. Blood products may also be administered to replace cellular and plasma losses with the added benefit of increasing venous return.

Crystalloids:
- Isotonic (or near isotonic) crystalloid solutions (eg, **lactated Ringer's** and **0.9% sodium chloride** [normal saline]) are the initial fluid of choice for resuscitation, and large volumes should be administered (except for patients with cardiogenic shock). Balanced salt solutions (eg, lactated Ringer's) and **multiple electrolytes injection** (eg, Plasma-Lyte A) and normal saline have similar efficacy in expanding plasma volume, but balanced salt solutions may be safer. Excess chloride administration with normal saline may be more likely to lead to hyperchloremic metabolic acidosis and possibly acute kidney injury (AKI). However, balanced salt solutions may aggravate preexisting hyperkalemia or exacerbate cerebral edema in brain-injured patients. If there are signs of tissue hypoperfusion and the clinical syndrome is consistent with a shock state that is fluid responsive (eg, hypovolemic), administer an initial fluid challenge of at least 500 mL of crystalloid.
- **3% sodium chloride** (hypertonic saline) causes redistribution of fluid from the intracellular space, resulting in rapid expansion of the intravascular compartment; however, its use is not associated with improved outcomes when used for initial fluid resuscitation in shock. In addition, potential dosing and administration errors can lead to adverse events, and dramatic fluid shifts may be associated with hypernatremia, metabolic acidosis from hyperchloremia, and peripheral vein damage due to high osmolality (1026 mOsm/L).

Colloids:
- **Albumin** (5% or 25%), **hydroxyethyl starch**, and **dextran** are large molecular weight solutions that have a prolonged intravascular retention time compared to crystalloid solutions; colloids remain in the intravascular space for hours or days, depending on the size of the colloid molecules and capillary permeability. However, colloids are expensive and have been associated with fluid overload, renal dysfunction, and bleeding. When compared with alternative resuscitation solutions, hydroxyethyl starch was associated with increased mortality, AKI, and need for renal replacement therapy. Consequently, the US product labeling was changed in 2013 to state that starch products are contraindicated in critically ill patients; therefore, they should not be used for fluid resuscitation.

Blood products:
- Some patients require blood products (**packed red blood cells, fresh frozen plasma, platelets,** or **cryoprecipitate**) to ensure maintenance of O_2-carrying capacity, as well as clotting factors and platelets for blood hemostasis. Blood products may be associated with circulatory overload, transfusion-related reactions, virus transmission (rarely), hypocalcemia from added citrate, increased blood viscosity from supranormal hematocrit elevations, and hypothermia from failure to appropriately warm solutions before administration.

Fluid Resuscitation in Distributive (Septic) Shock

- The initial fluid challenge volume is unclear; the Surviving Sepsis Campaign recommends 30 mL/kg crystalloids given within the first 3 hours of shock recognition, but supporting evidence for this specific volume is of low quality. Several approaches exist for fluid resuscitation during the first 6 hours: (1) liberal fluid administration (50–75 mL/kg) while reserving vasopressors; and (2) relatively restrictive initial fluid administration ($\leq$30 mL/kg) with earlier vasopressor use to maintain tissue perfusion. More than 30 mL/kg of crystalloid fluids may be needed to obtain goal MAP, reverse global hypoperfusion (lactate clearance, $SCVo_2$ $\geq$70% [0.70]), or achieve clinical indication of regional organ-specific perfusion (eg, urine production). An isolated bolus (eg, 250–500 mL) in an adult patient is unlikely to cause a substantial change in BP or acid–base balance. Therefore, multiple fluid boluses are often needed to achieve hemodynamic stability. However, excessive fluid administration has been associated with higher mortality, and overly aggressive fluid administration should be avoided, especially in patients with heart failure or impending pulmonary edema. Because intravenous medication diluents can contribute significantly to total fluid volume, the total fluid administration should be accounted for, and dynamic fluid response with clinical assessment should occur frequently after each fluid challenge.

Fluid Resuscitation in Hypovolemic (Hemorrhagic/Traumatic) Shock

- Immediate treatment of hemorrhagic shock with plasma expanders (crystalloids or colloids) seems logical, but no large, well-controlled clinical trials have supported this practice. In fact, some evidence suggests that fluid resuscitation beyond minimal levels (ie, MAP $\geq$60 mm Hg) is harmful in patients with abdominal trauma due to hemodilution and clot destabilization.
- Instead of immediate plasma expansion in all preoperative patients with circulatory insufficiency caused by hemorrhage, the initial priority should be surgical control of the bleeding source; until this is possible, fluids should be given in small aliquots to yield a palpable pulse and to maintain MAP values no more than 60 mm Hg and SBP no more than 90 mm Hg.
- Isotonic crystalloids are the fluid of choice because they are equal in efficacy to hypertonic sodium chloride solutions with a lower risk of adverse effects. Lactated Ringer's solution may be used as an alternative to normal saline but should be used cautiously in patients with traumatic brain injury because it may worsen cerebral edema. Hypotonic solutions should be avoided in this population given their relatively poor intravascular expansion and association with poor outcomes in animal models of closed head injury.
- Once hemostasis has been achieved in a patient with hemorrhage, a relatively restrictive transfusion strategy (ie, transfusion if hemoglobin $\leq$7 g/dL [70 g/L; 4.34 mmol/L]) is indicated unless a patient has active cardiac ischemia. Additional blood product administration should be guided by laboratory parameters (eg, PT/INR, platelets) or viscoelastic testing (eg, thromboelastography). Reversal of antithrombotic therapy (eg, prothrombin complex concentrates for warfarin) may also be used for severe bleeding.

Vasopressors and Inotropes

- Vasopressors and inotropes are required when volume resuscitation fails to maintain adequate BP (MAP $\geq$65 mm Hg) and organs and tissues remain hypoperfused. Vasopressors may also be needed temporarily to treat life-threatening hypotension when tissue perfusion is inadequate despite ongoing aggressive fluid resuscitation. Inotropes are frequently used to optimize Do_2 in septic shock and cardiac function in cardiogenic shock.
- **Table 12-1** lists the usual dosage range, receptor selectivity, and potential adverse effects of vasopressors and inotropes used in shock.
- **Norepinephrine** has combined strong α_1-agonist activity and less potent β_1-agonist effects while maintaining weak vasodilatory effects of β_2-receptor stimulation. It produces vasoconstriction primarily via its more prominent α-effects on all vascular beds, thus increasing SVR; it also produces a small (10%–15%) increase in stroke volume. Norepinephrine is the vasopressor of choice in patients in most shock states because (1) it may decrease mortality in septic shock; (2) it reverses inappropriate vasodilation and low global oxygen extraction; (3) it attenuates myocardial depression at unchanged or increased CO and increased coronary blood flow; (4) it improves renal perfusion pressure and renal filtration; (5) it enhances splanchnic perfusion; and (6) it is less likely than many other vasopressors to cause tachydysrhythmias. Norepinephrine 0.1–2 mcg/kg/min improves hemodynamic parameters to "normal" values in most patients with shock. As with other vasopressors, norepinephrine dosages exceeding those recommended by most references are frequently needed in critically ill patients with shock to achieve predetermined goals. A significant increase in MAP is caused by an increase in SVR. Heart rate generally decreases because of reflex bradycardia from increased SVR. Increasing doses to maintain higher MAPs may increase heart rate, cardiac index, Do_2, and cutaneous blood flow, but these results are inconsistent. Norepinephrine may be associated with tachydysrhythmias, which is more common with higher doses. The primary limitation to use is that norepinephrine is not commercially available as premixed ready-to-use solutions, so its use requires preparation time.

TABLE 12-1 Receptor Pharmacology and Adverse Events of Selected Vasopressor and Inotropic Agents Used in Shock[a]

Agent (Adverse Events)	α_1	α_2	β_1	β_2	D	V_1	V_2
Angiotensin II (5000–10,000 ng/mL NS)	Tachycardia, thrombosis, peripheral ischemia, lactic acidosis, bronchospasm, infection						
1.25–80 ng/kg/min	0	0	0	0	0	0	0
Dobutamine (500–4000 mcg/mL D$_5$W or NS)	Tachycardia, dysrhythmias, hypotension						
2–10 mcg/kg/min	+	0	++++	++	0	0	0
>10–20 mcg/kg/min	++	0	++++	+++	0	0	0
Dopamine (800–3200 mcg/mL D$_5$W or NS)	Tachycardia, dysrhythmias, decreased Pao$_2$, mesenteric hypoperfusion, gastrointestinal motility inhibition, T-cell inhibition						
1–3 mcg/kg/min	0	0	+	0	++++	0	0
3–10 mcg/kg/min	0/+	0	++++	+	++++	0	0
>10–20 mcg/kg/min	+++	0	++++	+	0	0	0
Epinephrine (8–16 mcg/mL D$_5$W or NS)	Tachycardia, dysrhythmias, decreased Pao$_2$, mesenteric hypoperfusion, increased lactate, hyperglycemia, immunomodulation						
0.01–0.05 mcg/kg/min	++	++	++++	+++	0	0	0
0.05–3 mcg/kg/min	++++	++++	+++	+	0	0	0
Norepinephrine (16–64 mcg/mL D$_5$W)	Mixed effects on myocardial performance and mesenteric perfusion, peripheral ischemia						
0.02–3 mcg/kg/min	+++	+++	+++	+/++	0	0	0
Phenylephrine (100–400 mcg/mL D$_5$W or NS)	Mixed effects on myocardial performance, peripheral ischemia						
0.5–9 mcg/kg/min	+++	+	+	0	0	0	0
Vasopressin (0.2–1 units/mL D$_5$W or NS)	Mixed effects on myocardial performance, mesenteric hypoperfusion, peripheral ischemia, hyponatremia, thrombocytopenia, hyperbilirubinemia						
0.01–0.1 units/min	0	0	0	0	0	+++	+++

AT, angiotensin; D, dopamine; D$_5$W, dextrose 5% in water; NS, normal saline; Pao$_2$, partial pressure of arterial oxygen; V, vasopressin.
[a]Activity ranges from no activity (0) to maximal (++++) activity. Angiotensin II has ++++ activity at AT-1 and AT-2 receptors but no activity at other receptors.

- **Epinephrine** has combined α- and β-agonist effects. At low doses (0.01–0.05 mcg/kg/min) β-adrenergic effects predominate with an increase in stroke volume and CO. For this reason, low doses may be used as an inotrope after cardiac surgery. When higher dosages are used, α-adrenergic effects are predominant and SVR and MAP are increased. Epinephrine is an acceptable choice for hemodynamic support of patients with shock because of its combined vasoconstrictor and inotropic effects. It is as effective as norepinephrine for MAP response in vasodilatory/distributive shock. Epinephrine doses of 0.04–1 mcg/kg/min alone increase hemodynamic and oxygen-transport variables to "supranormal" values in shock patients without coronary artery disease. Large doses (0.5–3 mcg/kg/min) are often required, particularly for patients with septic shock. Smaller doses (0.1–0.5 mcg/kg/min) are effective when epinephrine is added to other vasopressors and inotropes. In addition, younger patients appear to respond better to epinephrine, possibly due to greater β-adrenergic reactivity. Despite rapid improvement of hemodynamic variables and Do_2, it can have deleterious effects on the splanchnic circulation. Like norepinephrine, epinephrine is not commercially available as a premixed ready-to-use solution.
- **Phenylephrine** is a pure α_1-agonist and increases BP primarily through vasoconstriction. It improves MAP by increasing SVR and stroke index through enhanced venous return to the heart. Given the presence of cardiac α_1-receptors, phenylephrine may also increase contractility and CO. Tachydysrhythmias are infrequent, particularly when phenylephrine is used as a single agent or at higher doses because it exerts little activity on β_1-adrenergic receptors. Phenylephrine may be a useful alternative in patients who cannot tolerate tachycardia or tachydysrhythmias from norepinephrine or epinephrine and in patients who are refractory to those agents. Phenylephrine is also an attractive agent for vasodilatory/distributive shock because of its selective α-agonism with primarily vascular effects. As with other vasopressors, the doses required to achieve therapeutic goals are significantly higher than those traditionally recommended. Phenylephrine 0.5–9 mcg/kg/min, used alone or in combination with dobutamine or low dopamine doses, improves BP and myocardial performance in fluid-resuscitated patients with vasodilatory/distributive shock. In septic shock, phenylephrine does not significantly impair the cardiac index, pulmonary artery occlusion pressure (PAOP), or peripheral perfusion. Like norepinephrine and epinephrine, phenylephrine is not commercially available as a premixed ready-to-use solution.
- **Dopamine** has been described as having dose-related receptor activity at D_1-, D_2-, β_1-, and α_1-receptors, but this dose-response relationship has not been confirmed in critically ill patients. In patients with shock, great overlap of hemodynamic effects occurs, even at doses as low as 3 mcg/kg/min. Clinical trials and a meta-analysis indicate that low-dose dopamine does not enhance renal function or survival in critically ill patients. Dopamine is a natural precursor to norepinephrine and epinephrine but is generally not as effective for achieving goal MAP in patients with shock. Doses of 5–10 mcg/kg/min increase CO by improving contractility and heart rate, primarily from β_1 effects. At higher doses (>10 mcg/kg/min) it increases MAP as a result of both increased CO and SVR due to its combined β_1 and α_1 effects. The clinical utility of dopamine as a vasopressor in shock is limited because large doses are frequently necessary to maintain CO and MAP. At doses >20 mcg/kg/min, further improvement in cardiac performance and regional hemodynamics is limited. In addition, its clinical use is often hampered by tachycardia and tachydysrhythmias, which may lead to myocardial ischemia. For these reasons, dopamine is no longer considered a first-line therapy for shock. Dopamine is commercially available as premixed ready-to-use solution of various concentrations.
- **Dobutamine** is primarily a selective β_1-agonist with mild β_2- and vascular α_1-activity, resulting in strong positive inotropic activity without concomitant vasoconstriction. Compared to dopamine, dobutamine produces a larger increase in CO and is less arrhythmogenic. β_2-induced vasodilation and increased myocardial contractility with subsequent reflex reduction in sympathetic tone lead to decreased SVR. Optimal uses of dobutamine in shock are for patients with low CO

and high filling pressures (eg, left ventricular dysfunction on echocardiography) or ongoing signs of global or regional hypoperfusion despite adequate resuscitation; however, vasopressors may be needed to counteract arterial vasodilation. Dobutamine is an inotrope with vasodilatory properties (an "inodilator"). It is used for treatment of septic and cardiogenic shock to increase CO, typically by 25%–50%. Dobutamine increases stroke volume, left ventricular stroke work index, and thus cardiac index and Do_2 without increasing PAOP. Because dobutamine increases myocardial oxygen demand, it should be used cautiously in patients with cardiogenic shock. The combination of dobutamine and norepinephrine results in a lower increase in heart rate than use of epinephrine alone. Dobutamine is commercially available as a premixed ready-to-use solution.

- **Vasopressin** causes rapid and sustained vasoconstriction that increases SVR and BP, which allows for reductions in the dosage requirements of catecholamines and adrenergic agents in vasodilatory/distributive shock. These effects occur with doses up to 0.04 units/min. Doses >0.04 units/min may be associated with negative changes in CO and mesenteric mucosal perfusion. Cardiac ischemia occurs rarely with low doses; use of higher doses in septic shock patients with cardiac dysfunction warrants extreme caution. Vasopressin decreases heart rate after initiation because of reflex bradycardia from increased SVR. Unlike adrenergic agonists, the vasoconstrictive effects are preserved during hypoxemia and severe acidemia, and pulmonary arterial pressures do not increase. After treatment initiation, organ-specific vasodilation may preserve cardiac and renal function. Whereas V_2 stimulation promotes water retention from the distal kidney tubules and collecting ducts, V_1-receptors constrict efferent arterioles and dilate afferent arterioles to increase glomerular perfusion pressure and filtration rate, enhancing urine production. Vasopressin is not available as a premixed ready-to-use solution.

- **Angiotensin II** increases SVR and may be used for vasodilatory/distributive shock. BP rapidly increases after initiation in patients with low SVR. The starting dose is 10–20 ng/kg/min with rapid titration (as quickly as every 5 minutes) to MAP goal. In the first 3 hours of treatment, the dose may be increased up to 80 ng/kg/min; thereafter, the dose should not exceed 40 ng/kg/min. The effects of angiotensin II on myocardial performance, oxygen transport parameters, and regional organ perfusion are unclear. However, it may have a deleterious effect on regional tissue perfusion because its risk of lactic acidosis and delirium are higher. Angiotensin II has only been evaluated in patients without depressed CO so it should be used with extreme caution in patients with impaired left ventricular systolic function. Angiotensin II also increases glomerular perfusion pressure and filtration, but its effects on kidney function are unclear. Heart rate increases significantly after initiation, so it should be used cautiously in vulnerable patients (eg, older patients with coronary artery disease). Because it increases the risk of thromboembolic events, concurrent thromboembolism prophylaxis should be employed. Patients receiving angiotensin II have a higher risk for secondary infection. It has been associated with bronchospasm and should be avoided in patients with asthma or current bronchospasm.

Use of Vasopressors and Inotropes in Distributive (Septic) Shock

- Norepinephrine should be started when a MAP ≥65 mm Hg and/or adequate tissue perfusion are not achieved with fluid resuscitation. Infusions are initiated at 0.05–0.1 mcg/kg/min and rapidly titrated to preset BP goals (usually MAP ≥65 mm Hg) and/or improvement in global and regional peripheral perfusion (eg, decrease blood lactate or restore urine production).

- Epinephrine is second-line or adjunctive therapy to norepinephrine because it is associated with tachydysrhythmias, lactate elevation, and variable pH values.

- Phenylephrine improves myocardial performance in hyperdynamic, normotensive patients with sepsis but worsens myocardial performance in patients with cardiogenic shock because of decreased CO and increased SVR. Therefore, phenylephrine use warrants caution, and it should not be used as an initial vasopressor in shock patients with impaired myocardial performance.

- Dopamine is no longer recommended as a first-line vasopressor because of the limitations described previously.
- Current guidelines recommend a trial of dobutamine for patients with septic shock in the presence of myocardial dysfunction. However, administration of dobutamine purely to achieve a normal CO, Do_2, or $SCVo_2$ in the absence of other signs of tissue hypoperfusion (eg, low urine production) is not recommended. Dobutamine should be started at doses ranging from 2.5 to 5 mcg/kg/min up to a maximum of 20 mcg/kg/min. Doses >20 mcg/kg/min are limited by tachycardia, myocardial ischemia, hypertension, and tachydysrhythmias. Like other inotropes, dobutamine is usually given until improvement in myocardial function with resolution of the underlying etiology or dose-limiting side effects are observed.
- Vasopressin may be considered as add-on therapy to catecholamine adrenergic agents rather than as first-line therapy. Adjunctive use may obviate the need for dose escalation of adrenergic agents, decrease norepinephrine dosage, and increase MAP. In patients with septic shock, doses are generally fixed at 0.03–0.04 units/min, with higher doses reserved for salvage therapy. Increased arterial pressure should be evident within the first hour of vasopressin therapy, at which time the dose(s) of adrenergic agent(s) should be reduced while maintaining goal MAP.
- The role of angiotensin II is currently unclear, but it will most likely be used as an adjunctive therapy to catecholamines and vasopressin.
- Corticosteroid therapy in septic shock improves hemodynamic variables and allows lower catecholamine vasopressor dosages with minimal adverse effects on patient safety. Corticosteroids should be considered when fluids and moderate- to high-dose vasopressors are unable to restore hemodynamic stability, or when weaning of vasopressor therapy proves futile. They should also be started in cases of shock when adrenal insufficiency is suspected (eg, patients receiving long-term corticosteroid therapy for other indications prior to the onset of shock); however, assessment of adrenal function to guide therapy is not recommended. Adverse events are few because corticosteroids are administered for a short period, usually 7 days. Studies suggest that short-term, low-dose corticosteroids do not increase rates of gastrointestinal bleeding and superinfections but do increase the risk for hypernatremia, hyperglycemia, and perhaps neuromuscular weakness. Acutely elevated serum BUN and WBC count may also occur.

Use of Vasopressors and Inotropes in Hypovolemic (Hemorrhagic/Traumatic) Shock

- In contrast to other forms of shock, medications are a distant alternative to fluid resuscitation, which is the primary therapy for hypovolemic shock. In hypovolemic shock, peripheral resistance is high due to compensatory mechanisms aimed at maintaining tissue perfusion. Early or overzealous use of vasopressors in lieu of fluids may exacerbate this resistance to the point that flow is stopped.
- Vasopressors are only used as a temporizing measure or as a last resort when all other measures to maintain perfusion have been exhausted. Few studies have compared the various agents, but norepinephrine is considered the first-line vasopressor of choice.

EVALUATION OF THERAPEUTIC OUTCOMES

- The initial goals of therapy are to restore effective tissue and organ perfusion. Place priority on the ABCs of life support (ie, airway, breathing, and circulation), assessing vital signs and mental status, and determining tissue perfusion (eg, urine production after catheterization).
- Evaluate the underlying cause of tissue hypoperfusion to identify the correct treatment approach.
- For patients with sepsis, measure blood lactate concentration and administer 30 mL/kg of crystalloid for hypotension within 3 hours of presentation and obtain MAP ≥65 mm Hg with vasopressors, reassess volume status, and remeasure serum lactate

if the initial concentration was elevated within 6 hours of presentation. Usual care must include rapid (ie, within 1 hour of recognition) antibiotic administration and aggressive fluid resuscitation.

- Initial fluid resuscitation should include crystalloids if the patient is fluid responsive, vasopressors to achieve MAP at least 65 mm Hg (or SBP 80–90 mm Hg in trauma patients), and frequent clinical assessments to meet perfusion goals (eg, additional fluid challenge or inotropic therapy to achieve lactate clearance $\geq 20\%$, $SCVo_2 \geq 70\%$ (0.70), or urine production ≥ 0.5 mL/kg/hr).

- Initiate vasopressors/inotropes if tissue perfusion is not responding to fluid challenges. Titration and monitoring should be guided by the "best clinical response" and lactate clearance. Although doses required for efficacy may be much higher than recommended by most references, use the lowest effective dosage while minimizing evidence of global hypoperfusion (lactate, $SCVo_2$) and regional hypoperfusion such as myocardial (eg, tachydysrhythmias, electrocardiographic changes, troponin elevations), renal (decreased glomerular filtration rate and/or urine production), splanchnic/gastric (bowel ischemia, elevated transaminases), pulmonary (worsening Pao_2), or peripheral (cold extremities) ischemia. Continue vasopressors/inotropes until myocardial depression and/or BP improve, usually measured in hours to days.

- Monitor patients frequently for their response to therapy. If perfusion is not restored with the initial treatment approach, perform echocardiography with additional treatment options implemented based on the findings.

- Consider hemodynamic monitoring with a pulmonary artery (Swan-Ganz) catheter in complex patients (eg, mixed shock states) or when the validity of measurements from other monitoring devices is in question. The catheter provides multiple cardiovascular parameters, including CVP, pulmonary artery pressure, PAOP (wedge pressure), CO, SVR, and SVo_2. However, the pulmonary artery catheter should not be used routinely for patients with shock because it is more invasive (leading to a higher risk of complications) than a central venous catheter and is not associated with improved clinical outcomes.

- Laboratory tests for monitoring of shock include serum electrolytes, BUN, serum creatinine, and complete blood count to identify possible infection (WBC count), oxygen-carrying capacity of the blood (hemoglobin, hematocrit), and ongoing bleeding (hemoglobin, hematocrit, platelet count). Hepatic transaminases may be acutely elevated when blood flow to the liver is reduced because of sustained hypotension ("shock liver"), although the concentrations should decrease over time with recovery.

- In bleeding patients, monitor coagulation function via PT/INR, platelets, and perhaps viscoelastic tests (eg, thromboelastography) with initiation of appropriate support measures as indicated.

- Observe for an increasing blood lactate concentration and arterial base deficit or a decreasing bicarbonate concentration, which indicate inadequate perfusion leading to anaerobic metabolism.

- In patients responding to initial therapy, the goal is to discontinue vasopressors and inotropes as soon as the patient is hemodynamically stable. However, taper vasopressor/inotrope therapy slowly, and monitor the patient carefully to avoid worsening hemodynamics. Reevaluate fluid responsiveness frequently so the patient can be weaned from the vasopressor as soon as possible. Titrate doses downward approximately every 10 minutes to determine if the patient can tolerate gradual withdrawal and eventual discontinuation. Shock requiring vasopressor and/or inotropic support usually resolves within several days to 1 week.

See Chapter 41, Shock Syndromes, authored by Seth R. Bauer, Robert MacLaren, and Brian L. Erstad, for a more detailed discussion of this topic.

CHAPTER 13

Stroke

- *Stroke* involves the abrupt onset of focal neurologic dysfunction that lasts at least 24 hours and is caused by cerebral, spinal, or retinal infarction. Stroke can be either ischemic or hemorrhagic. Transient ischemic attacks (TIAs) are focal ischemic neurologic deficits lasting <24 hours and usually <30 minutes.

PATHOPHYSIOLOGY

ISCHEMIC STROKE

- Ischemic stroke (87% of all strokes) results from occlusion of a cerebral artery that reduces cerebral blood flow. Ischemic strokes are due either to local thrombus formation or emboli from a distant site. Atherosclerosis of large intracranial or extracranial arteries or small artery disease can result in ischemic stroke. Emboli can arise from the heart in patients with atrial fibrillation, valvular heart disease, or other prothrombotic heart problems and cause about 25% of ischemic strokes. The stroke cause is undetermined in some cases.
- Decreased cerebral blood flow can lead to infarction of cerebral tissue with a surrounding area that is ischemic but may maintain membrane integrity (the ischemic penumbra). This penumbra is an area of brain tissue that is potentially salvageable with urgent pharmacologic and endovascular treatment interventions.
- Insufficient oxygen supply in ischemic tissue leads to adenosine triphosphate (ATP) depletion with lactate buildup due to anaerobic metabolism and accumulation of intracellular sodium and water, leading to cytotoxic edema and eventual cell lysis. An influx of calcium intracellularly activates lipases and proteases, resulting in protein degradation and free fatty acid release from cellular membranes. Release of excitatory amino acids (eg, glutamate, aspartate) in ischemic tissue perpetuates neuronal damage and produces damaging prostaglandins, leukotrienes, and reactive oxygen species. These processes occur within 2–3 hours of the onset of ischemia and ultimately lead to cellular apoptosis and necrosis.
- The most common modifiable risk factors for ischemic stroke include hypertension, cigarette smoking, diabetes, atrial fibrillation, and dyslipidemia.

HEMORRHAGIC STROKE

- Hemorrhagic strokes (13% of strokes) include subarachnoid hemorrhage (SAH) and intracerebral hemorrhage (ICH). SAH may result from trauma or rupture of an intracranial aneurysm or arteriovenous malformation (AVM). ICH occurs when bleeding in the brain parenchyma results in hematoma formation.
- Intracranial hematoma causes mechanical compression of brain parenchyma. Early hematoma expansion often occurs within 3 hours of hemorrhage onset, contributing to worsened functional outcome and increased mortality.
- Secondary mechanisms of injury are mediated by the subsequent inflammatory response, cerebral edema, and damage from blood product degradation.

CLINICAL PRESENTATION

- Patients may be unable to provide a reliable history because of cognitive or language deficits. Family members or other witnesses may need to provide this information.
- Symptoms include unilateral weakness, inability to speak, loss of vision, vertigo, or falling. Ischemic stroke is not usually painful, but some patients complain of headache. Pain and headache are more common and severe in hemorrhagic stroke.
- Neurologic deficits on physical examination depend on the brain area involved. Hemi- or monoparesis and hemisensory deficits are common. Patients with posterior circulation involvement may have vertigo and diplopia. Anterior circulation strokes

commonly result in aphasia. Patients may experience dysarthria, visual field defects, and altered levels of consciousness.

DIAGNOSIS

- Blood glucose, platelet count, and coagulation parameters (eg, prothrombin time, aPTT) are used in stroke assessment to determine treatment eligibility.
- Tests for hypercoagulable states (protein C and S deficiency, antiphospholipid antibody) should be done only when the etiology cannot be determined based on presence of well-known risk factors.
- Computed tomography (CT) and magnetic resonance imaging (MRI) head scans can reveal areas of hemorrhage and infarction.
- Vascular imaging with computed tomography angiography (CTA) is recommended in patients with endovascular treatment indications.
- Carotid Doppler (CD), electrocardiogram (ECG), transthoracic echocardiogram (TTE), and transcranial Doppler (TCD) studies can each provide valuable diagnostic information.

TREATMENT

- <u>Goals of Treatment</u>: The goals are to: (1) reduce ongoing neurologic injury acutely to reduce mortality and long-term disability; (2) prevent complications secondary to immobility and neurologic dysfunction; and (3) prevent stroke recurrence.

GENERAL APPROACH

- Ensure adequate respiratory and cardiac support and determine quickly from CT scan whether the lesion is ischemic or hemorrhagic.
- Evaluate ischemic stroke patients presenting within hours of symptom onset for pharmacologic and mechanical reperfusion therapy.
- Patients with TIA require urgent assessment and intervention to reduce the risk of stroke, which is highest in the first few days after TIA.
- Assess patients with hemorrhagic stroke to determine whether they are candidates for surgical intervention.
- After the acute phase, focus on preventing progressive deficits, minimizing complications, and instituting secondary prevention strategies.

NONPHARMACOLOGIC THERAPY

Ischemic Stroke

- Endovascular intervention and thrombectomy with retrievable stents to reperfuse ischemic brain tissue is recommended by the American Heart Association (AHA) and American Stroke Association (ASA). Thrombectomy is strongly recommended for patients with anterior circulation occlusion in the internal carotid artery (ICA) or the M1 segment of the middle cerebral artery (MCA) who are within 6 hours of symptom onset and may be considered in select patients within 6–24 hours of symptom onset. The benefit of mechanical thrombectomy is less clear in posterior circulation occlusions and should be considered on a case-by-case basis.
- Decompressive hemicraniectomy is a surgical procedure to reduce intracranial pressure (typically due to cerebral edema) and can reduce mortality and improve functional outcome in select patients.
- For all ischemic stroke patients, coordinated care with a multidisciplinary approach to assessment and early rehabilitation reduces overall disability due to stroke.
- In secondary prevention, carotid endarterectomy of an ulcerated or stenotic carotid artery is effective in reducing stroke incidence and recurrence in appropriate patients and in centers where operative morbidity and mortality are low. In patients younger than age 70, carotid stenting is a less invasive alternative and can reduce recurrent stroke risk when combined with aspirin and clopidogrel therapy.

Hemorrhagic Stroke

- In SAH from ruptured intracranial aneurysm or AVM, early intervention with either surgical clipping or endovascular coiling of the vascular abnormality reduces mortality from rebleeding.
- Early surgical intervention and hematoma removal is recommended for patients with cerebellar hemorrhage and neurologic deterioration, brainstem compression, or hydrocephalus from ventricular obstruction. The usefulness of surgical hematoma evacuation is not well established for patients with cerebral hemorrhage.
- Ventricular drainage with an extraventricular drain (EVD) is reasonable in patients with hydrocephalus causing decreased consciousness.

Temperature Management

- Fever worsens outcomes in patients with both hemorrhagic and ischemic stroke. Identification of the source and pharmacologic and/or nonpharmacologic management is recommended to maintain normothermia range. Because of limited supporting data, induced hypothermia should be done only in the setting of controlled, clinical trials.

PHARMACOLOGIC THERAPY OF ISCHEMIC STROKE

- **Table 13-1** provides evidence-based recommendations for pharmacotherapy of ischemic stroke.
- **Alteplase** initiated within 4.5 hours of symptom onset improves functional ability after ischemic stroke. Adherence to a guideline-recommended protocol is essential to achieving positive outcomes: (1) activate the stroke team; (2) obtain CT scan to rule out hemorrhage; (3) treat as early as possible within 4.5 hours of symptom onset; (4) meet all inclusion criteria with no contraindications (**Table 13-2**); (5) administer alteplase 0.9 mg/kg IV total dose (maximum 90 mg), with 10% infused as an initial bolus over 1 minute and the remainder given over 1 hour; (6) avoid anticoagulant and antiplatelet therapy for 24 hours after alteplase; and (7) monitor the patient closely for elevated blood pressure (BP), neurologic status, and hemorrhage.
- **Aspirin** 160–325 mg/day started within 24–48 hours of symptom onset (and 24 hours after alteplase completion) reduces long-term death and disability. An alternate antiplatelet agent may be considered for patients with aspirin allergy or other severe contraindications.
- For patients with elevated BP who are eligible for alteplase, treatment to a goal BP <185/110 mm Hg is recommended before thrombolytic administration. While data are limited, it is also reasonable to maintain BP <185/110 mm Hg for patients undergoing mechanical thrombectomy. For patients not requiring IV thrombolysis or endovascular intervention, BP is often allowed to rise as high as 220/120 mm Hg for the first 48–72 hours because early BP reduction does not prevent death or improve the level of dependency. For patients with comorbid conditions requiring BP management, a reduction of 15% is probably safe. If BP is treated, short-acting and easily titrated IV agents are preferred:
  - ✓ **Labetalol:** 10–20 mg IV over 1–2 minutes; may repeat
  - ✓ **Nicardipine:** 5 mg/hr IV; titrate up by 2.5 mg/hr every 5–15 minutes; maximum 15 mg/hr
  - ✓ **Clevidipine:** 1–2 mg/hr IV; titrate by doubling the dose every 2–5 minutes; maximum 21 mg/hr
  - ✓ Other potential agents: **hydralazine, enalaprilat, nitroprusside** IV infusion, labetalol IV infusion

- Use of urgent anticoagulation (eg, unfractionated heparin or low-molecular-weight heparin) is not routinely recommended in the early phase of acute ischemic stroke treatment. Use of immediate anticoagulation for nonstroke indications (eg, prophylaxis of venous thromboembolism) should be weighed against the risk of intracranial hemorrhagic conversion.

TABLE 13-1	Recommendations for Pharmacotherapy of Ischemic Stroke	
	Recommendation	**Evidence[a]**
Acute treatment	Alteplase 0.9 mg/kg IV (maximum 90 mg), 10% as a bolus with remainder given over 1 hour in select patients within 3 hours of onset	IA
	Alteplase 0.9 mg/kg IV (maximum 90 mg), 10% as a bolus with remainder given over 1 hour in select patients between 3 and 4.5 hours of onset	IB
	Aspirin 160–325 mg daily started within 48 hours of onset	IA
Secondary prevention		
Noncardioembolic	Antiplatelet therapy	
	Aspirin 50–325 mg daily	IA
	Aspirin 25 mg + extended-release dipyridamole 200 mg twice daily	IB
	Clopidogrel 75 mg daily	IIaB
Cardioembolic (especially atrial fibrillation)	Anticoagulant therapy	
	Vitamin K antagonist (warfarin; target INR = 2.5)	IA
	Apixaban 5 mg twice daily	IA
	Dabigatran 150 mg twice daily	IB
	Edoxaban 60 mg daily	—[b]
	Rivaroxaban 20 mg daily	IIaB
Age ≤75 years	High-intensity statin therapy	IB
Age >75 years	Moderate- or high-intensity statin therapy	IIaB-R .
BP >140/90 mm Hg	BP reduction	IB-R

[a]Classes: I, evidence or general agreement about usefulness and effectiveness; II, conflicting evidence about usefulness; IIa, weight of evidence in favor of the treatment; IIb, usefulness less well established; III, not useful and maybe harmful. Levels of evidence: A, multiple randomized clinical trials; B, a single randomized trial or nonrandomized studies; C, expert opinion or case studies; B-R, moderate-quality evidence from one or more randomized controlled trials or meta-analyses of moderate-quality randomized controlled trials.
[b]Not graded in current guidelines.
INR, international normalized ratio; IV, intravenous.

- Secondary prevention of ischemic stroke:
  - ✓ All patients who have had an acute ischemic stroke or TIA should receive long-term antithrombotic therapy for secondary prevention. Antiplatelet therapy should be used in noncardioembolic stroke; **aspirin**, **extended-release dipyridamole plus aspirin**, and **clopidogrel** are all first-line agents (**Table 13-1**). Studies of the combination of clopidogrel plus ASA have shown conflicting results on reduction of recurrent stroke, and some found an increase in hemorrhagic events.
  - ✓ For patients with atrial fibrillation and a presumed cardiac source of embolism for stroke or TIA, oral anticoagulation with a vitamin K antagonist (**warfarin**), **apixaban**, **dabigatran**, **edoxaban**, or **rivaroxaban** is recommended.
  - ✓ Adults with previously treated hypertension who experience a stroke or TIA should be restarted on antihypertensive treatment after the first few days of the index event to reduce the risk of recurrent stroke and other vascular events. Useful options include a **thiazide diuretic**, **angiotensin-converting enzyme (ACE)**

TABLE 13-2 Inclusion Criteria and Contraindications to Alteplase Use in Acute Ischemic Stroke

Inclusion criteria
- Age 18 years or older
- Clinical diagnosis of ischemic stroke with neurologic deficit
- Time of symptom onset well established to be <4.5 hours before treatment would begin

Contraindications
- Symptoms/imaging consistent with SAH or acute intracerebral hemorrhage
- Current use of direct thrombin inhibitors or direct factor Xa inhibitors in prior 48 hours
- Use of treatment-dose low-molecular-weight heparin in prior 24 hours
- Infective endocarditis
- Intra-axial, intracranial neoplasm
- Aortic arch dissection
- Active internal bleeding or coagulopathy (platelets <100,000/mm³ [100 x 10⁹/L], INR>1.7, aPTT >40 sec, PT >15 sec)
- Severe head trauma in prior 3 months
- Gastrointestinal malignancy or bleeding within prior 21 days

Warnings/Use Clinical Judgment
- History of intracranial hemorrhage
- History of ischemic stroke within prior 3 months
- Unruptured/unsecured AVM or aneurysm >10 mm
- Major surgery or nonhead trauma
- History of bleeding diathesis
- Extensive regions of clear hypoattenuation on initial CT scan

aPTT, activated partial thromboplastin time; AVM, arteriovenous malformation; CT, computed tomography; INR, international normalized ratio; PT, prothrombin time; SAH, subarachnoid hemorrhage; TT, thrombin time.

inhibitor, **angiotensin receptor blocker**, or combination treatment with a thiazide plus ACE inhibitor. Selection of specific drugs should be individualized based on patient comorbidities. Adults not previously treated for hypertension who experience a stroke or TIA and have a BP ≥140/90 mm Hg should be prescribed antihypertensive treatment several days after the index event. A reasonable goal BP for patients who experienced a stroke or TIA is <130/80 mm Hg.

✓ **Statin** therapy is recommended to prevent stroke recurrence in all ischemic stroke patients regardless of baseline lipid levels. Patients ≤75 years of age experiencing ischemic stroke of presumed atherosclerotic origin should be treated with high-intensity statin therapy with a target of achieving ≥50% reduction in low-density lipoprotein (LDL) cholesterol. For patients older than age 75, moderate- or high-intensity statin therapy can be initiated as tolerated. **Ezetimibe** may be added for patients taking maximally tolerated statin therapy but with LDL cholesterol ≥70 mg/dL (1.81 mmol/L). A **proprotein convertase subtilisin/kexin type 9 (PCSK9) inhibitor** may be considered in very high-risk patients who are taking maximally tolerated statins and ezetimibe with LDL cholesterol ≥70 mg/dL (1.81 mmol/L).

PHARMACOLOGIC THERAPY OF HEMORRHAGIC STROKE

- The usefulness of pharmacotherapy is limited in spontaneous ICH.
- Because hypertension in hemorrhagic stroke increases the risk of hematoma expansion, it is reasonable for patients with a systolic BP >220 mm Hg to receive aggressive BP lowering with continuous IV infusion medications. Acute lowering of systolic BP to a goal of 140 mm Hg is safe and may improve functional outcome. For patients with SAH due to aneurysm rupture, BP control to at least a systolic BP <160 mm Hg is reasonable in the period from symptom onset to aneurysm obliteration.
- When intracranial hemorrhage occurs in a patient on anticoagulants, use of reversal agents to correct the medication-induced coagulopathy should be considered (**Table 13-3**).

TABLE 13-3	Select Anticoagulant Reversal	
Drug	**First-Line Reversal Recommendation**	**Alternate Treatment**
Warfarin	Vitamin K 10 mg IV × 1 -and- 4PCC INR 2 to <4: 25 units/kg, max 2500 units INR 4–6: 35 units/kg, max 3500 units INR >6: 50 units/kg, max 5000 units	Vitamin K 10 mg IV × 1 -and- FFP 10–15 mL/kg
Dabigatran	Idarucizumab 5 g IV × 1	Hemodialysis 4PCC 50 units/kg
Rivaroxaban ≤10 mg	Andexanet alfa 400 mg IV bolus at rate of 30 mg/min, followed by 4 mg/min IV infusion up to 120 min	4PCC 50 units/kg
Rivaroxaban >10 mg or unknown dose	If <8 hours since last dose or unknown time, andexanet alfa 800 mg IV bolus at rate of 30 mg/min, followed by 8 mg/min IV infusion up to 120 min If ≥8 hours since last dose, andexanet alfa 400 mg IV bolus at rate of 30 mg/min, followed by 4 mg/min IV infusion up to 120 min	4PCC 50 units/kg
Apixaban ≤5 mg	Andexanet alfa 400 mg IV bolus at rate of 30 mg/min, followed by 4 mg/min IV infusion up to 120 min	4PCC 50 units/kg
Apixaban >5 mg or unknown dose	If <8 hours since last dose or unknown time, andexanet alfa 800 mg IV bolus at rate of 30 mg/min, followed by 8 mg/min IV infusion up to 120 min If ≥8 hours since last dose, andexanet alfa 400 mg IV bolus at rate of 30 mg/min, followed by 4 mg/min IV infusion up to 120 min	4PCC 50 units/kg
Edoxaban	Andexanet alfa not studied	4PCC 50 units/kg

FFP, fresh frozen plasma; IV, intravenous; 4PCC, 4-factor prothrombin complex concentrate; INR, international normalized ratio.

EVALUATION OF THERAPEUTIC OUTCOMES

- Monitor patients with acute stroke intensely for development of neurologic worsening (recurrence or extension of stroke), complications (venous thromboembolism, infection), and adverse treatment effects.
- The most common reasons for clinical deterioration in stroke patients include: (1) extension of the original lesion in the brain; (2) development of cerebral edema and raised intracranial pressure; (3) hypertensive emergency; (4) infection (eg, urinary and respiratory tract); (5) venous thromboembolism; (6) electrolyte abnormalities and rhythm disturbances; and (7) recurrent stroke.

- For patients receiving alteplase therapy, monitor for bleeding with neurologic examination and BP every 15 minutes for 1 hour, then every half-hour for 6 hours, then every hour for 17 hours, then once every shift thereafter.
- For aspirin, clopidogrel, extended-release dipyridamole plus aspirin, warfarin, and other oral anticoagulants, monitor for bleeding daily.
- For patients receiving warfarin, check the PT/INR and hemoglobin/hematocrit daily.

See Chapter 38, Stroke, authored by Melody Ryan and Melisa Nestor, for a more detailed discussion of this topic.

Venous Thromboembolism

CHAPTER 14

- *Venous thromboembolism* (VTE) results from clot formation in the venous circulation and is manifested as deep vein thrombosis (DVT) and pulmonary embolism (PE).

PATHOPHYSIOLOGY

- Risk factors for VTE include increasing age, history of VTE, and aspects related to Virchow's triad: (1) blood stasis (eg, immobility and obesity); (2) vascular injury (eg, surgery, trauma, venous catheters); and (3) hypercoagulability (eg, malignancy, coagulation factor abnormalities, antiphospholipid antibodies, certain drugs).
- The most common inherited hypercoagulability disorder is activated protein C (aPC) resistance (Caucasian prevalence 2%–7%), which increases the risk of VTE three-fold. Most aPC resistance results from a factor V gene mutation (known as factor V Leiden) that renders it resistant to degradation by aPC.
- The prothrombin G20210A mutation is the second most frequent inherited hyper-coagulability disorder (Caucasian prevalence 2%–4%) and imparts a threefold increased risk of VTE. The mutation increases circulating prothrombin and may enhance thrombin generation.
- Inherited deficiencies of protein C, protein S, and antithrombin occur in <1% of the population and may increase the lifetime VTE risk by as much as sevenfold.
- Normal hemostasis maintains circulatory system integrity after blood vessel damage. Disruption of the endothelial cell lining with injury results in platelet activation and tissue-factor–mediated clotting factor cascade initiation, culminating in thrombin formation and ultimately a fibrin clot. In contrast to physiologic hemostasis, patho-logic VTE often occurs without gross vessel wall damage and may be triggered by tissue factor (TF) brought to the growing thrombus by circulating microparticles. Clots causing VTE impair blood flow and often cause complete vessel occlusion.
- Exposure of blood to damaged vessel endothelium causes platelets to become activated after binding to adhesion proteins (eg, von Willebrand factor, collagen). Activated platelets recruit additional platelets, causing growth of the platelet throm-bus. Activated platelets change shape and release components that sustain further thrombus formation at the site. Activated platelets express the adhesion molecule P-selectin, which facilitates capture of TF-bearing microparticles, resulting in fibrin clot formation via the coagulation cascade.
- The conceptual model for the coagulation cascade involves reactions that occur on cell surfaces in three overlapping phases (**Fig. 14-1**):
  - ✓ *Initiation*: A TF/VIIa complex (known as extrinsic tenase or X-ase) on cells bear-ing TF that have been exposed after vessel injury or captured via P-selectin acti-vates limited amounts of factors IX and X. Factor Xa then associates with factor Va to form the prothrombinase complex, which cleaves prothrombin (factor II) to generate a small amount of thrombin (factor IIa). Factor IXa moves to the surface of activated platelets in the growing platelet thrombus. Tissue factor pathway inhibitor (TFPI) regulates TF/VIIa-induced coagulation, rapidly terminating the initiation phase.
  - ✓ *Amplification*: Thrombin produced during the initiation phase activates factors V and VIII, which bind to platelet surfaces and support the large-scale thrombin generation occurring during the propagation phase. Platelet-bound factor XI is also activated by thrombin during amplification.
  - ✓ *Propagation*: A burst of thrombin generation occurs as factor VIIIa/IXa complex (known as intrinsic tenase) promotes factor Xa formation and prothrombinase complexes assemble on the surface of activated platelets, accelerating thrombin generation. Thrombin generation is further supported by factor XIa bound to platelet surfaces, which activates factor IX to form additional intrinsic tenase.

Platelet thrombus ⬤   P-selectin ⬤   Microparticle bearing tissue factor ⬤   Fibrin clot ∿

FIGURE 14-1. Model of pathologic thrombus formation: (A) activated platelets adhere to vascular endothelium; (B) activated platelets express P-selectin; (C) pathologic microparticles express active tissue factor and are present at a high concentration in the circulation—these microparticles accumulate, perhaps by binding to activated platelets expressing P-selectin; and (D) tissue factor can lead to thrombin generation, and thrombin generation leads to platelet thrombus formation and fibrin generation.

- Thrombin then converts fibrinogen to fibrin monomers that precipitate and polymerize to form fibrin strands. Factor XIIIa (also activated by thrombin) covalently bonds these strands to form an extensive meshwork that encases the aggregating platelet thrombus and red cells to form a stabilized fibrin clot.
- Hemostasis is controlled by antithrombotic substances produced by intact endothelium adjacent to damaged tissue. Thrombomodulin modulates thrombin activity by converting protein C to its activated form (aPC), which joins with protein S to inactivate factors Va and VIIIa. This prevents coagulation reactions from spreading to uninjured vessel walls. In addition, circulating antithrombin inhibits thrombin and factor Xa. Heparan sulfate is secreted by endothelial cells and accelerates antithrombin activity. These self-regulatory mechanisms limit fibrin clot formation to the zone of vessel injury.
- The fibrinolytic system dissolves formed blood clots; inactive plasminogen is converted to plasmin by tissue plasminogen activator (tPA). Plasmin is an enzyme that degrades the fibrin mesh into soluble end products (known as fibrin degradation products including D-dimer).
- Thrombi can form in any part of the venous circulation but usually begin in the leg(s). Isolated calf vein thrombi seldom embolize; those involving the popliteal and larger veins above it are more likely to embolize and lodge in the pulmonary artery or one of its branches, occluding blood flow to the lung and impairing gas exchange. Without treatment, the affected lung area becomes necrotic and oxygen delivery to other vital organs may decrease, potentially resulting in fatal circulatory collapse.

CLINICAL PRESENTATION

- Some patients with DVT are asymptomatic. Symptoms may include unilateral leg swelling, pain, tenderness, erythema, and warmth. Physical signs may include a palpable cord and a positive Homan sign.
- Symptoms of PE may include cough, chest pain or tightness, shortness of breath, palpitations, hemoptysis, dizziness, or lightheadedness. Signs of PE include tachypnea, tachycardia, diaphoresis, cyanosis, hypotension, shock, and cardiovascular collapse.
- Postthrombotic syndrome may produce chronic lower extremity swelling, pain, tenderness, skin discoloration, and ulceration.

DIAGNOSIS

- Assessment should focus on identifying risk factors (see section Pathophysiology).
- Compression ultrasound (CUS) and computed tomography pulmonary angiography (CTPA) are used most often for initial evaluation of suspected VTE.

- Radiographic contrast studies (venography, pulmonary angiography) are the most accurate and reliable diagnostic methods but are expensive, invasive, and difficult to perform and evaluate. The ventilation-perfusion (V/Q) scan is an alternative PE diagnostic test.
- Serum concentration of D-dimer is nearly always elevated; values <500 ng/mL (mcg/L) combined with clinical probability scores are useful in ruling out VTE.
- Clinical assessment checklists (eg, Wells score) can be used to determine whether a patient is likely or unlikely to have DVT or PE.

TREATMENT

- Goals of Treatment: The initial goal is to prevent VTE in at-risk populations. Treatment of VTE is aimed at preventing thrombus extension and embolization, reducing recurrence risk, and preventing long-term complications (eg, postthrombotic syndrome, chronic thromboembolic pulmonary hypertension).

PREVENTION OF VTE

- Nonpharmacologic methods improve venous blood flow by mechanical means and include early ambulation, graduated compression stockings, intermittent pneumatic compression (IPC) devices, and inferior vena cava filters.
- Hospitalized and acutely ill medical patients at high VTE risk and low bleeding risk should receive pharmacologic prophylaxis with **low-dose unfractionated heparin (LDUH)**, **low-molecular-weight heparin (LMWH)**, **fondaparinux**, or **betrixaban** during hospitalization or until fully ambulatory. Routine pharmacologic prophylaxis is not warranted in low-risk medical patients.
- In general, nonorthopedic surgery patients at high VTE risk but low bleeding risk should receive **LDUH** or **LMWH** prophylaxis plus graduated compression stockings or IPC. Low-risk patients able to ambulate early after surgery do not routinely require VTE prophylaxis.
- Recommended VTE prophylaxis following joint replacement surgery may include **aspirin**, adjusted-dose **warfarin, LDUH, LMWH, fondaparinux, dabigatran, apixaban**, or **rivaroxaban** for at least 10 days postsurgery.
- VTE prophylaxis after surgery should be given throughout the period of increased VTE risk. For general surgical procedures, prophylaxis can be discontinued when patients are able to ambulate and have no other VTE risk factors. Extended prophylaxis may be beneficial for patients undergoing lower extremity orthopedic procedures; most clinical trials support use of prophylaxis for 15–42 days after total knee or hip replacement surgery.
- Refer to *Antithrombotic Therapy and Prevention of Thrombosis, 9th edition: Evidence-Based Clinical Practice Guidelines* published by the American College of Chest Physicians for information on prophylaxis strategies based on clinical situation and risk level for VTE.

GENERAL APPROACH TO TREATMENT OF VTE

- Anticoagulation is the primary treatment for VTE; DVT and PE are treated similarly (**Fig. 14-2**).
- After VTE is confirmed objectively, therapy with a rapid-acting anticoagulant should be instituted as soon as possible. Anticoagulants can be administered in the outpatient setting in most patients with DVT and in carefully selected hemodynamically stable patients with PE.
- Stable patients with DVT or PE who have normal vital signs, low bleeding risk, and no other uncontrolled comorbid conditions requiring hospitalization can be discharged early or treated entirely on an outpatient basis (if considered appropriate candidates). Hemodynamically unstable patients with PE should be admitted for initiation of anticoagulation therapy.
- Three months is the appropriate initial duration of anticoagulation therapy for the acute first episode of VTE for all patients. This duration is also recommended when the initial thrombotic event was associated with a major transient or reversible risk factor (eg, surgery, hospitalization).

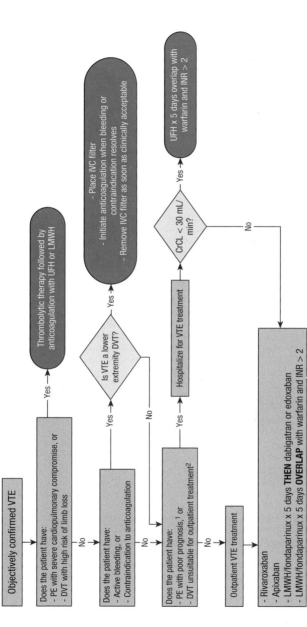

FIGURE 14-2. Acute treatment of venous thromboembolism (VTE).

[1]PESI score ≥86 points: age (1 pt for each year); male sex (10 pts); cancer (30 pts); heart failure (10 pts); COPD (10 pts); heart rate >110 bpm (20 pts); respiratory rate >30/min (20 pts); temperature <36°C (20 pts); altered mental status (60 pts); O₂ sat <90% (20 pts).

[2]Severe symptoms, renal impairment, inability to obtain or administer appropriate initial anticoagulant therapy, or high bleeding risk.

(CrCl, creatinine clearance via Cockcroft and Gault equation; DVT, deep vein thrombosis; INR, international normalized ratio; IVC, inferior vena cava; LMWH, low-molecular-weight heparin; PE, pulmonary embolism; UFH, unfractionated heparin; VTE, venous thromboembolism [includes DVT and PE].)

- Continuing anticoagulation is required to prevent new VTE episodes not directly related to the preceding episode. Consider extended therapy beyond 3 months for patients with a first provoked (idiopathic) VTE when feasible because of a relatively high recurrence rate. In patients with VTE and active cancer, extended therapy is rarely stopped because of a high recurrence risk.

NONPHARMACOLOGIC THERAPY

- Encourage patients to ambulate as much as symptoms permit.
- Ambulation in conjunction with graduated compression stockings results in faster reduction in pain and swelling than strict bedrest with no increase in embolization rate.
- Inferior vena cava filters should only be used when anticoagulants are contraindicated due to active bleeding.
- Elimination of the obstructing thrombus via thrombolysis or thrombectomy may be warranted in life- or limb-threatening DVT.

PHARMACOLOGIC THERAPY

Direct Oral Anticoagulants (DOACs)

- **Rivaroxaban**, **apixaban**, **edoxaban**, and **betrixaban** are oral selective inhibitors of both free and clot-bound factor Xa and do not require antithrombin to exert their anticoagulant effect. **Dabigatran** is an oral selective, reversible, direct factor IIa inhibitor.
- See **Table 14-1** for DOAC indications and dosing. Use DOACs with caution in patients with renal dysfunction.
- Single-drug oral therapy with rivaroxaban or apixaban produces similar rates of recurrent VTE compared to traditional therapy with warfarin overlapped with enoxaparin and perhaps less major bleeding. Both drugs are initiated with a higher dose and subsequently reduced to a maintenance dose. Until further data are available, these drugs should not be used in patients with creatinine clearance (CrCl) <25 mL/min (0.42 mL/s), active cancer, and patients requiring thrombolytic therapy. Neither drug requires routine anticoagulation monitoring, but the high acquisition cost may be a barrier for some patients.
- Edoxaban and dabigatran must be given only after at least 5 days of subcutaneous (SC) anticoagulation with UFH, LMWH, or fondaparinux. These regimens were noninferior to warfarin in patients with acute VTE for the outcome of recurrent VTE. Compared to warfarin, dabigatran caused similar major bleeding and edoxaban caused significantly less bleeding. Until further data are available, these agents should not be given to patients with hemodynamically unstable PE or at high bleeding risk.
- Bleeding is the most common adverse effect with DOAC therapy. Patients experiencing significant bleeding should receive routine supportive care and discontinuation of anticoagulant therapy. **Idarucizumab** (Praxbind) 5 g IV rapidly reverses the dabigatran anticoagulant effect when needed during emergency situations (eg, life-threatening bleeding) and when there is need for urgent surgical intervention. **Recombinant coagulation factor Xa** (also known as **andexanet alfa**; Andexxa) can reverse life-threatening bleeding in patients taking rivaroxaban or apixaban. Adding aspirin to DOAC therapy nearly doubles bleeding rates and should be avoided in most patients with VTE. All DOACs are P-gp substrates and subject to changes in anticoagulant effect when coadministered with P-gp inhibitors or inducers. Rivaroxaban and apixaban are subject to interactions involving inhibitors or inducers of CYP 3A4.

Low-Molecular-Weight Heparin

- LMWH fragments produced by either chemical or enzymatic depolymerization of UFH are heterogeneous mixtures of sulfated glycosaminoglycans with approximately one-third the mean UFH molecular weight. LMWH prevents thrombus propagation by accelerating the activity of antithrombin similar to UFH.

TABLE 14-1	Approved Indications and Dosing for the Direct Oral Anticoagulants		
Generic (Brand) Name	VTE Prophylaxis	Acute VTE Treatment	Reduction in Risk of Recurrent VTE in Patients at Continued Risk
Dabigatran (Pradaxa)	Hip replacement surgery: CrCl >30 mL/min: 110 mg the first day beginning 1–4 hours after surgery once hemostasis is achieved, then 220 mg once daily for 28–35 days CrCl ≤30 mL/min or on dialysis: Dosing recommendations cannot be provided	150 mg PO twice daily with or without food FOLLOWING at least 5 days of parenteral anticoagulant therapy	150 mg PO twice daily with or without food
Rivaroxaban (Xarelto)	Hip or knee replacement surgery: 10 mg PO once daily with or without food beginning 6–10 hours after surgery once hemostasis is achieved and continuing for 12 (knee) to 35 (hip) days	15 mg PO twice daily with food for days 1–21, then 20 mg PO once daily with food beginning on day 22	10 mg PO once daily with or without food
Apixaban (Eliquis)	Hip or knee replacement surgery: 2.5 mg PO twice daily with or without food beginning 12–24 hours after surgery and continuing for 12 (knee) or 35 (hip) days	10 mg PO twice daily with or without food on days 1–7, then 5 mg PO twice daily beginning on day 8	2.5 mg PO twice daily with or without food
Edoxaban (Savaysa)	Not approved for use	60 mg PO once daily with or without food FOLLOWING at least 5 days of parenteral anticoagulant therapy; 30 mg once daily with CrCl 15–50 mL/min (0.25–0.83 mL/sec) or body weight ≤60 kg or who use certain P-gp inhibitors	Not approved for use
Betrixaban (Bevyxxa)	Adults hospitalized for acute medical illness: Initial single dose of 160 mg PO with food, followed by 80 mg once daily with food for 35–42 days	Not approved for use	Not approved for use

PO, by mouth; CrCl, creatinine clearance; P-gp, P-glycoprotein; VTE, venous thromboembolism.

- LMWH given SC in fixed, weight-based doses is at least as effective as UFH given IV for VTE treatment. LMWH has largely replaced UFH for initial VTE treatment due to improved pharmacokinetic and pharmacodynamic profiles and ease of use. Advantages of LMWH over UFH include: (1) predictable anticoagulation dose response; (2) improved SC bioavailability; (3) dose-independent clearance; (4) longer biologic half-life; (5) lower incidence of thrombocytopenia; and (6) less need for routine laboratory monitoring.
- Recommended doses (based on actual body weight) include:
  ✓ **Enoxaparin** (Lovenox): For acute DVT treatment with or without PE, 1 mg/kg SC every 12 hours or 1.5 mg/kg every 24 hours;
  ✓ **Dalteparin** (Fragmin): For acute DVT treatment, 200 units/kg SC once daily or 100 units/kg SC twice daily (not FDA approved in the United States for this indication). For VTE in patients with cancer, 200 units/kg SC every 24 hours for 30 days, followed by 150 units SC every 24 hours. The maximum total daily dose is 18,000 units.
- In patients without cancer, acute LMWH treatment is generally transitioned to long-term warfarin therapy after 5–10 days.
- Routine laboratory monitoring is unnecessary because LMWH anticoagulant response is predictable when given SC. Prior to initiating therapy, obtain a baseline complete blood cell count (CBC) with platelet count and serum creatinine. Check the CBC every 5–10 days during the first 2 weeks of LMWH therapy and every 2–4 weeks thereafter to monitor for occult bleeding. Measuring anti–factor Xa activity is the most widely used method to monitor LMWH; routine measurement is unnecessary in stable, uncomplicated patients. Monitoring may be considered in patients who have significant renal impairment, are morbidly obese, or are pregnant.
- As with other anticoagulants, bleeding is the most common adverse effect of LMWH therapy, but major bleeding may be less common than with UFH. If major bleeding occurs, IV **protamine sulfate** can be administered, but it cannot neutralize the anticoagulant effect completely. The recommended protamine sulfate dose is 1 mg per 1 mg of enoxaparin or 1 mg per 100 anti–factor Xa units of dalteparin administered in the previous 8 hours. A second dose of 0.5 mg per 1 mg or 100 anti–factor Xa units can be given if bleeding continues. Smaller protamine doses can be used if the LMWH dose was given in the previous 8–12 hours. Protamine sulfate is not recommended if the LMWH was given more than 12 hours earlier.
- Thrombocytopenia can occur with LMWHs, but the incidence of heparin-induced thrombocytopenia (HIT) is one-third that of UFH. LMWH has been associated with osteopenia, but the risk of osteoporosis appears to be lower with LMWH than with UFH.

Fondaparinux

- **Fondaparinux** (Arixtra) prevents thrombus generation and clot formation by indirectly inhibiting factor Xa activity through its interaction with antithrombin. Unlike UFH or LMWH, fondaparinux inhibits only factor Xa activity.
- Fondaparinux is a safe and effective alternative to LMWH for acute VTE treatment and is likewise followed by long-term warfarin therapy.
- Fondaparinux is dosed once daily via weight-based SC injection: 5 mg if <50 kg, 7.5 mg if 50–100 kg, and 10 mg if >100 kg.
- Patients receiving fondaparinux do not require routine coagulation testing. Determine baseline kidney function before starting therapy because fondaparinux is contraindicated if CrCl is <30 mL/min (0.5 mL/s).
- Bleeding is the primary adverse effect associated with fondaparinux therapy. Measure CBC at baseline and periodically thereafter to detect occult bleeding. Monitor for signs and symptoms of bleeding daily. There is no specific antidote to reverse the antithrombotic activity of fondaparinux.

Unfractionated Heparin

- **Unfractionated heparin** binds to antithrombin, provoking a conformation change that makes it much more potent in inhibiting the activity of factors IXa, Xa, XIIa, and IIa.

This prevents thrombus growth and propagation allowing endogenous thrombolytic systems to lyse the clot. Because some patients fail to achieve an adequate response, IV UFH has largely been replaced by LMWH, fondaparinux, and DOACs. UFH continues to have a role in patients with CrCl <30 mL/min (0.5 mL/s) and unstable patients.

- When immediate and full anticoagulation is required, a weight-based IV loading dose followed by a continuous IV infusion is preferred (Table 14-2). Subcutaneous UFH (initial dose 333 units/kg followed by 250 units/kg every 12 hours) also provides adequate anticoagulation for treatment of acute VTE.

- The activated partial thromboplastin time (aPTT) is generally recommended for monitoring UFH, provided that institution-specific therapeutic ranges are defined. Measure aPTT prior to initiation of therapy and 6 hours after the start of therapy or a dose change. Adjust the UFH dose based on patient response and the institution-specific aPTT therapeutic range.

- Monitor patients closely for bleeding signs and symptoms during UFH therapy. If major bleeding occurs, discontinue UFH immediately, identify and treat the underlying bleeding source, and give **protamine sulfate** by slow IV infusion over 10 minutes (1 mg/100 units of UFH infused during the previous 4 hours; maximum 50 mg).

- HIT is a rare immunologic reaction requiring immediate intervention and that may be fatal. The most common complication of HIT is VTE; arterial thrombosis occurs less frequently. Thrombocytopenia is the most common clinical manifestation, but serologic confirmation of heparin antibodies is required to diagnose HIT. Use of a clinical prediction rule, such as the 4Ts score (Thrombocytopenia, Timing of platelet count fall or thrombosis, Thrombosis, oTher explanation for thrombocytopenia), can improve the predictive value of platelet count monitoring and heparin antibody testing. Discontinue all heparin if new thrombosis occurs in the setting of falling platelets in conjunction with a moderate or high 4Ts score. Alternative anticoagulation with a direct thrombin inhibitor should then be initiated.

- Using UFH doses of 20,000 units/day or more for longer than 6 months, especially during pregnancy, is associated with significant bone loss and may lead to osteoporosis.

TABLE 14-2	Weight-Based[a] Dosing for Unfractionated Heparin Administered by Continuous IV Infusion	
Indication	**Initial Loading Dose**	**Initial Infusion Rate**
Deep venous thrombosis/ pulmonary embolism	80–100 units/kg Maximum = 10,000 units	17–20 units/kg/hr Maximum = 2300 units/hr
Activated Partial Thromboplastin Time (seconds)	**Maintenance Infusion Rate**	
	Dose Adjustment	
<37 (or anti–factor Xa <0.20 unit/mL [kU/L])	80 units/kg bolus, and then increase infusion by 4 units/kg/hr	
37–47 (or anti–factor Xa 0.20–0.29 unit/mL [kU/L])	40 units/kg bolus, and then increase infusion by 2 units/kg/hr	
48–71 (or anti–factor Xa 0.30–0.70 unit/mL [kU/L])	No change	
72–93 (or anti–factor Xa 0.71–1 unit/mL [kU/L])	Decrease infusion by 1–2 units/kg/hr	
>93 (or anti–factor Xa >1 unit/mL [kU/L])	Hold infusion for 1 hour, and then decrease by 3 units/kg/hr	

[a]Use actual body weight for all calculations. Adjusted body weight may be used for obese patients (>130% of ideal body weight).

Warfarin

- **Warfarin** inhibits enzymes responsible for cyclic interconversion of vitamin K in the liver. Reduced vitamin K is a cofactor required for carboxylation of the vitamin K–dependent coagulation factors II (prothrombin), VII, IX, and X and the endogenous anticoagulant proteins C and S. By inhibiting the reduced vitamin K supply needed for production of these proteins, warfarin therapy produces coagulation proteins with less activity. By suppressing clotting factor production, warfarin prevents initial thrombus formation and propagation. The time required to achieve its anticoagulant effect depends on the elimination half-lives of the coagulation proteins (6 hours for factor VII and 72 hours for prothrombin). Full antithrombotic effect is not achieved for at least 6 days after warfarin therapy initiation.
- Because of its slow onset of effect, warfarin must be started concurrently with rapid-acting injectable anticoagulant therapy with an overlap of at least 5 days and until an international normalized ratio (INR) of 2 or greater has been achieved for at least 24 hours.
- Guidelines for initiating warfarin therapy are given in **Figure 14-3**. The initial dose should be 5–10 mg for most patients. Lower starting doses may be acceptable in patients with advanced age, malnutrition, liver disease, or heart failure. Starting doses more than 10 mg should be avoided.
- Monitor warfarin therapy by the INR; the recommended target INR for VTE treatment is 2.5, with an acceptable range of 2–3. After an acute thromboembolic event, obtain a baseline INR and CBC prior to initiating warfarin and every 1–3 days until stabilized. Once the patient's dose response is established, obtain an INR every 7–14 days until it stabilizes, then ideally every 4–12 weeks thereafter.
- In general, maintenance dose changes should not be made more frequently than every 3 days. Adjust maintenance doses by calculating the weekly dose and reducing or increasing it by 5%–25%. The full effect of a dose changes may not become evident for 5–7 days.
- Warfarin's primary adverse effect is bleeding that can range from mild to life threatening. It does not cause bleeding per se, but it exacerbates bleeding from existing lesions and enables massive bleeding from ordinarily minor sources. The likelihood of bleeding rises with increasing INR values; therefore, maintaining the INR within the target range is important to reduce bleeding risk:
  - ✓ When the INR is >4.5 without evidence of bleeding, the INR can be lowered by withholding warfarin, adjusting the warfarin dose, and/or providing a small dose of vitamin K to shorten the time to return to normal INR. Although vitamin K can be given parenterally or orally, the oral route is preferred in the absence of serious bleeding.
  - ✓ If the INR is between 5 and 10 and no bleeding is present, routine vitamin K use is not recommended because it has not been shown to affect the risk of developing subsequent bleeding or thromboembolism compared to simply withholding warfarin alone.
  - ✓ For INR >10 without evidence of bleeding, oral vitamin K (**phytonadione** 2.5 mg) is suggested. Use vitamin K with caution in patients at high risk of recurrent thromboembolism because of the possibility of INR overcorrection.
- Patients with warfarin-associated major bleeding require supportive care. Rapid reversal of anticoagulation with a four-factor prothrombin complex concentrate and 5–10 mg of vitamin K given by slow IV injection are also recommended.
- Nonhemorrhagic adverse effects of warfarin include the rare "purple toe" syndrome and skin necrosis.
- Because of the large number of food–drug and drug–drug interactions with warfarin, close monitoring and additional INR determinations may be indicated when other medications are initiated or discontinued or a change in consumption of vitamin K–containing foods occurs.

Thrombolytics

- Thrombolytic agents are proteolytic enzymes that enhance conversion of plasminogen to plasmin, which subsequently degrades the fibrin matrix.

(INR, international normalized ratio; PT, prothrombin time.)

FIGURE 14-3. Initiation of warfarin therapy.

- Most patients with VTE do not require thrombolytic therapy. Treatment should be reserved for patients who present with extensive proximal (eg, ileofemoral) DVT within 14 days of symptom onset, have good functional status, and are at low risk of bleeding.
- Patients with massive PE and evidence of hemodynamic compromise (hypotension or shock) should receive thrombolytic therapy unless contraindicated by bleeding risk.
- The same duration and intensity of anticoagulation therapy is recommended as for DVT patients not receiving thrombolysis. Patients with DVT involving the iliac and common femoral veins are at highest risk for postthrombotic syndrome and may receive the greatest benefit from thrombus removal strategies.

- For patients with massive PE manifested by shock and cardiovascular collapse (~5% of patients with PE), thrombolytic therapy is considered necessary in addition to aggressive interventions such as volume expansion, vasopressor therapy, intubation, and mechanical ventilation. Administer thrombolytic therapy in these patients without delay to reduce the risk of progression to multisystem organ failure and death. However, the risk of death from PE should outweigh the risk of serious bleeding associated with thrombolytic therapy.
- **Alteplase** (Activase) 100 mg by IV infusion over 2 hours is the most commonly used thrombolytic therapy for patients with PE.
- Before giving thrombolytic therapy for PE, IV UFH should be administered in full therapeutic doses. During thrombolytic therapy, IV UFH may be either continued or suspended; the most common practice in the United States is to suspend UFH.
- Measure the aPTT after completion of thrombolytic therapy. If the aPTT is <80 seconds, start UFH infusion and adjust to maintain the aPTT in the therapeutic range. If the posttreatment aPTT is >80 seconds, remeasure it every 2–4 hours and start UFH infusion when the aPTT is <80 seconds.

EVALUATION OF THERAPEUTIC OUTCOMES

- Monitor patients for resolution of symptoms, development of recurrent thrombosis, symptoms of postthrombotic syndrome, and adverse anticoagulant effects.
- Monitor hemoglobin, hematocrit, and blood pressure carefully to detect bleeding from anticoagulant therapy.
- Perform coagulation tests (aPTT, PT, INR) prior to initiating therapy to establish the patient's baseline values and guide later anticoagulation.
- Ask outpatients taking warfarin about medication adherence to prior dosing instructions, other medication use, changes in health status, and symptoms related to bleeding and thromboembolic complications. Any changes in concurrent medications should be carefully explored, and dietary intake of vitamin K-rich foods should be assessed.

See Chapter 37, Venous Thromboembolism, authored by Daniel M. Witt, Nathan P. Clark, and Sara R. Vazquez, for a more detailed discussion of this topic.

CHAPTER

15 | Acne Vulgaris

- *Acne* is a chronic skin disease characterized by open or closed comedones and inflammatory lesions, including papules, pustules, and nodules (cysts).

PATHOPHYSIOLOGY

- Acne usually begins during prepuberty and progresses as androgen production and sebaceous gland activity increase with gonad development.
- Acne progresses through four stages: (1) increased sebum production by sebaceous glands, (2) *Propionibacterium acnes* (renamed *Cutibacterium acnes*) follicular colonization (and bacterial lipolysis of sebum triglycerides to free fatty acids), (3) release of inflammatory mediators, and (4) increased follicular keratinization.
- Circulating androgens cause sebaceous glands to increase their size and activity. There is increased keratinization of epidermal cells and development of an obstructed sebaceous follicle, called a *microcomedone*. Cells adhere to each other, forming a dense keratinous plug. Sebum, produced in increasing amounts, becomes trapped behind the keratin plug and solidifies, contributing to open or closed comedone formation.
- Pooling of sebum in the follicle facilitates proliferation of the anaerobic bacterium *P. acnes*, which generates a T-cell response resulting in inflammation. *P. acnes* produces a lipase that hydrolyzes sebum triglycerides into free fatty acids that may increase keratinization and lead to microcomedone formation.
- *Noninflammatory acne* lesions include closed comedones (whiteheads) and open comedones (blackheads). Closed comedones are the first visible lesion in acne; they are almost completely obstructed to drainage and have a tendency to rupture. Open comedones are formed as the plug extends to the upper canal and dilates its opening.
- *Inflammatory acne* lesions include papules, pustules, and nodules. Pus formation occurs due to recruitment of neutrophils into the follicle during the inflammatory process and release of *P. acnes*–generated chemokines. *P. acnes* also produces enzymes that increase permeability of the follicular wall, causing it to rupture, thereby releasing keratin, lipids, and irritating free fatty acids into the dermis.

CLINICAL PRESENTATION

- Lesions usually occur on the face, back, neck, shoulders, and chest and may extend to the buttocks or extremities. One or more anatomic areas may be involved; once present, the pattern of involvement tends to remain constant. The skin, scalp, and hair are frequently oily.
- Lesions may take months to heal completely. Nodules and deep lesions may result in scarring. Resolution of inflammatory lesions may leave erythematous or pigmented macules (hyperpigmentation) that persist for months or longer, especially in dark-skinned individuals.

DIAGNOSIS

- Diagnosis is established by patient assessment, which includes observation of lesions and excluding other potential causes (eg, drug-induced acne). Several different systems are in use to grade acne severity.

TREATMENT

- <u>Goals of Treatment</u>: Reduce the number and severity of lesions, improve appearance, slow progression, limit duration and recurrence, prevent disfigurement from scarring and hyperpigmentation, and avoid psychologic suffering.

GENERAL APPROACH

- Acne is a chronic disease that warrants early and aggressive treatment (**Fig. 15-1**). Maintenance therapy is often needed for optimal outcomes. Patient adherence to lengthy treatment regimens is crucial to long-term control.
- Eliminating follicular occlusion will arrest the acne cascade. Nondrug and pharmacologic measures should be directed toward cleansing, reducing triggers, and combination therapy targeting all four pathogenic mechanisms.
- Combination therapy is often more effective than single therapy and may decrease side effects and minimize resistance or tolerance to individual treatments.
- Topical therapy is standard treatment for mild-to-moderate acne, whereas systemic therapy is required for moderate-to-severe acne.
- First-, second-, and third-line therapies should be selected and altered as appropriate for the severity and staging of the disease. Treatment is directed at control, not cure. Regimens should be tapered over time, adjusting to response.
- Combine the smallest number of agents at the lowest possible dosages to ensure efficacy, safety, avoidance of resistance, and patient adherence. Once control is achieved, simplify the regimen but continue with some suppressive therapy.

NONPHARMACOLOGIC THERAPY

- Encourage patients to avoid aggravating factors (eg, mechanical occlusion, cosmetics), maintain a balanced low-glycemic-load diet, and control stress.
- Patients should wash twice daily with a mild, nonfragranced opaque or glycerin soap or a soapless cleanser. Scrubbing should be minimized to prevent follicular rupture.
- Males using a safety razor for shaving should soften the beard with soap and warm water or shaving gel. Shaving should be done lightly and infrequently, using a sharp blade and being careful to avoid nicking lesions. Strokes should be in the direction of hair growth, shaving each area only once to minimize irritation.

© Debra Sibbald

FIGURE 15-1. Acne pathogenesis and drug mechanisms.

- Comedone extraction results in immediate cosmetic improvement but has not been widely tested in clinical trials.
- Light therapies are believed to work by killing *P. acnes* and by damaging and shrinking sebaceous glands, reducing sebum output with few or temporary adverse effects. Light therapies may be used once or twice weekly over a course of 6–10 treatments, with each irradiation lasting 10–20 minutes. Home-use blue light therapy is now available.

PHARMACOLOGIC THERAPY

- *Comedonal noninflammatory acne*: Select topical agents that target the increased keratinization by producing exfoliation. Topical retinoids (especially adapalene) or a fixed combination with a retinoid (eg, adapalene plus benzoyl peroxide) are drugs of choice. Benzoyl peroxide, azelaic acid, or salicylic acid are second-line alternatives.
- *Mild-to-moderate papulopustular inflammatory acne*: It is important to reduce the population of *P. acnes* in follicles. Either the fixed-dose combination of adapalene plus benzoyl peroxide or benzoyl peroxide, topical retinoid, or azelaic acid are recommended as first choice therapy. In moderate papulopustular inflammatory acne, the fixed-dose combination is preferred, with or without hormonal therapy and/or antibiotic, particularly if the trunk is involved. If there are limitations in use of first-choice agents, alternatives include blue light monotherapy, alternate combination therapy (such as fixed-dose combination of erythromycin plus tretinoin), or oral zinc. In cases of widespread disease, combining an oral antibiotic with topical benzoyl peroxide with or without adapalene can be considered.
- *Moderately severe or severe papulopustular or moderate nodular acne*: An oral antibiotic plus the fixed-dose topical combination is preferred. Alternatively, oral isotretinoin or oral hormonal therapy can be added. If there are limitations to use of these agents, consider oral antiandrogens in combination with oral antibiotics or topical treatments.
- *Nodular or conglobate acne*: Monotherapy with oral isotretinoin is first choice. As alternatives, a retinoid fixed combination or oral antibiotic can be recommended. For females, oral isotretinoin plus antiandrogenic hormonal therapy is preferred. Alternatively, a fixed combination retinoid with oral antibiotics and/or an oral antiandrogen can be recommended.
- *Maintenance acne therapy*: A topical retinoid alone or a retinoid plus benzoyl peroxide fixed-dose combination is most commonly recommended. Topical azelaic acid is an alternative. Maintenance is usually begun after a 12-week induction period and continues for 3–4 months. A longer duration may be necessary to prevent relapse upon discontinuation. Long-term therapy with antibiotics is not recommended to minimize antibiotic resistance.

Exfoliants (Peeling Agents)

- Exfoliants induce continuous mild drying and peeling by irritation, damaging superficial skin layers and inciting inflammation. This stimulates mitosis, thickening the epidermis and increasing horny cells, scaling, and erythema. Decreased sweating results in a dry, less oily surface and may resolve pustular lesions.
- **Resorcinol** is less keratolytic than salicylic acid and, when used alone, is classified by the Food and Drug Administration (FDA) as category II (not generally recognized as safe and effective). The FDA considers resorcinol 2% and resorcinol monoacetate 3% to be safe and effective when used in combination with sulfur 3%–8%. Resorcinol is an irritant and sensitizer and should not be applied to large areas or on broken skin. It produces a reversible dark brown scale on some dark-skinned individuals.
- **Salicylic acid** is a comedolytic agent available over the counter in 0.5%–2% strengths; concentrations between 3% and 6% are keratolytic, softening the horny layer and producing shedding of scales. It has mild antibacterial activity against *P. acnes* and offers slight anti-inflammatory activity at concentrations up to 5%. Salicylic acid is recognized by the FDA as safe and effective, but it offers no advantages over benzoyl peroxide or topical retinoids. Salicylic acid products are often used as first-line therapy

for mild acne because of their availability without a prescription in alcohol–detergent impregnated pads, washes, bars, and semisolid vehicles. Both wash-off and leave-on preparations are well tolerated. Lower concentrations are sometimes combined with sulfur to produce an additive keratolytic effect. Concentrations of 5%–10% can also be used by prescription, beginning with a low concentration and increasing as tolerance develops to the irritation. Salicylic acid is often used when patients cannot tolerate topical retinoids because of skin irritation.

- **Sulfur** is keratolytic and has antibacterial activity. It can quickly resolve pustules and papules, mask lesions, and produce irritation that leads to skin peeling. Sulfur is used in the precipitated or colloidal form in concentrations of 2%–10%. Although it is often combined with salicylic acid or resorcinol to increase effect, use is limited by offensive odor and availability of more effective agents.

Topical Retinoids

- Retinoids reduce obstruction within the follicle and are useful for both comedonal and inflammatory acne. They reverse abnormal keratinocyte desquamation and are active keratolytics. They inhibit microcomedone formation, decreasing the number of mature comedones and inflammatory lesions.
- Topical retinoids are safe, effective, and economical for treating all but the most severe cases of acne. They should be the first step in moderate acne, alone or with antibiotics and benzoyl peroxide, reverting to retinoids alone for maintenance once adequate results are achieved. Combination products containing benzoyl peroxide or topical antimicrobials are available.
- Retinoids can produce extended periods of remission if accompanying irritation does not impede patient adherence. Side effects of dryness, peeling, erythema, and irritation can be mitigated by reduced frequency of application.
- Retinoids should be applied at night, a half hour after cleansing, starting with every other night for 1–2 weeks to adjust to irritation. Doses can be increased only after 4–6 weeks of the lowest concentration and least irritating vehicle. Gels and creams are less irritating than solutions.
- **Tretinoin** (retinoic acid, vitamin A acid) is available in various strengths in creams, gels, and pumps. Tretinoin should not be used in pregnant women because of risk to the fetus.
- **Adapalene** (Differin) is the topical retinoid of first choice for both treatment and maintenance therapy because it is as effective but less irritating than other topical retinoids. Adapalene is available as 0.1% gel (nonprescription for once-daily application by patients age 12 years and older), cream, solution, lotion, and pads. A 0.3% gel is also available. It is also available in fixed-dose combinations with benzoyl peroxide to increase efficacy over monotherapies.
- **Tazarotene** (Tazorac) is as effective as adapalene in reducing noninflammatory and inflammatory lesion counts when applied half as frequently. Compared with tretinoin, it is as effective for comedonal and more effective for inflammatory lesions when applied once daily. The product is available as a 0.05% and 0.1% cream or gel and a 0.1% foam. Tazarotene is contraindicated in pregnancy.
- **Trifarotene** (Aklief) was approved in the United States in late 2019 for treatment of acne in patients age 9 years and older. The product is available as a 0.005% cream for application once daily in the evening.

Topical Antibacterial Agents

- **Benzoyl peroxide** is bactericidal to *P. acnes* and is also mildly comedolytic. It suppresses sebum production and reduces free fatty acids, which are comedogenic and trigger inflammation. No resistance has been reported, and addition of benzoyl peroxide to antibiotic therapy improves efficacy and may reduce resistance development.
  - ✓ Benzoyl peroxide is useful for both noninflammatory and inflammatory acne. It has a rapid onset and may decrease the number of inflamed lesions within 5 days. Used alone or in combination, benzoyl peroxide is the standard of care for mild-to-moderate papulopustular acne. It is an agent of first choice when combined

with adapalene for most patients with mild-to-moderate inflammatory acne and a second-line choice for patients with noninflammatory comedonal acne. It is often combined with a topical retinoid or antibiotic. For maintenance therapy, benzoyl peroxide can be added to a topical retinoid.

✓ Topical washes, foams, creams, or gels can be used as leave-on or wash-off agents. Strengths available range from 2.5% to 10%. All single-agent preparations are available without prescription.

✓ Therapy should be initiated with the weakest concentration (2.5%) in a water-based formulation in the evening. Once tolerance is achieved, the strength may be increased to 5% or the base changed to the acetone or alcohol gels, or to paste. It is important to wash the product off in the morning. A sunscreen should be applied during the day.

✓ Side effects of benzoyl peroxide include dryness, irritation, and, rarely, allergic contact dermatitis. It may bleach hair, clothing, and towels.

• **Topical clindamycin** and **erythromycin** are macrolide antibiotics that are effective and well-tolerated acne treatments. They are recommended for use in combination with topical benzoyl peroxide (wash-off or leave-on) or retinoids, which increases efficacy and decreases development of resistant organisms. Clindamycin is preferred over erythromycin because of better efficacy and lack of systemic absorption; it is available as a single-ingredient topical preparation or in combination with benzoyl peroxide. Erythromycin is available alone and in combination with retinoic acid or benzoyl peroxide, but it is seldom used in practice.

• **Azelaic acid** has antibacterial, anti-inflammatory, and comedolytic activity. It is used for mild-to-moderate inflammatory acne but has limited efficacy compared with other therapies. It is an alternative to first-choice therapy for comedonal and inflammatory acne, particularly in combination. It is also an alternative to topical retinoids for maintenance therapy. Azelaic acid is well tolerated, with adverse effects of pruritus, burning, stinging, and tingling occurring in 1%–5% of patients. Erythema, dryness, peeling, and irritation occur in fewer than 1% of patients. Azelaic acid is available in 20% cream (Azelex) and 15% gel (Finacea) formulations, which are usually applied twice daily (morning and evening) on clean, dry skin. Most patients experience improvement within 4 weeks, but treatment may be continued over several months if necessary.

• **Dapsone** (Aczone) is a sulfone that has antibacterial and anti-inflammatory properties and improves both inflammatory and noninflammatory acne. It may be particularly useful for patients with sensitivities or intolerance to conventional antiacne agents and may be used in sulfonamide-allergic patients. Dapsone 5% topical gel is applied twice daily; the 7.5% gel is applied once daily. Combination therapy with topical retinoids may be indicated if comedonal lesions are present. Topical dapsone 5% gel has also been used in combination with adapalene or benzoyl peroxide.

Oral Antibacterials

• Use of oral antibiotics is reserved for patients with moderate-to-severe inflammatory acne. Tetracyclines (**minocycline** and **doxycycline**) have both antibacterial and anti-inflammatory effects and are considered first-line therapy. Macrolides (**erythromycin**, **azithromycin**) and **trimethoprim/sulfamethoxazole** are acceptable alternative agents. Because of bacterial resistance, erythromycin should be limited to patients who cannot use a tetracycline (eg, pregnant women and children <8 years old).

• **Ciprofloxacin** and **trimethoprim** alone may be effective in cases where other antibiotics cannot be used or are ineffective.

• **Sarecycline** (Seysara) is a narrow-spectrum tetracycline derivative with anti-inflammatory properties approved for treatment of inflammatory lesions of non-nodular moderate-to-severe acne vulgaris in patients 9 years of age or older.

• Oral antibiotics should be accompanied by early use of combination therapy with retinoids. In such cases, the antibiotic may often be discontinued after 3–6 months of therapy.

- The incidence of significant adverse effects with oral antibiotic use is low. Vaginal candidiasis may complicate use of all oral antibiotics. Minocycline has been associated with pigment deposition in the skin, mucous membranes, and teeth; it may also cause dose-related dizziness, urticaria, hypersensitivity syndrome, autoimmune hepatitis, a systemic lupus erythematosus–like syndrome, and serum sickness–like reactions. Doxycycline is a photosensitizer, especially at higher doses.
- The choice of antibiotic should be determined based on the side effect profile, resistance, cost, and consensus guidelines.

Intralesional Corticosteroids

- Intralesional **triamcinolone acetonide** injections are effective for large individual inflammatory nodules. Intralesional injections may produce rapid improvement and decreased pain but may also be associated with local skin atrophy.

Antisebum Agents

- **Isotretinoin** is a metabolite of vitamin A that decreases sebum production, inhibits *P. acnes* growth, and reduces inflammation. It is approved for treatment of severe recalcitrant nodular acne in non-pregnant patients 12 years of age and older with multiple inflammatory nodules with a diameter of 5 mm or greater. It has also been used for moderate acne that is treatment resistant, relapses quickly after discontinuation of oral antibiotic therapy, or produces physical scarring or significant psychosocial distress. Isotretinoin is the only drug treatment for acne that produces prolonged remission.
  - ✓ The approved isotretinoin dose range is 0.5–2 mg/kg/day, usually given over a 20-week course. Drug absorption is greater when taken with food.
  - ✓ Guidelines recommend initiation at 0.5 mg/kg/day when appropriate, subsequently increasing to 1 mg/kg/day after the first month as tolerated, with a goal cumulative dose between 120 and 150 mg/kg.
  - ✓ Side effects include those of the mucocutaneous (most common), musculoskeletal, and ophthalmic systems, as well as headaches and central nervous system effects. Most adverse effects, such as cheilitis and dry nose, eyes, and mouth, are temporary and resolve after discontinuation. Laboratory monitoring during therapy should include triglycerides, cholesterol, transaminases, and complete blood counts. Mood disorders, depression, suicidal ideation, and suicides have been reported sporadically, but a causal relationship has not been established. The issue is complex because depression and suicidal ideation occur with severe acne in the absence of isotretinoin.
  - ✓ Because of teratogenicity, two different forms of contraception must be started in female patients of childbearing potential beginning 1 month before therapy, continuing throughout treatment, and for up to 4 months after discontinuation of therapy. All patients receiving isotretinoin must participate in the iPLEDGE program, which requires pregnancy tests and assurances by prescribers and pharmacists that they will follow required procedures.
- **Oral contraceptives** containing estrogen can be useful for acne in some women because of their antiandrogenic properties. Agents with FDA approval for acne in women who also desire contraception include **norgestimate with ethinyl estradiol** and **norethindrone acetate with ethinyl estradiol**; other estrogen-containing products may also be effective. They may be used alone or in combination with other acne treatments.
- **Spironolactone** in higher doses is an antiandrogen. Doses of 50–200 mg have been shown to be effective for acne in select women.
- **Cyproterone acetate** is an antiandrogen that may be effective for acne in females when combined with ethinyl estradiol (in the form of an oral contraceptive). No cyproterone/estrogen–containing oral contraceptives are available in the United States.

- **Oral corticosteroids** in high doses used for short courses may provide temporary benefit in patients with severe inflammatory acne. Low-dose **prednisone** (5–15 mg daily) given alone or with high estrogen-containing combination oral contraceptives has shown efficacy for acne and seborrhea. Long-term adverse effects preclude oral corticosteroid use as a primary therapy for acne.

EVALUATION OF THERAPEUTIC OUTCOMES

- Provide patients with acne with a monitoring framework that includes specific parameters and frequency of monitoring. Have them record the objective response to treatment in a diary. Contact patients within 2–3 weeks after the start of therapy to assess progress and then every 4–8 weeks thereafter.
- Good adherence to therapy is the key to treatment success.
- Lesion counts should decrease by 10%–15% within 4–8 weeks or by more than 50% within 2–4 months. Inflammatory lesions should resolve within a few weeks, and comedones should resolve by 3–4 months. If anxiety or depression is present at the outset, control or improvement should be achieved within 2–4 months.
- Long-term parameters should include no progression of severity, lengthening of acne-free periods throughout therapy, and no further scarring or pigmentation throughout therapy.
- Monitor patients regularly for adverse treatment effects with appropriate dose reduction, alternative therapy, preventative measures, or drug discontinuation as appropriate.

See Chapter 113, Acne Vulgaris, authored by Debra J. Sibbald, for a more detailed discussion of this topic.

Dermatologic Drug Reactions and Common Skin Conditions

16

- *Drug-induced skin reactions* can be irritant or allergic in origin. Allergic drug reactions are classified into exanthematous, urticarial, blistering, and pustular eruptions.
- Severe cutaneous adverse reactions to drugs (SCARs) include Stevens–Johnson syndrome (SJS), toxic epidermal necrolysis (TEN), and drug reaction with eosinophilia and systemic symptoms (DRESS).
- Skin disorders discussed in this chapter include contact dermatitis, diaper dermatitis, and atopic dermatitis.

PATHOPHYSIOLOGY

- *Exanthematous* drug reactions include maculopapular rashes and drug hypersensitivity syndrome. *Urticarial* reactions include urticaria, angioedema, and serum sickness-like reactions. *Blistering* reactions include fixed drug eruptions, Stevens–Johnson syndrome, and toxic epidermal necrolysis. *Pustular* eruptions include acneiform drug reactions and acute generalized exanthematous pustulosis (AGEP) (**Fig. 16-1**).
- Drug-induced *hyperpigmentation* may be related to increased melanin (eg, hydantoins), direct deposition (eg, silver, mercury, tetracyclines, and antimalarials), or other mechanisms (eg, fluorouracil).
- Drug-induced photosensitivity reactions may be *phototoxic* (a nonimmunologic reaction) or *photoallergic* (an immunologic reaction). Medications associated with phototoxicity include amiodarone, tetracyclines, sulfonamides, psoralens, and coal tar. Common causes of photoallergic reactions include sulfonamides, sulfonylureas, thiazides, nonsteroidal anti-inflammatory drugs (NSAIDs), chloroquine, and carbamazepine.
- *Contact dermatitis* is skin inflammation caused by irritants or allergic sensitizers. In *allergic contact dermatitis* (ACD), an antigenic substance triggers an immunologic response, sometimes several days later. *Irritant contact dermatitis* (ICD) is caused by an organic substance that usually results in a reaction within a few hours of exposure.
- *Diaper dermatitis* (diaper rash) is an acute, inflammatory dermatitis of the buttocks, genitalia, and perineal regions that are covered by the diaper. It is a type of contact dermatitis resulting from direct fecal and moisture contact with the skin in an occlusive environment.
- *Atopic dermatitis* (eczema) is an inflammatory condition with genetic, environmental, and immunologic mechanisms. Neuropeptides, irritation, or pruritus-induced scratching may cause release of proinflammatory cytokines from keratinocytes.

CLINICAL PRESENTATION

- *Maculopapular skin reaction* presents with erythematous macules and papules that may be pruritic. Lesions usually begin within 7–10 days after starting the offending medication and generally resolve within 7–14 days after drug discontinuation. Because of the delayed reaction, the offending agent could be discontinued (eg, a 7-day antibiotic treatment course) before the lesions appear. Lesions may spread and become confluent. Common culprits include penicillins, cephalosporins, sulfonamides, and some anticonvulsants.
- *Drug hypersensitivity syndrome* (also known as drug reaction with eosinophilia and systemic symptoms or DRESS) is an exanthematous eruption accompanied by fever, lymphadenopathy, and multiorgan involvement (kidneys, liver, lung, bone marrow, heart, and brain). Signs and symptoms begin 1–4 weeks after starting the offending drug, and the reaction may be fatal if not promptly treated. Drugs implicated include

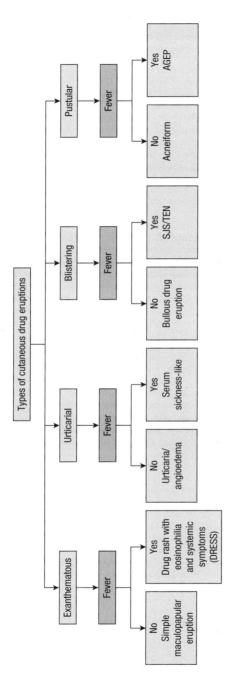

(AGEP, acute generalized exanthematous pustulosis; SJS, Stevens–Johnson syndrome; TEN, toxic epidermal necrolysis.)
(Adapted from Knowles, S. Drug-Induced Skin Reactions, Table 3, Description of Drug Eruptions. In: Compendium of Therapeutic Choices for Minor Ailments. 2nd ed. Ottawa, ON: Canadian Pharmacists Association; © 2016.)

FIGURE 16-1. Types of cutaneous drug eruptions.

allopurinol, sulfonamides, some anticonvulsants (barbiturates, phenytoin, carbamazepine, and lamotrigine), and dapsone.

- *Urticaria* and *angioedema* are simple eruptions that are caused by drugs in 5%–10% of cases. Other causes are foods (most common) and physical factors such as cold or pressure, infections, and latex exposure. Urticaria may be the first sign of an emerging anaphylactic reaction characterized by hives, extremely pruritic red raised wheals, angioedema, and mucous membrane swelling that typically occurs within minutes to hours. Offending drugs include penicillins and related antibiotics, aspirin, sulfonamides, radiograph contrast media, and opioids.

- *Serum sickness-like reactions* are complex urticarial eruptions presenting with fever, rash (usually urticarial), and arthralgias usually within 1–3 weeks after starting the offending drug.

- *Fixed drug eruptions* present as pruritic, red, raised lesions that may blister. Symptoms can include burning or stinging. Lesions may evolve into plaques. These so-called fixed eruptions recur in the same area each time the offending drug is given. Lesions appear and disappear within minutes to days, leaving hyperpigmented skin for months. Usual offenders include tetracyclines, barbiturates, sulfonamides, codeine, phenolphthalein, and NSAIDs.

- *Stevens–Johnson syndrome* (SJS) and *toxic epidermal necrolysis* (TEN) are blistering eruptions that are rare but severe and life-threatening. They are considered variants of the same disorder and are often discussed together as SJS/TEN. Onset occurs within 7–14 days after drug exposure. Patients present with generalized tender/painful bullous formation with fever, headache, and respiratory symptoms leading to rapid clinical deterioration. Lesions show rapid confluence and spread, resulting in extensive epidermal detachment and sloughing. This may result in marked fluid loss, hypotension, electrolyte imbalances, and secondary infections. Usual offending drugs include sulfonamides, penicillins, some anticonvulsants (hydantoins, carbamazepine, barbiturates, and lamotrigine), NSAIDs, and allopurinol.

- *Acneiform drug reactions* are pustular eruptions that induce acne. Onset is within 1–3 weeks. Common culprits include corticosteroids, androgenic hormones, some anticonvulsants, isoniazid, and lithium.

- *Acute generalized exanthematous pustulosis* (AGEP) has an acute onset (within days after starting the offending drug), fever, diffuse erythema, and many pustules. Generalized desquamation occurs 2 weeks later. Common offending drugs include β-lactam antibiotics, macrolides, and calcium channel blockers.

- *Sun-induced skin reactions* appear similar to a sunburn and present with erythema, papules, edema, and sometimes vesicles. They appear in areas exposed to sunlight (eg, ears, nose, cheeks, forearms, and hands).

- *Diaper dermatitis* results in an erythematous rash, and severe cases may have vesicles and oozing erosions. The rash may be infected by *Candida* species and present with confluent red plaques, papules, and pustules.

- *Atopic dermatitis* presents differently depending on age. In infancy, an erythematous, patchy, pruritic, papular skin rash may first appear on the cheeks and chin and progress to red, scaling, oozing lesions. The rash affects the malar region of the cheeks, forehead, scalp, chin, and behind the ears while sparing the nose and paranasal creases. Over several weeks, lesions may spread to extensor surfaces of the lower legs (due to the infant's crawling), and eventually the entire body may be involved except for the diaper area and nose. In childhood, the skin is often dry, flaky, rough, and cracked. Pruritus is a quintessential feature, and a diagnosis cannot be made if there is no history of itching. Scratching and rubbing itchy skin may result in bleeding and lichenification. In adulthood, lesions are more diffuse with underlying erythema. The face is commonly involved and may be dry and scaly. Lichenification may be seen.

DIAGNOSIS

- A comprehensive patient history is important to obtain the following information:
  - ✓ Signs and symptoms (onset, progression, timeframe, lesion location and description, presenting symptoms, and previous occurrence)
  - ✓ Urgency (severity, area, and extent of skin involvement; signs of a systemic/generalized reaction or disease condition)
  - ✓ Medication history (temporal correlation, previous exposure, and nonprescribed products)
  - ✓ Differential diagnosis
- Lesion assessment includes identifying macules, papules, nodules, blisters, plaques, and lichenification. Some skin conditions cause more than one type of lesions.
- Inspect lesions for color, texture, size, and temperature. Areas that are oozing, erythematous, and warm to the touch may be infected.

TREATMENT

- <u>Goals of Treatment</u>: Relieve bothersome symptoms, remove precipitating factors, prevent recurrences, avoid adverse treatment effects, and improve quality of life.

DRUG-INDUCED SKIN REACTIONS

- If a drug-induced skin reaction is suspected, the most important treatment is discontinuing the suspected drug as quickly as possible and avoiding use of potential cross-sensitizers.
- The next step is to control symptoms (eg, pruritus). Signs or symptoms of a systemic or generalized reaction may require additional supportive therapy. For high fevers, acetaminophen is more appropriate than aspirin or another NSAID, which may exacerbate some skin lesions.
- Most maculopapular reactions disappear within a few days after discontinuing the agent, so symptomatic control of the affected area is the primary intervention. Topical corticosteroids and oral antihistamines can relieve pruritus. In severe cases, a short course of systemic corticosteroids may be warranted.
- Treatment of fixed drug reactions involves removal of the offending agent. Other therapeutic measures include topical corticosteroids, oral antihistamines to relieve itching, and perhaps cool water compresses on the affected area.
- Photosensitivity reactions typically resolve with drug discontinuation. Some patients benefit from topical corticosteroids and oral antihistamines, but these are relatively ineffective. Systemic corticosteroids (eg, oral prednisone 1 mg/kg/day tapered over 3 weeks) are more effective.
- For life-threatening SJS/TEN, supportive measures such as maintenance of adequate blood pressure, fluid and electrolyte balance, broad-spectrum antibiotics and vancomycin for secondary infections, and IV immunoglobulin (IVIG) may be appropriate. Corticosteroid use is controversial; if used, employ relatively high doses initially, followed by rapid tapering as soon as disease progression stops.
- Inform patients about the suspected drug, potential drugs to avoid in the future, and which drugs may be used instead. Give patients with photosensitivity reactions information about preventive measures, such as use of sunscreens and sun avoidance.

CONTACT DERMATITIS

- The first intervention involves identification, withdrawal, and avoidance of the offending agent.
- The second treatment is symptomatic relief while decreasing skin lesions. Cold compresses help soothe and cleanse the skin; they are applied to wet or oozing lesions, removed, remoistened, and reapplied every few minutes for a 20- to 30-minute

period. If affected areas are already dry or hardened, wet dressings applied as soaks (without removal for up to 20–30 minutes) will soften and hydrate the skin; soaks should not be used on acute exudating lesions. **Calamine lotion** or **Burow solution (aluminum acetate)** may also be soothing.

- **Topical corticosteroids** help resolve the inflammatory process and are the mainstay of treatment. ACD responds better to topical corticosteroids than does ICD. Generally, use higher potency corticosteroids initially, switching to medium or lower potency corticosteroids as the condition improves (see Chapter 17, Table 17–1, for topical corticosteroid potencies).
- **Oatmeal baths** or oral **first-generation antihistamines** may provide relief for excessive itching.
- **Moisturizers** may be used to prevent dryness and skin fissuring.

DIAPER DERMATITIS

- Management involves frequent diaper changes, air drying (removing the diaper for as long as practical), gentle cleansing (preferably with nonsoap cleansers and lukewarm water), and use of barrier products. **Zinc oxide** has astringent and absorbent properties and provides an effective barrier. **Petrolatum** also provides a water-impermeable barrier but has no absorbent ability and may trap moisture.
- Candidal (yeast) diaper rash should be treated with a topical antifungal agent and then covered by a barrier product. **Imidazoles** are the treatment of choice. The antifungal agents should be stopped once the rash subsides and the barrier product continued to prevent recurrence.
- In severe inflammatory diaper rashes, a very low potency topical corticosteroid **(hydrocortisone 0.5%–1%)** may be used for short periods (1–2 weeks).
- Medical referral is indicated if the rash does not respond after a week of treatment, if pain or inflammation increases during therapy, if ulcerations develop, or if systemic signs or symptoms are present (eg, fever, diarrhea, skin lesions elsewhere).

ATOPIC DERMATITIS

- Nonpharmacologic measures for infants and children include the following:
  ✓ Apply moisturizers frequently throughout the day
  ✓ Give lukewarm baths
  ✓ Apply lubricants/moisturizers immediately after bathing
  ✓ Use nonsoap cleansers (which are neutral to low pH, hypoallergenic, fragrance free)
  ✓ Use wet-wrap therapy (with or without topical corticosteroid) during flare-ups for patients with moderate-to-severe disease. Wet-wrap involves applying damp tubular elasticized bandages and occlusive dressing to the limbs to promote skin hydration and absorption of emollients and topical corticosteroids.
  ✓ Keep fingernails filed short
  ✓ Select clothing made of soft cotton fabrics
  ✓ Consider sedating oral antihistamines to reduce scratching at night
  ✓ Keep the child cool; avoid situations that cause overheating
  ✓ Learn to recognize skin infections and seek treatment promptly
  ✓ Identify and remove irritants and allergens

- Topical corticosteroids are the drug treatment of choice. Low-potency agents (eg, **hydrocortisone 1%**) are suitable for the face, and medium-potency products (eg, **betamethasone valerate 0.1%**) may be used for the body. For longer-duration maintenance therapy, low-potency corticosteroids are recommended. Use mid-strength and high-potency corticosteroids for short-term management of exacerbations. Reserve ultra-high and high-potency agents (eg, **betamethasone dipropionate 0.05%** and **clobetasone propionate 0.05%**) for short-term treatment (1–2 weeks) of lichenified lesions in adults. After lesions have improved significantly, use a lower-potency corticosteroid for maintenance when necessary. Avoid potent fluorinated corticosteroids on the face, genitalia, and intertriginous areas and in infants.

- The topical immunomodulators **tacrolimus** (Protopic) and **pimecrolimus** (Elidel) inhibit calcineurin, which normally initiates T-cell activation. Both agents are approved for atopic dermatitis in adults and children older than age 2. Tacrolimus ointment 0.03% (for moderate-to-severe atopic dermatitis in patients ages 2 and older) and 0.1% (for ages 16 and older) is applied twice daily. Pimecrolimus cream 1% is applied twice daily for mild-to-moderate atopic dermatitis in patients older than age 2. The most common adverse effect is transient burning at the site of application. Both drugs are recommended as second-line treatments due to concerns about a possible risk of cancer. For this reason, sun protection factor (SPF) 30 or higher is recommended on all exposed skin areas.
- **Coal tar preparations** (**crude coal tar**, **liquor carbonis detergens**) have been widely used, but few controlled trials support their efficacy. These products are also staining and malodorous, although newer products may be more cosmetically acceptable. They are not recommended on acutely inflamed skin, since this may result in additional skin irritation.
- **Crisaborole** (Eucrisa) 2% ointment is a phosphodiesterase (PDE) 4 inhibitor approved for treatment of mild-to-moderate AD in adults and children 2 years of age or older. A thin layer of ointment is applied twice daily to affected areas. Burning or stinging may occur at the site of application.
- Phototherapy may be recommended when the disease is not controlled by topical corticosteroids and calcineurin inhibitors. It may also be steroid sparing, allowing for use of lower-potency corticosteroids, or even eliminating the need for corticosteroids in some cases.
- **Dupilumab** (dupixent) subcutaneous (SC) injection is an interleukin-4 receptor alpha antagonist FDA approved for treatment of patients aged 12 years and older with moderate-to-severe atopic dermatitis whose disease is not adequately controlled with topical prescription therapies or when those therapies are not advisable. It can be used with or without topical corticosteroids. Topical calcineurin inhibitors may be used but should be reserved for problem areas such as the face, neck, intertriginous, and genital areas. The recommended adult dose is 600 mg initially (given as two 300-mg SC injections), followed by 300-mg SC every other week. The dose for patients 12–17 years of age is based on body weight: <60 kg, 400 mg (two 200-mg injections) then 200 mg every other week; >60 kg, 600 mg (two 300-mg injections) then 300 mg every other week. The most common adverse reactions (≥1%) are injection site reactions, conjunctivitis, blepharitis, oral herpes, keratitis, eye pruritus, other herpes simplex virus infection, and dry eye.
- Other systemic therapies that have been used (but not FDA approved) for atopic dermatitis include other biologic agents, corticosteroids, cyclosporine, interferon-γ, azathioprine, methotrexate, mycophenolate mofetil, and IVIG.

EVALUATION OF THERAPEUTIC OUTCOMES

- Provide patients with information regarding causative factors, avoidance of substances that trigger skin reactions, and potential benefits and limitations of nondrug and drug therapy.
- Evaluate patients with chronic skin conditions periodically to assess disease control, the efficacy of current therapy, and the presence of possible adverse effects.

See Chapter e16, Skin Care and Minor Dermatologic Conditions, by Rebecca M. Law and Howard I. Maibach; Chapter 115, Atopic Dermatitis, by Rebecca M. Law, Wayne P. Gulliver, and Po Gin Kwa; and Chapter 117, Dermatologic Drug Reactions, Contact Dermatitis, and Common Skin Conditions, by Rebecca M. Law, David T.S. Law, and Howard I. Maibach, for more detailed discussions of these topics.

- *Psoriasis* is a chronic T-lymphocyte–mediated systemic inflammatory disease characterized by recurrent exacerbations and remissions of thickened, erythematous, and scaling plaques and multiple comorbidities, including psoriatic arthritis.

PATHOPHYSIOLOGY

- Genetic predisposition coupled with an unknown precipitating factor triggers an abnormal immune response mediated via T-lymphocytes, resulting in keratinocyte proliferation and the initial psoriatic skin lesions. Precipitating factors implicated in the development of psoriasis include skin injury, infection, drugs, smoking, alcohol consumption, obesity, and psychogenic stress.
- Psoriasis susceptibility genes and variants reside on various chromosomes. The psoriasis susceptibility locus 1 (*PSORS1*) on chromosome 6p is a key gene locus, accounting for up to 50% of disease heritability. The major histocompatibility complex antigen HLA-Cw6 and tumor necrosis factor (TNF)-α are major psoriasis susceptibility genes, along with interleukin (IL)-23 and many other loci. There appears to be a general role for T lymphocytes and a specific role for TH17 lymphocytes in psoriasis pathogenesis and as indicators of psoriasis risk.
- Interactions between dermal dendritic cells and activated Th-1 and Th-17 cells in concert with numerous growth factors and cytokines (eg, TNF-α, interferon gamma, IL-1) cause epidermal hyperplasia and dermal inflammation.

CLINICAL PRESENTATION

- Skin lesions in plaque psoriasis (psoriasis vulgaris) are erythematous, red-violet in color, at least 0.5 cm in diameter, well demarcated, and typically covered with silver flaking scales. They may appear as single lesions on predisposed areas (eg, knees and elbows) or generalized over a wide body surface area (BSA).
- Pruritus may be severe and require treatment to minimize excoriations from frequent scratching. Lesions may be physically debilitating or socially isolating.
- Preexisting psoriasis can be exacerbated by drugs (eg, lithium, nonsteroidal anti-inflammatory drugs [NSAIDs], antimalarials, β-adrenergic blockers, fluoxetine, and withdrawal of corticosteroids), times of stress, and seasonal changes.
- Potential comorbidities include psoriatic arthritis, depression, anxiety, hypertension, obesity, diabetes mellitus, Crohn disease, and alcoholism.
- Psoriatic arthritis develops in about 30% of patients with plaque psoriasis. It most commonly presents as polyarticular peripheral arthritis but can vary widely with peripheral and/or axial, monoarticular, or polyarticular patterns.

DIAGNOSIS

- Diagnosis is based on physical examination findings of characteristic lesions. Skin biopsies are not diagnostic of psoriasis.
- Classification of psoriasis as mild, moderate, or severe is based on BSA and Psoriasis Area and Severity Index (PASI) measurements. A 2011 European classification system defines severity of plaque psoriasis as either mild or moderate-to-severe.

TREATMENT

- <u>Goals of Treatment</u>: Minimize or eliminate skin lesions, alleviate pruritus, reduce frequency of flare-ups, treat comorbid conditions, screen for and manage lifestyle factors that may trigger exacerbations, avoid adverse treatment effects, provide

FIGURE 17-1. Treatment algorithm for mild-to-moderate psoriasis.

cost-effective treatment, provide appropriate counseling (eg, stress reduction), and maintain or improve quality of life.

- See **Figures 17-1** and **17-2** for psoriasis treatment algorithms based on disease severity.

NONPHARMACOLOGIC THERAPY

- Nonmedicated moisturizers help maintain skin moisture, reduce skin shedding, control scaling, and reduce pruritus.
- Oatmeal baths further reduce pruritus, and regular use may decrease need for systemic antipruritic drugs. Harsh soaps and detergents should be avoided. Cleansing should involve tepid water, preferably with lipid- and fragrance-free cleansers.
- Sunscreens (preferably sun protection factor [SPF] 30 or higher) should be used when outdoors.
- Stress management can improve extent and severity of psoriasis.

PHARMACOLOGIC THERAPY

Topical Therapies

- **Corticosteroids** (**Table 17-1**) have anti-inflammatory, antiproliferative, immuno-suppressive, and vasoconstrictive effects. They are recommended in U.S. treatment guidelines as first-line treatment for limited psoriasis either as monotherapy or with nonsteroidal topical agents; potency can be enhanced with different vehicles, and as needed by occlusion.
  - ✓ Lower-potency products should be used for infants and for lesions on the face, intertriginous areas, and areas with thin skin. Mid- to high-potency agents are recommended as initial therapy for other body areas in adults. Reserve the highest potency corticosteroids for patients with very thick plaques or recalcitrant disease, such as plaques on the palms and soles. Use potency class I corticosteroids for only 2–4 weeks.
  - ✓ Ointments are the most occlusive and most potent formulations because of enhanced penetration into the dermis. Patients may prefer the less greasy creams or lotions for daytime use.
  - ✓ Cutaneous adverse effects include skin atrophy, acne, contact dermatitis, hypertrichosis, folliculitis, hypopigmentation, perioral dermatitis, striae, telangiectasias, and traumatic purpura. Systemic adverse effects may occur with superpotent agents or with extended or widespread use of midpotency agents. Such effects

(MTX, methotrexate; PsA, psoriatic arthritis.)

FIGURE 17-2. Treatment algorithm for moderate-to-severe psoriasis.

include hypothalamic–pituitary–adrenal axis suppression and less commonly Cushing syndrome, osteonecrosis of the femoral head, cataracts, and glaucoma.

- **Calcipotriene** (Dovonex) and **calcitriol** (Vectical) are vitamin D_3 analogs that bind to vitamin D receptors, which inhibit keratinocyte proliferation and enhance keratinocyte differentiation. They also inhibit T-lymphocyte activity. These agents can be used as first-line monotherapy or in combination with a topical corticosteroid for mild plaque psoriasis. Calcipotriene 0.005% cream, ointment, foam, or gel is applied to affected areas twice daily. Calcitriol ointment 3 mcg/g is applied to affected areas twice daily. Adverse effects include mild irritant contact dermatitis, burning, pruritus, edema, peeling, dryness, and erythema.
- **Tazarotene** (Tazorac) is a topical retinoid that normalizes keratinocyte differentiation, diminishes keratinocyte hyperproliferation, and clears the inflammatory infiltrate in psoriatic plaques. It is available as a 0.05% or 0.1% gel and cream and is applied once daily (usually in the evening). It may be combined with a topical corticosteroid to enhance efficacy and reduce irritation. Adverse effects of tazarotene include a high incidence of dose-dependent irritation at application sites, resulting in burning, stinging, and erythema. Irritation may be reduced by using the cream formulation, lower concentration, alternate-day applications, or short-contact (30–60 minutes) treatment. Tazarotene is contraindicated in pregnancy and should not be used in women of childbearing potential unless effective contraception is being used.
- **Anthralin** has a direct antiproliferative effect on epidermal keratinocytes, normalizing keratinocyte differentiation. Short-contact anthralin therapy (SCAT) is the preferred regimen, with ointment applied only to the thick plaque lesions for 2 hours or less and then wiped off. Zinc oxide ointment or nonmedicated stiff paste should be applied to the surrounding normal skin to protect it from irritation. Use anthralin with caution, if at all, on the face and intertriginous areas due to potential for severe irritation. Anthralin concentrations for SCAT range from 1% to 4% or as tolerated. Concentrations for continuous therapy vary from 0.05% to 0.4%. Anthralin may cause severe skin irritation, folliculitis, and allergic contact dermatitis.
- **Coal tar** is keratolytic and may have antiproliferative and anti-inflammatory effects. Formulations include crude coal tar and tar distillates (liquor carbonis detergens) in ointments, creams, and shampoos. Coal tar is used infrequently due to limited efficacy and poor patient adherence and acceptance. It has a slower onset of action than

TABLE 17-1	Topical Corticosteroid Potency Chart
Potency Rating	**Topical Corticosteroid**
Class 1: Superpotent	Betamethasone dipropionate 0.05% ointment (Diprolene and Diprosone ointment) Clobetasol propionate 0.05% lotion/spray/shampoo/foam (Clobex lotion/spray/shampoo, OLUX and OLUX-E foam) Clobetasol propionate 0.05% cream, gel, solution (scalp), ointment (Cormax, Temovate, Dermovate) Diflorasone diacetate 0.05% ointment (Florone, Psorcon, ApexiCon) Flurandrenolide tape 4 mcg/cm^2 (Cordran) Halobetasol propionate 0.05% cream, lotion, ointment (Ultravate)
Class 2: Potent	Amcinonide 0.1% ointment (Cyclocort, Amcort) Betamethasone dipropionate 0.05% cream/gel (Diprolene cream, gel, and Diprosone cream) Desoximetasone 0.25% cream, gel, ointment (Topicort) Diflorasone diacetate 0.05% ointment (ApexiCon, Florone, Psorcon) Fluocinonide 0.05% cream, gel, ointment (Lidex) Halcinonide 0.1% cream (Halog)
Class 3: Upper mid-strength	Amcinonide 0.1% cream (Cyclocort) Betamethasone valerate 0.1% ointment (Betnovate/Valisone) Diflorasone diacetate 0.05% cream (Psorcon, Florone, ApexiCon) Fluticasone propionate 0.005% ointment (Cutivate) Mometasone furoate 0.1% ointment (Elocon) Triamcinolone acetonide 0.5% cream and ointment (Aristocort)
Class 4: Mid-strength	Betamethasone dipropionate 0.05% spray (Sernivo) Betamethasone valerate 0.12% foam (Luxiq) Clocortolone pivalate 0.1% cream (Cloderm) Desoximetasone 0.05% cream and gel (Topicort LP) Fluocinolone acetonide 0.025% ointment (Synalar) Fluocinolone acetonide 0.2% cream (Synalar-HP) Hydrocortisone valerate 0.2% ointment (Westcort) Mometasone furoate 0.1% cream, lotion, solution (Elocon) Triamcinolone acetonide 0.1% ointment (Kenalog)
Class 5: Lower mid-strength	Betamethasone dipropionate 0.05% lotion (Diprosone) Betamethasone valerate 0.1% cream and lotion (Betnovate/Valisone) Desonide 0.05% lotion, ointment, gel (DesOwen, Tridesilon) Fluocinolone acetonide 0.01% shampoo (Capex) Fluocinolone acetonide 0.01%, 0.025%, 0.03% cream (Synalar) Flurandrenolide 0.05% cream and lotion (Cordran) Fluticasone propionate 0.05% cream and lotion (Cutivate) Hydrocortisone butyrate 0.1% ointment, lotion, cream (Locoid, Locoid Lipocream) Hydrocortisone probutate 0.1% cream (Pandel) Hydrocortisone valerate 0.2% cream (Westcort) Prednicarbate 0.1% cream and ointment (Dermatop) Triamcinolone acetonide 0.1% cream, ointment and lotion (Kenalog)
Class 6: Mild (low potency)	Alclometasone dipropionate 0.05% cream and ointment (Aclovate) Betamethasone valerate 0.05% cream and ointment (Valisone) Desonide 0.05% cream, ointment, gel (DesOwen, Desonate, Tridesilon) Desonide 0.05% foam (Verdeso) Fluocinonide acetonide 0.01% cream and solution (Synalar) Fluocinonide acetonide 0.01% FS oil (Derma-Smoothe)
Class 7: Least Potent	Hydrocortisone 0.5%, 1%, 2%, 2.5% cream, lotion, spray, and ointment (various brands)

calcipotriene, has an unpleasant odor, and stains clothing. Adverse effects include folliculitis, acne, local irritation, and phototoxicity. Risk of teratogenicity is low when used in pregnancy.

- **Salicylic acid** has keratolytic properties and has been used in shampoos or bath oils for scalp psoriasis. It enhances penetration of topical corticosteroids, thereby increasing corticosteroid efficacy. Systemic absorption and toxicity can occur, especially when applied to >20% BSA or in patients with renal impairment. Salicylic acid should not be used in children. It may be used for limited and localized plaque psoriasis in pregnancy.

- **Pimecrolimus** 1% cream (Elidel) is a calcineurin inhibitor shown to be effective for plaque psoriasis when used under occlusion and for patients with moderate-to-severe inverse psoriasis (involving intertriginous areas). It may be a useful alternative for patients with intertriginous or facial lesions because it is less irritating than calcipotriene and does not have the topical adverse effects of corticosteroids (eg, skin atrophy).

Phototherapy and Photochemotherapy

- Phototherapy consists of nonionizing electromagnetic radiation, either ultraviolet A (UVA) or ultraviolet B (UVB), as light therapy for psoriatic lesions. UVB is given alone as either broadband or narrowband (NB-UVB). UVB is also given as photochemotherapy with topical agents such as crude coal tar (Goeckerman regimen) or anthralin (Ingram regimen) for enhanced efficacy. UVA is generally given with a photosensitizer such as an oral psoralen to enhance efficacy; this regimen is called PUVA (psoralen + UVA treatment). Adverse effects of phototherapy include erythema, pruritus, xerosis, hyperpigmentation, and blistering. Patients must be provided with eye protection during and for 24 hours after PUVA treatments. PUVA therapy may also cause nausea or vomiting, which may be minimized by taking the oral psoralens with food or milk. Long-term PUVA use can lead to photoaging and cataracts. PUVA is also associated with a dose-related risk of carcinogenesis.

Systemic Nonbiologic Agents

- **Acitretin** (Soriatane) is a retinoic acid derivative and the active metabolite of etretinate. Retinoids may be less effective than methotrexate or cyclosporine when used as monotherapy. Acitretin is more commonly used in combination with topical calcipotriene or phototherapy. Although low-dose acitretin (25 mg/day) is safer and better tolerated than higher-dose (50 mg/day) therapy, low-dose acitretin is not recommended as monotherapy. Therapy is continued until lesions have resolved. It is better tolerated when taken with meals. Adverse effects include hypertriglyceridemia and mucocutaneous effects such as dryness of the eyes, nasal and oral mucosa; chapped lips; cheilitis; epistaxis; xerosis; brittle nails; and burning skin. Ophthalmologic changes include photosensitivity, decreased color vision, and impaired night vision. Hepatitis and jaundice are rare and liver enzyme elevations are usually transient. All retinoids are teratogenic and are contraindicated in pregnancy. Acitretin should not be used in women of childbearing potential unless they use effective contraception for the duration of therapy and for at least 2 years after drug discontinuation. Blood donation (men and women) is not permitted during and for at least 1 year after treatment.

- **Cyclosporine** is a systemic calcineurin inhibitor that is effective for inducing remission and for maintenance therapy of moderate-to-severe plaque psoriasis. Intermittent short-course therapy (<12 weeks) is preferable to continuous therapy because it appears to reduce the risk of nephrotoxicity. Cyclosporine is significantly more effective than etretinate and has similar or slightly better efficacy than methotrexate. The usual oral dose is 2.5–5 mg/kg/day given in two divided doses. After inducing remission, maintenance therapy using low doses (1.25–3 mg/kg/day) may prevent relapse. When discontinuing cyclosporine, a gradual taper of 1 mg/kg/day each week may prolong the time before relapse compared to abrupt discontinuation. Because more than half of patients stopping cyclosporine relapse within 4 months, patients should be given appropriate alternative treatments shortly before or after discontinuing cyclosporine. Adverse effects include nephrotoxicity, hypertension, hypomagnesemia, hyperkalemia, hypertriglyceridemia, hypertrichosis, and gingival hyperplasia. The risk of skin cancer increases with the duration of treatment and with prior PUVA treatments.

- **Methotrexate** has anti-inflammatory effects due to its effects on T-cell gene expression and also has cytostatic effects. It is more effective than acitretin and has similar or slightly less efficacy than cyclosporine. Methotrexate can be administered orally, subcutaneously (SC), or intramuscularly. The starting dose is 7.5–15 mg once weekly, increased incrementally by 2.5 mg every 2–4 weeks until response; maximal doses are 25 mg weekly. Adverse effects include nausea, vomiting, stomatitis, macrocytic anemia, and hepatic and pulmonary toxicity. Nausea and macrocytic anemia may be reduced by giving oral folic acid 1–5 mg daily. It is an abortifacient and teratogenic and is contraindicated in pregnancy.

- **Tofacitinib** (Xeljanz, Xeljanz XR) is a small-molecule Janus Kinase (JAK) inhibitor that blocks signaling through common receptors for cytokines including IL-2, IL-4, IL-7, IL-9, IL-15, and IL-21. It is indicated for the treatment of adults with active psoriatic arthritis who have had an inadequate response or intolerance to methotrexate or other disease-modifying antirheumatic drugs (DMARDs). The recommended dose (in combination with nonbiologic DMARDs) is 5 mg orally twice daily or 11 mg (extended-release) once daily. The recommended dose is 5 mg once daily in patients with moderate-to-severe renal impairment or moderate hepatic impairment. Tofacitinib should not be used in combination with biologic DMARDs or potent immunosuppressants such as azathioprine and cyclosporine.

- **Apremilast** (Otezla) is a small-molecule inhibitor of phosphodiesterase 4 (PDE4), which increases intracellular cyclic AMP (cAMP) and reduces production of proinflammatory mediators. It is indicated for treatment of adults with active psoriatic arthritis and patients with moderate-to-severe plaque psoriasis who are candidates for phototherapy or systemic therapy. Recommended dosing is 10 mg orally on day 1, 10 mg twice daily on day 2, 10 mg in the morning and 20 mg in the evening on day 3, 20 mg twice daily on day 4, 20 mg in the morning and 30 mg in the evening on day 5, then 30 mg twice daily thereafter. The dosage regimen should be reduced in severe renal impairment. The most common adverse reactions (≥5%) are diarrhea, nausea, and headache.

Systemic Biologic Agents

- Biologic agents are considered for moderate-to-severe psoriasis when other systemic agents are inadequate or contraindicated or when comorbidities exist. Cost considerations tend to limit their use as first-line therapy.

TNF Inhibitors

- **Adalimumab** (Humira) is a monoclonal TNF-α antibody that provides rapid control of psoriasis. It is indicated for psoriatic arthritis and treatment of adults with moderate-to-severe chronic plaque psoriasis who are candidates for systemic therapy or phototherapy. The recommended dose for psoriatic arthritis is 40 mg SC every other week. The recommended dose for adults with plaque psoriasis is an initial dose of 80 mg SC, followed by 40 mg every other week starting 1 week after the initial dose. The most common adverse reactions are infections (eg, upper respiratory and sinusitis), injection site reactions, headache, and rash.

- **Etanercept** (Enbrel) is a fusion protein that binds TNF-α, competitively interfering with its interaction with cell-bound receptors. Unlike the chimeric infliximab, etanercept is fully humanized, minimizing the risk of immunogenicity. Etanercept is FDA approved for reducing signs and symptoms and inhibiting the progression of joint damage in patients with psoriatic arthritis; it can be used alone or in combination with methotrexate. It is also indicated for patients 4 years or older with chronic moderate-to-severe plaque psoriasis who are candidates for systemic therapy or phototherapy. The recommended dose for psoriatic arthritis is 50 mg SC once weekly. For plaque psoriasis, the dose is 50 mg SC twice weekly (administered 3 or 4 days apart) for 3 months, followed by a maintenance dose of 50 mg once weekly. Adverse effects include local reactions at the injection site (20% of patients), respiratory tract and GI infections, abdominal pain, nausea and vomiting, headaches, and rash.

- **Infliximab** (Remicade) is a chimeric monoclonal antibody directed against TNF-α. It is indicated for psoriatic arthritis and chronic severe plaque psoriasis. The recommended dose is 5 mg/kg by IV infusion at weeks 0, 2, and 6, then every 8 weeks thereafter. For psoriatic arthritis, it may be used with or without methotrexate. Adverse effects include headaches, fever, chills, fatigue, diarrhea, pharyngitis, and upper respiratory and urinary tract infections. Hypersensitivity reactions (urticaria, dyspnea, and hypotension) and lymphoproliferative disorders have been reported.
- **Certolizumab pegol** (Cimzia) is a humanized antigen-binding fragment of a monoclonal antibody that is further conjugated with a polyethylene glycol moiety. This binds to TNF-α, blocking its interaction with TNF receptors. It is indicated for treatment of adults with psoriatic arthritis or moderate-to-severe plaque psoriasis who are candidates for systemic therapy or phototherapy. Recommended dosing is 400 mg (as 2 × 200-mg SC injections) every 2 weeks, with a dose-reduced regimen for patients <90 kg: 400 mg (as 2 × 200-mg SC injections) initially and at weeks 2 and 4, followed by 200 mg SC every other week.

Interleukin-12/23 Inhibitors

- **Ustekinumab** (Stelara) is an IL-12/23 monoclonal antibody approved for the treatment of psoriasis in adults 18 years or older with moderate-to-severe plaque psoriasis. The recommended dose for patients weighing ≤100 kg is 45 mg SC initially and 4 weeks later, followed by 45 mg SC every 12 weeks. For patients weighing >100 kg, the dose is 90 mg SC initially and 4 weeks later, followed by 90 mg SC every 12 weeks. Common adverse effects include upper respiratory infections, headache, and tiredness. Serious adverse effects include those seen with other biologics, including tubercular, fungal, and viral infections and cancers. Reversible posterior leukoencephalopathy syndrome (RPLS) has also been reported.

Interleukin-17A Inhibitors

- **Secukinumab** (Cosentyx), **ixekizumab** (Taltz), and **brodalumab** (Siliq) are monoclonal antibodies that inhibit IL-17A, a proinflammatory cytokine that binds to receptors on keratinocytes, leading to inflammation and recruitment of inflammatory cell types, resulting in psoriatic plaques. These agents have comparable efficacy and similar adverse effects (eg, nasopharyngitis, upper respiratory tract infections, injection site reactions).
  - ✓ Secukinumab is a fully human IgG1κ monoclonal antibody that selectively binds and inhibits IL-17A. Recommended dosing for plaque psoriasis is 300 mg SC at weeks 0, 1, 2, 3, and 4 followed by 300 mg SC every 4 weeks.
  - ✓ Ixekizumab is a humanized IgG4 monoclonal antibody that neutralizes IL-17A. Recommended dosing is an initial dose of 160 mg SC followed by 80 mg every 2 weeks until week 12, followed by a maintenance phase of 80 mg SC every 4 weeks thereafter. Neutralizing anti-ixekizumab antibodies develop over time and are associated with reduced drug concentrations and loss of efficacy.
  - ✓ Brodalumab is a fully human IgG2 anti-IL-17RA monoclonal antibody that binds to the IL-17 receptor A and blocks the biologic activities of multiple IL-17 subtypes. The recommended dose is 210 mg SC on weeks 0, 1, and 2, then 210 mg every 2 weeks thereafter.

Interleukin-23 Inhibitors

- **Guselkumab** (Tremfya), **tildrakizumab** (Ilumya), and **risankizumab** (Skyrizi) inhibit IL-23, which induces a population of T-helper cells (TH17 cells) with a unique inflammatory gene signature important in the pathogenesis of psoriasis and other autoimmune diseases. Neutralizing antibodies to specific IL-17 inhibitors have been reported that may be associated with lower biologic serum concentrations and reduced efficacy.

✓ Guselkumab is a fully human IgG1 lambda monoclonal antibody that blocks the p19 subunit of IL-23. The recommended dose is 100 mg SC at weeks 0 and 4, and then every 8 weeks thereafter.

✓ Tildrakizumab is a humanized IgG1 monoclonal antibody designed to selectively block IL-23 by binding to the p19 subunit. The recommended dose is 100 mg SC administered only by a healthcare provider at weeks 0 and 4, and then every 12 weeks thereafter.

✓ Risankizumab is a humanized IgG1 monoclonal antibody that selectively inhibits IL-23 by binding to the p19 subunit. The recommended dose is 150 mg (two 75-mg SC injections) at weeks 0 and 4 and then every 12 weeks thereafter.

Combination Therapies

- Combination therapy may be used to enhance efficacy or minimize toxicity. Combinations can include two topical agents, a topical agent plus phototherapy, a systemic agent plus topical therapy, a systemic agent plus phototherapy, two systemic agents used in rotation, or a biologic agent with either a nonbiologic systemic or topical agent (see **Figs. 17-1** and **17-2**).
- The combination of a topical corticosteroid and a topical vitamin D_3 analogue is effective and safe with less skin irritation than monotherapy with either agent. The combination product containing calcipotriene and betamethasone dipropionate ointment (Taclonex) is effective for relatively severe psoriasis and may also be steroid sparing.
- The combination of retinoids with phototherapy (eg, tazarotene plus broadband UVB, acitretin plus broadband UVB or NB-UVB) also increases efficacy. Because retinoids may be photosensitizing and increase the risk of burning after UV exposure, doses of phototherapy should be reduced to minimize adverse effects. The combination of acitretin and PUVA (RE-PUVA) may be more effective than monotherapy with either treatment.
- Phototherapy has also been used with other topical agents, such as UVB with coal tar (Goeckerman regimen) to increase treatment response, because coal tar is also photosensitizing.
- Cyclosporine in combination with calcipotriene/betamethasone dipropionate is superior to cyclosporine alone. Cyclosporine may also be used with SCAT, but it should not be used with PUVA due to reduced efficacy and an increased risk of cutaneous malignancies.
- The combination of methotrexate and UVB appears to be synergistic. Low-dose methotrexate (eg, 7.5–10 mg once weekly) in combination with a biologic agent may be beneficial.

Alternative Drug Treatments

- **Mycophenolate mofetil** (CellCept) inhibits DNA and RNA synthesis and may have a lymphocyte antiproliferative effect. Although not FDA approved for psoriasis indications, oral mycophenolate mofetil may be effective in some cases of moderate-to-severe plaque psoriasis.
- **Hydroxyurea** inhibits cell synthesis in the S phase of the DNA cycle. It is occasionally used off-label for patients with recalcitrant severe psoriasis, but biologic agents may be a better option in these patients.

EVALUATION OF THERAPEUTIC OUTCOMES

- Help patients understand the general principles of therapy and the importance of medication adherence.
- A positive response involves normalization of involved areas of skin, as measured by reduced erythema and scaling, as well as reduction of plaque elevation.
- Successful management also includes control of itching and comorbid conditions such as dyslipidemia, hypertension, psoriatic arthritis, and depression.

- PASI is a uniform method to determine the extent of BSA affected, along with the degree of erythema, induration, and scaling. In the United States, severity of psoriasis is classified as mild, moderate, or severe:
  - ✓ Mild: ≤5% BSA involvement
  - ✓ Moderate: PASI ≥8 (higher in trials of biologics)
  - ✓ Severe: PASI ≥10 or Dermatology Life Quality Index (DLQI) ≥10 or BSA ≥10%
- The Physician Global Assessment can also be used to summarize erythema, induration, scaling, and extent of plaques relative to baseline assessment.
- Achievement of efficacy by any therapeutic regimen requires days to weeks. Initial dramatic response may be achieved with some agents, such as corticosteroids. However, sustained benefit with pharmacologically specific antipsoriatic therapy may require 2–8 weeks or longer for clinically meaningful response.

See Chapter 114, Psoriasis, authored by Rebecca M. Law and Wayne P. Gulliver, for a more detailed discussion of this topic.

CHAPTER 18 — Adrenal Gland Disorders

- Hyperfunction of the adrenal glands involves excess production of the adrenal hormones cortisol (resulting in Cushing syndrome) or aldosterone (resulting in hyperaldosteronism).
- Adrenal gland hypofunction is associated with primary (Addison disease) or secondary adrenal insufficiency.

Cushing Syndrome

PATHOPHYSIOLOGY

- Cushing syndrome results from effects of supraphysiologic glucocorticoid concentrations originating from either exogenous administration or endogenous overproduction by the adrenal gland (adrenocorticotropic hormone [ACTH] dependent) or by abnormal adrenocortical tissues (ACTH independent).
- ACTH-dependent Cushing syndrome (80% of all Cushing syndrome cases) is usually caused by overproduction of ACTH by the pituitary gland, causing bilateral adrenal hyperplasia. Pituitary adenomas account for about 85% of these cases (Cushing disease). Ectopic ACTH-secreting tumors and nonneoplastic corticotropin hypersecretion cause the remaining 20% of ACTH-dependent cases.
- Ectopic ACTH syndrome refers to excessive ACTH production resulting from an endocrine or nonendocrine tumor, usually of the pancreas, thyroid, or lung (eg, small-cell lung cancer).
- ACTH-independent Cushing syndrome is usually caused by adrenal adenomas and carcinomas.

CLINICAL PRESENTATION

- The most common findings in Cushing syndrome are central obesity and facial rounding (90% of patients). Peripheral obesity and fat accumulation occur in 50% of patients. Fat accumulation in the dorsocervical area (buffalo hump) is nonspecific, but increased supraclavicular fat pads are more specific for Cushing syndrome. Patients are often described as having moon facies and a buffalo hump.
- Other findings may include myopathy or muscular weakness, abdominal striae, hypertension, glucose intolerance, psychiatric changes, gonadal dysfunction, facial plethora (reddish complexion), and amenorrhea and hirsutism in women.
- Up to 60% of patients develop Cushing-induced osteoporosis; about 40% present with back pain; and 20% progress to spinal compression fractures.

DIAGNOSIS

- Hypercortisolism can be established with one or more of the following tests: 24-hour urinary free cortisol (UFC), midnight plasma cortisol, late-night (11 PM) salivary cortisol, and/or low-dose dexamethasone suppression test (DST).
- Other tests to determine etiology are plasma ACTH; adrenal vein catheterization; metyrapone stimulation test; adrenal, chest, or abdominal computed tomography

(CT); corticotropin-releasing hormone (CRH) stimulation test; inferior petrosal sinus sampling; and pituitary magnetic resonance imaging (MRI).
- Adrenal nodules and masses are identified using high-resolution CT scanning or MRI.

TREATMENT

- Goals of Treatment: Limit morbidity and mortality and return the patient to a normal functional state by removing the source of hypercortisolism while minimizing pituitary or adrenal deficiencies.
- Treatment plans in Cushing syndrome based on etiology are included in **Table 18-1**.

NONPHARMACOLOGIC THERAPY

- Treatment of choice for both ACTH-dependent and ACTH-independent Cushing syndrome is surgical resection of offending tumors.
- Transsphenoidal resection of the pituitary tumor is the treatment of choice for Cushing disease. Radiotherapy may be preferred for tumors invading the dura or cavernous sinus and provides clinical improvement in ~50% of patients within 3–5 years but increases the risk for pituitary-dependent hormone deficiencies (hypopituitarism).
- Laparoscopic adrenalectomy is often preferred for unilateral adrenal adenomas or when transsphenoidal surgery and pituitary radiotherapy have failed or cannot be used.

PHARMACOLOGIC THERAPY

- Pharmacotherapy is generally used as second-line treatments in patients who are not surgical candidates and may also be used preoperatively or as adjunctive therapy in postoperative patients awaiting response (**Table 18-1**). Rarely, monotherapy is used as a palliative treatment when surgery is not indicated.

Steroidogenesis Inhibitors

- **Metyrapone** inhibits 11 β-hydroxylase, thereby inhibiting cortisol synthesis. After administration, a sudden decrease in cortisol concentration prompts a compensatory rise in plasma ACTH levels. With cortisol synthesis blocked, adrenal steroidogenesis shunts toward androgen production, resulting in androgenic side effects such as acne and hirsutism. Inhibition of aldosterone synthesis can result in natriuresis and blood pressure changes. Nausea, vomiting, vertigo, headache, dizziness, abdominal discomfort, and allergic rash have been reported after oral administration. Metyrapone is currently available through the manufacturer only for compassionate use.
- **Ketoconazole** inhibits cytochrome P-450 enzymes, including 11 β-hydroxylase and 17 α-hydroxylase. It is effective in lowering serum cortisol levels after several weeks of therapy. It also has antiandrogenic activity, which may be beneficial in women but can cause gynecomastia and hypogonadism in men. The most common adverse effects are reversible elevation of hepatic transaminases, GI discomfort, and dermatologic reactions. Because of the risk of severe hepatotoxicity, monitoring should include liver function tests at baseline followed by weekly monitoring of serum ALT throughout therapy. Ketoconazole may be used concomitantly with metyrapone to achieve synergistic reduction in cortisol levels; in addition, ketoconazole's antiandrogenic actions may offset the androgenic potential of metyrapone.
- **Etomidate** is an imidazole derivative similar to ketoconazole that inhibits 11 β-hydroxylase and may have other mechanisms. Because it is only available in a parenteral formulation, use is limited to patients with acute hypercortisolemia requiring emergency treatment or in preparation for surgery. Frequent monitoring of serum cortisol is advised to prevent hypocortisolemia. Side effects include sedation, injection site pain, hypotension, myoclonus, nausea, and vomiting. The initial dose is 0.03 mg/kg by IV bolus followed by a continuous infusion of 0.1–0.3 mg/kg/hr.

TABLE 18-1 Treatment Options in Cushing Syndrome Based on Etiology

Etiology	Nondrug	Generic (Brand) Drug Name	Dosing		
			Initial Dose	Usual Range	Maximum
Ectopic ACTH syndrome	Surgery, chemotherapy, irradiation	Metyrapone (Metopirone) 250 mg capsules	0.5–1 g/day, divided every 4–6 hours	1–2 g/day, divided every 4–6 hours	6 g/day
		Ketoconazole (Nizoral) 200 mg tablets	200 mg once or twice a day	200–1200 mg/day, divided twice daily	1600 mg/day divided four times daily
Pituitary dependent	Surgery, irradiation	Mitotane (Lysodren) 500 mg tablets	0.5–1 g/day, increased by 0.5–1 g/day every 1–4 weeks	1–4 g daily, with food to decrease GI effects	12 g/day
		Metyrapone	See above	See above	See above
		Mifepristone (Korlym) 300 mg tablets	300 mg once daily, increased by 300 mg/day every 2–4 weeks	600–1200 mg/day	1200 mg/day or 20 mg/kg/day
		Cabergoline (Dostinex) 0.5 mg tablets	0.5 mg once weekly	0.5–7 mg once weekly	7 mg/week
		Pasireotide (Signifor) 0.3, 0.6, and 0.9 mg/mL solution	0.6–0.9 mg twice daily	0.3–0.9 mg twice daily	1.8 mg/day
Adrenal adenoma	Surgery, postoperative replacement	Ketoconazole	See above	See above	See above
Adrenal carcinoma	Surgery	Mitotane	See above	See above	See above

ACTH, adrenocorticotropic hormone.

Adrenolytic Agents

- **Mitotane** is a cytotoxic drug that inhibits the 11-hydroxylation of 11-deoxycortisol and 11-desoxycorticosterone in the adrenal cortex, reducing synthesis of cortisol and corticosterone. Similar to ketoconazole, mitotane takes weeks to months to exert beneficial effects. Sustained cortisol suppression occurs in most patients and may persist after drug discontinuation in up to one-third of patients. Mitotane degenerates cells within the zona fasciculata and reticularis, resulting in atrophy of the adrenal cortex; the zona glomerulosa is minimally affected during acute therapy but can be damaged during long-term treatment. Mitotane can cause significant neurologic and GI side effects, and patients should be monitored carefully or hospitalized when initiating therapy. Nausea and diarrhea are common at doses greater than 2 g/day and can be avoided by gradually increasing the dose and/or administering it with food. Lethargy, somnolence, and other CNS effects are also common. Reversible hypercholesterolemia and prolonged bleeding times can occur.

Neuromodulators of ACTH Release

- Pituitary secretion of ACTH is normally mediated by neurotransmitters such as serotonin, γ-aminobutyric acid (GABA), acetylcholine, and catecholamines. Although ACTH-secreting pituitary tumors (Cushing disease) self-regulate ACTH production to some degree, these neurotransmitters can still promote pituitary ACTH production. Consequently, agents that target these transmitters have been proposed for treatment of Cushing disease, including cyproheptadine, bromocriptine, cabergoline, valproic acid, octreotide, lanreotide, pasireotide, rosiglitazone, and tretinoin. With the exception of pasireotide, none of these drugs have demonstrated consistent clinical efficacy for treating Cushing disease.
- **Cyproheptadine**, a nonselective serotonin receptor antagonist and anticholinergic drug, can decrease ACTH secretion in some patients with Cushing disease. However, side effects such as sedation and weight gain significantly limit its use.
- **Pasireotide** (Signifor) is a somatostatin analogue that binds and activates somatostatin receptors, thereby inhibiting ACTH secretion, leading to decreased cortisol secretion. It is approved for treatment of adults with Cushing disease for whom pituitary surgery is not an option or has not been curative. Side effects include nausea, diarrhea, cholelithiasis, increased hepatic transaminases, hyperglycemia, sinus bradycardia, and QT prolongation.

Glucocorticoid-Receptor Blocking Agents

- **Mifepristone** (Korlym) is a progesterone- and glucocorticoid-receptor antagonist that inhibits dexamethasone suppression and increases endogenous cortisol and ACTH levels in normal subjects. Evidence suggests that mifepristone is highly effective in reversing the manifestations of hypercortisolism (hyperglycemia, hypertension, and weight gain). It is FDA approved for treatment of endogenous Cushing syndrome in patients who have type 2 diabetes or glucose intolerance and who are not eligible for, or have had poor response to, surgery. Common adverse effects include fatigue, nausea, headache, arthralgia, peripheral edema, endometrial hyperplasia, and hypokalemia.

EVALUATION OF THERAPEUTIC OUTCOMES

- Close monitoring of 24-hour UFC and serum cortisol is essential to identify adrenal insufficiency in patients with Cushing syndrome. Monitor steroid secretion with all drug therapy (except mifepristone) and give corticosteroid replacement if needed.

Hyperaldosteronism

PATHOPHYSIOLOGY

- Hyperaldosteronism involves excess aldosterone secretion and is categorized as either primary (stimulus arising from within the adrenal gland) or secondary (stimulus from extra-adrenal etiologies).
- *Primary hyperaldosteronism* (PA) is usually caused by bilateral adrenal hyperplasia and aldosterone-producing adenoma (Conn syndrome). Rare causes include unilateral (primary) adrenal hyperplasia, adrenal cortex carcinoma, renin-responsive adrenocortical adenoma, and three forms of familial hyperaldosteronism (FH): Type I (glucocorticoid-remediable aldosteronism); Type II (familial occurrence of adenoma or hyperplasia type II); and Type III.
- *Secondary hyperaldosteronism* results from excessive stimulation of the zona glomerulosa by an extra-adrenal factor, usually the renin–angiotensin system. Elevated aldosterone secretion can result from excessive potassium intake, oral contraceptives, pregnancy, and menses. Heart failure, cirrhosis, renal artery stenosis, and Bartter syndrome also can lead to elevated aldosterone concentrations.

CLINICAL PRESENTATION

- Patients may complain of muscle weakness, fatigue, paresthesias, headache, polydipsia, and nocturnal polyuria.
- Signs may include hypertension and tetany/paralysis.
- A plasma aldosterone concentration-to-plasma renin activity (PAC-to-PRA) ratio or aldosterone-to-renin ratio (ARR) >30 ng/dL per ng/(mL·hr) (830 pmol/L per mcg/(L·hr) and a PAC >15 ng/dL (420 pmol/L) is suggestive of PA.
- Other laboratory findings include suppressed renin activity, elevated plasma aldosterone, hypernatremia (>142 mEq/L), hypokalemia, hypomagnesemia, elevated serum bicarbonate (>31 mEq/L), and glucose intolerance.

DIAGNOSIS

- Initial diagnosis is made by screening patients with suspected PA. Any patient with a blood pressure >150/100 mm Hg measured on 3 separate days and those with resistant hypertension should be screened. Additional patients at risk for PA include those with diuretic-induced hypokalemia, hypertension and adrenal incidentaloma, hypertension and sleep apnea, hypertension and a family history of early onset hypertension or cerebrovascular accident at an age <40 years, and all patients with hypertension and a first-degree relative diagnosed with PA.
- Screening for PA is most often done using the PAC-to-PRA ratio (also known as the ARR). An elevated ARR is highly suggestive of PA.
- If the ARR is positive, confirmatory tests to exclude false-positives include the oral sodium-loading test, saline infusion test, fludrocortisone suppression test (FST), and captopril challenge test. A positive test indicates autonomous aldosterone secretion under inhibitory pressures and is diagnostic for PA.

TREATMENT

NONPHARMACOLOGIC THERAPY

- Aldosterone-producing adenomas are treated by laparoscopic resection of the tumor, leading to permanent cures in up to 72% of patients. Medical management with an aldosterone receptor antagonist is often effective if surgery is contraindicated.

PHARMACOLOGIC THERAPY

- Aldosterone-receptor antagonists are the treatment of choice for bilateral adrenal hyperplasia.
  - ✓ **Spironolactone** (Aldactone) is a nonselective aldosterone receptor antagonist that competes with aldosterone for binding at aldosterone receptors, thus preventing the negative effects of aldosterone receptor activation. The initial dose is 25 mg once daily titrated upward at 4- to 8-week intervals. Most patients respond to doses between 25 and 400 mg/day given in single or divided doses. Adverse effects include GI discomfort, impotence, gynecomastia, menstrual irregularities, and hyperkalemia.
  - ✓ **Eplerenone** (Inspra) is a selective aldosterone receptor antagonist with high affinity for aldosterone receptors and low affinity for androgen and progesterone receptors. Consequently, it elicits fewer sex-steroid–dependent effects than spironolactone. Dosing starts at 50 mg daily, with titration at 4- to 8-week intervals to 50 mg twice a day; some patients may require total daily doses as high as 200–300 mg.
  - ✓ **Amiloride** (Amiloride), a potassium-sparing diuretic, is less effective than spironolactone, and patients often require additional therapy to adequately control blood pressure. The initial dose is 5 mg twice daily, with a usual range of 20 mg/day given in two divided doses; doses up to 30 mg/day may be necessary.
  - ✓ Additional second-line options include calcium channel blockers, ACE inhibitors, and diuretics such as chlorthalidone, although all of these lack outcome data in PA.

- Treatment of secondary aldosteronism is dictated by etiology. Control or correction of the extra-adrenal stimulation of aldosterone secretion should resolve the disorder. Medical therapy with spironolactone is undertaken until the etiology is identified.

Adrenal Insufficiency

PATHOPHYSIOLOGY

- Primary adrenal insufficiency (Addison disease) usually involves destruction of all regions of the adrenal cortex. There are deficiencies of cortisol, aldosterone, and the various androgens, and levels of CRH and ACTH increase in a compensatory manner.
- Autoimmune dysfunction is responsible for 80%–90% of cases in developed countries, whereas tuberculosis is the predominant cause in developing countries.
- Medications that inhibit cortisol synthesis (eg, ketoconazole) or accelerate cortisol metabolism (eg, phenytoin, rifampin, phenobarbital) can also cause primary adrenal insufficiency.
- Secondary adrenal insufficiency most commonly results from exogenous corticosteroid use, leading to suppression of the hypothalamic–pituitary–adrenal axis and decreased ACTH release as well as impaired androgen and cortisol production. Mirtazapine and progestins (eg, medroxyprogesterone acetate, megestrol acetate) have also been reported to induce secondary adrenal insufficiency. Secondary disease typically presents with normal mineralocorticoid concentrations.

CLINICAL PRESENTATION

- Patients with adrenal insufficiency commonly complain of weakness, weight loss, GI symptoms, salt craving, headaches, memory impairment, depression, and postural dizziness.
- Early symptoms of acute adrenal insufficiency also include myalgias, malaise, and anorexia. As the situation progresses, vomiting, fever, hypotension, and shock develop.
- Signs of adrenal insufficiency include increased skin pigmentation, postural hypotension, fever, decreased body hair, vitiligo, amenorrhea, and cold intolerance.

DIAGNOSIS

- The short cosyntropin stimulation test can be used to assess patients with suspected hypercortisolism. An increase to a cortisol level of ≥18 mcg/dL (500 nmol/L) rules out adrenal insufficiency.
- Patients with Addison disease have an abnormal response to the short cosyntropin stimulation test. Plasma ACTH levels are usually elevated (400–2000 pg/mL or 88–440 pmol/L) in primary insufficiency versus normal to low (5–50 pg/mL or 1.1–11 pmol/L]) in secondary insufficiency. A normal cosyntropin-stimulation test does not rule out secondary adrenal insufficiency.
- Other tests include the insulin hypoglycemia test, the metyrapone test, and the CRH stimulation test.

TREATMENT

- Goals of Treatment: Limit morbidity and mortality, return the patient to a normal functional state, and prevent episodes of acute adrenal insufficiency.

NONPHARMACOLOGIC THERAPY

- Inform patients of treatment complications, expected outcomes, proper medication administration and adherence, and possible side effects.

PHARMACOLOGIC THERAPY

Corticosteroids

- The agents of choice are **hydrocortisone** and **cortisone acetate**, usually administered two times daily, with the goal of establishing the lowest effective dose while mimicking the normal diurnal adrenal rhythm. Once-daily **prednisolone** is an alternative when adherence to a multidose regimen is a concern.
- Recommended starting total daily doses are hydrocortisone 15–25 mg daily, which is approximately equivalent to cortisone acetate 20–35 mg daily, or prednisolone 3–5 mg daily (Table 18-2). For hydrocortisone or cortisone, two-thirds of the dose is given in the morning and one-third is given 6–8 hours later.
- Monitor the patient's symptoms every 6–8 weeks to assess proper glucocorticoid replacement. Measure body weight, postural blood pressures, subjective energy levels, and signs of glucocorticoid excess.
- In primary adrenal insufficiency, **fludrocortisone acetate** 0.05–0.2 mg orally once daily can be used to replace mineralocorticoid loss and maintain volume status. If

	Anti-inflammatory	Equivalent	Approximate	Sodium-Retaining
Glucocorticoid	**Potency**	**Potency (mg)**	**Half-Life (min)**	**Potency**
Cortisone	0.8	25	30	2
Hydrocortisone	1	20	90	2
Prednisone	3.5	5	60	1
Prednisolone	4	5	200	1
Triamcinolone	5	4	300	0
Methylprednisolone	5	4	180	0
Betamethasone	25	0.6	100–300	0
Dexamethasone	30	0.75	100–300	0

TABLE 18-2 Relative Potencies of Glucocorticoids

parenteral therapy is needed, 2–5 mg of **deoxycorticosterone trimethylacetate** in oil can be administered intramuscularly every 3–4 weeks. Mineralocorticoid replacement attenuates development of hyperkalemia, and patients on fludrocortisone therapy do not need to restrict salt intake. Mineralocorticoid therapy may be unnecessary in some cases because glucocorticoids (especially in large doses) also bind to mineralocorticoid receptors.

- Because most adrenal crises occur because of glucocorticoid dose reductions or lack of stress-related dose adjustments, patients receiving corticosteroid replacement therapy should add 5–10 mg hydrocortisone (or equivalent) to their normal daily regimen shortly before strenuous activities, such as exercise. During times of severe physical stress (eg, febrile illness, injury), patients should be instructed to double their daily dose until recovery.
- Treatment of secondary adrenal insufficiency is similar to primary disease treatment, except that mineralocorticoid replacement is usually not necessary.

PHARMACOLOGIC THERAPY OF ACUTE ADRENAL INSUFFICIENCY

- Acute adrenal insufficiency (adrenal crisis or addisonian crisis) represents a true endocrine emergency.
- Stressful situations, surgery, infection, and trauma are potential events that increase adrenal requirements, especially in patients with some underlying adrenal or pituitary insufficiency.
- The most common cause of adrenal crisis is HPA-axis suppression brought on by abrupt withdrawal of chronic glucocorticoid use.
- **Hydrocortisone** given parenterally is the corticosteroid of choice because of its combined glucocorticoid and mineralocorticoid activity. The starting dose is 100 mg IV by rapid infusion, followed by 200 mg over 24 hours as a continuous infusion or intermittent bolus every 6 hours. IV administration is continued for an additional day at a reduced dose of 100 mg over 24 hours. If the patient is stable at that time, oral hydrocortisone can be started at a dose of 50 mg every 6–8 hours, followed by tapering to the individual's chronic replacement needs.
- **Fluid replacement** often is required and can be accomplished with IV dextrose 5% in normal saline solution at a rate to support blood pressure.
- If therapy is needed for hypoglycemia, dextrose 25% in water can be infused at a dose of 2–4 mL/kg (maximum single dose of 25 g dextrose).
- If hyperkalemia is present after the hydrocortisone maintenance phase, additional mineralocorticoid supplementation can be achieved with **fludrocortisone acetate** 0.1 mg daily.
- Patients with adrenal insufficiency should carry a card or wear a bracelet or necklace that contains information about their condition. They should also have easy access to injectable hydrocortisone or glucocorticoid suppositories in case of an emergency or during times of physical stress, such as febrile illness or injury.

EVALUATION OF THERAPEUTIC OUTCOMES

- The end point of therapy for adrenal insufficiency is difficult to assess in most patients, but a reduction in excess pigmentation is a good clinical marker. Development of features of Cushing syndrome indicates excessive replacement.

See Chapter 93, Adrenal Gland Disorders, authored by Steven M. Smith, Scott G. Garland, and John G. Gums, for a more detailed discussion of this topic.

CHAPTER 19

Diabetes Mellitus

- *Diabetes mellitus* (DM) is a group of metabolic disorders characterized by chronically elevated blood glucose (BG) and abnormal carbohydrate, fat, and protein metabolism. Without effective treatment, DM can lead to acute complications such as diabetic ketoacidosis (DKA) and hyperosmolar hyperglycemic syndrome (HHS). Chronic hyperglycemia can cause microvascular, macrovascular, and neuropathic complications.

PATHOPHYSIOLOGY

- Type 1 DM (5%–10% of cases) usually results from autoimmune destruction of pancreatic β-cells, leading to absolute deficiency of insulin. It usually presents in children and adolescents but can occur at any age. The disorder is believed to be initiated by exposure to an unknown environmental trigger in a genetically susceptible individual. The autoimmune process is mediated by macrophages and T lymphocytes with autoantibodies to β-cell antigens (eg, islet cell antibody, insulin antibodies). Amylin (a hormone cosecreted from pancreatic β-cells with insulin) is also deficient in type 1 DM due to β-cell destruction. Amylin suppresses inappropriate glucagon secretion, slows gastric emptying, and causes central satiety.
  - ✓ After the initial diagnosis, a period of transient remission called the "honeymoon" phase may occur, during which insulin doses can be reduced or withdrawn before continued β-cell destruction requires lifelong insulin replacement therapy.
- Type 2 DM (90%–95% of cases) is characterized by multiple defects:
  - ✓ *Impaired insulin secretion*: β-cell mass and function are both reduced, and β-cell failure is progressive.
  - ✓ *Reduced incretin effect*: Normally, the gut incretin hormones glucagon-like peptide-1 (GLP-1) and glucose-dependent insulinotropic peptide (GIP) are released and stimulate insulin secretion in response to a meal. Patients with type 2 DM have a reduced incretin effect due to decreased concentrations of or resistance to the effects of incretin hormones.
  - ✓ *Insulin resistance*: This is manifested by excessive hepatic glucose production, decreased skeletal muscle uptake of glucose, and increased lipolysis and free fatty acid production.
  - ✓ *Excess glucagon secretion*: This occurs because type 2 DM patients fail to suppress glucagon in response to meals because of GLP-1 resistance/deficiency and insulin resistance/deficiency, which directly suppress glucagon.
  - ✓ *Sodium-glucose cotransporter-2 (SGLT-2) upregulation in the kidney*: This increases reabsorption of glucose by proximal renal tubular cells, which further contributes to hyperglycemia.
- *Gestational diabetes* (GDM) is DM that occurs in women during pregnancy.
- Less common causes of DM (1%–2%) include maturity onset diabetes of the young (MODY), genetic syndromes (eg, Down syndrome), endocrine disorders (eg, acromegaly, Cushing syndrome), pancreatic exocrine dysfunction, infections, and medications (eg, glucocorticoids, thiazides, niacin, atypical antipsychotics).
- Microvascular complications include retinopathy, neuropathy, and nephropathy. Macrovascular complications include coronary heart disease (CHD), stroke, and peripheral vascular disease.

CLINICAL PRESENTATION

TYPE 1 DIABETES MELLITUS

- Patients often have symptoms in the days or weeks preceding the diagnosis. The most common initial symptoms are polyuria, polydipsia, polyphagia, weight loss, fatigue, and lethargy.

- Individuals are often thin and are prone to develop DKA in the absence of an adequate insulin supply; many patients initially present with DKA. Symptom onset can be triggered by infection, trauma, or psychological stress.

TYPE 2 DIABETES MELLITUS

- Most patients are asymptomatic or have only mild fatigue at the time of diagnosis. Many patients are incidentally found to have type 2 DM after routine laboratory testing (eg, plasma glucose or A1C) or development of complications (eg, myocardial infarction, stroke).
- Because mild hyperglycemia may exist for years prior to the diagnosis, microvascular and macrovascular complications are often present at the time of diagnosis.
- Most patients are overweight or obese with an elevated waist:hip ratio.

DIAGNOSIS

- Normal fasting (no caloric intake for at least 8 hours) plasma glucose (FPG) is 70–99 mg/dL (3.9–5.5 mmol/L). Impaired fasting glucose (IFG) is FPG 100–125 mg/dL (5.6–6.9 mmol/L).
- Normal glucose tolerance based on a 2-hour post-load plasma glucose using the equivalent of 75 g anhydrous glucose dissolved in water (oral glucose tolerance test or OGTT) is <140 mg/dL (7.8 mmol/L). Impaired glucose tolerance (IGT) is OGTT 140–199 mg/dL (7.8–11.0 mmol/L).
- Normal A1C is 4%–5.6% (39–46 mmol/mol Hb). Increased risk of DM (prediabetes) is A1C 5.7%–6.4% (39–46 mmol/mol Hb).
- Criteria for diagnosis of DM include any one of the following:
  1. A1C ≥6.5% (48 mmol/mol Hb)
  2. FPG ≥126 mg/dL (7.0 mmol/L)
  3. OGTT ≥200 mg/dL (11.1 mmol/L)
  4. Random plasma glucose ≥200 mg/dL (11.1 mmol/L) with classic symptoms of hyperglycemia or hyperglycemic crisis

  In the absence of unequivocal hyperglycemia, a diagnosis using criteria 1 through 3 requires two abnormal test results from the same sample or in two separate test samples.
- *Prediabetes* is a condition of abnormal BG that is not sufficiently high to meet the thresholds that define DM but often progresses to the diagnosis.
- Screening for type 1 DM in asymptomatic children or adults is not recommended due to low disease prevalence and the acute onset of symptoms. Screening for type 2 DM is recommended for asymptomatic adults who are overweight (BMI ≥25 kg/m² or ≥23 kg/m² in Asian-Americans) and have at least one other risk factor for developing type 2 DM. All adults, even those without risk factors, should be screened every 3 years starting at 45 years old. Children at risk for developing type 2 DM should undergo screening every 3 years starting at age 10 years. Pregnant women should undergo risk assessment for GDM at the first prenatal visit; those with multiple risk factors for type 2 DM should be tested as soon as feasible. All women (even if the initial test was negative) should undergo testing at 24–28 weeks' gestation.

TREATMENT

- <u>Goals of Treatment</u>: The primary goal is to prevent or delay progression of long-term microvascular and macrovascular complications. Additional goals are to alleviate symptoms of hyperglycemia, minimize hypoglycemia and other adverse effects, minimize treatment burden, and maintain quality of life. General glycemic targets for most nonpregnant adults with DM are listed in **Table 19-1**.

INITIAL ASSESSMENT

- During the initial visit, perform a full medical evaluation to confirm the diagnosis, classify the type of diabetes, identify complications or potential comorbid conditions, and review previous treatments and risk factors in established patients.

TABLE 19-1	Glycemic Target Recommendations for Most Nonpregnant Adults with Diabetes	
Parameter	American Diabetes Association (ADA)	American Association of Clinical Endocrinologists (AACE)
A1C	<7.0% (53 mmol/mol Hb)	≤6.5% (48 mmol/mol Hb)
Fasting plasma glucose (FPG)	80–130 mg/dL (4.4–7.2 mmol/L)	<110 mg/dL (6.1 mmol/L)
Postprandial glucose (PPG)	<180 mg/dL (10 mmol/L)	<140 mg/dL (7.8 mmol/L)

Glycemic targets should be individualized. More stringent or less stringent goals may be appropriate for some patients.

- Review past medical, family, and social history as well as medication use, adherence, tolerability, and use of diabetes technology.
- Screen for psychosocial conditions, self-management education needs, and hypoglycemia.
- Perform a thorough physical exam (including height, weight, BMI, blood pressure, thyroid palpation, and foot exam) and laboratory evaluation (including A1C, lipid profile, liver function tests, serum creatinine, and eGFR).
- Calculate a 10-year ASCVD risk score.

NONPHARMACOLOGIC THERAPY

- Medical nutrition therapy (MNT) involves an individually tailored nutrition plan. Implement a healthy meal plan that is moderate in calories and carbohydrates and low in saturated fat with all of the essential vitamins and minerals. Target an initial weight loss goal of at least 5% in all type 2 DM patients who are overweight or obese through calorie restriction. For individuals with type 1 DM, focus on physiologically regulating insulin administration rather than the amount and type of carbohydrates ingested.
- Aerobic exercise can improve insulin sensitivity, modestly improve glycemic control, reduce cardiovascular (CV) risk, contribute to weight control, and improve well-being. Physical activity goals include at least 150 min/week of moderate (50%–70% maximal heart rate) intensity exercise spread over at least 3 days/week with no more than 2 days between activity. Resistance/strength training is recommended at least 2 times/week for patients without proliferative diabetic retinopathy.
- Offer access to diabetes self-management education and support (DSME/S) programs to all patients. Such programs target self-care behaviors of healthy eating, being active, monitoring glucose levels, taking medications, problem-solving, reducing risk of complications, and healthy coping. Patients must be involved in decision making and have strong knowledge of the disease and associated complications.

PHARMACOLOGIC THERAPY

Insulin

- The main advantage of insulin over other antihyperglycemic agents is that it can achieve a wide range of glucose targets and the dose can be individualized based on glycemic levels. Disadvantages include the risk of hypoglycemia, need for injections, weight gain, and treatment burden.
- All commercial insulin preparations are produced using recombinant DNA technology. "Human" insulins (NPH, regular) are recombinant DNA–derived human insulin, whereas insulin analogs have had amino acids substitutions in the insulin molecule that change the onset or duration of action.
- Most insulin products are administered subcutaneously (SC) for chronic diabetes management, except for inhaled human insulin, which is a dry powder of regular insulin that is inhaled and absorbed through pulmonary tissue.

- The most commonly used insulin concentration is 100 units/mL (U-100); more concentrated insulins (U-200, U-300, U-500) may be considered for patients requiring larger doses. U-500 regular insulin is reserved for patients with extreme insulin resistance and is usually given two or three times a day.
- The pharmacokinetics of insulin products is characterized by their onset, peak, and duration of action (Table 19-2).
- *Basal insulin* (or background insulin) refers to longer-acting insulins that regulate BG levels in between meals by suppressing hepatic glucose production and maintaining near-normal glycemic levels in the fasting state. Options include the following insulins:
  - ✓ **NPH** is the least ideal product because it has a distinct peak and a duration of action much less than 24 hours and usually requires twice-daily dosing.
  - ✓ **Detemir** also has a peak and often lasts <24 hours; it can be given once daily in some patients but should be dosed twice daily at low doses (<0.3 units/kg).

TABLE 19-2	Pharmacokinetics of Select Insulins Administered Subcutaneously		
Type of Insulin[a] by Generic (Brand) Name	**Onset**	**Peak[b]**	**Duration[b]**
Ultra-rapid acting			
Insulin aspart (Fiasp)	15–20 min[c]	90–120 min	5–7 hours
Insulin human—inhaled (Afrezza)	12 min	35–55 min	1.5–4.5 hours
Rapid-acting			
Insulin aspart (NovoLog)	10–20 min	30–90 min	3–5 hours
Insulin lispro U-100, U-200 (Humalog)			
Insulin glulisine (Apidra)			
Short-acting			
Regular (Humulin R, Novolin R)	30–60 min	2–4 hours	5–8 hours
Intermediate-acting			
NPH (Humulin N, Novolin N)	2–4 hours	4–10 hours	10–24 hours
Regular U-500 (Humulin R 500)	15 min	4–8 hours	13–24 hours
Long-acting			
Insulin detemir (Levemir)	1.5–4 hours	6–14 hours[d]	16–20 hours
Insulin glargine (Lantus, Basaglar)	2–4 hours	No peak	20–24 hours
Insulin glargine U-300 (Toujeo)	6 hours	No peak	36 hours
Insulin degludec U-100, U-200 (Tresiba)	1 hour	No peak	42 hours
Combination Products			
70% NPH/30% Regular (Humulin 70/30, Novolin 70/30)	30–60 min	Dual	10–16 hours
75% NPL, 25% lispro (Humalog 75/25)	5–15 min		10–16 hours
50% NPL, 50% lispro (Humalog 50/50)	5–15 min		10–16 hours
70% insulin aspart protamine, 30% insulin aspart (NovoLog 70/30)	5–15 min		15–18 hours

[a]U-100 unless otherwise noted.
[b]The peak and duration of insulin action are variable, depending on the injection site, duration of diabetes, renal function, smoking status, and other factors.
[c]Onset of appearance is 2.5 minutes compared to 5.2 minutes for insulin aspart (NovoLog).
[d]Long-acting insulins are considered "peakless" although they have exhibited peak effects during comparative testing.
NPH, neutral protamine Hagedorn; NPL, insulin lispro protamine suspension.

✓ **Glargine U-100** is considered to be peakless and can usually be given once daily.

✓ **Glargine U-300** and **degludec U-100 or U-200** are longer acting-agents that have no peak and are given once daily.

All basal insulins can achieve similar A1C reductions if dosed and titrated properly, but the longer-acting products have a lower risk of hypoglycemia (particularly nocturnal hypoglycemia) and may result in less glucose variability. However, they are more expensive.

- *Bolus insulin* refers to short- or rapid-acting insulins that cover meals (also called prandial insulin) or glycemic excursions (also called correction insulin). Basal insulin is the preferred and most convenient initial insulin formulation for patients with type 2 DM, whereas patients with type 1 DM require a combination of basal and bolus insulin to achieve adequate glycemic control. Bolus insulin options include:

  ✓ **Aspart**, **lispro**, and **glulisine**, the rapid-onset, short-duration insulins

  ✓ **Inhaled human insulin** and **fast-acting insulin aspart (Fiasp)**, the ultra-rapid onset insulins

  Rapid-acting insulins offer a faster onset and shorter duration of action than **regular insulin**, and ultra-rapid acting insulins offer an even faster onset; this may more closely mimic prandial endogenous insulin release. Rapid-acting insulins have a modestly lower risk of hypoglycemia than regular insulin. All prandial insulins can be used effectively, but cost differences can be substantial.

- Various premixed insulin products containing both a basal and a prandial component are also available for patients who require fewer injections or a simpler regimen (Table 19-2). However, these products are limited by fixed mixed formulations, which can make it challenging to tailor the dosing regimen.

- The insulin dose must be individualized. In type 1 DM, the average daily requirement is 0.5–0.6 units/kg, with approximately 50% given as basal insulin and the remaining 50% dedicated to meal coverage. During the honeymoon phase, requirements may fall to 0.1–0.4 units/kg. Higher doses are often needed during acute illness or with ketosis.

- Hypoglycemia is the most common adverse effects of insulin therapy. Insulin also causes dose-dependent weight gain, which occurs predominantly in truncal fat. Injection site reactions may include redness, pain, itching, urticaria, edema, and inflammation. SC administration can result in lipoatrophy or lipohypertrophy, which can be prevented by routinely rotating injection sites. Inhaled human insulin can cause cough and upper respiratory infections, and it is contraindicated in chronic obstructive pulmonary disease and asthma due to bronchospasm risk. Because inhaled insulin has been associated with a small decline in pulmonary function, patients should have spirometry tests performed at baseline, 6 months, and annually thereafter.

Biguanides

- **Metformin** decreases hepatic glucose production and enhances insulin sensitivity in peripheral (muscle) tissues, allowing for increased glucose uptake into muscle cells.

- Metformin is recommended as first-line pharmacotherapy in patients with type 2 DM (unless a contraindication or intolerability exists) due to extensive experience, high efficacy, minimal hypoglycemia risk, positive or neutral effects on weight, potential positive impact on CV risk, manageable side-effect profile, and low cost. It reduces A1C levels by 1.5%–2% (16–22 mmol/mol Hb) and FPG levels by 60–80 mg/dL (3.3–4.4 mmol/L) in drug-naïve patients with initial A1C values of approximately 9% (75 mmol/mol Hb). It does not cause weight gain and may lead to a modest (2–3 kg) weight loss. It has a low risk of hypoglycemia because it does not directly increase pancreatic insulin secretion. Metformin decreases plasma triglycerides and low-density lipoprotein cholesterol (LDL-C) by approximately 8%–15% and modestly increases high-density lipoprotein cholesterol (HDL-C) by 2%.

- Metformin frequently causes GI side effects (diarrhea, abdominal discomfort, stomach upset); these effects are usually dose-dependent, transient, mild, and can be minimized with slow dose titration and taking metformin with or immediately after meals. When initiating therapy, use a low dose (typically 500 mg) given with the largest meal. Then increase the dose in 500-mg increments over several weeks. Extended-release metformin may lessen some of the GI side effects, but a comparison of immediate-release vs extended-release metformin found no significant differences in rates of GI adverse effects.

- Metformin may cause a metallic taste and may lower vitamin B_{12} concentrations; B_{12} levels or methylmalonic acid should be measured annually or if a deficiency is suspected, with vitamin B_{12} supplementation given if indicated.
- Lactic acidosis occurs rarely, usually in the setting of severe illness or acute kidney injury. The risk may increase in moderate-to-severe renal insufficiency or tissue hypoperfusion states such as acute heart failure (HF), excessive alcohol intake, and hepatic impairment. Because symptoms are often nonspecific, the diagnosis must be confirmed by laboratory measurement of high lactic acid levels and acidosis.
- Metformin is renally excreted and accumulates in renal insufficiency; it is contraindicated in patients with eGFR <30 mL/min/1.73 m² and should be used with caution in patients with milder renal insufficiency. Metformin initiation is not recommended in patients with eGFR 30–45 mL/min/1.73 m² but can be continued with increased renal function monitoring; a reduction of 50% of maximal dose may be warranted. Due to the risk of acute renal failure with use of IV contrast dye, withhold metformin therapy starting the day of the procedure and resume it 2–3 days later if normal renal function has been documented.
- Metformin can be used in combination with any other antihyperglycemic therapy and is often continued when insulin therapy is initiated. The target metformin dose is 1000 mg twice daily or 2000 mg daily if the extended-release product is used. The minimal effective dose is 1000 mg/day. See Table 19-3 for metformin dosing recommendations.
- Numerous combination products containing metformin as well as combinations of other drug classes are available (Table 19-4).

Sulfonylureas

- Sulfonylureas enhance insulin secretion by binding to the sulfonylurea receptor SUR1 on pancreatic β-cells. First-generation agents (**chlorpropamide**, **tolazamide**, and **tolbutamide**) are lower in potency than second-generation drugs (**glyburide**, **glipizide**, and **glimepiride**), and are rarely used due to a higher risk of adverse effects.
- All sulfonylureas are equally effective in lowering BG when given in equipotent doses. On average, the A1C falls by 1.5%–2% (16–22 mmol/mol Hb) with FPG reductions of 60–70 mg/dL (3.3–3.9 mmol/L) in drug-naïve patients.
- Sulfonylureas are widely used because they have an extensive record of safety and effectiveness, are given orally, and are inexpensive. However, current treatment guidelines either discourage their use or suggest caution due to the risk of hypoglycemia and weight gain. In addition, tachyphylaxis to the insulin secretion effect occurs, leading to poor long-term durability of response in most patients.
- The most common side effect is hypoglycemia. Patients who skip meals, exercise vigorously, or lose a substantial amount of weight are more prone to hypoglycemia. Sulfonylureas with long durations of action and those with active metabolites should be used with extreme caution in older patients and those with renal insufficiency due to the high risk of hypoglycemia. Weight gain is common (typically 1–2 kg). Patients with sulfa allergy rarely experience crossreactivity with sulfonylureas.
- See Table 19-3 for sulfonylurea dosing information.

Thiazolidinediones (TZDs)

- TZDs bind to the peroxisome proliferator activator receptor-γ (PPAR-γ) located primarily on fat and vascular cells, enhancing insulin sensitivity in muscle, liver, and fat tissues.

TABLE 19-3 Dosing Recommendations for Oral Medications Used to Treat Type 2 Diabetes

Generic (Brand) Name	Starting Dose	Usual Recommended Dose	Maximal dose (mg/day)	Dosing/Use in Renal Insufficiency[a]
Biguanides				
Metformin (Glucophage)	500 mg once or twice daily or 850 mg once daily, titrate to target dose as tolerated	1000 mg twice daily	2550	Do not initiate if eGFR 30–45; Do not use if eGFR <30
Metformin XR	500–1000 mg once daily, titrate to target dose as tolerated	2000 mg once daily	2500	Do not initiate if eGFR 30–45; Do not use if eGFR <30
Sulfonylureas (first generation)				
Chlorpropamide	250 mg once daily (100 mg once daily in older adults)	100–500 mg once daily	750	Consider alternative agent or initiate conservatively at 100 mg in renal insufficiency to avoid hypoglycemia
Tolazamide	250 mg once daily (100 mg once daily in older adults or if FPG <200 mg/dL [11.1 mmol/L])	250–500 mg once daily	1000	Consider alternative agent or initiate conservatively at 100 mg in renal insufficiency to avoid hypoglycemia
Tolbutamide	1000–2000 mg once daily (250–500 mg once daily in older adults)	1000–2000 mg once daily	3000	Consider alternative agent or initiate conservatively in renal insufficiency to avoid hypoglycemia
Sulfonylureas (second generation)				
Glimepiride (Amaryl)	1–2 mg once daily (1 mg once daily in older adults)	4 mg once daily	8	Initiate conservatively at 1 mg in renal insufficiency to avoid hypoglycemia

(Continued)

TABLE 19-3 Dosing Recommendations for Oral Medications Used to Treat Type 2 Diabetes (*Continued*)

Generic (Brand) Name	Starting Dose	Usual Recommended Dose	Maximal dose (mg/day)	Dosing/Use in Renal Insufficiency[a]
Glipizide (Glucotrol)	5 mg once daily (2.5 mg daily in older adults)	5–10 mg once daily	40	Initiate conservatively at 2.5 mg in renal insufficiency to avoid hypoglycemia
Glipizide XL (Glucotrol XL)	5 mg once daily (2.5 mg once daily in older adults)	5–10 mg once daily	20	Initiate conservatively at 2.5 mg in renal insufficiency to avoid hypoglycemia
Glyburide (Diabeta)	2.5–5 mg once daily (1.25 mg once daily in older adults)	5–10 mg once daily	20	Consider alternative agent or initiate conservatively at 1.25 mg in renal insufficiency to avoid hypoglycemia
Glyburide micronized (Glynase)	1.5–3 mg once daily (0.75 mg once daily in older adults)	3–6 mg once daily	12	Consider alternative agent or initiate conservatively at 0.75 mg in renal insufficiency to avoid hypoglycemia
Meglitinides				
Nateglinide (Starlix)	120 mg three times daily before meals	120 mg three times daily before meals	360	No adjustment required
Repaglinide (Prandin)	1–2 mg three times daily before meals (0.5 mg before meals if A1C <8% [64 mmol/mol Hb])	2–4 mg three times daily before meals	16	Initiate conservatively at 0.5 mg before meals if CrCl 20–40 mL/ min (0.33–0.67 mL/sec)
Thiazolidinediones				
Pioglitazone (Actos)	15 mg once daily	30 mg once daily	45	No dose adjustment required
Rosiglitazone (Avandia)	4 mg once daily or in two divided doses	4 mg once daily or in two divided doses	8	No dose adjustment required

α-Glucosidase inhibitors

Acarbose (Precose)	25 mg once to three times daily with the first bite of a meal	50 mg once to three times daily with meals	300	Avoid if CrCl <25 mL/min (0.42 mL/sec)
Miglitol (Glyset)	25 mg once to three times daily with the first bite of a meal	50 mg once to three times daily with meals	300	Avoid if CrCl <25 mL/min (0.42 mL/sec)

Sodium-glucose transporter (SGLT)-2 inhibitors

Canagliflozin (Invokana)	100 mg once daily, taken before the first meal of the day	100–300 mg once daily	300	100 mg once daily if eGFR 45–60; Avoid if eGFR <45
Dapagliflozin (Farxiga)	5 mg once daily in the morning with or without food	5–10 mg once daily	10	Avoid if eGFR <60
Empagliflozin (Jardiance)	10 mg once daily in the morning with or without food	10–25 mg once daily	25	Avoid if eGFR <30
Ertugliflozin (Steglatro)	5 mg once daily in the morning with or without food	5–15 mg once daily	15	Avoid if eGFR<60

(Continued)

TABLE 19-3 Dosing Recommendations for Oral Medications Used to Treat Type 2 Diabetes *(Continued)*

Generic (Brand) Name	Starting Dose	Usual Recommended Dose	Maximal dose (mg/day)	Dosing/Use in Renal Insufficiency[a]
Dipeptidyl peptidase (DPP)-4 inhibitors				
Alogliptin (Nesina)	25 mg once daily with or without food	25 mg once daily	25	12.5 mg once daily if CrCl 30–60 mL/min (0.5–1.0 mL/sec); 6.25 mg once daily if CrCl <30 mL/min (0.5 mL/sec)
Linagliptin (Tradjenta)	5 mg once daily with or without food	5 mg once daily	5	No dose adjustment needed
Saxagliptin (Onglyza)	2.5–5 mg once daily with or without food	5 mg once daily	5	2.5 mg once daily if eGFR ≤50
Sitagliptin (Januvia)	100 mg once daily with or without food	100 mg once daily	100	50 mg once daily if eGFR 30–50; 25 mg once daily if eGFR <30
Bile acid sequestrants				
Colesevelam (Welchol)	1.875 g twice daily or 3.75 g once daily with meals	1.875 g twice daily or 3.75 g once daily with meals	3.75 g/day	No dose adjustment needed
Dopamine agonists				
Bromocriptine (Cycloset)	0.8 mg once daily, taken within 2 hours after waking in the morning with food	1.6–4.8 mg once daily	4.8	No dose adjustment needed

[a]eGFR units: mL/min/1.73 m²; CrCl units: mL/min.

TABLE 19-4	Combination Drug Products for Type 2 Diabetes		
Drug Classes	**Drug Combination**		**Brand Name**
Biguanide and sulfonylurea	Metformin	Glipizide	Metaglip[a]
	Metformin	Glyburide	Glucovance[a]
Biguanide and meglitinide	Metformin	Repaglinide	Prandimet[a]
Biguanide and thiazolidinedione	Metformin	Pioglitazone	Actoplus Met[a], Actoplus Met XR
	Metformin	Rosiglitazone	Avandamet[a]
Biguanide and DPP-4 inhibitor	Metformin	Alogliptin	Kazano
	Metformin	Linagliptin	Jentadueto, Jentadueto XR
	Metformin	Saxagliptin	Kombiglyze XR
	Metformin	Sitagliptin	Janumet, Janumet XR
Biguanide and SGLT-2 inhibitor	Metformin	Canagliflozin	Invokamet, Invokamet XR
	Metformin	Dapagliflozin	Xigduo XR
	Metformin	Empagliflozin	Synjardy, Synjardy XR
	Metformin	Ertugliflozin	Segluromet
Thiazolidinedione and sulfonylurea	Pioglitazone	Glimepiride	Duetact[a]
	Rosiglitazone	Glimepiride	Avandaryl
Thiazolidinedione and DPP-4 inhibitor	Pioglitazone	Alogliptin	Oseni
SGLT-2 inhibitor and DPP-4 inhibitor	Dapagliflozin	Saxagliptin	Qtern
	Empagliflozin	Linagliptin	Glyxambi
	Ertugliflozin	Sitagliptin	Steglujan
Basal insulin and GLP-1 receptor agonist	Insulin glargine U-100	Lixisenatide	Soliqua
	Insulin degludec U-100	Liraglutide	Xultophy

[a]Available as generic product.
XR, extended release.

- At maximal doses, **pioglitazone** and **rosiglitazone** reduce A1C by 1%–1.5% (11–22 mmol/mol Hb) and FPG by 60–70 mg/dL (3.3–3.9 mmol/L), and they have high durability over time. Maximum effects may not be seen until 3–4 months of therapy.
- TZDs are considered second or third-line agents and can be used in combination with metformin and other commonly prescribed medications for type 2 DM.
- Pioglitazone decreases plasma triglycerides by 10%–20%, whereas rosiglitazone tends to have no effect. Pioglitazone does not significantly increase LDL-C, whereas rosiglitazone may increase LDL-C by 5%–15%. Both drugs increase HDL-C, but the magnitude may be greater with pioglitazone.
- Fluid retention may occur due to peripheral vasodilation and improved insulin sensitization in the kidney with increased sodium and water retention. This may result

in peripheral edema (4%–5% of patients with monotherapy; 15% or more when combined with insulin), HF, hemodilution of hemoglobin and hematocrit, and weight gain. Edema is dose related and if not severe may be managed by dose reduction in most patients. TZDs are contraindicated in patients with New York Heart Association Class III or IV HF and should be used with caution in patients with Class I or II HF.

- Weight gain is dose related and results from both fluid retention and fat accumulation; a gain of 4 kg is not uncommon, and higher gains may require drug discontinuation. TZDs have also been associated with an increased fracture rate in the upper and lower limbs of postmenopausal women. An increased risk of bladder cancer is controversial.
- See Table 19-3 for TZD dosing information.

Glucagon-like Peptide 1 Receptor Agonists (GLP1-RAs)

- **Dulaglutide**, **exenatide, exenatide XR, lixisenatide, liraglutide**, and **semaglutide** stimulate insulin secretion and suppress inappropriately high postprandial glucagon secretion, decreasing hepatic glucose output. They also slow gastric emptying, increase satiety, and cause weight loss (average 1–3 kg).
- Short-acting agents (exenatide, lixisenatide) predominantly lower postprandial glucose (PPG) levels, whereas long-acting agents (dulaglutide, liraglutide, exenatide XR, semaglutide) lower both FPG and PPG, but with larger effects on FPG. Evidence suggests that liraglutide and semaglutide have the highest A1C and weight-lowering efficacy while exenatide and lixisenatide have the lowest.
- Liraglutide and semaglutide have demonstrated CV benefits in clinical trials. Liraglutide is FDA approved to reduce the risk of major adverse CV events in adults with type 2 DM and established atherosclerotic cardiovascular disease (ASCVD).
- GLP1-RAs are not currently recommended as first-line agents but can be used as monotherapy in patients who cannot tolerate or take first-line therapy. They are recommended second-line agents for patients with established ASCVD or chronic kidney disease (CKD) and those with a compelling need to avoid hypoglycemia or to avoid weight gain or induce weight loss. They can be used in combination with metformin, TZDs, sulfonylureas, SGLT-2 inhibitors, and basal insulin. They should not be used in combination with DPP-4 inhibitors due to similar mechanisms of action.
- The GLP1-RAs are administered SC and have important differences in efficacy, adverse effect rates, and dosing schedules (Table 19-5).
- The most common adverse effects of GLP1-RAs are nausea, vomiting, and diarrhea. These effects are dose related, so dose titration is recommended. They usually occur early in the treatment course and are mild and transient but may require drug discontinuation in some patients. Instruct patients to eat slowly and stop eating when satiated or nausea may worsen and cause vomiting. Injection site reactions and hypersensitivity reactions (including anaphylaxis and angioedema) have been reported.
- Because GLP1-RAs enhance insulin secretion in response to food intake, the risk of hypoglycemia is low when combined with metformin, SGLT-2 inhibitors, or a TZD. However, hypoglycemia may occur when combined with a sulfonylurea or insulin.

Dipeptidyl Peptidase-4 (DPP-4) Inhibitors

- **Alogliptin**, **linagliptin, saxagliptin**, and **sitagliptin** prolong the half-life of endogenously produced GLP-1 and GIP, thereby increasing glucose-dependent insulin secretion from the pancreas and reducing inappropriate postprandial glucagon secretion, resulting in lower glucose levels without an increase in hypoglycemia when used as monotherapy. They do not alter gastric emptying, cause nausea, have significant effects on satiety, or cause weight gain/loss.
- DPP-4 inhibitors produce average A1C reductions of 0.5%–0.9% (6–10 mmol/mol Hb) when used at maximum doses. There are no clear differences in efficacy among agents in the class.

TABLE 19-5	Dosing Recommendations for Subcutaneous GLP-1 Receptor Agonists		
Generic (Brand) Name	Dose[a]	Interval	Renal Dose/Use[b]
Exenatide (Byetta)	5–10 mcg	Twice daily (30–60 min before breakfast and dinner)	Avoid if eGFR <30
Lixisenatide (Adlyxin)	10–20 mcg	Once daily (1 hour before breakfast)	Limited experience in severe renal impairment; avoid if eGFR <15
Dulaglutide (Trulicity)	0.75–1.5 mg	Once weekly (at any time of day, with or without food)	Limited experience in severe renal impairment
Exenatide XR (Bydureon)	2 mg	Once weekly (at any time of day, with or without meals)	Avoid if eGFR <30
Liraglutide (Victoza)	0.6–1.8 mg	Once daily (with or without meals)	Limited experience in severe renal impairment
Semaglutide (Ozempic)	0.25–1 mg	Once weekly	No dose adjustment recommended

[a]All products require subcutaneous administration into the abdomen, thigh, or upper arm.
[b]eGFR units: mL/min/1.73 m^2.

- DPP-4 inhibitors are considered second- or third-line therapy. Advantages include once-daily dosing, oral administration, weight neutrality, low risk of hypoglycemia, and good tolerability. However, they have less A1C lowering efficacy than other second-line medication classes and are expensive.
- Adverse effects are uncommon and include stuffy, runny nose; headache; and upper respiratory tract infections. The labeling of saxagliptin and alogliptin includes information about increased risk of hospitalizations for HF. The FDA has also issued a warning on the risk of severe joint pain with DPP-4 inhibitors. Pancreatitis appears to be an established but rare safety concern.
- There is no need to titrate the dose of DPP-4 inhibitors; however, renal dose adjustments are required for alogliptin, saxagliptin, and sitagliptin (Table 19-3).

Sodium-Glucose Cotransporter-2 Inhibitors

- **Canagliflozin, dapagliflozin, empagliflozin,** and **ertugliflozin** reduce plasma glucose by preventing the kidneys from reabsorbing glucose back into the bloodstream, leading to increased glucose excretion in the urine. SGLT-2 inhibitors lower both FPG and PPG and are effective even in the absence of insulin.
- SGLT-2 inhibitors reduce A1C by 0.5%–1% (6–11 mmol/mol Hb) and appear to be more effective in patients with higher baseline A1C levels. Renal impairment decreases the efficacy of SGLT-2 inhibitors.
- SGLT-2 inhibitors are second-line agents that can be added to metformin or other second-line agents. They are not recommended as first-line agents but can be used as monotherapy in patients who cannot tolerate or take first-line therapy. They are recommended for patients with established ASCVD or CKD and those with a need to avoid hypoglycemia or weight gain or loss. They are unlikely to cause hypoglycemia unless combined with medications such as sulfonylureas, meglitinides, or insulin.

- Both empagliflozin and canagliflozin reduced major adverse CV events in large clinical trials, and empagliflozin is FDA approved to reduce the risk of CV death in adults with type 2 DM and established ASCVD.
- The most common adverse effect is genital mycotic infections, which are more common in women and uncircumcised men. There is also a slightly increased risk of urinary tract infections. Polyuria, dehydration, dizziness, or hypotension may occur because of the osmotic diuresis effects. Concomitant diuretic use may increase the risk of orthostatic hypotension and electrolyte abnormalities. Older adults and patients with stage 4 or 5 CKD are not optimal treatment candidates. Other potential safety concerns include ketoacidosis, amputations, fractures, and Fournier gangrene.
- The SGLT-2 inhibitors should be started at a low dose with assessment of volume status, adverse effects, and renal function. The dose may be titrated in patients who are tolerating the drug well and require additional glucose control (Table 19-3).

α-Glucosidase Inhibitors

- **Acarbose** and **miglitol** delay the breakdown of sucrose and complex carbohydrates in the small intestine, prolonging carbohydrate absorption. The net effect is reduction in PPG (40–50 mg/dL; 2.2–2.8 mmol/L) with relatively unchanged FBG. A1C lowering is modest, with average A1C reductions of 0.3%–1%.
- Good candidates for these drugs are patients who are near target A1C levels with near-normal FPG but high PPG levels.
- The most common side effects are flatulence, abdominal pain, and diarrhea, which can be reduced by slow dosage titration (Table 19-3).

Meglitinides

- **Nateglinide** and **repaglinide** stimulate insulin secretion from pancreatic β-cells by binding to a site adjacent to the sulfonylurea receptor. They are similar to sulfonylureas except that they have a faster onset and shorter duration of action. As monotherapy, they reduce PPG excursions and reduce A1C by 0.8%–1% (9–11 mmol/mol Hb).
- Similar to sulfonylureas, the main side effects are hypoglycemia and weight gain.
- Their role in therapy is unclear due to lack of clinical evidence. They are not included in the American Diabetes Association (ADA) treatment algorithm. They may be used in patients with renal insufficiency and may be a good option for patients with erratic meal schedules. However, multiple daily dosing may decrease adherence.
- Meglitinides should be taken by mouth with each meal, initiated at a low dose, and titrated over time until glycemic control is achieved (Table 19-3).

Bile Acid Sequestrants

- **Colesevelam** binds bile acid in the intestinal lumen, decreasing the bile acid pool for reabsorption. Its mechanism in lowering plasma glucose levels is unknown, and its role in therapy is unclear.
- A1C lowering efficacy is modest. It reduces LDL-C in patients with type 2 DM by 12%–16% but has not been proven to reduce CV morbidity or mortality. Colesevelam is weight neutral and has a low risk of hypoglycemia. Patients with type 2 DM who need a small reduction in A1C as well as additional LDL-C lowering may be candidates for this agent.
- The most common side effects are constipation and dyspepsia; colesevelam should be taken with a large amount of water. Colesevelam has multiple absorption-related drug–drug interactions. See Table 19-3 for dosing information.

Dopamine Agonists

- **Bromocriptine mesylate** is FDA approved for treatment of type 2 DM. The mechanisms by which it improves glycemic control are unknown but may involve improved hepatic insulin sensitivity and decreased hepatic glucose output.
- The A1C lowering efficacy is modest, and its role in the treatment of type 2 DM is unclear.

- Common side effects include nausea, vomiting, constipation, fatigue, headache, dizziness, and asthenia. Somnolence and orthostatic hypotension may also occur.

Amylin Analogs

- **Pramlintide** (Symlin) is a synthetic amylin analog that reduces glucagon secretion, slows gastric emptying, and increases satiety. It was the first noninsulin agent approved for patients with type 1 DM.
- Pramlintide lowers both PPG levels and A1C. The average A1C reduction is about 0.6% (7 mmol/mol Hb) in patients with type 2 DM and 0.4%–0.5% (5–6 mmol/mol Hb) in type 1 DM.
- It is used primarily in type 1 DM as adjunctive therapy for patients who are not achieving PPG goals despite maximizing mealtime insulin doses. It can also decrease weight and may allow for lower mealtime insulin doses.
- The most common adverse effects are nausea, vomiting, and anorexia. It does not cause hypoglycemia when used alone, but hypoglycemia can occur when used with insulin. To minimize the risk of severe hypoglycemia, empirically reduce the mealtime insulin dose by 30%–50% when pramlintide is initiated.
- In type 2 DM, the starting dose is 60 mcg SC prior to meals, titrated to the maximally recommended 120-mcg SC dose as tolerated and warranted based on PPG levels. In type 1 DM, dosing starts at 15 mcg SC prior to meals and can be titrated up in 15-mcg increments to a maximum of 60 mcg SC prior to each meal, if tolerated.

TREATMENT OF HYPERGLYCEMIA IN TYPE 2 DIABETES

- Upon diagnosis, assess the patient's current lifestyle, existing comorbidities, A1C, age, weight, presence or absence of symptoms, motivation, cultural preferences, health literacy level, and cost limitations. Set a patient-specific A1C target and discuss it with the patient.
- Implement comprehensive lifestyle modifications with MNT, physical activity, weight loss if obese, smoking cessation, and psychologic support upon diagnosis and reinforce them at every visit. All patients should be offered access to ongoing DSME/S programs.
- Initiate metformin as first-line therapy in patients without contraindications or tolerability issues. Start with a low dose and titrate to the maximum effective dose over time to improve tolerability.
- If the initial A1C is close to goal (eg, $\leq$7.5% [58 mmol/mol Hb]) consider initial treatment with lifestyle modifications alone if the patient is motivated.
- Consider starting two medications (metformin plus a second agent) if the initial A1C is >1.5% (16 mmol/mol Hb) higher than the target A1C.
- Consider early introduction of basal insulin in patients with very high A1C levels (>10% [86 mmol/mol Hb]), symptoms of hyperglycemia, or evidence of catabolism (eg, weight loss).
- See patients at least every 3 months if they are not meeting their goals and at least every 6 months if they are meeting goals. At those times, check an A1C level, assess medication adherence, and reinforce lifestyle recommendations. Add additional therapy if glucose targets have not been met.
- For patients maximized on metformin therapy but with A1C levels above the target, add a second-line antihyperglycemic agent. The ADA Standards of Care identify six drug classes to consider: (1) DPP-4 inhibitors, (2) GLP1-RAs, (3) SGLT-2 inhibitors, (4) sulfonylureas, (5) TZDs, and (6) basal insulin. Patient-specific factors to consider in medication selection include the individualized A1C target and presence of comorbidities (eg, ASCVD, HF, CKD, obesity). Drug-specific factors to consider include glucose-lowering efficacy, impact on comorbidities, effect on weight and hypoglycemia risk, side-effect profile, ease of use, and cost. Recommendations based on patient-specific comorbidities and other factors include:
  ✓ Established ASCVD or CKD: SGLT-2 inhibitor (eg, empagliflozin) or GLP1-RA (eg, liraglutide) with proven CV benefit.

- ✓ Established ASCVD and HF: SGLT-2 inhibitor with proven benefit in reducing HF progression. Avoid TZDs in patients with HF.
- ✓ CKD (with or without ASCVD): SGLT-2 inhibitor with proven benefit in reducing CKD progression.
- ✓ Need to minimize weight gain or promote weight loss in patients without ASCVD or CKD: GLP1-RA or SGLT-2 inhibitor. If these agents cannot be used, use a weight-neutral medication such as a DPP-4 inhibitor. Avoid sulfonylureas, insulin, and TZDs due to weight gain.
- ✓ Compelling need to minimize hypoglycemia: DPP-4 inhibitor, GLP1-RA, SGLT-2 inhibitor, or TZD could be added to metformin.

- If the A1C target is not achieved after 3 months of dual therapy or if the patient did not tolerate the selected drug(s), then triple therapy is warranted, adding a drug from another class.
- People with type 2 DM can often be managed with oral medications for years before injectable medications are needed. Insulin is recommended for extreme (A1C >10% [86 mmol/mol Hb]) or symptomatic hyperglycemia. Otherwise, GLP-1 RAs are preferred over basal insulin because they have equal or superior A1C lowering efficacy and lead to weight loss instead of weight gain with a low risk of hypoglycemia. Basal insulin can be initiated if additional glucose lowering is needed after the GLP-1 RA dose has been maximized.
- Basal insulin is started at a low dose (10 units once daily or 0.1–0.2 units/kg/day) and titrated slowly over time to a target FPG range (ie, 80–130 mg/dL [4.4-7.2 mmol/L] for patients targeting an A1C <7% [53 mmol/mol Hb]). If the A1C target is not reached by maximally titrating basal insulin, PPG levels are likely elevated and a GLP1-RA or SGLT-2 inhibitor should be considered if the patient is not already taking one. Prandial insulin is also an option, starting with 4 units or 10% of the basal dose with the largest meal of the day. If the A1C is <8% (64 mmol/mol Hb), the basal insulin dose can be decreased by the same amount to avoid hypoglycemia. Titrate the dose over time to achieve target PPG levels <180 mg/dL (10 mmol/L). A second or third injection can be added to the other meals if needed.
- Reevaluate the appropriateness of oral medications when injectable agents are started:

  - ✓ GLP-1 RAs can be used in combination with all oral agents except DPP-4 inhibitors.
  - ✓ Continue metformin when insulin is started. Stop TZDs and sulfonylureas or reduce the dose.
  - ✓ SGLT-2 inhibitors can be continued, but educate the patient about the risk of DKA.

TREATMENT OF HYPERGLYCEMIA IN TYPE 1 DIABETES

- All patients with type 1 DM require exogenous insulin. Achieving adequate glycemic control usually requires intensive insulin regimens designed to provide insulin in a manner that mimics normal physiologic insulin secretion, with consistent secretion of insulin throughout the day to manage glucose levels overnight and in between meals (ie, basal insulin), and bursts of insulin in response to glucose rises after ingestion of carbohydrates (ie, prandial insulin).
- Intensive insulin regimens can be given with either multiple daily injections (MDI) or use of continuous subcutaneous insulin infusion (CSII) via an insulin pump (Fig. 19-1).
- A common MDI approach is one injection of long-acting insulin (eg, insulin glargine U-100) for the basal component and three injections of rapid-acting insulin (eg, insulin lispro U-100) for the prandial component (Fig. 19-1A). A less expensive option consists of two injections of intermediate-acting insulin (eg, NPH insulin) and two injections of short-acting insulin (eg, regular insulin) (Fig. 19-1B). However, the ADA Standards of Care recommend that most patients should use rapid-acting insulins rather than regular insulin to reduce the risk of hypoglycemia.
- Insulin pump therapy or CSII infuses rapid-acting insulin to cover both the basal and prandial insulin needs (Fig. 19-1C). The pump infuses a basal rate constantly throughout the day and allows the patient to give bolus doses using a bolus dose calculator based on current glucose levels, carbohydrate intake, and insulin on board.

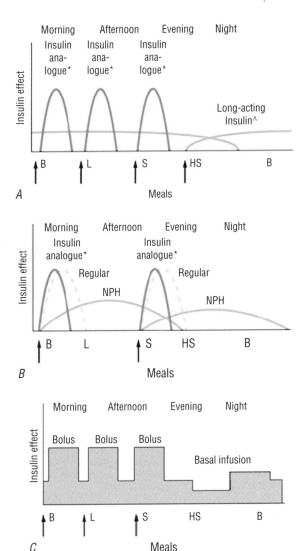

FIGURE 19-1. Common insulin regimens.
(A) Multiple-component insulin regimen consisting of one injection of long-acting insulin (^detemir, glargine degludec) to provide basal glycemic coverage and three injections of rapid-acting insulin (*aspart, lispro, glulisine) to provide glycemic coverage for each meal.
(B) Insulin regimen consisting of two injections of intermediate-acting insulin (NPH) and rapid-acting insulin (*aspart, lispro, glulisine [solid line]), or short-acting regular insulin (dashed line). Only one formulation of short-acting insulin is used.
(C) Insulin administration by insulin infusion device. The basal insulin rate is decreased during the evening and increased slightly prior to the patient awakening in the morning. Rapid-acting insulin (aspart, lispro, or glulisine) is used in the insulin pump.

Insulin pump therapy can provide more precise glucose control and allow greater flexibility and fine-tune tailoring.

- The starting insulin dose for someone with newly diagnosed type 1 DM is typically 0.4–1 units/kg/day of total insulin. The total daily insulin dose is then divided to give 50% as basal insulin and 50% as prandial insulin (distributed across meals). For example, an 80-kg patient started on 0.5 units/kg/day would start with a total daily dose of 40 units, with 20 units given as a long-acting insulin (eg, insulin detemir, glargine) and 7 units of rapid-acting insulin (eg, insulin aspart, lispro, or glulisine) with breakfast, lunch, and dinner. The insulin doses would then be adjusted based on SMBG data.

- Ideally, patients should learn to count carbohydrates so they can match their prandial insulin doses to their carbohydrate intake. Patients should also SMBG before each meal or use continuous glucose monitoring (CGM) to evaluate the insulin regimen and make treatment decisions. Bolus insulin doses can be better individualized by using carbohydrate-to-insulin ratios (C:I ratios) and correction factors (CF); refer to the textbook chapter for more detailed information.

- Pramlintide is indicated as adjunctive treatment in patients with type 1 DM who are not achieving glycemic targets despite optimization of mealtime insulin (refer to discussion earlier in this chapter). Pramlintide may improve glycemic control and minimize weight gain caused by insulin, but its use is limited by adverse effects such as nausea and vomiting, modest glucose improvements, increased injections and cost, and increased risk of hypoglycemia.

- Assess patients every 3 months if uncontrolled and every 6 months if controlled. Obtain an A1C and adjust treatment as needed. Patients on intensive insulin therapy should SMBG at least four times daily, before meals and at bedtime. Patients should also test before exercise, prior to critical tasks such as driving, and if symptoms of hypoglycemia occur. SMBG is crucial during times of intercurrent illness or stresses for early detection and prevention of DKA.

- Continuous glucose monitors report interstitial glucose levels in real time, provide insight into glucose trends, and can reduce A1C and reduce glucose variability in patients with type 1 DM. Current guidelines recommend CGM in patients with type 1 DM who are not meeting glycemic goals. They are also recommended in patients with hypoglycemia unawareness to better detect and prevent hypoglycemic events.

HYPOGLYCEMIA

- Hypoglycemia is a common complication of some diabetes medications and is associated with falls, injury, motor vehicle accidents, decreased quality of life, and increased risk of developing dementia, CV events, arrhythmias, and death.

- The severity of hypoglycemia is classified as follows:
  ✓ Level 1 (hypoglycemia alert value; ≤70 mg/dL [3.9 mmol/L]): May not cause symptoms but should be treated with a fast-acting carbohydrate and may need medication dose adjustment
  ✓ Level 2 (clinically significant hypoglycemia; <54 mg/dL [3.0 mmol/L]): Serious, clinically important hypoglycemia
  ✓ Level 3 (severe hypoglycemia): Associated with cognitive impairment requiring external assistance for recovery and can be life threatening

- Initial autonomic symptoms include tachycardia, palpitations, sweating, tremors, and hunger. Neuroglycopenic symptoms often occur with BG <60 mg/dL (3.3 mmol/L) and can include cognitive impairment, confusion, behavioral changes, anger, irritability, blurred vision, headaches, seizures, and loss of consciousness.

- Some patients have hypoglycemia unawareness and are unable to detect the early warning symptoms of hypoglycemia; they are at increased risk for the serious sequelae associated with severe hypoglycemia.

- SMBG and CGM can be useful in preventing hypoglycemia. Patients must be educated to understand situations that increase risk of hypoglycemia (eg, delaying meals, during or after exercising, or fasting).

- Treatment of hypoglycemia requires ingestion of carbohydrates, preferably glucose. Patients should carry a source of fast-acting glucose with them at all times and use the "rule of 15" for proper treatment:
  - ✓ First use SMBG to confirm BG <70 mg/dL (3.9 mmol/L) and then ingest 15 g of fast-acting carbohydrates such as 1/2 cup (4 oz or 125 mL) of milk, juice, or soda; 1 tablespoon of honey; hard candy; jelly beans; or glucose tablets.
  - ✓ Repeat SMBG in 15 minutes; if the BG is <70 mg/dL (3.9 mmol/L), repeat the process.
  - ✓ Once the BG is normalized, eat a snack or meal that includes complex carbohydrates and protein to prevent further hypoglycemic episodes.

- If the patient is unconscious, give IV glucose or glucagon injection. Glucagon increases glycogenolysis in the liver and may be given in any situation in which IV glucose cannot be rapidly administered. A glucagon kit should be prescribed and readily available to all patients on insulin who have a history of or high risk for severe hypoglycemia. It can take 10–15 minutes before glucose levels start to rise, and patients often vomit. Position the patient on the side with the head tilted slightly downward to avoid aspiration.

- Clinicians should monitor hypoglycemia at every visit. Ask the patient about the frequency, severity, and timing of hypoglycemic events, need for assistance by others, or the need to administer glucagon. Reevaluate the treatment regimen of patients with frequent or severe hypoglycemia to minimize future episodes.

COMPLICATIONS AND COMORBIDITIES

Diabetic Ketoacidosis (DKA)

- In patients with type 1 DM, DKA is usually precipitated by omitting insulin, infection, or acute illness with resultant increases in cortisol, catecholamines, glucagon, and growth hormone.
- Patients may be alert, stuporous, or comatose at presentation. Diagnostic laboratory values include hyperglycemia, anion gap acidosis, and large ketonemia or ketonuria.
- Patients have fluid deficits of several liters and significant sodium and potassium deficits. Treatment requires restoration of intravascular volume with normal saline followed by hypotonic saline to replace free water, potassium supplements, and insulin given by continuous IV infusion.
- Constant infusion of a fixed insulin dose and administration of IV glucose when the BG level decreases to <250 mg/dL (13.9 mmol/L) are preferred over titrating the insulin infusion based on the glucose level. Rapid correction of the glucose (a decrease >75–100 mg/dL/hr [4.2–5.6 mmol/L/hr]) is not recommended because it has been associated with cerebral edema, especially in children. Continue the insulin infusion until the urine ketones clear and the anion gap closes.
- Give long-acting insulin 1–3 hours before discontinuing the insulin infusion. Perform hourly bedside monitoring of glucose and frequent monitoring of potassium (every 2–4 hours).
- Treatment with bicarbonate to correct the acidosis is generally not needed and may be harmful.
- It is essential to correct the underlying situation or medical condition that precipitated DKA.
- Metabolic improvement is manifested by an increase in serum bicarbonate and pH. Because fluid administration alone reduces BG, reduced glucose values do not necessarily indicate improving metabolic status.

Hyperosmolar Hyperglycemic State (HHS)

- HHS is a potentially life-threatening acute complication of diabetes associated with very high glucose concentrations, typically >400 mg/dL (22.2 mmol/L). It usually occurs in older patients with type 2 DM or in younger patients with prolonged hyperglycemia and dehydration or significant renal insufficiency.

- The patient presentation is similar to DKA, but HHS patients usually have much higher BG, elevated serum osmolality, and little to no ketonuria or ketonemia.
- HHS typically evolves over several days to weeks, whereas DKA evolves much faster. Large ketonemia is not usually seen because residual insulin secretion suppresses lipolysis. Infection or another medical illness is the usual precipitant.
- Fluid deficits are often greater and BG levels higher—sometimes >1000 mg/dL (55.5 mmol/L)—in patients with HHS than in patients with DKA.
- BG should be lowered very gradually with hypotonic fluids and low-dose insulin infusions (1–2 units/hr).

Macrovascular Complications

- Macrovascular complications (eg, CHD, stroke) are the leading causes of death in people with diabetes.
- The ADA recommends low-dose **aspirin** therapy (75–162 mg daily) in all patients with established ASCVD. **Clopidogrel** may be used in patients allergic to aspirin. The role of antiplatelet therapy for primary CV prevention is unclear because the benefits may be offset by a higher risk of bleeding; some practice guidelines recommend aspirin if the 10-year risk of a CV event is >20%.
- In patients with established ASCVD, use of a GLP1-RA or an SGLT-2 inhibitor should be strongly considered.
- For all patients whose blood pressure (BP) exceeds 120/80 mm Hg, the ADA recommends dietary changes, physical activity, and weight loss in overweight or obese patients. Drug therapy using agents proven to reduce CV events should be started for BP >140/90 mm Hg. A combination of two medications should be used for BP >160/100 mm Hg.
- Initiate high-intensity statin therapy in all patients with diabetes and preexisting ASCVD regardless of baseline lipid levels. In the absence of ASCVD, prescribe a moderate-intensity statin to all patients with type 1 or type 2 DM over the age of 40. In patients <40 years of age, a moderate-intensity statin may be appropriate for patients with multiple CV risk factors. A fibrate (eg, **fenofibrate**), **omega-3 fatty acid**, or **niacin** can be added for patients with marked hypertriglyceridemia.
- Peripheral arterial disease can lead to claudication, nonhealing foot ulcers, and limb amputation. Smoking cessation, statin therapy, good glycemic control, and antiplatelet therapy are important strategies. **Cilostazol** may be useful in select patients to reduce symptoms. Revascularization surgery can be considered in some situations. Perform foot examinations during each face-to-face patient encounter and a yearly monofilament test to assess for loss of protective sensation to identify high-risk patients.

Microvascular Complications

- Efforts to improve glucose control significantly reduce the risk of developing microvascular complications and slow their progression.
- *Nephropathy*: Albuminuria is a marker of renal damage and can be predictive of end-stage renal disease. The ADA recommends screening for albuminuria upon diagnosis in persons with type 2 DM. Screening with type 1 DM should begin with puberty and after 5-years' disease duration. BP control is important for preventing and slowing progression of nephropathy. Angiotensin-converting enzyme (ACE) inhibitors and angiotensin receptor blockers (ARBs) can slow the progression of renal disease in patients with diabetes. Diuretics are often necessary due to volume-expanded states and are recommended second-line therapy. The ADA recommends a BP goal <140/90 mm Hg in patients with nephropathy but a lower target (eg, <130/80) if it can be achieved without undue burden or side effects. Three or more antihypertensives are often needed to reach goal BP.
- *Retinopathy*: Patients with diabetes should have routine dilated eye examinations to fully evaluate the retina. Early background retinopathy may reverse with improved glycemic control and optimal BP control. More advanced retinopathy will not fully regress with improved glycemia, and aggressive BG reductions may acutely worsen retinopathy. Laser photocoagulation has markedly improved sight preservation.

Intravitreal antivascular endothelial growth factor (VEGF) therapy is also highly effective for sight preservation. **Bevacizumab** (used off-label) and **ranibizumab** are anti-VEGF monoclonal antibodies, and **aflibercept** is a VEGF decoy receptor.

- *Neuropathy*:
  - ✓ Distal symmetrical peripheral neuropathy is the most common complication in patients with type 2 DM. Paresthesias, numbness, or pain are the predominant symptoms. The feet are involved far more often than the hands. Improved glycemic control is the primary treatment and may alleviate some symptoms. Pharmacologic therapy is symptomatic and includes low-dose tricyclic antidepressants (**nortriptyline** or **desipramine**), **duloxetine, gabapentin, pregabalin, venlafaxine, topical capsaicin,** and **tramadol.**
  - ✓ Gastroparesis can be severe and debilitating. Improved glycemic control, discontinuation of medications that slow gastric motility, and use of **metoclopramide** or low-dose **erythromycin** may be helpful.
  - ✓ Diabetic diarrhea is often nocturnal and frequently responds to a 10- to 14-day course of an antibiotic such as **doxycycline** or **metronidazole**. **Octreotide** may be useful in unresponsive cases.
  - ✓ Orthostatic hypotension may require mineralocorticoids (eg, **fludrocortisone**) or adrenergic agonists (**midodrine**).
  - ✓ Erectile dysfunction is common, and initial therapy should include a trial of an oral phosphodiesterase-5 inhibitor (eg, **sildenafil, vardenafil,** or **tadalafil**).

EVALUATION OF THERAPEUTIC OUTCOMES

- Measure A1C every 3–6 months to follow long-term glycemic control for the previous 2–3 months, even in patients who are stable on a therapeutic regimen and meeting treatment goals (**Table 19-1**).
- SMBG provides an opportunity to adjust medications, food intake, or physical activity and enables patients to detect hypoglycemia. For patients with type 1 DM, SMBG is typically performed 4–6 times per day—prior to food intake and physical activity and at bedtime. The optimal frequency of SMBG in patients with type 2 DM on oral agents is controversial.
- CGM should be considered in adults with type 1 DM who are at least 25 years of age and those younger than 25 years of age who can demonstrate adherence to its use.
- At each visit, ask patients with type 1 DM about the frequency and severity of hypoglycemia. Document any hypoglycemic episodes requiring assistance of another person, medical attention, or hospitalization and take steps to prevent future episodes.
- Screen for complications at the time of diagnosis and thereafter as follows:
  - ✓ Obtain yearly dilated eye exams in type 2 DM and an initial exam in the first 5 years in type 1 DM, then yearly.
  - ✓ Assess BP at each visit.
  - ✓ Examine the feet at each visit, including palpation of distal pulses and visual inspection for skin integrity, calluses, and deformities.
  - ✓ Screen for pedal sensory loss annually using a 10-g force monofilament.
  - ✓ Screen for albuminuria at the time of diagnosis in patients with type 2 DM and 5 years after diagnosis in type 1 DM. At least once a year, assess urinary albumin (urine albumin-to-creatinine ratio) and eGFR in all patients with type 2 DM and in patients with type 1 DM for at least 5 years.
  - ✓ Check fasting lipid panel annually if the patient is on lipid-lowering therapy.

- Administer an annual influenza vaccine and assess for administration of the pneumococcal vaccine and hepatitis B vaccine series along with management of other CV risk factors (eg, smoking).

See Chapter 91, Diabetes Mellitus, authored by Jennifer Trujillo and Stuart Haines, for a more detailed discussion of this topic.

Thyroid Disorders

20

CHAPTER

- *Thyroid disorders* involve thyroid hormone production or secretion and result in alterations in metabolic stability.

THYROID HORMONE PHYSIOLOGY

- The thyroid hormones thyroxine (T_4) and triiodothyronine (T_3) are formed within thyroglobulin, a large glycoprotein synthesized in the thyroid cell. Inorganic iodide enters the thyroid follicular cell and is oxidized by thyroid peroxidase and covalently bound (organified) to tyrosine residues of thyroglobulin.
- Iodinated tyrosine residues monoiodotyrosine (MIT) and diiodotyrosine (DIT) combine (couple) to form iodothyronines in reactions catalyzed by thyroid peroxidase. Thus, two molecules of DIT combine to form T_4, and MIT and DIT join to form T_3.
- Proteolysis within thyroid cells releases thyroid hormone into the bloodstream. T_4 and T_3 are transported by thyroid-binding globulin (TBG), transthyretin, and albumin. Only the unbound (free) thyroid hormone can diffuse into cells, elicit biologic effects, and regulate thyroid-stimulating hormone (TSH) secretion from the pituitary.
- T_4 is secreted solely from the thyroid, but <20% of T_3 is produced there; most T_3 is formed from breakdown of T_4 catalyzed by the enzyme 5′-monodeiodinase in peripheral tissues. T_3 is five times more active than T_4. T_4 may also be acted on by 5′-monodeiodinase to form reverse T_3, which has no significant biologic activity.
- Thyroid hormone production is regulated by TSH secreted by the anterior pituitary, which in turn is under negative feedback control by the circulating level of free thyroid hormone and the positive influence of hypothalamic thyrotropin-releasing hormone (TRH). Thyroid hormone production is also regulated by extrathyroidal deiodination of T_4 to T_3, which can be affected by nutrition, nonthyroidal hormones, drugs, and illness.

Thyrotoxicosis (Hyperthyroidism)

PATHOPHYSIOLOGY

- Thyrotoxicosis results when tissues are exposed to excessive levels of T_4, T_3, or both. Hyperthyroidism, which is one cause of thyrotoxicosis, refers to overproduction of thyroid hormone by the thyroid gland.
- TSH-secreting pituitary tumors occur sporadically and release biologically active hormone that is unresponsive to normal feedback control. The tumors may cosecrete prolactin or growth hormone; therefore, patients may present with amenorrhea, galactorrhea, or signs of acromegaly.
- Resistance to thyroid hormone occurs rarely and can be due to various molecular defects, including mutations in the TRβ gene. Pituitary resistance to thyroid hormone (PRTH) refers to selective resistance of the pituitary thyrotrophs to thyroid hormone.
- Graves' disease is the most common cause of hyperthyroidism, which results from the action of thyroid-stimulating antibodies (TSAb) directed against the thyrotropin receptor on the surface of thyroid cells. These immunoglobulins bind to the receptor and activate the enzyme adenylate cyclase in the same manner as TSH.
- An autonomous thyroid nodule (toxic adenoma) is a benign thyroid mass that produces thyroid hormone independent of pituitary and TSH control. Hyperthyroidism usually occurs with larger nodules (>3 cm in diameter).
- In multinodular goiter, follicles with autonomous function coexist with normal or even nonfunctioning follicles. Thyrotoxicosis occurs when autonomous follicles generate more thyroid hormone than is required.

218

- Painful subacute (granulomatous or de Quervain) thyroiditis often develops after a viral syndrome, but rarely has a specific virus been identified in thyroid parenchyma.
- Painless (silent, lymphocytic, or postpartum) thyroiditis is a common cause of thyrotoxicosis. Its etiology is not fully understood; autoimmunity may underlie most cases.
- Thyrotoxicosis factitia is hyperthyroidism due to ingestion of exogenous thyroid hormone. This may occur when thyroid hormone is used for inappropriate indications, excessive doses are used for accepted medical indications, there is accidental ingestion, or it is used surreptitiously.
- Amiodarone may induce thyrotoxicosis (2%–3% of patients), overt hypothyroidism (5% of patients), subclinical hypothyroidism (25% of patients), or euthyroid hyperthyroxinemia. Because of amiodarone's high iodine content (37% by weight), increased thyroid hormone synthesis commonly exacerbates thyroid dysfunction in patients with preexisting thyroid disease. Amiodarone also causes a destructive thyroiditis with leakage of thyroglobulin and thyroid hormones.

CLINICAL PRESENTATION

- Symptoms of thyrotoxicosis include nervousness, anxiety, palpitations, emotional lability, easy fatigability, heat intolerance, weight loss concurrent with increased appetite, increased frequency of bowel movements, proximal muscle weakness (noted on climbing stairs or arising from a sitting position), and scanty or irregular menses in women.
- Physical signs include warm, smooth, moist skin, and unusually fine hair; separation of the ends of the fingernails from the nail beds (onycholysis); retraction of the eyelids and lagging of the upper lid behind the globe upon downward gaze (lid lag); tachycardia at rest, widened pulse pressure, and systolic ejection murmur; occasional gynecomastia in men; fine tremor of the protruded tongue and outstretched hands; and hyperactive deep tendon reflexes. Thyromegaly is usually present.
- Graves' disease is manifested by hyperthyroidism, diffuse thyroid enlargement, and extrathyroidal findings of exophthalmos, pretibial myxedema, and thyroid acropachy. In severe disease, a thrill may be felt and a systolic bruit may be heard over the gland.
- In subacute thyroiditis, patients have severe pain in the thyroid region, which often extends to the ear. Systemic symptoms include fever, malaise, myalgia, and signs and symptoms of thyrotoxicosis. The thyroid gland is firm and exquisitely tender on physical examination.
- Painless thyroiditis has a triphasic course that mimics painful subacute thyroiditis. Most patients present with mild thyrotoxic symptoms; lid retraction and lid lag are present, but exophthalmos is absent. The thyroid gland may be diffusely enlarged without tenderness.
- Thyroid storm is a life-threatening medical emergency characterized by decompensated thyrotoxicosis, high fever (often >39.4°C [103°F]), tachycardia, tachypnea, dehydration, delirium, coma, nausea, vomiting, and diarrhea. Precipitating factors include infection, trauma, surgery, radioactive iodine (RAI) treatment, and withdrawal from antithyroid drugs.

DIAGNOSIS

- Elevated 24-hour radioactive iodine uptake (RAIU) indicates true hyperthyroidism: the patient's thyroid gland is overproducing T_4, T_3, or both (normal RAIU 10%–30%). A low RAIU indicates that excess thyroid hormone is not a consequence of thyroid gland hyperfunction but is likely caused by thyroiditis, struma ovarii, follicular cancer, or exogenous thyroid hormone ingestion.
- In thyrotoxic Graves' disease, there is an increase in the overall hormone production rate with a disproportionate increase in T_3 relative to T_4 (**Table 20-1**). Saturation of TBG is increased due to elevated serum levels of T_4 and T_3, which is reflected in elevated T_3 resin uptake. As a result, concentrations of free T_4, free T_3, and the free T_4 and T_3 indices are increased to an even greater extent than the measured serum

TABLE 20-1	Thyroid Function Tests in Different Thyroid Conditions			
	Total T_4	Free T_4	Total T_3	TSH
Normal	4.5–10.9 mcg/dL	0.8–2.7 ng/dL	60–181 ng/dL	0.5–4.7 milli-international units/L
Hyperthyroid	↑↑	↑↑	↑↑↑	↓↓*
Hypothyroid	↓↓	↓↓	↓	↑↑*
Increased TBG	↑	Normal	↑	Normal

*Primary thyroid disease.

total T_4 and T_3 concentrations. The TSH level is undetectable due to negative feedback by elevated levels of thyroid hormone at the pituitary. In patients with symptomatic disease, measurement of serum free T_4, total T_4, total T_3, and TSH will confirm the diagnosis of thyrotoxicosis. If the patient is not pregnant or lactating, an increased 24-hour RAIU indicates that the thyroid gland is inappropriately using iodine to produce more thyroid hormone when the patient is thyrotoxic.

- For toxic adenomas, because there may be isolated elevation of serum T_3 with autonomously functioning nodules, a T_3 level must be measured to rule out T_3 toxicosis if the T_4 level is normal. If autonomous function is suspected but the TSH is normal, the diagnosis can be confirmed by failure of the autonomous nodule to decrease iodine uptake during exogenous T_3 administration sufficient to suppress TSH.

- In multinodular goiters, a thyroid scan shows patchy areas of autonomously functioning thyroid tissue.

- TSH-induced hyperthyroidism is diagnosed by evidence of peripheral hypermetabolism, diffuse thyroid gland enlargement, elevated free thyroid hormone levels, and elevated serum immunoreactive TSH concentrations. Because the pituitary gland is extremely sensitive to even minimal elevations of free T_4, a "normal" or elevated TSH level in any thyrotoxic patient indicates inappropriate production of TSH.

- TSH-secreting pituitary adenomas are diagnosed by demonstrating lack of TSH response to TRH stimulation, inappropriate TSH levels, elevated TSH α-subunit levels, and radiologic imaging.

- In subacute thyroiditis, thyroid function tests typically run a triphasic course in this self-limited disease. Initially, serum T_4 levels are elevated due to release of preformed thyroid hormone. The 24-hour RAIU during this time is <2% because of thyroid inflammation and TSH suppression by the elevated T_4 level. As the disease progresses, intrathyroidal hormone stores are depleted, and the patient may become mildly hypothyroid with appropriately elevated TSH level. During the recovery phase, thyroid hormone stores are replenished, and serum TSH elevation gradually returns to normal.

- During the thyrotoxic phase of painless thyroiditis, the 24-hour RAIU is suppressed to <2%. Antithyroglobulin and antithyroid peroxidase antibody levels are elevated in more than 50% of patients.

- Thyrotoxicosis factitia should be suspected in a thyrotoxic patient without evidence of increased hormone production, thyroidal inflammation, or ectopic thyroid tissue. The RAIU is low because thyroid gland function is suppressed by exogenous thyroid hormone. Measurement of plasma thyroglobulin reveals presence of very low levels.

TREATMENT

- <u>Goals of Treatment</u>: Eliminate excess thyroid hormone; minimize symptoms and long-term consequences; and provide individualized therapy based on the type and severity of disease, patient age and gender, existence of nonthyroidal conditions, and response to previous therapy.

NONPHARMACOLOGIC THERAPY

- Surgical removal of the thyroid gland should be considered in patients with a large gland (>80 g), severe ophthalmopathy, or lack of remission on antithyroid drug treatment.
- If thyroidectomy is planned, **methimazole** is given until the patient is biochemically euthyroid (usually 6–8 weeks), followed by addition of **iodides** (500 mg/day) for 10–14 days before surgery to decrease vascularity of the gland.
- **Propranolol** has been used for several weeks preoperatively and 7–10 days after surgery to maintain pulse rate <90 beats/min. Combined pretreatment with propranolol and 10–14 days of **potassium iodide** also has been advocated.

PHARMACOLOGIC THERAPY

Thionamides

- **Methimazole** and **propylthiouracil (PTU)** block thyroid hormone synthesis by inhibiting the peroxidase enzyme system of the thyroid, preventing oxidation of trapped iodide and subsequent incorporation into iodotyrosines and ultimately iodothyronine ("organification"); and by inhibiting coupling of MIT and DIT to form T_4 and T_3. PTU (but not methimazole) also inhibits peripheral conversion of T_4 to T_3.
- Usual initial doses include methimazole 30–60 mg daily given in two or three divided doses or PTU 300–600 mg daily (usually in three or four divided doses). Evidence exists that both drugs can be given as a single daily dose.
- Improvement in symptoms and laboratory abnormalities should occur within 4–8 weeks, at which time a tapering regimen to maintenance doses can be started. Make dosage changes monthly because the endogenously produced T_4 will reach a new steady-state concentration in this interval. Typical daily maintenance doses are methimazole 5–30 mg and PTU 50–300 mg. Continue therapy for 12–24 months to induce long-term remission.
- Monitor patients every 6–12 months after remission. If a relapse occurs, alternate therapy with RAI is preferred over a second course of antithyroid drugs, because subsequent courses are less likely to induce remission.
- Minor adverse reactions include pruritic maculopapular rashes, arthralgias, fever, and benign transient leukopenia (white blood cell count <4000/mm³ or 4×10^9/L). The alternate thionamide may be tried in these situations, but cross-sensitivity occurs in about 50% of patients.
- Major adverse effects include agranulocytosis (with fever, malaise, gingivitis, oropharyngeal infection, and granulocyte count <250/mm³ or 0.25×10^9/L), aplastic anemia, lupus-like syndrome, polymyositis, GI intolerance, hepatotoxicity, and hypoprothrombinemia. If agranulocytosis occurs, it usually develops in the first 3 months of therapy; routine WBC count monitoring is not recommended because of its sudden onset.
- Because of the risk of serious hepatotoxicity, PTU should not be considered first-line therapy in either adults or children. Exceptions to this recommendation include (1) the first trimester of pregnancy (when the risk of methimazole-induced embryopathy may exceed that of PTU-induced hepatotoxicity), (2) intolerance to methimazole, and (3) thyroid storm.

Iodides

- **Iodide** acutely blocks thyroid hormone release, inhibits thyroid hormone biosynthesis by interfering with intrathyroidal iodide use, and decreases size and vascularity of the gland.
- Symptom improvement occurs within 2–7 days of initiating therapy, and serum T_4 and T_3 concentrations may be reduced for a few weeks.
- Iodides are often used as adjunctive therapy to prepare a patient with Graves' disease for surgery, to acutely inhibit thyroid hormone release and quickly attain the

euthyroid state in severely thyrotoxic patients with cardiac decompensation, or to inhibit thyroid hormone release after RAI therapy.

- **Potassium iodide** is available as a saturated solution (**SSKI**, 38 mg iodide per drop) or as **Lugol solution**, containing 6.3 mg of iodide per drop.
- Typical starting dose of SSKI is 3–10 drops daily (120–400 mg) in water or juice. When used to prepare a patient for surgery, it should be administered 7–14 days preoperatively.
- As an adjunct to RAI, SSKI should not be used before but rather 3–7 days after RAI treatment so that the RAI can concentrate in the thyroid.
- Adverse effects of iodide therapy include hypersensitivity reactions (skin rashes, drug fever, and rhinitis, conjunctivitis), salivary gland swelling, "iodism" (metallic taste, burning mouth and throat, sore teeth and gums, symptoms of a head cold, and sometimes stomach upset and diarrhea), and gynecomastia. Iodide is contraindicated in toxic multinodular goiter because the autonomous tissue utilizes the iodine for subsequent thyroid hormone synthesis.

Adrenergic Blockers

- β-Blockers are used to ameliorate symptoms such as palpitations, anxiety, tremor, and heat intolerance. They have no effect on peripheral thyrotoxicosis and protein metabolism and do not reduce TSAb or prevent thyroid storm. **Propranolol** and **nadolol** partially block conversion of T_4 to T_3, but this contribution to overall effect is small.
- β-Blockers are usually used as adjunctive therapy with antithyroid drugs, RAI, or iodides when treating Graves' disease or toxic nodules, in preparation for surgery, or in thyroid storm. The only conditions for which β-blockers are primary therapy for thyrotoxicosis are those associated with thyroiditis.
- **Propranolol** doses required to relieve adrenergic symptoms vary, but an initial dose of 20–40 mg orally four times daily is effective for most patients (heart rate <90 beats/min). Younger or more severely toxic patients may require 240–480 mg/day, perhaps because of increased clearance.
- β-Blockers are contraindicated in decompensated heart failure unless it is caused solely by tachycardia (high output). Other contraindications are sinus bradycardia, concomitant therapy with monoamine oxidase inhibitors or tricyclic antidepressants, and patients with spontaneous hypoglycemia. Side effects include nausea, vomiting, anxiety, insomnia, lightheadedness, bradycardia, and hematologic disturbances.
- Centrally acting sympatholytics (eg, **clonidine**) and calcium channel antagonists (eg, **diltiazem**) may be useful for symptom control when contraindications to β-blockade exist.

Radioactive Iodine

- **Sodium iodide–131** is an oral liquid that concentrates in the thyroid and initially disrupts hormone synthesis by incorporating into thyroid hormones and thyroglobulin. Over a period of weeks, follicles that have taken up RAI and surrounding follicles develop evidence of cellular necrosis and fibrosis of interstitial tissue.
- RAI is the agent of choice for Graves' disease, toxic autonomous nodules, and toxic multinodular goiters. Pregnancy is an absolute contraindication to use of RAI because radiation would be delivered to the fetal tissue.
- β-Blockers are the primary adjunctive therapy to RAI because they may be given anytime without compromising RAI therapy.
- If iodides are administered, they should be given 3–7 days after RAI to prevent interference with uptake of RAI in the thyroid gland.
- Patients with cardiac disease and elderly patients are often treated with thionamides prior to RAI ablation because thyroid hormone levels transiently increase after RAI treatment due to release of preformed thyroid hormone.
- Administering antithyroid drug therapy immediately after RAI may result in a higher rate of posttreatment recurrence or persistent hyperthyroidism.

- Use of lithium as adjunctive therapy to RAI has benefits of increased cure rate, shortened time to cure, and prevention of posttherapy increases in thyroid hormone levels.
- The goal of therapy is to destroy overactive thyroid cells, and a single dose of 4000–8000 rad results in a euthyroid state in 60% of patients at 6 months or sooner. A second dose of RAI should be given 6 months after the first RAI treatment if the patient remains hyperthyroid.
- Hypothyroidism commonly occurs months to years after RAI. The acute, short-term side effects include mild thyroidal tenderness and dysphagia. Long-term follow-up has not revealed an increased risk for development of mutations or congenital defects.

TREATMENT OF THYROID STORM

- Initiate the following therapeutic measures promptly: (1) suppression of thyroid hormone formation and secretion, (2) antiadrenergic therapy, (3) administration of corticosteroids, and (4) treatment of associated complications or coexisting factors that may have precipitated the storm (**Table 20-2**).
- **PTU** in large doses may be the preferred thionamide because it blocks peripheral conversion of T_4 to T_3 in addition to interfering with thyroid hormone production. However, β-blockers and corticosteroids serve the same purpose. **Methimazole** has a longer duration of action, which offers a theoretical advantage.
- **Iodides**, which rapidly block the release of preformed thyroid hormone, should be administered after a thionamide is initiated to inhibit iodide utilization by the overactive gland.
- Antiadrenergic therapy with the short-acting agent **esmolol** is preferred because it can be used in patients with pulmonary disease or at risk for cardiac failure and because its effects can be rapidly reversed.
- **Corticosteroids** are generally recommended, but there is no convincing evidence of adrenocortical insufficiency in thyroid storm; their benefits may be attributed to their antipyretic action and stabilization of blood pressure (BP).
- General supportive measures, including **acetaminophen** as an antipyretic (avoid aspirin or other nonsteroidal anti-inflammatory drugs, which may displace bound thyroid hormone), **fluid and electrolyte replacement, sedatives, digoxin, antiarrhythmics, insulin**, and **antibiotics** should be given as indicated.

TABLE 20-2	Drug Dosages Used in the Management of Thyroid Storm
Drug	**Regimen**
Propylthiouracil	900–1200 mg/day orally in four or six divided doses
Methimazole	90–120 mg/day orally in four or six divided doses
Sodium iodide	Up to 2 g/day IV in single or divided doses
Lugol solution	5–10 drops three times a day in water or juice
Saturated solution of potassium iodide	1–2 drops three times a day in water or juice
Propranolol	40–80 mg every 6 hours
Dexamethasone	5–20 mg/day orally or IV in divided doses
Prednisone	25–100 mg/day orally in divided doses
Methylprednisolone	20–80 mg/day IV in divided doses
Hydrocortisone	100–400 mg/day IV in divided doses

EVALUATION OF THERAPEUTIC OUTCOMES

- After therapy (surgery, thionamides, or RAI) for hyperthyroidism has been initiated, evaluate patients monthly until they reach a euthyroid condition.
- Assess for clinical signs of continuing thyrotoxicosis or development of hypothyroidism.
- If T_4 replacement is initiated, the goal is to maintain both the free T_4 level and the TSH concentration in the normal range. Once a stable dose of T_4 is identified, monitor the patient every 6–12 months.

Hypothyroidism

PATHOPHYSIOLOGY

- The vast majority of patients have primary hypothyroidism due to thyroid gland failure caused by chronic autoimmune thyroiditis (Hashimoto disease). Defects in suppressor T lymphocyte function lead to survival of a randomly mutating clone of helper T lymphocytes directed against antigens on the thyroid membrane. The resulting interaction stimulates B lymphocytes to produce thyroid antibodies.
- Iatrogenic hypothyroidism follows exposure to destructive amounts of radiation, after total thyroidectomy, or with excessive thionamide doses used to treat hyperthyroidism. Other causes of primary hypothyroidism include iodine deficiency, enzymatic defects within the thyroid, thyroid hypoplasia, and ingestion of goitrogens.
- Secondary hypothyroidism due to pituitary failure is uncommon. Pituitary insufficiency may be caused by destruction of thyrotrophs by pituitary tumors, surgical therapy, external pituitary radiation, postpartum pituitary necrosis (Sheehan syndrome), trauma, and infiltrative processes of the pituitary (eg, metastatic tumors, tuberculosis).

CLINICAL PRESENTATION

- Symptoms of hypothyroidism include dry skin, cold intolerance, weight gain, constipation, weakness, lethargy, depression, fatigue, exercise intolerance, loss of ambition or energy, muscle cramps, myalgia, and stiffness. Menorrhagia and infertility are common in women. In children, thyroid hormone deficiency may manifest as growth or intellectual retardation.
- Physical signs include coarse skin and hair, cold or dry skin, periorbital puffiness, bradycardia, and slowed or hoarse speech. Objective weakness (with proximal muscles affected more than distal muscles) and slow relaxation of deep tendon reflexes are common. Reversible neurologic syndromes such as carpal tunnel syndrome, polyneuropathy, and cerebellar dysfunction may also occur.
- Most patients with secondary hypothyroidism due to inadequate TSH production have clinical signs of generalized pituitary insufficiency, such as abnormal menses and decreased libido, or evidence of a pituitary adenoma, such as visual field defects, galactorrhea, or acromegaloid features.
- Myxedema coma is a rare consequence of decompensated hypothyroidism manifested by hypothermia, advanced stages of hypothyroid symptoms, and altered sensorium ranging from delirium to coma. Mortality rates of 60%–70% necessitate immediate and aggressive therapy.

DIAGNOSIS

- A rise in TSH level is the first evidence of primary hypothyroidism. Many patients have a free T_4 level within the normal range (compensated or subclinical hypothyroidism) and few, if any, symptoms of hypothyroidism. As the disease progresses, the free T_4 drops below normal. The T_3 concentration is often maintained in the normal range despite low T_4. Eventually, free and/or total T_4 and T_3 serum concentrations should be low.

- In secondary hypothyroidism in patients with pituitary disease, serum TSH concentrations are generally low or normal. A serum TSH in the normal range is inappropriate if the patient's T_4 is low.

TREATMENT OF HYPOTHYROIDISM (TABLE 20-3)

- <u>Goals of Treatment</u>: Restore thyroid hormone concentrations in tissue, provide symptomatic relief, prevent neurologic deficits in newborns and children, and reverse the biochemical abnormalities of hypothyroidism.
- **Levothyroxine** (L-thyroxine, T_4) is the drug of choice for thyroid hormone replacement and suppressive therapy because it is chemically stable, relatively inexpensive, active when given orally, free of antigenicity, and has uniform potency. Because T_3 (and not T_4) is the biologically active form, levothyroxine administration results in a pool of thyroid hormone that is readily and consistently converted to T_3.
- In patients with longstanding disease and older individuals without known cardiac disease, start therapy with levothyroxine 50 mcg daily and increase after 1 month.
- The recommended initial dose for older patients with known cardiac disease is 25 mcg/day titrated upward in increments of 25 mcg at monthly intervals to prevent stress on the cardiovascular system.
- The average maintenance dose for most adults is ~125 mcg/day, but there is a wide range of replacement doses, necessitating individualized therapy and appropriate TSH monitoring to determine an appropriate dose.
- Although treatment of subclinical hypothyroidism is controversial, patients presenting with marked elevations in TSH (>10 mIU/L) and high titers of thyroid peroxidase antibody or prior treatment with sodium iodide–131 may be most likely to benefit from treatment.
- Levothyroxine is the drug of choice for pregnant women, and the goal is to decrease TSH to the normal reference range for pregnancy.
- Cholestyramine, calcium carbonate, sucralfate, aluminum hydroxide, ferrous sulfate, soybean formula, dietary fiber supplements, and espresso coffee may impair the GI absorption of levothyroxine. Acid suppression with histamine blockers and proton pump inhibitors may also reduce levothyroxine absorption. Drugs that increase nondeiodinative T_4 clearance include rifampin, carbamazepine, and possibly phenytoin. Selenium deficiency and amiodarone may block conversion of T_4 to T_3.
- **Thyroid USP** (or desiccated thyroid) is usually derived from pig thyroid gland. It may be antigenic in allergic or sensitive patients. Inexpensive generic brands may not be bioequivalent.
- **Liothyronine** (synthetic T_3) has uniform potency but has a higher incidence of cardiac adverse effects, higher cost, and difficulty in monitoring with conventional laboratory tests. It must be administered three times a day and may require a prolonged adjustment period to achieve stable euthyroidism.
- **Liotrix** (synthetic T_4:T_3 in a 4:1 ratio) is chemically stable, pure, and has a predictable potency but is expensive. It also lacks therapeutic rationale because most T_3 is converted peripherally from T_4.
- Excessive doses of thyroid hormone may lead to heart failure, angina pectoris, and myocardial infarction (MI). Hyperthyroidism leads to reduced bone density and increased risk of fracture.

TREATMENT OF MYXEDEMA COMA

- Immediate and aggressive therapy with IV bolus **levothyroxine**, 300–500 mcg, has traditionally been used. Initial treatment with IV **liothyronine** or a combination of both hormones has also been advocated because of impaired conversion of T_4 to T_3.
- Give glucocorticoid therapy with IV **hydrocortisone** 100 mg every 8 hours until coexisting adrenal suppression is ruled out.

TABLE 20-3	Thyroid Preparations Used in the Treatment of Hypothyroidism		
Drug/Dosage Form	**Content**	**Relative Dose**	**Comments/Equivalency**
Thyroid USP Armour Thyroid, Nature-Throid, and Westhroid (T_4:T_3 ratio approximately 4.2:1); Armour, 1 grain = 60 mg; Nature-Throid and Westhroid, 1 grain = 65 mg. Doses include 1/4, 1/2, 1, 2, 3, 4, and 5 grain tablets	Desiccated pork thyroid gland	1 grain (equivalent to 74 mcg [~60–100] mcg of T_4)	High T_3:T_4 ratio; inexpensive
Levothyroxine Synthroid, Levothroid, Levoxyl, Levo-T, Unithroid, and other generics 25, 50, 75, 88, 100, 112, 125, 137, 150, 175, 200, 300 mcg tablets; Tirosint 13–150 mcg liquid in gelatin capsule; Tirosint-Sol liquid solution 13, 25, 50, 75, 88, 100, 112, 137, 150, 175, and 200 mcg in unit-dose ampules; 200 and 500 mcg per vial solution for injection	Synthetic T_4	100 mcg	Stable; predictable potency; generics may be bioequivalent; when switching from natural thyroid to L-thyroxine, lower dose by one half grain; variable absorption between products; half-life = 7 days, so daily dosing; considered to be drug of choice
Liothyronine Cytomel 5, 25, and 50 mcg tablets	Synthetic T_3	33 mcg (~equivalent to 100 mcg T_4)	Uniform absorption, rapid onset; half-life = 1.5 days, rapid peak and troughs
Liotrix Thyrolar 1/4, 1/2, 1, 2, and 3 grain tablets	Synthetic T_4:T_3 in 4:1 ratio	Thyrolar 1 = 50 mcg T_4 and 12.5 mcg T_3	Stable; predictable; expensive; risk of T_3 thyrotoxicosis because of high ratio of T_3 relative to T_4

- Consciousness, lowered TSH concentrations, and improvement in vital signs are expected within 24 hours.
- Maintenance levothyroxine doses are typically 75–100 mcg IV until the patient stabilizes and oral therapy is begun.
- Provide supportive therapy to maintain adequate ventilation, euglycemia, BP, and body temperature. Diagnose and treat underlying disorders such as sepsis and MI.

EVALUATION OF THERAPEUTIC OUTCOMES

- Serum TSH concentration is the most sensitive and specific monitoring parameter for adjustment of levothyroxine dose. Concentrations begin to fall within hours and are usually normalized within 2–6 weeks.
- Check both TSH and T_4 concentrations every 6 weeks until a euthyroid state is achieved. An elevated TSH level indicates insufficient replacement. Serum T_4 concentrations can be useful in detecting noncompliance, malabsorption, or changes in levothyroxine product bioequivalence. TSH may also be used to help identify noncompliance.
- In patients with hypothyroidism caused by hypothalamic or pituitary failure, alleviation of the clinical syndrome and restoration of serum T_4 to the normal range are the only criteria available for estimating the appropriate replacement dose of levothyroxine.

See Chapter 92, Thyroid Disorders, authored by Michael P. Kane and Gary Bakst, for a more detailed discussion of this topic.

CHAPTER 21

Cirrhosis and Portal Hypertension

- Chronic liver injury causes damage to normal liver tissue, resulting in development of regenerative nodules surrounded by dense fibrotic material, which are diagnostic hallmarks of cirrhosis.

PATHOPHYSIOLOGY

- The distorted architecture of the cirrhotic liver impedes portal blood flow, interferes with hepatocyte perfusion, and disrupts hepatic synthetic functions such as the production of albumin. Clinical consequences of cirrhosis include increased intrahepatic resistance leading to portal hypertension, varices, and variceal bleeding; ascites; infection; hepatic encephalopathy (HE); and hepatocellular carcinoma.

- Primary causes of cirrhosis in developed countries include hepatitis C, excessive alcohol intake, and nonalcoholic fatty liver disease (**Table 21-1**).

- Cirrhosis causes changes to the splanchnic vasculature and circulation. Splanchnic vasodilation and the formation of new blood vessels contribute to increased splanchnic blood flow, formation of gastroesophageal varices, and variceal bleeding. Additionally, splanchnic vasodilation leads to hypoperfusion of the renal system, which causes activation of the renin–angiotensin–aldosterone system and, subsequently, significant fluid retention. The pathophysiologic abnormalities that cause it often result in ascites, portal hypertension and esophageal varices, HE, and coagulation disorders.

TABLE 21-1	Etiology of Cirrhosis
Alcoholism	
Chronic hepatitis C	
Metabolic liver disease	
Hemochromatosis	
Wilson's disease	
Nonalcoholic fatty liver disease	
Immunologic disease	
Autoimmune hepatitis	
Primary biliary cirrhosis	
Primary biliary cholangitis	
Vascular disease	
Budd–Chiari	
Drugs	
Isoniazid, methyldopa, amiodarone, amoxicillin-clavulanate, nitrofurantoin, diclofenac, methotrexate, nevirapine, propylthiouracil, valproate	

- **Portal hypertension** is noted by elevated pressure gradient between the portal and central venous pressure and is characterized by hypervolemia, increased cardiac index, hypotension, and decreased systemic vascular resistance.
- Ascites is the pathologic accumulation of fluid within the peritoneal cavity. It is one of the earliest and most common presentations of cirrhosis.

PORTAL HYPERTENSION AND VARICES

- The most important sequelae of portal hypertension are the development of varices and alternative routes of blood flow resulting in acute variceal bleeding. Portal hypertension is defined by the presence of a gradient of >5 mm Hg (0.7 kPa) between the portal and central venous pressures.
- Progression to bleeding can be predicted by Child–Pugh score, size of varices, and the presence of red wale markings on the varices. First variceal hemorrhage occurs at an annual rate of about 15% and carries a mortality of 7%–15%.

HEPATIC ENCEPHALOPATHY

- HE is a functional disturbance of the brain caused by liver insufficiency or portal systemic shunting that presents on a wide spectrum of symptom severity ranging from subclinical alterations to coma.
- The symptoms of HE are thought to result from an accumulation of gut-derived nitrogenous substances in the systemic circulation as a consequence of decreased hepatic functioning and shunting through portosystemic collaterals bypassing the liver. These substances then enter the central nervous system (CNS) and result in alterations of neurotransmission that affect consciousness and behavior.
- Altered ammonia, glutamate, benzodiazepine receptor agonists, aromatic amino acids, and manganese are potential causes of HE. An established correlation between blood ammonia levels and mental status does not exist.
- Type A HE is induced by acute liver failure, type B results from portal-systemic bypass without intrinsic liver disease, and type C occurs with cirrhosis. HE may be classified as episodic, persistent, or minimal.

COAGULATION DEFECTS

- End-stage chronic liver disease is associated with decreased synthetic capability of the liver leading to decreased levels of most procoagulant factors as well as the naturally occurring anticoagulants antithrombin, protein C, and protein S.
- Antithrombin and protein C are decreased, but two procoagulant factors, factor VIII and von Willebrand factor, are actually elevated. The net effect of these events could be thrombosis or clinically significant bleeding.
- Both platelet number and function may be affected in cirrhosis. Thrombocytopenia, a common finding in cirrhosis, could promote bleeding.

CLINICAL PRESENTATION

- Initial symptoms of cirrhosis may be nonspecific including fatigue, loss of appetite, and weight loss (**Table 21-2**). Patients may also present with much more significant symptoms secondary to decompensation related to cirrhosis complications such as ascites (abdominal distention), spontaneous bacterial peritonitis (SBP) (abdominal discomfort with fever), hepatopulmonary syndrome (clubbing), hepatorenal syndrome (fluid overload, oliguria, renal failure), HE (confusion, lethargy), and/or variceal bleeding (secondary to esophageal or gastric varices from portal hypertension).
- Muscle wasting, palmar erythema, spider angiomas, parotid gland enlargement, white nails, Dupuytren contracture, peripheral neuropathy, and metabolic complications including gynecomastia, testicular atrophy, and axillary hair loss are all possibly related to cirrhosis.
- A thorough history including risk factors that predispose patients to cirrhosis should be taken. Diagnostics for cirrhosis include liver function tests, coagulation tests, complete blood count, and serologic tests for viral causes including hepatitis B and C.

TABLE 21-2	Clinical Presentation of Cirrhosis

Signs and Symptoms
- Asymptomatic
- Hepatomegaly and splenomegaly
- Pruritus, jaundice, palmar erythema, spider angiomata, and hyperpigmentation
- Gynecomastia and reduced libido
- Ascites, edema, pleural effusion, and respiratory difficulties
- Malaise, anorexia, and weight loss
- Encephalopathy

Laboratory Tests
- Hypoalbuminemia
- Elevated prothrombin time (PT)
- Thrombocytopenia
- Elevated alkaline phosphatase
- Elevated aspartate transaminase (AST), alanine transaminase (ALT), and γ-glutamyl transpeptidase (GGT)

LABORATORY ABNORMALITIES

- There are no laboratory or radiographic tests of hepatic function that can accurately diagnose cirrhosis. Serum or plasma chemistries called "liver function tests" can be grouped into two broad categories: (1) markers of liver injury such as aspartate transaminase (AST), alanine aminotransferase (ALT), γ-glutamyl transpeptidase (GGT), and alkaline phosphatase and (2) markers of hepatocellular function such as prothrombin time (PT), bilirubin, and albumin.
- The aminotransferases, AST and ALT, are enzymes that have increased concentrations in plasma after acute or chronic hepatocellular injury. The highest elevations (>10,000 units per liter) are most likely to occur in shock liver and drug- or toxin-induced hepatitis. The ratio of AST to ALT with AST>ALT is more likely when cirrhosis of any etiology exists but also occurs in alcoholic and ischemic liver disease.
- Elevated serum alkaline phosphatase and GGT occur in cases of liver injury with a cholestatic pattern and therefore often accompany conditions such as primary biliary cirrhosis, primary sclerosing cholangitis, drug-induced cholestasis, and bile duct obstruction.
- Elevations in serum conjugated (or direct) bilirubin indicate hepatocellular dysfunction or cholestasis. Indirect bilirubin elevations occur due to overproduction (as seen with hemolysis), decreased uptake, or decreased hepatic conjugation of bilirubin.
- Albumin and coagulation factors are markers of hepatic synthetic activity and are used to estimate hepatocyte function in cirrhosis. Reduction in albumin usually indicates a disease duration of more than 3 weeks whereas severe liver disease can cause PT elevation in less than 24 hours. Thrombocytopenia is a common feature in chronic liver disease.
- The Child–Pugh classification system uses a combination of physical and laboratory findings to assess and define the severity of cirrhosis and is a predictor of patient survival, surgical outcome, and risk of variceal bleeding (Table 21-3).
- The model for end-stage liver disease (MELD-Na) is a newer scoring system:

$$\text{MELD score} = 9.57 \times \log_e (\text{serum creatinine [mg/dL]}) + 3.78$$
$$\times \log_e (\text{bilirubin [mg/dL]}) + 11.20 \times \log_e (\text{INR}) + 6.43$$

or using SI units:
$$\text{MELD score} = 9.57 \times \log_e (\text{creatinine [µmol/L]} \times 0.01131) + 3.78$$
$$\times \log_e (\text{bilirubin [µmol/L]} \times 0.05848) + 11.20 \times \log_e (\text{INR}) + 6.43$$

TABLE 21-3	Criteria and Scoring for the Child–Pugh Grading of Chronic Liver Disease		
Score	**1**	**2**	**3**
Total bilirubin (mg/dL)	<2 (34.2 μmol/L)	2–3 (34.2–51.3 μmol/L)	>3 (51.3 μmol/L)
Albumin (g/dL)	>3.5 (35 g/L)	2.8–3.5 (28–35 g/L)	<2.8 (28 g/L)
Ascites	None	Mild	Moderate
Encephalopathy (grade)	None	1 and 2	3 and 4
Prothrombin time (seconds prolonged)	<4	4-6	>6

Grade A, <7 points; grade B, 7–9 points; grade C, 10–15 points.

where international normalized ratio (INR) is TK.
$$\text{MELD-Na score} = \text{MELD} - (\text{sodium [mEq/L]}) - (0.025 \times \text{MELD} \times (140 - \text{sodium [mEq/L]})) + 140$$

or using SI units:
$$\text{MELD-Na score} = \text{MELD} - (\text{sodium [mmol/L]}) - (0.025 \times \text{MELD} \times (140 - \text{sodium [mmol/L]})) + 140$$

- In MELD, laboratory values less than 1 are rounded up to 1. The formula's score is multiplied by 10 and rounded to the nearest whole number.

TREATMENT

- Goals of Treatment: *Resolution of acute complications* such as tamponade of bleeding and resolution of hemodynamic instability for an episode of acute variceal hemorrhage and *prevention of complications* through lowering of portal pressure with medical therapy using non-selective β-adrenergic blocker therapy or supporting abstinence from alcohol.

GENERAL APPROACH TO TREATMENT

- Approaches to treatment include the following:
  ✓ Identify and eliminate the causes of cirrhosis (eg, alcohol abuse).
  ✓ Assess the risk for variceal bleeding and begin pharmacologic prophylaxis where indicated, reserving endoscopic therapy for high-risk patients or acute bleeding episodes as well as patients with contraindications or intolerance to nonselective β-adrenergic blockers.
  ✓ Evaluate the patient for clinical signs of ascites and manage with pharmacologic treatment (eg, diuretics) and paracentesis. SBP should be carefully monitored in patients with ascites who undergo acute deterioration.
  ✓ HE is a common complication of cirrhosis and requires clinical vigilance and treatment with dietary restriction, elimination of CNS depressants, and therapy to lower ammonia levels.
  ✓ Frequent monitoring for signs of hepatorenal syndrome, pulmonary insufficiency, and endocrine dysfunction is necessary.

MANAGEMENT OF PORTAL HYPERTENSION AND VARICEAL BLEEDING

- The management of varices involves three strategies: (1) primary prophylaxis to prevent first bleeding episode, (2) treatment of variceal hemorrhage, and (3) secondary prophylaxis to prevent rebleeding in patients who have already bled.

Primary Prophylaxis

- All patients with cirrhosis and portal hypertension should be screened for varices on diagnosis.
- The mainstay of primary prophylaxis is the use of a nonselective β-adrenergic blocking agent such as **propranolol, nadolol,** or **carvedilol**. These agents reduce portal pressure by reducing portal venous inflow via two mechanisms: decrease in cardiac output and decrease in splanchnic blood flow.
- Patients with small varices plus risk factors for variceal hemorrhage including red wale marks or Child–Pugh grade C should receive prophylactic therapy with a nonselective β-adrenergic blocker.
- Therapy for medium or large varices that have not bled should be initiated with propranolol 20 mg twice daily, nadolol 20–40 mg once daily and titrate every 2–3 days to maximal tolerated dose or to a heart rates of 55–60 beats/min, or, rather than propranolol or nadolol, carvedilol could be chosen and started at 3.125 mg twice daily with slow titration at intervals of 1–2 weeks. β-Adrenergic blocker therapy should be continued indefinitely. Endoscopic vein ligation (EVL) is an alternative to β-adrenergic blockers. If EVL is chosen, it will be performed every 2–4 weeks until the obliteration of varices.
- Monitor patients for development of contraindications to β-adrenergic blockers such as renal impairment and hypotension that may accompany end-stage liver disease.

ACUTE VARICEAL HEMORRHAGE

- **Figure 21-1** presents an algorithm for managing variceal hemorrhage. Evidence-based recommendations for select treatments are presented in **Tables 21-4** and **21-5**.

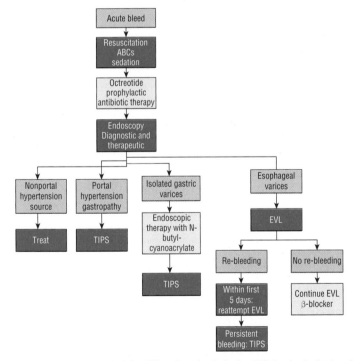

(ABCs, airway, breathing, and circulation; EVL, endoscopic vein ligation; TIPS, transjugular intrahepatic portosystemic shunt.)

FIGURE 21-1. Management of acute variceal hemorrhage.

TABLE 21-4	Evidence-Based Table of Select Treatment Recommendations: Variceal Bleeding in Portal Hypertension	
Recommendation		**Grade**
Prevention of variceal bleeding		
Nonselective β-blocker therapy should be initiated in:		
Patients with small varices and criteria for increased risk of hemorrhage		1b
Patients with medium/large varices		1a
EVL may be recommended for prevention in patients with medium/large varices at high risk of hemorrhage instead of nonselective β-blocker therapy		1a
Treatment of variceal bleeding		
Short-term antibiotic prophylaxis should be instituted on admission		1a
Vasoactive drugs should be started as soon as possible, prior to endoscopy, and maintained for up to 5 days		1a
Endoscopy should be performed to diagnose variceal bleeding and treat bleeding with EVL		1b
Endoscopy should be performed within 12 hours of presentation		5
Unless contraindicated, erythromycin 250 mg IV should be administered 30–120 minutes prior to endoscopy		1b
Secondary prophylaxis of variceal bleeding		
Nonselective β-blocker therapy plus EVL is the best therapeutic option for prevention of recurrent variceal bleeding		1a

Recommendation grading:
1a: Systematic review (with homogeneity) of randomized controlled trials.
1b: Individual randomized controlled trial with narrow confidence interval.
1c: All or none.
2a: Systematic review (with homogeneity) of cohort studies.
2b: Individual cohort study (including low-quality randomized controlled trial).
2c: Outcomes research; ecological studies.
3a: Systematic review (with homogeneity) of case-controlled studies.
3b: Individual case-control study.
4: Case-series (and poor quality cohort and case-control studies).
5: Expert opinion.

- Treatment of acute variceal bleeding includes general stabilizing and assessment measures as well as specific measures to control the acute hemorrhage and prevent complications.
- Initial treatment goals include: (1) adequate blood volume resuscitation, (2) protection of the airway from aspiration of blood, (3) prophylaxis against SBP and other infections, (4) control of bleeding, (5) prevention of rebleeding, (6) preservation of liver function of HE, and (7) prevention of acute kidney injury.
- Prompt stabilization of blood volume to maintain hemoglobin of 7 g/dL (70 g/L; 4.34 mmol/L) to 8 g/dL (80 g/L; 4.97 mmol/L) is recommended.
- Combination pharmacologic therapy plus EVL (preferred) or sclerotherapy (when EVL is not technically feasible) is the most rational approach to treatment of acute variceal bleeding.
- Vasoactive drug therapy is used to stop or slow bleeding as soon as a diagnosis of variceal bleeding is suspected and is started before endoscopy. Treatment with

TABLE 21-5	Evidence-Based Table of Selected Treatment Recommendations: Ascites and Spontaneous Bacterial Peritonitis
Recommendation	**Grade**

Recommendation	Grade
Ascites	
Paracentesis should be performed in patients with apparent new-onset ascites	IC
Sodium restriction of 2000 mg/day should be instituted as well as oral diuretic therapy with spironolactone and furosemide	IIaA
Diuretic-sensitive patients should be treated with sodium restriction and diuretics rather than serial paracentesis	IIaC
Refractory ascites	
Serial therapeutic paracenteses may be performed	IC
Postparacentesis albumin infusion of 6–8 g/L of fluid removed can be considered if more than 5 L is removed during paracentesis	IIaA
Treatment of SBP	
If ascitic fluid PMN counts are >250 cells/mm³ (0.25 × 10⁹/L), empiric antibiotic therapy should be instituted (cefotaxime 2 g every 8 hours)	IA
If ascitic fluid PMN counts are <250 cells/mm³ (0.25 × 10⁹/L), but signs or symptoms of infection exist, empiric antibiotic therapy should be initiated while awaiting culture results	IB
Ofloxacin 400 mg twice daily may be substituted for cefotaxime in patients without vomiting, shock, grade II or higher encephalopathy, or serum creatinine >3 mg/dL (265 μmol/L) and if there is no prior exposure to quinolones	IIaB
If ascitic fluid polymorphonuclear leukocyte counts are >250 cells/mm³ (0.25 × 10⁹/L), clinical suspicion of SBP is present, and the patient has a serum creatinine >1 mg/dL (88 μmol/L), blood urea nitrogen >30 mg/dL (10.7 mmol/L), or total bilirubin over 4 mg/dL (68.4 μmol/L), 1.5 g/kg albumin should be infused within 6 hours of detection and 1 g/kg albumin infusion should also be given on day 3	IIaB
Prophylaxis against SBP	
Short-term antibiotic prophylaxis should be used for 7 days to prevent SBP in cirrhosis patients with GI hemorrhage	IA
Patients who survive an episode of SBP should receive long-term prophylaxis with either daily ciprofloxacin or trimethoprim–sulfamethoxazole	IA
Patients with low-protein ascites (<1.5 g/dL [15 g/L]) plus at least one of the following: serum creatinine ≥1.2 mg/dL (106 μmol/L), blood urea nitrogen ≥25 mg/dL (8.9 mmol/L), serum sodium ≤130 mEq/L (mmol/L), or Child–Pugh score of ≥9 with bilirubin ≥3 mg/dL (51.3 μmol/L) may also justifiably receive long-term ciprofloxacin or sulfamethoxazole/trimethoprim as prophylaxis	IA

Recommendation grading: Class I—conditions for which there is evidence and/or general agreement; Class II—conditions for which there is conflicting evidence and/or a divergence of opinion; Class IIa—weight of evidence/opinion is in favor of efficacy; Class IIb—efficacy less well established; Class III—conditions for which there is evidence and/or general agreement that treatment is not effective and/or potentially harmful; Level A—data from multiple randomized trials or meta-analyses; Level B—data derived from single randomized trial or nonrandomized studies; Level C—only consensus opinion, case studies, or standard of care.

octreotide should be initiated early to control bleeding and facilitate endoscopy. Octreotide is administered as an IV bolus of 50 mcg followed by a continuous infusion of 50 mcg/hr. It should be continued for 2–5 days after acute variceal bleeding. Vasoactive therapy discontinuation can be considered once the patient is free of bleeding for at least 24 hours.

- Prophylactic antibiotic therapy to prevent SBP and other infections should be implemented upon admission. For all patients with cirrhosis and acute variceal bleeding, intravenous ceftriaxone 1 g/24 hours is recommended or oral **ciprofloxacin** 500 mg twice daily, or **trimethoprim–sulfamethoxazole** one double-strength tablet twice daily. A 250-mg dose of **erythromycin** intravenously prior to endoscopy may be used to accelerate gastric emptying of clots and improve visibility during the endoscopic procedure.
- Child–Pugh Class C patients and those in Class B with active hemorrhage at the time of diagnostic endoscopy are at high risk for failing standard therapy with EVL plus octreotide. In these patients early transjugular intrahepatic portosystemic shunt (TIPS) may be considered instead of standard therapy. The TIPS procedure involves the placement of one or more stents between the hepatic vein and the portal vein.

Prevention of Rebleeding

- A nonselective β-adrenergic blocker along with EVL is the best treatment option for prevention of rebleeding.
- **Propranolol** may be given at 20 mg twice daily (or **nadolol** 40 mg once daily) and titrated weekly to achieve a goal of heart rate 55–60 beats/min or the maximal tolerated dose. Patients should be monitored for evidence of bradycardia, bronchospasm, and hypoglycemia, particularly in patients with insulin-dependent diabetes, as well as symptoms of heart failure and excessive sodium and water retention.
- Patients who cannot tolerate or who fail pharmacologic and endoscopic interventions can be considered for tips or surgical shunting to prevent bleeding.

ASCITES

- The therapeutic goals for patients with ascites are to control the ascites, prevent or relieve ascites-related symptoms (dyspnea, abdominal pain, and distention), and prevent SBP and hepatorenal syndrome.
- For patients with ascites, a serum–ascites albumin gradient should be determined. If the gradient is ≥1.1 g/dL (11 g/L), the patient almost certainly has portal hypertension.
- The treatment of ascites secondary to portal hypertension includes abstinence from alcohol, sodium restriction (to 2 g/day), and diuretics. Fluid loss and weight change depend directly on sodium balance in these patients. A goal of therapy is to increase urinary excretion of sodium to >78 mmol/day.
- Diuretic therapy should be initiated with single morning doses of **spironolactone** 100 mg and **furosemide** 40 mg, titrated every 3–5 days (or spironolactone alone), using the 100:40 mg dose ratio (spironolactone to furosemide) with a goal of 0.5 kg maximum daily weight loss. The dose of each can be increased together, maintaining the 100:40 mg ratio, to a maximum daily dose of 400 mg spironolactone and 160 mg furosemide.
- Diuretic therapy should be discontinued in patients who experience uncontrolled or recurrent encephalopathy, severe hyponatremia (serum sodium <120 mEq/L [mmol/L]) despite fluid restriction, or renal insufficiency (serum creatinine >2 mg/dL [177 μmol/L]).
- If tense ascites is present, paracentesis should be performed prior to institution of diuretic therapy and salt restriction.
- Liver transplant should be considered in patients with refractory ascites.

SPONTANEOUS BACTERIAL PERITONITIS

- Patients with documented or suspected SBP should receive broad-spectrum antibiotic therapy to cover *Escherichia coli, Klebsiella pneumoniae,* and *Streptococcus pneumoniae.*

- **Cefotaxime** 2 g every 8 hours IV or a similar third-generation cephalosporin for 5 days is considered the drug of choice. Oral **ofloxacin** 400 mg every 12 hours for 8 days is an alternative for patients without vomiting, shock, significant HE, or serum creatinine >3 mg/dL (265 μmol/L).
- Patients who survive an episode of SBP should receive long-term antibiotic prophylaxis with daily ciprofloxacin 500 mg or double-strength trimethoprim–sulfamethoxazole.

HEPATIC ENCEPHALOPATHY

- The general approach to the management of HE is four pronged and includes the following: care for patients with altered consciousness, identify and treat any other causes besides HE for altered mental status, identify and treat any precipitating factors, and begin empirical HE treatment.
- The grading system for HE is shown in **Table 21-6**.
- Treatment approaches include: (1) reduction in blood ammonia concentrations by dietary restrictions, with drug therapy aimed at inhibiting ammonia production or enhancing its removal (non-absorbable disaccharides such as lactulose and antibiotics); and (2) inhibition of γ-aminobutyric acid-benzodiazepine receptors by **flumazenil**.
- To reduce blood ammonia concentrations in patients with episodic HE, protein intake is limited or withheld (while maintaining caloric intake) until the clinical situation improves. Protein intake can be titrated back up based on tolerance to a total of 1.2–1.5 g/kg/day. Vegetable-source and dairy-source protein may be preferable to meat-source protein because the latter contains a higher calorie-to-nitrogen ratio.
- To reduce blood ammonia concentrations in episodic HE, lactulose is initiated at a dose of 25 g (16.7 g) orally every 1–2 hours (or by retention enema: 300 mL lactulose syrup in 1 L water every 6–8 hours) until catharsis begins and the patient experiences one to two bowel movements. The dose is then decreased to 15–45 mL orally

TABLE 21-6	Grading System for Hepatic Encephalopathy		
Grade	Level of Consciousness	Personality/ Intellect	Neurologic Abnormalities
Unimpaired	Normal	Normal	Normal
Minimal	No clinical evidence of change	No clinical evidence of change/alterations identified on psychometric or neuropsychological testing	No clinical evidence of change
I	Trivial lack of awareness; shortened attention span	Euphoria or anxiety; impairment of addition or subtraction	Altered sleep rhythm
II	Lethargic	Obvious personality changes; inappropriate behavior; apathy	Asterixis; dyspraxia; disoriented for time
III	Somnolent but arousable	Bizarre behavior	Responsive to stimuli; confused; gross disorientation to time and space
IV	Coma/unarousable	None	Does not respond to stimuli

every 8–12 hours and titrated to produce two to three soft stools per day for chronic therapy.
• **Rifaximin** 550 mg twice daily plus lactulose is superior to lactulose alone in patients with a history of recurrent HE. Rifaximin is now considered the next line of therapy for recurrent HE over either metronidazole or neomycin.

EVALUATION OF THERAPEUTIC OUTCOMES

• **Table 21-7** summarizes the drug monitoring guidelines for patients with cirrhosis and portal hypertension, including monitoring parameters and therapeutic outcomes.

TABLE 21-7	Drug Monitoring Guidelines		
Drug	**Adverse Drug Reaction**	**Monitoring Parameter**	**Comments**
Nonselective β-adrenergic blocker	Heart failure, bronchospasm, glucose intolerance	BP, HR Goal HR: 55–60 beats/min or maximal tolerated dose	Nadolol, propranolol, carvedilol
Octreotide	Bradycardia, hypertension, arrhythmia, abdominal pain	BP, HR, EKG, abdominal pain	
Spironolactone/ furosemide	Electrolyte disturbances, dehydration, renal insufficiency, hypotension	Serum electrolytes (especially potassium), SCr, blood urea nitrogen, BP Goal sodium excretion: >78 mmol/day	Spot urine sodium concentration greater than potassium concentration correlates well with daily sodium excretion >78 mmol/day
Lactulose	Electrolyte disturbances	Serum electrolytes Goal number of soft stools per day: 2–3	
Neomycin	Ototoxicity, nephrotoxicity	SCr, annual auditory monitoring	
Metronidazole	Neurotoxicity	Sensory and motor neuropathy	
Rifaximin	Nausea, diarrhea		

BP, blood pressure; beats/min, beats per minute; EKG, electrocardiogram; HR, heart rate; SCr, serum creatinine; mmol, millimole.

See Chapter 54, Portal Hypertension and Cirrhosis, authored by Julie M. Sease and Alyson G. Wilder, for a more detailed discussion of this topic.

22 Constipation

- *Constipation* has been defined as difficult or infrequent passage of stool, at times associated with straining or a feeling of incomplete defecation. The condition is considered chronic if symptoms last for at least 3 months.

PATHOPHYSIOLOGY

- Constipation may be primary (occurs without an underlying identifiable cause) or secondary (the result of constipating drugs, lifestyle factors, or medical disorders).
- Constipation commonly results from a diet low in fiber, inadequate fluid intake, decreased physical activity, or from use of constipating drugs such as opioids.
- Diseases or conditions that may cause constipation include the following:
  - ✓ Gastrointestinal (GI) disorders: Irritable bowel syndrome (IBS), diverticulitis, upper and lower GI tract diseases, hemorrhoids, anal fissures, ulcerative proctitis, tumors, hernia, volvulus of the bowel, syphilis, tuberculosis, lymphogranuloma venereum, and Hirschsprung disease
  - ✓ Metabolic and endocrine disorders: Diabetes mellitus with neuropathy, hypothyroidism, panhypopituitarism, pheochromocytoma, hypercalcemia, and enteric glucagon excess
  - ✓ Pregnancy
  - ✓ Cardiac disorders (eg, heart failure)
  - ✓ Neurogenic constipation: Head trauma, CNS tumors, spinal cord injury, cerebrospinal accidents, and Parkinson disease
  - ✓ Psychogenic causes such as ignoring or postponing the urge to defecate and psychiatric diseases
- Causes of drug-induced constipation are listed in **Table 22-1**. All opioid derivatives are associated with constipation, but the degree of intestinal inhibitory effects seems

TABLE 22-1	Drugs Causing Constipation
Analgesics	
Inhibitors of prostaglandin synthesis	
Opioids	
Anticholinergics	
Antihistamines	
Antiparkinsonian agents (eg, benztropine or trihexyphenidyl)	
Phenothiazines	
Tricyclic antidepressants	
Antacids containing calcium carbonate or aluminum hydroxide	
Barium sulfate	
Calcium channel antagonists	
Clonidine	
Diuretics (non–potassium-sparing)	
Ganglionic blockers	
Iron preparations	
Muscle blockers (D-tubocurarine, succinylcholine)	
Nonsteroidal anti-inflammatory agents	
Polystyrene sodium sulfonate	

to differ among agents. Orally administered opioids appear to have a greater inhibitory effect than parenterally administered agents.

CLINICAL PRESENTATION

• **Table 22-2** shows the general clinical presentation of constipation. According to the Rome IV criteria patients should have at least two of the signs and symptoms listed in **Table 22-2** apply to a minimum of 25% of bowel movements.

TABLE 22-2	Clinical Presentation of Constipation

Signs and symptoms
- Infrequent bowel movements (<3 per week)
- Stools that are hard, small, or dry
- Straining
- Feeling of incomplete evacuation
- Feeling of anorectal obstruction or blockage
- Physical tactics needed for defecation
- Loose stools rarely occur without laxative use

Alarm signs and symptoms
- Hematochezia
- Melena
- Family history of colon cancer
- Family history of inflammatory bowel disease
- Anemia
- Weight loss
- Anorexia
- Nausea and vomiting
- Severe, persistent constipation that is refractory to treatment
- New-onset or worsening constipation in elderly without evidence of primary cause

Physical examination
- Perform rectal exam for presence of anatomical abnormalities (such as fistulas, fissures, hemorrhoids, rectal prolapse) or abnormalities of perianal descent
- Digital examination of rectum to check for fecal impaction, anal stricture, or rectal mass

Laboratory and other diagnostic tests
- No routine recommendations for lab testing—as indicated by clinical discretion
- In patients with signs and symptoms suggestive of organic disorder, specific testing may be performed (ie, thyroid function tests, electrolytes, glucose, complete blood count) based on clinical presentation
- In patients with alarm signs and symptoms or when structural disease is a possibility, select appropriate diagnostic studies:

1. Proctoscopy
2. Sigmoidoscopy
3. Colonoscopy
4. Barium enema

- A complete and thorough history should be obtained from the patient, including frequency of bowel movements and duration of symptoms. The patient should also be carefully questioned about usual diet and laxative regimens.
- General health status, signs of underlying medical illness (ie, hypothyroidism), and psychological status (eg, depression or other psychological illness) should be assessed.
- Patients with "alarm symptoms," a family history of colon cancer, or those older than 50 years with new symptoms may need further diagnostic evaluation.

TREATMENT

- <u>Goals of Treatment</u>: The major goals of treatment are to: (a) relieve symptoms; (b) reestablish normal bowel habits; and (c) improve quality of life by minimizing adverse effects of treatment.

GENERAL APPROACH TO TREATMENT

- If an underlying disease is recognized as the cause of constipation, attempts should be made to correct it. GI malignancies may be removed through a surgical resection. Endocrine and metabolic derangements are corrected by the appropriate methods.
- If a patient is consuming medications known to cause constipation, consideration should be given to alternative agents. If no reasonable alternatives exist to the medication thought to be responsible for constipation, consideration should be given to lowering the dose. If a patient must remain on constipating medications, more attention must be given to general measures for prevention of constipation.
- The proper management of constipation requires a combination of nonpharmacologic and pharmacologic therapies.

NONPHARMACOLOGIC THERAPY

- The most important aspect of the therapy for constipation is dietary modification to increase the amount of fiber consumed. Gradually increase daily fiber intake to 20–30 g, either through dietary changes or through fiber supplements. Fruits, vegetables, and cereals have the highest fiber content.
- A trial of dietary modification with high-fiber content should be continued for at least 1 month. Most patients begin to notice effects on bowel function 3–5 days after beginning a high-fiber diet.
- Abdominal distention and flatus may be particularly troublesome in the first few weeks, particularly with high bran consumption.

PHARMACOLOGIC THERAPY

- The laxatives are divided into three classifications: (1) those causing softening of feces in 1–3 days (bulk-forming laxatives, **docusates**, and low-dose **polyethylene glycol (PEG)**, **sorbitol**, and **lactulose**), (2) those resulting in soft or semifluid stool in 6–12 hours (**bisacodyl, senna**, and **magnesium sulfate**), and (3) those causing water evacuation in 1–6 hours (**magnesium salts, rectal bisacodyl**, and **PEG—electrolyte lavage solution**).
- Other agents include the calcium channel activator **lubriprosone**, the guanylate cyclase C agonist **linaclotide**, and **naldemedine**.
- Dosage recommendations for laxatives and cathartics are provided in **Table 22-3**.

Recommendations

- A constipation treatment algorithm is presented in **Figure 22-1**.
- Osmotic laxative therapy is considered the preferred first line for the treatment of constipation, in addition to increasing dietary fiber or using fiber supplementation.

TABLE 22-3	Dosage Recommendations for Pharmacologic Therapy
Agent	**Recommended Dose**
Agents that Cause Softening of Feces in 1–3 Days	
Bulk-forming agents	
Methylcellulose	4–6 g/day
Polycarbophil	4–6 g/day
Psyllium	Varies with product
Emollients	
Docusate sodium	50–360 mg/day
Docusate calcium	50–360 mg/day
Docusate potassium	100–300 mg/day
Osmotic laxatives	
Polyethylene glycol 3350	17 g/dose
Lactulose	15–30 mL orally
Sorbitol	30–50 g/day orally
Agents that Result in Soft or Semifluid Stool in 6–12 Hours	
Bisacodyl (oral)	5–15 mg orally
Senna	Dose varies with formulation
Magnesium sulfate (low dose)	<10 g orally
Agents that Cause Watery Evacuation in 1–6 Hours	
Magnesium citrate	18 g in 300 mL water
Magnesium hydroxide	2.4–4.8 g orally
Magnesium sulfate (high dose)	10–30 g orally
Sodium phosphates	Varies with salt used
Bisacodyl	10 mg rectally
Polyethylene glycol–electrolyte preparations	4 L
Intestinal Secretagogues	
Lubiprostone	24 mcg orally twice daily
Linaclotide	145 mcg orally daily
Plecanatide	3 mg orally daily
Opioid Antagonists	
Methylnaltrexone	450 mg orally daily or 12 mg subcutaneously daily
Naloxegol	25 mg daily
Naldemedine	0.2 mg daily

- Patients are often encouraged to increase daily fluid intake and physical activity as well as dedicate time to respond to the urge to defecate, although efficacy data are conflicting for these measures.

Emollient Laxatives (Docusates)

- **Docusates** are surfactant agents that increase water and electrolyte secretion in the small and large bowel and result in a softening of stools within 1–3 days.
- Emollient laxatives are not effective in treating constipation but are used mainly to prevent constipation. They may be helpful in situations where straining at stool

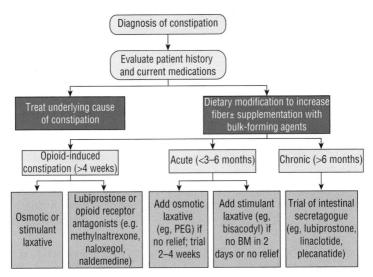

FIGURE 22-1. A general treatment algorithm for constipation.

should be avoided, such as after recovery from myocardial infarction, with acute perianal disease, or after rectal surgery.

- It is unlikely that these agents are effective in preventing constipation if major causative factors (eg, heavy opiate use, uncorrected pathology, and inadequate dietary fiber) are not concurrently addressed.

Lactulose and Sorbitol

- **Lactulose** is generally not recommended as a first-line agent for the treatment of constipation because it is costly and may cause flatulence, nausea, and abdominal discomfort or bloating. It may be justified as an alternative for acute constipation or in patients with an inadequate response to increased dietary fiber and bulking agents.
- **Sorbitol**, a monosaccharide, has been recommended as a primary agent in the treatment of functional constipation in cognitively intact patients. It is as effective as lactulose, may cause less nausea, and is much less expensive.

Magnesium Salts

- Magnesium salts, including hydroxide, phosphate, and citrate, and sodium phosphate are categorized as saline cathartics. These agents are frequently used as bowel preparations prior to diagnostic procedures such as colonoscopy.
- Milk of magnesia (an 8% suspension of magnesium hydroxide) may be used occasionally to treat constipation in otherwise healthy adults, but efficacy data are limited.
- Saline cathartics should not be used on a routine basis. These agents may cause fluid and electrolyte depletion. Also, magnesium or sodium accumulation may occur in patients with renal dysfunction or congestive heart failure. These risks increase with long-term use.
- **Glycerin** is usually administered as a suppository and with an onset of action usually less than 30 minutes. Glycerin is considered a safe laxative, although it may occasionally cause rectal irritation. Its use is acceptable on an intermittent basis for constipation, particularly in children.

Polyethylene Glycol–Electrolyte Lavage Solution

- Low doses of PEG solution (10–30 g or 17–34 g per 120–240 mL) once or twice daily may be used for treatment of constipation. Daily use in low dose (17 g) may be safe and effective for up to 6 months.
- The most common adverse effects are GI-related and include nausea, vomiting, flatulence, and abdominal cramping. PEG solutions with electrolytes are used as bowel cleansing regimens prior to GI-related procedures and should not be used routinely for treatment of constipation.

Stimulant Laxatives

- Stimulant laxatives such as diphenylmethane (bisacodyl) and anthraquinone (senna and others) derivates are expected to cause a bowel movement within 8–12 hours of administration.
- They are typically reserved for intermittent use or in patients who fail to respond adequately to bulking and osmotic laxatives. Some patients with severe chronic constipation and nonmodifiable risk factors may use these agents on a more regular basis.

Lubiprostone and Linaclotide

- **Lubiprostone** (Amitiza) is approved for chronic idiopathic constipation as well as for opioid-induced constipation (OIC). The dose is one 24-mg capsule twice daily with food. It appears safe for long-term treatment (up to 48 weeks). Lubiprostone may cause nausea, headache, and diarrhea.
- Lubiprostone is reserved for patients with chronic constipation who fail conventional first-line agents such as osmotic laxatives and fiber supplementation, or for those with OIC.
- **Linaclotide** (Linzess) is approved for the treatment of constipation and IBS-C. It is approved in a 145-mcg dose to be taken on an empty stomach at least 30 minutes before the first meal of the day. It should not be used in patients younger than 18 years of age.
- Plecanatide is approved for chronic idiopathic constipation in an adult dose of 3 mg given once daily without regard to food. It should not be used in patients under the age of 18.

Opioid-Receptor Antagonists

- Alvimopan is an oral GI-specific μ-receptor antagonist for short-term use in hospitalized patients to accelerate recovery of bowel function after large or small bowel resection. It is given as one 12-mg (capsule) 30 minutes–5 hours before surgery and then 12 mg twice daily for up to 7 days or until hospital discharge (maximum 15 doses). It is contraindicated in patients receiving therapeutic doses of opioids for more than 7 consecutive days prior to surgery.
- Methylnaltrexone is another μ-receptor antagonist approved for OIC in patients with advanced disease receiving palliative care or when response to laxative therapy has been insufficient for OIC with chronic noncancer pain.
- Other opioid-receptor antagonists include naloxegol and nalemedine.

See Chapter 53, Diarrhea, Constipation, and Irritable Bowel Syndrome, authored by Patricia H. Fabel and Kayce M. Shealy, for a more detailed discussion of this topic.

23 Diarrhea

- *Diarrhea* is an increased frequency and decreased consistency of fecal discharge as compared with an individual's normal bowel pattern. Diarrhea can be thought of as both a symptom and a sign of a systemic disease.
- Acute diarrhea is commonly defined as shorter than 14 days' duration, persistent diarrhea as longer than 14 days' duration, and chronic diarrhea as longer than 30 days' duration. Most cases of acute diarrhea are caused by infections with viruses, bacteria, or protozoa, and are generally self-limited.

PATHOPHYSIOLOGY

- Although viruses are more commonly associated with acute gastroenteritis, bacteria are responsible for more cases of acute diarrhea. Common causative bacterial organisms include *Shigella*, *Salmonella*, *Campylobacter*, *Staphylococcus*, and *Escherichia coli*. Acute viral infections are attributed mostly to the Norwalk and rotavirus groups.
- Diarrhea is an imbalance in absorption and secretion of water and electrolytes. It may be associated with a specific disease of the gastrointestinal (GI) tract or with a disease outside the GI tract.
- Four general pathophysiologic mechanisms disrupt water and electrolyte balance, leading to diarrhea: (1) a change in active ion transport by either decreased sodium absorption or increased chloride secretion, (2) a change in intestinal motility, (3) an increase in luminal osmolarity, and (4) an increase in tissue hydrostatic pressure. These mechanisms have been related to four broad clinical diarrheal groups: secretory, osmotic, exudative, and altered intestinal transit.
- Secretory diarrhea occurs when a stimulating substance (eg, vasoactive intestinal peptide [VIP] from a pancreatic tumor, unabsorbed dietary fat in steatorrhea, laxatives, hormones [such as secretion], bacterial toxins, and excessive bile salts) increases secretion or decreases absorption of large amounts of water and electrolytes.
- Inflammatory diseases of the GI tract can cause exudative diarrhea by discharge of mucus, proteins, or blood into the gut. With altered intestinal transit, intestinal motility is altered by reduced contact time in the small intestine, premature emptying of the colon, or bacterial overgrowth.

CLINICAL PRESENTATION

- Acute diarrhea is usually self-limiting and subsides within 72 hours of onset, whereas chronic diarrhea involves frequent attacks over extended time periods. However, infants, young children, the elderly, and debilitated persons are at risk for morbid and mortal events in prolonged or voluminous diarrhea.
- Signs and symptoms include:
  ✓ Abrupt onset of nausea, vomiting, abdominal pain, headache, fever, chills, and malaise
  ✓ Bowel movements are frequent and never bloody, and diarrhea lasts 12–60 hours
  ✓ Intermittent periumbilical or lower right quadrant pain with cramps and audible bowel sounds is characteristic of small intestinal disease
  ✓ When pain is present in large intestinal diarrhea, it is a gripping, aching sensation with tenesmus (straining, ineffective, and painful stooling)
  ✓ In chronic diarrhea, a history of previous bouts, weight loss, anorexia, and chronic weakness are important findings
- Physical examination typically demonstrates hyperperistalsis with borborygmi and generalized or local tenderness.

- Laboratory tests:
  - ✓ Stool analysis studies include examination for microorganisms, blood, mucus, fat, osmolality, pH, electrolyte and mineral concentration, and cultures
  - ✓ Stool test kits are useful for detecting GI viruses, particularly rotavirus
  - ✓ Antibody serologic testing shows rising titers over a 3- to 6-day period, but this test is not practical and is nonspecific
  - ✓ Occasionally, total daily stool volume is also determined
  - ✓ Direct endoscopic visualization and biopsy of the colon may be undertaken to assess for the presence of conditions such as colitis or cance
- Radiographic studies are helpful in neoplastic and inflammatory conditions.
- Many agents, including antibiotics and other drugs, cause diarrhea (Table 23-1). Laxative abuse for weight loss may also result in diarrhea.

TREATMENT

- Goals of Treatment: To manage the diet, prevent excessive water, electrolyte, and acid–base disturbances; provide symptomatic relief; treat curable causes of diarrhea; and manage secondary disorders causing diarrhea. Diarrhea, like a cough, may be a body defense mechanism for ridding itself of harmful substances or pathogens. The correct therapeutic response is not necessarily to stop diarrhea at all costs. If diarrhea is secondary to another illness, controlling the primary condition is necessary.

GENERAL APPROACH TO TREATMENT

- Management of the diet is a first priority for treatment of diarrhea (Figs. 23-1 and 23-2). Most clinicians recommend stopping solid foods for 24 hours and avoiding dairy products.
- Dietary management is a first priority in the treatment of diarrhea. Feeding should continue in children with acute bacterial diarrhea.
- If vomiting is present and is uncontrollable with antiemetics, nothing is taken by mouth. As bowel movements decrease, a bland diet is begun.
- Rehydration and maintenance of water and electrolytes are the primary treatment measures until the diarrheal episode ends. If vomiting and dehydration are not severe, enteral feeding is the less costly and preferred method. In the United States, many commercial oral rehydration preparations are available (Table 23-2). The WHO now recommends an oral rehydration solution (ORS) with a lower osmolarity, sodium content, and glucose load (see Table 23-2).
- Oral supplementation of zinc 20 mg daily for 10 days in addition to ORS significantly reduces the severity and duration of acute diarrhea in developing countries.

PHARMACOLOGIC THERAPY

- Drugs used to treat diarrhea (Table 23-3) are grouped into several categories: antimotility, adsorbents, antisecretory compounds, antibiotics, enzymes, and intestinal microflora. Usually, these drugs are not curative but palliative.
- Opiates and opioid derivatives delay the transit of intraluminal content or increase gut capacity, prolonging contact and absorption. The limitations of the opiates are addiction potential (a real concern with long-term use) and worsening of diarrhea in selected infectious diarrheas.
- **Loperamide** is often recommended for managing acute (including traveler's diarrhea) and chronic diarrhea. Diarrhea lasting 48 hours beyond initiating loperamide warrants medical attention.
- Diphenoxylate and difenoxin (a diphenoxylate derivative) are combined with **atropine** and have the same uses, precautions, and side effects.
- **Bismuth subsalicylate** is often used for treatment or prevention of diarrhea (traveler's diarrhea) and has antisecretory, anti-inflammatory, and antibacterial effects.

TABLE 23-1	Drugs Causing Diarrhea
Laxatives	Guanadrel
Antacids containing magnesium	Angiotensin-converting enzyme inhibitors
Antineoplastics	Cholinergics
Auranofin (gold salt)	Bethanechol
Antibiotics	Neostigmine
Clindamycin	Cardiac agents
Tetracyclines	Quinidine
Sulfonamides	Digitalis
Any broad-spectrum antibiotic	Digoxin
Antihypertensives	Nonsteroidal anti-inflammatory drugs
Reserpine	Misoprostol
Guanethidine	Colchicine
Methyldopa	Proton pump inhibitors
Guanabenz	H_2-receptor blockers

(RBC, red blood cells; WBC, white blood cells.)

FIGURE 23-1. Recommendations for treating acute diarrhea. Follow these steps: (1) Perform a complete history and physical examination. (2) Is the diarrhea acute or chronic? If chronic diarrhea, go to Figure 23-2. (3) If acute diarrhea, check for fever and/or systemic signs and symptoms (ie, toxic patient). If systemic illness (fever, anorexia, or volume depletion), check for an infectious source. If positive for infectious diarrhea, use the appropriate antibiotic/anthelmintic drug and symptomatic therapy. If negative for infectious cause, use only symptomatic treatment. (4) If no systemic findings, use symptomatic therapy based on severity of volume depletion, oral or parenteral fluid/electrolytes, antidiarrheal agents (see Table 23-3), and diet.

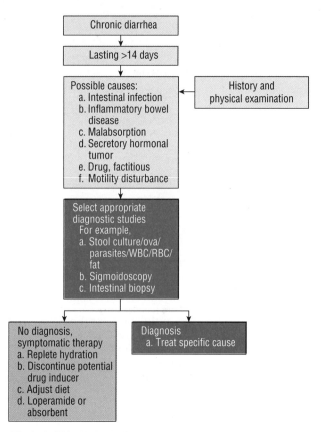

(RBC, red blood cells; WBC, white blood cells.)

FIGURE 23-2. Recommendations for treating chronic diarrhea. Follow these steps: (1) Perform a careful history and physical examination. (2) The possible causes of chronic diarrhea are many. These can be classified into intestinal infections (bacterial or protozoal), inflammatory disease (Crohn disease or ulcerative colitis), malabsorption (lactose intolerance), secretory hormonal tumor (intestinal carcinoid tumor or vasoactive intestinal peptide [VIP]–secreting tumors), drug (antacid), factitious (laxative abuse), or motility disturbance (diabetes mellitus, irritable bowel syndrome, or hyperthyroidism). (3) If the diagnosis is uncertain, appropriate diagnostic studies should be ordered. (4) Once diagnosed, treatment is planned for the underlying cause with symptomatic antidiarrheal therapy. (5) If no specific cause can be identified, symptomatic therapy is prescribed.

Bismuth subsalicylate contains multiple components that might be toxic if given in excess to prevent or treat diarrhea.

• **Probiotics**, including microorganisms such as *Saccharomyces boulardii*, *Lactobacillus* GG, and *Lactobacillus acidophilus* decrease the duration of infectious and antibiotic-induced diarrhea in adults and children. The dosage of probiotic preparations varies depending on the brand used. Intestinal flatus is the primary patient complaint experienced with this modality.

TABLE 23-2	Oral Rehydration Solutions			
	WHO-ORSYT[a]	Pedialyte[b] (Ross)	CeraLyte (Cera Products)	Enfalyte (Mead Johnson)
Osmolality (mOsm/ kg or mmol/kg)	245	250	220	167
Carbohydrates[b] (g/L)	13.5	25	40[c]	30[c]
Calories (cal/L [J/L])	65 (272)	100 (418)	160 (670)	126 (527)
Electrolytes (mEq/L; mmol/L)				
Sodium	75	45	50–90	50
Potassium	20	20	20	25
Chloride	65	35	40–80	45
Citrate	—	30	30	34
Bicarbonate	30	—	—	—
Calcium	—	—	—	—
Magnesium	—	—	—	—
Sulfate	—	—	—	—
Phosphate	—	—	—	—

[a]World Health Organization reduced osmolarity oral rehydration solution.
[b]Carbohydrate is glucose.
[c]Rice syrup solids are carbohydrate source.

TABLE 23-3	Selected Antidiarrheal Preparations	
	Dose Form	Adult Dose
Antimotility		
Diphenoxylate	2.5 mg/tablet 2.5 mg/5 mL	5 mg four times daily; do not exceed 20 mg/day
Loperamide	2 mg/capsule	Initially 4 mg, and then 2 mg after each loose stool; do not exceed 16 mg/day
Paregoric	2 mg/5 mL (morphine)	5–10 mL one to four times daily
Opium tincture	10 mg/mL (morphine)	0.6 mL four times daily
Difenoxin	1 mg/tablet	Two tablets, and then one tablet after each loose stool; up to eight tablets per day
Antisecretory		
Bismuth subsalicylate	1050 mg/30 mL 262 mg/15 mL 524 mg/15 mL 262 mg/tablet	Two tablets or 30 mL every 30 minutes to 1 hour as needed up to eight doses per day

(Continued)

TABLE 23-3	Selected Antidiarrheal Preparations (*Continued*)	
	Dose Form	**Adult Dose**
Enzymes (lactase)		
	1250 neutral lactase units/4 drops	Three to four drops taken with milk or dairy product
	3300 FCC lactase units per tablet	
Bacterial replacement (*Lactobacillus acidophilus, Lactobacillus bulgaricus*)		Two tablets or one granule packet three to four times daily; give with milk, juice, or water
Octreotide	0.05 mg/mL	Initial: 50 mcg subcutaneously
	0.1 mg/mL	One to two times per day
	0.5 mg/mL	and titrate dose based on indication up to 600 mcg/day in two to four divided doses

- **Octreotide**, a synthetic octapeptide analogue of endogenous somatostatin, is prescribed for the symptomatic treatment of carcinoid tumors and other peptide secreting tumors, dumping syndrome, and chemotherapy-induced diarrhea. The dosage range for managing diarrhea associated with carcinoid tumors is 100–600 mcg daily in two to four divided doses, subcutaneously, for 2 weeks. Octreotide is associated with adverse effects such as cholelithiasis, nausea, diarrhea, and abdominal pain.
- Vaccines. An oral vaccine for cholera (Vaxchora®) is licensed and available in the United States. The Advisory Committee for Immunization Practices (ACIP) recommends the vaccine for adults aged 18–64 years old who are traveling to an endemic area. Two orally administered rotavirus vaccines (RotaTeq and Rotarix) prevent gastroenteritis due to rotavirus infection in infants and children.

EVALUATION OF THERAPEUTIC OUTCOMES

- Therapeutic outcomes are directed to key symptoms, signs, and laboratory studies. The constitutional symptoms usually improve within 24–72 hours. Monitoring for changes in the frequency and character of bowel movements on a daily basis in conjunction with vital signs and improvement in appetite are of utmost importance.
- Monitor body weight, serum osmolality, serum electrolytes, complete blood cell count, urinalysis, and cultures (if appropriate). With an urgent or emergency situation, any change in the volume status of the patient is the most important outcome.
- In the urgent/emergent situation, restoration of the patient's volume status is the most important outcome. Toxic patients (fever dehydration, hematochezia, or hypotension) require hospitalization, IV fluids and electrolyte administration, and empiric antibiotic therapy while awaiting culture and sensitivity results. With timely management, these patients usually recover within a few days.

See Chapter 53, Diarrhea, Constipation, and Irritable Bowel Syndrome, authored by Patricia H. Fabel and Kayce M. Shealy, for a more detailed discussion of this topic.

CHAPTER 24

Gastroesophageal Reflux Disease

- *Gastroesophageal reflux disease* (GERD) is symptoms or complications resulting from refluxed stomach contents into the esophagus, oral cavity (including the larynx), or lungs. Episodic heartburn that is not frequent or painful enough to be bothersome is not included in the definition.

PATHOPHYSIOLOGY

- In some cases, reflux is associated with defective lower esophageal sphincter (LES) pressure or function. Patients may have decreased LES pressure from spontaneous transient LES relaxations, transient increases in intra-abdominal pressure, or an atonic LES. Some foods and medications decrease LES pressure (**Table 24-1**).
- Problems with other normal mucosal defense mechanisms may contribute to development of GERD, including abnormal esophageal anatomy, improper esophageal clearance of gastric fluids, reduced mucosal resistance to acid, delayed or ineffective gastric emptying, inadequate production of epidermal growth factor, and reduced salivary buffering of acid.
- Esophagitis occurs when the esophagus is repeatedly exposed to refluxed gastric contents for prolonged periods. This can progress to erosion of the squamous epithelium of the esophagus (erosive esophagitis).
- Substances that promote esophageal damage upon reflux into the esophagus include gastric acid, pepsin, bile acids, and pancreatic enzymes. Composition and volume of the refluxate and duration of exposure are the primary determinants of the consequences of gastroesophageal reflux.
- An "acid pocket" is thought to be an area of unbuffered acid in the proximal stomach that accumulates after a meal and may contribute to GERD symptoms postprandially. GERD patients are predisposed to upward migration of acid from the acid pocket, which may also be positioned above the diaphragm in patients with hiatal hernia, increasing the risk for acid reflux.
- Reflux and heartburn are common in pregnancy because of hormonal effects on LES tone and increased intra-abdominal pressure from an enlarging uterus.
- Obesity is a risk factor for GERD due to increased intra-abdominal pressure. Transient LES relaxations, an incompetent LES, and impaired esophageal motility have also been attributed to obesity.
- Complications from long-term acid reflux include esophagitis, esophageal strictures, Barrett esophagus, and esophageal adenocarcinoma.

CLINICAL PRESENTATION

- *Symptom-based GERD* (with or without esophageal tissue injury) typically presents with heartburn, usually described as a substernal sensation of warmth or burning rising up from the abdomen that may radiate to the neck. It may wax and wane in character and be aggravated by activities that worsen reflux (eg, recumbent position, bending-over, eating a high-fat meal). Other symptoms are water brash (hypersalivation), belching, and regurgitation. Alarm symptoms that may indicate complications include dysphagia, odynophagia, bleeding, and weight loss. The absence of tissue injury or erosions is termed nonerosive reflux disease (NERD).
- *Tissue injury–based GERD* (with or without esophageal symptoms) may present with esophagitis, esophageal strictures, Barrett esophagus, or esophageal carcinoma. Alarm symptoms may also be present.
- Extraesophageal symptoms may include chronic cough, laryngitis, wheezing, and asthma.

TABLE 24-1	Foods and Medications That May Worsen GERD Symptoms
Foods/Beverages	**Medications**
Decreased lower esophageal sphincter pressure	
Fatty meal	Anticholinergics
Carminatives (peppermint, spearmint)	Barbiturates
Chocolate	Caffeine
Coffee, cola, tea	Dihydropyridine calcium channel blockers
Garlic	Dopamine
Onions	Estrogen
Chili peppers	Nicotine
Alcohol	Nitrates
	Progesterone
	Tetracycline
	Theophylline
Direct irritants to the esophageal mucosa	
Spicy foods	Aspirin
Orange juice	Bisphosphonates
Tomato juice	Nonsteroidal anti-inflammatory drugs (NSAIDs)
Coffee	Iron
Tobacco	Quinidine
	Potassium choride

DIAGNOSIS

- Clinical history is sufficient to diagnose GERD in patients with typical symptoms.
- Perform diagnostic tests in patients who do not respond to therapy or who present with alarm symptoms. Endoscopy is preferred for assessing mucosal injury and identifying strictures, Barrett esophagus, and other complications.
- Ambulatory pH monitoring, combined impedance–pH monitoring, high-resolution esophageal pressure topography (HREPT), impedance manometry, and an empiric trial of a proton pump inhibitor (PPI) may be useful in some situations.

TREATMENT

- <u>Goals of Treatment</u>: The goals are to reduce or eliminate symptoms, decrease frequency and duration of gastroesophageal reflux, promote healing of injured mucosa, and prevent complications.

GENERAL APPROACH

- Therapy is directed toward decreasing acidity of the refluxate, decreasing the gastric volume available to be refluxed, improving gastric emptying, increasing LES pressure, enhancing esophageal acid clearance, and protecting the esophageal mucosa.
- Treatment is determined by disease severity and includes the following:
  ✓ Lifestyle changes and patient-directed therapy with **antacids** and/or nonprescription acid suppression therapy (**histamine 2–receptor antagonists [H₂RAs]** and/or **PPIs**)
  ✓ Pharmacologic treatment with prescription-strength acid suppression therapy
  ✓ Antireflux surgery
  ✓ Endoscopic therapies

- The initial intervention depends in part on the patient's condition (symptom frequency, degree of esophagitis, and presence of complications). A step-down approach is most often advocated, starting with a PPI instead of an H_2RA, and then stepping down to the lowest dose of acid suppression needed to control symptoms (**Table 24-2**).
- Patient-directed therapy (self-treatment with nonprescription medication) is appropriate for mild, intermittent symptoms. Patients with continuous symptoms for longer than 2 weeks should seek medical attention; such patients are generally started on empiric acid-suppression therapy. Patients not responding satisfactorily or those with alarm symptoms (eg, dysphagia) should undergo endoscopy.

NONPHARMACOLOGIC THERAPY

- Potential lifestyle changes depending on the patient situation:
  - ✓ Elevate head of the bed by placing 6- to 8-in blocks under the headposts. Sleep on a foam wedge.
  - ✓ Weight reduction for overweight or obese patients.
  - ✓ Avoid foods that decrease LES pressure (eg, fats, chocolate).
  - ✓ Include protein-rich meals to augment LES pressure.
  - ✓ Avoid foods with irritant effects on the esophageal mucosa (eg, citrus juices, coffee, pepper).
  - ✓ Eat small meals and avoid eating immediately prior to sleeping (within 3 hours if possible).
  - ✓ Stop smoking.
  - ✓ Avoid alcohol.
  - ✓ Avoid tight-fitting clothes.
  - ✓ For mandatory medications that irritate the esophageal mucosa, take in the upright position with plenty of liquid or food (if appropriate).
- Antireflux surgery (eg, laparoscopic Nissen fundoplication) should be considered when long-term pharmacotherapy is undesirable or when patients have complications. Bariatric surgery, specifically Roux-en-Y gastric bypass, should be considered in obese patients (BMI >35 kg/m^2) contemplating surgery.
- Two endoscopic therapies are: (1) radiofrequency ablation (for managing Barrett esophagus primarily when dysplasia is present), and (2) transoral incisionless fundoplication (for select patients with chronic GERD).
- Magnetic sphincter augmentation can improve lower esophageal resistance and reduce GERD symptoms. Five-year results showed long-term reduction in esophageal acid and symptom improvement with minimal complications.

PHARMACOLOGIC THERAPY

Antacids and Antacid-Alginic Acid Products

- Antacids provide immediate symptomatic relief for mild GERD and are often used concurrently with acid suppression therapies. Patients who require frequent use for chronic symptoms should receive prescription-strength acid suppression therapy instead.
- Some antacid products are combined with alginic acid, which is not a potent acid-neutralizing agent and does not enhance LES pressure, but it forms a viscous solution that floats on the surface of gastric contents. This serves as a protective barrier for the esophagus against reflux of gastric contents and reduces frequency of reflux episodes. The combination product may be superior to antacids alone in relieving GERD symptoms, but efficacy data indicating endoscopic healing are lacking.
- Antacids have a short duration, which necessitates frequent administration throughout the day to provide continuous acid neutralization. Taking antacids after meals can increase duration from approximately 1 hour to 3 hours; however, nighttime acid suppression cannot be maintained with bedtime doses. Antacids may cause diarrhea

TABLE 24-2 Therapeutics Approach to GERD in Adults

Recommended Treatment Regimen	Brand Name	Oral Dose	Comments
Intermittent, mild heartburn (individualized lifestyle modifications + patient-directed therapy with antacids and/or nonprescription H₂RAs or nonprescription PPI)			
Individualized lifestyle modifications			Lifestyle modifications should be individualized for each patient
Patient-directed therapy with antacids (≥12 years old)			
Magnesium hydroxide/Aluminum hydroxide with simethicone	Maalox	10–20 mL as needed or after meals and at bedtime	If symptoms are unrelieved with lifestyle modifications and nonprescription medications after 2 weeks, patient should seek medical attention; do not exceed 16 teaspoonfuls per 24 hours
Antacid/Alginic acid	Gaviscon	2–4 tablets or 10–20 mL after meals and at bedtime	Note: Content of alginic acid varies greatly among products; the higher the alginic acid the better (at least 500 mg)
Calcium carbonate	Tums	500 mg, 2–4 tablets as needed	
Patient-directed therapy with nonprescription H₂RAs (up to twice daily) (≥12 years old)			
Cimetidine	Tagamet HB	200 mg	If symptoms are unrelieved with lifestyle modifications and nonprescription medications after 2 weeks, patient should seek medical attention
Famotidine	Pepcid AC	10–20 mg	
Nizatidine	Axid AR	75 mg	
Ranitidine	Zantac	75–150 mg	
Patient-directed therapy (>18 years old) with nonprescription PPIs (taken once daily)			
Esomeprazole	Nexium 24HR	20 mg	If symptoms are unrelieved with lifestyle modifications and nonprescription medications after 2 weeks, patient should seek medical attention
Lansoprazole	Prevacid 24HR	15 mg	
Omeprazole	Prilosec OTC	20 mg	
Omeprazole/sodium bicarbonate	Zegerid OTC	20 mg/1100 mg	
Symptomatic relief of GERD (individualized lifestyle modifications + prescription-strength H₂RAs or prescription-strength PPIs)			
Individualized lifestyle modifications			Lifestyle modifications should be individualized for each patient

Prescription-strength H₂RAs (for 6–12 weeks)

Cimetidine (off-label use)	Tagamet	400 mg four times daily or 800 mg twice daily	For typical symptoms, treat empirically with prescription-strength acid suppression therapy: Note: Most patients
Famotidine	Pepcid	20 mg twice daily	If symptoms recur, consider maintenance therapy. Note: Most patients will require standard doses for maintenance therapy
Nizatidine	Axid	150 mg twice daily	
Ranitidine	Zantac	150 mg twice daily	

Prescription-strength PPIs (for 4–8 weeks)

Dexlansoprazole	Dexilant	30 mg once daily for 4 weeks	For typical symptoms, treat empirically with prescription-strength acid suppression therapy
Esomeprazole	Nexium	20–40 mg once daily	Patients with moderate-to-severe symptoms should receive a PPI as initial therapy
Lansoprazole	Prevacid	15 mg once daily	
Omeprazole	Prilosec	20 mg once daily	If symptoms recur, consider maintenance therapy
Omeprazole/Sodium bicarbonate	Zegerid	20 mg once daily	
Pantoprazole (off-label use)	Protonix	40 mg once daily	
Rabeprazole	Aciphex	20 mg once daily	

Healing of erosive esophagitis or treatment of patients with moderate-to-severe symptoms or complications (individualized lifestyle modifications + high-dose H₂RAs or PPIs or antireflux surgery)

Individualized lifestyle modifications			Lifestyle modifications should be individualized for each patient

(Continued)

TABLE 24-2 Therapeutics Approach to GERD in Adults *(Continued)*

Recommended Treatment Regimen	Brand Name	Oral Dose	Comments
PPIs (up to twice daily for up to 8 weeks)			
Dexlansoprazole	Dexilant	60 mg daily	For extraesophageal or alarm symptoms, obtain endoscopy with biopsy to evaluate mucosa
Esomeprazole	Nexium	20–40 mg daily	If symptoms are relieved, consider maintenance therapy. PPIs are the most effective maintenance therapy for patients with extraesophageal symptoms, complications, and erosive disease. Start with twice-daily PPI therapy if reflux chest syndrome present
Lansoprazole	Prevacid	30 mg once or twice daily	
Omeprazole	Prilosec	20 mg once or twice daily	
Rabeprazole	Aciphex	20 mg once or twice daily	
Pantoprazole	Protonix	40 mg once or twice daily	
			Patients not responding to pharmacologic therapy, including those with persistent extraesophageal symptoms, should be evaluated via manometry and/or ambulatory reflux monitoring
High-dose H_2RAs (for 8–12 weeks)			
Cimetidine	Tagamet	400 mg four times daily or 800 mg twice daily	If high-dose H_2RA needed, may consider using PPI to lower cost, increase convenience, and increase tolerability
Famotidine	Pepcid	20–40 mg twice daily	
Nizatidine	Aciphex	150 mg two to four times daily	Four times daily H_2RA is considered off-label use for nizatidine
Ranitidine	Zantac	150 mg four times daily	
Interventional therapy			
Antireflux surgery			
Bariatric surgery			
Endoscopic therapies			

H_2RA, histamine$_2$-receptor antagonist; PPI, proton pump inhibitor.

or constipation depending on the magnesium or aluminum content. These agents have significant drug interactions with tetracycline, ferrous sulfate, isoniazid, sulfonylureas, and quinolone antibiotics.

Proton Pump Inhibitors

- **Dexlansoprazole, esomeprazole, lansoprazole, omeprazole, pantoprazole,** and **rabeprazole** block gastric acid secretion by inhibiting hydrogen potassium adenosine triphosphatase in gastric parietal cells, resulting in profound and long-lasting antisecretory effects.
- PPIs provide more rapid symptom relief and higher healing rates than H_2RAs in patients with moderate-to-severe GERD and should be given empirically to patients with troublesome symptoms. Twice-daily use is indicated in patients not responding to standard once-daily therapy.
- Adverse effects include headache, diarrhea, nausea, and abdominal pain. Community-acquired pneumonia has occurred with short-term use. Potential long-term adverse effects include enteric infections, vitamin B_{12} deficiency, hypomagnesemia, and bone fractures. PPIs can decrease the absorption of **ketoconazole** and **itraconazole**, which require an acidic environment for absorption. Although some PPIs (especially omeprazole) inhibit cytochrome P450 2C19 and may reduce conversion of clopidogrel to its active metabolite, the only prospective randomized clinical trial conducted to date found no increased rate of clinical events in patients given clopidogrel plus omeprazole.
- PPIs degrade in acidic environments and are therefore formulated in delayed-release capsules or tablets. Dexlansoprazole, esomeprazole, lansoprazole, and omeprazole contain enteric-coated (pH-sensitive) granules in capsules. For patients unable to swallow the capsules, the contents can be mixed in applesauce or orange juice. In patients with nasogastric tubes, the contents can be mixed in 8.4% sodium bicarbonate solution. Esomeprazole granules can be dispersed in water. Esomeprazole, omeprazole, and pantoprazole are also available in a delayed-release oral suspension powder packet, and lansoprazole is available as a delayed-release, orally disintegrating tablet. Rabeprazole is available in a capsule sprinkle that can be opened and placed in a small amount of soft food such as applesauce. Patients taking delayed-release tablets of pantoprazole or rabeprazole should be instructed not to crush, chew, or split them. Dexlansoprazole is available in a dual delayed-release capsule, with the first release occurring 1–2 hours after the dose, and the second release occurring 4–5 hours after the dose.
- **Zegerid**® is a combination product containing omeprazole 20 or 40 mg with 1100 mg sodium bicarbonate in immediate-release oral capsules and powder for oral suspension. It should be taken on an empty stomach at least 1 hour before a meal. The capsules should be swallowed whole and not opened, sprinkled on food, or administered via nasogastric tube. The powder for oral suspension offers an alternative to delayed-release capsules or IV formulation in adults with nasogastric tubes.
- **Lansoprazole, esomeprazole,** and **pantoprazole** are available in IV formulations for patients who cannot take oral medications, but they are not more effective than oral preparations and are significantly more expensive.
- Patients should take oral PPIs in the morning 30–60 minutes before breakfast or their largest meal of the day to maximize efficacy, because these agents inhibit only actively secreting proton pumps. Dexlansoprazole can be taken without regard to meals. If dosed twice daily, the second PPI dose should be taken approximately 10–12 hours after the morning dose and prior to a meal or snack.

Histamine 2–Receptor Antagonists

- **Cimetidine, ranitidine, famotidine,** and **nizatidine** in divided doses are effective for treating mild-to-moderate GERD. Low-dose nonprescription H_2RAs or standard doses given twice daily may be beneficial for symptomatic relief of mild GERD. Patients not responding to standard doses may be hypersecretors of gastric acid and require higher doses (**Table 24-2**). However, when standard doses of H_2RAs do not adequately relieve symptoms, it is more cost-effective and clinically effective to switch to a PPI. The efficacy of H_2RAs for GERD treatment is highly variable and frequently less than desired. Prolonged courses are frequently required.

- The most common adverse effects include headache, fatigue, dizziness, and either constipation or diarrhea. Cimetidine may inhibit the metabolism of theophylline, warfarin, phenytoin, nifedipine, and propranolol, among other drugs.
- Because all H_2RAs are equally effective, selection of the specific agent should be based on differences in pharmacokinetics, safety profile, and cost.

Promotility Agents

- Promotility agents may be useful adjuncts to acid-suppression therapy in patients with a known motility defect (eg, LES incompetence, decreased esophageal clearance, delayed gastric emptying). However, these agents are not as effective as acid suppression therapy and have undesirable adverse effects.
- **Metoclopramide**, a dopamine antagonist, increases LES pressure in a dose-related manner and accelerates gastric emptying. However, it does not improve esophageal clearance. Metoclopramide provides symptomatic improvement for some patients, but evidence supporting endoscopic healing is lacking. Common adverse reactions include somnolence, nervousness, fatigue, dizziness, weakness, depression, diarrhea, and rash. In addition, extrapyramidal effects, tardive dyskinesia, and other CNS effects limit its usefulness.
- **Bethanechol** has limited value because of side effects (eg, urinary retention, abdominal discomfort, nausea, flushing). It is not routinely recommended for treatment of GERD.

Mucosal Protectants

- **Sucralfate** is a nonabsorbable aluminum salt of sucrose octasulfate. It has limited value for treatment of GERD but may be useful for management of radiation esophagitis and bile or nonacid reflux GERD.

Combination Therapy

- Combination therapy with an acid-suppressing agent and a promotility agent or mucosal protectant seems logical, but data supporting such therapy are limited. This approach is not recommended unless a patient has GERD with motor dysfunction. Using the omeprazole-sodium bicarbonate immediate-release product in addition to once daily PPI therapy offers an alternative for nocturnal GERD symptoms.

Maintenance Therapy

- Many patients with GERD relapse after medication is withdrawn, so maintenance treatment may be required. Consider long-term therapy to prevent complications and worsening of esophageal function in patients who have symptomatic relapse after discontinuation of therapy or dosage reduction, including patients with Barrett esophagus, strictures, or erosive esophagitis.
- Most patients require standard doses to prevent relapses. PPIs are the drugs of choice for maintenance treatment of moderate-to-severe esophagitis or symptoms. Usual once-daily doses are omeprazole 20 mg, lansoprazole 30 mg, rabeprazole 20 mg, or esomeprazole 20 mg. Low doses of a PPI or alternate-day regimen may be effective in some patients with milder symptoms. H_2RAs may be effective maintenance therapy in patients with mild disease.
- "On-demand" maintenance therapy, by which patients take their PPIs only when they have symptoms, may be effective for patients with endoscopy-negative GERD.

EVALUATION OF THERAPEUTIC OUTCOMES

- Monitor frequency and severity of GERD symptoms, and educate patients on symptoms that suggest presence of complications requiring immediate medical attention, such as dysphagia. Evaluate patients with persistent symptoms for presence of strictures or other complications.
- Monitor patients for adverse drug effects and the presence of extraesophageal symptoms such as laryngitis, asthma, or chest pain. These symptoms require further diagnostic evaluation.

See Chapter 49, Gastroesophageal Reflux Disease, authored by Dianne B. May, Michael Thiman, and Satish S.C. Rao, for a more detailed discussion of this topic.

- *Viral hepatitis* refers to the clinically important hepatotropic viruses responsible for hepatitis A (HAV), hepatitis B (HBV), delta hepatitis, hepatitis C (HCV), and hepatitis E.

Hepatitis A

- HAV infection usually produces a self-limited disease and acute viral infection, with a low fatality rate, and confers lifelong immunity. Outbreaks occur each year in the United States.
- HAV infection primarily occurs through transmission by the fecal-oral route, person-to-person, or by ingestion of contaminated food or water. The incidence of HAV correlates directly with low socioeconomic status, poor sanitary conditions, and overcrowding. Rates of HAV infection are increased among international travelers, injection drug users, the homeless population, and men who have sex with men.
- The disease exhibits three phases: 1) incubation (averaging 28 days, range 15–50 days), 2) acute hepatitis (generally lasting 2 months), and 3) convalescence. Acute hepatitis is marked by an abrupt onset of nonspecific symptoms; some very mild. Some patients may experience symptoms for up to 9 months. Nearly all individuals have clinical resolution within 6 months of the infection, and a majority have resolution by 2 months. HAV does not lead to chronic infections.
- The clinical presentation of HAV infection is given in Table 25-1. There are no specific symptoms unique to HAV. Children younger than 6 years of age are typically asymptomatic.
- The diagnosis of acute HAV infection is based on clinical criteria of acute onset of fatigue, abdominal pain, loss of appetite, intermittent nausea and vomiting, jaundice or elevated serum aminotransferase levels, and serologic testing for immunoglobulin (Ig) M anti-HAV. Detection of IgG anti-HAV replaces IgM and indicates host immunity following the acute phase of the infection.

PREVENTION

- The spread of HAV can be best controlled by avoiding exposure. The most important measures to avoid exposure include good handwashing techniques and personal hygiene practices.
- The current vaccination strategy in the United States includes vaccinating all children at 1 year of age. Groups who should receive HAV vaccine are shown in Table 25-2.
- Three inactivated virus vaccines are licensed in the United States: Havrix, Vaqta, and Twinrix. Approved dosing recommendations are shown in Table 25-3. Seroconversion rates of 94% or greater are achieved with the first dose.
- Common vaccine side effects include soreness and warmth at the injection site, headache, malaise, and pain.
- Ig is used when pre- or postexposure prophylaxis against HAV infection is needed in persons for whom vaccination is not an option. It is most effective if given during the incubation phase of infection. A single dose of Ig 0.02 mL/kg is given intramuscularly for postexposure prophylaxis or short-term (≤5 months) preexposure prophylaxis. For lengthy stays, a single dose of 0.06 mL/kg is used. HAV vaccine may also be given with Ig.
- For people recently exposed to HAV and not previously vaccinated, Ig is indicated for patients older than 40 years or with underlying medical conditions, when vaccine experience is limited, or the vaccine is contraindicated. Combined vaccine and immunoglobulin may be preferred for optimal protection.

TABLE 25-1	Clinical Presentation of Acute Hepatitis		
	Hepatitis A (HAV)	**Hepatitis B (HBV)**	**Hepatitis C (HCV)**
Signs and symptoms	>70% of patients are symptomatic with fever, jaundice, scleral icterus, hepatomegaly. Less common: splenomegaly, skin rash, arthralgia.	Approximately 70% of patients are anicteric or subclinical. Younger patients are most likely to be asymptomatic. If symptoms occur, jaundice, dark urine, white stool, abdominal pain, fatigue, fever, chills, loss of appetite, and pruritus are possible.	Approximately 70% of patients are asymptomatic. If symptoms occur, jaundice, dark urine, white stool, abdominal pain, fatigue, fever, chills, loss of appetite, and pruritus are possible.
Laboratory Findings			
Aminotransferase (ALT, AST) elevations	>1000 IU/L (6.7 μkat/L) ALT>AST	1000–2000 IU/L (16.7–33.3 μkat/L) ALT>AST	Highly variable, can be approximately 1000 IU/L (16.7 μkat/L) ALT>AST
Bilirubin	Elevated and preceded by aminotransferase elevations	Can be within normal or elevated	Elevated and preceded by aminotransferase elevations
Virus-specific tests	IgM anti-HAV	IgM anti-HBc (+), HBsAg (+)	HCV RNA (+) or quantifiable; HCV antibody reactive within 12 weeks of exposure

ALT, alanine aminotransferase; AST, aspartate aminotransferase; anti-, antibody to; HBc, hepatitis B core; HBsAg, hepatitis B surface antigen; IgM, immunoglobulin; IU, international units; L, liter; RNA, ribonucleic acid.

- Ig is recommended with vaccination if travel to an HAV high or intermediate risk country will begin in ≤2 weeks and the individual is an older adult, immunocompromised, or has chronic liver disease or other chronic medical condition.
- Anaphylaxis to Ig has been reported in patients with IgA deficiency.

TREATMENT

- <u>Goals of Treatment</u>: Complete clinical resolution, including reducing complications, normalization of liver function, and reducing infectivity and transmission. No specific treatment options exist for HAV. Management of HAV infection is primarily supportive. Corticosteroid use is not recommended.

Hepatitis B

- HBV is a leading cause of chronic hepatitis, cirrhosis, and hepatocellular carcinoma (HCC).
- Transmission of HBV occurs sexually, parenterally, and perinatally. In areas of high HBV prevalence, perinatal transmission from mother to child at birth is most common. In the United States, both homosexual and heterosexual contact are key routes of transmission.

TABLE 25-2	Recommendations for Hepatitis A Virus Vaccination

All children at 1 year of age

Any unvaccinated children ages 2–18 years

Persons traveling to or working in countries that have high or intermediate endemicity of infection[a]

Men who have sex with men

Users of injection and noninjection drugs

Persons with occupational risk for infection (eg, persons who work with HAV-infected primates or with HAV in a research laboratory)

Persons who have clotting factor disorders

Persons with chronic liver disease

All previously unvaccinated persons anticipating close personal contact (eg, household contact or regular babysitter) with an international adoptee from a country of high or intermediate endemicity within the first 60 days after the arrival of the adoptee

Anyone who would like to obtain immunity

[a]Travelers to Canada, Western Europe, Japan, Australia, or New Zealand are at no greater risk for infection than they are in the United States. All other travelers should be assessed for HAV risk.
HAV, hepatitis A virus.
Source: Centers for Disease Control and Prevention

TABLE 25-3	Recommended Dosing of Hepatitis A Vaccines			
Vaccine	Age (Years)	Dose of Hepatitis A Antigen (Volume)	No. of Doses	Schedule[a]
HAVRIX	1–18	720 ELISA units (0.5 mL)	2	0, 6–12 months
	≥19	1440 ELISA units (1 mL)	2	0, 6–12 months
VAQTA	1–18	25 units (0.5 mL)	2	0, 6–18 months
	≥19	50 units (1 mL)	2	0, 6–18 months
TWINRIX[b]	≥18	720 ELISA units (1 mL)	3	0, 1, 6 months
	≥18 (accelerate schedule)	720 ELISA units (1 mL)	4	0, 7 days, 21–30 days, +12 months

[a]Zero (0) denotes initial dose, subsequent numbers denote time after initial dose for timing of additional doses.
[b]Combination hepatitis A and B vaccine, also contains 20 mcg of hepatitis B surface antigen and requires a three-dose schedule for adequate HBV response.
ELISA, enzyme-linked immunosorbent assay.
Source: Centers for Disease Control and Prevention

- The hepatitis B surface antigen (HBsAg) is the most abundant of the three surface antigens and is detectable at the onset of clinical symptoms. Its persistence past 6 months after initial detection corresponds to chronic infection and indicates an increased risk for cirrhosis, hepatic decompensation, and hepatocellular carcinoma.
- The phases of chronic HBV, with patterns, are noted in Table 25-4.
- The interpretation of serologic markers for HBV is given in Table 25-5.
- The clinical presentation of HBV infection is given in Table 25-1.

TABLE 25-4	Patterns of Chronic Hepatitis B Virus Phases			
State	**HBeAg Status**	**ALT Level**	**HBV DNA IU/mL[a]**	**Other**
Phase 1 (immune tolerant)	+	WNL[b]	>1 million	
Phase 2 (immune active)	+	High	>20,000	ALT intermittently or persistently elevated
	−	WNL	>2000	ALT intermittently or persistently elevated
Phase 3 (inactive carrier)	−	WNL	<2000	Anti-HBe+
Phase 5 (occult infection)	−	WNL	Undetectable	Anti-HBc+, HBsAg−, with or without anti-HBs
Reactivation	±	High	>20,000	Associated with immunosuppressive states or therapies

[a]IU/mL is numerically equivalent to the SI unit of kIU/L.
[b]Per AASLD guidelines, ALT normal limits are defined as <35 IU/L (0.58 μkat/L) (men); <25 IU/L (0.42 μkat/L) (women).
ALT, alanine aminotransferase; DNA, deoxyribonucleic acid; HBeAg, hepatitis B e-antigen; HBV, hepatitis B virus; WNL, within normal limits.

TABLE 25-5	Interpretation of Serologic Tests in Hepatitis B Virus	
Tests	**Result**	**Interpretation**
HBsAg	(−)	Susceptible
Anti-HBc	(−)	
Anti-HBs	(−)	
HBsAg	(−)	Past HBV infection, resolved
Anti-HBc	(+)	No further management needed unless undergoing immunosuppressive therapy or chemotherapy
Anti-HBs	(+)	
HBsAg	(−)	Immune because of vaccination (valid only if test performed 1–2 months after third vaccine dose)
Anti-HBc	(−)	
Anti-HBs	(+)	
HBsAg	(+)	Acute infection
Anti-HBc	(+)	
IgM anti-HBc	(+)	
Anti-HBs	(−)	
HBsAg	(+)	Chronic infection. Further evaluation needed
Anti-HBc	(+)	
IgM anti-HBc	(−)	
Anti-HBs	(−)	
HBsAg	(−)	Possible interpretations: Resolved infection or false positive
Anti-HBc	(+)	Requires HBV DNA testing if immunocompromised patient
Anti-HBs	(−)	

Anti-, antibody to; HBsAg, hepatitis B surface antigen; HBc, hepatitis B core; HBs, hepatitis B surface; IgM, immunoglobulin M.
Note: Anti-HBc includes both IgM anti-HBc and IgG anti-HBc. IgM is present during acute phase of infection.
Source: Data from Hepatitis B Serology, Centers for Disease Control and Prevention. https://www.cdc.gov/hepatitis/hbv/pdfs/serologicchartv8.pdf.

PREVENTION

- Prophylaxis of HBV can be achieved by vaccination (HBV vaccine) or by passive immunity in postexposure cases with HBV Ig which provides temporary passive immunity.
- The goal of immunization against viral hepatitis is prevention of the short-term viremia that can lead to transmission of infection, clinical disease, and chronic HBV infection.
- Vaccination is the most effective strategy to prevent HBV infection, and a comprehensive vaccination strategy was implemented in the United States. Persons who should receive HBV vaccine are listed in **Table 25-6**.
- The most commonly reported adverse events for single-antigen vaccine are nausea/dizziness and fever/headache; for combination vaccines, fever, injection site erythema, and vomiting.

TREATMENT

- <u>Goals of therapy:</u> The goals of therapy are to suppress HBV replication and prevent disease progression to cirrhosis and HCC. HBeAg loss, with or without seroconversion to anti-HBeAg in patients who are HBeAg positive, indicates immune control.
- Some patients with chronic HBV infection should be treated. Recommendations for treatment consider the patient's age, serum HBV DNA and ALT levels, and histologic

TABLE 25-6	Recommendations for Hepatitis B Virus Vaccination
All infants	
All previously unvaccinated children <19 years	
All unvaccinated adults aged 19–59 with diabetes; those aged ≥60 should be vaccinated at the discretion of treating clinician	
Sex partners of persons who are HBsAg positive	
Sexually active persons not in a long-term monogamous relationship (>1 partner/6 months)	
Men who have sex with men	
STD clinic patients	
Persons with HIV	
Current or recent injection drug use	
Household contacts of persons with chronic hepatitis B infection	
Clients and staff of institutions for the developmentally disabled	
Healthcare and public safety workers with anticipated risk for exposure to blood or blood-contaminated fluid in the workplace	
Chronic dialysis/ESRD patients including predialysis, peritoneal dialysis, and home dialysis patients	
Correctional facilities inmates	
International travelers to regions with high or intermediate levels (HBsAg prevalence ≥2%) of endemic HBV infection	
Persons with chronic HCV infection	
Persons with chronic liver disease (eg, patients with alcoholic liver disease, cirrhosis, fatty liver disease, autoimmune hepatitis, etc.)	
All unvaccinated adults seeking vaccination (specific risk factor not required)	

ESRD, end-stage renal disease; HBsAg, hepatitis B surface antigen; HBV, hepatitis B virus; HIV, human immunodeficiency virus; MSM, men who have sex with men; STDs, sexually transmitted diseases.

TABLE 25-7	Generally Accepted Criteria for Treatment of HBV

Characteristics

Anyone with HBeAg (+) or HBeAg (−) active HBV defined as:

    HBV DNA >2000 IU/mL (kIU/L)

    ALT 2 × upper limit of normal[a] and/or with evidence of histological disease[b]

Anyone with compensated or decompensated cirrhosis with HBV DNA >2000 IU/mL (kIU/L)[c]

Anyone not fulfilling above criteria with ALT <2 × ULN and any detectable HBV DNA (<2000 IU/mL [kIU/L]), consider:

    Patient's age

    Family history of HCC

    Prior history of HBV treatment

    Extrahepatic manifestations of HBV

[a]Per European guidelines, any elevations in ALT.
[b]Moderate or greater fibrosis as determined by biopsy or noninvasive measures.
[c]Per European guidelines, any detectable HBV DNA.

evidence and clinical progression of the disease. Generally accepted criteria for treatment of HBV are given in **Table 25-7**.

- All patients with chronic HBV infection should be counseled on preventing disease transmission, avoiding alcohol, and on being immunized against HAV. Sexual and household contacts should be vaccinated against HBV.
- The immune-mediating agents approved for HBV treatment are interferon (**IFN**)-**alfa** and **pegylated (peg) IFN-alfa**. The nucleos(t)ide antiviral agents **lamivudine**, **telbivudine**, **adefovir**, **entecavir**, and **tenofovir diprovoxil** and **tenofovir alafenamide** are approved treatment options for chronic HBV.
- For HBeAg-positive patients, treatment is recommended until HBeAg seroconversion and an undetectable HBV viral load are achieved and for 6 months of additional treatment. In HBeAg-negative patients, treatment should be continued until HBsAg clearance.

Hepatitis C

- HCV is the most common blood-borne pathogen and is most often acquired through injection drug use. Screening for HCV infection is recommended in groups who are at high risk for infection (**Table 25-8**). The U.S. Preventive Services Task Force now recommends hepatitis C screening for everyone between the ages of 18 to 79 years.
- Transmission may occur by sexual contact; hemodialysis; or household, occupational, or perinatal exposure. Multiple sexual partners and coinfection with sexually transmitted diseases, including HIV, increase the risk for HCV sexual transmission.
- HCV is differentiated into six major genotypes (GT), numbered 1–6. GTs are further classified into subtypes (a, b, c, etc.). In the United States, GT1a and GT1b, followed by GT2 and GT3, cause most infections.
- In an acute HCV infection, most patients are asymptomatic and undiagnosed. HCV RNA is detectable within 1–2 weeks of exposure and levels rise quickly during the initial weeks.
- Patients with acute HCV are often asymptomatic and undiagnosed. One-third of adults will experience some mild and nonspecific symptoms, including fatigue,

TABLE 25-8 Recommendations for Hepatitis C Virus Screening

All persons between the ages of 18 to 79 years.

Current or past use of injection drugs

Persons with current or past intranasal illicit drug use

Patients who have ever been on hemodialysis

Persons with percutaneous/parenteral exposures in an unregulated setting

Healthcare and public safety workers after a needle-stick or mucosal exposure to HCV-positive blood

Children born to HCV-positive mothers

Received blood transfusions or organ transplantations before July 1992

Received clotting factors before 1987

Persons who were ever incarcerated

Coinfection with HIV

Sexually active persons about to start preexposure prophylaxis for HIV

Patients with unexplained elevated ALT levels or evidence of liver disease

Solid organ donors

ALT, alanine aminotransferase; HCV, hepatitis C virus; HIV, human immunodeficiency virus.

TABLE 25-9 AASLD/IDSA Recommended Treatment Regimens for Treatment-Naïve Patients with Hepatitis C Genotypes 1–3 (in Alphabetical Order)

HCV Genotype	No Cirrhosis	Compensated Cirrhosis (CTP Class A)
1a	Elbasvir/Grazoprevir × 12 weeks[a]	Elbasvir/Grazoprevir × 12 weeks[a]
	Glecaprevir/Pibrentasvir × 8 weeks	Glecaprevir/Pibrentasvir × 12 weeks
	Ledipasvir/Sofosbuvir × 12 weeks[b]	Ledipasvir/Sofosbuvir × 12 weeks
	Sofosbuvir/Velpatasvir × 12 weeks	Sofosbuvir/Velpatasvir × 12 weeks
1b	Elbasvir/Grazoprevir × 12 weeks	Elbasvir/Grazoprevir × 12 weeks
	Glecaprevir/Pibrentasvir × 8 weeks	Glecaprevir/Pibrentasvir × 12 weeks
	Ledipasvir/Sofosbuvir × 12 weeks[b]	Ledipasvir/Sofosbuvir × 12 weeks
	Sofosbuvir/Velpatasvir × 12 weeks	Sofosbuvir/Velpatasvir × 12 weeks
2	Glecaprevir/Pibrentasvir × 8 weeks	Glecaprevir/Pibrentasvir × 12 weeks
	Sofosbuvir/Velpatasvir × 12 weeks	Sofosbuvir/Velpatasvir × 12 weeks
3	Glecaprevir/Pibrentasvir × 8 weeks	Glecaprevir/Pibrentasvir × 12 weeks
	Sofosbuvir/Velpatasvir × 12 weeks	Sofosbuvir/Velpatasvir × 12 weeks[c]

[a]If no NS5A resistance detected.
[b]Eight-week duration may be considered for patients who are not black, not HIV coinfected, and with an HCV RNA <6 million IU/mL (kIU/L).
[c]Pretreatment resistance testing recommended.
CTP, Child—Turcotte—Pugh.

TABLE 25-10 AASLD/IDSA Recommended Treatment Regimens for Treatment-Experienced Patients with Hepatitis C Genotypes 1–3 (in Alphabetical Order)

HCV Genotype	Peg-Interferon/Ribavirin TE		NS3 PI + Peg-Interferon TE	
	Non-Cirrhotic	**Compensated Cirrhosis**	**Non-Cirrhotic**	**Compensated Cirrhosis**
1	Elbasvir/Grazoprevir × 12 weeks[a]	Elbasvir/Grazoprevir × 12 weeks[a]	Ledipasvir/Sofosbuvir × 12 weeks	Glecaprevir/Pibrentasvir × 12 weeks
	Glecaprevir/Pibrentasvir × 8 weeks	Glecaprevir/Pibrentasvir × 12 weeks	Glecaprevir/Pibrentasvir × 12 weeks	Sofosbuvir/Velpatasvir × 12 weeks
	Ledipasvir/Sofosbuvir × 12 weeks	Sofosbuvir/Velpatasvir × 12 weeks	Sofosbuvir/Velpatasvir × 12 weeks	
	Sofosbuvir/Velpatasvir × 12 weeks			
2	Glecaprevir/Pibrentasvir × 8 weeks	Sofosbuvir/Velpatasvir × 12 weeks		
	Sofosbuvir/Velpatasvir × 12 weeks	Glecaprevir/Pibrentasvir × 12 weeks		
3	Sofosbuvir/Velpatasvir × 12 weeks[b]	Elbasvir/Grazoprevir plus Sofosbuvir × 12 weeks		
		Sofosbuvir/Velpatasvir/ Voxilaprevir × 12 weeks		

[a]For GT 1a: Recommended treatment if no resistance for NS5A detected.
[b]Resistance testing for Y93 recommended before use; if Y93 present, add ribavirin or use different regimen.

anorexia, weakness, jaundice, abdominal pain, or dark urine. Additional symptoms include right upper quadrant pain, nausea, or poor appetite.

- Up to 85% of acutely infected patients go on to develop chronic HCV infection, defined as persistently detectable HCV RNA for 6 months or more.
- HCV cirrhosis poses a 30% risk of developing end-stage liver disease over 10 years as well as a 1%–2% risk per year of developing hepatocellular carcinoma.

TREATMENT

- <u>Goals of Treatment</u>: The goal is to eradicate HCV infection, which prevents the development of chronic HCV infection, end-stage liver disease, HCC, and death.
- Virologic cure, or sustained virologic response (SVR), is defined as a nondetectable HCV RNA at least 12 weeks after completing HCV therapy. Patients who achieve SVR will continue to have detectable HCV antibody, though this does not imply HCV immunity.
- Treatment is recommended for all HCV-infected persons. Patients with a short life expectancy (<12 months) are currently the only populations for whom treatment is not recommended.
- Before therapy is initiated, quantitative HCV testing and genotyping are performed.
- Recommended treatment regimens for treatment-naïve patients with hepatitis C genotypes 1–3 (in alphabetical order) are given in Table 25-9.
- Recommended treatment regimens for treatment-experienced patients with hepatitis C genotypes 1–3 (in alphabetical order) are given in Table 25-10.
- Patients with decompensated cirrhosis (CTP class B or C) often require concomitant ribavirin and have fewer treatment options due to the underlying level of liver disease and concerns for safety.
- Adherence to therapy is a crucial component in response, especially among genotype 1–infected patients.
- All patients with chronic HCV infection should be vaccinated for HAV and HBV.
- No HCV vaccine is currently available.

See Chapter 57, Viral Hepatitis, authored by Paulina Deming, for a more detailed discussion of this topic.

26 Inflammatory Bowel Disease

- There are two forms of idiopathic *inflammatory bowel disease* (IBD): ulcerative colitis (UC), a mucosal inflammatory condition confined to the rectum and colon, and Crohn disease (CD), a transmural inflammation of gastrointestinal (GI) mucosa that may occur in any part of the GI tract. The etiologies of both conditions are unknown, but they may have a common pathogenic mechanism.

ETIOLOGY AND PATHOPHYSIOLOGY

- Factors that cause IBD include infectious agents, genetics, the environment, and the immune system. This may involve abnormal regulation of the innate immune response or a reaction to various antigens. The microflora of the GI tract may provide an environmental trigger to activate inflammation in genetically susceptible individuals and is highly implicated in the development of IBD.
- Suspect infectious agents include viruses, protozoans, mycobacteria such as *Mycobacterium paratuberculosis* or *avium*, and other bacteria such as *Ruminococcus gnavus*, *Ruminococcus torques*, *Listeria monocytogenes*, *Chlamydia trachomatis*, and *Escherichia coli*.
- Th1 cytokine activity is excessive in CD, and increased expression of interferon-γ in the intestinal mucosa and production of IL-12 are features of the immune response in CD. In contrast, Th2 cytokine activity is excessive with UC (with excess production of IL-13). Tumor necrosis factor-α (TNF-α) is a pivotal proinflammatory cytokine that is increased in the mucosa and intestinal lumen of patients with CD and UC.
- Antineutrophil cytoplasmic antibodies are found in a high percentage of patients with UC and less frequently with CD.
- Smoking appears to be protective for UC but associated with increased frequency of CD. Use of nonsteroidal anti-inflammatory drugs (NSAIDs) may trigger disease occurrence or lead to disease flares.
- UC and CD differ in two general respects: anatomical sites and depth of involvement within the bowel wall. There is, however, overlap between the two conditions, with a small fraction of patients showing features of both diseases (Table 26-1).

ULCERATIVE COLITIS

- UC is confined to the colon and rectum and affects primarily the mucosa and the submucosa. The primary lesion occurs in the crypts of the mucosa (crypts of Lieberkühn) in the form of a crypt abscess.
- Local complications (involving the colon) occur in the majority of patients with UC. Relatively minor complications include hemorrhoids, anal fissures, and perirectal abscesses.
- A major complication is toxic megacolon, a severe condition that occurs in up to 7.9% of UC patients admitted to hospitals. Patients with toxic megacolon usually have a high fever, tachycardia, distended abdomen, elevated white blood cell count, and a dilated colon.
- The risk of colonic carcinoma is much greater in patients with UC than in the general population.
- Patients with UC may have hepatobiliary complications, including fatty liver, pericholangitis, chronic active hepatitis, cirrhosis, sclerosing cholangitis, cholangiocarcinoma, and gallstones.
- Arthritis commonly occurs in patients with IBD and is typically asymptomatic and migratory. Arthritis typically involves one or a few large joints, such as the knees, hips, ankles, wrists, and elbows.
- Ocular complications (iritis, episcleritis, and conjunctivitis) occur in some patients. Skin and mucosal lesions associated with IBD include erythema nodosum, pyoderma gangrenosum, aphthous ulceration, and Sweet syndrome.

TABLE 26-1	Comparison of the Clinical and Pathologic Features of Crohn Disease and Ulcerative Colitis	
Feature	**Crohn Disease**	**Ulcerative Colitis**
Clinical		
Malaise, fever	Common	Uncommon
Rectal bleeding	Common	Common
Abdominal tenderness	Common	May be present
Abdominal mass	Common	Absent
Abdominal pain	Common	Unusual
Abdominal wall and internal fistulas	Common	Absent
Distribution	Discontinuous	Continuous
Aphthous or linear ulcers	Common	Rare
Pathologic		
Rectal involvement	Rare	Common
Ileal involvement	Very common	Rare
Strictures	Common	Rare
Fistulas	Common	Rare
Transmural involvement	Common	Rare
Crypt abscesses	Rare	Very common
Granulomas	Common	Rare
Linear clefts	Common	Rare
Cobblestone appearance	Common	Absent

CROHN DISEASE

- CD is a transmural inflammatory process. The terminal ileum is the most common site, but it may occur in any part of the GI tract. Most patients have some colonic involvement. Patients often have normal bowel separating segments of diseased bowel; that is, the disease is often discontinuous.
- Complications of CD may involve the intestinal tract or organs unrelated to it. Small bowel stricture with subsequent obstruction is a complication that may require surgery. Fistula formation is common and occurs much more frequently than with UC.
- Systemic complications of CD are common and similar to those found with UC. Arthritis, iritis, skin lesions, and liver disease often accompany CD.
- Nutritional deficiencies are common with CD (including deficiencies of folate, vitamin B_{12}, vitamins A to D, calcium, magnesium, iron, and zinc).

CLINICAL PRESENTATION

ULCERATIVE COLITIS

- There is a wide range of presenting symptoms in UC, from mild abdominal cramping with frequent small-volume bowel movements to profuse diarrhea (Table 26-2). Many patients have disease confined to the rectum (proctitis).
- Most patients with UC experience intermittent bouts of illness after varying intervals of no symptoms.
- Mild disease, which afflicts two-thirds of patients, has been defined as fewer than four stools daily, with or without blood, with no systemic disturbance and a normal erythrocyte sedimentation rate (ESR <30 mm/hr).
- Patients with moderate disease have more than four stools per day but with minimal systemic disturbance.

TABLE 26-2	Clinical Presentation of Ulcerative Colitis

Signs and symptoms
- Abdominal cramping
- Frequent bowel movements, often with blood in the stool
- Weight loss
- Fever and tachycardia in severe disease
- Blurred vision, eye pain, and photophobia with ocular involvement
- Arthritis
- Raised, red, tender nodules that vary in size from 1 cm to several centimeters

Physical examination
- Hemorrhoids, anal fissures, or perirectal abscesses may be present
- Iritis, uveitis, episcleritis, and conjunctivitis with ocular involvement
- Dermatologic findings with erythema nodosum, pyoderma gangrenosum, or aphthous ulceration

Laboratory tests
- Decreased hematocrit/hemoglobin
- Increased ESR, CRP, and fecal calprotectin
- Leukocytosis and hypoalbuminemia with severe disease
- (+) perinuclear antineutrophil cytoplasmic antibodies

- With severe disease, the patient has more than six stools per day with blood, with systemic manifestations of fever, tachycardia, anemia, or ESR greater than 30 mm/hr (8.3 μm/sec). With fulminant disease there are more than 10 bowel movements per day with continuous bleeding, toxicity, abdominal tenderness, requirement for transfusion, and colonic dilation.

CROHN DISEASE

- As with UC, the presentation of CD is highly variable (Table 26-3). A patient may present with diarrhea and abdominal pain or a perirectal or perianal lesion. Patients with mild-to-moderate CD are typically ambulatory and have no evidence of dehydration, systemic toxicity, less than 10% loss of body weight, or abdominal tenderness, mass, or obstruction.
- The course of CD is characterized by periods of remission and exacerbation. Some patients may be free of symptoms for years, whereas others experience chronic problems despite medical therapy.
- The Crohn Disease Activity Index (CDAI) is used to gauge response to therapy and determine remission. Disease activity may be assessed and correlated by evaluation of serum C-reactive protein concentrations.

TREATMENT

- <u>Goals of Treatment</u>: Resolution of acute inflammatory processes, resolution of attendant complications (eg, fistulas or abscesses), alleviation of systemic manifestations (eg, arthritis), maintenance of remission from acute inflammation, or surgical palliation or cure.
- Treatment often involves use of specific targets, such as mucosal healing and endoscopic remission, or resolution of symptoms such as abdominal pain and diarrhea, as the main indicators of treatment efficacy (referred to as "Treat to Target").

NONPHARMACOLOGIC TREATMENT

- Protein–energy malnutrition and suboptimal weight are reported in up to 85% of patients with CD. The nutritional needs of the majority of patients can be adequately addressed with enteral supplementation.

TABLE 26-3	Clinical Presentation of Crohn Disease

Signs and symptoms
- Malaise and fever
- Abdominal pain
- Frequent bowel movements
- Hematochezia
- Fistula
- Weight loss and malnutrition
- Arthritis

Physical examination
- Abdominal mass and tenderness
- Perianal fissure or fistula

Laboratory tests
- Increased white blood cell count, ESR, CRP, and fecal calprotectin
- (+) anti–*Saccharomyces cerevisiae* antibodies

- Elimination of specific foods that appear to exacerbate symptoms can be tried; however, exclusion diets are generally not endorsed, even in the setting of severe disease.
- Parenteral nutrition is generally reserved for patients with severe malnutrition or those who fail enteral therapy or have a contraindication to receiving enteral therapy, such as perforation, protracted vomiting, short bowel syndrome, or severe intestinal stenosis.
- While probiotics are considered to be generally safe in patients with IBD, the added cost and requirement to often take multiple doses per day, coupled with the lack of quality data to support their use, should weigh into the decision to use them in IBD.
- Colectomy may be necessary for UC patients with disease uncontrolled by maximum medical therapy or when there are disease complications such as colonic perforation, toxic megacolon, uncontrolled colonic hemorrhage, or colonic strictures.
- Surgery in patients with CD is usually reserved for patients with intractable hemorrhage, perforation, persistent or recurrent obstruction, abscess, dysplasia, cancer, or medically refractory disease. CD has a high recurrence rate after surgery.

PHARMACOLOGIC THERAPY

- The major drug therapies used in IBD are **aminosalicylates; corticosteroids;** immunomodulators (**azathioprine, mercaptopurine,** and **methotrexate**); immunosuppressive agents (**cyclosporine** and **tacrolimus**); antimicrobials (**metronidazole** and **ciprofloxacin**); and agents to inhibit TNF-α (anti–TNF-α antibodies), leukocyte adhesion and migration (**natalizumab** and **vedolizumab**), interleukin function (**ustekinumab**), or Janus kinase function (**tofacitinib**).
- **Sulfasalazine** combines a sulfonamide (sulfapyridine) antibiotic and mesalamine (5-aminosalicylic acid) in the same molecule. Oral **mesalamine** derivatives are alternatives to sulfasalazine for treatment of mild-to-moderate UC with similar rates of efficacy. Mesalamine-based products are listed in **Table 26-4**.
- Oral corticosteroids in doses of 40–60 mg/day **prednisone** equivalent can be used for patients with moderate to extensive disease who are refractory to oral aminosalicylates or require more rapid control of symptoms.
- Immunomodulators such as azathioprine, mercaptopurine (a metabolite of azathioprine), methotrexate, or cyclosporine are used in the long-term treatment of IBD. These agents are generally reserved for patients who fail aminosalicylate therapy or are refractory to or dependent on corticosteroids.
- Cyclosporine has a short-term benefit in the treatment of acute, severe UC to avoid colectomy in patients failing corticosteroids but has little efficacy in CD.
- Methotrexate 15–25 mg intramuscularly or subcutaneously once weekly is useful for treatment and maintenance of CD and may be steroid sparing.

TABLE 26-4	Agents for the Treatment of Inflammatory Bowel Disease		
Drug	**Brand Name**	**Initial Dose (g)**	**Usual Range**
Sulfasalazine	Azulfidine	500 mg–1 g	4–6 g/day
	Azulfidine EN	500 mg–1 g	4–6 g/day
Mesalamine suppository	Rowasa	1 g	1 g daily to three times weekly
Mesalamine enema	Canasa	4 g	4 g daily to three times weekly
Mesalamine (oral)	Asacol HD	1.6 g/day	2.8–4.8 g/day
	Apriso	1.5 g/day	1.5 g/day once daily
	Lialda	1.2–2.4 g/day	1.2–4.8 g/day once daily
	Pentasa	2 g/day	2–4 g/day
	Delzicol	1.2 g/day	2.4–4.8 g/day
Olsalazine	Dipentum	1.5 g/day	1.5–3 g/day
Balsalazide	Colazal	2.25 g/day	2.25–6.75 g/day
Azathioprine	Imuran, Azasan	50–100 mg	1–2.5 mg/kg/day
Cyclosporine	Gengraf	2–4 mg/kg/day IV	2–4 mg/kg/day IV
	Neoral, Sandimmune	2–8 mg/kg/day oral	
Mercaptopurine	Purinethol	50–100 mg	1–2.5 mg/kg/day
Methotrexate	No branded IM injection	15–25 mg IM weekly	15–25 mg IM weekly
Adalimumab	Humira	160 mg SC day 1	80 mg SC 2 (day 15), and then 40 mg every 2 weeks
Adalimumab-atto	Amjevita		
Adalimumab-abdm	Cyltezo		
Certolizumab	Cimzia	400 mg SC	400 mg SC weeks 2 and 4, and then 400 mg SC monthly
Infliximab	Remicade	5 mg/kg IV	5 mg/kg weeks 2 and 6, 5–10 mg/kg every 8 weeks
Infliximab-dyyb	Inflectra		
Infliximab-abda	Renflexis		
Infliximab-qbtx	IXIFI		
Natalizumab	Tysabri	300 mg IV	300 mg IV every 4 weeks
Budesonide	Entocort EC capsule, Uceris tablet	9 mg orally once daily	6–9 mg daily
	Uceris rectal foam	2 mg twice daily	2 mg daily
Vedolizumab	Entyvio	300 mg IV	300 mg IV weeks 2 and 6 and then every 8 weeks

(Continued)

TABLE 26-4	Agents for the Treatment of Inflammatory Bowel Disease (*Continued*)		
Drug	**Brand Name**	**Initial Dose (g)**	**Usual Range**
Golimumab	Simponi	200 mg SC	100 mg SC weeks 2 and 4
Ustekinumab	Stelara	Weight-based initial IV dose <55 kg (260 mg), 55–85 kg (390 mg), >85 kg (520 mg)	90 mg SC every 8 weeks
Tofacitinib	Xeljanz	10 mg twice daily for 8 weeks; may continue for maximum of 16 weeks	5 mg twice daily

IM, intramuscular; SC, subcutaneous.

- Antimicrobial agents, particularly metronidazole and ciprofloxacin, are frequently used in attempts to control CD, particularly when it involves the perineal area or fistulas.
- **Infliximab** is an anti-TNFα antibody that is useful in moderate-to-severe active CD and UC as well as steroid-dependent or fistulizing disease, both as induction and maintenance therapy. **Adalimumab** is another anti-TNFα (fully humanized) antibody that is an option for patients with moderate-to-severe active CD or UC previously treated with infliximab who have lost response.
- Natalizumab and vedolizumab are leukocyte adhesion and migration inhibitors that are used for patients with CD who are unresponsive to other therapies.

Ulcerative Colitis

Mild-to-Moderate Disease

- Most patients with mild-to-moderate active UC can be managed on an outpatient basis with oral and/or topical aminosalicylates (**Fig. 26-1**). For patients with extensive disease, oral once-daily mesalamine is generally preferred in doses of 2–3 g/day. Doses greater than 3 g/day can be used in patients who are unresponsive to standard doses and generally should be combined with a rectal mesalamine formulation at a dose of 1 g/day.
- Oral mesalamine derivatives (see **Table 26-4**) are reasonable alternatives to sulfasalazine for treatment of UC because they are better tolerated. Topical mesalamine in an enema or suppository formulation is more effective than oral mesalamine or topical steroids for distal disease.
- **Budesonide** 9 mg/day is preferred for patients who are unresponsive to optimized doses of mesalamine.

Moderate-to-Severe Disease

- Oral mesalamine products may be effective for moderately severe UC, but budesonide is an alternative before using more systemic corticosteroids and is preferred for moderate disease.
- Steroids have a place in the treatment of moderate-to-severe UC or in patients who are unresponsive to maximal doses of oral and topical mesalamine. Oral corticosteroids in doses of 40–60 mg prednisone equivalent daily are recommended for adults.
- TNF-α inhibitors are an option for patients with moderate-to-severe disease who are unresponsive to aminosalicylates, corticosteroids, or other immunosuppressive agents. In general infliximab, adalimumab, and golimumab and their respective biosimilars have similar rates of efficacy when used as monotherapy in UC.

AZA, azathioprine; MMX, Multi-Matrix System; MP, mercaptopurine; TNF, tumor necrosis factor.

FIGURE 26-1. Treatment approaches for ulcerative colitis.

Severe or Intractable Disease

- Patients with uncontrolled severe UC or incapacitating symptoms require hospitalization for effective management. Most medications are given parenterally. Patients should be tested for *Clostridoidies difficile* infection and receive venous thromboembolism (VTE) prophylaxis.
- IV **hydrocortisone** 300 mg daily in three divided doses or **methylprednisolone** 60 mg once daily for 3–5 days is considered a first-line agent. A trial of corticosteroids is warranted in most patients before proceeding to colectomy, unless the condition is grave or rapidly deteriorating.
- Patients who are unresponsive to parenteral corticosteroids after 3–7 days can receive cyclosporine or infliximab. A continuous IV infusion of cyclosporine 2–4 mg/kg/day is the typical dose range used and may delay the need for colectomy.

Maintenance of Remission

- Once remission from active disease has been achieved, the goal of therapy is to maintain the remission.
- The major agents used for maintenance of remission are sulfasalazine and the newer mesalamine derivatives, infliximab, adalimumab and its biosimilars, golimumab, and azathioprine or mercaptopurine.

- Oral agents, including sulfasalazine, mesalamine, and **balsalazide**, are all effective options for maintenance therapy. The optimal dose to prevent relapse is 2–2.4 g/day of mesalamine equivalent, with rates of relapse over 6–12 months reported as 40%.
- Steroids do not have a role in the maintenance of remission with UC because they are ineffective. Steroids should be withdrawn gradually over 2–4 weeks after remission is induced.

Crohn Disease

Active Crohn Disease

- Mesalamine derivatives have not demonstrated significant efficacy in CD. They are often tried as an initial therapy for mild-to-moderate CD given their favorable adverse effect profile.
- Mesalamine derivatives that release mesalamine in the small bowel (eg, Pentasa) may be more effective than sulfasalazine for ileal involvement.
- Systemic corticosteroids are frequently used for treating moderate-to-severe active CD; however, controlled-release budesonide (Entocort) 9 mg daily is a preferred first-line option for patients with mild-to-moderate ileal or right-sided (ascending colonic) disease.
- Oral corticosteroids, such as prednisone 40–60 mg/day, are generally considered first-line therapy and are frequently used for moderate-to-severe CD unresponsive to aminosalicylates.
- Metronidazole 10–20 mg/kg/day orally in divided doses may be useful in some patients with CD, particularly for patients with colonic or ileocolonic involvement, those with perineal disease, or those who are unresponsive to sulfasalazine.
- Azathioprine, mercaptopurine, and methotrexate are not recommended to induce remission in moderate-to-severe CD; however, they are effective in maintaining steroid-induced remission and are generally limited to use for patients not achieving adequate response to standard medical therapy or in the setting of steroid dependency.
- Clinical response to azathioprine and mercaptopurine may be related to whole-blood concentrations of the metabolite 6-thioguanine (TGN). Concentrations of TGN greater than 230–450 pmol/8 × 10^8 erythrocytes have beneficial effects, but monitoring is not routinely performed or may not be available at some sites.
- Patients deficient in thiopurine S-methyltransferase (TPMT) are at greater risk of bone marrow suppression from azathioprine and mercaptopurine. Determination of TPMT or TPMT genotype is recommended to guide dosage.
- Methotrexate given weekly intramuscularly or subcutaneously in doses of 15–25 mg is effective in reducing steroid dependency and maintaining remission, and may be considered as an alternative to azathioprine or mercaptopurine.
- The TNF-α inhibitors are the most effective and thus the preferred agents in managing moderate to severe CD. All agents in this class, with the exception of golimumab, which is not approved for use in CD in the United States, have similar rates of efficacy. The use of TNF-α inhibitors in combination with thiopurines has quickly become the preferred approach to treatment of moderate-to-severe CD.
- The integrin antagonists are options for patients who do not respond to steroids or TNF-α inhibitors, and vedolizumab is also considered a first-line alternative to TNF-α inhibitors for moderate-to-severe disease.

Maintenance of Remission

- Prevention of recurrence of disease is more difficult with CD than with UC. There is minimal evidence that sulfasalazine and oral mesalamine derivatives are effective for maintenance of CD remission following medically induced remission, and therefore these agents are not preferred (**Fig. 26-2**).
- Systemic steroids have no role in the maintenance of remission or prevention of recurrence of CD; these agents do not appear to alter the long-term course of the disease. Budesonide can be considered for maintenance therapy for up to 4 months.

Disease severity

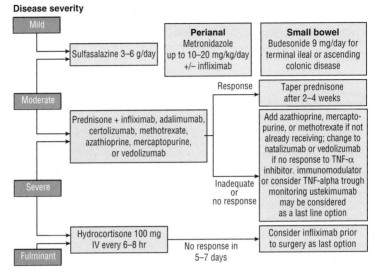

FIGURE 26-2. Treatment approaches for Crohn disease.

- All of the TNF-α inhibitors currently approved for use in CD are viable options for maintenance of remission. Combination therapy with a thiopurine should be highly considered to further improve efficacy and to extend the duration of TNF-α inhibitor efficacy by reducing immunogenicity.
- There is weak evidence to suggest that methotrexate is effective in maintaining remission in CD.

SELECT COMPLICATIONS

Toxic Megacolon

- The treatment required for toxic megacolon includes general supportive measures to maintain vital functions, consideration for early surgical intervention, and antimicrobials.
- Aggressive fluid and electrolyte management are required for dehydration. When the patient has lost significant amounts of blood (through the rectum), blood transfusion may be necessary.
- Steroids in high doses (eg, hydrocortisone 100 mg every 8 hours) should be administered IV to reduce acute inflammation.
- Broad-spectrum antimicrobials that include coverage for gram-negative bacilli and intestinal anaerobes should be used as preemptive therapy if perforation occurs.

Extraintestinal Manifestations

- For arthritis, **aspirin** or another NSAID may be beneficial, as are corticosteroids. However, NSAID use may exacerbate the underlying IBD and predispose patients to GI bleeding.
- Anemia secondary to blood loss from the GI tract can be treated with oral **ferrous sulfate**. **Vitamin B_{12}** or **folic acid** may also be required.
- If the patient is deemed high risk for osteoporosis or exhibits a reduced serum vitamin D concentration, **vitamin D** and **calcium** should be administered. If osteoporosis is present, then calcium, vitamin D, and a **bisphosphonate** or possibly **teriparatide** are recommended.

EVALUATION OF THERAPEUTIC OUTCOMES

- See Table 26-5 for drug monitoring guidelines.
- Patients receiving sulfasalazine should receive oral **folic acid** supplementation because sulfasalazine inhibits folic acid absorption.

TABLE 26-5	Drug Monitoring Guidelines		
Drug(s)	**Adverse Drug Reaction**	**Monitoring Parameters**	**Comments**
Sulfasalazine	Nausea, vomiting, headache	Folate, complete blood count	Increase the dose slowly, over 1−2 weeks
	Rash, anemia, pneumonitis	Liver function tests, Scr, BUN	
	Hepatotoxicity, nephritis		
	Thrombocytopenia, lymphoma		
Mesalamine	Nausea, vomiting, headache	GI disturbances	
Corticosteroids	Hyperglycemia, dyslipidemia	Blood pressure, fasting lipid panel	Avoid long-term use if possible or consider budesonide
	Osteoporosis, hypertension, acne	Glucose, vitamin D, bone density	
	Edema, infection, myopathy, psychosis		
Azathioprine/ Mercaptopurine	Bone marrow suppression, pancreatitis, Lymphoma	Complete blood count Scr, BUN, liver function tests, genotype/ phenotype	Check TPMT activity May monitor TGN
	Liver dysfunction, rash, arthralgia		
Methotrexate	Bone marrow suppression, pancreatitis	Complete blood count, Scr, BUN	Check baseline pregnancy test
	Pneumonitis, pulmonary fibrosis, hepatitis	Liver function tests	Chest x-ray
Infliximab Adalimumab Certolizumab Golimumab	Infusion-related reactions (infliximab), infection	Blood pressure/heart rate (infliximab)	Need negative PPD and viral serologies
	Heart failure, optic neuritis, demyelination, injection site reaction, signs of infection	Neurologic exam, mental status Trough concentrations (infliximab) Antidrug antibodies (all agents)	

(Continued)

TABLE 26-5	Drug Monitoring Guidelines (Continued)		
Drug(s)	**Adverse Drug Reaction**	**Monitoring Parameters**	**Comments**
Natalizumab Vedolizumab	Infusion-related reactions	Brain MRI, mental status, progressive multifocal leukoencephalopathy	Vedolizumab not associated with PML
Ustekinumab	Infections, skin cancers	Signs/symptoms of infection, annual skin exam	Rare instances of reversible posterior leukoencephalopathy syndrome (RPLS)
			Avoid live vaccines
Tofacitinib	Infection, thrombosis, lymphoma, elevated cholesterol, CK, LFTs, lymphopenia, neutropenia, anemia	Symptoms of infection or thrombosis	Avoid live vaccines
			Screen for baseline TB
			Do not initiate in patients with lymphocytes <500/mm³, ANC <1000/mm³, or hemoglobin <9 g/dL
			Monitor lipids and LFTs every 4–8 weeks
			Gastrointestinal perforation has been reported with use of the XR formulation
			Drug interactions with CYP3A4 and 2C19 inhibitors

ANC, absolute neutrophil count; BUN, blood urea nitrogen; CK, creatine kinase; GI, gastrointestinal; LFTs, liver function tests; MRI, magnetic resonance imaging; PML, progressive multifocal leukoencephalopathy; PPD, purified protein derivative; SCr, serum creatinine; TGN, thioguanine; TPMT, thiopurine methyltransferase; XR, extended-release.

- The success of therapeutic regimens to treat IBDs can be measured by patient-reported complaints, signs and symptoms, direct physician examination (including endoscopy), history and physical examination, select laboratory tests, and quality of life measures.
- Adverse effects of corticosteroids include hyperglycemia, hypertension, osteoporosis, acne, fluid retention, electrolyte disturbances, myopathies, muscle wasting, increased appetite, psychosis, infection, and adrenocortical suppression. To minimize corticosteroid effects, clinicians may use alternate-day steroid therapy; however, some patients do not do well clinically on the days when no steroid is given.
- To create more objective measures, disease-rating scales or indices have been created. CDAI is a commonly used scale, particularly for evaluation of patients during clinical trials. The scale incorporates eight elements: (1) number of stools in the past 7 days, (2) sum of abdominal pain ratings from the past 7 days, (3) rating of general

well-being in the past 7 days, (4) use of antidiarrheals, (5) body weight, (6) hematocrit, (7) finding of abdominal mass, and (8) a sum of symptoms present in the past week.

- Standardized assessment tools have also been constructed for UC. Elements in these scales include: (1) stool frequency; (2) presence of blood in the stool; (3) mucosal appearance (from endoscopy); and (4) physician's global assessment based on physical examination, endoscopy, and laboratory data.

See Chapter 51, Inflammatory Bowel Disease, authored by Brian A. Hemstreet, for a more detailed discussion of this topic.

- *Nausea* is usually defined as the inclination to vomit or as a feeling in the throat or epigastric region alerting an individual that vomiting is imminent. Vomiting is defined as the ejection or expulsion of gastric contents through the mouth, often requiring a forceful event.

ETIOLOGY AND PATHOPHYSIOLOGY

- Specific etiologies associated with nausea and vomiting are presented in **Table 27-1**.
- **Table 27-2** presents cytotoxic agents categorized by their emetogenic potential. Although some agents may have greater emetogenic potential than others, combinations of agents, high doses, clinical settings, psychological conditions, prior treatment experiences, and unusual stimuli to sight, smell, or taste may alter a patient's response to a drug treatment.

TABLE 27-1	Etiologies of Nausea and Vomiting

Intraperitoneal
Mechanical obstruction
   Gastric outlet obstruction
   Small-bowel obstruction
Altered sensorimotor function
   Gastroparesis
   Gastroesophageal reflux
   Intestinal pseudo-obstruction
   Irritable bowel syndrome
   Chronic idiopathic nausea
   Functional vomiting
   Cyclic vomiting syndrome
   Cannabinoid hyperemesis syndrome
   Rumination syndrome
Inflammatory diseases
   Pancreatitis
   Pyelonephritis
   Cholecystitis
   Appendicitis
   Hepatitis
Acute gastroenteritis
   Viral
   Bacterial
Biliary colic
Liver failure

Cardiovascular diseases
Myocardial infarction
Cardiomyopathy

(Continued)

TABLE 27-1	Etiologies of Nausea and Vomiting (*Continued*)

Neurologic processes

    Increased intracranial pressure

    Migraine headache

    Vestibular disorders

    Intracerebral hemorrhage

    Intracerebral malignancy

Metabolic disorders

    Diabetes mellitus (diabetic ketoacidosis)

    Addison's disease

    Renal disease (uremia)

Psychiatric causes

    Depression

    Anxiety disorders

    Anorexia and bulimia nervosa

Therapy-induced causes

    Antineoplastic agents

    Radiation therapy

    Anticonvulsant preparations

    Digoxin, cardiac antiarrhythmics

    Opioids

    Oral hypoglycemics

    Oral contraceptives

    Antibiotics

    Volatile general anesthetics

Drug withdrawal

    Opioids

    Benzodiazepines

Miscellaneous causes

    Pregnancy

    Noxious odors

    Postoperative vomiting

- The three consecutive phases of emesis are nausea, retching, and vomiting. Nausea, the imminent need to vomit, is associated with gastric stasis. Retching is the labored movement of abdominal and thoracic muscles before vomiting. The final phase of emesis is vomiting, the forceful expulsion of gastric contents due to GI retroperistalsis.
- Vomiting is triggered by afferent impulses to the vomiting center, a nucleus of cells in the medulla. Impulses are received from sensory centers, such as the chemoreceptor trigger zone, cerebral cortex, and visceral afferents from the pharynx and GI tract. The vomiting center integrates the afferent impulses, resulting in efferent impulses to the salivation center, respiratory center, and the pharyngeal, GI, and abdominal muscles, leading to vomiting.

TABLE 27-2	Emetic Risk of Agents Used in Oncology and Treatment Options	
Antiemetic Agent	**Antiemetic Dose on Day 1 of Chemotherapy**	**Antiemetic Dose on Subsequent Days**
High Risk (>90%): Anthracycline/Cyclophosphamide combination, carboplatin AUC >4, carmustine, cisplatin, cyclophosphamide >1500 mg/m², dacarbazine, mechlorethamine, streptozocin		
NK-1 Antagonist		
Aprepitant	125 mg oral	80 mg oral on days 2–3
Fosaprepitant	150 mg IV	
Netupitant/Palonosetron	300 mg/0.5 mg oral	
Rolapitant		
	180 mg oral	
5-HT3 Antagonist[a]		
Dolasetron	100 mg oral	
Granisetron	2 mg oral or 1 mg IV or 10 mcg/kg IV or 1 patch or 10 mg SQ	
Ondansetron	8 mg oral twice daily or 24 mg oral or 8 mg IV or 0.15 mg/kg IV	
	0.5 mg oral or 0.25 mg IV	
Palonosetron	0.3 mg IV	
Ramosetron	5 mg oral or 5 mg IV	
Tropisetron		
Dexamethasone[b]	12 mg or 20 mg oral/IV	8 mg oral/IV daily or twice daily on days 2–4
Olanzapine	10 mg oral	10 mg oral on days 2–4
Moderate Risk (30%–90%): Aldesleukin, alemtuzumab, arsenic trioxide, azacitidine, bendamustine, busulfan, carboplatin AUC <4, clofarabine, cyclophosphamide <1500 mg/m², cytarabine >1000 mg/m², dactinomycin, daunorubicin, daunorubicin/cytarabine liposomal, doxorubicin, epirubicin, idarubicin, ifosfamide, irinotecan (conventional and liposomal), melphalan, oxaliplatin, romidepsin, temozolomide, thiotepa, trabectedin		
5-HT3 Antagonist		
Dolasetron	100 mg oral	
Granisetron	2 mg oral or 1 mg IV or 10 mcg/kg IV or 1 patch or 10 mg SQ	
Ondansetron	8 mg oral twice daily or 8 mg IV or 0.15 mg/kg IV	
Palonosetron	0.5 mg oral or 0.25 mg IV	
Ramosetron	0.3 mg IV	
Tropisetron	5 mg oral or 5 mg IV	
Dexamethasone	8 mg oral/IV	8 mg oral/IV on days 2–3[c]

(Continued)

TABLE 27-2	Emetic Risk of Agents Used in Oncology and Treatment Options (Continued)

Low Risk (10%–30%): Aflibercept, atezolizumab, belinostat, blinatumomab, bortezomib, brentuximab, cabazitaxel, carfilzomib, cetuximab, cytarabine <1000 mg/m², docetaxel, doxorubicin, liposomal (Doxil®), elotuzumab, eribulin, etoposide, fluorouracil, gemcitabine, ipilimumab, ixabepilone, methotrexate, mitomycin, mitoxantrone, paclitaxel (conventional and albumin-bound), necitumumab, olaratumab, omacetaxine, panitumumab, pemetrexed, pentostatin, pertuzumab, talimogene-iaherparepvec, temsirolimus, topotecan, trastuzumab emtansine

Choose One

5-HT3 Antagonist

Dolasetron	100 mg oral
Granisetron	2 mg oral or 1 mg IV or 10 mcg/kg IV or 1 patch or 10 mg SQ
Ondansetron	8 mg oral twice daily or 8 mg IV or 0.15 mg/kg IV
Palonosetron	0.5 mg oral or 0.25 mg IV
Ramosetron	0.3 mg IV
Tropisetron	5 mg oral or 5 mg IV

OR

Dexamethasone	8 mg oral/IV

Minimal Risk (<10%): Avelumab, asparaginase (Erwinia and Pegaspargase), bevacizumab, bleomycin, cladribine, daratumumab, decitabine, durvalumab, fludarabine, nelerabine, nivolumab, obinutuzumab, ofatumumab, peginterferon, pembrolizumab, pralatrexate, ramucirumab, rituximab (IV and SQ), siltuximab, trastuzumab, valrubicin, vinblastine, vincristine (conventional and liposomal), vinorelbine

No routine prophylactic antiemetics are needed

[a]No additional 5-HT3-RA is needed if netupitant/palonosetron is used.
[b]Dexamethasone dose on day 1 should be reduced to 12 mg when given with aprepitant, fosaprepitant, and netupitant/palonosetron due to drug interactions. Dexamethasone dose on days 2–4 should be omitted when used as antiemetic with anthracycline/cyclophosphamide combination regimen or carboplatin AUC ≥4.
[c]Only if regimen is known to cause delayed nausea/vomiting (eg, cyclophosphamide, doxorubicin, oxaliplatin).

CLINICAL PRESENTATION

- The clinical presentation of nausea and vomiting is given in Table 27-3. Nausea and vomiting may be classified as either simple or complex.

TREATMENT

- <u>Goal of treatment</u>: Prevent or eliminate nausea and vomiting; ideally accomplished without adverse effects or with clinically acceptable adverse effects.

GENERAL APPROACH TO TREATMENT

- Treatment options for nausea and vomiting include drug and nondrug modalities such as biofeedback and hypnosis. For patients who are suffering due to excessive or disagreeable food or beverage consumption, avoidance or moderation in dietary intake may lead to symptom resolution.

TABLE 27-3	Clinical Presentation of Nausea and Vomiting

General

Depending on severity of symptoms, patients may present in mild-to-severe distress

Symptoms

Simple: Self-limiting, resolves spontaneously, and requires only symptomatic therapy

Complex: Not relieved after administration of antiemetics; progressive deterioration of patient secondary to fluid-electrolyte imbalances; usually associated with noxious agents or pyschogenic events

Signs

Simple: Patient complaint of queasiness or discomfort

Complex: Weight loss; fever; abdominal pain

Laboratory tests

Simple: None

Complex: Serum electrolyte concentrations; upper/lower GI evaluation

Other information

Fluid input and output

Medication history

Recent history of behavioral or visual changes, headache, pain, or stress

Family history positive for psychogenic vomiting

- Patients with symptoms of systemic illness may quickly improve as their underlying condition resolves. Patients in whom these symptoms result from labyrinthine changes produced by motion may benefit quickly by assuming a stable physical position.

- Changes in diet such as restricting oral intake, eating smaller meals, avoiding spicy or fried foods and instead eating bland foods such as with the BRAT diet (Bananas, Rice, Applesauce, and Toast) can help alleviate symptoms.

PHARMACOLOGIC MANAGEMENT

- Information concerning commonly available antiemetic preparations is compiled in **Table 27-4**. The treatment of simple nausea and vomiting often involves self-care from a list of nonprescription products. Nonprescription and prescription drugs are useful in the treatment of simple nausea and vomiting in small, infrequently administered doses and are associated with minimal side effects. As the symptoms persist or become worse, prescription medications may be chosen, either as single-agent therapy or in combination.

- For most conditions, a single-agent antiemetic is preferred; however, for patients not responding to such therapy and those receiving highly emetogenic chemotherapy, multiple-agent regimens are usually required.

- The management of complex nausea and vomiting, such as in patients who are receiving antineoplastic agents, may require initial combination therapy. In combination regimens, the goal is to achieve symptomatic control through administration of agents with different pharmacologic mechanisms of action.

CHEMOTHERAPY-INDUCED NAUSEA AND VOMITING (CINV)

- There are five categories of CINV: acute, delayed, anticipatory, breakthrough, and refractory. Nausea or vomiting that occurs within 24 hours of chemotherapy administration is defined as acute CINV, whereas when it starts more than 24 hours after chemotherapy administration, it is defined as delayed CINV.

TABLE 27-4 Common Antiemetic Preparations and Adult Dosage Regimens[a]

Drug	Adult Dosage Regimen	Dosage Form/Route	Availability
Antacids: Useful with simple nausea/vomiting			
Adverse drug reactions: Magnesium products—diarrhea; Aluminum or calcium products—constipation			
Antacids (various)	15–30 mL every 2–4 hours prn	Liquid/Oral	Nonprescription
Antihistaminic–Anticholinergic Agents: Especially problematic in the elderly; increased risk of complications in patients with BPH, narrow angle glaucoma, or asthma			
Adverse drug reactions: Drowsiness, confusion, blurred vision, dry mouth, urinary retention			
Dimenhydrinate (Dramamine)	50–100 mg every 4–6 hours prn	Tab, chew tab, cap	Nonprescription
Diphenhydramine (Benadryl)	25–50 mg every 4–6 hours prn 10–50 mg every 2–4 hours prn	Tab, cap, liquid IM, IV	Prescription/ nonprescription
Hydroxyzine (Vistaril, Atarax)	25–100 mg every 4–6 hours prn	Tab (unlabeled use)	Prescription
Meclizine (Bonine, Antivert)	12.5–25 mg 1 hour before travel; repeat every 12–24 hours prn	Tab, chew tab	Prescription/ nonprescription
Scopolamine (Transderm Scop)	1.5 mg every 72 hours	Transdermal patch	Prescription
Trimethobenzamide (Tigan)	300 mg three to four times daily 200 mg three to four times daily	Cap IM	Prescription
Benzodiazepine: Used for ANV but is contraindicated with olanzapine			
Adverse drug reactions: Dizziness, sedation, appetite changes, memory impairment; observe for additive sedation especially if used with narcotic analgesics			
Lorazepam (Ativan)	0.5–2 mg on night before and morning of chemotherapy	Tab, IV	Prescription (C-IV)
Butyrophenones: Used for breakthrough CINV; droperidol has limited use			
Adverse drug reactions: Haloperidol—sedation, constipation, hypotension, EPS; droperidol—QTc prolongation and/or torsade de pointes, 12-lead electrocardiogram prior to administration, followed by cardiac monitoring for 2–3 hours after administration			
Haloperidol (Haldol)	0.5–2 mg every 4–6 hours prn	Tab, liquid, IM, IV	Prescription
Droperidol (Inapsine)[b]	2.5 mg; additional 1.25 mg may be given	IM, IV	Prescription

(Continued)

TABLE 27-4	Common Antiemetic Preparations and Adult Dosage Regimens[a] *(Continued)*		
Cannabinoids: Used for breakthrough CINV			
Adverse drug reactions: Eurphoria, somnolence, xerostomia			
Dronabinol (Marinol)	5–15 mg/m^2 every 2–4 hours prn	Cap	Prescription (C-III)
		Oral solution	
	4.2–12.6 mg/m^2 every 2–4 hours prn		
Nabilone (Cesamet)	1–2 mg twice daily	Cap	Prescription (C-II)
Corticosteroids: Useful as a single agent or in combination therapy for prophylaxis of CINV or PONV			
Adverse drug reactions: Insomnia, GI symptoms, agitation, appetite stimulation, hypertension, and hyperglycemia			
Dexamethasone	See Table 27-2 for CINV dosing and Table 27-6 for PONV dosing	Tab, IV	Prescription
Histamine (H2) Antagonists: Useful with nausea secondary to heartburn or GERD			
Adverse drug reactions: Headache, constipation, or diarrhea			
Cimetidine (Tagamet HB)	200 mg twice daily prn	Tab	Nonprescription
Famotidine (Pepcid AC)	10 mg twice daily prn	Tab	Nonprescription
Nizatidine (Axid AR)	75 mg twice daily prn	Tab	Nonprescription
5-Hydroxytryptamine-3 Receptor Antagonists: Useful as a single-agent or combination therapy for prophylaxis of CINV or PONV			
Adverse drug reactions: Asthenia, constipation, headache			
	See Table 27-2 for CINV dosing and Table 27-6 for PONV dosing	Tab, IV	Prescription

Miscellaneous Agents

Metoclopramide: Prokinetic activity useful in diabetic gastroparesis. *Adverse drug reactions: Asthenia, headache, somnolence, EPS*

Olanzapine: Use with caution in elderly; contraindicated with benzodiazepines. *Adverse drug reactions: Sedation, prolonged QTc interval, EPS*

Pyridoxine: Used in NVP. May be used alone or in combination with doxylamine 12.5 mg. Combination product available as prescription. *Adverse drug reactions: Drowsiness, headache*

(Continued)

TABLE 27-4	Common Antiemetic Preparations and Adult Dosage Regimens[a] (Continued)		
Metoclopramide (Reglan)	10–20 mg (0.5–2 mg/kg) four times daily	Tab, IV	Prescription
Olanzapine (Zyprexa)	5–10 mg daily	Tab	Prescription
Pyridoxine (vitamin B$_6$)	10–25 mg orally three to four times daily	Tab, cap	Nonprescription

Phenothiazines: Useful in simple nausea/vomiting or breakthrough CINV

Adverse drug reactions: Prolonged QTc interval, constipation, dizziness, tachycardia, tardive dyskinesia, drowsiness

Chlorpromazine (Thorazine)	10–25 mg every 4–6 hours prn	Tab, liquid	Prescription
	25–50 mg every 4–6 hours prn	IM, IV	
Prochlorperazine (Compazine)	5–10 mg every 4–6 hours prn	Tab, liquid	Prescription
	5–10 mg every 3–4 hours prn	IM	
		IV	
	2.5–10 mg every 3–4 hours prn		Prescription
	25 mg twice daily prn	Supp	Prescription
Promethazine (Phenergan)	12.5–25 mg every 4–6 hours prn	Tab, liquid, IM, IV, supp	Prescription

Substance P/Neurokinin-1 Receptor Antagonist: Useful in combination therapy for prophylaxis of CINV and PONV

Adverse drug reactions: Constipation, diarrhea, headache, hiccups, dyspepsia, and fatigue

Aprepitant	See Table 27-2 for CINV dosing and Table 27-6 for PONV dosing	Cap, IV	Prescription
Fosaprepitant		IV	Prescription
Netupitant/ Palonosetron		Cap	Prescription
Rolapitant		Cap	Prescription

[a]All regimens should be monitored for resolution or occurrence of nausea and vomiting as well as maintaining an adequate hydration status.

[b]See text for warnings.

ANV, anticipatory nausea and vomiting; C-II, C-III, and C-IV, controlled substance schedule 2, 3, and 4, respectively; cap, capsule; chew tab, chewable tablet; CINV, chemotherapy-induced nausea and vomiting; GERD, gastroesophageal reflux disease; liquid, oral syrup, concentrate, or suspension; PONV, postoperative nausea and vomiting; prn, as needed; supp, rectal suppository; tab, tablet.

- Nausea or vomiting that occurs prior to receiving chemotherapy is termed anticipatory nausea and vomiting (ANV). Breakthrough nausea and vomiting is defined as emesis occurring despite prophylactic administration of antiemetics and requiring the use of rescue antiemetics. Breakthrough emesis occurs in 10%−40% treated with antiemetics.
- The emetogenic potential of the chemotherapeutic agent or regimen (see Table 27-2) is the primary factor to consider when selecting an antiemetic for prophylaxis of CINV. Recommendations for antiemetics in patients receiving chemotherapy are presented in Table 27-2.

Prophylaxis of CINV

- The primary goal of emesis prevention is no nausea and/or vomiting throughout the period of emetic risk.
- The duration of emetic risk is 2 days for patients receiving moderately emetogenic chemotherapy and 3 days for highly emetogenic chemotherapy. Emetic prophylaxis should be provided through the entire period of risk.
- The selection of the antiemetic regimen should be based on the chemotherapy drug with highest emetogenicity (see Table 27-2). Prior emetic experience and patient-specific factors should also be considered.
- When given in equipotent doses, oral and IV 5-HT3-RAs are equivalent in efficacy.
- The toxicities of antiemetics should be considered and managed appropriately.
- Patients receiving highly emetogenic chemotherapy should receive a four-drug antiemetic regimen that is initiated prior to the administration of chemotherapy on day 1, which includes an NK1 receptor antagonist, a 5-HT3-RA, dexamethasone, and olanzapine. Antiemetics administered on the subsequent days following completion of chemotherapy may include aprepitant (if aprepitant was used on day 1), dexamethasone, and olanzapine on days 2−4 as outlined in Table 27-2.
- Patients receiving moderately emetogenic chemotherapy should receive a two-drug regimen with a 5-HT3-RA and dexamethasone on day 1. Dexamethasone should be continued on days 2−3 only if the chemotherapy agent is known to cause delayed nausea and vomiting (eg, cyclophosphamide, doxorubicin, oxaliplatin). Depending on the dose given, patients receiving carboplatin may receive the three-drug combination of an NK1 receptor antagonist, a 5-HT3-RA, plus dexamethasone on day 1 of therapy. If aprepitant was used on day 1, it should be continued on days 2−3; otherwise, no additional antiemetics are required in the delayed emetic risk period.
- For chemotherapy regimens that are of low emetic risk, either dexamethasone or a 5-HT3-RA as a single agent may be used on day 1 only. For minimal emetic risk, no routine antiemetic prophylaxis is recommended.
- Nonpharmacologic interventions, such as behavioral therapy with systematic desensitization, hypnosis, acupuncture/acupressure or music therapy, may be of benefit for ANV. If ANV occurs, oral lorazepam 0.5−2 mg starting the evening prior to chemotherapy and then an additional dose 1−2 hours prior to chemotherapy administration may be used.

RADIATION-INDUCED NAUSEA AND VOMITING

- Radiotherapy-induced emesis risk groups include total-body irradiation (highest risk), upper body or abdomen and craniospinal radiotherapy (moderate risk), brain, head, and neck, thorax, and pelvic radiotherapy (low risk), and extremity or breast radiotherapy (minimal risk).
- Those at highest risk should receive preventive therapy with a 5-HT3-RA plus dexamethasone in patients who are receiving total-body irradiation (high emetic risk).
- Patients undergoing RT procedures with moderate emetic risk should receive a 5-HT3-RA prior to each fraction and optional dexamethasone prior to fractions 1 through 5.
- Those receiving low and minimal emetic risk radiotherapy may be offered rescue therapy with a 5-HT3-RA, dexamethasone, or dopamine receptor antagonist.

POSTOPERATIVE NAUSEA AND VOMITING (PONV)

- Risk factors for PONV are listed in **Table 27-5**. Those with 3−5 risk factors are at highest risk, 2−3 risk factors at moderate risk, and 0−1 at low risk.
- A variety of pharmacologic approaches are available and may be prescribed as single or combination therapy for prophylaxis of PONV. See **Table 27-6** for doses of specific agents.
- Patients at highest risk of vomiting should receive two or more prophylactic antiemetics from different pharmacologic classes, while those at moderate risk should receive one or two drugs. For prophylaxis of PONV scopolamine patches must be initiated the evening before the surgery or at least 2 hours prior, whereas NK1 antagonists should be given during the induction of anesthesia; all other agents are recommended to be given at the end of the surgery.
- Ondansetron is considered the "gold standard" 5-HT3-RA. Granisetron has similar results as ondansetron and is less effective than palonosetron.
- Patients who experience PONV after receiving prophylactic treatment with a combination of 5-HT3-RA plus dexamethasone should be given rescue therapy from a different drug class such as a phenothiazine, metoclopramide, or droperidol. If no prophylaxis was given initially, the recommended treatment is low-dose 5-HT3-RA such as ondansetron 1 mg.

DISORDERS OF BALANCE

- Beneficial therapy for patients with nausea and vomiting associated with disorders of balance can reliably be found among the antihistaminic–anticholinergic agents. Oral regimens of antihistaminic–anticholinergic agents given one to several times each day may be effective, especially when the first dose is administered prior to motion.
- Scopolamine (usually administered as a patch) is effective for the prevention of motion sickness and is considered first line for this indication.

ANTIEMETIC USE DURING PREGNANCY

- A prenatal vitamin started 1 month prior to becoming pregnant may help reduce the incidence and severity of nausea and vomiting of pregnancy (NVP). Eating smaller, more frequent meals every 1–2 hours, and avoiding foods or odors that trigger symptoms is recommended.
- Pyridoxine (10–25 mg one to four times daily) is recommended as first-line therapy with or without doxylamine (12.5–20 mg one to four times daily). Dimenhydrinate,

TABLE 27-5	Risk Factors for Postoperative Nausea and Vomiting (PONV)
Patient-related factors	
Age less than 50 years old	
Female gender (two to three times greater incidence of PONV vs males)	
Nonsmoker	
History of PONV or motion sickness (threefold increase in incidence of PONV)	
Hydration status	
Factors related to anesthesia	
Use of general anesthesia	
Use of volatile anesthetics	
Nitrous oxide	
Use of opioids (intraoperative or postoperative)	
Factors related to surgery	
Type of surgical procedure (laparoscopic, gynecological, cholecystectomy)	
Duration of surgery	

TABLE 27-6	Recommended Prophylactic Doses of Selected Antiemetics for Postoperative Nausea and Vomiting in Adults and Postoperative Vomiting in Children		
Drug	Adult Dose	Pediatric Dose (IV)	Timing of Dose[a]
Aprepitant[b]	40 mg orally	Not labeled for use in pediatrics	Within 3 hours prior to induction
Dexamethasone	4–5 mg IV	150 mcg/kg up to 5 mg	At induction
Dimenhydrinate	1 mg/kg IV	0.5 mg/kg up to 25 mg	Not specified
Dolasetron	12.5 mg IV	350 mcg/kg up to 12.5 mg	At end of surgery
Droperidol[c]	0.625–1.25 mg IV	10–15 mcg/kg up to 1.25 mg	At end of surgery
Granisetron	0.35–3 mg IV	40 mcg/kg up to 0.6 mg	At end of surgery
Haloperidol	0.5–2 mg (IM or IV)	N/A[d]	Not specified
Methylprednisolone	40 mg IV	N/A[d]	At induction
Ondansetron	4 mg IV, 8 mg orally disintegrating tablet	50–100 mcg/kg up to 4 mg	At end of surgery
Palonosetron[b]	0.075 mg IV	N/A[d]	At induction
Promethazine[c]	6.25–12.5 mg IV	N/A[d]	At induction
Scopolamine	Transdermal patch	N/A[d]	Prior evening or 4 hours before surgery

[a]Based on recommendations from consensus guidelines.
[b]Labeled for use in PONV but not included in consensus guidelines.
[c]See FDA "black box" warning.
[d]Pediatric dosing not included in consensus guidelines.

diphenhydramine, prochlorperazine, or promethazine may also be considered in the treatment of NVP.
• Patients with persistent NVP or who show signs of dehydration should receive IV fluid replacement with thiamine then dextrose.
• Ondansetron, promethazine, and metoclopramide have similar effectiveness for hyperemesis gravidarum, although ondansetron may be better tolerated due to less adverse effects.

ANTIEMETIC USE IN CHILDREN

• For children receiving highly emetogenic chemotherapy the three-drug combination of an NK-1 antagonist, a 5-HT3-RA, and dexamethasone is recommended. If an NK-1 antagonist cannot be used, a 5-HT3-RA and dexamethasone are recommended. If dexamethasone cannot be used, an NK-1 antagonist with a 5-HT3-RA should be used.

- Children treated with low emetic risk chemotherapy should receive single-agent 5-HT3-RA prior to chemotherapy, while minimal emetic risk chemotherapy regimens do not require routine antiemetics.
- For nausea and vomiting associated with pediatric gastroenteritis, there is greater emphasis on rehydration measures than on pharmacologic intervention.

See Chapter 52, Nausea and Vomiting, authored by Leigh Anne Hylton Gravatt, Krista L. Donohoe, and Mandy L. Gatesman, for a more detailed discussion of this topic.

28 Pancreatitis

- *Acute pancreatitis* (AP) is an inflammatory disorder of the pancreas characterized by upper abdominal pain and pancreatic enzyme elevations.
- *Chronic pancreatitis* (CP) is a progressive disease characterized by long-standing pancreatic inflammation leading to loss of pancreatic exocrine and endocrine function.

Acute Pancreatitis

PATHOPHYSIOLOGY

- Gallstones and alcohol abuse account for most cases in the United States. Diabetes mellitus and autoimmune disorders such as inflammatory bowel disease are also associated with an increase in AP. A cause cannot be identified in some patients (idiopathic pancreatitis).
- Many medications have been implicated (Table 28-1), but drug-induced AP is rare. A causal association is difficult to confirm because ethical and practical considerations preclude rechallenge.
- AP is initiated by premature activation of trypsinogen to trypsin within the pancreas, leading to activation of other digestive enzymes and autodigestion of the gland.
- Activated pancreatic enzymes within the pancreas and surrounding tissues produce damage and necrosis to pancreatic tissue, surrounding fat, vascular endothelium, and adjacent structures. Lipase damages fat cells, producing noxious substances that cause further pancreatic and peripancreatic injury.
- Release of cytokines by acinar cells injures those cells and enhances the inflammatory response. Injured acinar cells liberate chemoattractants that attract neutrophils, macrophages, and other cells to the area of inflammation, causing systemic inflammatory response syndrome (SIRS). Vascular damage and ischemia cause release of kinins, which make capillary walls permeable and promote tissue edema.
- Pancreatic infection may result from increased intestinal permeability and translocation of colonic bacteria.
- Local complications in severe AP include acute fluid collection, pancreatic necrosis, infection, abscess, pseudocyst formation, and pancreatic ascites.
- Systemic complications include respiratory failure and cardiovascular, renal, metabolic, hemorrhagic, and CNS abnormalities.

CLINICAL PRESENTATION

- Clinical presentation depends on severity of the inflammatory process and whether damage is confined to the pancreas or involves local and systemic complications.
- The initial presentation ranges from moderate abdominal discomfort to excruciating pain, shock, and respiratory distress. Abdominal pain occurs in 95% of patients and is usually epigastric, often radiating to the upper quadrants or back. Onset is usually sudden, and intensity is often described as "knife-like" or "boring." Pain usually reaches maximum intensity within 30 minutes and may persist for hours or days. Nausea and vomiting occur in 85% of patients and usually follow onset of pain.
- Signs include marked epigastric tenderness on palpation with rebound tenderness and guarding in severe cases. The abdomen is often distended and tympanic with decreased or absent bowel sounds in severe disease.

TABLE 28-1	Medications Associated with Acute Pancreatitis		
Well-Supported Association	**Probable Association**	**Possible Association**	
5-Aminosalicylic acid	Acetaminophen	Aldesleukin	Indinavir
Azathioprine	Itraconazole	Amiodarone	Indomethacin
Bortezomib	Ifosfamide	Calcium	Infliximab
Carbamazepine	Interferon α2b	Ceftriaxone	Ketoprofen
Cimetidine	Maprotiline	Capecitabine	Ketorolac
Corticosteroids	Methyldopa	Carboplatin	Lipid emulsion
Cisplatin	Oxaliplatin	Celecoxib	Liraglutide
Cytarabine		Clozapine	Lisinopril
Didanosine		Cholestyramine	Mefenamic acid
Enalapril		Ciprofloxacin	Metformin
Erythromycin		Clarithromycin	Metolazone
Estrogens		Clonidine	Metronidazole
Furosemide		Cyclosporine	Nitrofurantoin
Mercaptopurine		Danazol	Omeprazole
Mesalamine		Diazoxide	Ondansetron
Octreotide		Etanercept	Paclitaxel
Olsalazine		Ethacrynic acid	Pravastatin
Opioids		Exenatide	Propofol
Pentamidine		Famciclovir	Propoxyphene
Pentavalent antimonials		Glyburide	Rifampin
Sulfasalazine		Gold salts	Sertraline
Sulfamethoxazole and trimethoprim		Granisetron	Simvastatin
Sulindac		Ibuprofen	Sorafenib
Tamoxifen		Imatinib	Sulindac
Tetracyclines			Zalcitabine
Valproic acid/Salts			

- Vital signs may be normal, but hypotension, tachycardia, and low-grade fever are often observed, especially with widespread pancreatic inflammation and necrosis. Dyspnea and tachypnea are signs of acute respiratory complications.
- Jaundice and altered mental status may be present; other signs of alcoholic liver disease may be present in patients with alcoholic pancreatitis.

DIAGNOSIS

- Diagnosis of AP requires two of the following: (1) upper abdominal pain, (2) serum lipase or amylase at least three times the upper limit of normal, and (3) characteristic findings on imaging studies.
- Transabdominal ultrasound should be performed in all patients to detect dilated biliary ducts and gallstones. Contrast-enhanced computed tomography (CECT) is used if the diagnosis cannot be made from clinical and laboratory findings. Magnetic resonance cholangiopancreatography (MRCP) is used to grade severity of AP, identify bile duct problems not seen on CECT, or if there are contraindications to CECT.

- AP may be associated with leukocytosis, hyperglycemia, and hypoalbuminemia. Hepatic transaminases, alkaline phosphatase, and bilirubin are usually elevated in gallstone pancreatitis and in patients with intrinsic liver disease. Marked hypocalcemia indicates severe necrosis and is a poor prognostic sign.
- Serum amylase usually rises 4–8 hours after symptom onset, peaks at 24 hours, and returns to normal over the next 8–14 days. Concentrations greater than three times the upper limit of normal are highly suggestive of AP.
- Serum lipase is specific to the pancreas, and concentrations are elevated and parallel the serum amylase elevations. Increases persist longer than serum amylase elevations and can be detected after the amylase has returned to normal.
- Hematocrit may be normal, but hemoconcentration results from multiple factors (eg, vomiting). Hematocrit >47% predicts severe AP, and hematocrit <44% predicts mild disease.
- C-reactive protein levels >150 mg/dL at 48–72 hours predict severe AP.
- Thrombocytopenia and increased international normalized ratio (INR) occur in some patients with severe AP and associated liver disease.

TREATMENT (FIG. 28-1)

- <u>Goals of Treatment</u>: Relieve abdominal pain and nausea; replace fluids; correct electrolyte, glucose, and lipid abnormalities; minimize systemic complications; and manage pancreatic necrosis and infection.

NONPHARMACOLOGIC THERAPY

- Endoscopic retrograde cholangiopancreatography (ERCP) may be performed to remove biliary tract stones.
- Patients with alcohol-related pancreatitis should receive abstinence interventions during the inpatient stay.
- Nutritional support is important because AP creates a catabolic state that promotes nutritional depletion. Patients with mild AP can begin oral feeding when pain is decreasing and inflammatory markers are improving. Nutritional support should begin when it is anticipated that oral nutrition will be withheld for longer than 1 week. Enteral nutrition via nasogastric or nasojejunal tube is preferred over parenteral nutrition (PN) in severe AP, if tolerated. If enteral feeding is not possible or is inadequate, PN should be implemented before protein and calorie depletion become advanced.

PHARMACOLOGIC THERAPY

- Patients with AP often require IV antiemetics for nausea.
- Patients requiring ICU admission should be treated with antisecretory agents if they are at risk of stress-related mucosal bleeding.
- Vasodilation from the inflammatory response, vomiting, and nasogastric suction contribute to hypovolemia and fluid and electrolyte abnormalities, necessitating replacement. Patients should receive aggressive fluid replacement to reduce the risks of persistent SIRS and organ failure. Different guidelines recommend goal-directed IV fluid with either lactated Ringer's at an initial rate of 5–10 mL/kg/hr or crystalloids at a rate of 250–500 mL/hr.
- Intravenous potassium, calcium, and magnesium are used to correct electrolyte deficiency, and insulin is used to treat hyperglycemia.
- Parenteral opioid analgesics are used to control abdominal pain, although high-quality supporting evidence is lacking. Parenteral **morphine** is often used,

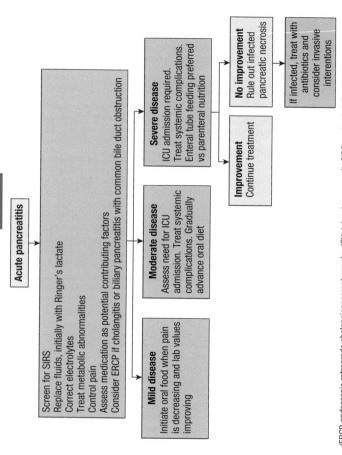

Acute pancreatitis

Screen for SIRS
Replace fluids, initially with Ringer's lactate
Correct electrolytes
Treat metabolic abnormalities
Control pain
Assess medication as potential contributing factors
Consider ERCP if cholangitis or biliary pancreatitis with common bile duct obstruction

Mild disease
Initiate oral food when pain is decreasing and lab values improving

Moderate disease
Assess need for ICU admission. Treat systemic complications. Gradually advance oral diet

Severe disease
ICU admission required. Treat systemic complications. Enteral tube feeding preferred vs parenteral nutrition

Improvement
Continue treatment

No improvement
Rule out infected pancreatic necrosis

If infected, treat with antibiotics and consider invasive interentions

(ERCP, endoscopic retrograde cholangiopancreatography; ICU, intensive care unit; SIRS, systemic inflammatory response syndrome.)

FIGURE 28-1. Algorithm of guidelines for evaluation and treatment of acute pancreatitis.

and patient-controlled analgesia should be considered in patients who require frequent opioid dosing (eg, every 2–3 hours). Nonsteroidal anti-inflammatory agents (NSAIDs) may be sufficient in patients with mild-to-moderate pain if not contraindicated.

- Selective digestive tract decontamination using minimally absorbed antibiotics may be effective in reducing the risk of pancreatic infection, but more studies are needed before this approach can be recommended.
- Prophylactic antibiotics are not recommended in patients with AP without signs or symptoms of infection, including those with necrosis, predicted severe AP, or necrotizing pancreatitis. However, empiric antimicrobial therapy may be considered in patients with necrosis who deteriorate or fail to improve within 7–10 days.
- Patients with known or suspected infected AP should receive broad-spectrum antibiotics that cover the range of enteric aerobic gram-negative bacilli and anaerobic organisms. **Imipenem–cilastatin** (500 mg IV every 8 hours) has been widely used but has been replaced on many formularies by newer carbapenems (eg, **meropenem**). A fluoroquinolone (eg, **ciprofloxacin** or **levofloxacin**) combined with **metronidazole** should be considered for penicillin-allergic patients.
- There are insufficient data to support routine use of somatostatin or octreotide for treatment of AP. Parenteral histamine2-receptor antagonists and proton pump inhibitors do not improve the overall outcome of patients with AP.

EVALUATION OF THERAPEUTIC OUTCOMES

- In patients with mild AP, assess pain control, fluid and electrolyte status, and nutrition periodically depending on the degree of abdominal pain and fluid loss.
- Goals for fluid therapy include one or more of the following: heart rate <120 bpm, mean arterial pressure 65–85 mm Hg, urinary output >0.5–1 mL/kg/hr, invasive measures of stroke volume or intrathoracic blood volume, or hematocrit 35%–44% with blood transfusion.
- Transfer patients with severe AP to an intensive care unit for close monitoring of vital signs, fluid and electrolyte status, white blood cell count, blood glucose, lactate dehydrogenase, aspartate aminotransferase, serum albumin, hematocrit, blood urea nitrogen, serum creatinine, and INR. Continuous hemodynamic and arterial blood gas monitoring is essential. Serum lipase, amylase, and bilirubin require less frequent monitoring. Monitor for signs of infection, relief of abdominal pain, and adequate nutritional status. Assess severity of disease and patient response using evidence-based methods.

Chronic Pancreatitis

PATHOPHYSIOLOGY

- CP results from long-standing pancreatic inflammation and leads to irreversible destruction of pancreatic tissue with fibrin deposition and loss of exocrine and endocrine function.
- Chronic ethanol consumption accounts for about two-thirds of cases in Western society. Most of the remaining cases are idiopathic, and a small percentage is due to rare causes such as autoimmune, hereditary, and tropical pancreatitis.
- The exact pathogenesis is unknown. Activation of pancreatic stellate cells by toxins, oxidative stress, and/or inflammatory mediators appears to be the cause of fibrin deposition.
- Abdominal pain may be caused by abnormal pain processing in the central nervous system and sensitization of visceral nerves. This may explain the hyperalgesia that CP patients often experience with the need for various methods of pain management. Impaired inhibition of somatic and visceral pain pathways may also cause pain in areas distant to the pancreas.

CLINICAL PRESENTATION

- The main features of CP are abdominal pain, malabsorption with steatorrhea, weight loss, and diabetes. Jaundice occurs in ~10% of patients.
- Patients typically report deep, penetrating epigastric or abdominal pain that may radiate to the back. Pain often occurs with meals and at night and may be associated with nausea and vomiting.
- Steatorrhea and azotorrhea occur in most patients. Steatorrhea is often associated with diarrhea and bloating. Weight loss may occur.
- Pancreatic diabetes is a late manifestation commonly associated with pancreatic calcification.

DIAGNOSIS

- Diagnosis is based primarily on clinical presentation and either imaging or pancreatic function studies. Noninvasive imaging includes abdominal ultrasound, CT, and MRCP. Invasive imaging includes endoscopic ultrasonography (EUS) and ERCP.
- Serum amylase and lipase are usually normal or only slightly elevated but may be increased in acute exacerbations.
- Total bilirubin, alkaline phosphatase, and hepatic transaminases may be elevated with ductal obstruction. Serum albumin and calcium may be low with malnutrition.
- Pancreatic function tests include:
  - ✓ Serum trypsinogen (<20 ng/mL is abnormal)
  - ✓ Fecal elastase (<200 mcg/g of stool is abnormal)
  - ✓ Fecal chymotrypsin (<3 units/g of stool is abnormal)
  - ✓ Fecal fat estimation (>7 g/day is abnormal; stool must be collected for 72 hours)
  - ✓ ^{13}C-mixed triglyceride breath test (not available in the United States)
  - ✓ Secretin stimulation (evaluates duodenal bicarbonate secretion)
  - ✓ Cholecystokinin stimulation (evaluates pancreatic lipase secretion)

TREATMENT

- <u>Goals of Treatment</u>: Major goals for uncomplicated CP are to relieve abdominal pain, treat complications of malabsorption and glucose intolerance, and improve quality of life. Secondary goals are to delay development of complications and treat associated disorders such as depression and malnutrition.

NONPHARMACOLOGIC THERAPY

- Lifestyle modifications should include abstinence from alcohol and smoking cessation.
- Advise patients with steatorrhea to eat smaller, more frequent meals and reduce dietary fat intake.
- Reduction in dietary fat may be needed if symptoms are uncontrolled with enzyme supplementation. Enteral nutrition via a feeding tube is recommended for patients who cannot consume adequate calories, have continued weight loss, experience complications, or require surgery.
- Invasive procedures and surgery are used primarily to treat uncontrolled pain and the complications of CP.

PHARMACOLOGIC THERAPY

- Pain may initially be treated with **acetaminophen** (eg, 500–650 mg every 4–6 hours) with or without NSAIDs (eg, **ibuprofen** 200–400 mg every 6–8 hours initially), with adjuvant agents added for inadequate pain relief or as the disease progresses.
- Analgesic regimens should be individualized and start with the lowest effective dose, with titration to maximum recommended or tolerated doses before adding or

TABLE 28-2	Commercially Available Pancreatic Enzyme (Pancrelipase) Preparations		
	Enzyme Content Per Unit Dose (USP Units)		
Product	**Lipase**	**Amylase**	**Protease**
Tablets			
Viokace™ 10,440 lipase units	10,440	39,150	39,150
Viokace™ 20,880 lipase units	20,880	78,300	78,300
Enteric-coated beads			
Zenpep® 3,000 lipase units	3,000	16,000	10,000
Zenpep® 5,000 lipase units	5,000	27,000	17,000
Zenpep® 10,000 lipase units	10,000	55,000	34,000
Zenpep® 15,000 lipase units	15,000	82,000	51,000
Zenpep® 20,000 lipase units	20,000	109,000	68,000
Zenpep® 25,000 lipase units	25,000	136,000	85,000
Zenpep® 40,000 lipase units	40,000	218,000	136,000
Enteric-coated microspheres with bicarbonate buffer			
Pertzye 4,000 lipase units	4,000	15,125	14,375
Pertzye 8,000 lipase units	8,000	30,250	28,750
Pertzye 16,000 lipase units	16,000	60,500	57,500
Enteric-coated microspheres			
Creon® 3,000 lipase units	3,000	15,000	9,500
Creon® 6,000 lipase units	6,000	30,000	19,000
Creon® 12,000 lipase units	12,000	60,000	38,000
Creon® 24,000 lipase units	24,000	120,000	76,000
Creon® 36,000 lipase units	36,000	180,000	114,000
Enteric-coated minitablets/microtablets			
Pancreaze® 4,200 lipase units	4,200	17,500	10,000
Pancreaze® 10,500 lipase units	10,500	43,750	25,000
Pancreaze® 16,800 lipase units	16,800	70,000	40,000
Pancreaze® 21,000 lipase units	21,000	61,000	37,000
Ultresa 4,000 lipase units	4,000	8,000	8,000
Ultresa 13,800 lipase units	13,800	27,600	27,600
Ultresa 20,700 lipase units	20,700	41,400	41,400
Ultresa 23,000 lipase units	23,000	46,000	46,000

USP, United States Pharmacopeia.

substituting agents. Schedule analgesics around the clock (rather than as needed) to maximize efficacy. Scheduling short-acting analgesics prior to meals may decrease postprandial pain.
- **Pregabalin** (75 mg twice daily initially; maximum 300 mg twice daily) has the best evidence as an adjuvant agent. Consider selective serotonin reuptake inhibitors (eg, **paroxetine**), serotonin/norepinephrine reuptake inhibitors (eg, **duloxetine**), and tricyclic antidepressants in patients with pain that is difficult to manage.
- **Tramadol** (50–100 mg every 4–6 hours, maximum 400 mg/day) may be tried before adding more potent opioid analgesics.

(H₂RA, histamine₂-receptor antagonist; PPI, proton pump inhibitor.)

FIGURE 28-2. Algorithm for the treatment of malabsorption and steatorrhea in chronic pancreatitis.

- Opioids should be reserved for severe or refractory pain:
  - ✓ **Codeine:** 30–60 mg every 6 hours
  - ✓ **Hydrocodone:** 5–10 mg every 4–6 hours
  - ✓ **Morphine sulfate (extended-release):** 30–60 mg every 8–12 hours
  - ✓ **Oxycodone:** 5–10 mg every 6 hours
  - ✓ **Methadone:** 2.5–10 mg every 8–12 hours
  - ✓ **Hydromorphone:** 0.5–1 mg every 4–6 hours
  - ✓ **Fentanyl patch:** 25–100 mcg/hr every 72 hours
- Adding pancreatic enzyme supplements or antioxidants for pain control has been studied but is not supported by high-quality evidence and is not recommended in current guidelines.
- Pancreatic enzyme supplementation is required for most patients with malabsorption to achieve adequate nutritional status and reduction in steatorrhea (**Fig. 28-2**). The enzyme dose required to minimize malabsorption is 25,000–50,000 units of lipase administered with each meal initially. Half of the necessary mealtime dose is recommended with snacks. The mealtime dose may be increased to a maximum of 90,000 units. Products containing enteric-coated microspheres are preferred (**Table 28-2**). Ideally, patients should eat 3–5 meals/day, and those who require more than one capsule/tablet per meal should distribute the doses throughout the meal.
- An antisecretory agent (eg, ranitidine, omeprazole) should be added when there is an inadequate response to enzyme therapy alone. The increased gastric and duodenal pH is thought to increase the amount of active enzymes available in the duodenum.
- Adverse effects from pancreatic enzyme supplements are generally benign, but high doses can cause nausea, diarrhea, and intestinal upset. A more serious but uncommon

adverse effect is fibrosing colonopathy, which has been reported mostly in children with cystic fibrosis who received high enzyme doses for prolonged periods.

- Assess patients with CP for deficiencies in fat-soluble vitamins and provide supplementation as required.
- Exogenous insulin is the primary means for treating diabetes mellitus associated with CP. Metformin may be initiated in early CP and has the added benefit of reducing the risk of pancreatic cancer.

EVALUATION OF THERAPEUTIC OUTCOMES

- Assess the severity and frequency of abdominal pain periodically using a standardized scale to determine analgesic efficacy. Patients receiving opioids should be prescribed laxatives on an as-needed or scheduled basis and be monitored for constipation.
- For patients receiving pancreatic enzymes for malabsorption, monitor body weight and stool frequency and consistency periodically.
- Monitor blood glucose carefully in diabetic patients.

See Chapter 56, Pancreatitis, authored by Scott Bolesta and Patricia A. Montgomery, for a more detailed discussion of this topic.

Peptic Ulcer Disease

- *Peptic ulcer disease* (PUD) refers to ulcerative disorders of the upper gastrointestinal (GI) tract that require acid and pepsin for their formation. The three common etiologies include (1) *Helicobacter pylori* infection, (2) nonsteroidal anti-inflammatory drug (NSAID) use, and (3) stress-related mucosal damage (SRMD).

PATHOPHYSIOLOGY

- Benign gastric ulcers, erosions, and gastritis can occur anywhere in the stomach, but the antrum and lesser curvature are the most common locations. Most duodenal ulcers occur in the first part of the duodenum (duodenal bulb).
- Pathophysiology is determined by the balance between aggressive factors (gastric acid and pepsin) and protective factors (mucosal defense and repair). Gastric acid, *H. pylori* infection, and NSAID use are independent factors that contribute to disruption of mucosal integrity. Increased acid secretion may be involved in duodenal ulcers, but patients with gastric ulcers usually have normal or reduced acid secretion (hypochlorhydria).
- Mucus and bicarbonate secretion, intrinsic epithelial cell defense, and mucosal blood flow normally protect the gastroduodenal mucosa from noxious endogenous and exogenous substances. Endogenous prostaglandins (PGs) facilitate mucosal integrity and repair. Disruptions in normal mucosal defense and healing mechanisms allow acid and pepsin to reach the gastric epithelium.
- *H. pylori* infection causes gastric mucosal inflammation in all infected individuals, but only a minority develops an ulcer or gastric cancer. Bacterial enzymes (urease, lipases, and proteases), bacterial adherence, and *H. pylori* virulence factors produce gastric mucosal injury. *H. pylori* induces gastric inflammation by altering the host inflammatory response and damaging epithelial cells.
- Nonselective NSAIDs (including aspirin) cause gastric mucosal damage by two mechanisms: (1) direct or topical irritation of the gastric epithelium, and (2) systemic inhibition of endogenous mucosal PG synthesis (the primary mechanism). COX-2 selective inhibitors have a lower risk of ulcers and related GI complications than nonselective NSAIDs. Addition of aspirin to a selective COX-2 inhibitor reduces its ulcer-sparing benefit and increases ulcer risk.
- Use of corticosteroids alone does not increase risk of ulcer or complications, but ulcer risk is doubled in corticosteroid users taking NSAIDs concurrently.
- Cigarette smoking has been linked to PUD, impaired ulcer healing, and ulcer recurrence. Risk is proportional to amount smoked per day.
- Psychological stress has not been shown to cause PUD, but ulcer patients may be adversely affected by stressful life events.
- Carbonated beverages, coffee, tea, beer, milk, and spices may cause dyspepsia but do not appear to increase PUD risk. Ethanol ingestion in high concentrations is associated with acute gastric mucosal damage and upper GI bleeding but is not clearly the cause of ulcers.

CLINICAL PRESENTATION

- Abdominal pain is the most frequent PUD symptom. Pain is often epigastric and described as burning but can present as vague discomfort, abdominal fullness, or cramping. Nocturnal pain may awaken patients from sleep, especially between 12 AM and 3 AM.
- Pain from duodenal ulcers often occurs 1–3 hours after meals and is usually relieved by food, whereas food may precipitate or accentuate ulcer pain in gastric ulcers. Antacids provide rapid pain relief in most ulcer patients.

- Heartburn, belching, and bloating often accompany pain. Nausea, vomiting, and anorexia are more common in gastric than duodenal ulcers and may be signs of an ulcer-related complication.
- Severity of symptoms varies among patients and may be seasonal, occurring more frequently in spring or fall.
- Presence or absence of epigastric pain does not define an ulcer, and ulcer healing does not necessarily render the patient asymptomatic. Conversely, absence of pain does not preclude an ulcer diagnosis, especially in older persons, who may present with a "silent" ulcer complication.
- Ulcer complications include upper GI bleeding, perforation into the peritoneal cavity, penetration into an adjacent structure (eg, pancreas, biliary tract, or liver), and gastric outlet obstruction. Bleeding may be occult or present as melena or hematemesis. Perforation is associated with sudden, sharp, severe pain, beginning first in the epigastrium but quickly spreading over the entire abdomen. Symptoms of gastric outlet obstruction typically occur over several months and include early satiety, bloating, anorexia, nausea, vomiting, and weight loss.

DIAGNOSIS

- Physical examination may reveal epigastric tenderness between the umbilicus and the xiphoid process that sometimes radiates to the back.
- Routine blood tests are not helpful in establishing a diagnosis of PUD. Hematocrit, hemoglobin, and stool guaiac tests are used to detect bleeding.
- Diagnosis of PUD depends on visualizing the ulcer crater; upper GI endoscopy has replaced radiography as the procedure of choice because it provides a more accurate diagnosis and permits direct visualization of the ulcer and implementation of maneuvers to control bleeding.
- Diagnosis of *H. pylori* infection can be made using endoscopic or nonendoscopic (urea breath test [UBT], serologic antibody detection, and fecal antigen) tests. Testing for *H. pylori* is only recommended if eradication therapy is planned. If endoscopy is not planned, serologic antibody testing is reasonable to determine *H. pylori* status. Endoscopic biopsy-based tests, UBT, and fecal antigen tests are the recommended tests to verify *H. pylori* eradication but must be delayed until at least 4 weeks after completion of antibiotic treatment and after proton pump inhibitor (PPI) therapy has been discontinued for 2 weeks to avoid confusing bacterial suppression with eradication.

TREATMENT

- <u>Goals of Treatment</u>: Overall goals are to relieve ulcer pain, heal the ulcer, prevent ulcer recurrence, and reduce ulcer-related complications. In *H. pylori*-positive patients with an active ulcer, previously documented ulcer, or history of an ulcer-related complication, goals are to eradicate *H. pylori*, heal the ulcer, and cure the disease with a cost-effective drug regimen. The primary goal for a patient with an NSAID-induced ulcer is to heal the ulcer as rapidly as possible.

NONPHARMACOLOGIC TREATMENT

- Lifestyle modifications including stress reduction and smoking cessation should be implemented. NSAIDs should be avoided if possible, and alternative agents such as acetaminophen or a nonacetylated salicylate (eg, salsalate) should be used for pain relief when feasible.
- There is no specific recommended diet, but patients should avoid foods and beverages that cause dyspepsia or exacerbate ulcer symptoms (eg, spicy foods, caffeine, and alcohol).
- Elective surgery is rarely performed because of highly effective medical management. Emergency surgery may be required for bleeding, perforation, or obstruction.

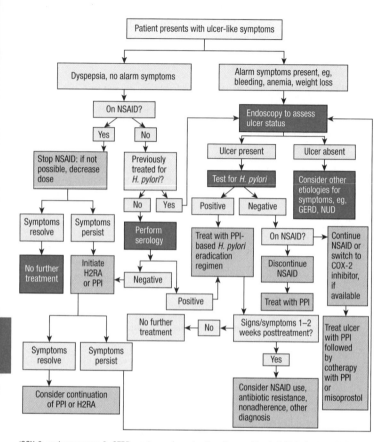

(COX-2, cyclooxygenase-2; GERD, gastroesophageal reflux disease; *H. pylori, Helicobacter pylori*; H2RA, histamine2-receptor antagonist; NSAID, nonsteroidal anti-inflammatory drug; NUD, nonulcer dyspepsia; PPI, proton pump inhibitor.)

FIGURE 29-1. **Guidelines for the evaluation and management of a patient who presents with dyspeptic or ulcer-like symptoms.**

PHARMACOLOGIC TREATMENT

- **Figure 29-1** depicts an algorithm for evaluation and management of a patient with dyspeptic or ulcer-like symptoms.
- Established indications for treatment of *H. pylori* infection include active PUD, past history of PUD (unless eradication was previously documented), mucosa-associated lymphoid tissue (MALT) lymphoma, and postendoscopic resection of gastric cancer. Treatment should be effective, well tolerated, convenient, and cost-effective. Drug regimens to eradicate *H. pylori* are shown in **Table 29-1**.
- *Clarithromycin triple therapy* (PPI, clarithromycin, amoxicillin) is no longer recommended in areas where *H. pylori* resistance exceeds 15%, which includes all of North America. This regimen given for 14 days remains an option in regions where clarithromycin resistance is <15% and no prior macrolide exposure is documented.

TABLE 29-1 Drug Regimens Used to Eradicate *Helicobacter pylori*

Regimen	Duration	Drug #1	Drug #2	Drug #3	Drug #4
Proton pump inhibitor–based triple therapy[a]	14 days	PPI once or twice daily[b]	Clarithromycin 500 mg twice daily	Amoxicillin 1 g twice daily or metronidazole 500 mg twice daily	
Bismuth quadruple therapy[a]	10–14 days	PPI or H2RA once or twice daily[b,c]	Bismuth subsalicylate[d] 525 mg four times daily	Metronidazole 250–500 mg four times daily	Tetracycline 500 mg four times daily
Non-bismuth quadruple or "concomitant" therapy[e]	10–14 days	PPI once or twice daily on days 1–10[b]	Clarithromycin 250–500 mg twice daily on days 1–10	Amoxicillin 1 g twice daily on days 1–10	Metronidazole 250–500 mg twice daily on days 1–10
Sequential therapy[e]	10 days	PPI once or twice daily on days 1–10[b]	Amoxicillin 1 g twice daily on days 1–5	Metronidazole 250–500 mg twice daily on days 6–10	Clarithromycin 250–500 mg twice daily on days 6–10
Hybrid therapy[e]	14 days	PPI once or twice daily on days 1–14[b]	Amoxicillin 1 g twice daily on days 1–14	Metronidazole 250–500 mg twice daily on days 7–14	Clarithromycin 250–500 mg twice daily on days 7–14
Levofloxacin triple	10–14 days	PPI twice daily	Levofloxacin 500 mg daily	Amoxicillin 1 g twice daily	
Levofloxacin sequential	10 days	PPI twice daily on days 1–10	Amoxicillin 1 g twice daily on days 1–10	Levofloxacin 500 mg once daily on days 6–10	Metronidazole 500 mg twice daily on days 6–10
LOAD	7–10 days	Levofloxacin 250 mg once daily	Omeprazole (or other PPI) at high dose once daily	Nitazoxanide (Alinia) 500 mg twice daily	Doxycycline 100 mg once daily

[a]Although treatment is minimally effective if used for 7 days, 10–14 days is recommended. The antisecretory drug may be continued beyond antimicrobial treatment for patients with a history of a complicated ulcer, for example, bleeding, or in heavy smokers.
[b]Standard PPI peptic ulcer healing dosages given once or twice daily.
[c]Standard H2RA peptic ulcer healing dosages may be used in place of a PPI.
[d]Bismuth subcitrate potassium (biskalcitrate) 140 mg, as the bismuth salt, is contained in a prepackaged capsule (Pylera), along with metronidazole 125 mg and tetracycline 125 mg; three capsules are taken with each meal and at bedtime; a standard PPI dosage is added to the regimen and taken twice daily. All medications are taken for 10 days.
[e]Requires validation as first-line therapy in the United States.
H2RA, H₂-receptor antagonist; PPI, proton pump inhibitor.

- *Bismuth quadruple therapy* (PPI or H2RA, bismuth subsalicylate, metronidazole, tetracycline) for 10–14 days is the preferred first-line therapy to eradicate *H. pylori* infection. PPIs generally produce higher *H. pylori* eradication rates and are preferred over H2RA. All medications except the PPI should be taken with meals and at bedtime. The PPI should be taken 30–60 minutes before a meal. The mean eradication rate for a 10-day course is ~90%, but limitations include the need for four-times-daily therapy (which can impair adherence), and frequent minor side effects.
- *Non-bismuth quadruple (or "concomitant") therapy* (PPI, clarithromycin, amoxicillin, metronidazole) for 10–14 days is another recommended first-line therapy. "Concomitant" therapy means that all four drugs are given at the same time twice daily for the entire duration of therapy. There is lack of evidence in North America for this regimen.
- *Sequential therapy* involves a PPI plus antibiotics given in sequence rather than together. The rationale is to treat initially with antibiotics that rarely promote resistance (eg, amoxicillin) to reduce bacterial load and preexisting resistant organisms and then to follow with different antibiotics (eg, clarithromycin and metronidazole) to kill any remaining organisms. The potential advantage of high eradication rates requires validation in the United States before this regimen can be recommended as first-line *H. pylori* eradication therapy.
- *Hybrid therapy* combines the strategies of concomitant and sequential therapy; it involves 7 days of dual therapy (PPI and amoxicillin) followed by 7 days of quadruple therapy (PPI, amoxicillin, clarithromycin, metronidazole). There is lack of evidence in North America with this regimen.
- *Levofloxacin-based regimens* include (1) triple therapy with amoxicillin and a PPI, (2) modified sequential therapy with 5–7 days of amoxicillin plus a PPI followed by 5–7 days of levofloxacin, and (3) quadruple therapy with levofloxacin, omeprazole or another PPI, nitazoxanide (Alinia), and doxycycline ("LOAD" therapy). The LOAD regimen is not currently recommended due to high cost and lack of efficacy data. In addition, concerns with fluoroquinolone use include development of resistance and adverse effects (eg, tendonitis, hepatotoxicity).
- If initial treatment fails to eradicate *H. pylori*, second-line (salvage) treatment should: (1) use antibiotics that were not included in the initial regimen, (2) be guided by region-specific or individual antibiotic resistance testing, and (3) use an extended treatment duration of 10–14 days. Patients failing clarithromycin triple therapy can be treated with either bismuth quadruple therapy or the levofloxacin triple regimen for 14 days. Other salvage regimens may also be successful. Penicillin allergy testing is recommended for patients who report penicillin allergy because many patients are not truly allergic.
- Patients with NSAID-induced ulcers should be tested to determine *H. pylori* status. If they are *H. pylori* positive, start treatment with a recommended first-line regimen (**Table 29-1**). If patients are *H. pylori* negative, discontinue the NSAID and treat with a PPI, H2RA, or sucralfate (**Table 29-2**). PPIs are generally preferred due to more rapid symptom relief and ulcer healing. If the NSAID must be continued, implement cotherapy with a PPI or misoprostol. Patients at highest risk of recurrent ulcers or ulcer-related complications should be switched to a COX-2 inhibitor.
- Limit maintenance therapy with a PPI or H2RA to high-risk patients with ulcer complications, patients who fail *H. pylori* eradication, and those with *H. pylori*-negative ulcers.
- Patients with ulcers refractory to treatment should undergo upper endoscopy to confirm a nonhealing ulcer, exclude malignancy, and assess *H. pylori* status. *H. pylori*-positive patients should receive eradication therapy. Refractory ulcers despite a complete standard PPI course should be retreated with double-dose of PPI, or consideration can be given to using a different PPI.

EVALUATION OF THERAPEUTIC OUTCOMES

- Monitor patients for symptomatic relief of ulcer pain, potential adverse drug effects, and drug interactions.

TABLE 29-2	Drug Dosing Table		
Drug	**Brand Name**	**Initial Dose**	**Usual Range**
Proton pump inhibitors			
Omeprazole	Prilosec, various	40 mg daily	20–40 mg/day
Omeprazole + sodium bicarbonate	Zegerid	40 mg daily	20–40 mg/day
Lansoprazole	Prevacid, various	30 mg daily	15–30 mg/day
Rabeprazole	Aciphex	20 mg daily	20–40 mg/day
Pantoprazole	Protonix, various	40 mg daily	40–80 mg/day
Esomeprazole	Nexium	40 mg daily	20–40 mg/day
Dexlansoprazole	Dexilant	30–60 mg daily	30–60 mg/day
H$_2$-receptor antagonists			
Cimetidine	Tagamet, various	300 mg four times daily, 400 mg twice daily, or 800 mg at bedtime	800–1600 mg/day in divided doses
Famotidine	Pepcid, various	20 mg twice daily, or 40 mg at bedtime	20–40 mg/day
Nizatidine	Axid, various	150 mg twice daily, or 300 mg at bedtime	150–300 mg/day
Ranitidine[a]	Zantac, various	150 mg twice daily, or 300 mg at bedtime	150–300 mg/day
Mucosal protectants			
Sucralfate	Carafate, various	1 g four times daily, or 2 g twice daily	2–4 g/day
Misoprostol	Cytotec	100–200 mcg four times daily	400–800 mcg/day

[a] In April 2020, the U.S. FDA asked manufacturers to withdraw all ranitidine products from the market. A contaminant known as N-Nitrosodimethylamine (NDMA) in some ranitidine products increases over time and when stored at higher than room temperatures and may result in exposure to unacceptable levels of NDMA, which is a probable human carcinogen.

- Ulcer pain typically resolves in a few days when NSAIDs are discontinued and within 7 days upon initiation of antiulcer therapy. Patients with uncomplicated PUD are usually symptom free after treatment with any of the recommended antiulcer regimens.
- Persistent or recurrent symptoms within 14 days after the end of treatment suggests failure of ulcer healing or *H. pylori* eradication or presence of an alternative diagnosis such as gastroesophageal reflux disease.
- Eradication of *H. pylori* should be confirmed after treatment in all patients, particularly those who are at risk for complications.
- Monitor patients taking NSAIDs closely for signs and symptoms of bleeding, obstruction, penetration, and perforation.
- Follow-up endoscopy is justified in patients with frequent symptomatic recurrence, refractory disease, complications, or suspected hypersecretory states.

See Chapter 50, Peptic Ulcer Disease and Related Disorders, authored by Bryan L. Love and Phillip L. Mohorn, for a more detailed discussion of this topic.

CHAPTER

30 | Contraception

- *Contraception* is the prevention of pregnancy by inhibiting sperm from reaching a mature ovum or by preventing a fertilized ovum from implanting in the endometrium.

MENSTRUAL CYCLE PATHOPHYSIOLOGY

- The median menstrual cycle length is 28 days (range 21–40 days). Day 1 is the first day of menses and marks the beginning of the follicular phase. Ovulation usually occurs on day 14, followed by the luteal phase that lasts until the beginning of the next cycle.
- The hypothalamus secretes gonadotropin-releasing hormone, which stimulates the anterior pituitary to secrete the gonadotropins follicle-stimulating hormone (FSH) and luteinizinig hormone (LH).
- In the follicular phase, FSH levels increase and cause recruitment of a small group of follicles for continued growth. Between days 5 and 7, one of these becomes the dominant follicle, which later ruptures to release the oocyte. The dominant follicle develops increasing amounts of estradiol and inhibin, providing a negative feedback on the secretion of gonadotropin-releasing hormone and FSH.
- The dominant follicle continues to grow and synthesizes estradiol, progesterone, and androgen. Estradiol stops the menstrual flow from the previous cycle, thickens the endometrial lining, and produces thin, watery cervical mucus. FSH regulates aromatase enzymes that induce conversion of androgens to estrogens in the follicle.
- The pituitary releases a midcycle LH surge that stimulates the final stages of follicular maturation and ovulation. Ovulation occurs 24–36 hours after the estradiol peak and 10–16 hours after the LH peak.
- The LH surge is the most clinically useful predictor of approaching ovulation. Conception is most successful when intercourse takes place from 2 days before ovulation to the day of ovulation.
- After ovulation, the remaining luteinized follicles become the corpus luteum, which synthesizes androgen, estrogen, and progesterone (**Fig. 30-1**).
- If pregnancy occurs, human chorionic gonadotropin prevents regression of the corpus luteum and stimulates continued production of estrogen and progesterone. If pregnancy does not occur, the corpus luteum degenerates, progesterone declines, and menstruation occurs.

TREATMENT

- <u>Goal of Treatment</u>: The prevention of pregnancy following sexual intercourse. Additional benefits from contraceptive use can also be realized (ie, sexually transmitted infections [STIs] prevention and menstrual cycle regulation).

NONPHARMACOLOGIC THERAPY

- A comparison of methods of nonhormonal contraception is shown in **Table 30-1**.
- The fertility awareness-based method includes avoiding intercourse on the days when contraception is likely to occur and is associated with relatively high pregnancy rates.

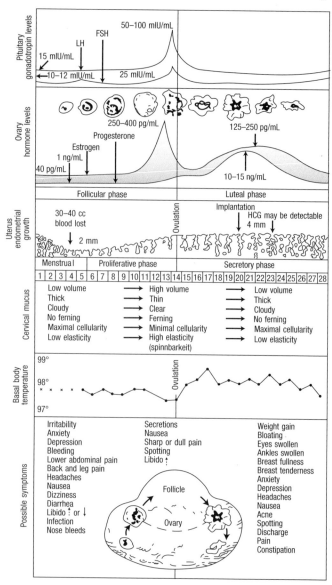

(FSH, follicle-stimulating hormone; HCG, human chorionic gonadotropin; LH, luteinizing hormone.)
LH: 15 mIU/mL = 15 IU/L; 50–100 mIU/mL = 50–100 IU/L.
FSH: 10–12 mIU/mL = 10–12 IU/L; 25 mIU/mL = 25 IU/L. Estrogen: 40 pg/mL = ~150 pmol/L; 250–400 pg/mL = ~920–1470 pmol/L; 125–250 pg/mL = ~460–920 pmol/L.
Progesterone: 1 ng/mL = 3 nmol/L; 10–15 ng/mL = ~30–50 nmol/L.
Temperatures: 99°F = 37.2°C; 98°F = 36.7°C; 97°F = 36.1°C.

FIGURE 30-1. Menstrual cycle events, idealized 28-day cycle. (Hatcher RA, Trussell J, Nelson AL, et al. *Contraceptive Technology.* 21st ed. Ardent, NY: Median, Inc.; 2015.)

TABLE 30-1 Comparison of Methods of Nonhormonal Contraception

Method	Absolute Contraindications	Advantages	Disadvantages	Percent of Women with Pregnancy[a] Perfect Use	Percent of Women with Pregnancy[a] Typical Use
Condoms, male	Allergy to latex or rubber	Inexpensive STI/STD protection, including HIV (latex only)	High user failure rate Poor acceptance Possibility of breakage Efficacy decreased by oil-based lubricants Possible allergic reactions to latex in either partner	2	13
Condoms, female	Allergy to polyurethane History of TSS	Can be inserted just before intercourse or ahead of time STI/STD protection, including HIV	High user failure rate Dislike ring hanging outside vagina Cumbersome	5	21
Diaphragm with spermicide	Allergy to latex, rubber, or spermicide Recurrent UTIs History of TSS Abnormal gynecologic anatomy	Low cost Decreased incidence of cervical neoplasia Some protection against STIs/STDs	High user failure rate Decreased efficacy with increased frequency of intercourse Increased incidence of vaginal yeast UTIs, TSS Efficacy decreased by oil-based lubricants Cervical irritation	16	17

(Continued)

TABLE 30-1 Comparison of Methods of Nonhormonal Contraception (Continued)

Method	Absolute Contraindications	Advantages	Disadvantages	Percent of Women with Pregnancy[a] Perfect Use	Percent of Women with Pregnancy[a] Typical Use
Cervical cap (FemCap)	Allergy to spermicide History of TSS Abnormal gynecologic anatomy Abnormal papanicolaou smear	Low cost Latex-free Some protection against STIs/STDs FemCap reusable for up to 2 years	High user failure rate Decreased efficacy with parity Cannot be used during menses	9	16[b]
Spermicides alone	Allergy to spermicide	Inexpensive	High user failure rate Must be reapplied before each act of intercourse May enhance HIV transmission No protection against STI/STDs	16	21
Sponge (Today)	Allergy to spermicide Recurrent UTIs History of TSS Abnormal gynecologic anatomy	Inexpensive	High user failure rate Decreased efficacy with parity Cannot be used during menses No protection against STIs/STDs	9[c]	14[d]

[a]Failure rate in the United States during first year of use.
[b]Failure rate with FemCap reported to be 24% per package insert.
[c]Failure rate with Today sponge reported to be 20% in parous women.
[d]Failure rate with Today sponge reported to be 27% in parous women.
HIV, human immunodeficiency virus; STI/STD, sexually transmitted infection/disease; TSS, toxic shock syndrome; UTI, urinary tract infection.

- **Diaphragms** and the **cervical cap** are effective barriers that should be used with spermicide before insertion. They should be inserted up to 6 hours before intercourse and must be left in place for at least 6 hours after. A diaphragm should not be left in place for more than 24 hours because of the risk of toxic shock syndrome (TSS), while the cervical cap should not remain in place for longer than 48 hours to reduce the risk of TSS. Condom use with diaphragms and cervical caps is necessary to protect against STIs including human immunodeficiency virus (HIV).
- Most **condoms** made in the United States are latex, which is impermeable to viruses, but ~5% are made from lamb intestine, which is not. Water-soluble lubricants (ie, Astroglide and K-Y Jelly) are preferred to prevent condom breakdown. Condoms with spermicides are not recommended, as they provide no additional protection against pregnancy or STIs and may increase vulnerability to HIV.
- The **female condom (Reality)** covers the labia as well as the cervix. While the pregnancy rate is higher than with male condoms, it will protect against many viruses, including HIV.

PHARMACOLOGIC THERAPY

- Table 30-2 compares unintended pregnancy rates and continuation rates for pharmacologic contraceptive methods.

Spermicides and Spermicide Implanted Barrier Techniques

- Most spermicides contain **nonoxynol-9**, a surfactant that destroys sperm cell walls and blocks entry into the cervical os. They offer no protection against STIs, and when used more than twice daily, nonoxynol-9 may increase the transmission of HIV.
- The **vaginal contraceptive sponge (Today)** is available over the counter and contains nonoxynol-9 and provides protection for 24 hours. After intercourse, the sponge must be left in place for at least 6 hours before removal. It should not be left in place for more than 24−30 hours to reduce the risk of TSS. It should not be reused after removal.

Hormonal Oral Contraceptives

- **Combined Hormonal Contraceptive** (CHC) is the most commonly used form of oral contraception (OC) and contains a combination of synthetic estrogen and synthetic progestin. Some OCs contain progestin alone.

TABLE 30-2	Pregnancy and Continuation Rates for Various Pharmacologic Contraceptive Methods		
Method	**Pregnancy Typical Use**	**Pregnancy Ideal Use**	**Continuation After 1 Year**
Combined oral contraceptive	7%	<1%	67%
Combined hormonal transdermal contraceptive patch	7%	<1%	—
Combined hormonal vaginal contraceptive ring	7%	<1%	—
Depot medroxyprogesterone acetate	4%	<1%	56%
Copper IUD	<1%	<1%	78%
Levonorgestrel IUD	<1%	<1%	80%
Progestin-only implant	<1%	<1%	89%

- Estrogens suppress FSH release (which may contribute to blocking the LH surge) and also stabilize the endometrial lining and provide cycle control. **Ethinyl estradiol** (EE) is the most common used synthetic estrogen.
- **Progestins** thicken cervical mucus, delay sperm transport, and induce endometrial atrophy. They also block the LH surge and thus inhibit ovulation. Progestins vary in their progestational activity and are metabolized to substances that differ in their inherent estrogenic, antiestrogenic, and androgenic effects. Androgenic activity depends on the presence of sex hormone (testosterone) binding globulin and the androgen-to-progesterone activity ratio. If sex hormone binding globulin decreases, free testosterone levels increase, and androgenic side effects are more prominent.
- **Table 30-3** lists available oral contraceptives by brand name and hormonal composition.
- With perfect use, OC efficacy is more than 99%, but with typical use, up to 7% of women experience unintended pregnancy.
- Monophasic CHCs contain a constant amount of estrogen and progestin for 21 days, followed by 7 days of placebo. Biphasic and triphasic pills contain variable amounts of estrogen and progestin for 21 days and are followed by a 7-day placebo phase.
- Extended-cycle pills and continuous combination regimens may offer some side effect and convenience benefits. With extended-cycle CHC the number of hormone-containing pills increases from 21 to 84 days, followed by a 7-day placebo phase, resulting in four menstrual cycles per year.
- The progestin-only "minipills" tend to be less effective than combination CHCs and are associated with irregular and unpredictable menstrual bleeding. They must be taken every day of the menstrual cycle at approximately the same time of day to maintain contraceptive efficacy. They are associated with more ectopic pregnancies than other hormonal contraceptives.
- In the first-day start method, women take the first pill on the first day of their menstrual cycle. In the Sunday start method, the first pill is taken on the first Sunday after starting the menstrual cycle. In the quick start method the first pill is taken the day of the office visit. Women should use a second contraceptive method for 7–30 days after OC initiation and resume hormonal contraception no sooner than 5 days after the use of emergency contraception (ie, ulipristal acetate).
- Women should be provided with guidance about what to do if a pill is missed or if vomiting and diarrhea occur.
- An important concern about OCs is their lack of protection against STIs, and condoms should be used to prevent STIs.
- The choice of an initial OC is based on hormonal content and dose, preferred formulation, and coexisting medical conditions.
- A complete medical examination and papanicolaou (Pap) smear are not necessary before a CHC is prescribed. Obtain a medical history and blood pressure measurement, and discuss the risks, benefits, and adverse effects with the patient before prescribing a CHC.
- **Table 30-4** shows graded eligibility criteria for contraceptive use.
- Noncontraceptive benefits of OCs include decreased menstrual cramps and ovulatory pain; decreased menstrual blood loss; improved menstrual regularity; decreased iron deficiency anemia; reduced risk of ovarian and endometrial cancer; and reduced risk of ovarian cysts, ectopic pregnancy, pelvic inflammatory disease, endometriosis, uterine fibroids, and benign breast disease.
  - ✓ Serious symptoms that may be associated with CHCs are given in **Table 30-5**.
  - ✓ Side effects occurring in the first cycle of OC use (eg, breakthrough bleeding, nausea, and bloating) improve by the third cycle of use. **Table 30-6** shows side effect monitoring of women taking CHCs.
  - ✓ Instruct women to immediately discontinue CHCs if they experience warning signs referred to by the mnemonic ACHES (Abdominal pain, Chest pain, Headaches, Eye problems, and Severe leg pain).

TABLE 30-3	Composition of Commonly Prescribed Oral Contraceptives[a]					
Product		Estrogen	Micrograms[b]	Progestin	Milligrams[b]	Spotting and Breakthrough Bleeding (%)
50 mcg Estrogen						
Ogestrel 0.5/50		Ethinyl estradiol	50	Norgestrel	0.5	4.5
Zovia 1/50		Ethinyl estradiol	50	Ethynodiol diacetate	1	13.9
Sub-50 mcg Estrogen Monophasic						
Afirmelle, Aubra, Aubra EQ, Aviane, Balcoltra, Delyla, Falmina, Larissia, Lessina, Lutera, Orsythia, Sronyx, Vienva, levonorgestrel/EE		Ethinyl estradiol	20	Levonorgestrel	0.1	26.5
Brevicon, Necon 0.5/35, Nortrel 0.5/35, Norminest Fe, Wera		Ethinyl estradiol	35	Norethindrone	0.5	24.6
Zovia 1/35, Kelnor 1/35		Ethinyl estradiol	35	Ethynodiol diacetate	1	37.4
Apri, Cyred, Desogen, desogestrel/EE, Emoquette, Enskyce, Isibloom, Juleber, Reclipsen		Ethinyl estradiol	30	Desogestrel	0.15	13.1
Altavera, Chateal, Kurvelo, Levora, Lillow, Marlissa, Portia		Ethinyl estradiol	30	Levonorgestrel	0.15	14
Aurovela 1/20, Aurovela Fe 1/20, Hailey Fe 1/20, Junel 1/20, Junel Fe 1/20, Loestrin 1/20; Fe 1/20, Melodetta 24 Fe (chewable), Microgestin 1/20, Microgestin Fe 1/20, norethindrone/EE, norethindrone/EE Fe, Tarina Fe 1/20		Ethinyl estradiol	20	Norethindrone	1	26.5
Aurovela 1.5/30-21, Aurovela 1.5/30-28, Aurovela Fe 1.5/30, Hailey Fe 1/20, Gildess Fe 1.5/30, Junel 1.5/30, Junel Fe 1.5/30, Larin (Fe) 1.5/30, Loestrin Fe 1.5/30, Microgestin 1.5/30, Microgestin Fe 1.5/30		Ethinyl estradiol	30	Norethindrone acetate	1.5	25.2
Cryselle, Elinest, Low-Ogestrel		Ethinyl estradiol	30	Norgestrel	0.3	9.6
Alyacen 1/35, Cyclafem 1/35, Dasetta 1/35, Necon 1/35, Norinyl 1+35, Nortrel 1/35, Ortho-Novum 1/35, Pirmella 1/35		Ethinyl estradiol	35	Norethindrone	1	14.7

(Continued)

TABLE 30-3 Composition of Commonly Prescribed Oral Contraceptives[a] *(Continued)*

Product	Estrogen	Micrograms[b]	Progestin	Milligrams[b]	Spotting and Breakthrough Bleeding (%)
Estarylla, Femynor, Norgestimate/ethinyl estradiol, Ortho-Cyclen, Mono-Linyah, Mononessa, Previfem, Sprintec	Ethinyl estradiol	35	Norgestimate	0.25	14.3
Balziva, Briellyn, Femcon Fe chewable, Zenchent, Gildagia, Nexesta Fe, Philith, Vyfemla, Wymzya Fe chewable, Zenchant, Zenchant Fe chewable	Ethinyl estradiol	35	Norethindrone	0.4	11
Drospirenone/EE, Ocella, Safyral[c], Syeda, Tydemy[c], Yasmin, Zarah	Ethinyl estradiol	30	Drospirenone	3	14.5
Generess Fe chewable, Layolis Fe, Kaitlib Fe, norethindrone/EE	Ethinyl estradiol	25	Norethindrone	0.8	14.5
Sub-50 mcg Estrogen Monophasic Extended Cycle (longer than 21 days of active tablets)					
Lo Loestrin-24 FE[d]	Ethinyl estradiol	10	Norethindrone	1	50[e]
Aurovela 24 Fe, Junel Fe 24, Larin (Fe) 1/20, Larin 24 Fe, Minastrin 24 Fe chewable, norethindrone/EE/Fe, Taytulla (capsules)	Ethinyl estradiol	20	Norethindrone	1	50[e]
Amethia Lo, Camrese Lo, levonorgestrel/EE, LoSeasonique	Ethinyl estradiol	20/10	Levonorgestrel	0.1	50[e]
Amethyst	Ethinyl estradiol	20	Levonorgestrel	0.09	52[e]
Introvale, levonorgestrel/EE, Jolessa, Quasense Setlakin[f]	Ethinyl estradiol	30	Levonorgestrel	0.15	58.5[e]
Amethia, Ashlyna, Camrese, Daysee, levonorgesterel/EE Seasonique	Ethinyl estradiol	30/10	Levonorgestrel	0.15	50[e]
Quartette, Rivelsa	Ethinyl estradiol	20/25/30/10	Levonorgestrel	0.15	50[e]
Beyaz[c], drospirenone/EE, Gianvi, Loryna, Nikki, Rajani[c], Vestura, Yaz[d]	Ethinyl estradiol	20	Drospirenone	3	52.5[e]
Sub-50 mcg Estrogen Multiphasic					
Caziant, Cyclessa, Velivet	Ethinyl estradiol	25 (7) 25 (7) 25 (7)	Desogestrel	0.1 (7) 0.125 (7) 0.15 (7)	11.1

Tilia Fe, Tri-Legest Fe	Ethinyl estradiol	20 (5)	Norethindrone acetate	1 (5)	21.7
	Ethinyl estradiol	30 (7)	Norethindrone acetate	1 (7)	
	Ethinyl estradiol	35 (9)	Norethindrone acetate	1 (9)	
Azurette, Bekyree, desogestrel/EE, Kariva, Kimidess, Mircette, Pimtrea, Viorele	Ethinyl estradiol	20 (21)	Desogestrel	0.15 (21)	19.7
Necon 10/11	Ethinyl estradiol	10 (5)	Desogestrel	1 (7)	
	Ethinyl estradiol	35 (10)	Norethindrone	0.5 (10)	17.6
	Ethinyl estradiol	35 (11)	Norethindrone	1 (11)	
Alyacen 7/7/7, Cyclafem 7/7/7, Dasetta 7/7/7, Necon 7/7/7, Nortrel 7/7/7, Ortho-Novum 7/7/7, Pirmella 7/7/7	Ethinyl estradiol	35 (7)	Norethindrone	0.5 (7)	14.5
	Ethinyl estradiol	35 (7)	Norethindrone	0.75 (7)	
	Ethinyl estradiol	35 (7)	Norethindrone	1 (7)	
Ortho Tri-Cyclen, Tri-Estarylla, Tri-Femynor, Tri-Linyah, TriNessa, Tri-Previfem, Tri-Sprintec, Norgestimate/EE	Ethinyl estradiol	35 (7)	Norgestimate	0.18 (7)	17.7
	Ethinyl estradiol	35 (7)	Norgestimate	0.215 (7)	
	Ethinyl estradiol	35 (7)	Norgestimate	0.25 (7)	
Ortho Tri-Cyclen Lo, Norgestimate/EE Tri-Lo Estarylla, Tri-Lo-Marzia, Tri-Lo-Sprintec, TriNessa Lo	Ethinyl estradiol	25 (7)	Norgestimate	0.18 (7)	11.5
	Ethinyl estradiol	25 (7)	Norgestimate	0.215 (7)	
	Ethinyl estradiol	25 (7)	Norgestimate	0.25 (7)	

(Continued)

TABLE 30-3   Composition of Commonly Prescribed Oral Contraceptives[a] *(Continued)*

Product	Estrogen	Micrograms[b]	Progestin	Milligrams[b]	Spotting and Breakthrough Bleeding (%)
Aranelle, Leena, Tri-Norinyl	Ethinyl estradiol	35 (7)	Norethindrone	0.5 (7)	25.5
	Ethinyl estradiol	35 (9)	Norethindrone	1 (9)	
	Ethinyl estradiol	35 (5)	Norethindrone	0.5 (5)	
Enpresse, Trivora, levonorgestrel/EE, Levonest, Myzilra	Ethinyl estradiol	30 (6)	Levonorgestrel	0.05 (6)	
	Ethinyl estradiol	40 (5)	Levonorgestrel	0.075 (5)	
	Ethinyl estradiol	30 (10)		0.125 (10)	
Natazia	Estradiol valerate	3 (2)	Dienogest	0 (2)	
		2 (22)		2 (5)	
		1 (2)		3 (17)	
				0 (4)	
Progestin Only					
Camila, Deblitane, Errin, Heather, Incassia, Jencycla Jolivette, Lyza, Ortho Micronor, Nora-BE, Norlyda, Norlyroc, Orthor Micronor, Sharobel,Tulana, norethindrone	Ethinyl estradiol	–	Norethindrone	0.35	42.3

[a]28-day regimens (21-day active pills, then 7-day pill-free interval) unless otherwise noted.
[b]Number in parentheses refers to the number of days the dose is received in multiphasic oral contraceptives.
[c]Also contains levomefolate calcium 0.451 mg in all 28 tablets.
[d]28-day regimen (24-day active pills, then 4-day pill-free interval).
[e]Percent reporting after 6–12 months of use.
[f]91-day regimen (84-day active pills, then 7-day pill-free interval).

TABLE 30-4	U.S. Medical Eligibility Criteria for Contraceptive Use: Classifications for Combined Hormonal Contraceptives

Category 4: Unacceptable health risk (method not to be used)

Breastfeeding or non-breastfeeding <21 days postpartum

Current breast cancer

Severe (decompensated) cirrhosis

Current deep venous thrombosis/pulmonary embolism

History/higher risk of deep venous thrombosis/pulmonary embolism (not on anticoagulant therapy)

History/higher risk of deep venous thrombosis/pulmonary embolism (established on anticoagulant therapy for 3 months or greater)

Thrombogenic mutations

Major surgery with prolonged immobilization

Migraines with aura, any age

Systolic blood pressure ≥160 mm Hg or diastolic ≥100 mm Hg

Hypertension with vascular disease

Current and history of ischemic heart disease

Benign hepatocellular adenoma or malignant liver tumor

Peripartum cardiomyopathy, moderately or severely impaired cardiac function; normal or mildly impaired cardiac function <6 months

Smoking ≥15 cigarettes per day and age ≥35

Complicated solid organ transplantation

History of cerebrovascular accident

SLE; positive or unknown antiphospholipid antibodies

Complicated valvular heart disease

Category 3: Theoretical or proven risks usually outweigh the advantages

Breastfeeding 21—30 days postpartum with or without risk factors for VTE

Breastfeeding 30—42 days postpartum with risk factors for VTE

Diabetes mellitus (type 1 or type 2), nonvascular disease

Gallbladder disease; symptomatic and treated by cholecystectomy or asymptomatic

Migraines without aura

History of pregnancy-related cholestasis

History of high blood pressure during pregnancy

Benign liver tumors; focal nodular hyperplasia

Obesity

Breastfeeding 30—42 days without other VTE risk factors

Breastfeeding 42 days or more postpartum

Non-breastfeeding 21—42 days postpartum without risk factors for VTE

Rheumatoid arthritis on or off immunosuppressive therapy

Smoking and <35 years old

Uncomplicated sold organ transplantation

Stable SLE without antiphospholipid antibodies

Unexplained vaginal bleeding before evaluation

Uncomplicated valvular heart disease

Use of antiretrovirals other than fosamprenavir (*category 1 or 2 depending on agent*)

Use of St. John's wort

Inflammatory bowel disease (*possibly category 3 for those with increased risk of VTE*)

(Continued)

TABLE 30-4	U.S. Medical Eligibility Criteria for Contraceptive Use: Classifications for Combined Hormonal Contraceptives (Continued)

Non-breastfeeding 21—42 days postpartum with other risk factors for VTE

Past breast cancer and no evidence of disease for 5 years

History of DVT/PE (not on anticoagulant therapy or established on anticoagulant therapy for at least 3 months), but lower risk for recurrent DVT/PE

Current gallbladder disease, symptomatic, and medically treated

History of bariatric surgery; malabsorptive procedures (COCs only, vaginal ring/transdermal patch category 1)

History of cholestasis, past COC-related

Hypertension; systolic blood pressure 140—159 mm Hg or diastolic 90—99 mm Hg

Adequately controlled hypertension

Peripartum cardiomyopathy, normal or mildly impaired cardiac function ≥6 months

Smoking <15 cigarettes per day and age ≥35

Use of fosamprenavir

Use of certain anticonvulsants (phenytoin, carbamazepine, barbiturates, primidone, topiramate, oxcarbazepine, and lamotrigine)

Use of rifampicin or rifabutin therapy

Diabetes with vascular disease or >20 years duration (possibly category 4 depending upon severity)

Multiple risk factors for arterial cardiovascular disease (older age, smoking, diabetes, low HDL, high LDL, or high triglycerides and hypertension) (possibly category 4 depending on category and severity)

Acute flare of viral hepatitis (possibly category 4 depending on severity[initiation])

Multiple sclerosis with prolonged immobility

Current or history of superficial venous thrombosis

Acute flare of viral hepatitis occurring during use of product (continuation, category 3 or 4 for initiation of product)

Category 1: No restriction (method can be used)

Thalassemia, iron deficiency anemia

Mild compensated cirrhosis

Benign ovarian tumors

Benign breast disease or family history of cancerFamily history of cancer

Schistosomiasis

Cystic fibrosis

Cervical ectropion

Viral hepatitis (carrier/chronic)

Minor surgery without immobilization

Depression

Endometrial cancer/hyperplasia, endometriosis

Epilepsy

Gestational trophoblastic disease

Nonmigrainous headaches

History of bariatric surgery; restrictive procedures

History of pelvic surgery

HIV infected or high risk

Malaria

Multiple sclerosis without prolonged immobility

Ovarian cancer

Past ectopic pregnancy

Parity, parous, or nulliparous

PID

Postabortion

Non-breastfeeding >42 days postpartum

Severe dysmenorrhea

Sexually transmitted infections

(Continued)

TABLE 30-4	U.S. Medical Eligibility Criteria for Contraceptive Use: Classifications for Combined Hormonal Contraceptives *(Continued)*
Category 2: Advantages generally outweigh theoretical or proven risks	Varicose veins
Age ≥40 (in the absence of other comorbid conditions that increase CVD risk)	Vaginal bleeding—irregular pattern without heavy bleeding or heavy, prolonged bleeding
Sickle cell disease	Thyroid disorders
Undiagnosed breast mass	Tuberculosis
Cervical cancer and awaiting treatment; cervical intraepithelial neoplasia	Uterine fibroids
Family history (first-degree relatives) of DVT/PE	Use of SSRIs
Major surgery without prolonged immobilization	Use of broad-spectrum antibiotics, antifungals, and antiparasitics

CHC, combined hormonal contraception; CVD, cardiovascular disease; HIV, human immunodeficiency virus; PE, pulmonary embolism; PID, pelvic inflammatory disease; VTE, venous thromboembolism.

TABLE 30-5	Symptoms of a Serious or Potentially Serious Nature Associated with Combined Hormonal Contraception
Symptom	**Possible Cause**
SERIOUS: Stop immediately	
Loss of vision, proptosis, diplopia, papilledema	Retinal artery thrombosis
Unilateral numbness, weakness, or tingling	Hemorrhagic or thrombotic stroke
Severe pains in chest, left arm, or neck	Myocardial infarction
Hemoptysis	Pulmonary embolism
Severe pains, tenderness or swelling, warmth or palpable cord in legs	Thrombophlebitis or thrombosis
Slurring of speech	Hemorrhagic or thrombotic stroke
Hepatic mass or tenderness	Liver neoplasm
POTENTIALLY SERIOUS: May continue with caution while being evaluated	
Absence of menses	Cervical endometrial or vaginal cancer
Spotting or breakthrough bleeding	Cholecystitis, cholelithiasis, or liver neoplasm
Breast mass, pain, or swelling	Pituitary adenoma
Right upper-quadrant pain	Cholestatic jaundice
Mid-epigastric pain	B_6 deficiency
Migraine headache	Leiomyomata, adenomyosis
Severe nonvascular headache	
Galactorrhea	
Jaundice, pruritus	
Depression, sleepiness	
Uterine size increase	

Transdermal Contraceptives

- A combination contraceptive is available as a **transdermal patch** (Xulane) that includes 0.75 mg of EE and 6 mg of norelgestromin. It is as effective as CHCs in women weighing less than 90 kg (198 lb) but is not first line in women weighing more than 90 kg.
  - ✓ The patch should be applied to the abdomen, buttocks, upper torso, or upper arm at the beginning of the menstrual cycle and replaced every week for 3 weeks. The fourth week is patch-free. Women should be counseled on the steps to follow should the patch detach or is forgotten.
  - ✓ Approved labeling includes a warning regarding VTE risk.

Vaginal Rings

- **NuvaRing** releases ~15 mcg/day of EE and 120 mcg/day of etonogestrel over a 3-week period. On first use, the ring should be inserted on or prior to the fifth day of the cycle, remain in place for 3 weeks, and then be removed. One week should lapse before the new ring is inserted on the same day of the week as it was for the last cycle. A second form of contraception should be used for the first 7 days of ring use or if the ring has been expelled for more than 3 hours.

Long-Acting Injectable and Implantable Contraceptives

- Women who particularly benefit from progestin-only methods, including minipills, are those who are breastfeeding, intolerant of estrogens, and those with concomitant medical conditions in which estrogen is not recommended (Table 30-4).
- Injectable and implantable contraceptives are also beneficial for women with adherence issues as failure rates are lower than with CHC.

Injectable Progestins

- **Depot medroxyprogesterone acetate (DMPA)** 150 mg is administered by deep intramuscular injection in the gluteal or deltoid muscle within 5 days of onset of menstrual bleeding, and the dose should be repeated every 12 weeks. Another formulation contains 104 mg of DMPA (Depo-SubQ Provera 104), which is injected subcutaneously into the thigh or abdomen. Exclude pregnancy in women more than 1 week late for repeat injection of the intramuscular formulation or 2 weeks late for repeat injection of the subcutaneous formulation. Return of fertility may be delayed after discontinuation.
- DMPA can be given immediately postpartum in women who are not breastfeeding, and at 6 weeks postpartum in women breastfeeding. The median time to conception from the first omitted dose is 10 months.
  - ✓ DMPA is contraindicated in women with a current diagnosis of breast cancer and should be used cautiously in those with a history of breast cancer, cardiovascular disease, or lupus.
  - ✓ The most frequent adverse effect of DMPA is menstrual irregularity, which decreases after the first year. Breast tenderness, weight gain, and depression occur less frequently.
  - ✓ DMPA is associated with reduced bone mineral density (BMD), and has a black box warning, but this is controversial as data do not demonstrate increased fracture risk. Loss of BMD seems to be greater with increasing duration of use, and effects on BMD may not be completely reversible upon discontinuation. DMPA should not be continued beyond 2 years unless other contraceptive methods are inadequate.

Subdermal Progestin Implants

- **Etonogestrel implant** (Nexplanon) is a radiopaque, 4-cm implant containing 68 mg of etonogestrel that is placed under the skin of the upper arm. It releases 60 mcg daily for the first month, decreasing gradually to 30 mcg/day at the end of the 3 years of recommended use. Efficacy exceeds 99%, but it may be less in women who weigh more than 130% of their ideal body weight.

TABLE 30-6	Drug Monitoring Table for Hormonal Contraception		
Drug (or Drug Class)	**Adverse Drug Reactions**	**Monitoring Parameter**	**Comments**
Combined hormonal contraception	Nausea/vomiting	Patient symptoms	Typically improves after two to three cycles; consider changing to lower estrogenic
	Breast tenderness	Patient symptoms	
	Weight gain	Weight	
	Acne, oily skin	Visual inspection	
	Depression, fatigue	Depression screening	Consider changing to lower androgenic
	Breakthrough bleeding/ spotting	Menstrual symptoms	Data are limited and conflicting
	Application site reaction (transdermal)	Visual inspection	Consider changing to higher estrogenic
		Patient symptoms	
	Vaginal irritation (vaginal ring)		
Depo-medroxyprogesterone acetate	Menstrual irregularities[a]	Menstrual symptoms	Typically improves after 6 months
	Weight gain	Weight	Data are limited and conflicting
	Acne	Visual inspection	
	Hirsutism	Visual inspection	Do not routinely screen with DXA
	Depression	Depression screening	
	Decreased bone density	BMD	
Levonorgestrel IUD	Menstrual irregularities[a]	Menstrual symptoms	Typically spotting, amenorrhea
	Insertion-related complications	Cramping, pain	Prophylactic nonsteroidal anti-inflammatory drugs (NSAIDs) or local anesthetic may reduce occurrence
	Expulsion	Cramping, pain, spotting, dyspareunia, missing strings	
	Pelvic inflammatory disease	Lower abdominal pain, unusual vaginal discharge, fever	IUD strings should be checked regularly by women to ensure IUD properly placed
			Overall risk of developing is rare, but counseling on STI/STD prevention is important

(Continued)

TABLE 30-6	Drug Monitoring Table for Hormonal Contraception (Continued)		
Drug (or Drug Class)	**Adverse Drug Reactions**	**Monitoring Parameter**	**Comments**
Copper IUD	See levonorgestrel IUD above	See levonorgestrel IUD above	Menstrual irregularities are typically heavier menses with copper IUD
Progestin-only implant	Menstrual irregularities[a]	Menstrual symptoms	Typically well-tolerated and resolve without treatment; infection is rare
	Insertion-site reactions	Pain, bruising, skin irritation, erythema, pus, fever	

[a]Suggested management of irregular bleeding may include use of NSAIDs for 5—7 days; hormonal treatment (if medically eligible) with COC or estrogen therapy for 10—20 days of treatment.

- Need for backup contraception varies based on prior contraceptive use and where in the menstrual cycle the implant is inserted. Fertility returns 30 days after removal.
  - ✓ The major adverse effect is irregular menstrual bleeding. Other side effects are headache, vaginitis, weight gain, acne, and breast and abdominal pain. It does not appear to decrease BMD. Fertility returns within 30 days of removal.

Intrauterine Devices (IUDs)

- The contraceptive activity occurs before implantation. Endometrial suppression is caused by progestin-releasing IUDs. Efficacy rates are greater than 99%.
- Strong consideration of an IUD is appropriate in nulliparous and adolescent women due to high efficacy rates and low complication rates. Need for backup contraception varies based on prior contraceptive use and where in the menstrual cycle the implant is inserted.
- The risk of pelvic inflammatory disease among users is low with no long-term effects on fertility.
- ParaGard (copper) can be left in place for 10 years. Mirena, Liletta, Skyla, and Kyleena release levonorgestrel and must be replaced after 5 years (Mirena, Liletta, and Kyleena) and 3 years (Skyla).
  - ✓ Major adverse effects include increased menstrual blood flow and dysmenorrhea with ParaGard, while levonorgestrel IUDs are associated with reduced menstrual blood loss and possible amenorrhea.

Special Consideration for Contraceptive Use

Women Over 35 Years of Age

- Use of CHCs containing less than 50 mcg estrogen may be considered in healthy nonsmoking women older than 35 years.
- CHCs are not recommended for women older than 35 years with migraine, uncontrolled hypertension, smoking, or diabetes with vascular disease.
- Studies have not demonstrated an increased risk of cardiovascular disease with low-dose CHCs in healthy, nonobese women.
- Smoking 15 or more cigarettes per day by women over 35 years is a contraindication to the use of CHCs. Progestin-only methods should be considered in this group.

Smoking

- Use of a CHC with less than 50 mcg EE should be used in women under the age of 35 who smoke to reduce the risk of myocardial infarction (MI).

Hypertension

- CHCs, regardless of estrogen dose, can cause small increases in blood pressure (6–8 mm Hg). Use of low-dose CHCs is acceptable in women younger than 35 years with well-controlled and monitored hypertension to reduce the risk of MI and stroke.
- Women with a systolic blood pressure of 140−159 or a diastolic blood pressure of 90−99 mm Hg should avoid CHCs. Their use is contraindicated for women with blood pressure ≥160/100 mm Hg.
- Monitor potassium in women taking potassium-sparing diuretics, angiotensin-converting enzyme inhibitors, angiotensin-receptor blockers, or aldosterone antagonists if they are also using an OC-containing drospirenone.

Diabetes

- Women younger than 35 years with diabetes but no vascular disease who do not smoke can safely use CHCs. Women who have had diabetes for more than 20 years or have vascular disease should not use CHCs.

Dyslipidemia

- Generally, synthetic progestins decrease high-density lipoprotein (HDL) and increase low-density lipoprotein (LDL). Estrogens decrease LDL but increase HDL and may moderately increase triglycerides. Most low-dose CHCs have no significant impact on HDL, LDL, triglycerides, or total cholesterol.
- The mechanism for the increased cardiovascular disease in CHC users is believed to be thromboembolic and thrombotic changes, not atherosclerosis.
- CHCs use in women with dyslipidemia as the single cardiovascular risk factor is generally acceptable; however, care should be taken in women with dyslipidemia and other cardiovascular risk factors. An alternative method of contraception may be recommended.

Thromboembolism

- The risk of venous thromboembolism (VTE) in women using OCs is three times the risk in nonusers. However, this risk is less than the risk of thromboembolic events during pregnancy.
- Estrogens increase hepatic production of factors involved in the coagulation cascade. Risk for thromboembolic events is increased in women with underlying hypercoagulable states or those with acquired conditions (eg, obesity, pregnancy, immobility, trauma, surgery, and certain malignancies) that predispose them to coagulation abnormalities.
- OCs containing the newer progestins (eg, drospirenone, desogestrel, norgestimate) carry a slightly increased risk of thrombosis compared to other progestins due to unknown mechanisms.
- The transdermal patch and vaginal ring provide continuous higher exposure to estrogen and have an increased thromboembolic risk.
- For women at increased risk of thromboembolism (older than 35 years, obesity, smoking, personal or family history of venous thrombosis, prolonged immobilization), consider low-dose oral estrogen contraceptives containing older progestins or progestin-only methods.

Obesity

- OCs have lower efficacy in obese women, and low-dose OCs may be especially problematic. IUDs, implants, and DMPA have very low failure rates, and progestin-only contraceptives are considered safe in obese women.
- Obese women are at increased risk for VTE, and progestin-only contraception may be better for obese women over 35 years.

Migraine Headache

- CHCs may decrease or increase migraine frequency.

- CHCs may be considered for healthy, nonsmoking women (less than 35 years old) with migraines without aura. Discuss continued use of CHC risks and benefits with women developing migraines without aura.
- Women of any age who have migraine with aura should not use CHCs due to the risk of stroke. Women who develop migraines with aura while receiving CHCs should discontinue their use and consider a progestin-only option.

Breast Cancer

- There is a small increase in the relative risk of having breast cancer while CHCs are taken and for up to 10 years following discontinuation.
- For women over the age of 40 or those who have an elevated risk of breast cancer because of family history or other factors, alternatives may be considered.
- The choice to use CHCs should not be influenced by the presence of benign breast disease or a family history of breast cancer. For women with either *BRCA1* or *BRCA2* mutation, CHC use is controversial, and women with a current or past history of breast cancer should not use CHCs.

Systemic Lupus Erythematosus (SLE)

- OCs with less than 50 mcg EE do not increase the risk of flare among women with stable SLE and without antiphospholipid/anticardiolipin antibodies. CHCs should be avoided in women with SLE and antiphospholipid antibodies or vascular complications. The copper IUD may be the best option in this situation.
- For women with SLE without antiphospholipid antibodies or vascular complications, progestin-only contraceptives or the copper IUD may be an alternative. Copper IUD and DMPA injection should be avoided in those with SLE and severe thrombocytopenia.

Postpartum

- In the first 21 days postpartum (when the risk of thrombosis is higher), estrogen-containing hormonal contraceptives should be avoided due to increased VTE risk. Progestin-only methods should be used if contraception is necessary.
- CHC should be avoided in the first 42 days postpartum in women with VTE risk factors and for 30 days for those without VTE risk factors who are breastfeeding.

Drug Interactions

- Tell women to use an alternative method of contraception if there is a possibility of a drug interaction compromising OC efficacy.
- Rifampin reduces the efficacy of OCs. Additional nonhormonal contraception should be used for at least 7−28 days after rifampin therapy.
- There is a small risk of interaction with other antimicrobials, and additional nonhormonal contraceptives can be considered if desired. An alternate method of contraception should be used when receiving an antimicrobial for more than 2 months.
- Phenobarbital, carbamazepine, and phenytoin potentially reduce the efficacy of OCs, and many anticonvulsants are known teratogens. IUDs, injectable medroxyprogesterone, or nonhormonal options may be considered for women taking these drugs.
- Combined OCs may decrease the efficacy of lamotrigine and increase the risk of seizures.
- Certain antiretroviral therapies and St. John's Wort may decrease the efficacy of OCs.
- Monitor potassium in patients taking drospirenone and concomitant medications that increase potassium levels or those taking strong CYP3A4 inhibitors.

Return of Fertility After Discontinuation

- There is no evidence that OCs, patches, or vaginal rings use decreases subsequent fertility.
- There is no greater chance of miscarriage or a birth defect in the first month after an OC discontinuation compared to the general population.

Emergency Contraception (EC)

- EC is used to prevent unintended pregnancy after unprotected or inadequately protected sexual intercourse.
- FDA-approved progestin-only and progesterone receptor modulator products are recommended as first-line EC options. They will not disrupt the fertilized egg if implantation has already occurred.
- Progestin-only EC formulations containing one 1.5 mg tablet of levonorgestrel are a regimen of choice and are available without a prescription in the United States. They may be less effective in women weighing greater than 75 kg.
- **Ulipristal** (Ella) is a prescription selective progesterone receptor modulator. It is taken as a single dose of 30 mg within 120 hours (5 days) of unprotected intercourse. It is considered noninferior to levonorgestrel-containing ECs and is not recommended in breastfeeding women.
- Common adverse effects of EC include nausea, vomiting, and irregular bleeding.
- Insertion of a copper IUD or prescribing higher doses of combined OCs (Yuzpe method) are other EC options.
- EC should be given within 72 hours (3 days) of unprotected intercourse, but the sooner it is taken, the greater the efficacy. There is some evidence that it may be effective for up to 5 days after unprotected intercourse, but in this situation ulipristal or a copper IUD may be a better option.
- Backup non-hormonal contraceptive methods should be used after EC for at least 7 days.

Pregnancy Termination

- Medications used in early pregnancy (≤70 days) termination include **mifepristone, misoprostol**, and **methotrexate**. Misoprostol can be used alone or more effectively in combination with mifepristone and methotrexate. The FDA has approved mifepristone 600 mg on day 1 and then misoprostol 400 mcg administered orally 48 hours after the mifepristone dose as a pregnancy termination regimen.
- Mifepristone binds progesterone receptors to block progesterone, resulting in cervical softening and increasing prostaglandin synthesis, leading to contraction stimulation. Mifepristone is usually administered orally, and prescribing is limited to trained prescribers who also dispense the medication. It is contraindicated in patients with bleeding disorders or those on anticoagulants.
- Misoprostol is a prostaglandin 1 analog that may be given orally, vaginally, bucally, or sublingual resulting in cervical ripening and contractions.
- Methotrexate is an immunomodulator that inhibits cell replication. It is effective in the first 7 weeks of pregnancy.
  ✓ Side effects of misoprostol and methotrexate may include stomach upset, diarrhea, headache, dizziness, and fever. Mifepristone has a boxed warning regarding infection and bleeding and women experiencing bleeding that soaks two maxi pads per hour for 2 consecutive hours should contact their healthcare provider.

EVALUATION OF THERAPEUTIC OUTCOMES

- Monitor blood pressure annually in all CHC users.
- Monitor glucose levels closely when CHCs are started or stopped in women with a history of glucose intolerance or diabetes mellitus.
- For all contraceptive users do annual cytologic screening (more often if they are at risk for STIs), pelvic and breast examination, and well woman consultation. Also, regularly evaluate for problems that may relate to the CHCs (eg, breakthrough bleeding, amenorrhea, weight gain, and acne). These screenings do not have to occur before prescribing hormonal contraceptives.
- Annually monitor women using Nexplanon for menstrual cycle disturbances, weight gain, local inflammation or infection at the implant site, acne, breast tenderness, headaches, and hair loss.

- Evaluate women using DMPA every 3 months for weight gain, menstrual cycle disturbances, and fractures.
- Monitor women with IUDs at 1- to 3-month intervals for proper positioning of the IUD, changes in menstrual bleeding patterns, upper genital tract infection, and protection against STIs.
- Clinicians should monitor and when indicated screen for HIV and STIs. Counsel all women about healthy sexual practices, including the use of condoms to prevent transmission of STIs when necessary.

See Chapter 18, Contraception, authored by Shareen Y. El-Ibiary, Sarah P. Shrader, and Kelly R. Ragucci, for a more detailed discussion of this topic.

31 Hormone Therapy in Women

- *Perimenopause* begins with the onset of menstrual irregularity and ends 12 months after the last menstrual period, which marks the beginning of menopause. *Menopause* is the permanent cessation of menses caused by the loss of ovarian follicular activity. Women spend about 40% of their lives in postmenopause.

PHYSIOLOGY

- The hypothalamic–pituitary–ovarian axis controls reproductive physiology. Follicle-stimulating hormone (FSH) and luteinizing hormone (LH), produced by the pituitary in response to gonadotropin-releasing hormone from the hypothalamus, regulate ovarian function. Gonadotropins are also influenced by negative feedback from the sex steroids estradiol (produced by the dominant follicle) and progesterone (produced by the corpus luteum). Other sex steroids are androgens, primarily testosterone and androstenedione, secreted by the ovarian stroma.
- As women age, circulating FSH progressively rises, and ovarian inhibin-B and anti-Mullerian hormone declines. In menopause, there is a 10- to 15-fold increase in circulating FSH, a 4- to 5-fold increase in LH, and a greater than 90% decrease in circulating estradiol concentrations.

CLINICAL PRESENTATION

- Symptoms of perimenopause and menopause include vasomotor symptoms (hot flushes and night sweats), sleep disturbances, depression, anxiety, poor concentration and memory, vaginal dryness and dyspareunia, headache, sexual dysfunction, and arthralgia.
- Signs include urogenital atrophy in menopause and dysfunctional uterine bleeding in perimenopause. Other potential causes of dysfunctional uterine bleeding should be ruled out.
- Additionally, loss of estrogen production results in metabolic changes; increase in central abdominal fat; and effects on lipids, vascular function, and bone metabolism.

DIAGNOSIS

- Menopause is determined retrospectively after 12 consecutive months of amenorrhea. FSH on day 2 or 3 of the menstrual cycle greater than 10–12 IU/L indicates diminished ovarian reserve.
- The diagnosis of menopause should include a comprehensive medical history and physical examination, complete blood count, and measurement of serum FSH. When ovarian function has ceased, serum FSH concentrations exceed 40 IU/L. Altered thyroid function and pregnancy must be excluded.

TREATMENT

- <u>Goals of Treatment</u>: The goals are to relieve symptoms, improve quality of life, and minimize medication adverse effects.

NONPHARMACOLOGIC THERAPY

- Mild vasomotor and/or vaginal symptoms can often be alleviated by lowering the room temperature; decreasing intake of caffeine, spicy foods, and hot beverages; smoking cessation; exercise; and a healthy diet.
- Mild vaginal dryness can sometimes be relieved by nonestrogenic vaginal creams, but significant vaginal dryness often requires local or systemic estrogen therapy.

PHARMACOLOGIC THERAPY

- **Figure 31-1** outlines the pharmacologic treatment of women with menopausal symptoms. Food and Drug Administration (FDA)-approved indications and contraindications for menopausal hormone therapy (MHT) are shown in **Table 31-1**.
- The decision to use MHT and the type of formulation used must be individualized based on several factors, including personal preference, age, menopause onset, the severity of menopausal symptoms, and MHT-associated risks.
- Combined hormonal contraceptives (CHCs) provide contraception and vasomotor symptom relief but should not be used in perimenopausal women if they smoke or have a history of estrogen-dependent cancer, cardiovascular or cerebrovascular disease, hypertension, diabetes with vascular disease, or risk factors for thromboembolism, liver disease, or migraine headaches (see **Chapter 30**).
- MHT remains the most effective treatment for moderate and severe vasomotor symptoms, impaired sleep quality, and vulvovaginal symptoms of menopause.
- Several national and international guidelines and consensus statements on the management of menopause are available (eg, United States Preventive Services Task Force, American Association of Clinical Endocrinologists, North American Menopause Society).
- When urogenital symptoms, such as vaginal dryness and dyspareunia, are the only menopausal complaint, **intravaginal estrogen cream, tablet**, or **ring** should be considered before oral therapy. Intravaginal estrogen minimizes systemic absorption and is more effective for vaginal symptoms than oral therapy. **Ospemifene**, a selective estrogen receptor modulator, is another option. Intravaginal estrogen reduces the risk of recurrent urinary tract infections and may improve urge incontinence and overactive bladder.
- MHT is the most effective treatment for moderate-to-severe vasomotor symptoms, and impaired sleep quality. **Estrogen-only** therapy may decrease heart disease and all-cause mortality in 50- to 59-year-old women with a history of hysterectomy.
- MHT is effective and appropriate for prevention of osteoporosis-related fractures in recently menopausal women at risk.
- In women with an intact uterus, MHT consists of an **estrogen plus a progestogen** or **estrogen agonist/antagonist** (eg, **bazedoxifene** see **Fig. 31-1**). In women who have undergone hysterectomy, estrogen therapy is given unopposed by a progestogen. Concomitant progestogen therapy is unnecessary when low-dose vaginal estrogen is used.
- Women with vasomotor symptoms taking MHT have better mental health and fewer depressive symptoms compared with those taking placebo, but hormone therapy may worsen quality of life in women without vasomotor symptoms.

Estrogens

- Estrogen products and doses for MHT are shown in **Table 31-2**. The oral and transdermal routes are used most frequently and are considered equally effective.
- **Conjugated equine estrogens** are composed of estrone sulfate (50%–60%) and other estrogens such as equilin and 17α-dihydroequilin.
- **Estradiol** is the predominant and most active form of endogenous estrogens. Given orally, it is metabolized by the intestinal mucosa and liver, and resultant estrone concentrations are three to six times those of estradiol.
- **Ethinyl estradiol** is a semisynthetic estrogen that has similar activity following oral or parenteral administration.
- **Non-Oral estrogens**, including transdermal, intranasal, and vaginal products, avoid first-pass metabolism and result in a more physiologic estradiol:estrone ratio (ie, estradiol concentrations greater than estrone concentrations). Transdermal estrogen is also less likely to increase sex hormone–binding globulin, triglycerides, blood pressure, or C-reactive protein levels. Transdermal dosage forms may also have a lower risk for deep vein thrombosis, stroke, and myocardial infarction.

TABLE 31-1	FDA-approved Indications and Contraindications for Menopausal Hormone Therapy with Estrogens and Progestins
Indications	
For systemic use	Treatment of moderate-to-severe vasomotor symptoms (ie, moderate-to-severe hot flashes)
For intravaginal use (low systemic exposure)	Treatment of moderate-to-severe symptoms of vulvar and vaginal atrophy (ie, moderate-to-severe vaginal dryness, dyspareunia, and atrophic vaginitis)
Contraindications	
Absolute contraindications	Undiagnosed abnormal genital bleeding
	Known, suspected, or history of cancer of the breast
	Known or suspected estrogen- or progesterone-dependent neoplasia
	Active deep vein thrombosis, pulmonary embolism, or a history of these conditions
	Active or recent (eg, within the past year) arterial thromboembolic disease (eg, stroke, myocardial infarction)
	Liver dysfunction or disease
Relative contraindications	Elevated blood pressure
	Hypertriglyceridemia
	Impaired liver function and past history of cholestatic jaundice
	Hypothyroidism
	Fluid retention
	Severe hypocalcemia
	Ovarian cancer
	Exacerbation of endometriosis
	Exacerbation of asthma, diabetes mellitus, migraine, systemic lupus erythematosus, epilepsy, porphyria, and hepatic hemangioma

- Variability in absorption is common with the percutaneous preparations (gels, creams, and emulsions).
- **Estradiol pellets** (unavailable in the United States) contain pure crystalline 17β-estradiol and are placed subcutaneously (abdomen or buttock). They are difficult to remove.
- **Vaginal creams**, **tablets**, and **rings** are used for treatment of urogenital atrophy. Most tablets and rings provide local estrogen, but Femring is designed to achieve systemic estrogen concentrations and is indicated for moderate-to-severe vasomotor symptoms.
- New evidence indicates that lower doses of estrogens are effective in controlling postmenopausal symptoms and reducing bone loss. Low-dose estrogen regimens include 0.3–0.45 mg conjugated estrogens, 0.5 mg micronized 17β-estradiol, and 0.014–0.0375 mg transdermal 17β-estradiol patch. Topical gels, creams, and sprays are also available in low doses. Lower doses typically have fewer adverse effects, and may have better benefit to risk profiles than standard doses. The lowest effective dose should be used.

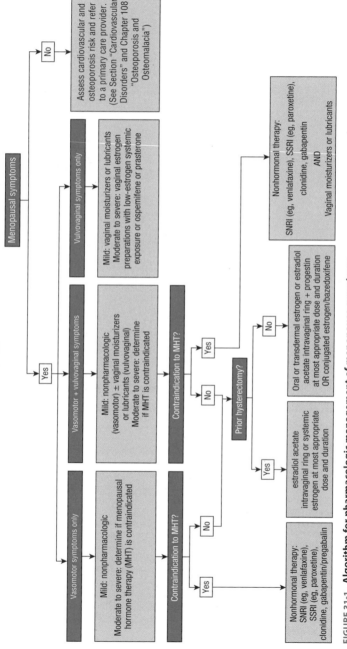

FIGURE 31-1. Algorithm for pharmacologic management of menopause symptoms.

TABLE 31-2 FDA-Approved Estrogen Products for Menopausal Hormone Therapy

Drug	Brand Name[a]	Initial Dose/Low Dose	Usual Dose Range	Comments
Systemic Estrogen Products (for the treatment of moderate and severe vasomotor symptoms ± urogenital symptoms)				
Oral estrogens[b]				
Conjugated equine estrogens	Premarin	0.3 or 0.45 mg once daily	0.3–1.25 mg once daily	Dosage form available as 0.3, 0.45, 0.625, 0.9, 1.25 mg
Esterified estrogens (75%–85% estrone + 6%–15% equilin)	Menest	0.3 mg once daily	0.3–1.25 mg once daily	Administer 3 weeks on and 1 week off Dosage form available as 0.3, 0.625, 1.25 mg
Estradiol acetate	Femtrace	0.45 once daily	0.45–1.8 mg once daily	Dosage form available as 0.45, 0.9, 1.8 mg
Micronized 17β-estradiol	Estrace Generics	1 mg once daily	1 or 2 mg once daily	Administer 3 weeks on and 1 week off Dosage form available as 0.5, 1, 2 mg
Transdermal estrogens patches				
17β-estradiol	Alora	0.025 mg/day (patch applied twice weekly)[c]	0.025–0.1 mg/day (patch applied twice weekly)[c]	Dosage form available as 0.025, 0.05, 0.075, 0.1 mg/day
	Climara	0.025 mg/day (patch applied once weekly)[c]	0.025–0.1 mg/day (patch applied once weekly)[c]	Dosage form available as 0.025, 0.0375, 0.05, 0.06, 0.075, 0.1 mg/day
	Menostar	0.014 mg/day (patch applied once weekly)[c,d]	0.014 mg/day (patch applied once weekly)[c,d]	Dosage form available as 0.014 mg/day

(Continued)

TABLE 31-2 FDA-Approved Estrogen Products for Menopausal Hormone Therapy (Continued)

Drug	Brand Name[a]	Initial Dose/Low Dose	Usual Dose Range	Comments
Transdermal estrogens patches (continued)				
	Estraderm	–	0.05 or 0.1 mg/day (patch applied twice weekly)[c]	Dosage form available as 0.05, 0.1 mg/day
	Minivelle, Vivelle, Vivelle Dot	0.025 mg/day (patch applied twice weekly)[c]	0.025–0.1 mg/day, 0.05 is standard dose (patch applied twice weekly)[c]	Dosage form available as 0.025, 0.0375, 0.05 (standard dose), 0.075, 0.1 mg/day
Other topical forms of estrogen				
17β-estradiol topical emulsion	Estrasorb 0.25% emulsion	–	Two pouches once daily (which delivers 0.05 mg of estradiol per day)	Apply to legs
17β-estradiol topical gel	EstroGel 0.06% metered-dose pump	–	1.25 g/day once daily (contains 0.75 mg estradiol)	Apply from wrist to shoulder
	Elestrin 0.06% metered-dose pump	–	1–2 unit doses once daily (1 unit dose: 0.87 g, which contains 0.52-mg estradiol)	Apply to upper arm
	Divigel 0.1% (topical once daily)	0.25 g once daily	0.25–1 g (provides 0.25–1 mg of estradiol)	Apply to upper thigh; dosage form available as 0.25, 0.5, 0.75, 1 mg
17β-estradiol transdermal spray	Evamist	1 spray once daily	1–3 sprays once daily (1.53 mg of estradiol per spray)	Apply to inner surface of forearm
Implanted estrogens[e]				
Implanted 17β-estradiol	Estradiol pellets	25-mg implanted subcutaneously every 6 months	50–100 mg implanted subcutaneously every 6 months	

Vaginal estrogens

Estradiol acetate vaginal ring	Femring	12.4 mg every 3 months	12.4-, 24.8-mg ring (delivers 0.05- or 0.1-mg estradiol/day)	Administer 21 days on and 7 days off

Intravaginal Estrogen Products (for the treatment of urogenital symptoms only/low systemic exposure)

Conjugated equine estrogens (CEE) vaginal cream	Premarin		0.5–2 g/day (contains 0.625 mg CEE per g)	Dosage form available as tube containing 1½ oz with calibrated applicator for delivery of 1, 2, 3, or 4 g
17β-estradiol vaginal cream	Estrace	2–4 g daily for 1 or 2 weeks then gradually reduced to ½ initial dosage for similar period	Maintenance dose of 1 g, one to three times weekly	
17β-estradiol vaginal ring	Estring	2 mg replaced every 90 days	2 mg ring (delivers 0.0075 mg/day) replaced every 90 days	
17β-estradiol vaginal insert	Imvexxy	1 vaginal insert daily for 2 weeks, then 1 insert twice weekly	4 or 10 mcg twice weekly	
Estradiol hemihydrate vaginal tablet	Vagifem Yuvafem Generics	10 mcg once weekly for 2 weeks, then twice weekly	10 mcg twice weekly	

aUS brand names.
bOrally administered estrogens stimulate synthesis of hepatic proteins and increase circulating concentrations of sex hormone-binding globulin, which in turn may compromise the bioavailability of androgens and estrogens. Women with elevated triglyceride concentrations or significant liver function abnormalities are candidates for nonoral estrogen therapy.
cDo not apply estrogen patches on or near breasts. Avoid waistline as patch may rub off with tight-fitting clothing.
dFDA-approved for prevention of postmenopausal osteoporosis only.
eNot available in the United States.

✓ Adverse effects of estrogen include nausea, headache, breast tenderness, and heavy bleeding. More serious adverse effects include increased risk for stroke, venous thromboembolism (VTE), and gall bladder disease. Transdermal estrogen is less likely to cause breast tenderness, gallbladder disease, and deep vein thrombosis.

✓ The Women's Health Initiative (WHI) trial showed an overall increase in the risk of coronary heart disease in healthy postmenopausal women ages 50−79 years taking estrogen–progestogen therapy compared to placebo. The estrogen-alone arm showed no effect (either increase or decrease) in the risk of coronary heart disease.

✓ The more recent Early versus Late Intervention Trial with Estradiol (ELITE) trial suggests that the benefits of hormone therapy are dependent on the timing of initiation and hormone therapy may be cardioprotective if started around the time of menopause (within 6 years) and therapy may be harmful when initiated in late postmenopausal women (after 10 years). MHT should not be initiated or continued solely for prevention of cardiovascular disease.

✓ Risk of VTE and stroke increases with oral MHT containing estrogen, but the absolute risk is low in women below 60 years of age. Transdermal MHT and low-dose oral estrogen therapy appear to have a lower risk of VTE and stroke compared to standard-dose oral estrogen regimens. The norpregnane progestogens also appear to be thrombogenic. MHT should be avoided in women at high risk for thromboembolic events (eg, those with Factor V Leiden mutation, obesity, or history of previous thromboembolic events).

✓ MHT is contraindicated in women with a personal history of breast cancer. In the WHI, the risk of MHT-related breast cancer appears to be associated with the addition of progestogen to estrogen after 3 years of combined use.

✓ The WHI trial suggests that combined oral MHT does not increase endometrial cancer risk compared with placebo, but estrogen alone given to women with an intact uterus significantly increases uterine cancer risk.

✓ While the WHI trial suggested that oral combined MHT does not increase the risk of ovarian cancer, more recent research now suggests that MHT are associated with an increased risk of ovarian cancer regardless of the type or the regimen used. More research is needed.

✓ The WHI study found that postmenopausal women 65 years or older taking estrogen plus progestogen therapy had twice the rate of dementia, including Alzheimer disease, than those taking placebo. Combined therapy did not prevent mild cognitive impairment. The estrogen-alone arm showed similar findings.

Progestogens

• In women who have not undergone hysterectomy, a **progestogen** or tissue-selective estrogen complex (estrogen/bazedoxifene) should be added for endometrial protection.

• Several progestogen regimens to prevent endometrial hyperplasia are shown in Table 31-3. **Combination estrogen–progestogen** regimens are shown in Table 31-4.

TABLE 31-3	Progestogen Dosing for Endometrial Protection (Cyclic Administration)
Progestogen	**Dosage**
Medroxyprogesterone acetate	5−10 mg/day for 12−14 days per calendar month (oral dosage form available as 2.5-, 5-, 10-mg tablets)
Micronized progesterone	200 mg/day for 12−14 days per calendar month (oral dosage form available as 100- and 200-mg tablets)
Norethindrone acetate	5 mg/day for 12−14 days per calendar month (oral dosage form available as 2.5-, 5-mg tablets)

TABLE 31-4	Common Combination Menopausal Hormone Therapy Regimens	
Regimen	**Brand name**	**Dosage**
Oral Regimens		
Conjugated equine estrogen (CEE) + medroxyprogesterone acetate (MPA)	Prempro (continuous)	0.625 mg CEE/2.5 mg MPA, 0.625 mg CEE/5 mg MPA daily
		Low-dose: 0.3 mg CEE/1.5 mg MPA, 0.45 mg CEE/1.5 mg MPA daily
	Premphase (continuous sequential)	0.625 mg CEE daily only in the first 2 weeks of a 4-week cycle, then 0.625 mg daily, CEE + 5 mg MPA daily in the last 2 weeks of a 4-week cycle
Conjugated equine estrogen (CEE) + bazedoxifene	Duavee (continuous)	0.45/20 mg daily
Ethinyl estradiol (EE) + norethindrone acetate (NETA)	Generic, Femhrt (continuous)	Femhrt: 2.5 mcg EE/0.5 mg NETA daily
	Fayvolv (continuous)	Fyavolv: 2.5 mcg EE/0.5 mg NETA daily, 5 mcg EE/1 mg NETA daily
Estradiol (E) + drospirenone (DRSP)	Angeliq (continuous)	1 mg E/0.5 mg DRSP daily
		Low dose: 0.5 mg E/0.25 mg DRSP daily
Estradiol (E) + norgestimate	Prefest (estrogen/ intermittent progestogen)	1 mg E daily for first 3 days, then 1 mg E/0.09 mg norgestimate daily for next 3 days; this pattern is repeated continuously
Estradiol (E) + norethindrone acetate (NETA)	Activella (continuous)	1 mg E/0.5 mg NETA daily
	Mimvey (continuous)	Low-dose: 0.5 mg E/0.1 mg NETA daily
	Mimvey Lo (continuous)	
	Amabelz (continuous)	
	Lopreeza (continuous)	
Estradiol (E) + progesterone	Bijuva (continuous)	1 mg E/100 mg progesterone daily
Transdermal Regimens		
Estradiol + norethindrone acetate patch	CombiPatch (continuous)	Continuous: 0.05/0.14 mg, 0.05/0.25 mg (apply 1 patch twice weekly)
	CombiPatch (continuous sequential)	Continuous sequential: 0.05 mg of an estradiol only patch (apply 1 patch twice weekly) in the first 2 weeks of a 4-week cycle, then either dose of the CombiPatch (apply 1 patch twice weekly) in the last 2 weeks of a 4-week cycle
Estradiol (E) + levonorgestrel patch	Climara Pro (continuous)	0.045 mg E/0.015 mg/day (apply 1 patch once weekly)

CEE, conjugated equine estrogen; DRSP, drospirenone; E, estradiol; EE, ethinyl estradiol; NETA, norethindrone acetate; MPA, medroxyprogesterone acetate.

Methods of administration include the following:

- **Continuous-cyclic estrogen-progestogen (sequential)** results in scheduled vaginal withdrawal bleeding in approximately 90% of women. The progestogen is administered 12−14 days of the 28-day cycle.
- **Continuous-combined estrogen-progestogen** causes endometrial atrophy but prevents monthly bleeding. It may initially cause unpredictable spotting or bleeding. Use of conjugated equine estrogens [0.625 mg/day] plus medroxyprogesterone acetate [2.5 mg/day]) lead to a decreased risk of endometrial cancer in the WHI study.
- **Continuous long-cycle estrogen-progestogen (cyclic withdrawal).** Estrogen is given daily, and progestogen is given six times yearly (every other month) for 12−14 days, resulting in six periods per year. Bleeding may be heavier and last for more days than with sequential use.
- **Intermittent-combined estrogen-progestogen (continuous pulsed)** consists of 3 days of estrogen therapy alone, followed by 3 days of combined estrogen and progestogen, repeated without interruption. It causes fewer side effects than regimens with higher progestogen doses and lowers the incidence of uterine bleeding.
    ✓ Adverse effects of progestogens include irritability, headache, mood swings, fluid retention, and sleep disturbance. See previous estrogen section for additional adverse effects associated with estrogen and progesterone in combination.

Compounded Bioidentical Hormone Therapy (CBHT)

- CBHTs are hormone therapy formulations custom-prepared (ie, compounded) for individual patients, often involving the use of measuring and monitoring hormone levels in blood and/or other body fluids such as saliva. Hormones commonly used in CBHT include estrone, estradiol, estriol, progesterone, testosterone, DHEA, and thyroid hormone. Bioidentical hormones appear to carry the same risks as traditional hormone therapy products and several major medical organizations have released statements against this practice.

Non-Hormonal Treatments

- For women with contraindications to or who cannot tolerate estrogens and/or progestogens, other treatment options for hot flushes can be considered (Table 31-5). Some clinicians consider selective serotonin reuptake inhibitors (eg, **paroxetine, fluoxetine, citalopram, escitalopram**) or serotonin-norepinephrine reuptake inhibitors (eg, **venlafaxine** and **desvenlafaxine**) to be first-line agents. **Clonidine** can be effective, but side effects are often problematic (eg, sedation, dry mouth, hypotension). **Gabapentin** has beneficial effects for reducing the frequency and severity of vasomotor symptoms but side effects may limit dosing. It may be a reasonable option for women with disrupted sleep and hot flashes when administered in the evening.

Androgens

- **Testosterone** use in women, although controversial, is becoming more common, even in the absence of androgen deficiency. Testosterone, with or without estrogen, may improve the quality of the sexual experience in postmenopausal women.
- Absolute contraindications to androgen therapy include pregnancy or lactation and known or suspected androgen-dependent neoplasia.
- Excessive dosage may cause virilization, fluid retention, and adverse lipoprotein lipid effects, which are more likely with oral administration. Evidence on the efficacy and safety of testosterone in women is lacking, and its use is currently not recommended.
- Adverse effects include virilization, fluid retention, and potentially adverse lipoprotein lipid effects, which are more likely with oral administration.
- **Dehydroepiandrosterone** (DHEA) is a precursor hormone in the synthesis of estrone, estradiol, and testosterone. Intravaginal DHEA (Prasterone) has FDA approval for the treatment of moderate-to-severe dyspareunia at a dose of 6.5 mg once daily at bedtime, which does not appear to convey the same systemic risks seen from other oral hormonal products.

TABLE 31-5	Alternatives to Estrogen for Treatment of Hot Flashes[a]			
Drug	**Brand Name[b]**	**Initial Dose**	**Usual Dose Range**	**Comments**
Tibolone[c]	Livial (not available in the United States)	2.5 mg	2.5 mg/day	Tibolone is not recommended during the perimenopause period because it may cause irregular bleeding
Venlafaxine	Effexor, Effexor XR	37.5 mg	37.5—150 mg/day	Adverse effects include nausea, headache, somnolence, dizziness, insomnia, nervousness, xerostomia, anorexia, constipation, diaphoresis, weakness, and hypertension
Desvenlafaxine	Pristiq	100—150 mg	100—150 mg/day	Adverse effects include nausea, headache, somnolence, dizziness, insomnia, xerostomia, anorexia, constipation, diaphoresis, and weakness
Paroxetine[d]	Brisdelle[e], Paxil, Paxil CR, Pexeva	7.5 mg/day (paroxetine)[e], 10 mg/day (paroxetine), or 12.5 mg/day (paroxetine CR)	7.5 mg/day[e], 10[e]—20 mg/day or 12.5—25 mg/day	Adverse effects include nausea, somnolence, insomnia, headache, dizziness, xerostomia, constipation, diarrhea, weakness, and diaphoresis
Citalopram		10 mg/day	10—20 mg/day	Adverse effects include drowsiness, insomnia, diaphoresis, nausea, xerostomia, dose-dependent QTc prolongation

(Continued)

TABLE 31-5	Alternatives to Estrogen for Treatment of Hot Flashes[a] *(Continued)*			
Drug	Brand Name[b]	Initial Dose	Usual Dose Range	Comments
Escitalopram		10 mg/day, start with 5 mg/day in sensitive or older women and titrate up	10–20 mg/day	Adverse effects include headache, insomnia, nausea, increased sweating, fatigue, and somnolence; decreased libido and anorgasmia
Clonidine	Catapres and generic tablets (oral) Catapres-TTS (transdermal) Kapvay tablets (extended release; oral)	0.1 mg/day	0.1 mg/day	Adverse effects include drowsiness, dizziness, hypotension, and dry mouth, especially with higher doses
Pregabalin	Lyrica	150 mg/day	150–300 mg/day	Adverse effects include drowsiness, dizziness, dry mouth, edema, blurred vision, weight gain, impaired concentration
Gabapentin	Gralise, Neurontin	300 mg at bedtime	900 mg/day (divided in three daily doses), doses up to 2400 mg/day (divided in three daily doses) have been studied	Adverse effects include somnolence and dizziness; these symptoms often can be obviated with a gradual increase in dosing

[a]Treatment of postmenopausal hot flashes is an off-label indication in the United States for all medications listed except for one formulation of paroxetine (paroxetine mesylate).
[b]US brand names.
[c]Not available in the United States.
[d]Other selective serotonin reuptake inhibitors (eg, citalopram, escitalopram, fluoxetine, and sertraline) have also been studied and may be used for the treatment of hot flashes.
[e]The brand Brisdelle contains 7.5 mg of paroxetine and is FDA-approved to treat moderate-to-severe vasomotor symptoms of menopause. This specific product is not FDA-approved for treating psychiatric conditions.
CR, controlled release; XR, extended release.

Selective Estrogen Receptor Modulators (SERMs)

- SERMs are nonsteroidal compounds that act as estrogen agonists in some tissues such as bone and as estrogen antagonists in other tissues such as breast through high-affinity binding to the estrogen receptor.
- **Tamoxifen** is an antagonist in breast tissue and an agonist on the bone and endometrium (see Chapter 60).
- **Raloxifene** is approved for prevention and treatment of postmenopausal osteoporosis and reduction in risk of invasive breast cancer. The dose is 60 mg once daily.
- The third-generation SERM, **bazedoxifene**, is used in conjunction with **conjugated estrogen**, and is FDA-approved for moderate-to-severe vasomotor symptoms and prevention of osteoporosis.
- **Ospemifene** is approved for moderate-to-severe dyspareunia from menopausal vulvar and vaginal atrophy. It has a boxed warning for increased risk of endometrial cancer in women with a uterus who use ospemifene (an estrogen agonist in the endometrium) without a progestogen to reduce endometrial hyperplasia. It also has a boxed warning about the possible risk of stroke and VTE.
    - ✓ Depending on tissue selectively, the SERMs are associated with hot flashes and leg cramps. They can also increase the risk of VTE and stroke similar to oral estrogen, but the degree of risk is agent specific. Additional side effects of bazedoxifene include muscle spasms, nausea, diarrhea, dyspepsia, upper abdominal pain, oropharyngeal pain, dizziness, and neck pain. Adverse effects of ospemifene include hot flashes, vaginal discharge, muscle spasm, genital discharge, and hyperhidrosis.

Tibolone

- Tibolone (unavailable in the United States) has combined estrogenic, progestogenic, and androgenic activity and improves mood, libido, menopausal symptoms, and vaginal atrophy. It protects against bone loss and reduces the risk of vertebral fractures. It reduces total cholesterol and triglycerides, but may decrease high-density lipoprotein concentrations. It decreases the risk of breast and colon cancer in women ages 60–85 years.
    - ✓ Adverse effects include weight gain and bloating, increased risk of stroke in older women, and possible breast cancer recurrence. It may increase endometrial cancer risk.

Complementary and Alternative Agents

Phytoestrogens

- Phytoestrogens are plant compounds with estrogen-like biologic activity and relatively weak estrogen receptor-binding properties, resulting in physiologic effects in humans.
- Although some data support their use, clarity regarding, dosing, biological activity, safety, and efficacy is needed before they can be considered as an alternative to MHT in postmenopausal women.
    - ✓ Common adverse effects include constipation, bloating, and nausea.

Others

- Other herbals and alternative treatments that may be used by women include **black cohosh, dong quai, red clover leaf** (contains phytoestrogens), and **ginseng**. Complementary and alternative therapies should not be recommended to treat menopausal symptoms as their efficacy and safety have not been completely established.

EVALUATION OF THERAPEUTIC OUTCOMES

- Management of patients taking hormone therapy is summarized in **Table 31-6**.
- In order to adequately assess treatment effect, women should be encouraged to continue their MHT regimen for at least 1 month with dosages being modified to

balance adverse effects and efficacy. Women receiving MHT should be seen annually for monitoring.
- Many women have no difficulty stopping MHT, while some develop vasomotor symptoms after discontinuation, regardless of discontinuation rate (ie, gradual or sudden withdrawal).

TABLE 31-6	Management of Patients Taking Hormone Therapy Regimens

Initiation of Hormone Therapy

Hormone therapy should be used only as long as vasomotor symptom control is necessary

Six-Week Follow-up Visit

To discuss patient concerns about hormone therapy

To evaluate the patient for symptom relief, adverse effects, and patterns of withdrawal bleeding (if continuous sequential hormone therapy is given)

Drug	Adverse Drug Reaction	Monitoring Parameter	Suggested Change
Estrogen		Persistence of hot flashes	Increase estrogen dose
Estrogen	Breast tenderness		Reduce estrogen dose; switch to a transdermal regimen
Progestogen	Bloating Premenstrual-like symptoms		Switch to another progestogen or bazedoxifene

Annual Follow-up Visit

Annual monitoring: Medical history, physical examination (including pelvic examination), blood pressure measurement, and routine endometrial cancer surveillance (as indicated). Additional follow-up is determined based on the patient's initial response to therapy and the need for any modification of the regimen.

Breast examinations: Annual mammograms (scheduled based on patient's age and risk factors).

Osteoporosis prevention: BMD should be measured in women 65 years and older and in women younger than 65 years with risk factors for osteoporosis. Repeat testing should be performed as clinically indicated.

In women taking sequential hormone therapy	Transvaginal ultrasound, and where indicated an endometrial biopsy should be performed if vaginal bleeding occurs at any time other than the expected time of withdrawal bleeding or when heavier or more prolonged withdrawal bleeding occurs (if endometrial pathology cannot be excluded by endovaginal ultrasonography, further evaluation may be required, such as hysteroscopy).
In women taking continuous combined hormone therapy	Endometrial evaluation should be considered when irregular bleeding persists for more than 6 months after initiating therapy.

BMD, bone mineral density.

See Chapter 98, Hormone Therapy in Women, authored by Devra K. Dang, Kathryn E. Wheeler, and Judy T. Chen, for a more detailed discussion of this topic.

- Resources on the use of *drugs in pregnancy and lactation* include the Food and Drug Administration (FDA) product labeling, the primary literature, tertiary compendia, textbooks, and computerized databases (eg, www.motherisk.org and www.toxnet. nlm.nih.gov).

PREGNANCY PHYSIOLOGY

- The duration of pregnancy is approximately 280 days (measured from the first day of the last menstrual period to birth). Pregnancy is divided into three periods of three calendar months (ie, trimesters).
- Drug absorption during pregnancy may be altered by delayed gastric emptying and vomiting. An increased gastric pH may affect absorption of weak acids and bases. Hepatic perfusion increases. Higher estrogen and progesterone levels may alter liver enzyme activity and increase elimination of some drugs but cause accumulation of others.
- Maternal plasma volume, cardiac output, and glomerular filtration increase by 30%−50% or higher during pregnancy, possibly lowering the plasma concentration of renally cleared drugs. Body fat increases; thus, volume of distribution of fat-soluble drugs may increase. Plasma albumin concentrations decrease; thus volume of distribution of highly protein-bound drugs may increase. However, there may be little change in serum concentration, as these unbound drugs are more rapidly cleared by the liver and kidneys.
- The placenta is the organ of exchange between the mother and fetus for drugs. Drugs with molecular weights less than 500 Dalton (Da) transfer readily, drugs with molecular weights from 600 to 1000 Da cross more slowly, and drugs with molecular weights greater than 1000 Da (eg, insulin and heparin) do not cross in significant amounts.
- Lipophilic drugs (eg, opiates and antibiotics) cross more easily than do water-soluble drugs. Certain protein-bound drugs may achieve higher plasma concentrations in the fetus than in the mother.

DRUG SELECTION DURING PREGNANCY

- The incidence of congenital malformation is approximately 3%−6%, with less than 1% of all birth defects caused by medication exposure.
- Principles for drug use during pregnancy include: (1) selecting drugs that have been used safely for a long time; (2) prescribing doses at the lower end of the dosing range; (3) eliminating nonessential medication and discouraging self-medication; and (4) avoiding medications known to be harmful.
- Adverse effects on the fetus depend on drug dosage, route of administration, and stage of pregnancy when the exposure occurred.
- Fetal exposure to a teratogen in the first 2 weeks after conception may have an "all or nothing" effect (ie, could destroy the embryo or have no ill effect). Exposure during organogenesis (18−60 days postconception) may cause structural anomalies (eg, **methotrexate, cyclophosphamide, diethylstilbestrol, lithium, retinoids, thalidomide**, some **antiepileptic drugs [AEDs]**, and **coumarin derivatives**).
- Exposure after this point may result in growth retardation, central nervous system (CNS) or other abnormalities, or death. **Nonsteroidal anti-inflammatory drugs (NSAIDs)** and **tetracycline derivatives** are more likely to exhibit effects in the second or third trimester.

PRECONCEPTION PLANNING

- **Folic acid** supplementation between 0.4 and 0.9 mg daily is recommended throughout the reproductive years to reduce the risk for neural tube defects (NTDs) in offspring. Women of childbearing potential who take AED medications should take prenatal vitamins with folic acid 0.4–5 mg/day. Higher folate doses should be used in women who have previously delivered a child with an NTD and those taking valproic acid.
- Reduction in the use of alcohol, tobacco, and other substances prior to pregnancy improves outcomes. For smoking cessation, behavioral interventions are preferred. Use of **nicotine replacement therapy** during pregnancy is controversial.

PREGNANCY-INFLUENCED ISSUES

GASTROINTESTINAL TRACT

- Constipation commonly occurs during pregnancy. Institute education, physical exercise, and increased intake of dietary fiber and fluid. If additional therapy is warranted, give **supplemental fiber** and/or a stool softener. **Polyethylene glycol, lactulose**, and **sorbitol**, can be used intermittently. **Senna** and **bisacodyl** can also be used occasionally. Magnesium and sodium salts can cause electrolyte imbalance. Avoid **castor oil** and **mineral oil**.
- Therapy for gastroesophageal reflux disease includes lifestyle and dietary modifications, for example, small, frequent meals; alcohol, tobacco, and caffeine avoidance; food avoidance before bedtime; and elevation of the head of the bed. If necessary, initiate **aluminum, calcium**, or **magnesium antacids; sucralfate; cimetidine** or **ranitidine**. Proton pump inhibitors are options if response to histamine 2 (H_2)–receptor blockers is inadequate. Avoid **sodium bicarbonate** and **magnesium trisilicate**.
- Therapy for hemorrhoids includes high intake of dietary fiber, adequate oral fluid intake, and use of sitz baths. If response is inadequate, laxatives and stool softeners can be used. Topical anesthetics, skin protectants, and astringents may help irritation and pain. Topical hydrocortisone may reduce inflammation and pruritus.
- Nonpharmacologic treatments for nausea and vomiting include eating small, frequent meals; avoiding fatty and spicy foods; and acupressure. Pharmacotherapy may include ginger, antihistamines (eg, **doxylamine**), and **pyridoxine**. The American College of Obstetricians and Gynecologists (ACOG) considers pyridoxine alone or in combination with doxylamine to be first-line treatment. Metoclopramide and phenothiazines are considered safe, but may cause sedation and extrapyramidal effects. **Ondansetron** may cause oral clefts.
- **Corticosteroids** have been effective for hyperemesis gravidarum (ie, severe nausea and vomiting causing weight loss >5% of prepregnancy weight, dehydration, and ketonuria), but the risk of oral clefts is increased. They should not be used during the first trimester.

GESTATIONAL DIABETES MELLITUS (GDM)

- All high-risk women should be screened for overt diabetes at their first prenatal visit.
- **Table 32-1** summarizes the screening and diagnosis of GDM which should occur during weeks 24–28.
- First-line therapy for GDM includes exercise, dietary modification, and caloric restrictions for obese women. Daily self-monitoring of blood glucose is required. If lifestyle interventions fail to achieve glycemic control, drug therapy is indicated. Glycemic control is preprandial capillary glucose concentrations at or below 95 mg/dL (5.3 mmol/L) along with one of the following: a 1-hour postprandial glucose at or below 140 mg/dL (7.8 mmol/L), or a 2-hour postprandial glucose of 120 mg/dL (6.7 mmol/L) or below. **Human insulin** is the drug of choice for diabetes management during pregnancy, because it does not cross the placenta. **Glyburide** and **metformin** are alternatives, but long-term safety data are limited and they may not be as effective as insulin.

TABLE 32-1	Screening and Diagnosis of Gestational Diabetes Mellitus		
One-Step Method		**Two-Step Method**	
Give	75-g OGTT[a]	*Step 1*	Give 50-g OGTT[b]
	If any plasma glucose levels are met or exceeded, GDM is diagnosed		
Fasting	≥92 mg/dL (5.1 mmol/L)	1-hour	≥130 mg/dL (7.2 mol/L), ≥135 mg/dL (7.5 mmol/L), or ≥140 mg/dL (7.8 mmol/L)[c]
			If plasma glucose level is met or exceeded, proceed to Step 2[d]
1-hour	≥180 mg/dL (10 mmol/L)	*Step 2*	Give 100-g OGTT[a]
			If two or more plasma glucose levels are met or exceeded, GDM is diagnosed
2-hour	≥153 mg/dL (8.5 mmol/L)		Carpenter–Coustan Method[e]
		Fasting	95 mg/dL (5.3 mmol/L)[d]
		1-hour	180 mg/dL (10 mmol/L)
		2-hour	155 mg/dL (8.6 mmol/L)
		3-hour	140 mg/dL (7.8 mmol/L)

[a]Perform with plasma glucose measurement in a fasting state. Should be performed in the morning after fasting at least 8 hours.
[b]Perform with plasma glucose measurement in a fasting or nonfasting state.
[c]Threshold set by individual practices; lower thresholds equate to higher false-positive results.
[d]If >200 mg/dL (11.1 mmol/L), diagnosis of GDM is made; do not proceed to step 2.
[e]Carpenter and Coustan developed diagnostic criteria for gestational diabetes that lowered diagnostic plasma glucose levels compared to the National Diabetes Data Group.
OGTT, oral glucose tolerance test.

- Screening with a 2-hour OGTT at 6 weeks postpartum is recommended for those diagnosed with GDM to diagnose type 2 diabetes not recognized prior to pregnancy.

HYPERTENSION (HTN)

- Hypertensive disorders of pregnancy (HDP) include: (1) preeclampsia–eclampsia, (2) chronic hypertension (HTN; preexisting HTN or developing before 20 weeks' gestation), (3) chronic HTN with superimposed preeclampsia, and (4) gestational HTN (ie, HTN without proteinuria developing after 20 weeks' gestation).
- Eclampsia, a medical emergency, is preeclampsia with seizures. HTN in pregnancy is either systolic blood pressure above 140 mm Hg or diastolic blood pressure above 90 mm Hg based on two or more measurements at least 4 hours apart. Severe HTN is two measurements of systolic blood pressure >160 mm Hg and/or diastolic blood pressure >110 mm Hg at least 15 minutes apart.
- Nondrug management of HDP includes stress reduction and light exercise or activity restriction. Exercise >50 minutes 3 days a week can reduce the incidence of HTN threefold over women who are more sedentary.

- For women at risk for preeclampsia, low-dose **aspirin** (60–81 mg/day) beginning weeks 12–28 of gestation reduces the risk for preeclampsia. Aspirin also reduces the risk of preterm birth by 14% and intrauterine grown restriction by 20%. Calcium and/or vitamin D supplementation may decrease the relative risk of HTN and pre-eclampsia. ACOG states that these recommendations do not apply to populations with adequate calcium intake, such as the United States.
- Antihypertensive drug therapy is discussed later under Chronic Illnesses in Pregnancy below.
- **Magnesium sulfate** (4–6 g IV over 15–20 minutes followed by a 2 g/hr continuous infusion) decreases the risk of progression of preeclampsia to eclampsia by almost 60%, and it also treats eclamptic seizures. Avoid **diazepam** and **phenytoin**.

THYROID ABNORMALITIES

- Gestational transient thyrotoxicosis usually resolves by 20 weeks' gestation. Antithyroid medication is usually not needed.
- Pregnant women with overt hyperthyroidism should be treated with **methimazole** or **propylthiouracil** (PTU), and those with overt hypothyroidism should receive thyroid replacement therapy (ie, **levothyroxine**).

VENOUS THROMBOEMBOLISM (VTE)

- For treatment of acute thromboembolism during pregnancy, **low-molecular-weight heparin (LMWH)** is preferred over **unfractionated heparin** or **warfarin**. Continue treatment throughout pregnancy and for 6 weeks after delivery. Duration of therapy should not be less than 3 months. Avoid fondaparinux, lepirudin, and bivalirudin unless a severe allergy to heparin exists. Dabigatran, rivaroxaban, and apixaban are not recommended. Avoid warfarin because it may cause fetal bleeding, nasal hypoplasia, stippled epiphyses, or CNS anomalies.
- For women at intermediate or high risk for recurrent VTE, provide antepartum prophylaxis with LMWH plus 6-week postpartum prophylaxis with LMWH or warfarin. For women with prosthetic heart valves, thrombophilias, and those at very high risk for VTE, consult current guidelines.

ACUTE CARE ISSUES IN PREGNANCY

HEADACHE

- For tension and migraine headaches during pregnancy, first-line therapies are non-pharmacologic, including relaxation, stress management, and biofeedback.
- For tension headache, **acetaminophen** or **ibuprofen** can be used if necessary. All NSAIDs and aspirin are contraindicated in the third trimester because of the potential for closure of the ductus arteriosus. Aspirin may also cause maternal and fetal bleeding, and decreased uterine contractility. **Opioids** are rarely used.
- For migraine headache, acetaminophen and ibuprofen can be used. Opioids have been used, but they can contribute to nausea, and long-term use can cause neonatal withdrawal. For nonresponsive migraines, **sumatriptan** can be used. **Ergotamine** and **dihydroergotamine** are contraindicated. For migraine-associated nausea, **promethazine**, **prochlorperazine**, and **metoclopramide** can be used.
- For pregnant women with severe headaches (usually migraine) not responsive to other treatments, **propranolol**, at the lowest effective dose, can be used as preventive treatment. Alternatives include **amitriptyline** or **nortriptyline**, 10–25 mg daily by mouth.

URINARY TRACT INFECTION

- The principal infecting organism is *Escherichia coli*, but *Proteus mirabilis*, *Klebsiella pneumoniae*, and group B *Streptococcus* cause some infections. Untreated bacteriuria may result in pyelonephritis, preterm labor, HTN, anemia, transient renal failure, and low birth weight.

- Treatment of asymptomatic bacteriuria is necessary to reduce the risk of pyelonephritis and premature delivery. Treatment of asymptomatic bacteriuria and cystitis for 7–14 days is common.
- The most commonly used antibiotics for asymptomatic bacteriuria and cystitis are the β-lactams (penicillins and cephalosporins) and nitrofurantoin. *E. coli* resistance to ampicillin and amoxicillin is problematic. **Nitrofurantoin** is not active against *Proteus* and should not be used after week 37 in patients with glucose-6-phosphate dehydrogenase deficiency due to concern for hemolytic anemia in the newborn. **Sulfa-containing drugs** may increase the risk for kernicterus in the newborn and should be avoided during the last weeks of gestation. **Folate antagonists**, such as **trimethoprim**, are relatively contraindicated during the first trimester because of their association with cardiovascular malformations. Regionally, increased rates of *E. coli* resistance to trimethoprim-sulfa limit its use. **Fluoroquinolones** and **tetracyclines** are contraindicated.
- Inpatient therapy for pyelonephritis has included parenteral administration of second- or third-generation cephalosporins, ampicillin plus gentamicin, or ampicillin-sulbactam. Switching to oral antibiotics can occur after the woman is afebrile for 48 hours, but avoid nitrofurantoin. The total duration of antibiotic therapy for pyelonephritis is 10–14 days.

SEXUALLY TRANSMITTED INFECTIONS (STIs)

- Pharmacotherapy for selected STIs is shown in **Table 32-2**.
- Complications of *Chlamydia trachomatis* include pelvic inflammatory disease, ectopic pregnancy, and infertility. *Chlamydia* infection can be transmitted at birth to the neonate and cause conjunctivitis and a subacute, afebrile pneumonia.
- **Benzathine penicillin G** is the drug of choice for all stages of syphilis except neurosyphilis, which is treated with **aqueous penicillin G**. Penicillin is effective for preventing transmission to the fetus and treating the already infected fetus.
- *Neisseria gonorrhoeae* is a risk factor for pelvic inflammatory disease and preterm delivery. Symptoms in the neonate (eg, rhinitis, vaginitis, urethritis, ophthalmia neonatorum, and sepsis) usually start within 2–5 days of birth. Blindness can occur. Oral cephalosporins have been removed as a preferred treatment option for gonorrhea because of antimicrobial resistance. Coinfection with *Chlamydia* is common, so usually treatment of gonorrhea includes treatment for *Chlamydia*.
- The overriding concern with genital herpes is transmission of the virus to the neonate during birth. Maternal use of **acyclovir** during the first trimester is not associated with an increased risk of birth defects. **Valacyclovir** is an alternative.
- Bacterial vaginosis is caused by anaerobic bacteria, mycoplasmas, and *Gardnerella vaginalis*. It is a risk factor for premature rupture of membranes, preterm labor, preterm birth, intra-amniotic infection, and postpartum endometritis.
- Trichomoniasis is associated with an increased risk of premature rupture of membranes, premature delivery, and low birth weight. Treatment may prevent respiratory or genital infection in the neonate.

CHRONIC ILLNESSES IN PREGNANCY

- **Table 32-3** shows treatment of some chronic illnesses in pregnancy.

ALLERGIC RHINITIS AND ASTHMA

- Diagnosis and staging of asthma during pregnancy is the same as in nonpregnant women, but more frequent follow-up is necessary. The risks of medication use to the fetus are lower than the risks of untreated asthma.
- Treatment of asthma follows a stepwise approach. As step 1, all pregnant patients with asthma should have access to a short-acting inhaled β_2-agonist (**albuterol** is the preferred agent). For persistent asthma (step 2 or higher), low, medium, or high doses of controller corticosteroids are foundational. **Budesonide** is preferred, but corticosteroids used before pregnancy can be continued. Long-acting β_2-agonists

TABLE 32-2	Management of Sexually Transmitted Infections in Pregnancy			
STI	Drug Name (Brand Name)	Usual Dose	Monitoring	Comments
Bacterial vaginosis	*Recommended:* Metronidazole (Flagyl) **OR**	500 mg by mouth two times daily × 7 days	Follow-up testing not required if symptoms resolve	No link between intravaginal clindamycin and newborn complications
	Metronidazole 0.75% gel	5 g intravaginally once daily × 5 days		Oral or vaginal preparations can be used
	Alternatives[a]: Clindamycin (Cleocin)			
Chlamydia	*Recommended:* Azithromycin (Zithromax)	1 g by mouth × 1 dose	Test-of-cure at 3–4 weeks after therapy completion; retest all after 3 months	Gonorrheal coinfection common; both are treated concurrently
	Alternatives[a]: Amoxicillin (Amoxil)			*Chlamydia* is asymptomatic in men and women
	Erythromycin base			Women below age 25 years and those at high risk should be retested in the third trimester
	Erythromycin ethylsuccinate			
Genital herpes	*Recommended:* Acyclovir (Zovirax) **OR**	400 mg by mouth three times a day	Routine serologic testing for HSV-2 is not recommended	Start treatment at 36 weeks of gestation
	Valacyclovir	500 mg by mouth twice a day		
Gonorrhea	*Recommended:* Ceftriaxone (Rocephin) *PLUS*	250 mg IM × 1 dose	Because of high reinfection rate, repeat testing for gonorrhea 3 months after treatment	Chlamydial coinfection common; both are treated concurrently
	Azithromycin (Zithromax)	1 g by mouth × 1 dose		Consult with infectious disease specialist in case of cephalosporin allergy

Syphilis[a]

Primary, secondary, early latent	*Recommended:* Benzathine penicillin G (Bicillin L-A)	2.4 million units IM × 1 dose; a second dose can be given 1 week after initia dose	Nontreponemal serologic evaluation[c] at 6 and 12 months	For treatment failure or reinfection, use same drug and dose but increase to 3 weekly doses unless neurosyphilis is present
Tertiary, late latent	*Recommended:* Benzathine penicillin G (Bicillin L-A)	2.4 million units IM × 3 doses at 1-week intervals	Nontreponemal serologic evaluation[b] at 6, 12, and 24 months. CSF examination may be required	Use this regimen for late latent or latent syphilis of unknown duration
Neurosyphilis	*Recommended:* Aqueous penicillin G (Pfizerpen)	3–4 million units IV every 4 hours or 18–24 million units IV continuously × 10–14 days	If initial elevation of leukocytes in CSF, repeat CSF examination every 6 months until normalization	Consider repeat treatment if CSF leukocytes or protein do not normalize after 2 years
	Alternative:[c] Procaine penicillin (Wycillin, Pfizerpen-AS) PLUS Probenecid	2.4 million units IM daily × 10–14 days 500 mg by mouth four times daily × 10–14 days		Use alternative regimen only if compliance can be ensured
Trichomoniasis	*Recommended:* Metronidazole	2 g by mouth × 1 dose	Rescreen HIV patients at 3 months after treatment	While tinidazole is an alternative for nonpregnant women, avoid during pregnancy

[a]Pregnant women with history of penicillin allergy should undergo penicillin desensitization as no proven alternatives exist.
[b]Nontreponemal evaluation consists of VDRL (Venereal Disease Research Laboratory) and RPR (rapid plasma regain).
[c]Refer to Reference 50 for specific dosing recommendations.
CSF, cerebrospinal fluid; IM, intramuscular; STI, sexually transmitted infection.

TABLE 32-3	Treatment of Chronic Illnesses in Pregnancy	
Chronic Illness	**Treatment**	**Comments**
Allergic rhinitis	• Intranasal corticosteroids • Intranasal cromolyn • Antihistamines (chlorpheniramine, diphenhydramine, hydroxyzine)	Budesonide and beclomethasone most widely studied intranasal corticosteroids
		Second-generation antihistamines do not appear to increase fetal risk, but are less extensively studied than first-generation products
		Use of external nasal dilator, short-term topical oxymetazoline, or ICS is preferable to oral decongestants
Asthma		Budesonide is the preferred ICS, but any may be used
Step 1 (intermittent)	• SABA (albuterol)	
Step 2 and above (persistent)	• SABA (albuterol) • Step-appropriate ICS • LABA	Alternatives are cromolyn (less effective), leukotriene receptor antagonists (less experience in pregnancy), and theophylline (more potential toxicity)
		Systemic corticosteroids recommended to gain control in patients with most severe disease
Epilepsy	Probably safest AEDs • Carbamazepine • Lamotrigine • Levetiracetam • Phenytoin Lower risk than VPA • Gabapentin • Oxcarbazepine • Zonisamide Significant risk greater than other AEDs • Phenobarbital • Topiramate • VPA	Polytherapy carries higher risk of major malformations than monotherapy
		Rates of major malformation with AEDs range between 0.7 and 10 per 100 exposures
		Phenytoin, phenobarbital, and topiramate may cause cleft palate
		Phenobarbital is associated with cardiac malformations
		Risk for most AED-associated malformations is dose-dependent

(continued)

TABLE 32-3	Treatment of Chronic Illnesses in Pregnancy (*Continued*)	
Chronic Illness	**Treatment**	**Comments**
HIV	Currently receiving ART: • Continue current regimen if viral load is suppressed ART-naïve, no evidence of resistance, preferred regimen: • Dual NRTI backbone PLUS • Ritonavir-boosted PI • Integrase inhibitor	ARV drug resistance testing should be performed to guide ART if HIV RNA is >500 copies/mL (0.5 x 10^6/L) for ART-naïve women For women already receiving ART with virologic failure and HIV RNA >1000 copies/mL (1.0 x 10^6/L), ARV drug-resistance testing should be performed to inform change in ARV therapy
Hypertension, chronic	Initial treatment: • Labetalol • Nifedipine • Methyldopa	ACE inhibitors, ARBs, renin inhibitors, mineralocorticoid receptor antagonists are not recommended Atenolol has been associated with fetal growth restriction Thiazide diuretics theoretically lower the increase in plasma volume during pregnancy, but are considered second-line
Thyroid disorders	Hypothyroid • Levothyroxine	For hypothyroidism, attain a TSH of 0.1–2.5, 0.2–3, and 0.3–3 milli-international units/L (mIU/L) in the first, second, and third trimester, respectively
	Hyperthyroid • PTU • Methimazole	Use PTU in first trimester followed by switch to methimazole in second and third trimester to balance the risk of PTU-induced hepatotoxicity and methimazole embryopathy

ACE, angiotensin converting enzyme; AED, antiepileptic drug; ARB, angiotensin receptor blocker; ART, antiretroviral therapy; ARV, antiretroviral; ICS, inhaled corticosteroid; LABA, long-acting beta agonist; NNRTI, nonnucleoside reverse transcriptase inhibitor; NRTI, nucleoside reverse transcriptase inhibitor; NTDs, neural tube defects; PI, protease inhibitor; PTU, propylthiouracil; SABA, short-acting beta agonist; TSH, thyroid-stimulating hormone; VPA, valproic acid.

are safe. **Cromolyn, leukotriene receptor antagonists**, and **theophylline** are considered alternative agents, but they are not preferred. For patients with the most severe disease, systemic corticosteroids are recommended.

- First-line medications for allergic rhinitis during pregnancy include intranasal **corticosteroids, nasal cromolyn**, and first-generation antihistamines (eg, **chlorpheniramine, diphenhydramine**, and **hydroxyzine**). **Intranasal corticosteroids** are the most effective treatment and have a low risk for systemic effect. **Beclomethasone** and **budesonide** have been used most. **Loratadine** and **cetirizine** do not appear to increase fetal risk, but they have not been extensively studied.
- Use of an external nasal dilator, short-term **topical oxymetazoline**, or **inhaled corticosteroids** may be preferred over oral decongestants, especially during early pregnancy.

DIABETES MELLITUS

- Glycemic control can change dramatically during pregnancy, and frequent adjustments may be needed. Self-monitored blood glucose should occur before and after meals, and sometimes between 2 and 4 AM. Patients with type 1 or 2 diabetes may continue human insulin. Data have not shown that the use of insulin analogs (eg, insulin aspart, insulin detemir, insulin glargine, insulin lispro) to cause major safety concerns in pregnancy. Metformin (and to lesser extent glyburide) can be considered, however, safety data are limited.

EPILEPSY

- Major malformations are two to three times more likely in children born to women taking AEDs than to those who do not, but the risks of untreated epilepsy to the fetus are considered to be greater than those associated with the AEDs.
- When possible, avoid valproic acid during pregnancy to minimize the risk of NTDs, facial clefts, and cognitive teratogenicity. Phenobarbital and topirimate should also be avoided. If either is used during pregnancy, the lowest effective dose should be used.
- Drug therapy should be optimized prior to conception, and AED monotherapy is recommended when possible.
- If drug withdrawal is planned, it should be fully completed prior to conception.
- All women taking AEDs should take folic acid, 4–5 mg daily, starting before pregnancy and continuing through at least the first trimester and preferably through the entire pregnancy.

HUMAN IMMUNODEFICIENCY VIRUS (HIV) INFECTION

- In women newly diagnosed with HIV, or who have not previously received antiretroviral therapy (ART), it should be initiated as soon as pregnancy is determined, since risk of perinatal transmission is lower with earlier viral suppression. ART therapy is selected from those recommended for nonpregnant adults (with consideration given to the teratogenic profiles of each drug). Women already taking ART therapy should continue their regimen provided that viral suppression below the level of detection is documented.
- Recommendations regarding combination ART change frequently and the most recent clinical guidelines can be found at https://aidsinfo.nih.gov.
- Pregnant women with HIV RNA levels above 1000 copies/mL (1000 × 10³/L) approaching delivery should have cesarean section at 38 weeks' gestation to reduce the risk of perinatal HIV transmission. Cesarean section is not recommended if HIV RNA levels are at or below that level. If maternal viral load is greater than that level or unknown, IV zidovudine should be initiated with a 1-hour load (2 mg/kg) followed by a continuous infusion (1 mg/kg/hr) for 2 hours (cesarean) or until vaginal delivery. Women with a viral load at or below 1000 copies/mL (1000 × 10³/L) near delivery do not require zidovudine IV, but should continue their ART.

HYPERTENSION

- HTN occurring before 20 weeks of gestation, the use of antihypertensive medications before pregnancy, or the persistence of HTN beyond 12 weeks postpartum defines chronic HTN in pregnancy. It is classified as mild/nonsevere (systolic blood pressure [sBP] 140–159 mm Hg or diastolic blood pressure [dBP] 90–109 mm Hg), or severe (sBP 160 mm Hg or higher or dBP 110 mm Hg or higher). Chronic HTN can cause maternal complications, fetal growth restriction, and hospital admission.
- ACOG recommends drug therapy for pregnant women with persistent chronic HTN with a blood pressure of 160/105 mm Hg and above. When antihypertensive therapy is used, maintenance of sBP between 120 and 160 mm Hg and dBP between 80 and 105 mm Hg is recommended. If there is no evidence of end-organ damage, and sBP is below 160 mm Hg and dBP is below 105 mm Hg, drug therapy is not suggested.
- Severe HTN in pregnancy requires treatment, and lowering of BP should occur over a period of hours to prevent compromise of uteroplacental blood flow. Recommended agents are parenteral **labetalol** and **hydralazine**, but hydralazine is associated with more maternal and fetal adverse effects. Oral **nifedipine** may also be used. Limited evidence supports the use of **magnesium sulfate**, except when it is being used concomitantly for preeclampsia. **Nitroprusside, diazoxide**, and **nitroglycerin** should be reserved for refractory HTN in an appropriately monitored environment.

DEPRESSION

- Antidepressants should be used at the lowest possible dose for the shortest possible time to minimize adverse fetal and maternal pregnancy outcomes. Monotherapy is preferred over polytherapy even if higher doses are required.
- Pregnant women who stopped taking antidepressants are more likely to relapse than women who completed treatment.
- The **selective serotonin reuptake inhibitors (SSRIs)** are not considered major teratogens with the exception of paroxetine. Initiation of paroxetine, for women who intend to become pregnant, or are in their first trimester of pregnancy, should be considered only after other treatment options have been evaluated because of the risk for cardiovascular malformations in the fetus. The **serotonin/norepinephrine reuptake inhibitors (SNRIs)** are less well defined. Use of SSRIs and SNRIs in the latter part of pregnancy is associated with persistent pulmonary HTN of the newborn and prenatal antidepressant exposure syndrome (ie, cardiac, respiratory, neurologic, gastrointestinal, and metabolic complications from drug toxicity or withdrawal of drug therapy). Tricyclic antidepressants are not considered major teratogens but have been associated with neonatal withdrawal syndrome when used late in pregnancy.

THYROID DISORDERS

- For hypothyroidism in pregnancy, initiate **levothyroxine** 0.1 mg/day. Women receiving thyroid replacement therapy before pregnancy may require increased dosage during pregnancy. Monitor thyroid-stimulating hormone (TSH) levels every 4–6 weeks during pregnancy to allow for dose titration according to TSH levels.
- Hyperthyroidism therapy includes the thioamides (eg, **methimazole, PTU**). The goal of therapy is to attain free thyroxine concentrations near the upper limit of normal.

LABOR AND DELIVERY

PRETERM LABOR

- Preterm labor is labor that occurs between 20 and 37 weeks of gestation when changes in cervical dilations and/or effacement happen along with regular uterine contractions or when the initial presentation includes regular contractions and cervical dilation of at least 2 cm.

Tocolytic Therapy

- Tocolytic therapy is used to postpone delivery long enough to allow for maximum effect of antenatal steroids, for transportation of the mother to a facility equipped to deal with high-risk deliveries, and to prolong pregnancy when there are underlying self-limited conditions that can cause labor. Tocolytics can be started when there are regular uterine contractions with cervical change. They are not generally used beyond 34 weeks of gestation. Do not use them in cases of previability, intrauterine fetal demise, a lethal fetal anomaly, intrauterine infection, fetal distress, severe pre-eclampsia, vaginal bleeding, or maternal hemodynamic instability.
- There are four classes of tocolytics in the United States: **β-agonists**, **magnesium sulfate**, **prostaglandin inhibitors** (ie, NSAIDs), and **calcium channel blockers**. Prolongation of pregnancy with tocolytics is not associated with significant reduction in rates of respiratory distress syndrome, neonatal death, or birth before 37 weeks of gestation. Prostaglandin inhibitors and calcium channel blockers may be preferable, based on delaying delivery and improving neonatal outcomes.
- β-Agonists (**terbutaline** and **ritodrine** [unavailable in the United States]) have a higher risk for maternal side effects. A common dose of terbutaline is 250 mcg sub-cutaneously which may be repeated in 15–30 minutes for inadequate response, with a maximum of 500 mcg given in a 4-hour period.
  ✓ An FDA black box warning cautions against oral dosing or prolonged parenteral use (beyond 48–72 hours) because of maternal cardiotoxicity and death.
- A Cochrane review does not support the effectiveness of **magnesium sulfate** for tocolysis. However, it can be used IV during preterm labor to decrease the occurrence of moderate-to-severe cerebral palsy.
- **Nifedipine** is associated with fewer side effects than magnesium or β-agonist therapy and decreases risk of delivery within 7 days compared to β-agonist. Nifedipine loading doses range between 10 and 40 mg, with subsequent dosing of 10–20 mg every 4–6 hours, with dose adjustment based on patterns of preterm contractions. Five to 10 mg nifedipine may be administered sublingually every 15–20 minutes for three doses. Once stabilized, 10–20 mg may be administered orally every 4–6 hours for preterm contractions.
  ✓ It can cause hypotension and a change in uteroplacental blood flow.
- **Indomethacin**, 50–100 mg orally or rectally, followed by 25–50 mg orally every 6 hours for 48 hours has been used.
  ✓ Premature constriction of the ductus arteriosus has been reported.

Antenatal Glucocorticoids

- A Cochrane review shows the benefit of antenatal **corticosteroids** for fetal lung maturation to prevent respiratory distress syndrome, intraventricular hemorrhage, and death in infants delivered prematurely.
- Current recommendations are **betamethasone**, 12 mg IM every 24 hours for two doses, or **dexamethasone**, 6 mg IM every 12 hours for four doses, to pregnant women between 24 and 34 weeks' gestation who are at risk for preterm delivery within the next 7 days. Benefits from antenatal glucocorticoid administration are believed to begin within 24 hours.

GROUP B *STREPTOCOCCUS* INFECTION

- Prenatal screening (vaginal/rectal cultures) for group B *Streptococcus* colonization of all pregnant women at 35–37 weeks' gestation is recommended. If cultures are positive, or if the woman had a previous infant with invasive group B *Streptococcus* disease, or if the woman had group B *Streptococcus* bacteriuria, antibiotics are given.
- The currently recommended regimen for group B *Streptococcus* disease is **penicillin G**, 5 million units IV, followed by 2.5 million units IV every 4 hours until delivery. Alternatives include **ampicillin**, 2 g IV, followed by 1 g IV every 4 hours; **cefazolin**, 2 g IV, followed by 1 g every 8 hours; **clindamycin**, 900 mg IV every 8 hours; or **erythromycin**, 500 mg IV every 6 hours. In penicillin-allergic women in whom sensitivity

testing shows resistance to clindamycin and erythromycin, **vancomycin**, 1 g IV every 12 hours until delivery, can be used.

CERVICAL RIPENING AND LABOR INDUCTION

- Prostaglandin E_2 analogues (eg, **dinoprostone** [Prepidil Gel and Cervidil Vaginal Insert]) are commonly used for cervical ripening. Fetal heart rate monitoring is required when Cervidil Vaginal Insert is used and for 15 minutes after its removal. **Misoprostol**, a prostaglandin E_1 analogue, is effective and inexpensive.
  ✓ It has been associated with uterine rupture.
- **Oxytocin** is the most commonly used agent for labor induction after cervical ripening.

LABOR ANALGESIA

- Nonpharmacologic options for labor analgesia include continuous support from nurses, midwives, childbirth educators, or doulas (lay women trained in labor support) as well as warm water baths and acupuncture.
- The IV or IM administration of narcotics is commonly used for pain associated with labor. Compared with epidural analgesia, parenteral **opioids** are associated with lower rates of oxytocin augmentation, shorter stages of labor, and fewer instrumental deliveries.
- Epidural analgesia involves administering an opioid and/or an anesthetic (eg, **fentanyl** and/or **bupivacaine**) through a catheter into the epidural space to provide pain relief. Patient-controlled epidural analgesia results in a lower total dose of local anesthetic.
  ✓ Epidural analgesia is associated with longer stages of labor, more instrumental deliveries, and maternal fever compared to parenteral narcotic analgesia. Complications of epidural analgesia include hypotension, itching, and urinary retention.
- Other options for labor analgesia include spinal analgesia, combined spinal-epidural analgesia, and nerve blocks.

POSTPARTUM HEMORRHAGE (PPH)

- PPH is an obstetrical emergency and is a major cause of morbidity and mortality worldwide.
- A stepwise approach to the treatment is advised starting with exclusion of retained products of contraception.
- Oxytocin administration results in reduced maternal blood loss, fewer cases of PPH, and a shorter third stage of labor. Other agents to use include **methylergonovine, carboprost**, and **tranexamic acid**.

DRUG USE DURING LACTATION

- Medications enter breast milk via passive diffusion of nonionized and non-protein-bound medication. Drugs with high molecular weights, lower lipid solubility, and higher protein binding are less likely to cross into breast milk, or they transfer more slowly or in smaller amounts. The higher the maternal serum concentration of drug, the higher the concentration will be in breast milk. Drugs with longer half-lives are more likely to maintain higher levels in breast milk. The timing and frequency of feedings and the amount of milk ingested by the infant are also important.
- Strategies for reducing infant risk from drugs transferred into breast milk include selecting medications for the mother that would be considered safe for use in the infant and choosing medications with shorter half-lives, higher protein binding, lower bioavailability, and lower lipid solubility.
- Penicillin-resistant *Staphylococcus aureus* is the most common bacterial cause of mastitis. Treatment with penicillinase-resistant penicillins or cephalosporins may be indicated. Application of heat and direct massage along with NSAIDs may be used for pain relief.

POSTPARTUM DEPRESSION

- Postpartum depression affects up to 13% of women, with almost 5% experiencing major depression
- Nonpharmacologic treatment may include interpersonal psychotherapy, cognitive behavioral therapy, and group/family therapy.
- Sertraline, paroxetine, fluoxetine, and nortriptyline are the most studied in the postpartum period and selection of medication with low transfer to breast milk is desirable.

RELACTATION

- For relactation use **metoclopramide**, 10 mg three times daily for 7–14 days only if nondrug therapy is ineffective.

See Chapter 95, Pregnancy and Lactation: Therapeutic Considerations, authored by Kristina E. Ward, for a more detailed discussion of this topic.

CHAPTER 33

Anemias

- *Anemia* is a group of diseases characterized by a decrease in either hemoglobin (Hb) or the volume of red blood cells (RBCs), resulting in decreased oxygen-carrying capacity of blood. The World Health Organization defines anemia as Hb less than 13 g/dL (130 g/L; 8.07 mmol/L) in men or less than 12 g/dL (120 g/L; 7.45 mmol/L) in women.

PATHOPHYSIOLOGY

- The functional classification of anemias is found in **Fig. 33-1**. The most common anemias are included in this chapter.
- Morphologic classifications are based on cell size. Macrocytic cells are larger than normal and are associated with deficiencies of vitamin B_{12} or folic acid. Microcytic cells are smaller than normal and are associated with iron deficiency, whereas normocytic anemia may be associated with recent blood loss or chronic disease.
- Iron-deficiency anemia (IDA), characterized by decreased levels of ferritin (most sensitive marker) and serum iron, and decreased transferrin saturation, can be caused by inadequate dietary intake, inadequate gastrointestinal (GI) absorption, increased iron demand (eg, pregnancy), blood loss, and chronic diseases.
- Vitamin B_{12}– and folic acid–deficiency anemias, macrocytic in nature, can be caused by inadequate dietary intake, malabsorption syndromes, and inadequate utilization. Deficiency of intrinsic factor causes decreased absorption of vitamin B_{12} (ie, pernicious anemia). Folic acid–deficiency anemia can be caused by hyperutilization due to pregnancy, hemolytic anemia, myelofibrosis, malignancy, chronic inflammatory disorders, long-term dialysis, or growth spurt. Drugs can cause anemia by reducing absorption of folate (eg, phenytoin) or through folate antagonism (eg, methotrexate).
- Anemia of inflammation (AI) is a newer term used to describe both anemia of chronic disease and anemia of critical illness. A diagnosis of exclusion, AI is an anemia that traditionally has been associated with malignant, infectious, or inflammatory processes, tissue injury, and conditions associated with release of proinflammatory cytokines. Serum iron is decreased but in contrast to IDA, the serum ferritin concentration is normal or increased. See **Table 33-1** for diseases associated with AI. For information on anemia of chronic kidney disease, see Chapter 75.
- Age-related reductions in bone marrow reserve can render elderly patients more susceptible to anemia caused by multiple minor and often unrecognized diseases (eg, nutritional deficiencies) that negatively affect erythropoiesis.
- Pediatric anemias are often due to a primary hematologic abnormality. The risk of IDA is increased by rapid growth spurts and dietary deficiency.

CLINICAL PRESENTATION

- Signs and symptoms depend on rate of development and age and cardiovascular status of the patient. Acute-onset anemia is characterized by cardiorespiratory symptoms such as palpitations, angina, orthostatic light-headedness, and breathlessness. Chronic anemia is characterized by weakness, fatigue, headache, orthopnea, dyspnea on exertion, vertigo, faintness, cold sensitivity, pallor, and loss of skin tone.

FIGURE 33-1. Functional classification of anemia. Each of the major categories of anemia (hypoproliferative, maturation disorders, and hemorrhage/hemolysis) can be further subclassified according to the functional defect in the several components of normal erythropoiesis.

- IDA is characterized by glossal pain, smooth tongue, reduced salivary flow, pica (compulsive eating of nonfood items), and pagophagia (compulsive eating of ice).
- Neurologic effects (eg, numbness and paraesthesisas) of vitamin B_{12} deficiency may precede hematologic changes. Psychiatric findings, including irritability, depression, and memory impairment, may also occur with vitamin B_{12} deficiency. Anemia with folate deficiency is not associated with neurologic symptoms.

DIAGNOSIS

- Rapid diagnosis is essential because anemia is often a sign of underlying pathology. Severity of symptoms does not always correlate with the degree of anemia.
- Initial evaluation of anemia involves a complete blood cell count (CBC), reticulocyte index, and examination of the stool for occult blood. Figure 33-2 shows a broad, general algorithm for the diagnosis of anemia based on laboratory data.
- The earliest and most sensitive laboratory change for IDA is decreased serum ferritin (storage iron), which should be interpreted in conjunction with decreased transferrin saturation and increased total iron-binding capacity (TIBC). Hb, hematocrit (Hct), and RBC indices usually remain normal until later stages of IDA.
- In macrocytic anemias, mean corpuscular volume is usually elevated to greater than 100 fL. Vitamin B_{12} and folate concentrations can be measured to differentiate between the two deficiency anemias. A vitamin B_{12} value less than 200 pg/mL (148 pmol/L), together with appropriate peripheral smear and clinical symptoms, is diagnostic of vitamin B_{12}–deficiency anemia. A decreased RBC folate concentration (less than 150 ng/mL [340 nmol/L]) appears to be a better indicator of folate-deficiency anemia than a decreased serum folate concentration (less than 3 ng/mL [7 nmol/L]).
- The diagnosis of AI is usually one of exclusion, with consideration of coexisting iron and folate deficiencies. Serum iron is usually decreased, but, unlike IDA, serum ferritin is normal or increased, and TIBC is decreased. The bone marrow reveals an abundance of iron; the peripheral smear reveals normocytic anemia.

TABLE 33-1	Diseases Causing Anemia of Inflammation

Common causes

Chronic infections
  Tuberculosis
  Other chronic lung infections (eg, lung abscess, bronchiectasis)
  Human immunodeficiency virus
  Subacute bacterial endocarditis
  Osteomyelitis
  Chronic urinary tract infections
Chronic inflammation
  Rheumatoid arthritis
  Systemic lupus erythematosus
  Inflammatory bowel disease
  Inflammatory osteoarthritis
  Gout
  Other (collagen vascular) diseases
  Chronic inflammatory liver diseases
Malignancies
  Carcinoma
  Lymphoma
  Leukemia
  Multiple myeloma

Less common causes

Alcoholic liver disease
Congestive heart failure
Thrombophlebitis
Chronic obstructive pulmonary disease
Ischemic heart disease

- Elderly patients with symptoms of anemia should undergo a CBC with peripheral smear and reticulocyte count and other laboratory studies as needed to determine the etiology of anemia.
- The diagnosis of anemia in pediatric populations requires use of age- and sex-adjusted norms for laboratory values.

TREATMENT

- <u>Goals of Treatment</u>: The goals are to return hematologic parameters to normal, restore normal function and quality of life, and prevent long-term complications.

IRON-DEFICIENCY ANEMIA

- **Oral iron** therapy with soluble ferrous iron salts, which are not enteric coated and not slow or sustained release, is recommended at a daily dosage of 150–200 mg elemental iron in two or three divided doses (see **Table 33-2**).

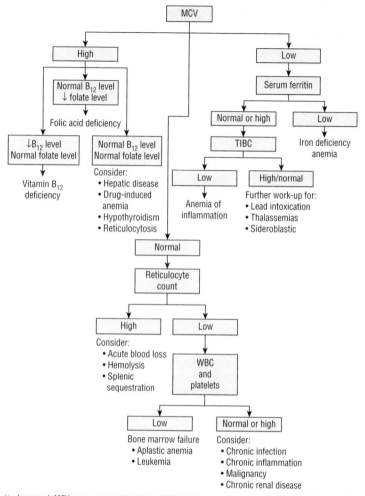

(↓, decreased; MCV, mean corpuscular volume; TIBC, total iron-binding capacity; WBC, white blood cells.)

FIGURE 33-2. General algorithm for diagnosis of anemias.

- Iron is best absorbed from meat, fish, and poultry. Administer iron at least 1 hour before meals because food interferes with absorption, but administration with food may be needed to improve tolerability.
- Consider **parenteral iron** for patients with iron malabsorption, intolerance of oral iron therapy, or nonadherence. The following formula can be used to estimate the total dose of parenteral iron needed to correct anemia:

  Dose of iron (mg) = whole blood hemoglobin deficit (g/dL) × body weight (lb) or Dose of iron (mg) = whole blood hemoglobin deficit (g/L) × body weight (kg) × 0.22

- An additional quantity of iron to replenish stores should be added (about 600 mg for women and 1000 mg for men).

TABLE 33-2	Oral Iron Products	
Iron Salt	**Percent Elemental Iron**	**Common Formulations and Elemental Iron Provided**
Ferrous sulfate	20	60–65 mg/324–325 mg tablet
		60 mg/5 mL syrup
		44 mg/5 mL elixir
		15 mg/1 mL drops
Ferrous sulfate (exsiccated)	30	65 mg/200 mg tablet
		50 mg/160 mg tablet
Ferrous gluconate	12	38 mg/325 mg tablet
		28–29 mg/240–246 mg tablet
Ferrous fumarate	33	66 mg/200 mg tablet
		106 mg/324–325 mg tablet

- **Iron dextran, sodium ferric gluconate, iron sucrose, ferumoxytol,** and **ferric carboxymaltose** are available parenteral iron preparations with similar efficacy but different molecular size, pharmacokinetics, bioavailability, and adverse effect profiles (see **Table 75–2**).

VITAMIN B$_{12}$–DEFICIENCY ANEMIA

- Oral vitamin B$_{12}$ supplementation is as effective as parenteral, even in patients with pernicious anemia, because the alternate vitamin B$_{12}$ absorption pathway is independent of intrinsic factor. Initiate oral **cobalamin** at 1–2 mg daily for 1–2 weeks, followed by 1 mg daily.
- Parenteral therapy acts more rapidly than oral therapy and is recommended if neurologic symptoms are present. A popular regimen is IM **cyanocobalamin**, 1000 mcg daily for 1 week, then weekly for 1 month, and then monthly for maintenance therapy. Initiate daily oral cobalamin administration after symptoms resolve.
- Continue vitamin B$_{12}$ for life in patients with pernicious anemia.

FOLATE-DEFICIENCY ANEMIA

- Oral **folic acid**, 1 mg daily for 4 months, is usually sufficient for treatment of folic acid–deficiency anemia, unless the etiology cannot be corrected. If malabsorption is present, a dose of 1–5 mg daily may be necessary. Parenteral folic acid is available but rarely necessary.

ANEMIA OF INFLAMMATION

- Treatment of AI is less specific than that of other anemias and should focus on correcting reversible causes. Reserve iron therapy for an established IDA; iron is not effective when inflammation is present. RBC transfusions are effective but should be limited to episodes of inadequate oxygen transport and Hb of 7–8 g/dL (70–80 g/L; 4.34–4.97 mmol/L).
- **Erythropoiesis-stimulating agents (ESAs)** can be considered, but response can be impaired in patients with AI. The initial dosage for **epoetin alfa** is 50–100 units/kg three times weekly and **darbepoetin alfa** 0.45 mcg/kg once weekly. Iron, cobalamin, and folic acid supplementation may improve response to ESA treatment.
- Potential toxicities of exogenous ESA administration include increases in blood pressure, nausea, headache, fever, bone pain, and fatigue. Hb must be monitored during

ESA therapy. An increase in Hb greater than 12 g/dL (120 g/L; 7.45 mmol/L) with treatment or a rise of greater than 1 g/dL (10 g/L; 0.62 mmol/L) every 2 weeks has been associated with increased mortality and cardiovascular events.

- In patients with anemia of critical illness, parenteral iron is often used but is associated with a theoretical risk of infection.

ANEMIA IN PEDIATRIC POPULATIONS

- Infants aged 9–12 months: Administer ferrous sulfate 3–6 mg/kg/day (elemental iron) divided once or twice daily between meals for 4 weeks. Continue for two additional months in responders to replace storage iron pools. The dose and schedule of vitamin B_{12} should be titrated according to clinical and laboratory response. The daily dose of folic acid is 1 mg.

EVALUATION OF THERAPEUTIC OUTCOMES

- IDA: Positive response to oral iron therapy is characterized by modest reticulocytosis in a few days with an increase in Hb seen at 2 weeks. Reevaluate the patient if reticulocytosis does not occur. Hb should return to normal after 2 months; continue iron therapy until iron stores are replenished and serum ferritin normalized (up to 12 months).
- Megaloblastic anemia: Signs and symptoms usually improve within a few days after starting vitamin B_{12} or folic acid therapy. Neurologic symptoms can take longer to improve or can be irreversible, but should not progress during therapy. Reticulocytosis should occur within 3–5 days. Hb begins to rise a week after starting vitamin B_{12} therapy and should normalize in 1–2 months. Hct should rise within 2 weeks after starting folic acid therapy and should normalize within 2 months.
- ESAs: Reticulocytosis should occur within a few days. Monitor iron, TIBC, transferrin saturation, and ferritin levels at baseline and periodically during therapy. The optimal form and schedule of iron supplementation are unknown. Discontinue ESAs if a clinical response does not occur after 8 weeks.
- Pediatrics: Monitor Hb, Hct, and RBC indices 4–8 weeks after initiation of iron therapy. Monitor Hb or Hct weekly in premature infants.

See Chapter 100, Anemias, authored by Kristen Cook and Devon M. Greer, for a more detailed discussion of this topic.

34 Sickle Cell Disease

- *Sickle cell syndromes*, which can be divided into sickle cell trait (SCT) and sickle cell disease (SCD), are hereditary conditions characterized by the presence of sickle hemoglobin (HbS) in red blood cells (RBCs).
- SCT is the heterozygous inheritance of one normal β-globin gene producing hemoglobin A (HbA) and one sickle gene producing HbS (HbAS) gene. Individuals with SCT are asymptomatic.
- SCD can be of homozygous or compounded heterozygous inheritance. Homozygous HbS (HbSS) has historically been referred to as sickle cell anemia (SCA), which now also includes HbSβ⁰-thal due to similarities in clinical severity. The heterozygous inheritance of HbS with another qualitative or quantitative β-globin mutation results in sickle cell hemoglobin C (HbSC), sickle cell β-thalassemia (HbSβ⁺-thal and HbSβ⁰-thal), and some other rare phenotypes.

PATHOPHYSIOLOGY

- Clinical manifestations of SCD are due to impaired circulation, RBC destruction, and stasis of blood flow and ongoing inflammatory responses. These changes result from disturbances in RBC polymerization and membrane damage. In addition to sickling, other factors contributing to the clinical manifestations include functional asplenia (and increased risk of infection by encapsulated organisms), deficient opsonization, and coagulation abnormalities.
- Polymerization allows deoxygenated hemoglobin to exist as a semisolid gel that protrudes into the cell membrane, distorting RBCs into sickle shapes. Sickle-shaped RBCs increase blood viscosity and encourage sludging in the capillaries and small vessels, leading to local tissue hypoxia that accentuates the pathologic process.
- Repeated cycles of sickling, upon deoxygenation, and unsickling, upon oxygenation, damage the RBC membrane and cause irreversible sickling. Rigid, sickled RBCs are easily trapped, resulting in shortened circulatory survival and chronic hemolysis.

CLINICAL PRESENTATION

- SCD involves multiple organ systems. Clinical manifestations depend on the genotype (**Table 34-1**).
- Cardinal features of SCD are hemolytic anemia and vasoocclusion. Symptoms are delayed until 4–6 months of age when HbS replaces fetal hemoglobin (HbF). Common findings include pain with fever, pneumonia, splenomegaly, and, in infants, pain and swelling of the hands and feet (eg, hand-and-foot syndrome or dactylitis).
- Usual clinical signs and symptoms of SCD include chronic anemia; fever; pallor; arthralgia; scleral icterus; abdominal pain; weakness; anorexia; fatigue; enlarged liver, spleen, and heart; and hematuria.
- Acute complications of SCD include fever and infection (eg, sepsis caused by encapsulated pathogens such as *Streptococcus pneumoniae*), stroke, acute chest syndrome, and priapism. Acute chest syndrome is characterized by pulmonary infiltration, respiratory symptoms, and equivocal response to antibiotic therapy.
- Acute episodes of pain can be precipitated by fever, infection, dehydration, hypoxia, acidosis, and sudden temperature changes. The most common type is vasoocclusive pain, which is manifested by pain over the involved areas without change in Hb. Aplastic crisis is characterized by acute decrease in Hb with decreased reticulocyte count manifested as fatigue, dyspnea, pallor, and tachycardia. Acute splenic sequestration is the sudden massive enlargement of the spleen due to sequestration of sickled RBCs. The trapping of sickled RBCs by the spleen leads to hypotension and

TABLE 34-1	Clinical Features of Sickle Cell Trait and Common Types of Sickle Cell Disease
Type	**Clinical Features**
Sickle cell trait (SCT)	Rare painless hematuria; heavy exercise under extreme conditions can provoke gross hematuria and complications (normal Hb)
Sickle cell anemia (SCA-HbSS)	Pain episodes, microvascular disruption of organs (spleen, liver, bone marrow, kidney, brain, and lung), gallstones, priapism, leg ulcers; anemia (Hb 6–9 g/dL [60–90 g/L; 3.72–5.59 mmol/L])
Sickle cell hemoglobin C (HbSC)	Painless hematuria and rare aseptic necrosis of bone; pain episodes are less common and occur later in life; other complications are ocular disease and pregnancy-related problems; mild anemia (Hb 9–14 g/dL [90–140 g/L; 5.59–8.69 mmol/L])
Sickle cell β⁺-thalassemia (HbSβ⁺-thal)	Rare pain; milder severity than HbSS because production of some HbA; Hb 9–12 g/dL (90–120 g/L; 5.59–7.45 mmol/L) with microcytosis
Sickle cell β⁰-thalassemia (HbSβ⁰-thal)	No HbA production; severity similar to SCA; Hb 7–9 g/dL (70–90 g/L; 4.34–5.59 mmol/L) with microcytosis

Hb, hemoglobin; HbA, hemoglobin A.

shock, and can cause sudden death in young children. Repeated infarctions lead to autosplenectomy; therefore, incidence declines as adolescence approaches.

- Chronic complications involve many organs and include pulmonary hypertension, airway inflammation and hyperresponsiveness, bone and joint destruction, ocular problems, cholelithiasis, cardiovascular abnormalities, depression, hematuria, and other renal complications. Children experience delayed growth and sexual maturation.
- Patients with SCT are usually asymptomatic, except for rare painless hematuria. Other reported complications associated with SCT are delayed hemorrhage after eye trauma, venous thromboembolism, particularly pulmonary embolism, and chronic kidney disease.

DIAGNOSIS

- SCD is usually identified by routine neonatal screening programs using isoelectric focusing, high-performance liquid chromatography, or electrophoresis.
- Laboratory findings include low hemoglobin; increased reticulocyte, platelet, and white blood cell counts; and sickled red cell forms on the peripheral smear.

TREATMENT

- <u>Goals of Treatment</u>: The goals are to reduce hospitalizations, complications, and mortality.

GENERAL PRINCIPLES

- Patients with SCD require lifelong interprofessional care that combines general symptomatic supportive care, preventative medical therapies, and specific disease-modifying therapies.
- Routine immunizations plus influenza, meningococcal, and pneumococcal vaccinations are recommended.

- Prophylactic **penicillin** is recommended until at least 5 years of age. An effective regimen is penicillin V potassium, 125 mg orally twice daily until 3 years of age and then 250 mg orally twice daily until age 5 years.

DISEASE-MODIFYING THERAPIES

- HbF directly affects polymer formation. Increases in HbF correlate with decreased RBC sickling and adhesion. Patients with low HbF levels have more frequent pain and higher mortality. HbF levels of 20% or greater reduce the risk of acute sickle cell complications.
- **Hydroxyurea**, a chemotherapeutic agent, stimulates HbF production and increases the number of HbF-containing reticulocytes and intracellular HbF. It is indicated for patients 2 years of age and older with recurrent moderate to severe painful crises to reduce the frequency of pain crises and the need for blood transfusions. The recommended single daily dose for adults is 15 mg/kg and 20 mg/kg for children (**Fig. 34-1**).
- **ʟ-Glutamine** is approved for SCD patients age 5 and older to reduce the acute complications of SCD. Dose is weight-based: 5 g twice a day for <30 kg; 10 g twice a day for 30–65 kg and 15 g twice a day for >65 kg.
- Chronic RBC transfusions are indicated for primary and secondary stroke prevention and amelioration of organ damage. Transfusions are usually given every 3–4 weeks or as needed to maintain desired HbS levels. The optimal duration of primary prophylactic transfusion therapy in children is unknown. Risks include alloimmunization, hyperviscosity, viral transmission (requiring hepatitis A and B vaccination), volume and iron overload, and transfusion reactions.
- Allogeneic hematopoietic stem cell transplantation is the only curative therapy for SCD. The best candidates are younger than 16 years, have severe complications, and have human leukocyte antigen–matched donors. Risks must be carefully considered and include mortality, graft rejection, and secondary malignancies.

TREATMENT OF COMPLICATIONS

- Educate patients to recognize conditions that require urgent evaluation. Balanced fluid status and oxygen saturation of at least 92% are important to avoid exacerbation during acute illness.
- RBC transfusions are indicated for acute exacerbation of baseline anemia (eg, aplastic crisis, hepatic or splenic sequestration, or severe hemolysis), severe vasoocclusive episodes, and procedures requiring general anesthesia.
- Promptly evaluate fever of 38.5°C (101.3°F) or higher. Empiric antibiotic therapy should provide coverage against encapsulated organisms (eg, **ceftriaxone** for outpatients and **cefotaxime** for inpatients; **clindamycin** for cephalosporin-allergic patients).
- For acute chest syndrome, initiate incentive spirometry; appropriate fluid therapy; broad-spectrum antibiotics, including a **macrolide** or **quinolone**; and, for hypoxia or acute distress, oxygen therapy. Other potential therapies include steroids and nitric oxide.
- Priapism has been treated with analgesics, antianxiety agents, and vasoconstrictors to force blood out of the corpus cavernosum (eg, **phenylephrine** and **epinephrine**), and vasodilators to relax smooth muscle (eg, **terbutaline** and **hydralazine**).
- Treatment of aplastic crisis is primarily supportive. Blood transfusions may be indicated for severe or symptomatic anemia.
- Hydration and blood transfusions are indicated to treat hypovolemia associated with splenic sequestration. Manage recurrent episodes with observation and splenectomy. Consider chronic transfusions in children younger than 2 years of age to delay splenectomy until the age of 2 years. Splenectomy is an option for chronic hypersplenism.
- Hydration and analgesics are mainstays of treatment for vasoocclusive (painful) crisis. Administer fluids IV or orally at 1–1.5 times the maintenance requirement; monitor closely to avoid volume overload. Consider an infectious etiology and initiate empiric therapy if indicated.

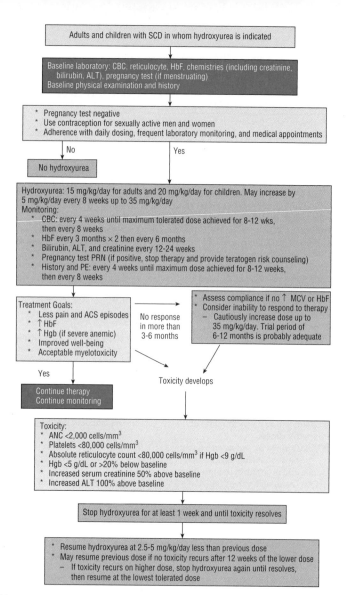

Adults and children with SCD in whom hydroxyurea is indicated

Baseline laboratory: CBC, reticulocyte, HbF, chemistries (including creatinine, bilirubin, ALT), pregnancy test (if menstruating)
Baseline physical examination and history

* Pregnancy test negative
* Use contraception for sexually active men and women
* Adherence with daily dosing, frequent laboratory monitoring, and medical appointments

No → No hydroxyurea

Yes

Hydroxyurea: 15 mg/kg/day for adults and 20 mg/kg/day for children. May increase by 5 mg/kg/day every 8 weeks up to 35 mg/kg/day
Monitoring:
* CBC: every 4 weeks until maximum tolerated dose achieved for 8-12 wks, then every 8 weeks
* HbF every 3 months × 2 then every 6 months
* Bilirubin, ALT, and creatinine every 12-24 weeks
* Pregnancy test PRN (if positive, stop therapy and provide teratogen risk counseling)
* History and PE: every 4 weeks until maximum dose achieved for 8-12 weeks, then every 8 weeks

Treatment Goals:
* Less pain and ACS episodes
* ↑ HbF
* ↑ Hgb (if severe anemic)
* Improved well-being
* Acceptable myelotoxicity

No response in more than 3-6 months →

* Assess compliance if no ↑ MCV or HbF
* Consider inability to respond to therapy
  – Cautiously increase dose up to 35 mg/kg/day. Trial period of 6-12 months is probably adequate

Yes

Continue therapy
Continue monitoring

Toxicity develops

Toxicity:
* ANC <2,000 cells/mm³
* Platelets <80,000 cells/mm³
* Absolute reticulocyte count <80,000 cells/mm³ if Hgb <9 g/dL
* Hgb <5 g/dL or >20% below baseline
* Increased serum creatinine 50% above baseline
* Increased ALT 100% above baseline

Stop hydroxyurea for at least 1 week and until toxicity resolves

* Resume hydroxyurea at 2.5-5 mg/kg/day less than previous dose
* May resume previous dose if no toxicity recurs after 12 weeks of the lower dose
  – If toxicity recurs on higher dose, stop hydroxyurea again until resolves, then resume at the lowest tolerated dose

(ACS, acute chest syndrome; ALT, alanine aminotransferase; ANC, absolute neutrophil count; CBC, complete blood cell count; Hb, hemoglobin; HbF, fetal hemoglobin; HbSS, homozygous sickle cell hemoglobin; HbSSβ⁰, sickle cell β⁰-thalassemia; MCV, mean corpuscular volume; PE, physical examination; PRN, as needed; RBC, red blood cell.)

FIGURE 34-1. Hydroxyurea use in sickle cell disease. (*Data from Alrayyes S, Baghdan D, Haddad RY, et al. Sickle cell disease: An overview of the disease and its systemic effects. Dis Mon. 2018;64:283–289; Ware RE, de Montalembert M, Tshilolo L, Abboud MR. Sickle cell disease. Lancet. 2017;390:311–323; Quinn CT. Sickle cell disease in childhood: From newborn screening through transition to adult medical care. Pediatr Clin North Am. 2013;60:1363–1381; National Institutes of Health, National Heart Lung and Blood Institute. Evidence-Based Management of Sickle Cell Disease: Expert Panel Report.* http://www.nhlbi.nih.gov/health-pro/guidelines/sickle-cell-disease-guidelines/. *Accessed, October 15, 2018.*)

- Tailor analgesic therapy to the individual because of the variable frequency and severity of pain. Pain scales should be used to quantify the degree of pain.
- Use **nonsteroidal anti-inflammatory drugs (NSAIDs)** or **acetaminophen** for mild to moderate pain. Consider adding an opioid if mild to moderate pain persists. (eg, **codeine** or **hydrocodone**).
- Treat severe pain aggressively with an opioid, such as **morphine**, **hydromorphone**, **fentanyl**, or **methadone**. Avoid **meperidine** due to accumulation of the normeperidine metabolite, which can cause neurotoxicity, especially in patients with impaired renal function.
- Treat severe pain with an IV opioid titrated to pain relief and then administered on a scheduled basis with as-needed dosing for breakthrough pain. Patient-controlled analgesia is commonly utilized.
- Treatment of chronic pain in SCD requires an interprofessional team approach. Guidelines for chronic pain management are available.

EVALUATION OF THERAPEUTIC OUTCOMES

- Evaluate patients on a regular basis to establish baseline symptoms, monitor changes, and provide age-appropriate education.
- Evaluate CBC and reticulocyte counts every 3–6 months up to 2 years of age, then every 6–12 months. Screen HbF level annually until 2 years of age. Evaluate renal, hepatobiliary, and pulmonary function annually. Screen patients for retinopathy.
- Assess efficacy of hydroxyurea by monitoring the number, severity, and duration of sickle cell crises.

See Chapter 120, Sickle Cell Disease, authored by C. Y. Jennifer Chan and Melissa Frei-Jones, for a more detailed discussion of this topic.

CHAPTER 35

Antimicrobial Regimen Selection

- A systematic approach to the selection and evaluation of an antimicrobial regimen is shown in **Table 35-1**. An *empiric* antimicrobial regimen is begun before the offending organism is identified and sometimes before documentation of the presence of infection, whereas a *definitive* regimen is instituted when the causative organism is known.

CONFIRMING THE PRESENCE OF INFECTION

FEVER

- *Fever* is defined as a controlled elevation of body temperature above the expected 37°C (98.6°F) (measured orally) and is a manifestation of many disease states other than infection.
- Many drugs have been identified as causes of fever. Drug-induced fever is defined as persistent fever in the absence of infection or other underlying condition. The fever must coincide temporally with the administration of the offending agent and disappear promptly upon its withdrawal, after which the temperature remains normal.

WHITE BLOOD CELL COUNT

- Most infections result in elevated white blood cell (WBC) counts (leukocytosis) because of the mobilization of granulocytes and/or lymphocytes to destroy invading microbes. Normal values for WBC counts are between 4000 and 10,000 cells/mm^3 (4×10^9 and 10×10^9/L).

TABLE 35-1	Systematic Approach for Selection of Antimicrobials
Confirm the presence of infection	
Careful history and physical examination	
Signs and symptoms	
Predisposing factors	
Identification of the pathogen (see Pharmacotherapy textbook Chapter e122.)	
Collection of infected material	
Stains	
Serologies	
Culture and sensitivity	
Selection of presumptive therapy considering every infected site	
Host factors	
Drug factors	
Monitor therapeutic response	
Clinical assessment	
Laboratory tests	
Assessment of therapeutic failure	

- Bacterial infections are associated with elevated granulocyte counts (neutrophils and basophils), often with increased numbers of immature forms (band neutrophils) seen in peripheral blood smears. With infection, peripheral leukocyte counts may be high, but they are rarely higher than 10,000 to 40,000 cells/mm^3 (10×10^9/L to 40×10^9/L). Low neutrophil counts (neutropenia) after the onset of infection indicate an abnormal response and are generally associated with a poor prognosis for bacterial infection.
- Relative lymphocytosis, even with normal or slightly elevated total WBC counts, is generally associated with tuberculosis and viral or fungal infections. Many types of infections, however, may be accompanied by a completely normal WBC count and differential.

LOCAL SIGNS

- Pain and inflammation may accompany infection and are sometimes manifested by swelling, erythema, tenderness, and purulent drainage. Unfortunately, these signs may be apparent only if the infection is superficial or in a bone or joint.
- The manifestations of inflammation with deep-seated infections such as meningitis, pneumonia, endocarditis, and urinary tract infection must be ascertained by examining tissues or fluids. For example, the presence of polymorphonuclear leukocytes (neutrophils) in spinal fluid, lung secretions (sputum), and urine is highly suggestive of bacterial infection.

IDENTIFICATION OF THE PATHOGEN

- Identification and antimicrobial susceptibility of a suspected pathogen are the most important factors in determining the choice of antimicrobial therapy.
- Infected body materials must be sampled, if at all possible or practical, before the institution of antimicrobial therapy. A Gram stain of the material may reveal bacteria, or an acid-fast stain may detect mycobacteria or actinomycetes. Premature use of antimicrobials can suppress the growth of pathogens that might result in false-negative culture results or alterations in the cellular and chemical composition of infected fluids.
- Blood cultures should be performed in the acutely ill, febrile patient. Infected materials produced by the patient (eg, blood, sputum, urine, stool, and wound or sinus drainage) and less accessible fluids or tissues are obtained when needed to assess localized signs or symptoms. Abscesses and cellulitic areas should also be aspirated.
- After a positive Gram stain, culture results, or both are obtained, the clinician must be cautious in determining whether the organism recovered is a true pathogen, a contaminant, or a part of the normal flora. Cultures of specimens from purportedly infected sites that are obtained by sampling from or through a contaminated areas might contain significant numbers of the normal flora.

SELECTION OF PRESUMPTIVE THERAPY

- A variety of factors must be considered to select rational antimicrobial therapy for a given clinical situation. These include the severity and acuity of the disease, local epidemiology and antibiogram, patient history, host factors, factors related to the drugs used, and the necessity for using multiple agents. Choice of antimicrobial is influenced by local antimicrobial susceptibility data rather than information published by other institutions or national compilations.
- The drugs of choice for the treatment of most pathogens are compiled from a variety of sources and are intended as guidelines rather than specific rules for antimicrobial use (Table 35-2).
- Important considerations when selecting empiric antimicrobial therapy include: (1) prior knowledge of colonization or infections, (2) previous antimicrobial use, (3) the site of infection and the organisms most likely pathogens, and (4) local antibiogram and resistance patterns for important pathogens.

TABLE 35-2 Drugs of Choice, First Choice, *Alternative(s)*

Gram-Positive Cocci

Enterococcus faecalis (generally not as resistant to antibiotics as *Enterococcus faecium*)
• Serious infection (endocarditis, meningitis, pyelonephritis with bacteremia)
  • Ampicillin (or penicillin G) + (gentamicin or streptomycin)
  • *Vancomycin + (gentamicin or streptomycin), daptomycin, linezolid, tedizolid, telavancin, tigecycline[a]*
• Urinary tract infection
  • Ampicillin, amoxicillin
  • *Fosfomycin or nitrofurantoin*

E. faecium (generally more resistant to antibiotics than *E. faecalis*)
• Recommend consultation with infectious disease specialist
  • *Linezolid, quinupristin/dalfopristin, daptomycin, tigecycline[a]*

Staphylococcus aureus/Staphylococcus epidermidis
• Methicillin (oxacillin)-sensitive
  • Nafcillin or oxacillin
  • *FGC,[b,c] trimethoprim–sulfamethoxazole, clindamycin, BL/BLI[d]*
• Hospital-acquired methicillin (oxacillin)–resistant
  • Vancomycin ± (gentamicin or rifampin)
  • *Ceftaroline, daptomycin, linezolid, telavancin, tigecycline,[a] trimethoprim–sulfamethoxazole, quinupristin–dalfopristin*
• Community-acquired methicillin (oxacillin)–resistant
  • Clindamycin, trimethoprim–sulfamethoxazole, doxycycline[a]
  • *Ceftaroline, dalbavancin, daptomycin, linezolid, oritivancin, tedizolid, telavancin, tigecycline,[a] or vancomycin*

Streptococcus (groups A, B, C, G, and *Streptococcus bovis*)
• Penicillin G or V or ampicillin
• *FGC,[b,c] erythromycin, azithromycin, clarithromycin*

Streptococcus pneumoniae
• Penicillin-sensitive (minimal inhibitory concentration [MIC] <0.1 mcg/mL [mg/L])
  • Penicillin G or V or ampicillin
  • *FGC,[b,c] doxycycline,[a] azithromycin, clarithromycin, erythromycin*
• Penicillin intermediate (MIC 0.1–1 mcg/mL [mg/L])
  • High-dose penicillin (12 million units/day for adults) or ceftriaxone[c] or cefotaxime[c]
  • *Levofloxacin,[a] moxifloxacin,[a] gemifloxacin,[a] or vancomycin*
• Penicillin-resistant (MIC ≥1.0 mcg/mL [mg/L])
  • Recommend consultation with infectious disease specialist.
    – Vancomycin ± rifampin
    – *Per sensitivities: ceftaroline, cefotaxime, ceftriaxone,[c] levofloxacin,[a] moxifloxacin,[a] or gemifloxacin[a]*

Streptococcus, viridans group
• Penicillin G ± gentamicin[e]
• *Cefotaxime,[c] ceftriaxone,[c] erythromycin, azithromycin, clarithromycin, or vancomycin ± gentamicin*

Gram-Negative Cocci

Moraxella (Branhamella) catarrhalis
• Amoxicillin–clavulanate, ampicillin–sulbactam
• *Trimethoprim–sulfamethoxazole, erythromycin, azithromycin, clarithromycin, doxycycline,[a] SGC,[c,f] cefotaxime,[c] ceftriaxone,[c] or TGCPO[c,g]*

(Continued)

| **TABLE 35-2** | Drugs of Choice, First Choice, *Alternative(s)* (Continued) |

Neisseria gonorrhoeae (also give concomitant treatment for *Chlamydia trachomatis*)
- Disseminated gonococcal infection
  - Ceftriaxone[c] or cefotaxime[c]
  - Oral follow-up: cefpodoxime,[c] ciprofloxacin,[a] or levofloxacin[a]
- Uncomplicated infection
  - Ceftriaxone,[c] cefotaxime,[c] or cefpodoxime[c]
  - Ciprofloxacin[a] or levofloxacin[a]

Neisseria meningitides
- Penicillin G
- Cefotaxime[c] or ceftriaxone[c]

Gram-Positive Bacilli

Clostridium perfringens
- Penicillin G ± clindamycin
- Metronidazole,[a] clindamycin, doxycycline,[a] cefazolin,[c] carbapenem[h,j]

Clostridioides (formerly *Clostridium*) *difficile*
- Oral vancomycin or fidaxomicin
- Oral metronidazole

Gram-Negative Bacilli

Acinetobacter spp.
- Doripenem, imipenem, or meropenem ± aminoglycoside[j] (amikacin usually most effective)
- Ampicillin–sulbactam, polymyxins,[i] or tigecycline[a]

Bacteroides fragilis (and others)
- Metronidazole[a]
- BL/BLI,[d] clindamycin, cefoxitin,[c] cefotetan,[c] ceftolozane-azobactam, ceftazidime-avibactam, or carbapenem[h,j]

Enterobacter spp.
- Carbapenem[h] or cefepime ± aminoglycoside[j]
- Ceftolozane-tazobactam, ceftazidime-avibactam, ciprofloxacin,[a] levofloxacin,[a] piperacillin–tazobactam, ticarcillin–clavulanate

Escherichia coli
- Meningitis
  - Cefotaxime,[c] ceftriaxone,[c] meropenem
- Systemic infection
  - Cefotaxime[c] or ceftriaxone[c]
  - BL/BLI,[d] fluoroquinolone,[a,k] carbapenem[h,j]
- Urinary tract infection
  - Most oral agents: check sensitivities
  - Ampicillin, amoxicillin–clavulanate, doxycycline,[a] or cephalexin[c]
  - Aminoglycoside,[j] FGC,[b,c] nitrofurantoin, fluoroquinolone[a,k]

Gardnerella vaginalis
- Metronidazole[a]
- Clindamycin

Haemophilus influenzae
- Meningitis
  - Cefotaxime[c] or ceftriaxone[c]
  - Meropenem[i]
- Other infections
  - BL/BLI,[d] or if β-lactamase-negative, ampicillin or amoxicillin
  - Trimethoprim–sulfamethoxazole, cefuroxime,[c] azithromycin, clarithromycin, or fluoroquinolone[a,k]

(Continued)

TABLE 35-2	Drugs of Choice, First Choice, *Alternative(s)* *(Continued)*

Klebsiella pneumoniae
- BL/BLI,[d] cefotaxime,[c] ceftriaxone,[c] cefepime[c]
- *Carbapenem,[h,j] ceftolozane-tazobactam, ceftazidime-avibactam, fluoroquinolone[a,k]*

Legionella spp.
- Azithromycin, erythromycin ± rifampin, or fluoroquinolone[a,k]
- *Trimethoprim–sulfamethoxazole, clarithromycin, or doxycycline[a]*

Pasteurella multocida
- Penicillin G, ampicillin, amoxicillin
- *Doxycycline,[a] BL/BLI,[d] trimethoprim–sulfamethoxazole or ceftriaxone[c]*

Proteus mirabilis
- Ampicillin
- *Trimethoprim–sulfamethoxazole*

Proteus (indole-positive) (including *Providencia rettgeri, Morganella morganii,* and *Proteus vulgaris*)
- Cefotaxime,[c] ceftriaxone,[c] or fluoroquinolone[a,k]
- *BL/BLI,[d] aztreonam,[l] aminoglycosides,[j] carbapenem,[h,j] ceftolozane-tazobactam, ceftazidime-avibactam*

Providencia stuartii
- Amikacin, cefotaxime,[c] ceftriaxone,[c] fluoroquinolone[a,k]
- *Trimethoprim–sulfamethoxazole, aztreonam,[l] carbapenem[h,j]*

Pseudomonas aeruginosa
- Urinary tract infection only
  - Aminoglycoside[j]
  - *Ciprofloxacin,[a] levofloxacin[a]*
- Systemic infection
  - Cefepime,[c] ceftazidime,[c] doripenem,[l] imipenem,[l] meropenem,[l] piperacillin–tazobactam, or ticarcillin–clavulanate + aminoglycoside[j]
  - *Aztreonam,[l] ceftolozane-tazobactam, ceftazidime-avibactam, ciprofloxacin,[a] levofloxacin,[a] polymyxin[j]*

Salmonella typhi
- Ciprofloxacin,[a] levofloxacin,[c] ceftriaxone,[c] cefotaxime[c]
- *Trimethoprim–sulfamethoxazole*

Serratia marcescens
- Ceftriaxone,[c] cefotaxime,[c] cefepime,[c] ciprofloxacin,[a] levofloxacin[a]
- *Aztreonam,[l] carbapenem,[h,j] piperacillin–tazobactam, ticarcillin–clavulanate*

Stenotrophomonas (Xanthomonas) maltophilia (generally very resistant to all antimicrobials)
- Trimethoprim–sulfamethoxazole.
- *Check sensitivities to ceftazidime,[c] doxycycline,[a] minocycline,[a] and ticarcillin–clavulanate*

Miscellaneous Microorganisms

Chlamydia pneumoniae
- Doxycycline[a]
- *Azithromycin, clarithromycin, erythromycin, or fluoroquinolone[a,k]*

C. trachomatis
- Azithromycin or doxycycline[a]
- *Levofloxacin,[a] erythromycin*

Mycoplasma pneumoniae
- Azithromycin, clarithromycin, erythromycin, fluoroquinolone[a,k]
- *Doxycycline[a]*

(Continued)

TABLE 35-2	Drugs of Choice, First Choice, *Alternative(s)* *(Continued)*

Spirochetes

Treponema pallidum
- Neurosyphilis
  - Penicillin G
  - Ceftriaxone[c]
- Primary or secondary
  - Benzathine, penicillin G
  - Ceftriaxone[c] or doxycycline[a]

Borrelia burgdorferi (choice depends on stage of disease)
- Ceftriaxone[c] or cefuroxime axetil,[c] doxycycline,[a] amoxicillin
- High-dose penicillin, cefotaxime[c]

[a]Not for use in pregnant patients or children.
[b]First-generation cephalosporins—IV: cefazolin; orally: cephalexin, cephradine, or cefadroxil.
[c]Some penicillin-allergic patients may react to cephalosporins.
[d]β-Lactam/β-lactamase inhibitor combination—IV: ampicillin–sulbactam, piperacillin–tazobactam, and ticarcillin–clavulanate; orally: amoxicillin–clavulanate.
[e]Gentamicin should be added if tolerance or moderately susceptible (MIC >0.1 mcg/mL [mg/L]) organisms are encountered; streptomycin is used but can be more toxic.
[f]Second-generation cephalosporins—IV: cefuroxime; orally: cefaclor, cefditoren, cefprozil, cefuroxime axetil, and loracarbef.
[g]Third-generation cephalosporins—orally: cefdinir, cefixime, cefetamet, cefpodoxime proxetil, and ceftibuten.
[h]Carbapenem: doripenem, ertapenem, imipenem/cilastatin, and meropenem.
[i]Reserve for serious infection.
[j]Aminoglycosides: gentamicin, tobramycin, and amikacin; use per sensitivities.
[k]Fluoroquinolones IV/orally: ciprofloxacin, levofloxacin, and moxifloxacin.
[l]Generally reserved for patients with hypersensitivity reactions to penicillin.

HOST FACTORS

- When a patient for initial or empiric therapy is evaluated, the following factors should be considered:
  - ✓ Allergy or history of adverse drug reactions.
  - ✓ Age of patient.
  - ✓ Pregnancy.
  - ✓ Metabolic or genetic variation.
  - ✓ *Renal and hepatic function*: Patients with diminished renal and/or hepatic function will accumulate certain drugs unless the dosage is adjusted.
  - ✓ *Concomitant drug therapy*: Any concomitant therapy the patient is receiving may influence the selection of drug therapy, the dose, and monitoring. A list of selected drug interactions involving antimicrobials is provided in **Table 35-3**.
  - ✓ Concomitant disease states.

DRUG FACTORS

- Integration of both pharmacokinetic and pharmacodynamic properties of an agent is important when choosing antimicrobial therapy to ensure efficacy and prevent resistance. Antibiotics may demonstrate concentration-dependent (aminoglycosides and fluoroquinolones) or time-dependent (β-lactams) bactericidal effects.
- The importance of tissue penetration varies with the site of infection. The central nervous system (CNS) is one body site where the importance of antimicrobial penetration is relatively well defined, and correlations with clinical outcomes are established. Drugs that do not reach significant concentrations in CSF should either be avoided or instilled directly when treating meningitis.

TABLE 35-3	Major Drug Interactions with Antimicrobials		
Antimicrobial	**Other Agent(s)**	**Mechanism of Action/Effect**	**Clinical Management**
Aminoglycosides	Neuromuscular blocking agents	Additive adverse effects	Avoid
	Nephrotoxins (N) or ototoxins (O) (eg, amphotericin B [N], cisplatin [N/O], cyclosporine [N], furosemide [O], NSAIDs [N], radiocontrast [N], vancomycin [N])	Additive adverse effects	Monitor aminoglycoside SDC and renal function
Amphotericin B	Nephrotoxins (eg, aminoglycosides, cidofovir, cyclosporine, foscarnet, pentamidine)	Additive adverse effects	Monitor renal function
Azoles	See Chapter 38		
Chloramphenicol	Phenytoin, tolbutamide, ethanol	Decreased metabolism of other agents	Monitor phenytoin SDC, blood glucose
Foscarnet	Pentamidine IV	Increased risk of severe nephrotoxicity/ hypocalcemia	Monitor renal function/serum calcium
Isoniazid	Carbamazepine, phenytoin	Decreased metabolism of other agents (nausea, vomiting, nystagmus, ataxia)	Monitor drug SDC
Macrolides/ Azalides	Digoxin	Decreased digoxin bioavailability and metabolism	Monitor digoxin SDC; avoid if possible
	Theophylline	Decreased metabolism of theophylline	Monitor theophylline SDC
Metronidazole	Ethanol (drugs containing ethanol)	Disulfiram-like reaction	Avoid
Penicillins and cephalosporins	Probenecid, aspirin	Blocked excretion of β-lactams	Use if prolonged high concentration of β-lactam desirable
Ciprofloxacin/ Norfloxacin	Theophylline	Decreased metabolism of theophylline	Monitor theophylline

(Continued)

TABLE 35-3	Major Drug Interactions with Antimicrobials (*Continued*)		
Antimicrobial	**Other Agent(s)**	**Mechanism of Action/Effect**	**Clinical Management**
Quinolones	Classes Ia and III antiarrhythmics	Increased Q-T interval	Avoid
	Multivalent cations (antacids, iron, sucralfate, zinc, vitamins, dairy, citric acid), didanosine	Decreased absorption of quinolone	Separate by 2 hours
Rifampin	Azoles, cyclosporine, methadone propranolol, PIs, oral contraceptives, tacrolimus, warfarin	Increased metabolism of other agent	Avoid if possible
Sulfonamides	Sulfonylureas, phenytoin, warfarin	Decreased metabolism of other agent	Monitor blood glucose, SDC, PT
Tetracyclines	Antacids, iron, calcium, sucralfate	Decreased absorption of tetracycline	Separate by 2 hours
	Digoxin	Decreased digoxin bioavailability	Monitor digoxin SDC; avoid if possible

PI, protease inhibitor; PT, prothrombin time; SDC, serum drug concentrations.
Azalides: azithromycin; azoles: fluconazole, itraconazole, ketoconazole, and voriconazole; macrolides: erythromycin and clarithromycin; protease inhibitors: amprenavir, indinavir, lopinavir/ritonavir, nelfinavir, ritonavir, and saquinavir; quinolones: ciprofloxacin, gemifloxacin, levofloxacin, and moxifloxacin.

- Apart from the bloodstream, other body fluids in which drug concentration data are clinically relevant are cerebrospinal fluid, urine, synovial fluid, and peritoneal fluid.
- Pharmacokinetic parameters such as area under the drug concentration-time curve (AUC) and maximal plasma concentration can be predictive of treatment outcome when specific ratios of AUC or maximal plasma concentration to the minimum inhibitory concentration (MIC) are achieved. For some agents, the ratio of AUC to MIC, peak-to-MIC ratio, or the time that the drug concentration is above the MIC may predict efficacy.
- The most important pharmacodynamic relationship for antimicrobials that display time-dependent bactericidal effects (such as penicillins and cephalosporins) is the duration that drug concentrations exceed the MIC.

COMBINATION ANTIMICROBIAL THERAPY

- Combinations of antimicrobials are generally used to broaden the spectrum of coverage for empiric therapy, achieve synergistic activity against the infecting organism, and prevent the emergence of resistance.
- Increasing the coverage of antimicrobial therapy is generally necessary in mixed infections in which multiple organisms are likely to be present, such as intra-abdominal and female pelvic infections in which a variety of aerobic and anaerobic bacteria may produce disease. Combination antimicrobial therapy is also used in critically ill patients with presumed healthcare-associated infections in which an increased spectrum of activity is desirable.

Synergism

- The achievement of synergistic antimicrobial activity is advantageous for infections caused by gram-negative bacilli in immunosuppressed patients.

- Traditionally, combinations of aminoglycosides and β-lactams have been used because these drugs together generally act synergistically against a wide variety of bacteria. However, the data supporting superior efficacy of synergistic over nonsynergistic combinations are weak.
- Synergistic combinations may produce better results in infections caused by *Pseudomonas aeruginosa*, as well as in certain infections caused by *Enterococcus* spp.
- The use of combinations to prevent the emergence of resistance is widely applied but not often realized. The only circumstance in which this has been clearly effective is in the treatment of tuberculosis.

Disadvantages of Combination Therapy

- Although there are potentially beneficial effects from combining drugs, there are also potential disadvantages, including increased cost, greater risk of drug toxicity, and superinfection with even more resistant bacteria.
- Some combinations of antimicrobials are potentially antagonistic. For example, agents that are capable of inducing β-lactamase production in bacteria (eg, cefoxitin) may antagonize the effects of enzyme-labile drugs such as penicillins or imipenem.

MONITORING THERAPEUTIC RESPONSE

- After antimicrobial therapy has been instituted, the patient must be monitored carefully for a therapeutic response. Culture and sensitivity reports from specimens sent to the microbiology laboratory must be reviewed and the therapy changed accordingly.
- Use of agents with the narrowest spectrum of activity against identified pathogens is recommended.
- Patient monitoring should include a variety of parameters, including WBC count, body temperature, signs and symptoms of infection, appetite, radiologic studies as appropriate, and determination of antimicrobial concentrations in body fluids.
- As the patient improves, the route of antibiotic administration should be reevaluated. Streamlining therapy from parenteral to oral (switch therapy) has become an accepted practice for many infections. Criteria favoring the switch to oral therapy include the following:

  ✓ Overall clinical improvement
  ✓ Lack of fever for 8–24 hours
  ✓ Decreased WBC
  ✓ A functioning gastrointestinal (GI) tract

FAILURE OF ANTIMICROBIAL THERAPY

- A variety of factors may be responsible for the apparent lack of response to therapy. It is possible that the disease is not infectious or nonbacterial in origin, or there is an undetected pathogen in a polymicrobial infection. Other factors include those directly related to drug selection, the host, or the pathogen. Laboratory error in identification and/or susceptibility testing errors are rare.

Failures Caused by Drug Selection

- Factors directly related to the drug selection include an inappropriate selection of drug, dosage, or route of administration. Malabsorption of a drug product due to GI disease (eg, short-bowel syndrome) or a drug interaction (eg, complexation of fluoroquinolones with multivalent cations resulting in reduced absorption) may lead to potentially subtherapeutic serum concentrations.
- Accelerated drug elimination is also a possible reason for failure and may occur in patients with cystic fibrosis or during pregnancy, when more rapid clearance or larger volumes of distribution may result in low serum concentrations, particularly for aminoglycosides.
- A common cause of failure of therapy is poor penetration into the site of infection. This is especially true for the so-called privileged sites, such as the CNS, the eye, and the prostate gland.

Failures Caused by Host Factors

- Patients who are immunosuppressed (eg, granulocytopenia from chemotherapy and acquired immunodeficiency syndrome) may respond poorly to therapy because their own defenses are inadequate to eradicate the infection despite seemingly adequate drug regimens.
- Other host factors are related to the necessity for surgical drainage of abscesses or removal of foreign bodies and/or necrotic tissue. If these situations are not corrected, they result in persistent infection and, occasionally, bacteremia, despite adequate antimicrobial therapy.

Failures Caused by Microorganisms

- Factors related to the pathogen include the development of drug resistance during therapy. Primary resistance refers to the intrinsic resistance of the pathogens producing the infection. However, acquisition of resistance during treatment has become a major problem as well.
- The increase in resistance among pathogenic organisms is believed to be due, in large part, to continued overuse of antimicrobials in the community, as well as in hospitals, and the increasing prevalence of immunosuppressed patients receiving long-term suppressive antimicrobials for the prevention of infections.

See Chapter 123, Antimicrobial Regimen Selection, authored by Grace C. Lee and David S. Burgess, for a more detailed discussion of this topic.

CHAPTER 36

Central Nervous System Infections

- Central nervous system (CNS) infections include a wide variety of clinical conditions and etiologies: meningitis, meningoencephalitis, encephalitis, brain and meningeal abscesses, and shunt infections. The focus of this chapter is meningitis.

PATHOPHYSIOLOGY

- The development of bacterial meningitis involves four main processes: (1) mucosal colonization and bacterial invasion of the host and CNS, (2) bacterial replication in the subarachnoid space, (3) pathophysiologic alterations resulting in progressive inflammation, and (4) increased intracranial pressure (ICP) and cerebral edema leading to neuronal damage.
- The critical first step in the acquisition of acute bacterial meningitis is nasopharyngeal colonization of the host by the bacterial pathogen. Most cases of acute bacterial meningitis probably occur following bacteremia, but the high incidence of pneumococcal meningitis in patients with sinusitis and otitis media suggests that direct spread to the CNS can also occur.
- CNS infections may be caused by a variety of bacteria, fungi, viruses, and parasites. The most common causes of bacterial meningitis are *Streptococcus pneumoniae*, group B *Streptococcus*, *Neisseria meningitidis*, *Haemophilus influenzae*, and *Listeria monocytogenes*.
- A common characteristic of most CNS bacterial pathogens (eg, *H. influenzae*, *Escherichia coli*, *N. meningitidis*) is the presence of an extensive polysaccharide capsule that is resistant to neutrophil phagocytosis and complement opsonization.
- The neurologic sequelae of meningitis occur due to the activation of host inflammatory pathways. Bacterial cell lysis causes the release of cell wall components such as lipopolysaccharide, lipid A (endotoxin), lipoteichoic acid, teichoic acid, and peptidoglycan, depending on whether the pathogen is gram-positive or gram-negative.
- These cell wall components cause capillary endothelial cells and CNS macrophages to release cytokines (interleukin-1, tumor necrosis factor, and other inflammatory mediators). Proteolytic products and toxic oxygen radicals cause an alteration of the blood–brain barrier, whereas platelet-activating factor activates coagulation, and arachidonic acid metabolites stimulate vasodilation. These events lead to cerebral edema, elevated intracranial pressure, cerebrospinal fluid (CSF) pleocytosis, decreased cerebral blood flow, cerebral ischemia, and death.
- Passive and active exposure to cigarette smoke and the presence of a cochlear implant that includes a positioner both increase the risk of bacterial meningitis.

CLINICAL PRESENTATION

- Signs and symptoms of acute bacterial meningitis include fever, nuchal rigidity, altered mental status, chills, vomiting, photophobia, and severe headache. Up to 95% of patients exhibit at least two of the following symptoms: fever, nuchal rigidity, headache, and altered mental status. Kernig and Brudzinski signs may be present but are poorly sensitive and frequently absent in children.
- Clinical signs and symptoms in young children may include bulging fontanelle, apnea purpuric rash, and convulsions.
- Purpuric and petechial skin lesions typically indicate meningococcal involvement, although the lesions may be present with *H. influenzae* meningitis. Rashes rarely occur with pneumococcal meningitis.
- Meningitis causes changes in CSF fluid, and these changes can be used as diagnostic markers of infection (**Table 36-1**).

TABLE 36-1	Mean Values of the Components of Normal and Abnormal Cerebrospinal Fluid				
Type	Normal	Bacterial	Viral	Fungal	Tuberculosis
WBC (cells/ mm³ or 10⁶/L)	<5 (<30 in newborns)	1000–5000	50–1000	20–500	25–500
Differentialᵃ	Monocytes	Neutrophils	Lymphocytes	Lymphocytes	Lymphocytes
Protein (mg/dL)	<50 (<500 mg/L)	Elevated	Mild elevation	Elevated	Elevated
Glucose (mg/dL)	45–80 (2.5–4.4 mmol/L)	Low	Normal	Low	Low
CSF/blood glucose ratio	50%–60%	Decreased	Normal	Decreased	Decreased

ᵃInitial cerebrospinal fluid (CSF), while blood cell (WBC) count may reveal a predominance of polymorphonuclear neutrophils (PMNs). In CNS infection due to tuberculosis, "therapeutic paradox" may occur in which a lymphocytic predominance becomes neutrophilic during antituberculous treatment.

- CSF culture is the gold standard for diagnosis of bacterial meningitis and is positive in 80%–90% of patients with community-acquired bacterial meningitis if the CSF sample is obtained before the start of antimicrobial therapy.
- Gram stain is a rapid, inexpensive, and accurate method to assess the presence of bacteria in CSF. However, prior antibiotic therapy may cause the Gram stain and CSF culture to be negative, but the antibiotic therapy rarely affects CSF protein or glucose. The sensitivity of the Gram stain depends on the causative microorganism, so that its aggregate diagnostic yield is 90% in pneumococcal meningitis, 70%–90% in meningococcal, 50% in *H. influenza*, and only 25%–35% in *L. monocytogenes* meningitis.
- Polymerase chain reaction (PCR) techniques can rapidly diagnose CNS infections and may be particularly useful in patients who have received antimicrobial therapy before lumbar puncture, have negative cultures, or when the organism is fastidious or fails to grow in conventional culture.

TREATMENT

- Goals of Treatment: Eradication of infection with amelioration of signs and symptoms preventing morbidity and mortality.
- Key elements include initiating appropriate antimicrobials, providing supportive care, and preventing disease through timely introduction of vaccination and chemoprophylaxis.
- Administration of fluids, electrolytes, antipyretics, and analgesics may be indicated for patients presenting with a possible CNS infection. Additionally, venous thromboembolism prophylaxis, antiepileptic therapy, and ICP monitoring may be needed.

PHARMACOLOGIC TREATMENT

- Empiric antimicrobial therapy should be instituted as soon as possible to eradicate the causative organism (Table 36-2). Antimicrobial therapy should last at least 48–72 hours or until the diagnosis of bacterial meningitis can be ruled out. The first dose of antibiotic should not be withheld even when lumbar puncture is delayed or neuroimaging is being performed. The time period from suspected diagnosis to initiation of antibiotic treatment should not exceed 1 hour.
- Continued therapy should be based on the assessment of clinical improvement, cultures, and susceptibility testing results. Once a pathogen is identified, antibiotic therapy should be tailored to the specific pathogen.

TABLE 36-2	Bacterial Meningitis: Most Likely Etiologies and Empiric Therapy by Age Group

Age	Most Likely Organisms	Empirical Therapy[a]
<1 month	S. agalactiae Gram-negative enterics[b] L. monocytogenes	Ampicillin + cefotaxime or ampicillin + aminoglycoside
1–23 months	S. pneumoniae N. meningitidis H. influenzae S. agalactiae	Vancomycin[c] + 3rd generation cephalosporin (cefotaxime or ceftriaxone)
2–50 years	N. meningitidis S. pneumoniae	Vancomycin[c] + 3rd generation cephalosporin (cefotaxime or ceftriaxone)
>50 years	S. pneumoniae N. meningitidis Gram-negative enterics[b] L. monocytogenes	Vancomycin[c] + ampicillin + 3rd generation cephalosporin (cefotaxime or ceftriaxone)

[a]All recommendations are A-III.
[b]E. coli, Klebsiella spp., Enterobacter spp. common.
[c]Vancomycin use should be based on local incidence of penicillin-resistant S. pneumoniae and until cefotaxime or ceftriaxone minimum inhibitory concentration results are available.

Strength of recommendation: (A) Good evidence to support a recommendation for use; should always be offered. (B) Moderate evidence to support a recommendation for use; should generally be offered.

Quality of evidence: (I) Evidence from one or more properly randomized, controlled trial. (II) Evidence from one or more well-designed clinical trial, without randomization; from cohort or case-controlled analytic studies (preferably from one or more center) or from multiple time-series. (III) Evidence from opinions of respected authorities, based on clinical experience, descriptive studies, or reports of expert committees.

- With increased meningeal inflammation, there will be greater antibiotic penetration (**Table 36-3**). Problems of CSF penetration can be overcome by direct instillation of antibiotics intrathecally or intraventricularly. Advantages of direct instillation, however, must be weighed against the risks of invasive CNS procedures and adverse effects. Intraventricular delivery may be necessary in patients who have shunt infections that are difficult to eradicate or who cannot undergo the surgical components of therapy.
- See **Table 36-4** for antimicrobial agents of first choice and alternatives for treatment of meningitis caused by gram-positive and gram-negative microorganisms.
- Meningitis caused by S. pneumoniae has been treated successfully with 10–14 days of antibiotic therapy, while cases caused by N. meningitidis or H. influenzae usually can be treated with a 7-day course. In contrast, a longer duration (21 days or more) has been recommended for patients with L. monocytogenes, Gram-negative or pseudo-monal meningitis. Nonetheless, antibiotic treatments for bacterial meningitis should be individualized, and some patients may require enduring courses.

Dexamethasone as an Adjunctive Treatment for Meningitis

- In addition to antibiotics, dexamethasone is a commonly used adjunctive therapy in the treatment of acute bacterial meningitis to immunomodulate the inflammatory response.
- Recommendations by the Infectious Diseases Society of America (IDSA) call for the use of adjunctive dexamethasone in infants and children (6 weeks of age and older) with H. influenzae meningitis. The recommended intravenous dose is 0.15 mg/kg

TABLE 36-3	Penetration of Anti-infective Agents into the CSF[a]
Therapeutic Levels in CSF With or Without Inflammation of Meninges	
Acyclovir	Levofloxacin
Chloramphenicol	Linezolid
Ciprofloxacin	Metronidazole
Fluconazole	Moxifloxacin
Flucytosine	Pyrazinamide
Foscarnet	Rifampin
Fosfomycin	Sulfonamides
Ganciclovir	Trimethoprim
Isoniazid	Voriconazole
Therapeutic Levels in CSF With Inflammation of Meninges	
Ampicillin ± sulbactam	Imipenem
Aztreonam	Meropenem
Cefepime	Nafcillin
Cefotaxime	Ofloxacin
Ceftazidime	Penicillin G
Ceftriaxone	Piperacillin/Tazobactam[b]
Cefuroxime	Pyrimethamine
Colistin	Quinupristin/Dalfopristin
Daptomycin	Ticarcillin ± clavulanic acid[b]
Ethambutol	Vancomycin
Nontherapeutic Levels in CSF With or Without Inflammation of Meninges	
Aminoglycosides	Cephalosporins (second generation)[d]
Amphotericin B	Doxycycline[e]
β-Lactamase inhibitors[c]	Itraconazole[f]
Cephalosporins (first generation)	

[a]Using recommended CNS dosing and compared to MIC of target pathogens.
[b]May not achieve therapeutic levels against organisms with higher MIC, as in *P. aeruginosa.*
   Tazobactam does not penetrate the blood-brain barrier.
[c]Includes clavulanic acid, sulbactam, and tazobactam.
[d]Cefuroxime is an exception.
[e]Documented effectiveness for *B. burgdorferi.*
[f]Achieves therapeutic concentrations for *Cryptococcus neoformans* therapy.

every 6 hours for 2–4 days, initiated 10–20 minutes prior to or concomitant with the first dose of antibiotics. In infants and children with pneumococcal meningitis, adjunctive dexamethasone may be considered after weighing the potential benefits and possible risks. If pneumococcal meningitis is suspected or proven, adults should receive dexamethasone 0.15 mg/kg (up to 10 mg) every 6 hours for 2–4 days with the first dose administered 10–20 minutes prior to first dose of antibiotics.

Neisseria meningitidis (Meningococcus)

- *N. meningitidis* is a leading cause of bacterial meningitis among children and young adults in the United States and around the world. It is spread by direct person-to-person close contact, including respiratory droplets and pharyngeal secretions.

TABLE 36-4	Antimicrobial Agents of First Choice and Alternative Choice for Treating Meningitis Caused by Gram-Positive and Gram-Negative Microorganisms		
Organism	Antibiotics of First Choice	Alternative Antibiotics	Recommended Duration of Therapy
Gram-Positive Organisms			
Streptococcus pneumoniae[a]			10–14 days
Penicillin susceptible MIC ≤0.06 mcg/mL (mg/L)	Penicillin G or ampicillin (A-III)	Cefotaxime (A-III), ceftriaxone (A-III), cefepime (B-II), or meropenem (B-II)	
Penicillin resistant MIC >0.06 mcg/mL (mg/L)	Vancomycin[b,c] + cefotaxime or ceftriaxone (A-III)	Moxifloxacin (B-II)	
Ceftriaxone resistant MIC >0.5 mcg/mL (mg/L)	Vancomycin[b,c] + cefotaxime or ceftriaxone (A-III)	Moxifloxacin (B-II)	
Staphylococcus aureus			14–21 days
Methicillin susceptible	Nafcillin or oxacillin (A-III)	Vancomycin (A-III) or meropenem (B-III)	
Methicillin resistant	Vancomycin[b,c] (A-III)	Trimethoprim-sulfamethoxazole or linezolid (B-III)	
Group B *Streptococcus*	Penicillin G or ampicillin (A-III) ± gentamicin[b,c]	Ceftriaxone or cefotaxime (B-III)	14–21 days
S. epidermidis	Vancomycin[b,c] (A-III)	Linezolid (B-III)	14–21 days[d]
L. monocytogenes	Penicillin G or ampicillin ± gentamicin[b,c,e] (A-III)	Trimethoprim-sulfamethoxazole (A-III), meropenem (B-III)	≥21 days
Gram-Negative Organisms			
Neisseria meningitis			7–10 days
Penicillin susceptible	Penicillin G or ampicillin (A-III)	Cefotaxime or ceftriaxone (A-III)	
Penicillin resistant	Cefotaxime or ceftriaxone (A-III)	Meropenem or moxifloxacin (A-III)	
Haemophilus influenzae			7–10 days
β-lactamase negative	Ampicillin (A-III)	Cefotaxime (A-III), ceftriaxone (A-III), cefepime (A-III) or moxifloxacin (A-III)	

(Continued)

383

TABLE 36-4	Antimicrobial Agents of First Choice and Alternative Choice for Treating Meningitis Caused by Gram-Positive and Gram-Negative Microorganisms (*Continued*)		
Organism	Antibiotics of First Choice	Alternative Antibiotics	Recommended Duration of Therapy
β-lactamase positive	Cefotaxime or ceftriaxone (A-I)	Cefepime (A-I) or moxifloxacin (A-III)	
Enterobacteriaceaeᶠ	Cefotaxime or ceftriaxone (A-II)	Cefepime (A-III), moxifloxacin (A-III), meropenem (A-III) or aztreonam (A-III)	21 days
Pseudomonas aeruginosa	Cefepime or ceftazidime (A-II) ± tobramycinᵇ,ᶜ (A-III)	Ciprofloxacin (A-III), meropenem (A-III), piperacillin plus tobramycinᵃ,ᵇ (A-III), colistin sulfomethateᵍ (B-III), aztreonam (A-III)	21 days

ᵃEuropean Guidelines recommend considering the addition of rifampin to vancomycin therapy.
ᵇDirect CNS administration may be considered if failed conventional treatment.
ᶜMonitor serum drug levels.
ᵈBased on clinical experience; no clear recommendations.
ᵉEuropean guidelines recommend adding gentamicin for the first 7 days of treatment.
ᶠIncludes *E. coli* and *Klebsiella* spp.
ᵍShould be reserved for multidrug-resistant pseudomonal or *Acinetobacter* infections for which all other therapeutic options have been exhausted.
See Table 36-2 footnotes for rating scale of evidence.

- The presence of petechiae may be the primary clue that the underlying pathogen is *N. meningitidis*. Patients may also have an obvious or subclinical picture of disseminated intravascular coagulation (DIC).
- Deafness unilaterally, or more commonly bilaterally, may develop early or late in the disease course.
- Third-generation cephalosporins (ie, cefotaxime and ceftriaxone) are the recommended empiric treatment for meningococcal meningitis. Penicillin G or ampicillin is recommended for penicillin-susceptible isolates. The recommended duration of therapy is typically 7 days if there is good clinical response.
- Antimicrobial chemoprophylaxis of close contacts should be started as soon as possible (ideally <24 hours after identification of the index patient). In general, rifampin, ceftriaxone, and ciprofloxacin are recommended for prophylaxis; however, there is an increase in rifampin-resistant and ciprofloxacin-resistant isolates.
- For full details on vaccine availability and vaccination recommendations in various age groups and for those with significant risk factors, readers are referred to the current recommendations from the Advisory Committee on Immunization Practices.

Streptococcus pneumoniae (Pneumococcus or Diplococcus)

- *Streptococcus* group B (GBS) is a leading cause of neonatal meningitis in the United States and around the world.
- Neurologic sequelae include sight or hearing loss and cerebral palsy.
- Universal prenatal screening and intrapartum antimicrobial prophylaxis of GBS-colonized pregnant women decreases the rate of early onset invasive disease.

Recommended agents for intrapartum prophylaxis are penicillin or ampicillin, cefazolin (if penicillin allergy and not at high risk for anaphylaxis), or vancomycin (if penicillin allergy and at high risk for anaphylaxis).

- Ampicillin plus an aminoglycoside is the treatment of choice for a newborn infant with presumptive early-onset GBS meningitis. For empirical therapy of late-onset meningitis, ampicillin and an aminoglycoside or cefotaxime is recommended. Ampicillin or penicillin G is the recommended agent in adults. Addition of an aminoglycoside could also be considered. For infants with uncomplicated meningitis, 14 days of treatment is satisfactory, but longer periods of treatment may be necessary for patients with prolonged or complicated courses. For adults, the recommended duration of antibiotics is 14–21 days.
- Refer to Chapter 52 for information on pneumococcal vaccines.

Haemophilus influenzae

- Widespread vaccination of infants and children has effectively decreased the incidence of bacterial meningitis due to Hib in children between the ages of 1 month and 5 years, resulting in a significant decline in all cases of bacterial meningitis.
- Third-generation cephalosporins (cefotaxime and ceftriaxone) are the drugs of choice for empirical therapy for *H. influenzae* type b meningitis as they are active against β-lactamase–producing and non-β-lactamase–producing strains. Cefepime and fluoroquinolones are suitable alternatives regardless of β-lactamase activity.
- Recommended duration of treatment is 7 days (adults) or 7–10 days (children).
- Dexamethasone is beneficial for treatment of infants and children with Hib meningitis to diminish the risk of hearing loss, if given before or concurrently with the first dose of antimicrobial agent(s).
- Chemoprophylaxis with rifampin is indicated to reduce the risk of secondary invasive Hib disease in close contacts by eliminating nasopharyngeal and oropharyngeal carriages of *H. influenzae*. Rifampin should be administered orally, once a day for 4 days (20 mg/kg/dose; maximum, 600 mg). For information on who should receive prophylaxis (adults and children), refer to the recommendations of the American Academy of Pediatrics.
- Refer to Chapter 52 for information on *H. influenzae* vaccination.

Listeria monocytogenes

- *L. monocytogenes* is implicated in approximately 10% of meningitis cases in patients older than 65 years of age and carries a case-fatality rate of approximately 18% in the United States.
- Treatment of *L. monocytogenes* meningitis should consist of penicillin G or ampicillin. The addition of aminoglycoside is also recommended in proven infection in both children and adults. Patients should be treated a minimum of 21 days.
- **Trimethoprim–sulfamethoxazole** and **meropenem** may be effective alternatives because adequate CSF penetration is achieved with these agents.

See Chapter 124, Central Nervous System Infections, authored by Christina Koutsari, Thomas J. Dilworth, Jessica S. Holt, Ramy H. Elshaboury, and John C. Rotschafer, for a more detailed discussion of this topic.

Endocarditis

CHAPTER 37

- *Endocarditis* is an inflammation of the endocardium, the membrane lining the chambers of the heart and covering the cusps of the heart valves. *Infective endocarditis* (IE) refers to infection of the heart valves by microorganisms, primarily bacteria.
- Endocarditis is often referred to as either acute or subacute depending on the clinical presentation. Acute bacterial endocarditis is a fulminating infection associated with high fevers, systemic toxicity, and death within days to weeks if untreated. Subacute infectious endocarditis is a more indolent infection, usually occurring in a setting of prior valvular heart disease.

ETIOLOGY

- Most patients with IE have risk factors, such as preexisting cardiac valve abnormalities. Many types of structural heart disease resulting in turbulence of blood flow will increase the risk for IE. Some of the most important risk factors include the following:
  ✓ Highest risk: presence of a prosthetic valve or previous IE
  ✓ Congenital heart disease (CHD), chronic intravenous (IV) access, diabetes mellitus, acquired valvular dysfunction (eg, rheumatic heart disease), cardiac implantable device, chronic heart failure, mitral valve prolapse with regurgitation, IV drug abuse (IVDA), HIV infection, and poor dentition and/or oral hygiene.
- Three groups of organisms cause most cases of IE: staphylococci, streptococci, and enterococci (Table 37-1). Staphylococci (*S. aureus* and coagulase-negative staphylococci) are the most common cause of prosthetic valve endocarditis (PVE) within the first year after valve surgery, and *S. aureus* is common in those with a history of IVDA.

CLINICAL PRESENTATION

- The clinical presentation of patients with IE is highly variable and nonspecific. Fever is the most common finding (more than 90% of patients). The mitral and aortic valves are most often affected.
- IE usually begins insidiously and worsens gradually. Patients may present with nonspecific findings such as fever, chills, weakness, dyspnea, cough, night sweats, weight loss, or malaise.
- Important clinical signs, especially prevalent in subacute illness, may include the following peripheral manifestations ("stigmata") of endocarditis: Osler nodes, Janeway lesions, splinter hemorrhages, petechiae, clubbing of the fingers, Roth spots, and emboli. The patient may also have a heart murmur (sometimes new or changing), congestive heart failure, cardiac conduction abnormalities, cerebral manifestations, embolic phenomenon, and splenomegaly.
- Without appropriate antimicrobial therapy and surgery, IE is usually fatal. With proper management, recovery can be expected in most patients.
- Factors associated with increased mortality include: congestive heart failure, culture-negative endocarditis, endocarditis caused by resistant organisms such as fungi and gram-negative bacteria, left-sided endocarditis caused by *Staphylococcus aureus*, PVE.
- Ninety to 95% of patients with IE have a positive blood culture. The hallmark laboratory finding is continuous bacteremia; three sets of blood cultures should be collected over 24 hours. The patient's white blood cell count may be normal or only slightly elevated. Anemia, leukocytosis, and thrombocytopenia may be present. The erythrocyte sedimentation rate (ESR) and C-reactive protein (CRP) may be elevated in approximately 60% of patients. Urinalysis may reveal proteinuria and microscopic hematuria.

TABLE 37-1	Etiologic Organisms in Infective Endocarditis[a]
Agent	**Percentage of Cases**
Staphylococci	30–70
Coagulase positive *S. aureus*	20–68
Coagulase negative	3–26
Streptococci	9–38
Viridans streptococci	10–28
Other streptococci	3–14
Enterococci	5–18
Gram-negative aerobic bacilli	1.5–13
Fungi	1–9
Miscellaneous bacteria	<5
Polymicrobial infections	1–2
Culture negative	<5–17

[a]Values encompass community-acquired, healthcare-associated, native valve, and prosthetic valve infective endocarditis.

- Transesophageal echocardiography is important in identifying and localizing valvular lesions in patients suspected of having IE. It is more sensitive for detecting vegetations (90%–100%), compared with transthoracic echocardiography (40%–65%).
- The Modified Duke criteria, encompassing major findings of persistent bacteremia and echocardiographic findings and other minor findings, are used to categorize patients as "definite IE" or "possible IE."

TREATMENT

- <u>Goals of Treatment</u>: relieve the signs and symptoms of disease. Decrease morbidity and mortality associated with infection. Eradicate the causative organism with minimal drug exposure. Provide cost-effective antimicrobial therapy. Prevent IE in high-risk patients with appropriate prophylactic antimicrobials.
- The most important approach to treatment of IE is isolation of the infecting pathogen and determination of antimicrobial susceptibilities, followed by high-dose, bactericidal antibiotics for an extended period.
- Treatment usually is started in the hospital, but in select patients, it may be completed in the outpatient setting as long as defervescence has occurred and follow-up blood cultures show no growth.
- Large doses of parenteral antimicrobials as opposed to oral antimicrobials are currently recommended to achieve bactericidal concentrations within vegetations. An extended duration of therapy is required, even for susceptible pathogens, because microorganisms are enclosed within valvular vegetations and fibrin deposits.
- Outpatient antimicrobial therapy should be considered early in the treatment of IE, after the patient is stable clinically and responds favorably to initial antibiotics.
- Drug dosing for treatment of IE is given in **Table 37-2**. β-Lactam antibiotics, such as penicillin G (or ceftriaxone), nafcillin (or oxacillin), and ampicillin, remain the drugs of choice for streptococcal, staphylococcal, and enterococcal endocarditis, respectively.

TABLE 37-2	Drug Dosing Table for Treatment of Infective Endocarditis[a]			
Drug	Brand Name	Recommended Dose	Pediatric (Ped) Dose[b]	Additional Information
Ampicillin	NA	2 g IV every 4 hours	50 mg/kg every 4 hours or 75 mg/kg every 6 hours	24-hour total dose may be administered as a continuous infusion: 12 g IV every 24 hours
Ampicillin–sulbactam	Unasyn®	3 g IV every 6 hours	50 mg/kg every 4 hours or 75 mg/kg every 6 hours	
Aqueous crystalline penicillin G sodium	NA			
• MIC <0.12 mcg/mL (mg/L) (native valve only)		3 million units IV every 4 hours or every 6 hours	50,000 units/kg IV every 6 hours	24-hour total dose may be administered as a continuous infusion: 12–18 million units IV every 24 hours (Ped: 200,000 units/kg IV/24 hours)
• All other indications		4 million units IV every 4 hours or 6 million units IV every 6 hours	50,000 units/kg IV every 4 hours or 75,000 units/kg IV every 6 hours	24 million units IV every 24 hours (Ped: 300,000 units/kg IV every 24 hours)
Cefazolin	N/A	2 g IV every 8 hours	33 mg/kg IV every 8 hours	
Cefepime	Maxipime®	2 g IV every 8 hours	50 mg/kg IV every 8 hours	
Ceftriaxone sodium	N/A	2 g IV or IM every 24 hours 2 g IV or IM every 12 hours (E. faecalis only)	100 mg/kg IV or IM every 24 hours	
Ciprofloxacin	Cipro®	400 mg IV every 12 hours or 500 mg orally every 12 hours	20–30 mg/kg IV or orally every 12 hours	Avoid use if possible in patients <18 years of age

Drug	Brand	Dose	Dose	Comments
Daptomycin	Cubicin®	≥8 mg/kg IV every 24 hours	6 mg/kg IV every 24 hours	Doses as high as 10–12 mg/kg IV every 24 hours have been used in adults with enterococcus resistant to penicillin, aminoglycosides, and vancomycin; doses should be calculated using actual body weight
Doxycycline	Vibramycin®	100 mg IV or orally every 12 hours	1–2 mg/kg IV or orally every 12 hours	
Gentamicin sulfate	NA	3 mg/kg IV or IM every 24 hours or 1 mg/kg IV or IM every 8 hours^c	1 mg/kg IV or IM every 8 hours	Once-daily dosing is only recommended for treatment of streptococcal infections
Linezolid	Zyvox®	600 mg IV or orally every 12 hours	10 mg/kg IV every 8 hours	
Nafcillin or oxacillin	NA	2 g IV every 4 hours	50 mg/kg IV every 6 hours	
Rifampin	Rifadin®	300 mg IV or orally every 8 hours	5–7 mg/kg IV or orally every 8 hours	24-hour total dose may be administered as a continuous infusion: 12 g IV every 24 hours
Streptomycin	NA	7.5 mg/kg IV or IM every 8 hours or every 12 hours		
Vancomycin	Vancocin®	15–20 mg/kg IV every 8 hours or every 12 hours	15 mg/kg IV every 6 hours	A loading dose of 25–30 mg/kg may be administered in adults; doses should be calculated using actual body weight; single doses should not exceed 2 g

^a All doses assume normal renal function.
^b Should not exceed adult dosage.
^c Actual body weight should be used when the full aminoglycoside dose is administered once daily; when administered in three divided doses, use ideal body weight or adjusted body weight when actual body weight is >120% ideal body weight.

NONPHARMACOLOGIC THERAPY

- Surgical intervention to remove the infectious foci and repair valves and/or valvular structures is an important adjunct in the management of both NVE and PVE In most cases, valvectomy and valve replacement are performed to remove infected tissues and restore hemodynamic function. Indications for surgery include heart failure, persistent bacteremia, persistent vegetation, an increase in vegetation size, or recurrent emboli despite prolonged antibiotic treatment, valve dysfunction, paravalvular extension (eg, abscess), or endocarditis caused by resistant organisms.

STREPTOCOCCAL ENDOCARDITIS

- Streptococci are a common cause of IE, with most isolates being viridans group streptococci.
- Most viridans group streptococci are highly sensitive to penicillin G with minimum inhibitory concentrations (MICs) of 0.12 mcg/mL (mg/L) or less. The MIC should be determined for all viridans streptococci and the results used to guide therapy. Approximately 10%–20% are moderately susceptible (MIC 0.12–0.5 mcg/mL [mg/L]).
- Recommended therapy in the uncomplicated case caused by fully susceptible strains in native valves is 4 weeks of either high-dose **penicillin G** or **ceftriaxone**, or 2 weeks of combined penicillin G or ceftriaxone therapy plus **gentamicin** (Table 37-3).
- Shorter-course antimicrobial regimens are advocated when possible. With susceptible streptococcal endocarditis (MICs ≤0.12 mcg/mL [mg/L]), a 2-week regimen of high-dose parenteral penicillin G or ceftriaxone in combination with an aminoglycoside is as effective as 4 weeks of penicillin alone.
- When a patient has a history of an immediate-type hypersensitivity to penicillin, vancomycin should be chosen for IE caused by viridans group streptococci. When vancomycin is used, the addition of gentamicin is not recommended.
- For patients with complicated infection (eg, extracardiac foci) or when the organism is relatively resistant (MIC = 0.12–0.5 mcg/mL [mg/L]), combination therapy with an aminoglycoside and penicillin (higher dose) or ceftriaxone for the first 2 weeks is recommended followed by penicillin or ceftriaxone alone for an additional 2 weeks.
- In patients with endocarditis of prosthetic valves or other prosthetic material caused by viridans streptococci and *Streptococcus bovis*, treatment courses are extended to 6 weeks (Table 37-4).

STAPHYLOCOCCAL ENDOCARDITIS

- Endocarditis is most commonly caused by staphylococci, in particular *S. aureus*, mainly because of increased IVDA, more frequent use of peripheral and central venous catheters, and increased frequency of valve replacement surgery. Coagulase-negative staphylococci (usually *S. epidermidis*) are prominent causes of PVE.
- The recommended therapy for patients with left-sided IE caused by methicillin-susceptible *S. aureus* (MSSA) is 6 weeks of **nafcillin** or **oxacillin** (see Table 37-3).
- If a patient has a mild, delayed allergy to penicillin, first-generation cephalosporins (such as **cefazolin**) are effective alternatives but should be avoided in patients with an immediate-type hypersensitivity reaction.
- In a patient with a positive penicillin skin test or a history of immediate hypersensitivity to penicillin, **vancomycin** is an option. Vancomycin, however, kills *S. aureus* slowly and is generally regarded as inferior to penicillinase-resistant penicillins for MSSA. Penicillin-allergic patients who fail on vancomycin therapy should be considered for penicillin desensitization. **Daptomycin** (at a dose of 6 mg/kg/day) is a recommended alternative.
- **Vancomycin** is the drug of choice for methicillin-resistant staphylococci because most methicillin-resistant *S. aureus* (MRSA) and most coagulase-negative staphylococci are susceptible. Reports of *S. aureus* strains resistant to vancomycin are increasing. Daptomycin (at a dose of 6 mg/kg/day) is now a recommended alternative.

TABLE 37-3 Treatment Options for Native Valve Endocarditis by Causative Organism

Agent[a]	Duration	Strength of Recommendation	Comments
Highly Penicillin-Susceptible (MIC ≤ 0.12 mcg/mL [mg/L]) Viridans Group Streptococci and S. gallolyticus			
Aqueous crystalline penicillin G sodium[b]	4 weeks	IIaB	2-week regimens are not intended for the following patients:
Ceftriaxone	4 weeks	IIaB	• Most patients >65 years of age
Aqueous crystalline penicillin G sodium[b] plus gentamicin	2 weeks	IIaB	• Children • Impairment of the eighth cranial nerve function • Renal function with a creatinine clearance <20 mL/min
Ceftriaxone plus gentamicin	2 weeks	IIaB	(0.33 mL/sec) • Known cardiac or extracardiac abscess • Infection with *Abiotrophia, Granulicatella,* or *Gemella* species
Vancomycin	4 weeks	IIaB	Recommended only for patients unable to tolerate penicillin or ceftriaxone
Viridans Group Streptococci and S. Gallolyticus Relatively Resistant to Penicillin (MIC >0.12 to ≤0.5 mcg/mL [mg/L])			
Aqueous crystalline penicillin G sodium[b] plus gentamicin	4 weeks 2 weeks	IIaB	
Ceftriaxone plus gentamicin	4 weeks 2 weeks	IIbC	
Vancomycin	4 weeks	IIaB	Recommended only for patients unable to tolerate penicillin or ceftriaxone
Oxacillin-Susceptible Staphylococci[c]			
Nafcillin or oxacillin	6 weeks	IC	
Cefazolin	6 weeks	IB	For use in patients with nonanaphylactoid-type penicillin allergies; patients with an unclear history of immediate-type hypersensitivity to penicillin should be considered for skin testing

(Continued)

TABLE 37-3 Treatment Options for Native Valve Endocarditis by Causative Organism (*Continued*)

Agent[a]	Duration	Strength of Recommendation	Comments
Vancomycin	6 weeks	IB	For use in patients with anaphylactoid-type hypersensitivity to penicillin and/or cephalosporins
Daptomycin	6 weeks	IIaB	For use in patients with immediate-type hypersensitivity reactions to penicillin
Oxacillin-Resistant Staphylococci			
Vancomycin	6 weeks	IB	
Daptomycin	6 weeks	IIbB	

[a]See Table 37-2 for appropriate dosing, administration, and monitoring information.

[b]May use ampicillin in the event of a penicillin shortage.

[c]Regimens indicate treatment for left-sided endocarditis or complicated right-sided endocarditis; uncomplicated right-sided endocarditis may be treated for shorter durations and is described in the text.

Please refer to Table 37-5 for treatment of NVE caused by enterococci.

| TABLE 37-4 | Treatment Options for Prosthetic Valve Endocarditis (PVE) by Causative Organism | | |

Agent[a]	Duration	Strength of Recommendation	Comments
Highly Penicillin-Susceptible (MIC ≤0.12 mcg/mL [mg/L]) Viridans Group Streptococci and _S. gallolyticus_			
Aqueous crystalline penicillin G sodium[b] with or without gentamicin	6 weeks 2 weeks	IIaB	Combination therapy with gentamicin has not demonstrated superior cure rates compared with monotherapy with a penicillin or cephalosporin and should be avoided in patients with CrCl <30 mL/min (0.50 mL/sec)
Ceftriaxone with or without gentamicin	6 weeks 2 weeks	IIaB	
Vancomycin	6 weeks	IIaB	Recommended only for patients unable to tolerate penicillin or ceftriaxone
Relatively Resistant or Fully Resistant (MIC >0.12 mcg/mL [mg/L]) Viridans Group Streptococci and _S. gallolyticus_			
Aqueous crystalline penicillin G sodium[b] plus gentamicin	6 weeks	IIaB	
Ceftriaxone plus gentamicin	6 weeks	IIaB	
Vancomycin[c]	6 weeks	IIaB	Recommended only for patients unable to tolerate penicillin or ceftriaxone
Oxacillin-Susceptible Staphylococci			
Nafcillin or oxacillin plus rifampin plus gentamicin	≥6 weeks ≥6 weeks 2 weeks	IB	Cefazolin may be substituted for nafcillin or oxacillin in patients with nonimmediate-type hypersensitivity
Vancomycin plus rifampin plus gentamicin	≥6 weeks ≥6 weeks 2 weeks	IB	Recommended only for patients with anaphylactoid-type hypersensitivity to penicillin and/or cephalosporins
Oxacillin-Resistant Staphylococci			
Vancomycin plus rifampin plus gentamicin	≥6 weeks ≥6 weeks 2 weeks	IB	

[a]See Table 37-2 for appropriate dosing, administration, and monitoring information.
[b]May use ampicillin in the event of a penicillin shortage.
[c]The ESC 2015 guidelines recommend gentamicin (3 mg/kg/day) be administered with vancomycin for the initial 2 weeks of therapy in patients with relatively resistant strains to penicillin.
Please refer to Table 37-5 for treatment of PVE caused by enterococci.

Treatment of *Staphylococcus* Endocarditis in IV Drug Abusers

- IE in IV drug abusers is most frequently (60%–70%) caused by *S. aureus*, although other organisms may be more common in certain geographic locations.
- A 2-week course of **nafcillin, oxacillin,** or **daptomycin** without an aminoglycoside is recommended. If vancomycin is selected, the standard 6-week regimen should therefore be used.

Treatment of Staphylococcal Prosthetic Valve Endocarditis

- PVE that occurs within 2 months of cardiac surgery is usually caused by staphylococci implanted at the time of surgery. Methicillin-resistant organisms are common. Vancomycin is the cornerstone of therapy.
- Because of the high morbidity and mortality associated with PVE and refractoriness to therapy, combinations of antimicrobials are usually recommended.
- For methicillin-resistant staphylococci (both MRSA and coagulase-negative staphylococci), **vancomycin** is used with rifampin for 6 weeks or more (see Table 37-4). An **aminoglycoside** is added for the first 2 weeks if the organism is susceptible. Due to the risk of developing on therapy resistance, rifampin should not be started until blood cultures have cleared.
- For methicillin-susceptible staphylococci, a **penicillinase-resistant penicillin** is used in place of vancomycin. If an organism is identified other than staphylococci, the treatment regimen should be guided by susceptibilities and should be at least 6 weeks in duration.

ENTEROCOCCAL ENDOCARDITIS

- Enterococci are the third leading cause of endocarditis and are noteworthy for the following reasons: (1) no single antibiotic is bactericidal; (2) MICs to penicillin are relatively high (1–25 mcg/mL [mg/L]); (3) they are intrinsically resistant to all cephalosporins and relatively resistant to aminoglycosides (ie, "low-level" aminoglycoside resistance); (4) combinations of a cell wall–active agent, such as a penicillin or vancomycin, plus an aminoglycoside are necessary for killing; and (5) resistance to all available drugs is increasing.
- Enterococcal endocarditis ordinarily requires 4–6 weeks of high-dose **penicillin G** or **ampicillin**, plus **gentamicin** for cure (Table 37-5). Ampicillin plus ceftriaxone is as effective as ampicillin plus gentamicin and should be considered as a treatment option. A 6-week course is recommended for patients with symptoms lasting longer than 3 months and those with PVE. Relatively low serum concentrations of aminoglycosides appear adequate for successful therapy, such as a gentamicin peak concentration of approximately 3–4 mcg/mL (mg/L; 6.3–8.4 µmol/L).
- In addition to isolates with high-level aminoglycoside resistance, β-lactamase–producing enterococci (especially *Enterococcus faecium*) are increasingly reported. If these organisms are discovered, use of vancomycin or ampicillin–sulbactam in combination with gentamicin should be considered.

EVALUATION OF THERAPEUTIC OUTCOMES

- The evaluation of patients treated for IE includes assessment of signs and symptoms, blood cultures, microbiologic tests (eg, MIC, minimum bactericidal concentration [MBC], or serum bactericidal titers), serum drug concentrations, and other tests to evaluate organ function.
- Persistence of fever beyond 1 week may indicate ineffective antimicrobial therapy, emboli, infections of intravascular catheters, or drug reactions. In some patients, fever may persist even with appropriate antimicrobial therapy.
- With effective therapy, blood should sterilize with negative cultures within a few days, although microbiologic response to vancomycin may be unusually slower. After the initiation of therapy, blood cultures should be rechecked until they are negative. During the remainder of the therapy, frequent blood culturing is not necessary.

| TABLE 37-5 | Treatment Options for Native or Prosthetic Valve Endocarditis Caused by Enterococci |

Agent[a]	Duration[b]	Strength of Recommendation	Comments
Ampicillin-, Penicillin-, and Vancomycin-Susceptible Strains			
Ampicillin plus gentamicin	4–6 weeks	IIaB	Native valve plus symptoms present for <3 months: use 4-week regimen
Aqueous crystalline penicillin G sodium plus gentamicin	4–6 weeks	IIAB	Prosthetic valve or native valve plus symptoms present for >3 months: use 6-week regimen
Ampicillin plus ceftriaxone	6 weeks	IIaB	Recommended regimen if creatinine clearance is <50 mL/min (0.83 mL/sec; at baseline or due to therapy with a gentamicin-containing regimen)
Vancomycin plus gentamicin	6 weeks	IIaB	Recommended only for patients unable to tolerate penicillin or ampicillin
Gentamicin-Resistant Strains			
If susceptible, use streptomycin in place of gentamicin in the regimens listed above if creatinine clearance is >50 mL/min (0.83 mL/sec), cranial nerve VIII function is intact and there is laboratory capability for rapid streptomycin serum concentrations.			
Penicillin-Resistant Strains			
Ampicillin–sulbactam plus gentamicin (β-lactamase–producing strain)	6 weeks	IIbC	
Vancomycin plus gentamicin (intrinsic penicillin resistance[c])	6 weeks	IIbC	May also use in patients with β-lactamase–producing strains who have known intolerance to ampicillin–sulbactam
***Enterococcus faecium* Strains Resistant to Penicillin, Aminoglycosides, and Vancomycin[d]**			
Linezolid	>6 weeks	IIbC	Antimicrobial cure rates may be <50%; bacteriologic cure may only be achieved with cardiac valve replacement
Daptomycin	>6 weeks	IIbC	

[a]See Table 37-2 for appropriate dosing, administration, and monitoring information.
[b]All patients with prosthetic valves should be treated for at least 6 weeks.
[c]Infectious diseases consult highly recommended.
[d]Patients should be managed by a multidisciplinary team that includes specialists in cardiology, cardiovascular surgery, infectious diseases, and clinical pharmacy.

- If bacteria continue to be isolated from blood beyond the first few days of therapy, it may indicate that the antimicrobials are inactive against the pathogen or that the doses are not producing adequate concentrations at the site of infection.
- For all isolates from blood cultures, MICs (not MBCs) should be determined.

PREVENTION OF ENDOCARDITIS

- Antimicrobial prophylaxis is used to prevent IE in patients believed to be at high risk.
- The use of antimicrobials for this purpose requires consideration of the types of patients who are at risk; the procedures causing bacteremia; the organisms that are likely to cause endocarditis; and the pharmacokinetics, spectrum, cost, and ease of administration of available agents. The objective of prophylaxis is to diminish the likelihood of IE in high-risk individuals who are undergoing procedures that cause transient bacteremia.
- The literature lacks adequate evidence to prove the effectiveness or ineffectiveness of antibiotic prophylaxis, and the common practice of using antimicrobial therapy in this setting remains controversial.

TABLE 37-6	Prophylaxis of Infective Endocarditis	
Highest Risk Cardiac Conditions	Presence of a prosthetic heart valve	
	Prosthetic material used for cardiac valve repair	
	Prior diagnosis of infective endocarditis	
	Cardiac transplantation with subsequent valvulopathy	
	Congenital heart disease (CHD)[a]	
Types of Procedures	Dental procedures that require perforation of the oral mucosa or manipulation of the periapical region of the teeth of gingival tissue	
	Invasive respiratory procedures involving an incision or biopsy	
	Invasive procedures involving infected skin, skin structures, or musculoskeletal tissue	
Antimicrobial Options	**Adult Doses[b]**	**Pediatric Doses[b] (mg/kg)**
Oral amoxicillin	2 g	50
IM or IV ampicillin[c]	2 g	50
IM or IV cefazolin or ceftriaxone[c,d,e]	1 g	50
Oral cephalexin[d,e,f]	2 g	50
Oral clindamycin[e]	600 mg	20
Oral azithromycin or clarithromycin[e]	500 mg	15
IV or IM clindamycin[c,e]	600 mg	20

[a]Includes only the following: unrepaired cyanotic CHD, prophylaxis within the first 6 months of implanting prosthetic material to repair a congenital heart defect, and repaired CHD with residual defects at or adjacent to prosthetic material.
[b]All one-time doses administered 30–60 minutes prior to initiation of the procedure.
[c]For patients unable to tolerate oral medication.
[d]Should be avoided in patients with immediate-type hypersensitivity reaction to penicillin or ampicillin (eg, anaphylaxis, urticaria, or angioedema).
[e]Option for patients with nonimmediate hypersensitivity reaction to penicillin or ampicillin.
[f]May substitute with an alternative first- or second-generation cephalosporin at an equivalent dose.

- IE prophylaxis should be recommended only for patients with underlying cardiac conditions associated with the highest risk, which includes presence of a prosthetic heart valve, prosthetic material used for cardiac valve repair, prior diagnosis of IE, cardiac transplantation with subsequent valvulopathy, CHD, for dental procedures involving manipulation of gingival tissue or the periapical region of teeth or perforation of the oral mucosa, invasive respiratory procedures involving an incision or biopsy, or invasive procedures involving infected skin, skin structures, or musculoskeletal tissues.
- Antibiotic regimens for a dental procedure are given in **Table 37-6.**

See Chapter 129, Infective Endocarditis, authored by Daniel B. Chastain and Angie Veverka, for a more detailed discussion of this topic.

Histoplasmosis

- *Histoplasmosis* is caused by inhalation of dust-borne microconidia of the dimorphic fungus *Histoplasma capsulatum*. In the United States, most disease is localized along the Ohio and Mississippi river valleys.

CLINICAL PRESENTATION AND DIAGNOSIS

- In the vast majority of patients, low-inoculum exposure to *H. capsulatum* results in mild or asymptomatic pulmonary histoplasmosis. The course of disease is generally benign, and symptoms usually abate within a few weeks of onset. Patients exposed to a higher inoculum during a primary infection or reinfection may experience an acute, self-limited illness with flu-like pulmonary symptoms, including fever, chills, headache, myalgia, and nonproductive cough.
- Chronic pulmonary histoplasmosis generally presents as an opportunistic infection imposed on a preexisting structural abnormality, such as lesions resulting from emphysema. Patients demonstrate chronic pulmonary symptoms and apical lung lesions that progress with inflammation, calcified granulomas, and fibrosis. Progression of disease over a period of years, seen in 25%–30% of patients, is associated with cavitation, bronchopleural fistulas, extension to the other lung, pulmonary insufficiency, and often death.
- In patients exposed to a large inoculum and in immunocompromised hosts, progressive illness, disseminated histoplasmosis, occurs. The clinical severity of the diverse forms of disseminated histoplasmosis (Table 38-1) generally parallels the degree of macrophage parasitization observed.
- Acute (infantile) disseminated histoplasmosis is seen in infants and young children and (rarely) in adults with Hodgkin disease or other lymphoproliferative disorders. It is characterized by unrelenting fever; anemia; leukopenia or thrombocytopenia; enlargement of the liver, spleen, and visceral lymph nodes; and GI symptoms, particularly nausea, vomiting, and diarrhea.
- If untreated it is uniformly fatal in 1-2 months. A less severe "subacute" form of the disease, which occurs in both infants and immunocompetent adults, is characterized by focal destructive lesions in various organs, weight loss, weakness, fever, and malaise.
- Most adults with disseminated histoplasmosis demonstrate a mild, chronic form of the disease. Untreated patients are often ill for 10–20 years, with long asymptomatic periods interrupted by relapses characterized by weight loss, weakness, and fatigue.
- Adult patients with acquired immunodeficiency syndrome (AIDS) demonstrate an acute form of disseminated disease that resembles the syndrome seen in infants and children. Progressive disseminated histoplasmosis can occur as the direct result of initial infection or because of reactivation of dormant foci.
- In most patients, serologic evidence (complement fixation test or immunodiffusion testing) remains the primary method in the diagnosis of histoplasmosis. Detection of histoplasma antigen by enzyme immunoassay (EIA) in the urine, blood, or bronchoalveolar lavage fluid of infected patients provides rapid diagnostic information and is particularly useful in patients who are severely ill.

TREATMENT

- The goals of therapy are resolution of clinical abnormalities, prevention of relapse, and eradication of infection whenever possible, although chronic suppression of infection can be adequate in immunosuppressed patients, including those with HIV disease.

TABLE 38-1	Clinical Manifestations and Therapy of Histoplasmosis	
Type of Disease and Common Clinical Manifestations	**Approximate Frequency (%)[a]**	**Therapy/Comments**
Nonimmunosuppressed Host		
Acute pulmonary histoplasmosis		
Asymptomatic or mild-to-moderate disease	50–99	*Asymptomatic, mild, or symptoms <4 weeks:* No therapy generally required; itraconazole (200 mg three times daily for 3 days and then 200 mg once or twice daily for 6–12 weeks) is recommended for patients who continue to have symptoms for 11 months *Symptoms >4 weeks:* Itraconazole 200 mg once daily × 6–12 weeks[b]
Self-limited disease	1–50	Amphotericin B[c] 0.3–0.5 mg/kg/day IV × 2–4 weeks (total dose 500 mg) or ketoconazole 400 mg orally daily × 3–6 months can be beneficial in patients with severe hypoxia following inhalation of large inocula; antifungal therapy generally not useful for arthritis or pericarditis; NSAIDs or corticosteroids can be useful in some cases
Mediastinal granulomas	1–50	Most lesions resolve spontaneously; surgery or antifungal therapy with amphotericin B 40–50 mg/day IV × 2–3 weeks or itraconazole 400 mg/day orally × 6–12 months can be beneficial in some severe cases; mild-to-moderate disease can be treated with itraconazole for 6–12 months
Moderately severe to severe diffuse pulmonary disease		Lipid amphotericin B 3–5 mg/kg/day IV followed by itraconazole 200 mg twice daily for 3 days then twice daily for a total of 12 weeks of therapy; alternatively, in patients at low risk for nephrotoxicity, amphotericin B deoxycholate 0.7–1 mg/kg/day IV can be utilized; methylprednisolone (0.5–1 mg/kg daily IV) during the first 1–2 weeks of antifungal therapy is recommended for patients who develop respiratory complications, including hypoxemia or significant respiratory distress
Inflammatory/fibrotic disease	0.02	*Fibrosing mediastinitis:* The benefit of antifungal therapy (itraconazole 200 mg orally twice daily × 3 months) is controversial but should be considered, especially in patients with elevated ESR or CF titers ≤1:32; surgery can be of benefit if disease is detected early; late disease cannot respond to therapy *Sarcoid-like:* NSAIDs or corticosteroids[d] can be of benefit for some patients *Pericarditis:* Severe disease: Prednisone (0.5–1.0 mg/kg daily [maximum, 80 mg daily] in tapering doses over 1–2 weeks) or pericardial drainage procedure *(Continued)*

TABLE 38-1	Clinical Manifestations and Therapy of Histoplasmosis (*Continued*)	
Type of Disease and Common Clinical Manifestations	**Approximate Frequency (%)[a]**	**Therapy/Comments**
Chronic cavitary pulmonary histoplasmosis	0.05	Antifungal therapy generally recommended for all patients to halt further lung destruction and reduce mortality *Mild–moderate disease:* Itraconazole 200 mg three times daily for 3 days and then one or two times daily for at least 1 year; some clinicians recommend therapy for 18–24 months due to the high rate of relapse; itraconazole plasma concentrations should be obtained after the patient has been receiving this agent for at least 2 weeks *Severe disease:* Amphotericin B 0.7 mg/kg/day for a minimum total dose of 25–35 mg/kg is effective in 59%–100% of cases and should be used in patients who require hospitalization or are unable to take itraconazole because of drug interactions, allergies, failure to absorb drug, or failure to improve clinically after a minimum of 12 weeks of itraconazole therapy
Histoplasma endocarditis		Amphotericin B (lipid formulations may be preferred, due to their lower rate of renal toxicity) plus a valve replacement is recommended; if the valve cannot be replaced, lifelong suppression with itraconazole is recommended
CNS histoplasmosis		Amphotericin B should be used as initial therapy (lipid formulations at 5 mg/kg/day IV, for a total dosage of 175 mg/kg may be preferred, due to their lower rate of renal toxicity) for 4–6 weeks, followed by an oral azole (fluconazole or itraconazole 200 mg two or three times daily) for at least a year; some patients may require lifelong therapy; response to therapy should be monitored by repeat lumbar punctures to assess *Histoplasma* antigen levels, WBC, and CF antibody titers; blood levels of itraconazole should be obtained to ensure adequate drug exposure
Immunosuppressed Host		
Disseminated histoplasmosis	0.02–0.05	Untreated mortality 83%–93%; relapse 5%–23% in non-AIDS patients; therapy is recommended for all patients

(*Continued*)

TABLE 38-1	Clinical Manifestations and Therapy of Histoplasmosis (*Continued*)
Type of Disease and Common Clinical Manifestations	**Approximate Frequency (%)[a]** **Therapy/Comments**

Type of Disease and Common Clinical Manifestations	Approximate Frequency (%)[a]	Therapy/Comments
Acute (infantile)		*Nonimmunosuppressed patients:* Ketoconazole 400 mg/day orally or deoxycholate amphotericin B >35 mg/day IV × 6–12 months
Subacute		*Immunosuppressed patients (non-AIDS) or endocarditis or CNS disease:* Deoxycholate amphotericin B >35 mg/day IV × 3 months followed by fluconazole or itraconazole 200 mg orally twice daily × 12 months
Progressive histoplasmosis (immuno-competent patients and immuno-suppressed patients without AIDS)		*Mild to moderate:* Itraconazole (200 mg orally twice daily for at least 12 months) *Moderately severe to severe:* Liposomal amphotericin B (3 mg/kg daily) IV, amphotericin B lipid complex (ABLC, 5 mg/kg daily) IV, or deoxycholate amphotericin B (0.7–1 mg/kg daily) for 1–2 weeks IV, followed by itraconazole (200 mg twice daily for at least 12 months)
Progressive disease of AIDS	25–50[e]	Deoxycholate amphotericin B 15–30 mg/day IV (1–2 g over 4–10 weeks)[f] or itraconazole 200 mg orally three times daily for 3 days then twice daily for 12 weeks, followed by lifelong suppressive therapy with itraconazole 200–400 mg orally daily; although patients receiving secondary prophylaxis (chronic maintenance therapy) might be at low risk for recurrence of systemic mycosis when their CD4+ T-lymphocyte counts increase to >100 cells/μL (0.1 × 10⁹/L) in response to HAART, the number of patients who have been evaluated is insufficient to warrant a recommendation to discontinue prophylaxis

[a]As a percentage of all patients presenting with histoplasmosis.
[b]Itraconazole plasma concentrations should be measured during the second week of therapy to ensure that detectable concentrations have been achieved. If the concentration is below 1 mcg/mL (mg/L; 1.4 μmol/L), the dose may be insufficient or drug interactions can be impairing absorption or accelerating metabolism, requiring a change in dosage. If plasma concentrations are greater than 10 mcg/mL (mg/L; 14 μmol/L), the dosage can be reduced.
[c]Deoxycholate amphotericin B.
[d]Effectiveness of corticosteroids is controversial.
[e]As a percentage of AIDS patients presenting with histoplasmosis as the initial manifestation of their disease.
[f]Liposomal amphotericin B (AmBisome) may be more appropriate for disseminated disease.
AIDS, acquired immunodeficiency syndrome; CF, complement fixation; ESR, erythrocyte sedimentation rate; HAART, highly active antiretroviral therapy; NSAIDs, nonsteroidal anti-inflammatory drugs; PO, orally.

- Recommended therapy for the treatment of histoplasmosis is summarized in **Table 38-1**.
- Patients with mild, self-limited disease, chronic disseminated disease, or chronic pulmonary histoplasmosis who have no underlying immunosuppression usually can be treated with either oral **itraconazole** or IV **amphotericin B**.
- In AIDS patients, intensive 12-week primary antifungal therapy (induction and consolidation therapy) is followed by lifelong suppressive (maintenance) therapy with itraconazole. Amphotericin B dosages of 50 mg/day (up to 1 mg/kg per day) should

be administered IV to a cumulative dose of 15–35 mg/kg (1–2 g) in patients who require hospitalization.

- Amphotericin B can be replaced with itraconazole 200 mg orally twice daily when the patient no longer requires hospitalization or IV therapy to complete a 12-week total course of induction therapy. In patients who do not require hospitalization, itraconazole therapy for 12 weeks can be used.
- Response to therapy should be measured by resolution of radiologic, serologic, and microbiologic parameters and improvement in signs and symptoms of infection.
- After the initial course of therapy for histoplasmosis is completed, lifelong suppressive therapy with oral azoles or amphotericin B (1–1.5 mg/kg weekly or biweekly) is recommended, because of the frequent recurrence of infection.
- Relapse rates in AIDS patients not receiving preventive maintenance are 50%–90%.

Blastomycosis

- North American *blastomycosis* is a systemic fungal infection caused by *Blastomyces dermatitidis*. Pulmonary disease can be acute or chronic and can mimic infection with tuberculosis, pyogenic bacteria, other fungi, or malignancy.

CLINICAL PRESENTATION AND DIAGNOSIS

- Acute pulmonary blastomycosis is generally an asymptomatic or self-limited disease characterized by fever, shaking chills, and a productive, purulent cough, with or without hemoptysis in immunocompetent individuals.
- Sporadic pulmonary blastomycosis may present as a more chronic or subacute disease, with low-grade fever, night sweats, weight loss, and a productive cough resembling that of TB rather than bacterial pneumonia. Chronic pulmonary blastomycosis is characterized by fever, malaise, weight loss, night sweats, chest pain, and productive cough.
- The simplest and most successful method of diagnosing blastomycosis is by direct microscopic visualization of the large, multinucleated yeast with single, broad-based buds in sputum or other respiratory specimens, following digestion of cells and debris with 10% potassium hydroxide. Histopathologic examination of tissue biopsies and culture of secretions should be used to identify *B. dermatitidis*, although it can require up to 30 days to isolate and identify a small inoculum.

TREATMENT

- In the immunocompetent host, acute pulmonary blastomycosis can be mild and self-limited and may not require treatment. However, consideration should be given to treating all infected individuals to prevent extrapulmonary dissemination. All individuals with moderate-to-severe pneumonia, disseminated infection, or those who are immunocompromised require antifungal therapy (Table 38-2).
- Some authors recommend azole therapy for the treatment of self-limited pulmonary disease, with the hope of preventing late extrapulmonary disease.
- **Itraconazole**, 200–400 mg/day, demonstrated 90% efficacy as a first-line agent in the treatment of non-life-threatening, non-CNS blastomycosis and 95% success rate for compliant patients who completed at least 2 months of therapy.
- All patients with disseminated blastomycosis, as well as those with extrapulmonary disease, require therapy.

Coccidioidomycosis

- *Coccidioidomycosis* is caused by infection with *Coccidioides immitis*. The endemic regions encompass the semiarid areas of the southwestern United States from California to Texas, known as the Lower Sonoran Zone. It encompasses a spectrum of illnesses ranging from primary uncomplicated respiratory tract infection that resolves spontaneously to progressive pulmonary or disseminated infection.

TABLE 38-2	Therapy of Blastomycosis
Type of Disease	**Preferred Treatment**
Pulmonary[a]	
Moderately severe to severe disease	Lipid formulation of amphotericin B 3–5 mg/kg IV daily or amphotericin B[b] 0.7–1 mg/kg IV daily (total dose 1.5–2.5 g) × 1–2 weeks or until improvement is noted, followed by itraconazole[c,d] 200 mg orally three times daily for 3 days, then 200 mg twice daily, × total of 6–12 months
Mild-to-moderate disease	Itraconazole[b,d] 200 mg orally three times daily for 3 days, then 200 mg twice daily, for a total of 6 months[b]
CNS Disease	*Induction:* Lipid formulation of amphotericin B 5 mg/kg IV daily × 4–6 weeks, followed by an oral azole as consolidation therapy
	Consolidation: Fluconazole[d] 800 mg orally daily, or itraconazole[d] 200 mg two or three times orally daily, or voriconazole[d] 200–400 mg orally twice daily, for ≥12 months and until resolution of CSF abnormalities
Disseminated or Extrapulmonary Disease	
Moderately severe to severe disease	Lipid formulation of amphotericin B 3–5 mg/kg IV daily or amphotericin B[b] 0.7–1 mg/kg IV daily × 1–2 weeks or until improvement is noted, followed by itraconazole[c,d] 200 mg orally three times daily for 3 days, then 200 mg twice daily × 6–12 months; treat osteoarticular disease with 12 months of antifungal therapy
	Most clinicians prefer to step-down to itraconazole[d] therapy once the patient's condition improves
Mild to moderate	Itraconazole[c,d] 200 mg orally three times daily for 3 days, then 200 mg once or twice daily × ≥12 months; treat osteoarticular disease with 12 months of antifungal therapy
Immunocompromised Host (Including Patients with AIDS, Transplants, or Receiving Chronic Glucocorticoid Therapy)	
Acute disease	Lipid formulation of amphotericin B 3–5 mg/kg IV daily or amphotericin B[a] 0.7–1 mg/kg IV daily × 1–2 weeks or until improvement is noted, then give suppressive therapy for a total of at least 12 months of therapy
Suppressive therapy	Itraconazole[c,d] 200 mg orally three times daily for 3 days, then 200 mg twice daily for a total of at least 12 months of therapy; lifelong suppressive therapy with oral itraconazole[d] 200 mg daily may be required for immunosuppressed patients in whom immunosuppression cannot be reversed, and in patients who experience relapse despite appropriate therapy

[a]In the immunocompetent host, acute pulmonary blastomycosis can be mild and self-limited and may not require treatment.
[b]Desoxycholate amphotericin B.
[c]Serum levels of itraconazole should be determined after the patient has received itraconazole for ≥2 weeks to ensure adequate drug exposure.
[d]Azoles should not be used during pregnancy.
AIDS, acquired immunodeficiency syndrome.

CLINICAL PRESENTATION AND DIAGNOSIS

- Approximately 60% of infected patients have an asymptomatic, self-limited infection without clinical or radiological manifestations. The remaining 40% of patients exhibit nonspecific symptoms that are often indistinguishable from ordinary upper respiratory infections, including fever, cough, headache, sore throat, myalgias, and fatigue that occur 1–3 weeks after exposure to the pathogen. A fine, diffuse rash may appear during the first few days of illness.
- Chronic, persistent pneumonia or persistent pulmonary coccidioidomycosis (primary disease lasting >6 weeks) is complicated by hemoptysis, pulmonary scarring, and the formation of cavities or bronchopleural fistulas.
- Disseminated infection occurs in less than 1% of infected patients. Dissemination may occur to the skin, lymph nodes, bone, meninges, spleen, liver, kidney, and adrenal gland. CNS infection occurs in ~16% of patients with disseminated infection.
- The diagnoses of coccidioidomycosis generally includes identification or recovery of *Coccidioides* spp. from clinical specimens and detection of specific anticoccidioidal antibodies in serum or other body fluids.

TREATMENT

- Desired outcomes of treatment are resolution of signs and symptoms of infection, reduction of serum concentrations of anticoccidioidal antibodies, and return of function of involved organs.
- Therapy of coccidioidomycosis is difficult, and the results are unpredictable. Only 5% of infected persons require therapy.
- Azole antifungals, primarily fluconazole and itraconazole, have replaced amphotericin B as initial therapy for most chronic pulmonary or disseminated infections. Specific antifungals (and their usual dosages) for the treatment of coccidioidomycosis include **amphotericin B** IV (0.5–1.5 mg/kg/day), **ketoconazole** (400 mg orally daily), IV or oral **fluconazole** (usually 400–800 mg daily, although dosages as high as 1200 mg/day have been used without complications), and **itraconazole** (200–300 mg orally twice daily as either capsules or solution). If itraconazole is used, measurement of serum concentrations may be helpful to ascertain whether oral bioavailability is adequate.
- Therapy often ranges from many months to years in duration, and in some patients, lifelong suppressive therapy is needed to prevent relapses.
- Amphotericin B is generally preferred as initial therapy in patients with rapidly progressive disease, whereas azoles are generally preferred in patients with subacute or chronic presentations. Lipid formulations of amphotericin B have not been extensively studied for coccidioidomycosis but can offer a means of giving more drugs with less toxicity.
- Patients with disease outside the lungs should be treated with 400 mg/day of an oral azole. For meningeal disease, fluconazole 400 mg/day orally should be used; however, some clinicians initiate therapy with 800 or 1000 mg/day, and itraconazole doses of 400–600 mg/day are comparable.

Cryptococcosis

- *Cryptococcosis* is a noncontagious, systemic mycotic infection caused by the ubiquitous encapsulated soil yeast *Cryptococcus neoformans*.

CLINICAL PRESENTATION AND DIAGNOSIS

- Primary cryptococcosis in humans almost always occurs in the lungs. Symptomatic infections are usually manifested by cough, rales, and shortness of breath that generally resolve spontaneously. Infection is acquired by inhalation of the organism.
- Disease may remain localized in the lungs or disseminate to other tissues, particularly the CNS, although the skin can also be affected.

- In the non-AIDS patient, the symptoms of cryptococcal meningitis are nonspecific. Symptomatic infections usually are manifested by cough, rales, and shortness of breath that generally resolve spontaneously. Headache, fever, nausea, vomiting, mental status changes, and neck stiffness are generally observed. In AIDS patients, fever and headache are common, but meningismus and photophobia are much less common than in non-AIDS patients.
- Examination of cerebrospinal fluid (CSF) in patients with cryptococcal meningitis generally reveals an elevated opening pressure, CSF pleocytosis (usually lymphocytes), leukocytosis, a decreased CSF glucose, an elevated CSF protein, and a positive cryptococcal antigen by latex agglutination.
- *C. neoformans* can be detected in ~60% of patients by India ink smear of CSF and cultured in more than 96% of patients.

TREATMENT

- Treatment of cryptococcosis is detailed in **Table 38-3**. For asymptomatic, immunocompetent persons with isolated pulmonary disease and no evidence of CNS disease, careful observation may be warranted. With symptomatic infection, **fluconazole** for 6–12 months is warranted.
- The use of intrathecal **amphotericin B** is not recommended for the treatment of cryptococcal meningitis except in very ill patients or in those with recurrent or progressive disease despite aggressive IV amphotericin B therapy. The dosage of amphotericin B employed is usually 0.5 mg administered via the lumbar, cisternal, or intraventricular (via an Ommaya reservoir) route two or three times weekly.
- Amphotericin B with **flucytosine** is the initial treatment of choice for acute therapy of cryptococcal meningitis in AIDS patients, although 1 week of amphotericin B plus flucytosine and 2 weeks of fluconazole plus flucytosine were effective as induction therapy for cryptococcal meningitis in resource limited settings. After the initially successful 2-week induction period, consolidation therapy with fluconazole can be administered for 8 weeks or until CSF cultures are negative.
- Immunocompromised patients with CNS infection require more prolonged therapy; treatment regimens are based on those used in the HIV-infected population and follow induction therapy with amphotericin B and consolidation therapy with 6–12 months of suppressive therapy with fluconazole.
- Relapse of *C. neoformans* meningitis occurs in ~50% of AIDS patients after completion of primary therapy. After the completion of induction/consolidation phases of therapy, long-term chronic suppression with fluconazole (200 mg orally daily) should be continued for a minimum of 1 year.

Candida Infections

- Eight species of *Candida* are regarded as clinically important pathogens in human disease: *C. albicans*, *C. tropicalis*, *C. parapsilosis*, *C. krusei*, *C. stellatoidea*, *C. guilliermondii*, *C. lusitaniae*, and *C. glabrata*. *C. albicans* is a normal commensal of the skin, female genital tract, and entire GI tract of humans.

HEMATOGENOUS CANDIDIASIS

- Dissemination of *C. albicans* can result in infection in single or multiple organs, particularly the kidney, brain, myocardium, skin, eye, bone, and joints.
- *Candida* is generally acquired via the gastrointestinal (GI) tract, although organisms may also enter the bloodstream via indwelling IV catheters.
- Immunosuppressed patients, including those with lymphoreticular or hematologic malignancies, diabetes, immunodeficiency diseases, or those receiving immunosuppressive therapy with high-dose corticosteroids, immunosuppressants, antineoplastic agents, or broad-spectrum antimicrobial agents are at high risk for invasive fungal infections.

TABLE 38-3 Therapy of Cryptococcosis[a,b]

Type of Disease and Common Clinical Manifestations	Therapy/Comments
Nonimmunocompromised Patients (Non–HIV-Infected, Nontransplant)	
Meningoencephalitis *without* neurological complications, in patients in whom CSF yeast cultures are negative after 2 weeks of therapy	*Induction:* Amphotericin B[c] IV 0.7–1 mg/kg/day *plus* flucytosine 100 mg/kg/day orally in four divided doses × ≥4 weeks A lipid formulation of amphotericin B may be substituted for amphotericin B in the second 2 weeks
Follow all regimens with suppressive therapy	*Consolidation:* Fluconazole 400–800 mg orally daily × 8 weeks *Maintenance:* Fluconazole 200 mg orally daily × 6–12 months
Meningoencephalitis *with* neurological complications	*Induction:* Same as for patients without neurologic complications, but consider extending the induction therapy for a total of 6 weeks; a lipid formulation of amphotericin B may be given for the last 4 weeks of the prolonged induction period *Consolidation:* Fluconazole 400 mg orally daily × 8 weeks
Mild-to-moderate pulmonary disease (nonmeningeal disease)	Fluconazole 400 mg orally daily × 6–12 months
Severe pulmonary cryptococcosis	*Same as CNS disease × 12 months*
Cryptococcemia (nonmeningeal, nonpulmonary disease)	*Same as CNS disease × 12 months*
Immunocompromised Patients	
Severe pulmonary cryptococcosis	*Same as CNS disease × 12 months*
HIV-Infected Patients	
Primary therapy; induction and consolidation[d]	*Preferred regimen:* *Induction:* Amphotericin B[e] IV 0.7–1 mg/kg IV daily *plus* flucytosine 100 mg/kg/day orally in four divided doses for ≥2 weeks
Follow all regimens with suppressive therapy	*Consolidation:* Fluconazole 400 mg (6 mg/kg) orally daily × ≥8 weeks Liposomal amphotericin B 3–4 mg/kg IV daily, or amphotericin B lipid complex (ABLC) 5 mg/kg IV daily, for ≥2 weeks can be substituted for amphotericin B[e] in patients with or at risk for renal dysfunction *Alternative regimens, in order of preference:* Amphotericin B[e] IV 0.7–1 mg/kg IV daily × 4–6 weeks *or* liposomal amphotericin B 3–4 mg/kg IV daily[f] × 4–6 weeks *or* ABLC 5 mg/kg IV daily × 4–6 weeks *or* Amphotericin B[e] IV 0.7 mg/kg IV daily, *plus* fluconazole 800 mg (12 mg/kg) orally daily × 2 weeks, followed by fluconazole 800 mg (12 mg/kg) orally daily × ≥8weeks *or* Fluconazole ≥800 mg (1200 mg/day is preferred) orally daily *plus* flucytosine 100 mg/kg/day orally in four divided doses × 6 weeks

(Continued)

TABLE 38-3	Therapy of Cryptococcosis[a,b](Continued)
Type of Disease and Common Clinical Manifestations	**Therapy/Comments**
	or
	Fluconazole 800–1200 mg/day orally daily × 10–12 weeks (a dosage ≥1200 mg/day is preferred when fluconazole is used alone)[g]
	or
	Itraconazole 200 mg orally twice daily × 10–12 weeks (use of itraconazole, which produces minimal concentrations of active drug in the CSF, is discouraged)[h]
Suppressive/Maintenance therapy[i]	Preferred: Fluconazole 200 mg orally daily × ≥1 year
	or
	Itraconazole[h] 200 mg orally twice daily × ≥1 year
	or
	Amphotericin B[j] IV 1 mg/kg weekly × ≥1 year
Organ Transplant Recipients	
Mild-to-moderate non-CNS disease or mild-to-moderate symptoms without diffuse pulmonary infiltrates	Fluconazole 400 mg (6 mg/kg) orally daily × 6–12 months
CNS disease, moderately severe or severe CNS disease or disseminated disease without CNS disease, or severe pulmonary disease without evidence of extrapulmonary or disseminated disease	*Induction:* Liposomal amphotericin B 3–4 mg/kg IV daily,[f] or ABLC 5 mg/kg IV daily *plus* flucytosine 100 mg/kg/day orally in four divided doses × ≥2 weeks
	If induction therapy does not include flucytosine, consider a lipid formulation of amphotericin B for ≥4–6 weeks of induction therapy; consider the use of a lipid formulation of amphotericin B[j] lipid formulation (6 mg/kg IV daily) in patients with a high-fungal burden disease or relapse of disease
	Consolidation: Fluconazole 400–800 mg (6–12 mg/kg) per day orally for 8 weeks
	Maintenance: Fluconazole 200–400 mg per day orally for 6–12 months

[a]When more than one therapy is listed, they are listed in order of preference.
[b]See the text for definitions of induction, consolidation, suppressive/maintenance therapy, and prophylactic therapy.
[c]Deoxycholate amphotericin B.
[d]Initiate HAART therapy 2–10 weeks after commencement of initial antifungal treatment.
[e]In patients with significant renal disease, lipid formulations of amphotericin B can be substituted for deoxycholate amphotericin B during the induction.
[f]Liposomal amphotericin B has been given safely up to 6 mg/kg daily; could be considered in treatment failure or in patients with a high-fungal burden.
[g]Or until cerebrospinal fluid (CSF) cultures are negative.
[h]Drug level monitoring is strongly advised.
[i]Consider discontinuing suppressive therapy during HAART in patients with a CD4 cell count ≥100 cells/μL (0.1 × 10^9/L) and an undetectable or very low HIV RNA level sustained for ≥3 months (with a minimum of 12 months of antifungal therapy). Consider reinstitution of maintenance therapy if the CD4 cell count decreases to <100 cells/μL (0.1 × 10^9/L).
[j]Use is discouraged except in azole intolerant patients, since it is less effective than azole therapy, and is associated with a risk of IV catheter-related infections.
HIV, human immunodeficiency virus; IT, intrathecal.

| TABLE 38-4 | Antifungal Therapy of Invasive Candidiasis |

Type of Disease and Common Clinical Manifestations	Therapy/Comments
Prophylaxis of Candidemia	
Non-neutropenic patients[a]	Not recommended except for severely ill/ high-risk patients in whom fluconazole IV/oral 400 mg daily should be used
Neutropenic patients[a]	The optimal duration of therapy is unclear but at a minimum should include the period at risk for neutropenia: fluconazole IV/oral 400 mg daily *or* itraconazole solution 2.5 mg/kg every 12 hours orally *or* micafungin 50 mg (1 mg/kg in patients under 50 kg) IV daily
Solid-organ transplantation, liver transplantation	*Patients with two or more key risk factors[b]:* Amphotericin B IV 10–20 mg daily *or* liposomal amphotericin B (AmBisome) 1 mg/kg/day *or* fluconazole 400 mg orally daily
Empirical (Preemptive) Antifungal Therapy	
Suspected disseminated candidiasis in febrile non-neutropenic patients	None recommended; data are lacking defining subsets of patients who are appropriate for therapy
Initial Antifungal Therapy (Documented Candidemia with Unknown *Candida* Species)	
Febrile neutropenic patients with prolonged fever despite 4–6 days of empirical antibacterial therapy	*Treatment duration:* Until resolution of neutropenia An echinocandin[c] is a reasonable alternative; voriconazole can be used in selected situations (see the text)
Less critically ill patients with no recent azole exposure	An echinocandin[c] or fluconazole (loading dose of 800 mg [12 mg/kg], then 400 mg [6 mg/kg] daily)
Additional mold coverage is desired	Voriconazole
Antifungal Therapy of Documented Candidemia and Acute Hematogenously Disseminated Candidiasis, Unknown Species	
Nonimmunocompromised host[d]	*Treatment duration:* 2 weeks after the last positive blood culture and resolution of signs and symptoms of infection *Remove existing central venous catheters when feasible plus fluconazole (loading dose of 800 mg [12 mg/kg], then 400 mg [6 mg/kg] daily) or an echinocandin[d]*
Patients with recent azole exposure, moderately severe or severe illness, or who are at high risk of infection due to *C. glabrata* or *C. krusei*	An echinocandin[c] Transition from an echinocandin to fluconazole is recommended for patients who are clinically stable and have isolates (eg, *C. albicans*) likely to be susceptible to fluconazole
Patients who are less critically ill and who have had no recent azole exposure	Fluconazole

(Continued)

TABLE 38-4 Antifungal Therapy of Invasive Candidiasis (*Continued*)

Type of Disease and Common Clinical Manifestations	Therapy/Comments
Antifungal Therapy of Specific Pathogens	
C. albicans, C. tropicalis, and *C. parapsilosis*	Fluconazole IV/oral 6 mg/kg/day *or* an echinocandin[c] or amphotericin B IV 0.7 mg/kg/day *plus* fluconazole IV/orally 800 mg/day; amphotericin B deoxycholate 0.5–1 mg/kg daily or a lipid formulation of amphotericin B (3–5 mg/kg daily) are alternatives in patients who are intolerant to other antifungals; transition from amphotericin B deoxycholate or a lipid formulation of amphotericin B to fluconazole is recommended in patients who are clinically stable and whose isolates are likely to be susceptible to fluconazole (eg, *C. albicans*); voriconazole (400 mg [6 mg/kg] twice daily × two doses then 200 mg [3 mg/kg] twice daily thereafter) is efficacious, but offers little advantage over fluconazole; it may be utilized as step-down oral therapy for selected cases of candidiasis due to *C. krusei* or voriconazole-susceptible *C. glabrata* *Patients intolerant or refractory to other therapy*[e]: Amphotericin B lipid complex IV 5 mg/kg/day Liposomal amphotericin B IV 3–5 mg/kg/day Amphotericin B colloid dispersion IV 2–6 mg/kg/day
C. krusei	Amphotericin B IV ≤1 mg/kg/day *or* an echinocandin[c]
C. lusitaniae	Fluconazole IV/orally 6 mg/kg/day
C. glabrata	An echinocandin[c] (transition to fluconazole or voriconazole therapy is not recommended without confirmation of isolate susceptibility)
Neutropenic host[f]	*Treatment duration:* Until resolution of neutropenia *Remove existing central venous catheters when feasible, plus:* Amphotericin B IV 0.7–1 mg/kg/day (total dosages 0.5–1 g) *or patients failing therapy with traditional amphotericin B:* Lipid formulation of amphotericin B IV 3–5 mg/kg/day
Chronic disseminated candidiasis (hepatosplenic candidiasis)	*Treatment duration:* Until calcification or resolution of lesions *Stable patients:* Fluconazole IV/orally 6 mg/kg/day *Acutely ill or refractory patients:* Amphotericin B IV 0.6–0.7 mg/kg/day

(*Continued*)

TABLE 38-4	Antifungal Therapy of Invasive Candidiasis (*Continued*)
Type of Disease and Common Clinical Manifestations	**Therapy/Comments**
Urinary candidiasis	*Asymptomatic disease:* Generally no therapy is required
	Symptomatic or high-risk patients[g]: Removal of urinary tract instruments, stents, and Foley catheters, +7–14 days therapy with fluconazole 200 mg orally daily *or* amphotericin B IV 0.3–1 mg/kg/day

[a]Patients at significant risk for invasive candidiasis include those receiving standard chemotherapy for acute myelogenous leukemia, allogeneic bone marrow transplants, or high-risk autologous bone marrow transplants. However, among these populations, chemotherapy or bone marrow transplant protocols do not all produce equivalent risk, and local experience should be used to determine the relevance of prophylaxis.

[b]Risk factors include retransplantation, creatinine of more than 2 mg/dL (177 μmol/L), choledochojejunostomy, intraoperative use of 40 units or more of blood products, and fungal colonization detected within the first 3 days after transplantation.

[c]Echinocandin = caspofungin 70 mg loading dose, then 50 mg IV daily maintenance dose, or micafungin 100 mg daily, or anidulafungin 200 mg loading dose, then 100 mg daily maintenance dose.

[d]Therapy is generally the same for acquired immunodeficiency syndrome (AIDS)/non-AIDS patients except where indicated and should be continued for 2 weeks after the last positive blood culture and resolution of signs and symptoms of infection. All patients should receive an ophthalmologic examination. Amphotericin B can be switched to fluconazole (IV or oral) for the completion of therapy. Susceptibility testing of the infecting isolate is a useful adjunct to species identification during selection of a therapeutic approach because it can be used to identify isolates that are unlikely to respond to fluconazole or amphotericin B. However, this is not currently available at most institutions.

[e]Often defined as failure of $\geq$500 mg amphotericin B, initial renal insufficiency (creatinine $\geq$2.5 mg/dL [221 μmol/L] or creatinine clearance <25 mL/min [0.42 mL/sec]), a significant increase in creatinine (to 2.5 mg/dL [221 μmol/L] for adults or 1.5 mg/dL [133 μmol/L] for children), or severe acute administration-related toxicity.

[f]Patients who are neutropenic at the time of developing candidemia should receive a recombinant cytokine (granulocyte colony–stimulating factor or granulocyte–monocyte colony-stimulating factor) that accelerates recovery from neutropenia.

[g]Patients at high risk for dissemination include neutropenic patients, low-birth-weight infants, patients with renal allografts, and patients who will undergo urologic manipulation.

- Major risk factors for hematogenous candidiasis include the use of central venous catheters, total parenteral nutrition, receipt of multiple antibiotics, extensive surgery and burns, renal failure and hemodialysis, mechanical ventilation, and prior fungal colonization.
- Treatment of candidiasis is presented in **Table 38-4**.

Aspergillus Infections

- *Aspergillus fumigatus* is the most commonly observed pathogen, followed by *Aspergillus flavus*.
- Invasive aspergillosis commonly affects immunocompromised patients and patients with acute myeloid leukemia (AML) and those who undergo allogeneic HSCT who have prolonged durations (more than 10 days) of neutropenia. Aspergillosis is generally acquired by inhalation of airborne conidia that are small enough (2.5–3 mm) to reach the alveoli or the paranasal sinuses.
- Superficial or locally invasive infections of the ear, skin, or appendages can often be managed with topical antifungal therapy.

ALLERGIC BRONCHOPULMONARY ASPERGILLOSIS

- Allergic manifestations of *Aspergillus* range in severity from mild asthma to allergic bronchopulmonary aspergillosis characterized by severe asthma with wheezing, fever, malaise, weight loss, chest pain, and a cough productive of blood-streaked sputum.
- Therapy is aimed at minimizing the quantity of antigenic material released in the tracheobronchial tree.
- Antifungal therapy is generally not indicated in the management of allergic manifestations of aspergillosis, although some patients have demonstrated a decrease in their glucocorticoid dose following therapy with itraconazole.

ASPERGILLOMA

- In the nonimmunocompromised host, *Aspergillus* infections of the sinuses most commonly occur as saprophytic colonization (aspergillomas, or "fungus balls") of previously abnormal sinus tissue. Treatment consists of removal of the aspergilloma. Therapy with glucocorticoids and surgery is generally successful.
- Although IV **amphotericin B** is generally not useful in eradicating aspergillomas, intracavitary instillation of amphotericin B has been used successfully in a limited number of patients.

INVASIVE ASPERGILLOSIS

- Patients with invasive aspergillosis generally have blunted or nonspecific signs and symptoms of infection due to impaired inflammatory responses. Patients often present with classic signs and symptoms of acute pulmonary embolus: pleuritic chest pain, fever, hemoptysis, and friction rubs.
- Demonstration of *Aspergillus* by repeated culture and microscopic examination of tissue provides the most firm diagnosis.

TREATMENT

- **Voriconazole** is the drug of choice for primary therapy of most patients with invasive aspergillosis as it provided improved survival and fewer side effects.
- In patients who cannot tolerate voriconazole, amphotericin B can be used. Full doses (1–1.5 mg/kg/day) are generally recommended, with response measured by defervescence and radiographic clearing. The lipid-based formulations may be preferred as initial therapy in patients with marginal renal function or in patients receiving other nephrotoxic drugs. The optimal duration of treatment is unknown.
- **Caspofungin** is indicated for treatment of invasive aspergillosis in patients who are refractory to or intolerant of other therapies such as amphotericin B.
- The use of prophylactic antifungal therapy to prevent primary infection or reactivation of aspergillosis during subsequent courses of chemotherapy is controversial.

See Chapter 139, Invasive Fungal Infections, authored by Peggy L. Carver, for a more detailed discussion of this topic.

39 CHAPTER

Vulvovaginal Candidiasis

- Vulvovaginal candidiasis (VVC) refers to infections in individuals with or without symptoms who have positive vaginal cultures for *Candida* species. It may be sporadic or recurrent.
- By 25 years of age, approximately 50% of college-age women will have had at least one episode of VVC.

PATHOPHYSIOLOGY

- *C. albicans* is the major pathogen responsible for VVC, accounting for 80%–92% of symptomatic episodes. The remainder are caused by non–*C. albicans* species, with *Candida glabrata* dominating.
- Changes in the host's vaginal environment or response are necessary to induce a symptomatic infection. In most cases of symptomatic VVC, no precipitating factor can be identified.

CLINICAL PRESENTATION

- There is a dramatic increase in the frequency of VVC when women become sexually active.
- Antibiotic use can increase the risk of VVC, but it is significant in only a small number of women.
- Symptoms include intense vulvar itching, soreness irritation, burning on urination, and dyspareunia.
- Signs include erythema, fissuring, curdy "cheese"-like discharge, satellite lesions, and edema.
- Laboratory tests: Vaginal pH—normal saline, and 10% potassium hydroxide (KOH) microscopy for blastospores or pseudohyphae.
- *Candida* cultures are not recommended unless classic signs and symptoms with normal vaginal pH and microscopy are inconclusive or recurrence is suspected.
- The diagnosis should be based on both clinical presentation and investigations, including vaginal pH, saline microscopy, and 10% KOH microscopy of vaginal discharge.

TREATMENT

- <u>Goals of Treatment</u>: Complete resolution of symptoms in patients who have symptomatic VVC.

GENERAL APPROACH

- Remove or improve any predisposing factors if they can be identified.
- Avoid harsh soaps and perfumes that can cause or worsen vulvar irritation. The genital area must be kept clean and dry by avoiding constrictive clothing and frequent or prolonged exposure to hot tub use. Douching is not recommended for either prevention or treatment.

NONPHARMACOLOGIC THERAPY

- The value of oral use of lactobacillus remains unclear. Daily ingestion of 240 mL yogurt containing *Lactobacillus acidophilus* decreased colonization and symptomatic infections of VVC in women with recurrent infections.

• A trial of an oral mixture of bee-honey and yogurt showed some efficacy with mycotic cure rates of 76.9% compared to cure rates with antifungal agents of 91.5%.

PHARMACOLOGIC THERAPY

• Effective antimycotic agents should have limited local and systemic side effects, a high cure rate, and easy administration.
• Table 39-1 lists treatments for uncomplicated VVC. There are no significant differences in in-vitro activity or clinical efficacy among the topical azole agents. Oral azoles (such as **fluconazole** or **itraconazole**) are therapeutically equivalent to topical therapies.
• Patients with complicated VVC (immunocompromised or uncontrolled diabetes mellitus) should be treated for 10–14 days.
• Pregnant patients with VVC should be treated with topical agents.
• Patients with recurrent VVC should receive a 10-day initial treatment (such as with oral **fluconazole** 150 mg) followed by 6 months of prolonged treatment (with oral fluconazole once weekly 150 mg).
• Treatment of VVC is considered to have positive outcomes if the symptoms are resolved within 24–48 hours and no adverse medication events are experienced. Self-assessment of symptom relief is appropriate for most cases of VVC. If symptoms remain unresolved or recur, then further testing and treatment can be required.

TABLE 39-1	Treatment for Uncomplicated Vulvovaginal Candidiasis	
Active Ingredient	**Preparation**	**Regimen**
Nonprescription/Topical vaginal products		
Butoconazole	2% cream	One applicator × 3 days
Clotrimazole	1% cream	One applicator × 1 day
	100 mg tablet	One 100 mg tablet × 7 days
	2% cream	One applicator × 1 day
	200 mg tablet	One 200 mg tablet × 3 days
	10% cream	One applicator × 1 day
	500 mg tablet	One 500 mg tablet × 1 day
Miconazole[a]	2% cream	One applicator × 1 day
	100 mg suppository	One 100 mg suppository × 7 days
	200 mg suppository	One 200 mg suppository × 3 days
	1200 mg ovule	One ovule × 1 day
Ticonazole	2% cream	One applicator × 3 days
	6.5% cream	One applicator × 1 day
Prescription/Topical		
Nystatin	100,000 unit tablet	One tablet × 14 days
Terconazole	0.4% cream	One applicator × 7 days
	0.8% cream	One applicator × 3 days
Oral products		
Fluconazole	150 mg	One tablet × 1 day

[a]The FDA warns of the possible increase in the anticoagulant effects of warfarin with concomitant use.

O](**Orophyryngeal and Esophageal Candidiasis**

- Oropharyngeal candidiasis (OPC), often referred to as thrush, is caused by the yeast *Candida,* most often *C. albicans.*

PATHOPHYSIOLOGY

- A variety of host and exogenous factors can lead to the transformation of asymptomatic colonization to symptomatic disease, such as oropharyngeal and esophageal candidiasis.
- Endocrine disorders besides diabetes mellitus, such as hypothyroidism, hypoparathyroidism, and hypoadrenalism, also can predispose patients to *Candida* species overgrowth.
- Patients with primary immune deficiencies such as lymphocytic abnormalities, phagocytic dysfunction, immunoglobulin A (IgA) deficiency, viral-induced immune paralysis, and severe congenital immunodeficiencies are also at risk for OPC as well as disseminated candidiasis.
- OPC remains the most common opportunistic infection in patients with HIV disease. The CD4 T-cell count is the hallmark predictor for development of OPC; however, HIV viral load may have a stronger association with OPC than CD4 cell number.

CLINICAL PRESENTATION

- Various classifications of OPC are given in **Table 39-2**. The clinical presentation of OPC and esophageal candidiasis is presented in **Table 39-3**.
- A presumptive diagnosis of OPC usually is made by the characteristic appearance on the oral mucosa, with resolution of signs and symptoms after antifungal therapy.

TREATMENT

- The primary desired outcome in the management of OPC is a clinical cure; that is, elimination of clinical signs and symptoms. Efficacy end points for oropharyngeal and esophageal candidiasis include rapid relief of symptoms and prevention of complications without early relapse after completion of the course of therapy.
- Minimizing toxicities and drug–drug interactions of systemic antifungal agents, as well as maximizing adherence by ensuring that the patient understands the importance of therapy and the directions to take the medication appropriately, are important secondary outcomes of therapy.

GENERAL APPROACH

- Whenever feasible, it is desirable to minimize all predisposing factors, such as administration of corticosteroids, chemotherapeutic agents, and antimicrobials, as well as to institute proper oral hygiene and resolve concurrent conditions, such as denture stomatitis.

PHARMACOLOGIC THERAPY

- Topical agents, such as **nystatin** and **clotrimazole**, are the standard treatment for uncomplicated OPC and generally are effective for treatment in otherwise healthy adults and infants with no underlying immunodeficiencies (**Table 39-4**).
- Systemic therapy is necessary in patients with OPC that is refractory to topical treatment, those who cannot tolerate topical agents, have moderate-to-severe disease, and those at high risk for disseminated systemic or invasive candidiasis.
- When patients become unresponsive to topical agents or **fluconazole** and **itraconazole**, alternative agents include **amphotericin B** and other triazoles such as **voriconazole** and **posaconazole** and echinocandins (**caspofungin, micafungin,** and **anidulafungin**).

TABLE 39-2	Clinical Classification of Oropharyngeal Candidiasis	
Types	**Population at Risk**	**Clinical Signs and Appearance**
Pseudomembranous (thrush)	Neonates, patients with HIV or cancer, the debilitated elderly, patients on broad-spectrum antibiotics or steroid inhalers, patients with dry mouth from various causes, and smokers	Classic "cottage cheese" appearance, yellowish white, soft plaques (or milk curds) overlying areas of erythema on the buccal mucosa, tongue, gums, and throat; plaques are easily removed by vigorous rubbing but can leave red or bleeding sites when removed; lesions on the tongue dorsum give it a bald, depapillated appearance
Erythematous (atrophic)	Patients with HIV, patients on broad-spectrum antibiotics or steroid inhalers	Sensitive and painful erythematous mucosa with few, if any, white plaques; lesions are generally on the dorsal surface of the tongue or the hard palate, occasionally on the soft palate, but any part of the mucosa can be involved; appear as flat red patches on the palate or atrophic patches on the tongue dorsum with loss of papillae. Can be acute or chronic
Hyperplastic (candidal leukoplakia)	Smokers; uncommon in patients with HIV	Thick white and adherent keratotic plaques commonly seen on the buccal mucosa and lateral border of the tongue; can also be seen on the lips and the bottom of the mouth; plaques cannot be easily scraped off or only partially removed; this condition is distinct from oral hairy leukoplakia, and it can progress to severe dysplasia or malignancy
Angular cheilitis	Patients with HIV, denture wearers	Painful red, ulcerative, cracking, or fissuring lesion at one or both corners of the mouth because of an inflammatory reaction; usually lesions are small and rather punctate, but occasionally they can extend in a linear fashion from the angles onto the facial skin
Denture stomatitis (chronic atrophic)	Denture wearers who tend to be elderly and have poor oral hygiene	Red, flat lesions on the mucosa beneath the denture and extend right up to the denture border; more commonly located beneath a maxillary denture, although they can be encountered beneath a mandibular denture
Central papillary atrophy (median rhomboid glossitis)	Uncommon (<1% prevalence), men more commonly infected than women (3:1)	Rhomboid-shaped hypertrophic or atrophic plaque in the mid-DORSAL tongue. Lesions may not resolve completely

HIV, human immunodeficiency virus.

TABLE 39-3	Clinical Presentation of Oropharyngeal and Esophageal Candidiasis
Oropharyngeal Candidiasis	**Esophageal Candidiasis**
General	**General**
The clinical features can be quite diverse (see Table 39-2)	This usually occurs as an extension of OPC; however, the esophagus can be the only site involved; the distal two-thirds, rather than the proximal one-third, is the most common site
Symptoms	**Symptoms**
Symptoms are diverse and range from none to a sore, painful mouth, burning tongue, metallic taste, and dysphagia and odynophagia with involvement of the hypopharynx	Typically, the symptoms are dysphagia, odynophagia, and retrosternal chest pain but can be asymptomatic in some patients; although rare, epigastric pain can be the dominant symptom
Signs	**Signs**
Signs are variable and can include diffuse erythema and white patches on the surfaces of the buccal mucosa, throat, tongue, or gums; constitutional signs are absent	Constitutional signs, including fever, occasionally occur; physical findings can range from a few to numerous white or beige plaques of variable size
	Plaques can be hyperemic or edematous, with ulceration in more severe cases
	Most advanced cases can occur with increased mucosal friability and narrowing of lumen
	Uncommon complications include perforation and aortic–esophageal fistula formation
Laboratory tests	**Laboratory tests**
Scraping of an active lesion for microscopic examination can help confirm the diagnosis (presence of pseudohyphae and budding yeast) but is usually not necessary	The best test is upper GI endoscopy (more useful than barium swallow); helps exclude other causes of esophagitis (eg, viral, aphthous ulcers); diagnosis is confirmed by the histologic presence of *Candida* species in biopsy lesions taken during endoscopy
Cultures are not necessary because isolation of *Candida* species does not distinguish between colonization and true infection; cultures can be taken in patients responding poorly to therapy to determine the infecting species and to predict likely drug resistance	Cultures to look for drug-resistant *Candida* species are warranted in patients who require endoscopy

GI, gastrointestinal; OPC, oropharyngeal candidiasis.

- Long-term suppressive therapy with fluconazole is effective in preventing recurrences or new infections of OPC in HIV disease and in patients with cancer. However, the indications for antifungal prophylaxis and the best long-term management strategy still have not been well established.
- Patients with a history of one or more episodes of documented esophageal candidiasis and a CD4 T-cell count <200 cells/mm³ (<0.2 × 10⁹/L) despite being on highly active antiretroviral therapy (HAART) are candidates for secondary prophylaxis. Oral **fluconazole** 100 mg three times weekly is the regimen recommended for patients deemed in need of chronic suppressive therapy.

| **TABLE 39-4** | Therapeutic Options for Mucosal Candidiasis |

Initial Episodes of OPC[a]: Treat for 7–14 Days (Strength of Recommendation and Level of Evidence)	Common/Significant Side Effects
Clotrimazole 10 mg troche: hold 1 troche in mouth for 15–20 minutes for slow dissolution 5 times daily (B-2)[b]	Altered taste, mild nausea, vomiting
Nystatin 100,000 units/mL suspension: 5 mL swish and swallow orally 4 times daily (B-2)	Mild nausea, vomiting, diarrhea
Miconazole 50 mg mucoadhesive buccal tablets 50 mg orally daily (A-1)	Diarrhea, headache, nausea, dysgeusia, upper abdominal pain, and vomiting
Fluconazole 100 mg tablets[c]: 100–200 mg orally daily (A-1)	GI upset, hepatitis not common
Itraconazole 10 mg/mL solution[d]: 200 mg orally daily (A-2)	GI upset, not common: hepatotoxicity, CHF, pulmonary edema with long-term use[e]
Posaconazole 40 mg/mL suspension: 400 mg orally daily with a full meal (A-2)	GI upset, fever, headache, increased hepatic transaminases not common
Fluconazole-refractory OPC: Treat for ≥14 days	
Itraconazole 10 mg/mL solution: 200 mg orally daily (A-3)	See above
Voriconazole 200 mg tablets: 200 mg orally twice daily (>40 kg), taken on empty stomach (A-3)	GI upset, rash, reversible visual disturbance (altered light perception, photopsia, chromatopsia, photophobia), increased hepatic transaminases, hallucinations, or confusion
Posaconazole 40 mg/mL suspension: 400 mg orally twice daily × 3 days, then 400 mg daily × 28 days (A-2)	See above
Amphotericin B 100 mg/mL suspension[f]: 1–5 mL swish and swallow orally 4 times daily (B-2)	Oral: nausea, vomiting, diarrhea with higher dose
Amphotericin B deoxycholate 50 mg injection: 0.3–0.7 mg/kg/day IV daily (B-2)	IV: fever, chills, sweats, nephrotoxicity, electrolyte disturbances, bone marrow suppression
Caspofungin 50 mg IV daily (B-2)	Fever, headache, infusion-related reactions (<5%) (eg, rash, facial swelling, pruritus, vasodilation), hypokalemia, increased hepatic transaminases, anemia, neutropenia
Micafungin 150 mg IV daily (B-2)	Similar to caspofungin
Anidulafungin 200 mg IV daily (B-2)	Similar to caspofungin
Esophageal candidiasis[a]: Treat for 14–21 days	
Fluconazole 100 mg tablets: 200–400 mg orally (3–6 mg/kg) daily (A-1)	See above
Echinocandin: see above (B-2)	See above

(Continued)

417

TABLE 39-4 Therapeutic Options for Mucosal Candidiasis (*Continued*)	
Initial Episodes of OPC[a]: Treat for 7–14 Days (Strength of Recommendation and Level of Evidence)	**Common/Significant Side Effects**
Amphotericin B deoxycholate 50 mg injection: 0.3–0.7 mg/kg/day IV daily (B-2)	See above
Posaconazole 40 mg/mL suspension: 400 mg orally twice daily (A-3)	See above
Itraconazole 10 mg/mL solution[d]: 200 mg orally daily (A-3)	See above
Voriconazole 200 mg tablets: 200 mg orally twice daily (>40 kg) (A-3)	See above
Voriconazole IV and echinocandins (A-1): generally reserved for refractory cases	See above
Fluconazole-refractory EC: Treat for 21–28 days	
Itraconazole 10 mg/mL solution: 200 mg orally daily (A-2)	See above
Posaconazole 40 mg/mL suspension: 400 mg orally twice daily (A-3)	See above
Voriconazole 200 mg tablets: 200 mg orally twice daily (>40 kg), taken on empty stomach (A-3)	See above
Caspofungin 50 mg IV daily (B-2)	See above
Micafungin 150 mg IV daily (B-2)	Similar to caspofungin
Anidulafungin 100 mg IV on day 1, then 50 mg IV daily (B-2)	Similar to caspofungin
Amphotericin B deoxycholate: 0.3–0.7 mg/kg/day IV, or lipid-based amphotericin 3–5 mg/kg/day IV (B-2)	See above

[a]Initial episodes of OPC can be adequately treated first with topical agents before resorting to systemic therapy (B-2), but systemic therapy is required for effective treatment of esophageal candidiasis. (A-2) Suppressive therapy is recommended for patients with frequent or severe recurrences (A-1).
[b]Fluconazole is more effective than ketoconazole (A-1).
[c]Strength of Recommendation and Level of Evidence
[d]Solution is more effective than capsule (A-1); solution is better taken on an empty stomach.
[e]Suspension is not marketed; can be prepared extemporaneously by pharmacy.
[f]See discussion under onychomycosis.
CHF, congestive heart failure; EC, esophageal candidiasis; GI, gastrointestinal; IV, intravenous; OPC, oropharyngeal candidiasis.
Recommendation grades: Strength of recommendation: **A**—Both strong evidence for efficacy and substantial clinical benefit to support recommendation for use. *Should always be offered.* **B**—Moderate evidence for efficacy but only limited clinical benefit, to support recommendation for use. *Should generally be* offered. **C**—Evidence for efficacy is insufficient to support recommendation for or against use; or evidence for efficacy might not outweigh adverse consequences or cost of the treatment under consideration. *Optional.* **D**—Moderate evidence for lack of efficacy or adverse outcome supports a recommendation against use. *Should generally not be offered.* Quality of evidence: 1—Evidence from at least one properly designed randomized, controlled trial. 2—Evidence from at least one well-designed trial without randomization, from cohort or case-controlled analytic studies (preferably from more than one center), or from multiple time-series studies, or dramatic results from uncontrolled experiments. 3—Evidence from opinions of respected authorities based on clinical experience, descriptive studies, or reports of expert committees. (UR) Evidence currently unrated.

EVALUATION OF THERAPEUTIC OUTCOMES

- Patient counseling tips for managing OPC are given in **Table 39-5.**

TABLE 39-5	Patient Counseling Tips for Managing Oropharyngeal Candidiasis
1.	Clean the oral cavity prior to administering the topical antifungal agent. Daily fluoride rinses can help reduce the risk of caries when using an agent containing sucrose or dextrose.
2.	Use the topical antifungal agent after meals, as saliva flow and mouth movements can reduce the contact time.
3.	Dissolve troches slowly in the mouth and swallow the saliva; do not chew or swallow them whole.
4.	Swish the suspension, around the mouth in the oral cavity to cover all areas for as long as possible, ideally at least 1 minute, then gargled and swallowed.
5.	Remove dentures while medication is being applied to the oral tissues.
6.	Use a suspension or buccal mucoadhesive tablet instead of a troche if xerostomia is present; if a troche is preferred, rinse or drink water prior to dosing. For xerostomia, you may use nonpharmacologic measures for symptomatic relief (eg, ice chips, sugarless gum or hard candy, citrus beverages).
7.	Remove dentures and disinfect overnight using an antiseptic solution (eg, chlorhexidine 0.12%–0.2%). Disinfect oral tissues in addition to dental prosthesis.
8.	Complete treatment course even though symptomatic improvement can occur in 48–72 hours.
9.	Maintain good oral hygiene. Brush teeth daily (twice daily) and floss, rinse mouth, or brush teeth after eating sweets.
10.	Stop smoking; avoid alcohol.

Mycotic Infections of the Skin, Hair, and Nails

PATHOPHYSIOLOGY

- Superficial cutaneous mycoses affect up to 20%–25% of the population globally. The usual pathogens are the dermatophytes classified by genera: *Trichophyton, Epidermophyton,* and *Microsporum.*
- Dermatophytes have the ability to penetrate keratinous structures of the body and therefore infections are limited to hair, nails, and skin. These infections affect both male and female genders and all races. Reservoirs of mycotic infections include humans, animals, and soil.
- Risk factors for the development of an infection include prolonged exposure to sweat or soaking in water, maceration, intertriginous folds, sharing personal belongings such as combs, close living quarters (dormitories, barracks).

CLINICAL PRESENTATION

- Mycotic infections of the skin have a classic appearance that consists of a central clearing surrounded by an advancing red, scaly, elevated border, also referred to as an "active" border.
- Diagnosis usually is based on patient history, as well as the physical examination. Diagnostic tests include direct microscopic examination of a specimen after the addition of KOH or fungal cultures. The KOH test is quick, inexpensive, and easy to perform.

TREATMENT

GENERAL APPROACH

- A general approach to treatment of superficial mycotic infections includes keeping the infected area dry and clean and limiting exposure to the infected reservoir. Topical agents generally are considered to be first-line therapy for infections of the skin. Oral therapy is preferred when the infection is extensive or severe or when treating *tinea capitis* or onychomycosis.
- Treatment of mycoses of the skin, hair, and nails is given in **Table 39-6**.

TABLE 39-6	Treatment of Mycoses of the Skin, Hair, and Nails	
	Topical[a,b]	**Oral Regimen**[c]
Tinea pedis	Butenafine, daily	Fluconazole 150 mg 1 per week × 1–4 weeks
	Sertaconazole, twice daily	
	Luliconazole, daily	
	Naftifine cream daily, gel daily	
Tinea manuum	Ciclopirox, twice daily	Ketoconazole 200 mg daily × 4 weeks
Tinea cruris	Clotrimazole, twice daily	Itraconazole 200–400 mg/day × 1 week
	Luliconazole, daily	
	Naftifine cream, daily	
Tinea corporis	Econazole, daily	Terbinafine 250 mg/day × 2 weeks
	Haloprogin, twice daily	
	Ketoconazole cream, daily	
	Luliconazole, daily	
	Miconazole, twice daily	
	Naftifine cream, daily	
	Oxiconazole, twice daily	
	Sulconazole, twice daily	
	Terbinafine, twice daily	
	Tolnaftate, twice daily	
	Triacetin cream, solution, three times daily	
	Undecylenic acid, various preparations: apply as directed	
Tinea capitis	Shampoo only in conjunction with oral therapy **or** for treatment of asymptomatic carriers	Terbinafine 250 mg/day × 4–8 weeks
Tinea barbae	Ketoconazole twice weekly × 4 weeks	Ketoconazole 200 mg daily × 4 weeks
	Selenium sulfide daily × 2 weeks	Itraconazole 100–200 mg/day × 4–6 weeks
		Griseofulvin 500 mg/day × 4–6 weeks

(Continued)

TABLE 39-6	Treatment of Mycoses of the Skin, Hair, and Nails (*Continued*)	
	Topical[a,b]	**Oral Regimen**[c]
Pityriasis versicolor	Clotrimazole, twice daily Econazole, daily	Fluconazole 300 mg once weekly × 2 weeks.
	Haloprogin, twice daily Ketoconazole, daily	Itraconazole 200 mg daily × 3–7 days
	Miconazole, twice daily	
	Oxiconazole cream only, twice daily	
	Sulconazole, twice daily	
	Tolnaftate, three times daily	
Onychomycosis	Ciclopirox 8% nail lacquer: apply solution at night for up to 48 weeks (fingernails and toenails)	Terbinafine 250 mg/day × 6 weeks (fingernail), 12 weeks (toenail)
	Efinaconazole 10% topical solution daily for 48 weeks (toenails)	Itraconazole 200 mg twice daily × 1 week/month for 2 months (fingernail); 200 mg daily × 12 weeks (toenail)
	Tavaborole 5% topical solution daily for 48 weeks (toenails)	Fluconazole 50 mg daily or 300 mg once weekly for ≥6 months (fingernail) or 12 months (toenail)

[a]Other products are available, including combination products.
[b]Length of therapy depends on mycotic sensitivity and severity of infection.
[c]Only capsule formulation studied; give with food for increased absorption.

See Chapter 138, Superficial Fungal Infections, authored by Thomas E.R. Brown and Linda Dresser, for a more detailed discussion of this topic.

- *Gastrointestinal* (GI) infections are among the more common causes of morbidity and mortality around the world. Most are caused by viruses, and some are caused by bacteria or other organisms. In underdeveloped and developing countries, acute gastroenteritis involving diarrhea is the leading cause of mortality in infants and children younger than 5 years of age. In the United States, there are 179 million episodes of acute gastroenteritis each year, causing nearly 500,000 hospitalizations and over 5000 deaths.
- Viruses are now the leading global cause of infectious diarrhea. Noroviruses, previously known as Norwalk-like viruses, account for greater than 90% of viral gastroenteritis among all age groups, and 50% of outbreaks worldwide.
- Public health measures such as clean water supply and sanitation facilities, as well as quality control of commercial products, are important for the control of most enteric infections. Sanitary food handling and preparation practices significantly decrease the incidence of enteric infections.

Rehydration, Antimotility, And Probiotic Therapy

- The cornerstone of management for all GI infections and enterotoxigenic poisonings is to prevent dehydration by correcting fluid and electrolyte imbalances. In mild, self-limiting acute gastroenteritis, a diet of oral fluids and easily digestible foods is recommended. In patients with severe dehydrating watery diarrhea and dysenteric diarrhea, IV rehydration therapy, antibiotics, and/or antimotility treatments are needed.
- Initial assessment of fluid loss is essential for rehydration. Weight loss is the most reliable means of determining the extent of water loss. Clinical signs such as changes in skin turgor, sunken eyes, dry mucous membranes, decreased tearing, decreased urine output, altered mentation, and changes in vital signs can be helpful in determining approximate deficits (**Table 40-1**).

TABLE 40-1	Clinical Assessment of Degree of Dehydration in Children Based on Percentage of Body Weight Loss[a]		
Variable	**Minimal or No Dehydration (<3% Loss of Body Weight)**	**Mild-to-Moderate (3%-9% Loss of Body Weight)**	**Severe (≥10% Loss of Body Weight)**
Blood pressure	Normal	Normal	Normal to reduced
Quality of pulses	Normal	Normal or slightly decreased	Weak, thready, or not palpable
Heart rate	Normal	Normal to increased	Increased (bradycardia in severe cases)
Breathing	Normal	Normal to fast	Deep
Mental status	Normal	Normal to listless	Apathetic, lethargic, or comatose
Eyes	Normal	Sunken orbits/ decreased tears	Deeply sunken orbits/ absent tears
Mouth and tongue	Moist	Dry	Parched

(*Continued*)

TABLE 40-1	Clinical Assessment of Degree of Dehydration in Children Based on Percentage of Body Weight Loss[a] (Continued)		
Variable	Minimal or No Dehydration (<3% Loss of Body Weight)	Mild-to-Moderate (3%-9% Loss of Body Weight)	Severe (≥10% Loss of Body Weight)
Thirst	Normal	Eager to drink	Drinks poorly; too lethargic to drink
Skin fold	Normal	Recoil in <2 seconds	Recoil in >2 seconds
Extremities	Warm, normal capillary refill	Cool, prolonged capillary refill	Cold, mottled, cyanotic, prolonged capillary refill
Urine output	Normal to decreased	Decreased	Minimal
Hydration therapy	None	ORS 50–100 mL/kg over 3–4 hours	Lactated Ringer's solution or normal saline 20 mL/kg over 15–30 minutes IV until mental status or perfusion improves Followed by 5% dextrose/0.45% sodium chloride IV at higher maintenance rates or ORS 100 mL/kg over 4 hours
Replacement of ongoing losses	For each diarrheal stool or emesis <10 kg body weight: 60–120 mL ORS >10 kg body weight: 120–240 mL ORS	Same as minimal dehydration	If unable to tolerate ORS, administer through nasogastric tube or administer 5% dextrose/0.45% sodium chloride with 20 mEq/L (mmol/L) potassium chloride IV

[a]Percentages vary among patients for each dehydration category; hemodynamic and perfusion status is most important; when unsure of category, therapy for more severe category is recommended. ORS, oral rehydration solution.

- The necessary components of **oral rehydration solution** (ORS) include glucose, sodium, potassium chloride, and water (Table 40-2). ORS should be given in small frequent volumes (5 mL every 2–3 minutes) in a teaspoon or oral syringe.
- Severely dehydrated patients should be resuscitated initially with lactated Ringer's solution or normal intravenous (IV) saline. Guidelines for rehydration therapy based on the degree of dehydration and replacement of ongoing losses are outlined in Table 40-1. After rehydration, maintenance fluid is given based on accurate recording of intake and output volumes. ORS should be instituted as soon as it can be tolerated.
- Early refeeding with age-appropriate unrestricted diet is recommended in children and shortens the course of diarrhea. Initially, easily digested foods, such as bananas, applesauce, and cereal may be added as tolerated. Foods high in fiber, sodium, and sugar should be avoided.
- Antimotility drugs such as **diphenoxylate** and **loperamide** offer symptomatic relief in patients with watery diarrhea by reducing the number of stools. Antimotility drugs should be avoided if possible and are not recommended in patients with many toxin-mediated dysenteric diarrheas (ie, enterohemorrhagic *Escherichia coli* [EHEC], pseudomembranous colitis, shigellosis).

TABLE 40-2	Comparison of Common Solutions Used in Oral Rehydration and Maintenance

Product	Na (mEq/L)[b]	K (mEq/L)[b]	Base (mEq/L)	Carbohydrate (mmol/L)	Osmolarity (mOsm/L)
WHO/ UNICEF (2002)	75	20	30	75	245
Pedialyte	45	20	30	140	250
Infalyte	50	25	30	70	200
Oralyte	60	20	0	90	260
Rehydralyte	75	20	30	140	250
Cola[a]	2	0	13	700	750
Apple juice[a]	5	32	0	690	730
Chicken broth[a]	250	8	0	0	500
Sports beverage[a]	20	3	3	255	330

[a]These solutions should be avoided in dehydration.
[b]Concentration of monovalent ions expressed in mEq/L is numerically equivalent to mmol/L concentration.

- Individual studies have not shown significant benefit from probiotics, and meta-analyses have shown conflicting results. Probiotics should not be recommended for prophylaxis or treatment of initial antibiotic-associated diarrhea.

Bacterial Infections

- Antibiotic therapy is recommended in severe cases of diarrhea, moderate-to-severe cases of traveler's diarrhea, most cases of febrile dysenteric diarrhea, and culture-proven bacterial diarrhea. Antibiotics are not essential in the treatment of most mild diarrheas, and empirical therapy for acute GI infections may result in unnecessary antibiotic courses. Antibiotic choices for bacterial infections are given in **Table 40-3**. Antimicrobial therapy is not recommended in EHEC diarrhea as it may increase risk of hemolytic-uremic syndrome.
- Common pathogens responsible for watery diarrhea in the United States are norovirus and enterotoxigenic *Escherichia coli* (ETEC), while those most commonly associated with dysentery diarrhea are *Campylobacter* spp., EHEC, *Salmonella* spp., and *Shigella* spp. ETEC is also the most common cause of traveler's diarrhea and a common cause of food- and water-associated outbreaks. Cholera is caused by toxigenic *V. cholera*.

TRAVELER'S DIARRHEA

- Traveler's diarrhea describes the clinical syndrome caused by contaminated food or water that is manifested by malaise, anorexia, and abdominal cramps followed by the sudden onset of diarrhea that incapacitates many travelers.
- The most common pathogens are bacterial in nature and include ETEC, *Shigella*, *Campylobacter*, and *Salmonella*. Viruses are also potential causes.
- Patient education in avoiding high-risk food and beverages should be the best method for minimizing the risk. High-risk foods and beverages include raw or undercooked meat and seafood, moist foods served at room temperature, fruits that cannot be peeled, vegetables, milk from a questionable source, hot sauces on the table, tap water, unsealed bottled water, iced drinks, and food from street vendors.

TABLE 40-3	Recommendations for Antibiotic Therapy	
Pathogen	**Children**	**Adults**
Watery Diarrhea		
Enterotoxigenic *Escherichia coli*	Azithromycin 10 mg/kg/day given orally once daily × 3 days; ceftriaxone 50 mg/kg/day given IV once daily × 3 days	Ciprofloxacin 750 mg orally once daily × 1–3 days; alternatives: rifaximin 200 mg orally three times daily × 3 days; azithromycin 1000 mg orally × 1 day *or* 500 mg orally daily × 3 days
Vibrio cholerae O1	Erythromycin 30 mg/kg/day divided every 8 hours orally × 3 days; azithromycin 10 mg/kg/day given orally once daily × 3 days	Doxycycline 300 mg orally × 1 day Alternatives: azithromycin 500 mg orally once daily × 3 days; ciprofloxacin 750 mg orally once daily × 3 days; ceftriaxone IV
Dysenteric Diarrhea		
Campylobacter species[a]	Azithromycin 10 mg/kg/day given orally once daily × 3–5 days; erythromycin 30 mg/kg/day divided into two to four doses orally × 3–5 days	Azithromycin 500 mg orally once daily × 3 days Alternatives: ciprofloxacin 750 mg orally once daily × 7 days
Salmonella Nontyphoidal[a]	Ceftriaxone 100 mg/kg/day divided IV every 12 hours × 7–10 days; azithromycin 20 mg/kg/day orally once daily × 7 days	Ceftriaxone 2 g IV/IM once; ciprofloxacin 750 mg orally once daily × 7–10 days Alternatives: ampicillin 250–500 mg orally every 6 hours × 7 days; azithromycin 500 mg orally once daily × 7 days; trimethoprim-sulfamethoxazole 160/800 mg twice daily × 7 days For immunocompromised patients, duration should be increased to 14 days for both fluoroquinolones and azithromycin
Shigella species[a]	Azithromycin 10 mg/kg/day given orally once daily × 3 days; ceftriaxone 50 mg/kg/day given IV once daily × 3 days	Azithromycin 500 mg orally once daily × 3 days; ceftriaxone 2 g IV/IM once; ciprofloxacin 750 mg orally once daily × 3 days Alternatives: ampicillin 250–500 mg orally every 6 hours × 7 days; trimethoprim-sulfamethoxazole 160/800 mg twice daily × 7 days

(Continued)

TABLE 40-3	Recommendations for Antibiotic Therapy *(Continued)*	
Pathogen	**Children**	**Adults**
Yersinia species[a]	Treat as children with shigellosis	Trimethoprim-sulfamethoxazole160/800 mg twice daily × 7 days Alternatives: cefotaxime IV or ciprofloxacin 750 mg orally once daily × 7 days
Traveler's Diarrhea		
Prophylaxis[a]		Norfloxacin 400 mg or ciprofloxacin 750 mg orally daily; rifaximin 200 mg one to three times daily up to 2 weeks
Treatment		Ciprofloxacin 750 mg orally × 1 day or 500 mg orally every 12 hours × 3 days; levofloxacin 1000 mg orally × 1 day or 500 mg orally daily × 3 days; rifaximin 200 mg three times daily × 3 days; azithromycin 1000 mg orally × 1 day or 500 mg orally daily × 3 days

[a]For high-risk patients only. See the preceding text for the high-risk patients in each infection.

- Prophylactic antibiotic use is not recommended for most travelers due to the potential side effects of antibiotics, predisposition to other infections such as *Clostridioides difficile* infection or vaginal candidiasis, the increased risk of selection of drug-resistant organisms, cost, lack of data on the safety and efficacy of antibiotics given for more than 2 or 3 weeks, and availability of rapidly effective antibiotics for treatment.
- Prophylactic antibiotics are recommended only in high-risk individuals or in situations in which short-term illness could ruin the purpose of the trip, such as a military mission. A fluoroquinolone is the drug of choice when traveling to most areas of the world. Azithromycin can be considered when traveling to South and Southeast Asia.

TREATMENT

- The goals of treatment of traveler's diarrhea are to avoid dehydration, reduce the severity and duration of symptoms, and prevent interruption to planned activities.
- Fluid and electrolyte replacement should be initiated at the onset of diarrhea.
- Antibiotics used for treatment are found in **Table 40-3**.
- For symptom relief, **loperamide** (preferred because of its quicker onset and longer duration of relief relative to bismuth) may be taken (4 mg orally initially and then 2 mg with each subsequent loose stool to a maximum of 16 mg/day in patients without bloody diarrhea and fever). Loperamide should be discontinued if symptoms persist for more than 48 hours.

CLOSTRIOIDES DIFFICILE

- *C. difficile* is the most commonly recognized cause of infectious diarrhea in healthcare settings with high rates of disease in the elderly and those exposed to antibiotic agents. The antibiotics most commonly associated with *C. difficile* infection (CDI) include fluoroquinolones, clindamycin, carbapenems, and third-/fourth-generation cephalosporins.
- Other risk factors for acquisition of *C. difficile* include recent healthcare exposure, chemotherapy, patients undergoing GI surgery or receiving tube feeding, and potentially those receiving acid suppressive medications.

- The spectrum of disease ranges from mild diarrhea to life-threatening toxic. The diarrhea is typically watery and nonbloody, and is often associated with abdominal discomfort, fever, and leukocytosis.
- Diagnosis of CDI is confirmed by identification of *C. difficile* organisms/toxin in stool or pseudomembranous colitis visualized during endoscopy.
- Supportive care of CDI includes fluid and electrolyte replacement therapy, in addition to discontinuation of the offending antimicrobial if possible.

TREATMENT

- Once determination of disease severity has been made, treatment should be initiated with an antibiotic effective against *C. difficile*. **Metronidazole, vancomycin,** and **fidaxomicin** are the most commonly prescribed agents. Initial therapy should also include discontinuation of the offending agent. The patient should be supported with fluid and electrolyte replacement.
- Classification of CDI severity and recommended treatment for adults is given in **Table 40-4**. In patients with severe/complicated or fulminant CDI the preferred regimen is combination therapy with IV **metronidazole** and **vancomycin**.
- Recurrence of CDI can occur in 25%–35% of patients. If metronidazole was used initially, then a standard vancomycin course can be utilized for the first recurrence. If vancomycin was used initially, then **fidaxomicin** can be used for the first recurrence. Alternatively, a tapered and pulsed dose of vancomycin can be used for the first recurrence and is the recommended treatment strategy for second or subsequent recurrences.
- Treatment with fecal microbiota transplant (FMT) has gained popularity among many practitioners. Multiple randomized controlled trials have shown efficacy of FMT with resolution rates of 80%–90% in most studies, yet the specific preparation and route of administration are not well established.

VIRAL INFECTIONS

- Viruses are now recognized as the leading cause of diarrhea in the world.
- In infants and children rotavirus, a double-stranded, wheel-shaped RNA virus is the most common cause of diarrhea worldwide, and 1 million people die annually from the infection.

TABLE 40-4   *Clostridioides difficile* Infection Severity and Treatment

Severity	Markers of Disease Severity	Recommended Treatment
Nonsevere	WBC ≤15,000 cells/mm³ (15 × 10⁹/L) SCr <1.5 mg/dL (133 μmol/L)	Vancomycin 125 mg orally 4 times daily for 10 days, OR fidaxomicin 200 mg orally twice daily for 10 days, OR metronidazole 500 mg orally every 8 hours for 10 days[a]
Severe	WBC >15,000 cells/mm³ (15 × 10⁹/L) SCr >1.5 mg/dL (133 μmol/L)	Vancomycin 125 mg orally 4 times daily for 10 days, OR fidaxomicin 200 mg orally twice daily for 10 days
Fulminant	Hypotension or shock Ileus and/or megacolon	Metronidazole 500 mg IV every 8 hours *PLUS* vancomycin 500 mg every 6 hours via NG or orally (if ileus present use rectally)

[a]Metronidazole is an alternative therapy if other agents are unavailable or too costly.
NG, nasogastric; SCr, serum creatinine; WBC, white blood cell.

TABLE 40-5	Characteristics of Agents Responsible for Acute Viral Gastroenteritis				
Virus	**Peak Age of Onset**	**Time of Year**	**Duration**	**Mode of Transmission**	**Common Symptoms**
Rotavirus	6 months–2 years	October–April	3–7 days	Fecal–oral, water, food	Nausea, vomiting, diarrhea, fever, abdominal pain, lactose intolerance
Norovirus	All age groups	Peak in winter	2–3 days	Fecal–oral, food, water, environment	Nausea, vomiting, diarrhea, abdominal cramps, myalgia
Astrovirus	<7 years	Winter	1–4 days	Fecal–oral, water, shellfish	Diarrhea, headache, malaise, nausea
Enteric adenovirus	<2 years	Year-round	7–9 days	Fecal–oral	Diarrhea, respiratory symptoms, vomiting, fever
Pestivirus	<2 years	NR	3 days	NR	Mild
Coronavirus-like particles	<2 years	Fall and early winter	7 days	NR	Respiratory disease
Enterovirus	NR	NR	NR	NR	Mild diarrhea, secondary organ damage

NR, not reported.

- In the United States, routine rotavirus vaccination is recommended for all infants beginning at age 2 months. There are two vaccines, RotaTeq (RV5) and Rotarix (RV1), available for reducing rotaviral gastroenteritis.
- Characteristics of agents responsible for viral gastroenteritis are given in Table 40-5.

See Chapter 131, Gastrointestinal Infections and Enterotoxigenic Poisonings, authored by Andrew Roecker and Brittany Bates, for a more detailed discussion of this topic.

CHAPTER 41

Human Immunodeficiency Virus Infection

- **Table 41-1** presents the case definition for adult, adolescent, and children, respectively, for *human immunodeficiency virus* (HIV) infection.

ETIOLOGY AND PATHOGENESIS

- Infection with HIV occurs through three primary modes: sexual, parenteral, and perinatal. Sexual intercourse, primarily anal and vaginal intercourse, is the most common vehicle for transmission. The highest risk appears to be from receptive ano-rectal intercourse at about 1.4 transmissions per 100 sexual acts. Condom use reduces the risk of transmission by approximately 80%. Individuals with genital ulcers or sexually transmitted diseases are at great risk for contracting HIV.
- Heterosexual transmission is the most common mode of transmission in sub-Saharan Africa and worldwide (~80% of cases).
- The risk of HIV transmission from sharing needles is approximately 0.67 per 100 episodes.
- Healthcare workers have a small risk of occupationally acquiring HIV, mostly through accidental injury, most often percutaneous needlestick injury. Mucocutaneous exposures (eg, tainted blood splash in eyes, mouth, or nose) carry a transmission risk of approximately 0.09%.
- Perinatal infection, or vertical transmission, is the most common cause of pediatric HIV infection. The risk of mother-to-child transmission is ~25% in the absence of antiretroviral therapy. Breast-feeding can also transmit HIV.

CLINICAL PRESENTATION

- The natural history of HIV infection exhibits three general phases: acute, chronic, and terminal (AIDS).
- Primary HIV infection also presents with high viral load (may exceed 1,000,000 copies/mL or 10^9/L) and a persistent decrease in CD4 lymphocytes.
- The most common signs and symptoms of primary HIV infection are fever, headache, sore throat, fatigue, GI upset (diarrhea, nausea, vomiting), weight loss, myalgia, morbilliform or maculopapular rash usually involving the trunk, lymphadenopathy, and night sweats. Less common signs and symptoms are aseptic meningitis, oral ulcers, and leukopenia.
- Clinical presentations of primary HIV infection vary, but patients often have a viral syndrome or mononucleosis-like illness with fever, pharyngitis, and adenopathy. Symptoms may last for 2 weeks.
- Most children born with HIV are asymptomatic. On physical examination, they often present with unexplained physical signs such as lymphadenopathy, hepatomegaly, splenomegaly, failure to thrive, weight loss or unexplained low birth weight, and fever of unknown origin. Laboratory findings include anemia, hypergammaglobulinemia, altered mononuclear cell function, and altered T-cell subset ratios. The normal range for CD4 cell counts in children is much different than for adults.
- The probability of progression to AIDS is related to RNA viral load; viral load is a major prognostic factor for disease progression, CD4 count decline, and death.
- The presence of HIV infection is screened with an enzyme-linked immunosorbent assay (ELISA), which detects antibodies against HIV-1. ELISA tests are generally highly sensitive (greater than 99%) and highly specific (greater than 99%), but rare false-positive results can occur particularly in those with autoimmune disorders. Positive screening tests are confirmed with another enzyme immunoassay to specify if the antibodies are to HIV-1 versus HIV-2. False-negative results also occur and

TABLE 41-1	Surveillance Case Definition for HIV Infection Stage Based on CD4+ T-Lymphocyte Counts, United States, 2014

Age on Date of CD4+ T-Lymphocyte Test[a]

	<1 year		1–5 years		≥6 years	
Stage	Cells/μL (×10⁶/L)	%	Cells/μL (×10⁶/L)	%	Cells/μL (×10⁶/L)	%
1	≥1500	≥34	≥1000	≥30	≥500	≥26
2	750–1499	26–33	500–999	22–29	200–499	14–25
3 (AIDS)	<750	<26	<500	<22	<200	<14

AIDS Indicator Conditions

Bacterial infections, multiple or recurrent (specific to children <6 years)

Candidiasis of bronchi, trachea, or lungs

Candidiasis, esophageal

Cervical cancer, invasive (specific to adults, adolescents, children >6 years)

Coccidioidomycosis, disseminated or extrapulmonary

Cryptococcosis, extrapulmonary

Cryptosporidiosis, chronic intestinal (duration >1 month)

Cytomegalovirus disease (other than liver, spleen, or nodes), onset at age >1 month

Cytomegalovirus retinitis (with loss of vision)

Encephalopathy, HIV-related

Herpes simplex: chronic ulcer(s) (duration >1 month); or bronchitis, pneumonitis, or esophagitis, onset at age >1 month

Histoplasmosis, disseminated or extrapulmonary isosporiasis, chronic intestinal (duration >1 month) Kaposi's sarcoma

Lymphoma, Burkitt

Lymphoma, immunoblastic

Lymphoma, primary, or brain

Mycobacterium avium complex or *Mycobacterium kansasii*, disseminated or extrapulmonary

Mycobacterium tuberculosis, any site (pulmonary or extrapulmonary)

Mycobacterium, other species or unidentified species, disseminated or extrapulmonary

Pneumocystis jirovecii pneumonia (PCP)

Pneumonia, recurrent (specific to adults, adolescents, children >6 years)

Progressive multifocal leukoencephalopathy

Salmonella septicemia, recurrent

Toxoplasmosis of brain, onset at age >1 month

Wasting syndrome due to HIV

[a]Age-specific CD4+ T-lymphocyte count or CD4+ T-lymphocyte percentage of total lymphocytes

may be attributed to the "window-period" before adequate production of antibodies or antigen.

- Once diagnosed, HIV disease is monitored primarily by two surrogate biomarkers, viral load and CD4 cell count. The viral load test quantifies viremia by measuring the amount of viral RNA. There are several methods used for determining the amount of HIV RNA: reverse transcriptase–coupled polymerase chain reaction, branched DNA, transcription-mediated amplification, and nucleic acid sequence–based assay.
- The number of CD4 lymphocytes in the blood is a surrogate marker of disease progression. The normal adult CD4 lymphocyte count ranges between 500 and 1600 cells/mm³ (500 and 1600 × 10⁶/L), or 40%–70% of all lymphocytes.

TREATMENT

- <u>Goal of Treatment</u>: The central goal of antiretroviral therapy is to decrease morbidity and mortality, improve quality of life, restore and preserve immune function, and prevent further transmission through maximum suppression of HIV replication (HIV RNA level that is less than the lower limit of quantitation (ie, undetectable; usually less than 20 or 50 copies/mL [20×10^3 or 50×10^3/L]).

GENERAL APPROACH

- Contemporary combinations of three active antiretroviral agents from two pharmacologic classes potently inhibit HIV replication to undetectable plasma levels, prevent and reverse immune deficiency, and substantially decrease morbidity and mortality—constituting the modern ART era.
- Regular, periodic measurement of plasma HIV RNA levels and CD4 cell counts is necessary to determine the risk of disease progression in an HIV-infected individual and to determine when to initiate or modify antiretroviral treatment regimens.
- The use of potent combination antiretroviral therapy to suppress HIV replication to below the levels of detection of sensitive plasma HIV RNA assays limits the potential for selection of antiretroviral-resistant HIV variants, the major factor limiting the ability of antiretroviral drugs to inhibit virus replication and delay disease progression. Maximum achievable suppression of HIV replication should be the goal of therapy.
- The most effective means to accomplish durable suppression of HIV replication is the simultaneous initiation of combinations of effective anti-HIV drugs with which the patient has not been previously treated and that are not cross-resistant with antiretroviral agents with which the patient has been treated previously.
- Each of the antiretroviral drugs used in combination therapy regimens should always be used according to optimum schedules and dosages. Combinations of three active antiretroviral agents from two pharmacologic classes profoundly inhibit HIV replication to undetectable plasma levels, prevent and reverse immune deficiency, and substantially decrease morbidity and mortality.
- Women should receive optimal antiretroviral therapy regardless of pregnancy status.
- The same principles of antiretroviral therapy apply to both HIV-infected children and adults, although the treatment of HIV-infected children involves unique pharmacologic, virologic, and immunologic considerations.
- Persons with acute primary HIV infections should be treated with combination antiretroviral therapy to suppress virus replication to levels below the limit of detection of sensitive plasma HIV RNA assays.
- HIV-infected persons, even those with viral loads below detectable limits, should be considered infectious and should be counseled to avoid sexual and drug-use behaviors that are associated with transmission or acquisition of HIV and other infectious pathogens.
- An excellent source for information on treatment guidelines can be found at http://aidsinfo.nih.gov/.
- Untreated HIV is harmful even at high CD4 counts, and immediate ART confers individual- and population-level benefit compared with delayed ART. Major policymakers now recommend immediate ART regardless of CD4 count.

PHARMACOLOGIC THERAPY

Antiretroviral Agents

- Systemic delivery of antiretroviral agents for direct inhibition of viral replication has been the most clinically successful strategy for both treatment and prophylaxis.
- Inhibiting viral replication with a combination of potent antiretroviral therapy has been the most clinically successful strategy in the treatment of HIV infection. There have been four primary groups of drugs used: entry inhibitors, reverse transcriptase

inhibitors, integrase strand transfer inhibitors (InSTIs), and HIV protease inhibitors (PIs) (**Table 41-2**).

- Significant drug interactions can occur with many antiretroviral agents. The latest information on drug interactions of antiretroviral drugs should be consulted. Many clinically significant antiretroviral-associated drug interactions involve CYP3A-mediated first-pass metabolism and clearance.
  - ✓ **Ritonavir** and **cobicistat** are potent inhibitors of cytochrome P450 enzyme 3A and are now used exclusively at lower doses as pharmacokinetic enhancers of other HIV PI.
  - ✓ **Rifampin**, a potent inducer of CYP3A metabolism and conjugation enzymes, is contraindicated with use of most HIV PIs, **etravirine**, **rilpivirine**, and **maraviroc** because concentrations are reduced substantially even with ritonavir enhancement.

TREATMENT DURING PREGNANCY

- Generally, pregnant women should be treated as would nonpregnant women, with the goal of maximally suppressing HIV RNA, with some exceptions. **Efavirenz** should be avoided in women planning to become pregnant or who are not using effective contraception as efavirenz has been associated with neural tube defects in the first trimester, in some but not all studies.
- **Dolutegravir** use at the time of conception was associated with neural tube defects in infants and until more is known, dolutegravir should be avoided if possible in women who are planning to become pregnant or are not using effective contraception.
- Intravenous (IV) **zidovudine** is recommended intrapartum depending on the mother's viral load, based on early studies demonstrating clear prophylactic effectiveness as well as extensive familiarity with the side-effect profile. Infants born to HIV-infected mothers should also receive zidovudine (±several doses of **nevirapine**) prophylaxis for 4–6 weeks after birth.

CHEMOPROPHYLAXIS

- Post-exposure prophylaxis (PEP) with conventional ART regimens (eg, **tenofovir disoproxil fumarate–emtricitabine–rategravir**) should be initiated as soon as possible (ideally within 1–2 hours) after high-risk exposures to prevent HIV infection. The optimal duration of treatment is unknown, but at least 4 weeks of therapy is advocated.
- Preexposure prophylaxis (PrEP) involves daily tenofovir disoproxil fumarate–emtricitabine in HIV-negative persons at high risk of HIV acquisition to prevent infection should an HIV-exposure occur.

EVALUATION OF THERAPEUTIC OUTCOMES

- Following the initiation of therapy, patients are generally monitored at 3-month intervals until HIV RNA reaches undetectable levels. An assessment at 2–8 weeks is warranted to document early response. Monitoring may be increased to every 6 months in stabilized patients.
- There are two general indications to change therapy: significant toxicity and treatment failure.
- Specific criteria to indicate treatment failure have not been established through controlled clinical trials. As a general guide, the following events should prompt consideration for changing therapy: the inability to achieve less than 200 copies/mL $(200 \times 10^3/L)$ HIV RNA by 24 weeks of therapy initiation (repeat testing is suggested to confirm), or, after HIV RNA suppression, repeated detection of greater than 200 copies/mL $(200 \times 10^3/L)$ of HIV RNA.

THERAPEUTIC FAILURE

- The most important measure of therapeutic failure is suboptimal suppression of viral replication.
- Therapeutic failure may be the result of factors such as pre-ART disease factors (eg, high viral load or preexisting drug resistance), nonadherence to medication,

TABLE 41-2	Treatment of Human Immunodeficiency Virus Infection: Antiretroviral Regimens Recommended in Antiretroviral-Naïve Persons	
	Preferred Regimens[a]	**Selected Limitations**
InSTI-based	Bictegravir + tenofovir alafenamide fumarate + emtricitabine (coformulated) (AI)	Only if CrCl ≥30 mL/min (0.5 mL/sec); interactions with polyvalent antacids; bictegravir inhibits creatinine secretion increasing serum creatinine (distinguish vs. renal dysfunction)
	Raltegravir + tenofovir + emtricitabine (AI for tenofovir disoproxil fumarate; AII for tenofovir alafenamide fumarate)	Can be dosed once or twice daily; interactions with polyvalent antacids; creatine kinase increases
	Dolutegravir + abacavir + lamivudine (coformulated) (AI)	Only if HLA-B5701 negative; interactions with polyvalent antacids; possible increased risk of neural tube defects in infants if used at the time of conception; dolutegravir inhibits creatinine secretion increasing Scr—distinguish vs. renal dysfunction
	Dolutegravir + tenofovir disoproxil fumarate (or tenofovir alafenamide fumarate) + emtricitabine (AI)	Same as above without HLA-B5701 negative requirement
Selected Alternative Regimens (Some Potential Disadvantages vs. Preferred Regimens)		
InSTI-based	Elvitegravir + cobicistat + tenofovir disoproxil fumarate + emtricitabine (coformulated) (AI)	Only if CrCl ≥70 mL/min (1.17 mL/sec); food requirement; interactions with polyvalent antacids; CYP3A4 drug interactions; cobicistat inhibits creatinine secretion increasing Scr— distinguish vs. renal dysfunction
	Elvitegravir + cobicistat + tenofovir alafenamide fumarate + emtricitabine (coformulated) (AI)	Only if CrCl ≥30 mL/min (0.5 mL/sec); same as above
	Raltegravir + abacavir + lamivudine (BI)	Only if HLA-B5701 negative and HIV RNA <100,000 copies/mL (100 × 10^6/L); can be dosed once or twice daily; interactions with polyvalent antacids; creatine kinase increases

(Continued)

TABLE 41-2	Treatment of Human Immunodeficiency Virus Infection: Antiretroviral Regimens Recommended in Antiretroviral-Naïve Persons (*Continued*)	
	Preferred Regimens[a]	**Selected Limitations**
HIV PI-based	Atazanavir + ritonavir (or cobicistat) + tenofovir disoproxil fumarate (or tenofovir alafenamide fumarate) + emtricitabine (BI)	GI; food requirement; CYP3A4 drug interactions; hyperbilirubinemia leading to drug discontinuation, especially in those with Gilbert's; only for CrCl ≥70 mL/min (1.17 mL/sec) as cobicistat inhibits creatinine secretion increasing Scr— distinguish vs. renal dysfunction
	Atazanavir + ritonavir (or cobicistat) + abacavir + lamivudine (CI for ritonavir and CIII for cobicistat)	Only if HLA-B5701 negative; see issues above
	Darunavir + ritonavir (or cobicistat) + tenofovir disoproxil fumarate (or tenofovir alafenamide fumarate) + emtricitabine (AI for ritonavir and AII for cobicistat)	Rash (darunavir has sulfonamide moiety); GI; food requirement; CYP3A4 drug interactions; only for CrCl ≥70 mL/min (1.17 mL/sec) as cobicistat inhibits creatinine secretion increasing serum creatinine (distinguish vs. renal dysfunction); see issues above
	Darunavir + ritonavir (or cobicistat) + abacavir + lamivudine (BII)	Only if HLA-B5701 negative; see issues above
NNRTI-based	Doravirine + tenofovir disoproxil fumarate + lamivudine (coformulated) (BI)	Only if CrCl ≥50 mL/min (0.83 mL/sec)
	Doravirine + tenofovir alafenamide + emtricitabine (BIII)	
	Efavirenz + tenofovir disoproxil fumarate + emtricitabine (coformulated) (BI)	CNS side effects with efavirenz; CYP450 drug interactions; empty stomach dosing; teratogenic in nonhuman primates—controversial in humans—consider avoiding in women planning to conceive
	Efavirenz + tenofovir alafenamide fumarate + emtricitabine (BII)	
	Rilpivirine + tenofovir disoproxil fumarate (or tenofovir alafenamide fumarate) + emtricitabine (coformulated) (BI)	Not recommended when HIV RNA >100,000 copies/mL (100 × 10^6/L) or CD4 <200 cells/μL (0.2 × 10^9/L); no proton pump inhibitors (rilpivirine); food requirement; antacid interactions
If abacavir and tenofovir cannot be used	Dolutegravir + lamivudine (CI)	Only if HIV RNA <500,000 copies/mL (500 × 10^6/L); possible increased risk of neural tube defects in infants if used at the time of conception

(*Continued*)

TABLE 41-2	Treatment of Human Immunodeficiency Virus Infection: Antiretroviral Regimens Recommended in Antiretroviral-Naïve Persons (*Continued*)
Preferred Regimens[a]	**Selected Limitations**
Darunavir + ritonavir + raltegravir (CI)	Only if HIV RNA <100,000 copies/mL (100 × 10⁶/L)and CD4 >200 cells/mm³ (0.2 × 10⁹/L); raltegravir must be dosed twice daily
Darunavir + ritonavir + lamivudine (CI)	

Selected Regimens or Components that Should Not be Used at Any Time

Regimen or Component	Comment
Monotherapy with any single agent (AI)	Inferior virologic efficacy
Any NRTI regimen (AI)	Inferior virologic efficacy
Atazanavir + indinavir (AIII)	Additive adverse effects, including hyperbilirubinemia and jaundice
Didanosine + tenofovir (AII)	Inferior virologic efficacy, CD4 declines
Didanosine + stavudine (AII)	Toxicity including subcutaneous fat loss, peripheral neuropathy, and lactic acidosis
2 NNRTI combinations (AI)	Higher adverse events, drug interactions
Emtricitabine + lamivudine or zidovudine + stavudine (AIII, AII)	Analogs of same nucleobase, no additive benefit (or antagonistic)
Unboosted PIs (ie, darunavir, saquinavir, tipranavir) (AII)	Inadequate bioavailability
Etravirine + selected boosted PIs (AII)	Possible induction of PI metabolism, doses not established
Nevirapine in ARV naïve with higher CD4 counts (>250 cells/μL [0.25 × 10⁹/L] for women, >400 cells/μL [0.4 × 10⁹/L] for men) (BI)	High incidence of symptomatic hepatotoxicity

[a]Evidence-based rating definition. Rating strength of recommendation—A, strong recommendation; B, moderate recommendation; C, optional recommendation. Rating quality of evidence supporting the recommendation—I, evidence from at least one correctly randomized, controlled trial with clinical outcomes and/or validated laboratory; II, evidence from at least one well-designed clinical trial without randomization or observational cohorts with long-term clinical outcomes; III, expert opinion. Lamivudine and emtricitabine are considered interchangeable endpoints.

development of new drug resistance, intolerance to one or more medications, adverse drug–drug or drug–food interactions, or pharmacokinetic–pharmacodynamic variability.

- Drug resistance testing is recommended while the patient is undergoing the failing regimen or within 4 weeks after stopping the regimen as long as the HIV RNA count is greater than 500 copies/mL (500 × 10³/L), which is the threshold for resistance assays (~500–1000 copies/mL [~500 × 10³–1000 × 10³/L]). Patients should be treated with at least two (preferably three) fully active antiretroviral drugs based on medication history and resistance tests. The goal of therapy is to suppress HIV RNA to undetectable levels. In cases when less than 50 copies/mL (<50 × 10³/L) cannot be attained, maintenance on the regimen is preferred over drug discontinuation so as to prevent rapid immunological and clinical decline.

INFECTIOUS COMPLICATIONS OF HUMAN IMMUNODEFICIENCY VIRUS

- The probability of developing specific opportunistic infections (OIs) is closely related to CD4 count thresholds. The principle in the management of OIs is treating HIV infection to enable CD4 cells to recover and be maintained above protective levels. Other important principles are:
  ✓ Preventing exposure to opportunistic pathogens
  ✓ Using vaccinations to prevent first-episode of disease (consult HIV-specific guidelines)
  ✓ Use primary chemoprophylaxis at certain CD4 thresholds to prevent first-episode of disease
  ✓ Treating emergent OIs
  ✓ Use secondary chemoprophylaxis to prevent disease recurrence
  ✓ Discontinuing prophylaxis with sustained immune recovery
- The spectrum of infectious diseases observed in HIV-infected individuals and recommended first-line therapies are shown in **Table 41-3.**

PNEUMOCYSTIS JIROVECII PNEUMONIA

- *P. jirovecii* pneumonia (PCP) is the most common life-threatening OI in patients with AIDS. The taxonomy of the organism is unclear, having been classified as both protozoan and fungal.

Clinical Presentation

- Characteristic symptoms include fever and dyspnea. Clinical signs are tachypnea with or without rales or rhonchi and a nonproductive or mildly productive cough occurring over a period of weeks, although more fulminant presentations can occur. Chest radiographs may show florid or subtle infiltrates or may occasionally be normal, although infiltrates are usually interstitial and bilateral. Arterial blood gases may show minimal hypoxia (partial pressure of oxygen [PaO$_2$] 80–95 mm Hg [10.6–12.6 kPa]) but in more advanced disease may be markedly abnormal.
- The onset of PCP is often insidious, occurring over a period of weeks. Clinical signs are tachypnea with or without rales or rhonchi and a nonproductive or mildly productive cough occurring over a period of weeks, although more fulminant presentations can occur. The diagnosis of PCP usually is made by identification of the organism in induced sputum or in specimens obtained from bronchoalveolar lavage.

Treatment

- The treatment of choice is **trimethoprim–sulfamethoxazole,** which is associated with a 60%–100% response rate.
- Trimethoprim–sulfamethoxazole is given in doses of 15–20 mg/kg/day (based on the trimethoprim component) as three or four divided doses for the treatment of PCP. Treatment duration is typically 21 days but must be based on clinical response.
- Trimethoprim–sulfamethoxazole is usually initiated by the IV route, although oral therapy (as oral absorption is high) may suffice in mildly ill and reliable patients

	TABLE 41-3 Selected Therapies for Common Opportunistic Pathogens in HIV-Infected Individuals	
Clinical Disease	Preferred Initial Therapies for Acute Infection in Adults (Strength of Recommendation in Parentheses)	Common Drug- or Dose-Limiting Adverse Reactions
Fungi		
Candidiasis, oral	Fluconazole 100 mg orally for 7–14 days (AI)	Elevated liver function tests, hepatotoxicity, nausea, and vomiting
	or	
	Nystatin 500,000 units oral swish (~5 mL) four times daily for 7–14 days (BII)	Taste, patient acceptance
Candidiasis, esophageal	Fluconazole 100–400 mg orally or IV daily for 14–21 days (AI)	Same as above
	or	
	Itraconazole 200 mg/day orally for 14–21 days (AI)	Elevated liver function tests, hepatotoxicity, nausea, and vomiting
Pneumocystis jirovecii pneumonia	*Moderate-to-severe episodes* Trimethoprim–sulfamethoxazole IV or orally 15–20 mg/kg/day as trimethoprim component in three to four divided doses for 21 days[a] (AI) moderate or severe therapy should be started IV	Skin rash, fever, leucopenia, thrombocytopenia
	Mild-to-moderate episodes Trimethoprim–sulfamethoxazole 15–20 mg/kg/day as trimethoprim component orally in three divided doses or trimethoprim– sulfamethoxazole double strength tablets, two tablets three times daily	
Cryptococcal meningitis	Liposomal amphotericin B 3–4 mg/ kg/day IV with flucytosine 100 mg/ kg/day orally in four divided doses for a minimum of 2 weeks (AI) *followed by*	Nephrotoxicity, hypokalemia, anemia, fever, chills Bone marrow suppression
	Fluconazole 400 mg/day, orally for 8 weeks or until CSF cultures are negative (AI)[a]	Same as above
Histoplasmosis	Liposomal amphotericin B 3 mg/kg/ day IV for 2 weeks (AI) *followed by*	Same as above
	Itraconazole 200 mg orally thrice daily for 3 days then twice daily, for 12 months (AII)[a]	

(Continued)

TABLE 41-3	Selected Therapies for Common Opportunistic Pathogens in HIV-Infected Individuals (*Continued*)	
Clinical Disease	**Preferred Initial Therapies for Acute Infection in Adults (Strength of Recommendation in Parentheses)**	**Common Drug- or Dose-Limiting Adverse Reactions**
Coccidioidomycosis	Liposomal amphotericin B 3–5 mg/kg/day IV until clinical improvement (usually after 500–1000 mg) then switch to azole (AIII)[a]	Same as above
	or	
	Fluconazole 400–800 mg once daily (meningeal disease) (AII)[a]	Same as above
Protozoa		
Toxoplasmic encephalitis	Pyrimethamine 200 mg orally once, then 50–75 mg/day	Bone marrow suppression
	plus	
	Sulfadiazine 1–1.5 g orally four times daily	Rash, drug fever
	and	
	Leucovorin 10–25 mg orally daily for 6 weeks (AI)[a]	
Isosporiasis	Trimethoprim and sulfamethoxazole: 160 mg trimethoprim and 800 mg sulfamethoxazole orally or IV times daily for 10 days (AII)[a]	Same as above
Bacteria		
Mycobacterium avium complex	Clarithromycin 500 mg orally twice daily, *plus* ethambutol 15 mg/kg/day orally (AI) for at least 12 months	GI intolerance, optic neuritis, peripheral neuritis, elevated liver tests
Salmonella enterocolitis or bacteremia	Ciprofloxacin 500–750 mg orally (or 400 mg IV) twice daily for 14 days (longer duration for bacteremia or advanced HIV) (AIII)	GI intolerance, headache, dizziness
Campylobacter enterocolitis (mild-to-moderate)	Ciprofloxacin 500–750 mg orally (or 400 mg IV) twice daily for 7–10 days (or longer with bacteremia) (BIII)	Same as above
Shigella enterocolitis	Ciprofloxacin 500–750 mg orally (or 400 mg IV) twice daily for 7–10 days (or 14 days for bacteremia) (AIII)	Same as above
Viruses		
Mucocutaneous herpes simplex	Acyclovir 5 mg/kg IV every 8 hours until lesions regress, then acyclovir 400 mg orally three times daily until complete healing (famciclovir or valacyclovir is alternative) (AIII)	GI intolerance, crystalluria

(Continued)

TABLE 41-3	Selected Therapies for Common Opportunistic Pathogens in HIV-Infected Individuals (*Continued*)	
Clinical Disease	**Preferred Initial Therapies for Acute Infection in Adults (Strength of Recommendation in Parentheses)**	**Common Drug- or Dose-Limiting Adverse Reactions**
Primary varicella-zoster	Acyclovir 10–15 mg/kg every 8 hours IV for 7–10 days (severe cases), then switch to oral valacyclovir 1 g three times daily after defervescence (famciclovir or acyclovir is alternative) (AIII)	Obstructive nephropathy, CNS symptoms
Cytomegalovirus (retinitis)	Intravitreal ganciclovir (2 mg) or foscarnet (2.4 mg) for 1–4 doses over 7–10 days (for sight threatening lesions) *plus* valganciclovir 900 mg twice daily for 14–21 days then once daily until immune recovery from ART (AIII)[a]	Neutropenia, thrombocytopenia
Cytomegalovirus esophagitis or colitis	Ganciclovir 5 mg/kg IV every 12 hours for 21–42 days; may switch to valganciclovir 900 mg orally every 12 hours when oral therapy can be tolerated (BI)	Same as above

[a]Maintenance therapy is recommended.
ART, antiretroviral therapy; CSF, cerebrospinal fluid; HIV, human immunodeficiency virus.
See Table 41-3 for levels of evidence-based recommendations.

or to complete a course of therapy after a response has been achieved with IV administration.

- The more common adverse reactions seen with trimethoprim–sulfamethoxazole are rash (including Stevens–Johnson syndrome), fever, leukopenia, elevated serum transaminases, and thrombocytopenia. The incidence of these adverse reactions is higher in HIV-infected individuals than in those not infected with HIV. Mild rashes should be watched closely for progression to more severe reactions but are not an absolute contraindication to continuing therapy.

- For pentamidine, side effects include hypotension, tachycardia, nausea, vomiting, severe hypoglycemia or hyperglycemia, pancreatitis, irreversible diabetes mellitus, elevated transaminases, nephrotoxicity, leukopenia, and cardiac arrhythmias.

Prophylaxis

- Primary prophylaxis of PCP is recommended for any HIV-infected person who has a CD4 lymphocyte count less than 200 cells/mm^3 (200 × 10^6/L) (or CD4 percentage of total lymphocytes <14%) or a history of oropharyngeal candidiasis. Secondary prophylaxis is recommended for all HIV-infected individuals who have had a previous episode.

- Trimethoprim–sulfamethoxazole is the preferred therapy for both primary and secondary prophylaxis of PCP in adults and adolescents. The recommended dose in adults and adolescents is one double-strength tablet daily.

See Chapter 143, Human Immunodeficiency Virus Infection, authored by Peter L. Anderson, Jenna Yager, and Courtney V. Fletcher, for a more detailed discussion of this topic.

Influenza

- *Influenza* is a viral illness associated with high mortality and high hospitalization rates. The highest rates of severe illness, hospitalization, and death occur among those older than age 65 years, young children (younger than 2 years old), and those who have underlying medical conditions, including pregnancy and cardiopulmonary disorders.
- The route of influenza transmission is person-to-person via inhalation of respiratory droplets, which can occur when an infected person coughs or sneezes. The incubation period for influenza ranges between 1 and 7 days, with an average incubation of 2 days. Adults are considered infectious from the day before their symptoms begin through 7 days after the onset of illness, whereas children can be infectious for longer than 10 days after the onset of illness. Viral shedding can persist for weeks to months in severely immunocompromised people.

CLINICAL PRESENTATION

- The presentation of influenza is similar to a number of other respiratory illnesses.
- The clinical course and outcome are affected by age, immunocompetence, viral characteristics, smoking, comorbidities, pregnancy, and the degree of preexisting immunity.
- Complications of influenza may include exacerbation of underlying comorbidities, primary viral pneumonia, secondary bacterial pneumonia or other respiratory illnesses (eg, sinusitis, bronchitis, and otitis), encephalopathy, transverse myelitis, myositis, myocarditis, pericarditis, and Reye's syndrome.

SIGNS AND SYMPTOMS

- Classic signs and symptoms of influenza include rapid onset of fever, myalgia, headache, malaise, nonproductive cough, sore throat, and rhinitis.
- Nausea, vomiting, and otitis media are also commonly reported in children.
- Signs and symptoms typically resolve in 3–7 days, although cough and malaise may persist for more than 2 weeks.

LABORATORY TESTS

- The gold standard for diagnosis of influenza is reverse-transcription polymerase chain reaction (RT-PCR) or viral culture.
- Rapid influenza diagnostic tests (RIDTs), also known as point-of-care (POC) tests, direct (DFA) or indirect (IFA) fluorescence antibody tests, and the RT-PCR assay may be used for rapid detection of virus.
- Chest radiograph should be obtained if pneumonia is suspected.

PREVENTION

- The best means to decrease the morbidity and mortality associated with influenza is to prevent infection through vaccination. Appropriate infection control measures, such as hand hygiene, basic respiratory etiquette (cover your cough and throw tissues away), and contact avoidance, are also important in preventing the spread of influenza. Additionally, chemoprophylaxis is useful in certain situations.
- Annual vaccination is recommended for all persons age 6 months or older and caregivers (eg, parents, teachers, babysitters, nannies) of children less than 6 months of age.
- Vaccination is also recommended for those who live with and/or care for people who are at high risk, including household contacts and healthcare workers.

- The Advisory Committee on Immunization Practices (ACIP) has made the following recommendations regarding the vaccinations of persons with reports of egg allergy: (a) vaccination with any age appropriate IIV or RIV3 vaccine, for persons with a history of egg allergy that involves only hives; (b) Persons with severe allergic reactions (ie, symptoms other than hives), such as angioedema, respiratory distress, light-headedness, or recurrent emesis or required epinephrine after an egg exposure may be immunized with any licensed IIV or RIV3 that is appropriate for age and health status; (c) Severe allergic reaction to influenza vaccine is a contraindication to receiving future vaccinations; (d) Vaccine providers should consider observing all patients for 15 minutes after vaccination to decrease the risk for injury should a patient experiences syncope.

  ✓ The ideal time for vaccination is October or November to allow for the development and maintenance of immunity during the peak of the influenza season.

  ✓ The two vaccines currently available for prevention of influenza are the inactivated vaccine IIV and the LAIV. The specific strains included in the vaccine each year change based on antigenic drift.

  ✓ IIV is FDA approved for use in people over 6 months of age, regardless of their immune status. Several commercial products are available and are approved for different age groups (Table 42-1). Because the vaccine content can change each year, vaccination providers should consult the most recent recommendations of the ACIP regarding use of seasonal influenza vaccines in the United States.

  ✓ Adults older than 65 years benefit from influenza vaccination, including prevention of complications and decreased risk of influenza-related hospitalization and death. However, people in this population may not generate a strong antibody response to the vaccine and may remain susceptible to infection.

  ✓ The most frequent adverse effect associated with IIV is soreness at the injection site that lasts for less than 48 hours. IIV may cause fever and malaise in those who have not previously been exposed to the viral antigens in the vaccine. Allergic-type reactions (hives and systemic anaphylaxis) rarely occur after influenza vaccination and are likely a result of a reaction to residual egg protein in the vaccine.

  ✓ Vaccination should be avoided in persons who are not at high risk for influenza complications and who have experienced Guillain–Barré syndrome within 6 weeks of receiving a previous influenza vaccine.

  ✓ LAIV is made with live, attenuated viruses and is approved for intranasal administration in healthy people between 2 and 49 years of age (Table 42-2). Advantages of LAIV include its ease of administration, intranasal rather than intramuscular administration, and the potential induction of broad mucosal and systemic immune response.

  ✓ The adverse effects typically associated with LAIV administration include runny nose, congestion, sore throat, and headache.

  ✓ LAIV should not be given to immunosuppressed patients or given by healthcare workers who are severely immunocompromised. LAIV is not recommended in several populations, including people older than 50 years and pregnant women.

POSTEXPOSURE PROPHYLAXIS

- Antiviral drugs available for prophylaxis of influenza should be considered adjuncts but are not replacements for annual vaccination.

- **Amantadine** and **rimantadine** are currently not recommended for prophylaxis or treatment in the United States because of the rapid emergence of resistance.

- The neuraminidase inhibitors **oseltamivir** and **zanamivir** are effective prophylactic agents against influenza in terms of preventing laboratory-confirmed influenza when used for seasonal prophylaxis and preventing influenza illness among persons exposed to a household contact who were diagnosed with influenza. Table 42-3 gives dosing recommendations. **Peramivir** is not approved for chemoprophylaxis.

- In those patients who did not receive the influenza vaccination and are receiving an antiviral drug for prevention of disease during the influenza season, the medication should optimally be taken for the entire duration of influenza activity in the community.

TABLE 42-1 Approved Influenza Vaccines for Different Age Groups—United States, 2019–2020 Season

Vaccine	Trade Name	Manufacturer	Dose/Presentation	Thimerosal Mercury Content (mcg Hg/0.5-mL dose)	Age Group	Number of Doses
Trivalent IIV (IIV3s)—adjuvanted and high dose						
aIIV3	Fluad	Seqirus	0.5-mL single dose prefilled syringe	0	≥65 years	1
IIV3 High dose	Fluzone HD	Sanofi Pasteur	0.5-mL prefilled syringe	0	≥65 years	1
Quadrivalent IIVs (IIV4s)						
IIV4	Afluria	Seqirus	0.25-mL prefilled syringe	0	6–35 months	1 or 2[a]
			0.5-mL prefilled syringe	0	≥3 years	1 or 2[a]
			5-mL multidose vial	24.5	≥6 months via needle/syringe or 18–64 years via jet injector	1 or 2[a]
IIV4	Fluarix Quadrivalent	GlaxoSmithKline	0.5-mL prefilled syringe	0	≥6 months	1 or 2[a]
IIV4	FluLaval Quadrivalent	GlaxoSmithKline	0.5-mL prefilled syringe	0	≥6 months	1 or 2[a]
			5-mL multidose vial	<25	≥6 months	1 or 2[a]
IIV4	Fluzone Quadrivalent[b]	Sanofi Pasteur	0.25-mL prefilled syringe	0	6–35 months	1 or 2[a]
			0.5-mL prefilled syringe	0	≥6 months	1 or 2[a]
			0.5-mL single-dose vial	0	≥6 months	1 or 2[a]
			5-mL multidose vial	25	≥6 months	1 or 2[a]

Quadrivalent IIV high dose (IIV4-HD)

| IIV4 High dose | Fluzone HD Quadrivalent | Sanofi Pasteur | 0.7-mL prefilled syringe | 0 | ≥65 years | 1 |

Cell culture–based quadrivalent IIVs (ccIIV4)

| ccIIV4 | Flucelvax Quadrivalent | Seqirus | 0.5-mL prefilled syringe | 0 | ≥4 years | 1 or 2[a] |
| | | | 5-mL multidose vial | 25 | ≥4 years | 1 or 2[a] |

Recombinant quadrivalent IIVs (RIV4)

| RIV4 | Flublok Quadrivalent | Sanofi Pasteur | 0.5-mL prefilled syringe | 0 | ≥18 years | 1 |

LAIV quadrivalent (LAIV4)

| LAIV | FluMist Quadrivalent | AstraZeneca | 0.2-mL sprayer | 0 | 2–49 years | 1 or 2[c] |

[a]Two doses administered at least 4 weeks apart are recommended for children aged 6 months to less than 9 years who are receiving influenza vaccine for the first time or received one dose in first year of vaccination during the previous influenza season.

[b]Fluzone Quadrivalent may be given to children aged 6 through 35 months as either 0.25 mL per dose or 0.5 mL per dose. No preference is expressed for one or the other dose volume for this age group. Persons aged ≥3 years should receive 0.5-mL dose volume.

[c]Two doses administered.

IIV, inactivated influenza vaccine; IIV3, inactivated influenza trivalent vaccine; aIIV3, adjuvanted inactivated influenza vaccine, trivalent, standard dose; IIV4, inactivated influenza quadrivalent vaccine; IIV4-HD, inactivated influenza quadrivalent vaccine—high dose; ccIIV3, cell culture–based trivalent influenza vaccine; RIV4, recombinant quadrivalent influenza vaccine; LAIV, live-attenuated influenza vaccine.

Note: IIVs and RIV4 may be administered concomitantly or sequentially with other inactivated vaccines or live vaccines. LAIV4 may be administered simultaneously with other live or inactivated vaccines. However, after administration of a live vaccine (such as LAIV4), at least 4 weeks should elapse before another live vaccine is administered.

Influenza antiviral medications might reduce the effectiveness of LAIV4 if given within 48 hours before, to 14 days after administration of LAIV4. Persons who receive influenza antiviral medications within this period of LAIV4 vaccination can be revaccinated with another appropriate influenza vaccine (eg, IIV or RIV4).

TABLE 42-2	Comparison of Inactivated Influenza Vaccine (IIV) and Live-Attenuated Influenza Vaccine (LAIV)	
Characteristic	IIV (IIV3/IIV4)	LAIV
Age groups approved for use	≥6 months	2–49 years
Immune status requirements	Immunocompetent or immunocompromised	Immunocompetent
Viral properties	Inactivated (killed) influenza A (H3N2), A (H1N1), and B viruses	Live-attenuated influenza A (H3N2), A (H1N1), and B viruses
Route of administration	Intramuscular	Intranasal
Immune system response	High serum IgG antibody response	Lower IgG response and high serum IgA mucosal response

TABLE 42-3	Recommended Daily Dosage of Influenza Antiviral Medications for Treatment and Prophylaxis—United States			
Drug	Adult Treatment	Adult Prophylaxis[a]	Pediatric Treatment	Pediatric Prophylaxis[a]
CAP-dependent endonuclease inhibitor				
Baloxavir[b,c]	12 years and older: 40–<80 kg: One 40 mg dose >80 kg: One 80 mg dose	None	FDA approved and recommended for use in children 12 years or older weighing at least 40 kg; see adult dosage	None
Neurominidase inhibitors				
Oseltamivir[d,e,f]	75-mg capsule twice daily × 5 days	75-mg capsule daily × 10 days	Term infants 0–8 months: 3 mg/kg/dose twice daily 9–11 months[g]: 3.5 mg/kg/dose twice daily or 3 mg/kg/dose twice daily ≥1 year: ≤15 kg: 30 mg twice daily >15–23 kg: 45 mg twice daily >23–40 kg: 60 mg twice daily >40 kg: 75 mg twice daily Duration: All for 5 days	Not recommended if <3 months 3–<12 months: 3 mg/kg/dose daily 9–11 months: 3.5 mg/kg/dose daily ≥1 year: ≤15 kg: 30 mg daily >15–23 kg: 45 mg daily >23–40 kg: 60 mg daily >40 kg: 75 mg daily Duration: All for 10 days

(*Continued*)

Drug	Adult Treatment	Adult Prophylaxis[a]	Pediatric Treatment	Pediatric Prophylaxis[a]
	TABLE 42-3 Recommended Daily Dosage of Influenza Antiviral Medications for Treatment and Prophylaxis—United States (Continued)			
Zanamivir	10 mg (2 of 5 mg inhalations) twice daily × 5 days	10 mg (2 of 5 mg inhalations) daily × 10 days	10 mg (2 of 5 mg inhalations) twice daily × 5 days for ≥7 years old	10 mg (2 of 5 mg inhalations) daily for ≥5 years old × 10 days
Peramivir[c,e]	13 years and older: One 600 mg dose via intravenous infusion for 15–30 minutes	None	2–12 years of age: One 12 mg/kg dose, up to 600 mg maximum, via intravenous infusion for a minimum of 15–30 minutes	None

[a]If influenza vaccine is administered, prophylaxis can generally be stopped 14 days after vaccination for noninstitutionalized persons. When prophylaxis is being administered following an exposure, prophylaxis should be continued for 10 days after the last exposure. In persons at high risk for complications from influenza for whom vaccination is contraindicated or expected to be ineffective, chemoprophylaxis should be continued for the duration that influenza viruses are circulating in the community during influenza season.

[b]Time to peak = 4 hours. Food and cations (calcium, aluminum, magnesium, iron) can decrease peak concentration by 48%. Long half-life (79.1 hours) and is metabolized by UDP-glucuronosyltransferase (UGT1A3) and CYP3A4.

[c]For the treatment of uncomplicated influenza with oral baloxavir or intravenous peramivir, a single dose is recommended. Longer daily dosing (oral oseltamivir or intravenous peramivir) can be considered for patients who remain severely ill after 5 days of treatment.

[d]Oseltamivir dosing for preterm infants using their postmenstrual age (ie, gestational age + chronological age): <38 weeks: 1.0 mg/kg/dose twice daily; 38–40 weeks: 1.5 mg/kg/dose twice daily; >40 weeks: 3.0 mg/kg/dose twice daily.

[e]In patients with renal insufficiency, the dose should be adjusted on the basis of creatinine clearance. See https://www.cdc.gov/flu/professionals/antivirals/summary-clinicians.htm.

[f]Some experts recommend 150 mg twice daily for severe illness in pregnant women. Optimal dosing for prophylaxis in pregnant women is unknown.

[g]The American Academy of Pediatrics recommends 3.5 mg/kg per dose twice daily; CDC and US Food and Drug Administration (FDA)–approved dosing is 3 mg/kg per dose twice daily for children aged 9–11 months.

Note: Although amantadine and rimantadine have been used historically for the treatment and prophylaxis of influenza A viruses, due to high resistance, the CDC no longer recommends the use of these agents for the treatment and/or prophylaxis of influenza.

• Prophylaxis should be considered during influenza season for the following groups of patients:

✓ Persons at high risk of serious illness and/or complications who cannot be vaccinated.

✓ Persons at high risk of serious illness and/or complications who are vaccinated after influenza activity has begun in their community because the development of sufficient antibody titers after vaccination takes ~2 weeks.

✓ Persons with severe immune deficiency or who may have an inadequate response to vaccination (eg, advanced human immunodeficiency virus [HIV] disease, persons receiving immunosuppressive medications), after exposure to an infectious person.

✓ Long-term care facility residents, regardless of vaccination status, when an outbreak has occurred in the institution.

- LAIV should not be administered until 48 hours after influenza antiviral therapy has stopped, and influenza antiviral drugs should not be administered for 2 weeks after the administration of LAIV because the antiviral drugs inhibit influenza virus replication.
- Pregnant women, regardless of trimester, should receive annual influenza vaccination with IIV but not with LAIV.
- The adamantanes and neuraminidase inhibitors are not recommended during pregnancy because of concerns regarding the effects of the drugs on the fetus.
- Immunocompromised hosts should receive annual influenza vaccination with IIV but not LAIV.

TREATMENT

- Goals of Therapy: To shorten the duration of illness and provide symptom control.
- Antiviral drugs are most effective if started within 48 hours of the onset of illness. Adjunct agents, such as acetaminophen for fever or an antihistamine for rhinitis, may be used concomitantly with the antiviral drugs.
- Patients suffering from influenza should get adequate sleep and maintain a low level of activity. They should stay home from work and/or school in order to rest and prevent the spread of infection. Appropriate fluid intake should be maintained. Cough/throat lozenges, warm tea, or soup may help with symptom control (cough and sore throat).

PHARMACOLOGIC THERAPY

- The neuraminidase inhibitors (**oseltamivir, zanamivir**, and **peramivir**) are the only antiviral drugs available for treatment and prophylaxis of influenza. Peramivir is the only intravenous formulation commercially available. The adamantanes (**amantadine** and **rimantadine**) are no longer recommended due to high resistance among influenza viruses.
- Oseltamivir, zanamivir, and peramivir have activity against both influenza A and influenza B viruses. When administered within 48 hours of the onset of illness, oseltamivir and zanamivir may reduce the duration of illness by ~1 day versus placebo. Benefits are highly dependent on the timing of initiation of treatment, ideally being within 12 hours of illness onset, up to 48 hours after onset of illness.
- Oseltamivir is approved for treatment in those older than 14 days, zanamivir is approved for treatment in those older than 7 years, and peramivir for those 18 years and older. The recommended dosages vary by agent and age (see **Table 42-3**), and the recommended duration of treatment for both agents is 5 days for oseltamivir and zanamivir and one dose for 1 day for peramivir.
- Neuropsychiatric complications consisting of delirium, seizures, hallucinations, and self-injury in pediatric patients have been reported following treatment with oseltamivir and peramivir.
- Oseltamivir and zanamivir have been used in pregnancy, but solid clinical safety data are lacking. Oseltamivir is preferred for the treatment of pregnant women because of its systemic activity; however, the drug of choice for chemoprophylaxis is not yet defined.
- Both the adamantanes and the neuraminidase inhibitors are excreted in breast milk and should be avoided by mothers who are breast-feeding their infants.

EVALUATION OF THERAPEUTIC OUTCOMES

- Patients should be monitored daily for resolution of signs and symptoms associated with influenza, such as fever, myalgia, headache, malaise, nonproductive cough, sore throat, and rhinitis. These signs and symptoms will typically resolve within ~1 week. If the patient continues to exhibit signs and symptoms of illness beyond 10 days or a worsening of symptoms after 7 days, a physician visit is warranted, as this may be an indication of a secondary bacterial infection.

See Chapter 127, Influenza, authored by Jessica C. Njoku, for a more detailed discussion of this topic.

43 Intra-Abdominal Infections

- Intra-abdominal infections are those contained within the peritoneum or retroperitoneal space. Two general types of intra-abdominal infections are discussed throughout this chapter: peritonitis and abscess.
- Peritonitis is defined as the acute, inflammatory response of peritoneal lining to microorganisms, chemicals, irradiation, or foreign body injury. It may be classified as either primary, secondary, or tertiary. With primary peritonitis, an intra-abdominal focus of disease may not be evident. In secondary peritonitis, a focal disease process is evident within the abdomen. Tertiary peritonitis occurs in critically ill patients and is infection that persists or recurs at least 48 hours after apparently adequate management of primary or secondary peritonitis.
- An abscess is a purulent collection of fluid separated from surrounding tissue by a wall consisting of inflammatory cells and adjacent organs. It usually contains necrotic debris, bacteria, and inflammatory cells.

PATHOPHYSIOLOGY

- **Table 43-1** summarizes many of the potential causes of bacterial peritonitis. Appendicitis is the most common cause of intra-abdominal infection. Intra-abdominal infection results from entry of bacteria into the peritoneal or retroperitoneal spaces or from bacterial collections within intra-abdominal organs. When peritonitis results from peritoneal dialysis, skin surface flora are introduced via the peritoneal catheter.
- In primary peritonitis, bacteria may enter the abdomen via the bloodstream or the lymphatic system, by transmigration through the bowel wall, through an indwelling peritoneal dialysis catheter, or via the fallopian tubes in female patients.
- In secondary peritonitis, bacteria most often enter the peritoneum or retroperitoneum as a result of disruption of the integrity of the gastrointestinal (GI) tract caused by diseases or traumatic injuries.
- When bacteria become dispersed throughout the peritoneum, the inflammatory process involves the majority of the peritoneal lining. Fluid and protein shift into the abdomen (called "third spacing") may decrease circulating blood volume and cause shock.
- Peritonitis often results in death because of the effects on major organ systems. Fluid shifts, cytokines, and microorganism toxins may result in hypovolemia, hypoperfusion, and shock.
- An abscess begins by the combined action of inflammatory cells (eg, neutrophils), bacteria, fibrin, and other inflammatory components. Within the abscess, oxygen tension is low, and anaerobic bacteria thrive.

MICROBIOLOGY

- Primary bacterial peritonitis is often caused by a single organism. In children, the pathogen is usually group A *Streptococcus, Escherichia coli, Streptococcus pneumoniae,* or *Bacteroides* species. When peritonitis occurs in association with cirrhotic ascites, *E. coli* is isolated most frequently.
- Peritonitis in patients undergoing peritoneal dialysis is most often caused by common skin organisms: coagulase negative staphylococci, *Staphylococcus aureus,* streptococci, and enterococci. Gram-negative bacteria associated with peritoneal dialysis infections include *E. coli, Klebsiella,* and *Pseudomonas.*

TABLE 43-1	Causes of Bacterial Peritonitis

Primary (spontaneous) bacterial peritonitis

Cirrhosis with ascites

Nephrotic syndrome

Peritoneal dialysis (may be secondary to catheter site infection)

Secondary bacterial peritonitis

Miscellaneous causes

    Divertic ulitis

    Appendicitis

    Inflammatory bowel diseases

    Salpingitis

    Biliary tract infections

    Necrotizing pancreatitis

    Neoplasms

    Intestinal obstruction

    Perforation

Mechanical GI problems

    Any cause of small bowel obstruction (adhesions, hernia)

Vascular causes

    Mesenteric arterial or venous occlusion (atrial fibrillation)

    Mesenteric ischemia without occlusion

Trauma

    Blunt abdominal trauma with rupture of intestine

    Penetrating abdominal trauma

Iatrogenic intestinal perforation (endoscopy)

Intraoperative events

    Solid organ transplant in the abdomen

Peritoneal contamination during abdominal operation

Leakage from GI anastomosis

GI, gastrointestinal.

- Secondary intra-abdominal infections are often polymicrobial. The mean number of isolates of microorganisms from infected intra-abdominal sites has ranged from 2.9–3.7, including an average of 1.3–1.6 aerobes and 1.7–2.1 anaerobes. The frequencies with which specific bacteria were isolated in intra-abdominal infections are given in Table 43-2.
- The combination of aerobic and anaerobic organisms appears to greatly the severity of infection. In intra-abdominal infections, facultative bacteria may provide an environment conducive to the growth of anaerobic bacteria.
- Aerobic enteric bacteria and anaerobic bacteria are both pathogens in intra-abdominal infection. Aerobic bacteria, particularly *E. coli*, appear responsible for the early mortality from peritonitis, whereas anaerobic bacteria are major pathogens in abscesses, with *Bacteroides fragilis* predominating.

TABLE 43-2	Pathogens Isolated from Patients with Intra-Abdominal Infection		
	Secondary Peritonitis (%)	Community-Acquired Infection (%)	Nosocomial Infection (%)
Gram-negative bacteria			
Escherichia coli	32–61	29	22.5
Enterobacter	8–26	5.2	8.0
Klebsiella	6–26	2.8	4.5
Proteus	4–23	1.7	2.4
Pseudomonas	5–13	5	13
Gram-positive bacteria			
Enterococcus	18–24	10.6	18
Streptococcus	6–55	13.7	10
Staphylococcus	6–16	3.1	4.8
Anaerobic bacteria			
Bacteroides	25–80	13.7	10.3
Clostridium	5–18	3.5	3.4
Fungi	2–5	3	4

- The role of *Enterococcus* as a pathogen is not clear. Enterococcal infection occurs more commonly in postoperative peritonitis, in the presence of specific risk factors indicating failure of the host defenses, or with the use of broad-spectrum antibiotics.

CLINICAL PRESENTATION

- Intra-abdominal infections have a wide spectrum of clinical features often depending on the specific disease process, the location and the magnitude of bacterial contamination, and concurrent host factors. Patients with primary and secondary peritonitis present quite differently (Table 43-3).
- If peritonitis continues untreated, the patient may experience hypovolemic shock from fluid loss into the peritoneum, bowel wall, and lumen. This may be accompanied by sepsis. Intra-abdominal abscess may pose a diagnostic challenge, as the symptoms are neither specific nor dramatic.
- The overall outcome from intra-abdominal infection depends on five key factors: inoculum size, virulence of the organisms, the presence of adjuvants within the peritoneal cavity that facilitate infection, the adequacy of host defenses, and the adequacy of initial treatment.

TREATMENT

- Goals of Treatment: Correction of intra-abdominal disease processes or injuries that have caused infection and the drainage of collections of purulent material (eg, abscess). A secondary objective is to achieve resolution of infection without major organ system complications or adverse treatment effects.
- The three major modalities for the treatment of intra-abdominal infection are prompt surgical control and drainage of the infected site, hemodynamic resuscitation and support of vital functions, and early administration of appropriate antimicrobial therapy to treat infection not removed by surgery.

TABLE 43-3	Clinical Presentation of Peritonitis

Primary Peritonitis

General

The patient may not be in acute distress, particularly with peritoneal dialysis

Signs and symptoms

The patient may complain of loss of appetite, bloating, nausea, vomiting (sometimes with diarrhea), and abdominal tenderness

Temperature may be only mildly elevated or not elevated in patients undergoing peritoneal dialysis

Bowel sounds are hypoactive

The cirrhotic patient may have worsening encephalopathy

Cloudy dialysate fluid with peritoneal dialysis

Laboratory tests

The patient's WBC count may be only mildly elevated

Ascitic fluid usually contains greater than 250 leukocytes/mm³ (0.25 × 10⁹/L), and bacteria may be evident on gram stain of a centrifuged specimen

In 60%–80% of patients with cirrhotic ascites, the gram stain is negative

Other diagnostic tests

Culture of peritoneal dialysate or ascitic fluid should be positive, particularly if collected prior to initiation of antibiotics

Procalcitonin in conjunction with clinical findings is a sensitive test for bacterial peritonitis

Secondary Peritonitis

Signs and symptoms

Generalized abdominal pain

Tachypnea

Tachycardia

Nausea and vomiting

Temperature is normal initially then increases to 37.8–38.9°C (100–102°F) within the first few hours and may continue to rise for the next several hours

Hypotension, hypoperfusion, and shock if volume is not restored

Decreased urine output due to vascular volume depletion

Physical examination

Voluntary abdominal guarding changing to involuntary guarding and a "board-like abdomen"

Abdominal tenderness and distension

Faint bowel sounds that cease over time

Laboratory tests

Leukocytosis (15,000–20,000 WBC/mm³ [15 × 10⁹ to 20 × 10⁹/L]), with neutrophils predominating and an elevated percentage of immature neutrophils (bands)

Elevated hematocrit and blood urea nitrogen because of dehydration

Patient progresses from early alkalosis because of hyperventilation and vomiting to metabolic acidosis

Other diagnostic tests

Abdominal radiographs may be useful because free air in the abdomen (indicating intestinal perforation) or distension of the small or large bowel is often evident

WBC, white blood cell.

- Antimicrobials are an important adjunct to drainage procedures in the treatment of intra-abdominal infections; however, the use of antimicrobial agents without surgical source control is usually inadequate. For most cases of primary peritonitis, drainage procedures may not be required, and antimicrobial agents become the mainstay of therapy.
- In the early phase of serious intra-abdominal infections, attention should be given to the maintenance of organ system functions. With generalized peritonitis, large volumes of IV fluids are required to restore vascular volume, to improve cardiovascular function, and to maintain adequate tissue perfusion and oxygenation.
- An important component of therapy is nutrition. Enteral or parenteral nutrition as indicated facilitates improved immune function and wound healing to ensure recovery.

NONPHARMACOLOGIC THERAPY

- Secondary peritonitis is treated surgically; this is called "source control," which refers to the physical measures undertaken to eradicate the focus of infection. Abdominal laparotomy may be used to correct the cause of peritonitis. After an abscess is located, it must be drained.
- Aggressive fluid repletion and management are required for the purposes of achieving or maintaining proper intravascular volume to ensure adequate cardiac output, tissue perfusion, and correction of acidosis.
- The Surviving Sepsis Campaign recommends that resuscitation should be guided by normalization of lactate (weak recommendation, low quality of evidence). Furthermore, in patients with septic shock requiring vasopressors, an initial mean arterial pressure (MAP) of 65 mm Hg should be targeted (strong recommendation, moderate quality of evidence). Urine output should equal or exceed 0.5 mL/kg of body weight per hour.
- In patients with sepsis hypoperfusion or septic shock, IV fluids should consist of a 30 mL/kg bolus of crystalloids with additional fluids targeting predefined therapeutic goals. Initial fluid resuscitation should be completed within 3 hours of hypoperfusion recognition. Thereafter, fluids may be required at a rate of 1 L/hr or higher. Once targeted therapeutic goals are reached, judicious use of fluids should be used as a sustained positive fluid balance after initial resuscitation may be harmful.
- Maintenance fluids should be instituted with 0.9% sodium chloride and potassium chloride (20 mEq/L [mmol/L]) or 5% dextrose and 0.45% sodium chloride with potassium chloride (20 mEq/L [mmol/L]). The administration rate should be based on estimated daily fluid loss through urine and nasogastric suction, including 0.5–1 L for insensible fluid loss.
- In patients with significant blood loss (hematocrit $\leq 25\%$), blood should be given. This is generally in the form of packed red blood cells.
- Enteral or parenteral nutrition facilitates improved immune function and wound healing to ensure recovery.

PHARMACOLOGIC THERAPY

- The goals of antimicrobial therapy are: (a) to eliminate the intra-abdominal infection and prevent the establishment of metastatic foci of infection or bacteremia, (b) to reduce suppurative complications (eg, abscess formation) after bacterial contamination, and (c) to prevent local spread of existing infection.
- An empiric antimicrobial regimen should be started as soon as the presence of intra-abdominal infection is suspected on the basis of likely pathogens. Antimicrobial therapy should be administered within 1 hour of the recognition of sepsis or septic shock (strong recommendation, moderate quality of evidence).

TABLE 43-4	Recommended Agents for the Treatment of Community-Acquired Complicated Intra-Abdominal Infections in Adults

Agents Recommended for Mild-to-Moderate Infections	Agents Recommended for High Severity Infections
Single agent	
Cefoxitin[a]	Piperacillin–tazobactam
Moxifloxacin[b]	Imipenem–cilastatin,[c] meropenem,[c] doripenem[c]
Ertapenem[c]	
Combination regimens	
Cefazolin,[a] cefuroxime,[a] ceftriaxone, or cefotaxime each in combination with metronidazole	Cefepime, ceftazidime, ceftazidime/avibactam,[d] or ceftolozane/tazobactam[e] each in combination with metronidazole
Ciprofloxacin[b] or levofloxacin[b] each in combination with metronidazole	Ciprofloxacin[b] or levofloxacin[b] each in combination with metronidazole

[a]Empiric first- and second-generation cephalosporin use should be avoided unless local antibiograms show >80%–90% susceptibility of *E. coli* to these agents.

[b]Use of quinolones may be associated with treatment failure due to increasing resistance of enteric pathogens including *E. coli*. Empiric quinolone use should be avoided unless local antibiograms show >80%–90% susceptibility of *E. coli* to quinolones.

[c]Carbapenems should be reserved for settings where there is a high risk of resistance to other agents (ie, extended-spectrum β-lactamase [ESBL]-producing pathogens).

[d]Ceftazidime/Avibactam should be reserved for patients infected with *Enterobacteriaceae* that are resistant to all other β-lactams including carbapenems, and in particular, *Klebsiella pneumoniae* carbapenemase (KPC)-producing pathogens.

[e]Ceftolozane/Tazobactam should be reserved for patients infected with gram-negative bacteria that are resistant to all other β-lactams. Ceftolozane/tazobactam may have activity against multidrug-resistant *Pseudomonas*, however susceptibility must be confirmed.

Recommendations

- For most Intra-abdominal infections, the antimicrobial regimen should be effective against both aerobic and anaerobic bacteria. Table 43-4 presents recommended and alternative regimens for community-acquired complicated intra-abdominal infections. Guidelines for initial antimicrobial treatment of specific intra-abdominal infections are presented in Table 43-5.
- Evidence-based treatment principles for complicated intra-abdominal infections are given in Table 43-6.
- For established intra-abdominal infections, most patients are adequately treated with 4–7 days of antimicrobial therapy.
- For peritonitis that occurs from chronic peritoneal dialysis the selection of a specific agent or combination should be based on culture and susceptibility data. If microbiologic data are unavailable, empiric therapy should be initiated.
- Intraperitoneal administration of antibiotics is preferred over IV therapy in the treatment of peritonitis that occurs in patients undergoing continuous ambulatory peritoneal dialysis. For empiric intraperitoneal therapy, **cefazolin** or **vancomycin** in cases of high prevalence of methicillin-resistant *S. aureus* (MRSA) or β-lactam allergy may be used for gram-positive coverage.
- Antimicrobial therapy should typically be continued for 14–21 days.

EVALUATION OF THERAPEUTIC OUTCOMES

- The patient should be continually reassessed to determine the success or failure of therapies.
- Once antimicrobials are initiated and other important therapies described earlier in the Treatment section are used, most patients should show improvement within

TABLE 43-5	Guidelines for Empiric Antimicrobial Agents for Intra-abdominal Infections	
	Primary Agents	**Alternatives**
Primary (spontaneous) bacterial peritonitis		
Cirrhosis	Ceftriaxone, cefotaxime	1. Piperacillin–tazobactam, carbapenems
		2. Aztreonam combined with an agent active against *Streptococcus* spp. (eg, vancomycin) or quinolones with significant *Streptococcus* spp. activity (levofloxacin, moxifloxacin)
Peritoneal dialysis	Initial empiric regimens should be active against both gram-positive (including *S. aureus*) and gram-negative pathogens: gram-positive agent (first-generation cephalosporin or vancomycin) plus a gram-negative agent (third-generation cephalosporin or aminoglycoside)	1. Cefepime or carbapenems may be used alone
		2. Aztreonam or an aminoglycoside may be used in place of ceftazidime or cefepime as long as combined with a gram-positive agent
		3. Quinolones may be used in place of gram-negative agents if local susceptibilities allow
	1. *Staphylococcus* spp.: oxacillin/ nafcillin or first-generation cephalosporin	1. Vancomycin should be used for methicillin-resistant *Staphylococcus* spp.
		2. May consider addition of rifampin for 5–7 days with vancomycin for methicillin-resistant *S. aureus*
	2. *Streptococcus* or *Enterococcus*: ampicillin	1. Daptomycin or linezolid should ideally be used to treat vancomycin-resistant *Enterococcus* spp. not susceptible to ampicillin
	3. Aerobic gram-negative bacilli: ceftazidime or cefepime	1. The regimen should be based on in vitro sensitivity tests
	4. *Pseudomonas aeruginosa*: two agents with differing mechanisms of action, such as an intraperitoneal ceftazidime or cefepime each combined with either tobramycin or oral ciprofloxacin	
Secondary bacterial peritonitis		
Perforated peptic ulcer	First-generation cephalosporins	1. Ceftriaxone, cefotaxime, or antianaerobic cephalosporins[a]

(Continued)

TABLE 43-5	Guidelines for Empiric Antimicrobial Agents for Intra-abdominal Infections (*Continued*)	
	Primary Agents	**Alternatives**
Other	Third- or fourth-generation cephalosporin with metronidazole, piperacillin–tazobactam or carbapenem	1. Ciprofloxacin[b] or levofloxacin[b] each with metronidazole or moxifloxacin[b] alone 2. Aztreonam with vancomycin and metronidazole 3. Antianaerobic cephalosporins[a]
Abscess		
General	Third- or fourth-generation cephalosporin with metronidazole or piperacillin–tazobactam	1. Imipenem–cilastatin, meropenem, doripenem, or ertapenem 2. Ciprofloxacin[b] or levofloxacin[b] each with metronidazole or moxifloxacin alone
Liver	As above	Use metronidazole if amoebic liver abscess is suspected
Spleen	Ceftriaxone or cefotaxime	Moxifloxacin[b] or levofloxacin[b]
Other intra-abdominal infections		
Appendicitis	Same management as for community-acquired complicated intra-abdominal infections as listed in Table 43-4	
Community-acquired acute cholecystitis	Ceftriaxone or cefotaxime	Severe infection, piperacillin/tazobactam, antipseudomonal carbapenem, aztreonam with metronidazole
Cholangitis	Ceftriaxone or cefotaxime each with or without metronidazole	Vancomycin with aztreonam with or without metronidazole
Acute contamination from abdominal trauma	Antianaerobic cephalosporins[a] or metronidazole with either ceftriaxone or cefotaxime	1. Piperacillin/tazobactam or a carbapenem 2. Ciprofloxacin[b] or levofloxacin[b] each with metronidazole or moxifloxacin alone

[a]Cefoxitin or ceftizoxime; these agents should be avoided empirically unless local antibiograms show >80%–90% susceptibility of *E. coli* to these agents.

[b]Use of quinolones may be associated with treatment failure due to increasing resistance of enteric pathogens including *E. coli*. Empiric quinolone use should be avoided unless local antibiograms show >80%–90% susceptibility of *E. coli* to quinolones.

2–3 days. Usually, temperature will return to near normal, vital signs should stabilize, and the patient should not appear in distress, with the exception of recognized discomfort and pain from incisions, drains, and nasogastric tube.

- Within 24–48 hours, aerobic bacterial culture results should return. If a suspected pathogen is not sensitive to the antimicrobial agents being given, the regimen should typically be changed to active therapy. If the isolated pathogen is susceptible to a narrower spectrum agent, therapy should be deescalated.

- With present anaerobic culturing techniques and the slow growth of these organisms, anaerobes are often not identified until 4–7 days after culture, and sensitivity information is difficult to obtain. A report indicating that anaerobes were not isolated should not be the sole justification for discontinuing antianaerobic drugs.

TABLE 43-6	Evidence-Based Recommendations for Treatment of Complicated Intra-Abdominal Infections

	Grade of Recommendation[a]

Elements of appropriate intervention

| An appropriate source control procedure to drain infected foci, control ongoing peritoneal contamination by diversion or resection, and restore anatomic and physiological function to the extent feasible is recommended for nearly all patients with intra-abdominal infection | B-2 |

Community-acquired infections of mild-to-moderate severity in adults

Antibiotics used for empiric treatment of community-acquired intra-abdominal infections should be active against enteric gram-negative aerobic and facultative bacilli and enteric gram-positive streptococci	A-1
For patients with mild-to-moderate community-acquired infections, regimens with substantial anti-pseudomonal activity are not required (Table 43-4)	A-1
Empiric coverage of *Enterococcus* is not necessary in patients with mild-to-moderate community-acquired intra-abdominal infection	A-1
The use of agents listed as appropriate for high-severity community-acquired infection and healthcare-associated infection is not recommended for patients with mild-to-moderate community-acquired infection, because such regimens may carry a greater risk of toxicity and facilitate acquisition of more resistant organisms	B-2

High-severity community-acquired infections in adults[b]

| The empiric use of antimicrobial regimens with broad-spectrum activity against gram-negative organisms including *Pseudomonas* spp., such as meropenem, imipenem–cilastatin, doripenem, piperacillin–tazobactam, ciprofloxacin or levofloxacin in combination with metronidazole, or ceftazidime or cefepime in combination with metronidazole, is recommended for patients with high-severity community-acquired intra-abdominal infection (Table 43-4) | A-1 |
| Aztreonam plus metronidazole is an alternative, but addition of an agent effective against gram-positive cocci is recommended | B-3 |

Healthcare-associated infections in adults[c]

| Empiric antibiotic therapy for healthcare-associated intra-abdominal infection should be driven by local microbiologic results | A-2 |
| To achieve empiric coverage of likely pathogens, multidrug regimens that include agents with expanded spectra of activity against gram-negative aerobic and facultative bacilli may be needed. These agents include meropenem, imipenem–cilastatin, doripenem, piperacillin–tazobactam, or metronidazole combined with either cefepime or ceftazidime. For multidrug-resistant aerobic gram-negative pathogens, aminoglycosides, colistin, polymyxin B, ceftazidime/avibactam, or ceftolozane/tazobactam may be required | B-3 |

(Continued)

TABLE 43-6 Evidence-Based Recommendations for Treatment of Complicated Intra-Abdominal Infections *(Continued)*	
	Grade of Recommendation[a]

Antimicrobial agents not recommended

Ampicillin–sulbactam is not recommended for use because of high rates of resistance to this agent among community-acquired *E. coli*	B-2
Quinolone-resistant *E. coli* have become common in some communities, and quinolones should not be used unless hospital surveys indicate 90% susceptibility of *E. coli* to quinolones	A-2
Cefotetan and clindamycin are not recommended for use because of increasing prevalence of resistance to these agents among *Bacteroides fragilis*	B-2
Because of the availability of less toxic agents demonstrated to be at least equally effective, aminoglycosides are not recommended for routine use in adults with community-acquired intra-abdominal infection	B-2

Oral completion therapy

For adults recovering from intra-abdominal infection, completion of the antimicrobial course with oral forms of moxifloxacin, ciprofloxacin plus metronidazole, levofloxacin plus metronidazole, an oral cephalosporin with metronidazole, or amoxicillin–clavulanic acid is acceptable in patients able to tolerate an oral diet and in patients in whom susceptibility studies do not demonstrate resistance	B-2

Duration of therapy

Antimicrobial therapy of established infection should be limited to 4 days, unless it is difficult to achieve adequate source control. Longer durations of therapy have not been associated with improved outcome	A-1
For acute stomach and proximal jejunum perforations, in the absence of acid-reducing therapy or malignancy and when source control is achieved within 24 hours, prophylactic anti-infective therapy directed at aerobic gram-positive cocci for 24 hours is adequate	B-2
Bowel injuries attributable to penetrating, blunt, or iatrogenic trauma that are repaired within 12 hours and any other intraoperative contamination of the operative field by enteric contents should be treated with antibiotics for ≤24 hours	A-1
Acute appendicitis without evidence of perforation, abscess, or local peritonitis requires only prophylactic administration of narrow spectrum regimens active against aerobic and facultative and obligate anaerobes; treatment should be discontinued within 24 hours	A-1
The administration of prophylactic antibiotics to patients with severe necrotizing pancreatitis prior to the diagnosis of infection is not recommended	A-1

Anaerobic coverage

Coverage for obligate anaerobic bacilli should be provided for distal small bowel, appendiceal, and colon-derived infection and for more proximal GI perforations in the presence of obstruction or paralytic ileus	A-1

(Continued)

TABLE 43-6	Evidence-Based Recommendations for Treatment of Complicated Intra-Abdominal Infections (*Continued*)	
		Grade of Recommendation[a]
Antifungal therapy		
Antifungal therapy for patients with high-severity community-acquired or healthcare-associated infection is recommended if *Candida* is grown from intra-abdominal cultures		B-2
Anti-MRSA therapy		
Empiric antimicrobial coverage directed against MRSA should be provided to patients with healthcare-associated intra-abdominal infection who are known to be colonized with the organism or who are at risk of having an infection due to this organism because of prior treatment failure and significant antibiotic exposure		B-2
Vancomycin is recommended for treatment of suspected or proven intra-abdominal infection due to MRSA		A-3
Antienterococcal therapy		
Antimicrobial therapy for enterococci should be given when enterococci are recovered from patients with high-severity community-acquired or healthcare-associated infection		B-III
Empiric antienterococcal therapy is recommended for patients with high-severity community-acquired infections and healthcare-associated intra-abdominal infections, particularly those with postoperative infection, those who have previously received cephalosporins or other antimicrobial agents selected for *Enterococcus* species, immunocompromised patients, and those with valvular heart disease or prosthetic intravascular materials		B-II
Initial empiric antienterococcal therapy should be directed against *Enterococcus faecalis*. Antibiotics that can potentially be used against this organism, on the basis of susceptibility testing of the individual isolate, include ampicillin, piperacillin/tazobactam, and vancomycin		B-III
Empiric therapy directed against vancomycin-resistant *Enterococcus faecium* is not recommended unless the patient is at very high risk for an infection due to this organism, such as a liver transplant recipient with an intra-abdominal infection originating in the hepatobiliary tree or a patient known to be colonized with vancomycin-resistant *E. faecium*		B-III

[a]Strength of recommendations: A, B, C, good, moderate, and poor evidence to support recommendation, respectively. Quality of evidence: 1, evidence from ≥1 properly randomized, controlled trial; 2, evidence from ≥1 well-designed clinical trial without randomization, from cohort or case-controlled analytic studies, from multiple time series, or from dramatic results from uncontrolled experiments; 3, evidence from opinions of respected authorities, based on clinical experience, descriptive studies, or reports of expert communities.
[b]Criteria for high-severity community-acquired infection: sepsis or septic shock, APACHE II score ≥15, delay in initial intervention >24 hours, advanced age, comorbidity and degree of organ dysfunction, low albumin level, poor nutritional status, degree of peritoneal involvement or diffuse peritonitis, inability to achieve adequate debridement or control of drainage, and presence of malignancy.
[c]Criteria for classification of intra-abdominal infections as healthcare-associated infection varies. However, patients who develop an infection after surgery, reside in a long-term care facility, who were recently hospitalized, or who have other significant healthcare exposure can be considered to have a healthcare-associated intra-abdominal infection.
MRSA, methicillin-resistant *Staphylococcus aureus*.

- Superinfection in patients being treated for intra-abdominal infection is often due to *Candida*; however, enterococci or opportunistic gram-negative bacilli such as *Pseudomonas* may be involved.
- Treatment regimens for intra-abdominal infection can be judged successful if the patient recovers from the infection without recurrent peritonitis or intra-abdominal abscess and without the need for additional antimicrobials. A regimen can be considered unsuccessful if a significant adverse drug reaction occurs, if reoperation is necessary, or if patient improvement is delayed beyond 1 or 2 weeks.

See Chapter 132, Intra-abdominal Infections, authored by Alan E. Gross and Keith M. Olsen, for a more detailed discussion of this topic.

Acute Bronchitis

- Bronchitis is frequently classified as either acute or chronic. Acute bronchitis is characterized by inflammation of the epithelium of the large airways resulting from infection or exposure to irritating environmental triggers (eg, air pollution and cigarette smoke).
- Acute bronchitis occurs year-round, but more commonly during the winter months. Viral infections, cold, damp climates, and/or the presence of high concentrations of irritating environmental triggers such as air pollution or cigarette smoke may precipitate attacks.
- Respiratory viruses are the predominant infectious agents associated with acute bronchitis. The most common infecting agents include influenza A and B, respiratory syncytial virus (RSV), and parainfluenza virus. Bacterial pathogens are involved in a minority of cases and involve pathogens often associated with community-acquired pneumonia (CAP).
- Infection of the trachea and bronchi causes hyperemic and edematous mucous membranes and an increase in bronchial secretions. Destruction of respiratory epithelium can range from mild to extensive and may affect bronchial mucociliary function. In addition, the increase in desquamated epithelial cells and bronchial secretions, which can become thick and tenacious, further impairs mucociliary activity.
- Recurrent acute respiratory infections may be associated with increased airway hyperreactivity and possibly the pathogenesis of asthma and chronic obstructive lung disease.

CLINICAL PRESENTATION

- Acute bronchitis usually begins as an upper respiratory infection with nonspecific complaints. Cough is the hallmark of acute bronchitis and occurs early. The onset of cough may be insidious or abrupt, and the symptoms persist despite resolution of nasal or nasopharyngeal complaints; cough may persist for up to 3 or more weeks. Frequently, the cough initially is nonproductive, but then progresses, yielding mucopurulent sputum.
- Fever, when present, rarely exceeds 39°C (102.2°F) and appears most commonly with adenovirus, influenza virus, and *Mycoplasma pneumoniae* infections.
- Bacterial cultures of expectorated sputum are generally of limited utility because of the inability to avoid normal nasopharyngeal flora by the sampling technique. For the vast majority of affected patients, an etiologic diagnosis is unnecessary and will not change the prescribing of routine supportive care for the management of these patients.

TREATMENT

- Goals of Treatment: The goal is to provide comfort to the patient and, in the unusually severe case, to treat associated dehydration and respiratory compromise.
- The treatment of acute bronchitis is symptomatic and supportive. Reassurance and antipyretics alone are often sufficient. Bedrest for comfort may be instituted as desired. Patients should be encouraged to drink fluids to prevent dehydration and possibly to decrease the viscosity of respiratory secretions.
- **Aspirin** or **acetaminophen** (650 mg in adults or 10–15 mg/kg per dose in children with a maximum daily adult dose of <4 g and 60 mg/kg for children) or **ibuprofen**

(200–800 mg in adults or 10 mg/kg per dose in children with a maximum daily dose of 3.2 g for adults and 40 mg/kg for children) is administered every 6–8 hours.

- In children under 19 years of age, aspirin should be avoided and acetaminophen used as the preferred agent because of the possible association between aspirin use and the development of Reye syndrome.
- In otherwise healthy patients, no meaningful benefits have been described with the use of oral or aerosolized β_2-receptor agonists and/or oral or aerosolized corticosteroids.
- Persistent, mild cough, which may be bothersome, may be treated with **dextromethorphan**; more severe coughs may require intermittent **codeine** or other similar agents. Codeine is no longer recommended for use in pediatric patients.
- Routine use of antibiotics in the treatment of acute bronchitis is strongly discouraged; however, in patients who exhibit persistent fever or respiratory symptomatology for more than 5–7 days, the possibility of a concurrent bacterial infection should be suspected.
- When possible, antibiotic therapy is directed toward anticipated respiratory pathogen(s) (ie, *Streptococcus pneumoniae* and *Haemophilus influenzae*).
- *M. pneumoniae*, if suspected by history or if confirmed by culture, serology, or PCR may be treated with **azithromycin**. Also, a fluoroquinolone with activity against these pathogens (**levofloxacin** or **moxifloxacin**) may be used empirically, but reserved for patients not responding adequately to supportive care and deemed at risk of associated complications.
- See Chapter 42 for recommendations to treat influenza.

Chronic Bronchitis

- Chronic bronchitis is a result of several contributing factors, including cigarette smoking; exposure to occupational dusts, fumes, and environmental pollution; host factors (eg, genetic factors); and bacterial or viral infections.
- Chronic bronchitis is defined clinically as the presence of a chronic cough productive of sputum lasting more than 3 consecutive months of the year for 2 consecutive years without an underlying etiology of bronchiectasis or tuberculosis.

CLINICAL PRESENTATION

- The hallmark of chronic bronchitis is a cough that may range from a mild to severe, incessant coughing productive of purulent sputum. Expectoration of the largest quantity of sputum usually occurs upon arising in the morning, although many patients expectorate sputum throughout the day. The expectorated sputum is usually tenacious and can vary in color from white to yellow-green.
- On physical examination, patients with advanced disease may have cyanosis and clubbing of digits.
- Chest auscultation usually reveals inspiratory and expiratory rales, rhonchi, and mild wheezing with an expiratory phase that is often prolonged. There may be hyperresonance on percussion with obliteration of the area of cardiac dullness. Normal vesicular breathing sounds are diminished.
- Chest radiograph may show increased anteroposterior diameter of the thoracic cage (barrel chest) and depressed diaphragm with limited mobility.
- Laboratory findings may include erythrocytosis (ie, increased hematocrit) in advanced disease.
- Pulmonary function tests may reveal decreased vital capacity and prolonged expiratory flow.
- The diagnosis of chronic bronchitis is based primarily on clinical assessment and history.

TABLE 44-1	Common Bacterial Pathogens Isolated from Sputum of Patients with Acute Exacerbation of Chronic Bronchitis
Pathogen	**Percent of Cultures**
H. influenzae[a,b]	45
M. catarrhalis[a]	30
S. pneumoniae[c]	20
E. coli, Enterobacter species, Klebsiella species, P. aeruginosa	5

[a]Often β-lactamase positive.
[b]Vast majority are nontypeable strains.
[c]More than 25% of strains may have intermediate or high resistance to penicillin.

- The most common bacterial isolates (expressed in percentages of total cultures) identified from sputum culture in patients experiencing an acute exacerbation of chronic bronchitis are given in Table 44-1.

TREATMENT

- <u>Goals of Treatment</u>: Reduce the severity of symptoms, to ameliorate acute exacerbations, and to achieve prolonged infection-free intervals.
- A complete occupational/environmental history for the determination of exposure to noxious and irritating gases, as well as cigarette smoking must be assessed.
- Attempts must be made to reduce the patient's exposure to known bronchial irritants (eg, reduce smoking and workplace pollution).
- Pulmonary rehabilitation programs (including exercise-training program with resistance and aerobic exercise) individualized for patients with chronic respiratory impairment can improve quality of life by optimizing each patient's physical and social performance and autonomy.
- Chest physiotherapy (pulmonary toilet) can be instituted. Humidification of inspired air may promote the hydration (liquefaction) of tenacious secretions, allowing for more effective sputum production. The use of mucolytic aerosols (eg, N-acetylcysteine and deoxyribonuclease) is of questionable therapeutic value.
- For patients with moderate-to-severe chronic obstructive pulmonary disease (COPD), combination therapy with a long-acting β_2-agonist and inhaled corticosteroid led to decreased exacerbations and rescue medication use while it also improved quality of life, lung function, and symptom scores compared with long-acting β_2–agonist monotherapy.

PHARMACOLOGIC THERAPY

- Patients should be up-to-date with vaccinations, particularly pneumococcal and an annual influenza vaccine.
- For patients who consistently demonstrate clinical limitation in airflow, a therapeutic challenge of a short-acting β_2–agonist bronchodilator (eg, as **albuterol** aerosol) should be considered. Regular use of a long-acting β-receptor agonist (LABA) aerosol (eg, **salmeterol** and **formoterol**) in responsive patients are more effective and probably more convenient than short-acting β_2-receptor agonists. Chronic inhalation of a combination LABA and a corticosteroid (eg, **salmeterol-fluticasone** and **formoterol-mometasone**) improved pulmonary function and quality of life.
- Long-term use of aerosolized corticosteroid is associated with increased side effects including hoarseness, sore throat, thrush, pneumonia, and osteoporosis; however,

caution should be exercised in withdrawing inhaled glucocorticoid administration in patients with severe COPD receiving triple inhalation therapy.

- Long-term inhalation of **ipratropium** (or **tiotropium**) decreases the frequency of cough, severity of cough, and volume of expectorated sputum.
- Inhaled long-acting muscarinic antagonists (LAMAs) alone or more frequently, in combination with a LABA, improve lung function and symptom control and reduce the number of acute exacerbations.
- Long-acting **theophylline** remains an effective "add on" therapy, particularly for severe chronic bronchitis/COPD, due to the drug's beneficial effects of bronchodilation, improved ciliary function and increased beat frequency, possibly increased mucus hydration, and low cost.
- The role of **roflumilast** in chronic lung disease is evolving but many guidelines suggest its greatest use is in the more severely affected patients.
- Use of antimicrobials for treatment of chronic bronchitis has been controversial but is becoming more accepted. The goal is to select the most effective antibiotic drug for the patient based on their history of previous exacerbations and response to drug therapy (see **Fig. 44-1**).
- The Anthonisen criteria can be used to determine if antibiotic therapy is indicated. The patient will most likely benefit from antibiotic therapy if two or three of the following are present: (1) increase of shortness of breath, (2) increase in sputum volume, or (3) production of purulent sputum.
- Selection of antibiotics should consider that up to 30%–40% of *H. influenzae* and 95%–100% of *Moraxella catarrhalis* are β-lactamase producers; up to 40% of *S. pneumoniae* demonstrate intermediate susceptibility or resistance to penicillin, with 20% being highly resistant.
- Antibiotics commonly used in the treatment of these patients and their respective adult starting doses are outlined in **Table 44-2**. Duration of symptom-free periods may be enhanced by antibiotic regimens using the upper limit of the recommended daily dose for 5–7 days.

Bronchiolitis

- Bronchiolitis is an acute viral infection of the lower respiratory tract of infants that affects ~50% of children during the first year of life and 100% by 2 years.
- RSV is the most common cause of bronchiolitis, accounting for up to 75% of all cases. Other detectable viruses include parainfluenza, adenovirus, and influenza. Bacteria serve as secondary pathogens in a minority of cases.

CLINICAL PRESENTATION

- The most common clinical signs of bronchiolitis. A prodrome suggesting an upper respiratory tract infection, usually lasting from 1–4 days, precedes the onset of clinical symptoms. As a result of limited oral intake due to coughing combined with fever, vomiting, and diarrhea, infants are frequently dehydrated.
- The diagnosis of bronchiolitis is based primarily on history and clinical findings. Identification of *respiratory syncytial virus* by PCR should be available routinely from most clinical laboratories, but its relevance to the clinical management of bronchiolitis remains obscure and routine testing is not recommended.

SIGNS AND SYMPTOMS

- Prodrome with irritability, restlessness, and mild fever.
- Cough and coryza.
- Vomiting, diarrhea, noisy breathing, and increased respiratory rate as symptoms progress.
- Labored breathing with retractions of the chest wall, nasal flaring, and grunting.

aSee Table 44–2 for commonly used antibiotics and doses.
(AECB, acute exacerbation of chronic bronchitis; COPD, chronic obstructive pulmonary disease; CB, chronic bronchitis; TMP/SMX, trimethoprim/sulfamethoxazole.)

FIGURE 44-1. Clinical algorithm for the diagnosis and treatment of chronic bronchitic patients with an acute exacerbation incorporating the principles of the clinical classification system.

PHYSICAL EXAMINATION

- Tachycardia and respiratory rate of 40–80 per minute in hospitalized infants.
- Wheezing and inspiratory rales.
- Mild conjunctivitis in one-third of patients.
- Otitis media in 5%–10% of patients.

LABORATORY TESTS

- Peripheral white blood cell count normal or slightly elevated.
- Abnormal arterial blood gases (hypoxemia and, rarely, hypercarbia).

463

TABLE 44-2 Oral Antibiotics Commonly Used for the Treatment of Acute Respiratory Exacerbations in Chronic Bronchitis

Antibiotic	Brand Name	Usual Adult Oral Dose (mg)	Dose Schedule (Doses/Day)
Preferred drugs			
Ampicillin	–	250–500	3–4
Amoxicillin	–	500–875	2–3
Amoxicillin–clavulanate	Augmentin*	500–875	2–3
Ciprofloxacin	Cipro*	500–750	2
Levofloxacin	Levaquin*	500–750	1
Moxifloxacin	Avelox*	400	1
Doxycycline	Monodox*	100	2
Minocycline	Minocin*	100	2
Tetracycline HCl	–	500	4
Trimethoprim–sulfamethoxazole	Bactrim DS*/ Septra DS*	1 DS	2
Supplemental drugs			
Azithromycin	Zithromax*	250–500	1
Erythromycin	Ery-Tab*/ Erythrocin*	500	4
Clarithromycin	Biaxin*	250–500	2
Cephalexin	Keflex*	500	4

DS, double-strength tablet (160-mg trimethoprim/800-mg sulfamethoxazole).

TREATMENT

- Bronchiolitis is a self-limiting illness and usually requires no therapy (other than reassurance, antipyretics, and adequate fluid intake) unless the infant is hypoxic or dehydrated. Otherwise healthy infants can be treated for fever, provided generous amounts of oral fluids, and observed closely for evidence of respiratory deterioration.
- In severely affected children, the mainstays of therapy for bronchiolitis are oxygen therapy and intravenous (IV) fluids.
- Aerosolized β-adrenergic therapy appears to offer little benefit for the majority of patients but may be useful in the child with a predisposition toward bronchospasm. The routine use of systemically administered corticosteroids is not recommended.
- The American Academy of Pediatrics guidelines support the use of nebulized hypertonic saline (eg, 3% saline) for the treatment of bronchiolitis in hospitalized infants and children.
- The American Academy of Pediatrics does not recommend the routine use of **ribavirin** in children with bronchiolitis and most experts recommend reserving use of ribavirin for severely ill patients. Use of ribavirin requires special equipment (small-particle aerosol generator) and specifically trained personnel for administration via oxygen hood or mist tent.

Pneumonia

- Pneumonia remains one of the most common causes of severe sepsis and infectious cause of death in children and adults in the United States, with a mortality rate as high as 50%. Table 44-3 presents the classification of pneumonia and risk factors.

TABLE 44-3	Pneumonia Classifications and Risk Factors	
Type of Pneumonia	**Definition**	**Risk Factors**
Community-acquired pneumonia (CAP)	Pneumonia developing outside the hospital or <48 hours after hospital admission	• Age >65 years • Diabetes mellitus • Asplenia • Chronic cardiovascular, pulmonary, renal, and/or liver disease • Smoking and/or alcohol abuse
Hospital-acquired pneumonia (HAP)	Pneumonia developing >48 hours after hospital admission	• Witnessed aspiration • COPD, ARDS, or coma • Administration of antacids, H_2-antagonists, or proton pump inhibitor • Supine position • Enteral nutrition, nasogastric tube • Reintubation, tracheostomy, or patient transport • Head trauma, ICP monitoring • Age >60 years • MDR risk (eg, MRSA, MDR *Pseudomonas*) if IV antibiotic use within 90 days
Ventilator-associated pneumonia (VAP)	Pneumonia developing >48 hours after endotracheal intubation	• Same as hospital acquired • MDR risk with IV antibiotics in past 90 days, septic shock, ARDS preceding VAP, acute renal replacement therapy preceding VAP, or 5+ days of hospitalization preceding VAP

ARDS, acute respiratory distress syndrome; CAP, community-acquired pneumonia; COPD, chronic obstructive pulmonary disease; HAP, hospital-acquired pneumonia; ICP, intracranial pressure; MDR, multidrug-resistant; MRSA, methicillin-resistant *S. aureus*; VAP, ventilator-associated pneumonia.

PATHOPHYSIOLOGY

• Respiratory pathogens enter the lower respiratory tract by one of three routes: (1) direct inhalation of infectious droplets; (2) aspiration of oropharyngeal contents; or (3) hematogenous spread from another infection site.

• Pneumonia is caused by a variety of viral and bacterial pathogens.

• Pneumonia is categorized as either community-acquired or hospital-acquired. Pneumonia onset outside of the hospital or within 48 hours of hospital admission have CAP. Pneumonia onset in the hospital after at least 48 hours of hospitalization have hospital-acquired pneumonia (HAP). Pneumonia onset following 48 hours of endotracheal intubation have ventilator-associated pneumonia (VAP).

• The causative pathogen in CAP in adult patients is most commonly viral, with human rhinovirus and influenza most common. The most prominent bacterial pathogen causing CAP in otherwise healthy adults is *S. pneumoniae* accounting for up to 35% (12%–68%) of all acute cases. Other common bacterial causes are *H. influenzae*, the "atypical" pathogens including *M. pneumoniae*, *Legionella* species, *C. pneumoniae*.

• Viral pathogens (RSV and human rhinovirus) predominate in CAP among pediatric patients with a prevalence of up to 80% in those less than 2 years of age.

• HAP is predominantly caused by gram-negative aerobic bacilli and *S. aureus* and is much more likely to be caused by a multidrug-resistant isolate. *P. aeruginosa* and *Acinetobacter* spp. are the most common cause of HAP (about 25%–45%) while *K. pneumoniae* and *E. coli* are also common.

• Aspiration pneumonia has a bacteriology similar to CAP or HAP and anaerobic pathogens are less common and typically seen in patients with specific risk factors such as periodontal disease or alcoholism.

CLINICAL PRESENTATION

GRAM-POSITIVE AND GRAM-NEGATIVE BACTERIAL PNEUMONIA

- Classifications of pneumonia are given in Table 44-3.
- Blood cultures and noninvasive sputum cultures (ie, expectorated sputum, sputum induction, or nasotracheal suctioning) are recommended for all adult patients with suspected HAP or VAP.
- The chest radiograph and sputum examination and culture are the most useful diagnostic tests for gram-positive and gram-negative bacterial pneumonia. Typically, the chest radiograph reveals a dense lobar or lobular consolidated infiltrates.
- Signs and symptoms: Abrupt onset of fever, chills, dyspnea, and productive cough; Rust-colored sputum or hemoptysis; Pleuritic chest pain; and Dyspnea.
- Physical examination findings: Tachypnea and tachycardia; dullness to percussion; increased tactile fremitus, whispered pectoriloquy, and egophony; Chest wall retractions and grunting respirations; Diminished breath sounds over affected area; and Inspiratory crackles during lung expansion.
- Chest radiograph findings: Dense lobar or segmental infiltrate.
- Laboratory tests: Leukocytosis with predominance of polymorphonuclear cells. Low oxygen saturation on arterial blood gas or pulse oximetry.

ATYPICAL PNEUMONIA (*M. PNEUMONIAE* AND *C. PNEUMONIAE*)

- Pneumonia caused by the atypical pathogens, such as *M. pneumoniae* and *C. pneumoniae*, often has a more gradual onset and overall lower severity compared with other bacterial causes. Patients with atypical pneumonia also commonly have extrapulmonary, constitutional symptoms.

HOSPITAL-ACQUIRED PNEUMONIA

- The strongest predisposing factor for HAP is mechanical ventilation. Factors predisposing patients to HAP include severe illness, long duration of hospitalization, supine positioning, witnessed aspiration, coma, acute respiratory distress syndrome, patient transport, and prior antibiotic exposure. HAP is exacerbated by the wide use of acid-reducing drugs (eg, H_2-receptor blocking agents and proton pump inhibitors) which increases the pH of gastric secretions and may promote the proliferation of microorganisms in the upper GI tract.
- The diagnosis of nosocomial pneumonia is usually established by the presence of a new infiltrate on chest radiograph, fever, worsening respiratory status, and the appearance of thick, neutrophil-laden respiratory secretions.

TREATMENT

- <u>Goal of Treatment</u>: Eradication of the offending organism and complete clinical cure. Secondary goals include minimization of the unintended consequences of therapy, including toxicities and selection for secondary infections such a *Clostridioides difficile* or antibiotic-resistant pathogens, and minimizing costs through outpatient and oral therapy when the patient's severity of illness and clinical considerations permit.
- The supportive care of the patient with pneumonia includes the use of humidified oxygen for hypoxemia, fluid resuscitation, administration of bronchodilators (**albuterol**) when bronchospasm is present, and chest physiotherapy with postural drainage if there is evidence of retained secretions.
- Important therapeutic adjuncts include adequate hydration (by IV route if necessary), optimal nutritional support, and fever control.
- Severity scoring systems such as CURB-65 are used to guide treatment. For CURB-65, patients receive 1 point for each criterion present: **C**onfusion, **U**remia (BUN >20 mg/dL [7.1 mmol/L]), **R**espiratory rate ≥30 breaths/min, **B**lood pressure (systolic <90 mm Hg,

diastolic $\leq$60 mm Hg), age $\geq$65 years. Patients with CURB-65 score <2 are generally candidates for outpatient treatment. Patients with a score of 2 are typically admitted to the general ward of the hospital with ICU admission considered for patients with scores $\geq$3.

- The treatment of bacterial pneumonia initially involves the empiric use of a relatively broad-spectrum antibiotic therapy effective against probable pathogens after appropriate cultures and specimens for laboratory evaluation have been obtained. Therapy should be narrowed to cover specific pathogens once the results of cultures are known. The minimum duration of therapy for CAP is 5 days although CAP is commonly treated for 7–10 days.
- Appropriate empiric choices for the treatment of bacterial pneumonias relative to a patient's underlying disease are shown in **Table 44-4** for adults and **Table 44-5** for children. Dosages for antibiotics to treat pneumonia are provided in **Table 44-6**. Pathogen-directed antimicrobial therapy for common pneumonia pathogens in adult patients is given in **Table 44-7**.
- Antibiotic concentrations in respiratory secretions in excess of the pathogen minimum inhibitory concentration (MIC) are necessary for successful treatment of pulmonary infections.

EVALUATION OF THERAPEUTIC OUTCOMES

- For patients with pneumonia of mild-to-moderate clinical severity, the time to resolution of cough, decreasing sputum production, and fever, as well as other constitutional symptoms of malaise, nausea, vomiting, and lethargy, should be noted. Progress should be observed in the first 2 days, with complete resolution in 5–7 days.
- When discontinuing therapy, patients should be afebrile for 48–72 hours and have no more than one CAP-related sign of clinical instability (ie, tachycardia, tachypnea, hypotension, hypoxia, altered mental status).
- With HAP some resolution of symptoms should be observed within 2 days of instituting antibiotic therapy. If no resolution of symptoms is observed within 2 days of starting seemingly appropriate antibiotic therapy or if the patient's clinical status is deteriorating, the appropriateness of initial antibiotic therapy should be critically reassessed. The clinician should consider the possibility of changing the initial antibiotic therapy to expand antimicrobial coverage not included in the original regimen if the patient's clinical status is worsening or failing to improve after 48–72 hours of therapy.

TABLE 44-4	Evidence-Based Empirical Antimicrobial Therapy for Pneumonia in Adults[a]	
Clinical Setting and/or Patient Characteristics	**Usual Pathogens**	**Empirical Therapy**
Outpatient/Community-acquired		
No at-risk comorbidity (diabetes, heart/lung/liver/renal disease, alcoholism, malignancy, asplenia) AND no antimicrobial use in past 3 months	S. pneumoniae, M. pneumoniae, H. influenzae, C. pneumoniae, M. catarrhalis	Macrolide[b] OR doxycycline
At-risk comorbidity (diabetes, heart/lung/liver/renal disease, alcoholism, malignancy, aspelnia) OR immunosuppressive condition/drugs OR antimicrobial use in past 3 months	S. pneumoniae (including drug-resistant), M. pneumoniae, H. influenzae, C. pneumoniae, M. catarrhalis	Antipneumococcal fluoroquinolone[c] OR β-lactam[d] + EITHER macrolide[b] OR doxycycline

(Continued)

TABLE 44-4	Evidence-Based Empirical Antimicrobial Therapy for Pneumonia in Adults[a] (Continued)	
Clinical Setting and/or Patient Characteristics	**Usual Pathogens**	**Empirical Therapy**
Regions with more than 25% rate of macrolide-resistant *S. pneumoniae*	*S. pneumoniae* (including drug-resistant), *M. pneumoniae*, *H. influenzae*, *C. pneumoniae*, *M. catarrhalis*	Antipneumococcal fluoroquinolone[c] OR β-lactam[d] + EITHER macrolide[b] OR doxycycline
Inpatient/Community-acquired		
Non-ICU	*S. pneumoniae* (including drug-resistant), *H. influenzae*, *M. pneumoniae*, *C. pneumoniae*, *Legionella* spp.	Antipneumococcal fluoroquinolone[c] OR β-lactam[e] + EITHER macrolide[b] OR doxycyline
ICU	*S. pneumoniae* (including drug-resistant), *S. aureus, Legionella* spp., gram-negative bacilli, *H. influenzae*	β-lactam[e] + EITHER azithromycin OR Antipneumococcal fluoroquinolone[c]
	If MRSA suspected	Add vancomycin or linezolid to above regimen
	If *P. aeruginosa* suspected	Antipseudomonal, antipneumococcal β-lactam[f] + EITHER (1) ciprofloxacin OR (2) levofloxacin OR (3) aminoglycoside + azithromycin OR (4) aminoglycoside + moxifloxacin
	If influenza suspected	Add oral oseltamivir or intravenous peramivir (when oral medications not possible)
Hospital-acquired pneumonia		
Low mortality risk[g] AND No MDR HAP[h] risk factors AND Local MRSA prevalence <20%	Non-fermenting gram-negative bacilli, enteric gram-negative bacilli, MSSA	Piperacillin–tazobactam, cefepime, levofloxacin, imipenem OR meropenem
Low mortality[g] risk AND No MDR HAP[h] risk factors AND Local MRSA ≥20% OR unknown	Non-fermenting gram-negative bacilli, enteric gram-negative bacilli, MRSA	Piperacillin–tazobactam, cefepime, levofloxacin, ciprofloxacin, imipenem, meropenem, OR aztreonam + vancomycin OR linezolid
High mortality risk[g] OR MDR risk factor(s)[h]	Non-fermenting gram-negative bacilli, enteric gram-negative bacilli, MRSA	Double cover *P. aeruginosa* with two of the following, avoiding two from the same class: piperacillin–tazobactam, cefepime, levofloxacin, ciprofloxacin, imipenem, meropenem, aztreonam, gentamicin, tobramycin, amikacin + vancomycin OR linezolid

(Continued)

TABLE 44-4	Evidence-Based Empirical Antimicrobial Therapy for Pneumonia in Adults[a] (Continued)	
Clinical Setting and/or Patient Characteristics	**Usual Pathogens**	**Empirical Therapy**
Ventilator-associated pneumonia		
No MDR VAP risk factors[i] AND Local MRSA and gram-negative bacilli-resistance both <10%[j]	Non-fermenting gram-negative bacilli, enteric gram-negative bacilli, MSSA	Piperacillin–tazobactam, cefepime, levofloxacin, imipenem OR meropenem
No MDR VAP risk factors[i] AND Local MRSA ≥10% or unknown AND gram-negative bacilli-resistance <10%[j]	Non-fermenting gram-negative bacilli, enteric gram-negative bacilli, MRSA	Piperacillin–tazobactam, cefepime, levofloxacin, ciprofloxacin, imipenem, meropenem, OR aztreonam + vancomycin OR linezolid
MDR VAP risk factor(s)[i] OR local MRSA and gram-negative bacilli-resistance >10%[j] or unknown	MDR non-fermenting gram-negative bacilli, MDR enteric gram-negative bacilli, MRSA	Double cover P. aeruginosa with two of the following, avoiding two from the same class : piperacillin–tazobactam, cefepime, levofloxacin, ciprofloxacin, imipenem, meropenem, aztreonam, gentamicin, tobramycin, amikacin, colistin, polymyxin B + vancomycin OR linezolid
Aspiration pneumonia		
Community-acquired	S. pneumoniae, M. pneumoniae, H. influenzae, C. pneumoniae	Treat as above for CAP
Hospital-acquired	S. aureus, P. aeruginosa enteric gram-negative bacilli	Treat as above for HAP
	If anaerobes suspected	Treat as above for CAP/HAP using antibiotic with anaerobic coverage OR add clindamycin OR metronidazole

[a]See the section Selection of Antimicrobial Agents.
[b]Macrolide: erythromycin, clarithromycin, and azithromycin.
[c]Antipneumococcal fluoroquinolone: levofloxacin and moxifloxacin.
[d]Infectious Diseases Society of America recommended outpatient β-lactams: high-dose amoxicillin or amoxicillin/clavulanate preferred, cefpodoxime, cefuroxime, ceftriaxone (intramuscular) alternatives.
[e]Infectious Diseases Society of America recommended inpatient β-lactams: ceftriaxone (intravenous), cefotaxime, ampicillin.
[f]Infectious Diseases Society of America recommended antipneumococcal, antipseudomonal β-lactams: piperacillin/tazobactam, cefepime, meropenem, imipenem.
[g]Indicators of high HAP mortality risk: need for ventilator support due to pneumonia; septic shock.
[h]MDR HAP risk factors: receipt of IV antibiotics in previous 90 days; structural lung disease (bronchiectasis or cystic fibrosis).
[i]MDR VAP risk factors: receipt of IV antibiotics in previous 90 days; septic shock; acute respiratory distress syndrome preceding VAP; ≥5 days hospitalization preceding VAP; acute renal replacement therapy preceding VAP.
[j]Resistance to antibiotic being considered for empiric gram-negative monotherapy.
MDR, multidrug resistant; MRSA, methicillin-resistant Staphylococcus aureus; MSSA, methicillin-sensitive Staphylococcus aureus.

TABLE 44-5	Empirical Antimicrobial Therapy for Pneumonia in Pediatric Patients[a]	
Clinical Setting and/or Patient Characteristics	**Usual Pathogen(s)**	**Empirical Therapy**
Outpatient/Community-acquired		
<1 month	Group B *Streptococcus, H. influenzae* (nontypeable), *E. coli, S. aureus, Listeria* CMV, RSV, adenovirus	Ampicillin–sulbactam, cephalosporin,[b] carbapenem[c] Ribavirin for RSV[d]
1–3 months	*C. pneumoniae,* possibly *Ureaplasma,* CMV, *Pneumocystis carinii* (afebrile pneumonia syndrome) *S. pneumoniae, S. aureus*	Macrolide/azalide,[e] trimethoprim–sulfamethoxazole Semisynthetic penicillin[f] OR cephalosporin[g]
Preschool-aged children	Viral (rhinovirus, RSV, influenza A and B, parainfluenzae, adenovirus, human metapneumovirus, coronavirus)	Antimicrobial therapy not routinely required
Previously healthy, fully immunized infants and preschool children with suspected mild–moderate bacterial CAP	*S. pneumonia* *M. pneumoniae,* other atypical	Amoxicillin, cephalosporin[b,g] Macrolide/Azalide or fluoroquinolone
Previously healthy, fully immunized school-aged children and adolescents with mild–moderate CAP	*S. pneumonia* *M. pneumoniae,* other atypical	Amoxicillin, cephalosporin,[b,g] or fluoroquinolone Macrolide/Azalide, fluoroquinolone, or tetracycline
Moderate–severe CAP during influenza virus outbreak	Influenza A and B, other viruses	Oseltamivir or zanamivir
Inpatient/Community-acquired		
Fully immunized infants and school-aged children	*S. pneumonia* CA-MRSA *M. pneumoniae, C. pneumoniae*	Ampicillin, penicillin G, cephalosporin[b] β-Lactam + vancomycin/ clindamycin β-Lactam + macrolide/ fluoroquinolone/doxycycline

(Continued)

TABLE 44-5	Empirical Antimicrobial Therapy for Pneumonia in Pediatric Patients[a] (Continued)

Clinical Setting and/or Patient Characteristics	Usual Pathogen(s)	Empirical Therapy
Not fully immunized infants and children; regions with invasive penicillin-resistant pneumococcal strains; patients with life-threatening infections	S. pneumoniae, PCN-resistant MRSA M. pneumoniae, other atypical pathogens	Cephalosporin[b] Add vancomycin/clindamycin Macrolide/azalide[e] + β-lactam/doxycycline/fluoroquinolone

[a]See the section Selection of Antimicrobial Agents.
[b]Third-generation cephalosporin: ceftriaxone and cefotaxime. Note that cephalosporins are not active against *Listeria*.
[c]Carbapenem: imipenem–cilastatin and meropenem.
[d]See text for details regarding possible ribavirin treatment for RSV infection.
[e]Macrolide/Azalide: erythromycin and clarithromycin/azithromycin.
[f]Semisynthetic penicillin: nafcillin and oxacillin.
[g]Second-generation cephalosporin: cefuroxime and cefprozil.
CAP, community-acquired pneumonia; CMV, cytomegalovirus; MRSA, methicillin resistant *Staphylococcus aureus*; RSV, respiratory syncytial virus.

TABLE 44-6	Antibiotic Doses for Treatment of Bacterial Pneumonia

| Antibiotic Class | Antibiotic | Antibiotic Dose[a] | |
		Pediatric	Usual Adult Dose
Penicillin	Ampicillin ± sulbactam	150–200 mg/kg/day IV	2 g IV every 4–6 h (6 h if ampicillin/sulbactam)
	Amoxicillin ± clavulanate[b]	45–100 mg/kg/day orally	875–2000 mg orally twice daily
	Piperacillin–tazobactam	200–300 mg/kg/day IV	3.375–4.5 g IV every 6–8 h
	Penicillin	100,000–250,000 units/kg/day IV	12–24 million units/day in divided doses IV every 4–6 h
Extended-spectrum cephalosporins	Ceftriaxone	50–75 mg/kg/day IV	1–2 g IV daily
	Cefotaxime	150 mg/kg/day IV	1–2 g IV every 8 h
	Ceftazidime	90–150 mg/kg/day IV	1–2 g IV every 8 h
	Cefepime	100–150 mg/kg/day IV	1–2 g IV every 6–8 h
	Ceftolozane–tazobactam	–	3 g IV every 8 h
	Ceftazidime–avibactam	–	2.5 g IV every 8 h
Monobactam	Aztreonam	90–120 mg/kg/day IV	1–2 g IV every 8 h

(Continued)

TABLE 44-6	Antibiotic Doses for Treatment of Bacterial Pneumonia (*Continued*)		
		Antibiotic Dose[a]	
Antibiotic Class	**Antibiotic**	**Pediatric**	**Usual Adult Dose**
Macrolide/Azalide	Clarithromycin	15 orally mg/kg/day	0.5–1 g orally once or twice daily
	Erythromycin	30–50 IV or orally mg/kg/day	500 mg IV or orally every 6–8 h
	Azithromycin	10 mg/kg × 1 day (×2 days if parenteral), and then 5 mg/kg days 2–5 IV or orally	500 mg × 1 day (×2 days if parenteral), and then 250 mg days 2–5 IV or orally
Fluoroquinolones[c]	Moxifloxacin	–	400 mg IV or orally daily
	Levofloxacin	8–20 mg/kg/day IV or orally	750 mg IV or orally daily
	Ciprofloxacin	30 mg/kg/day IV or orally	400 mg IV every 8 h / 750 mg orally twice daily
Tetracycline[d]	Doxycycline	2–5 mg/kg/day IV or orally	100 mg IV or orally twice daily
	Tetracycline HCl	25–50 mg/kg/day orally	–
Aminoglycosides	Gentamicin	7.5–10 mg/kg/day IV	7.5 mg/kg IV daily
	Tobramycin	7.5–10 mg/kg/day IV	7.5 mg/kg IV daily
	Amikacin	15–20 mg/kg/day IV	15–20 mg/kg IV daily
Carbapenems	Imipenem	60–100 mg/kg/day IV	500–1000 mg IV every 6 to 8 h
	Meropenem	30–60 mg/kg/day IV	500–2000 mg IV every 6 to 8 h
	Meropenem–vaborbactam		2 g/2 g IV every 8 h
Polymyxins	Colistin	2.5–5 mg/kg/day IV	IV: 300 mg × 1, then 150 mg daily/Neb: 150 mg every 8 h
	Polymyxin B	15,000–30,000 units/kg/day IV	IV: 2–2.5 mg/kg × 1, then 1.25–1.5 mg/kg every 12 h
Other	Vancomycin	45–60 mg/kg/day IV	15–20 mg/kg IV every 8–12 h
	Linezolid	20–30 mg/kg/day IV or orally	600 mg IV or orally every 12 h
	Clindamycin	30–40 mg/kg/day IV or orally	600 mg IV or orally every 8 h or 450 mg orally every 6 h

[a]Doses can be increased for more severe disease and may require modification for patients with organ dysfunction.

[b]Higher-dose amoxicillin and amoxicillin/clavulanate (eg, 90 mg/kg/day) are used for penicillin-resistant *S. pneumoniae*.

[c]Fluoroquinolones have been avoided for pediatric patients because of the potential for cartilage damage; however, they have been used for MDR bacterial infection safely and effectively in infants and children (see text).

[d]Tetracyclines are rarely used in pediatric patients, particularly in those younger than 8 years because of tetracycline-induced permanent tooth discoloration.

TABLE 44-7	Directed Antimicrobial Therapy for Common Pneumonia Pathogens in Adult Patients	
Pathogen	**Preferred Antibiotic Therapy**	**Alternative Antibiotic Therapy**
Penicillin-susceptible *S. pneumoniae* (MIC ≤2 mg/L)	Ampicillin, amoxicillin, penicillin G	Ceftriaxone, cefotaxime, macrolide, levofloxacin, moxifloxacin, doxycycline, clindamycin, vancomycin
Penicillin-resistant *S. pneumoniae* (MIC >2 mg/L)	Ceftriaxone, cefotaxime, levofloxacin, moxifloxacin	High-dose amoxicillin (3 g/day), linezolid, clindamycin, vancomycin
Non-β-lactamase-producing *H. influenzae*	Ampicillin (IV), amoxicillin	Fluoroquinolone, doxycycline, azithromycin, clarithromycin
β-Lactamase-producing *H. influenzae*	Ceftriaxone, cefotaxime, ampicillin–sulbactam, amoxicillin–clavulanate	Fluoroquinolone, doxycycline, azithromycin, clarithromycin
Mycoplasma pneumoniae	Macrolide, doxycycline	Fluoroquinolone
Chlamydophila pneumoniae	Macrolide, doxycycline	Fluoroquinolone
Legionella pneumophila	Fluoroquinolone or azithromycin	Doxycycline
MSSA	Cefazolin, antistaphylococcal penicillin	Clindamycin, vancomycin
MRSA	Vancomycin, linezolid	Telavancin, ceftaroline, quinupristin/dalfopristin, clindamycin, sulfamethoxazole/trimethoprim
P. aeruginosa	Antipseudomonal β-lactam[a] or fluoroquinolone[b] based on antimicrobial susceptibility testing results. Can consider adding aminoglycoside if patient in septic shock or at high mortality risk	IV colistin or polymyxin B + inhaled colistin for isolates resistant to all preferred therapies
Acinetobacter spp.	Carbapenem OR ampicillin–sulbactam based on antimicrobial susceptibility testing results	IV colistin or polymyxin B + inhaled colistin for isolates resistant to all preferred therapies
Extended-spectrum β-lactamase-producing gram-negative bacilli	Carbapenem	Piperacillin–tazobactam or cefepime potential options depending on susceptibility/adequate dosing

(Continued)

TABLE 44-7	Directed Antimicrobial Therapy for Common Pneumonia Pathogens in Adult Patients (*Continued*)	
Pathogen	**Preferred Antibiotic Therapy**	**Alternative Antibiotic Therapy**
Carbapenem-resistant organisms	New β-lactam/β-lactamase inhibitors[c] based on antimicrobial susceptibility testing OR IV colistin or polymyxin B + inhaled colistin	

[a]Antipseudomonal β-lactam: piperacillin/tazobactam, cefepime, ceftazidime, meropenem, imipenem/cilastatin, doripenem, aztreonam.
[b]Antipseudomonal fluoroquinolone: ciprofloxacin and levofloxacin
[c]New β-lactam/ β-lactamase inhibitors: ceftazidime/avibactam, meropenem/vaborbactam, ceftolozane/tazobactam.
MIC, minimum inhibitory concentration; MRSA, methicillin-resistant *Staphylococcus aureus*; MSSA, methicillin-sensitive *Staphylococcus aureus*; PCN, penicillin.

- De-escalation of antibiotic therapy to be more narrow spectrum in patients with HAP/VAP is strongly recommended. Evidence suggests this approach does not affect clinical outcomes while reducing excess antibiotic use. The recommended duration of therapy for HAP/VAP is 7 days, as the clinical benefit of longer durations of therapy (≥10 days) is not clear based on available clinical evidence.

See Chapter 125, Lower Respiratory Tract Infections, authored by Evan J. Zasowski and Martha G. Blackford, for a more detailed discussion of this topic.

Acute Otitis Media

- *Otitis media* is an inflammation of the middle ear that is most common in infants and children. There are three subtypes of otitis media: acute otitis media, otitis media with effusion, and chronic otitis media. The three are differentiated by (a) acute signs of infection, (b) evidence of middle ear inflammation, and (c) presence of fluid in the middle ear.

PATHOPHYSIOLOGY

- Bacteria have been found in more than 90% of cases of otitis media. Common bacterial pathogens include *Streptococcus pneumoniae*, nontypeable *Haemophilus influenzae*, and *Moraxella catarrhalis*.
- Acute otitis media usually follows a viral upper respiratory tract infection that impairs the mucociliary apparatus and causes eustachian tube dysfunction in the middle ear.
- Many *S. pneumoniae* isolates in the United States are penicillin nonsusceptible, and most nonsusceptible strains have high-level penicillin resistance.
- Many *H. influenzae* isolates and nearly all *M. catarrhalis* isolates, from the upper respiratory tract, produce β-lactamases.

CLINICAL PRESENTATION

- Acute otitis media is characterized as acute onset of otalgia (ear pain). Irritability and tugging on the ear are often the first clues that a child has acute otitis media.
- Children should be diagnosed with acute otitis media if they have middle ear effusion and either (1) moderate-to-severe bulging of the tympanic membrane or new onset otorrhea not due to acute otitis externa or (2) mild bulging of the tympanic membrane and onset of ear pain within the last 48 hours or intense erythema of the tympanic membrane.
- Nonverbal children with ear pain might hold, rub, or tug their ear. Very young children might cry, be irritable, and have difficulty sleeping. Signs and symptoms include bulging of the tympanic membrane, otorrhea, otalgia (considered to be moderate or severe if pain lasts at least 48 hours), and fever (considered to be severe if temperature is 39°C [102.2°F] or higher).

TREATMENT

- <u>Goals of Treatment:</u> Pain management, prudent antibiotic use, and secondary disease prevention. Acute otitis media should first be differentiated from otitis media with effusion or chronic otitis media.
- Primary prevention of acute otitis media with pneumococcal conjugate vaccine and annual influenza vaccine are recommended for all children.
- Pain of otitis media should be addressed with oral analgesics. **Acetaminophen** or a nonsteroidal anti-inflammatory agent, such as **ibuprofen**, should be offered early to relieve pain of acute otitis media.
- Children 6 months–12 years of age, with moderate-to-severe ear pain or temperature of 39°C (102.2°F) or higher should receive antibiotics. Children 6–23 months of age, with nonsevere bilateral acute otitis media should also receive antibiotics. Children 6–23 months, with nonsevere unilateral acute otitis media, and children 24 months–12 years of age, with nonsevere acute otitis media, may receive initial antibiotics or initial observation without antibiotics.
- The central principle is to administer antibiotics quickly when the diagnosis is certain, but to withhold antibiotics, at least initially, when the diagnosis is uncertain.

- High-dose **amoxicillin** (80–90 mg/kg/day) is recommended for most children. Children who have received amoxicillin in the last 30 days, have concurrent purulent conjunctivitis, or have a history of recurrent infection unresponsive to amoxicillin should receive high-dose **amoxicillin–clavulanate** (90 mg/kg/day of amoxicillin, with 6.4 mg/kg/day of clavulanate, in two divided doses) instead of amoxicillin.
- Antibiotic treatment recommendations for acute otitis media are given in Table 45-1.
- If treatment failure occurs with amoxicillin, an agent should be chosen with activity against β-lactamase-producing *H. influenzae* and *M. catarrhalis*, as well as drug-resistant *S. pneumoniae*, such as high-dose amoxicillin–clavulanate (recommended) or **cefuroxime, cefdinir, cefpodoxime**, or intramuscular or intravenous **ceftriaxone**.
- Traditional recommendations call for 10 days of antibiotic therapy. In children at least 6 years old who have mild-to-moderate acute otitis media, a 5- to 7-day course

TABLE 45-1 Antibiotics and Doses for Acute Otitis Media

Antibiotic	Brand Name	Dose	Comments[a]
Initial diagnosis			
Amoxicillin	Amoxil®	80–90 mg/kg/day orally divided twice daily	First line
Amoxicillin–clavulanate	Augmentin®	90 mg/kg/day orally of amoxicillin plus 6.4 mg/kg/day orally of clavulanate, divided twice daily	First line if certain criteria are present[b]
Cefdinir, cefuroxime, cefpodoxime	Omnicef®, Ceftin®, Vantin®	Cefdinir (14 mg/kg/day orally in 1–2 doses), cefuroxime (30 mg/kg/day orally in two divided doses), cefpodoxime (10 mg/kg/day orally in two divided doses)	Second line or nonsevere penicillin allergy
Ceftriaxone (1–3 days)	Rocephin®	50 mg/kg/day IM or IV for 3 days	Second line or nonsevere penicillin allergy
Failure at 48–72 hours			
Amoxicillin–clavulanate[b]	Augmentin®	90 mg/kg/day orally of amoxicillin plus 6.4 mg/kg/day orally of clavulanate, divided twice daily	First line
Ceftriaxone (1–3 days)	Rocephin®	50 mg/kg/day IM or IV for 3 days	First line or nonsevere penicillin allergy
Clindamycin	Cleocin®	30–40 mg/kg/day orally in three divided doses ± second- or third-generation cephalosporin	Second line or nonsevere penicillin allergy

[a]Amoxicillin–clavulanate 90:6.4 or 14:1 ratio is available in the United States; 7:1 ratio is available in Canada (use amoxicillin 45 mg/kg for one dose, amoxicillin 45 mg/kg with clavulanate 6.4 mg/kg for second dose).
[b]If a patient has received amoxicillin in the last 30 days, has concurrent purulent conjunctivitis, or has a history of recurrent infection unresponsive to amoxicillin.
IM, intramuscular; IV, intravenous; po, orally.

of antibiotics may be used. Short-course treatment is not recommended in children younger than 2 years of age.

- Surgical insertion of tympanostomy tubes (T tubes) is an effective method for preventing recurrent otitis media. Patients with acute otitis media should be reassessed after 48–72 hours, with most children being asymptomatic at 7 days.

Pharyngitis

- *Pharyngitis* is an acute infection of the oropharynx or nasopharynx that is responsible for 6% of visits by children to their primary care provider annually. Although viral causes are most common, group A β-hemolytic *Streptococcus* (GABHS) is the primary bacterial cause.
- Viruses (eg, rhinovirus, coronavirus, and adenovirus) cause most of the cases of acute pharyngitis. A bacterial etiology for acute pharyngitis is far less likely. Of all of the bacterial causes, GABHS is the most common (10%–30% of cases in pediatric patients and 5%–15% in adults).
- Suppurative and nonsuppurative complications include acute rheumatic fever, acute glomerulonephritis, reactive arthritis, peritonsillar abscess, retropharyngeal abscess, cervical lymphadenitis, mastoiditis, otitis media, rhinosinusitis, and necrotizing fasciitis.

CLINICAL PRESENTATION

- The most common symptom of pharyngitis is sore throat of sudden onset that is mostly self-limited.
- Fever and constitutional symptoms resolve in about 3–5 days.
- Signs and symptoms of GABHS pharyngitis include sore throat; pain on swallowing; fever; headache; nausea; vomiting; and abdominal pain (especially in children); erythema/inflammation of the tonsils and pharynx with or without patchy exudates; enlarged; tender lymph nodes; red swollen uvula; petechiae on the soft palate; and a scarlatiniform rash.
- Signs suggestive of viral origin for pharyngitis include conjunctivitis, coryza, and cough.
- Diagnosis can be confirmed by throat swab and culture and a rapid antigen-detection test (RADT).

TREATMENT

- <u>Goals of Treatment</u>: Improve clinical signs and symptoms, minimize adverse drug reactions, prevent transmission to close contacts, and prevent acute rheumatic fever and suppurative complications such as peritonsillar abscess, cervical lymphadenitis, and mastoiditis.
- Antimicrobial therapy should be limited to those who have clinical and epidemiologic features of GABHS pharyngitis, preferably with a positive laboratory test.
- Because pain is often the primary reason for visiting a physician, emphasis on analgesics such as **acetaminophen** and nonsteroidal anti-inflammatory drugs (NSAIDs) to aid in pain relief is strongly recommended.
- **Penicillin** and **amoxicillin** are the treatments of choice. Antimicrobial treatment should be limited to those who have clinical and epidemiologic features of GABHS pharyngitis with a positive laboratory test (Table 45-2). Table 45-3 presents antibiotics and doses for eradication of GABHS in chronic carriers. The duration of therapy for GABHS pharyngitis is 10 days, except for **benzathine penicillin** and **azithromycin**, to maximize bacterial eradication. However, 3–6 days of oral antibiotics has comparable efficacy to oral **penicillin** for 10 days.
- **Amoxicillin–clavulanate, clindamycin, penicillin/rifampin** combination, and **benzathine penicillin G/rifampin** combination may be considered for recurrent

episodes of pharyngitis to maximize bacterial eradication in potential carriers and to counter copathogens that produce β-lactamases.

• Most cases of pharyngitis are self-limited; however, antimicrobial therapy will hasten resolution when given early to proven cases of GABHS. Symptoms generally resolve by 3 or 4 days even without antibiotics; however, symptoms will improve 0.5–2.5 days earlier with antibiotic therapy. Follow-up testing is generally not necessary for index cases or in asymptomatic contacts of the index patient; however, throat cultures 2–7 days after completion of antibiotics are warranted for patients who remain symptomatic or when symptoms recur despite completion of treatment.

TABLE 45-2	Antibiotics and Doses for Group A β-Hemolytic Streptococcal Pharyngitis			
Antibiotic	Brand Name	Dose	Duration	Rating
Preferred antibiotics if no penicillin allergy				
Penicillin V	Pen-V	Children: 250 mg twice daily or three times daily orally; adult: 250 mg four times daily or 500 mg twice daily orally	10 days	IB
Penicillin G benzathine	Bicillin L-A	<27 kg: 0.6 million units; 27 kg or greater: 1.2 million units intramuscularly	One dose	IB
Amoxicillin[a]	Amoxil	50 mg/kg once daily (maximum 1000 mg); 25 mg/kg (maximum 500 mg) twice daily	10 days	IB
Penicillin allergy				
Cephalexin	Keflex	20 mg/kg/dose orally twice daily (maximum 500 mg/dose)	10 days	IB
Cefadroxil	Duricef	30 mg/kg orally once daily (maximum 1 g)	10 days	IB
Clindamycin	Cleocin	7 mg/kg/dose orally thrice daily (maximum 300 mg/dose)	10 days	IIaB
Azithromycin[b]	Zithromax	12 mg/kg orally once daily (maximum 500 mg) for 1 day, then 6 mg/kg orally once daily (maximum 250 mg) for 4 days	5 days	IIaB
Clarithromycin[b]	Biaxin	15 mg/kg orally per day divided in two doses (maximum 250 mg twice daily)	10 days	IIaB

[a]Standard formulation, not extended release.
[b]Resistance of group A β-hemolytic *Streptococcus* (GABHS) to these agents may vary and local susceptibilities should be considered with these agents.

These guidelines provide a systematic weighting of the strength of the recommendation (Class I, conditions for which there is evidence and/or general agreement that a given procedure or treatment is beneficial, useful, and effective; Class II, conditions for which there is conflicting evidence and/or a divergence of opinion about the usefulness/efficacy of a procedure or treatment; Class IIa, weight of evidence/opinion is in favor of usefulness/efficacy; Class IIb, usefulness/efficacy is less well established by evidence/opinion; Class III, conditions for which there is evidence and/or general agreement that a procedure/treatment is not useful/effective and in some cases may be harmful) and quality of evidence (A, data derived from multiple randomized clinical trials or meta-analyses; B, data derived from a single-randomized trial or nonrandomized studies; C, only consensus opinion of experts, case studies, or standard of care).

TABLE 45-3	Antibiotics and Doses for Eradication of Group A β-Hemolytic Streptococcal Pharyngitis in Chronic Carriers	
Antibiotic	**Brand Name**	**Dose**
Clindamycin	Cleocin	20–30 mg/kg/day orally in three divided doses (maximum 300 mg/dose)
Amoxicillin–clavulanate	Augmentin	40 mg/kg/day orally in three divided doses (maximum 2000 mg/day of amoxicillin)
Penicillin V and rifampin	Pen-V, Rifadin	Penicillin V: 50 mg/kg/day orally in four doses for 10 days (maximum 2000 mg/day); *and* rifampin: 20 mg/kg/day orally in one dose for the last 4 days of treatment (maximum 600 mg/day)
Penicillin G benzathine and rifampin	Bicillin L-A, Rifadin	Penicillin G benzathine: <27 kg—0.6 million units; 27 kg or greater: 1.2 million units intramuscularly; *and* rifampin: 20 mg/kg/day orally in two doses during last 4 days of treatment with penicillin (maximum 600 mg/day)

Acute Bacterial Rhinosinusitis

- *Sinusitis* is an inflammation and/or infection of the paranasal sinuses, or membrane-lined air spaces, around the nose. The term *rhinosinusitis* is now preferred, because sinusitis typically also involves the nasal mucosa. The majority of these infections are viral in origin. It is important to differentiate between viral and bacterial sinusitis to aid in optimizing treatment decisions.
- Acute bacterial sinusitis is most often caused by the same bacteria implicated in acute otitis media: *S. pneumoniae* and *H. influenzae.* These organisms are responsible for ~50%–70% of bacterial causes of acute sinusitis in both adults and children.

CLINICAL PRESENTATION

- There are three clinical presentations that are most consistent with acute bacterial vs viral rhinosinusitis: 1) Onset with *persistent* signs or symptoms compatible with acute rhinosinusitis, lasting for ≥10 days without any evidence of clinical improvement; 2) Onset with severe signs or symptoms of high fever (≥39°C [102.2°F]) and purulent nasal discharge or facial pain lasting for at least 3–4 consecutive days at the beginning of illness; 3) Onset with *worsening* signs or symptoms characterized by new-onset fever, headache, or increase in nasal discharge following a typical viral URI that lasted 5–6 days and were initially improving ("double sickening").
- Signs and symptoms of bacterial rhinosinusitis include purulent anterior nasal discharge, purulent or discolored posterior nasal discharge, nasal congestion or obstruction, facial congestion or fullness, facial pain or pressure, fever, headache, ear pain/pressure/fullness, halitosis, dental pain, cough, and fatigue.

TREATMENT

- <u>Goals of Treatment</u>: Reducing signs and symptoms, achieving and maintaining patency of the ostia, limiting antimicrobial treatment to those who may benefit, eradicating bacterial infection with appropriate antimicrobial therapy, minimizing the duration of illness, preventing complications, and preventing progression from acute disease to chronic disease.

TABLE 45-4	Antibiotics and Doses for Acute Bacterial Rhinosinusitis in Children		
Antibiotic	**Brand Name**	**Dose**	**Comments**
Initial empirical therapy			
Amoxicillin–clavulanate	Augmentin	45 mg/kg/day orally twice daily	First line
Amoxicillin–clavulanate	Augmentin	90 mg/kg/day orally twice daily	Second line
β-Lactam allergy			
Clindamycin plus cefixime or cefpodoxime	Cleocin Suprax, Vantin	Clindamycin (30–40 mg/kg/day orally three times daily) plus cefixime (8 mg/kg/day orally twice daily) or cefpodoxime (10 mg/kg/day orally twice daily)	Non-type 1 allergy
Levofloxacin	Levaquin	10–20 mg/kg/day orally every 12–24 hours	Type 1 allergy
Risk for antibiotic resistance or failed initial therapy			
Amoxicillin–clavulanate	Augmentin	90 mg/kg/day orally twice daily	
Clindamycin plus cefixime or cefpodoxime	Cleocin, Suprax, Vantin	Clindamycin (30–40 mg/kg/day orally three times daily) plus cefixime (8 mg/kg/day orally twice daily) or cefpodoxime (10 mg/kg/day orally twice daily)	
Levofloxacin	Levaquin	10–20 mg/kg/day orally every 12–24 hours	
Severe infection requiring hospitalization			
Ampicillin–sulbactam	Unasyn	200–400 mg/kg/day IV every 6 hours	
Ceftriaxone	Rocephin	50 mg/kg/day IV every 12 hours	
Cefotaxime	Claforan	100–200 mg/kg/day IV every 6 hours	
Levofloxacin	Levaquin	10–20 mg/kg/day IV every 12–24 hours	

- Nasal decongestant sprays such as **phenylephrine** and **oxymetazoline** that reduce inflammation by vasoconstriction are often used in nonbacterial rhinosinusitis. Use should be limited to the recommended duration of the product (no more than 3 days) to prevent development of tolerance and/or rebound congestion. Oral decongestants may also aid in nasal or sinus patency. Irrigation of the nasal cavity with saline and steam inhalation may be used to increase mucosal moisture, and mucolytics (eg, guaifenesin) may be used to decrease the viscosity of nasal secretions. Antihistamines and oral decongestants should not be used for acute bacterial sinusitis in view of their anticholinergic effects that can dry mucosa and disturb clearance of mucosal secretions.
- **Amoxicillin–clavulanate** is first-line treatment for acute bacterial rhinosinusitis. The approach to treating acute bacterial rhinosinusitis in children and adults is given in **Tables 45-4** and **45-5**.
- High-dose amoxicillin–clavulanate is preferred in the following situations: (a) geographic regions with high endemic rates (10% or greater) of invasive penicillin-nonsusceptible *S. pneumoniae*, (b) severe infection, (c) attendance at daycare, (d) age

TABLE 45-5	Antibiotics and Doses for Acute Bacterial Rhinosinusitis in Adults		
Antibiotic	**Brand Name**	**Dose**	**Comments**
Initial empirical therapy			
Amoxicillin–clavulanate	Augmentin®	500 mg/125 mg orally three times daily, or 875 mg/125 mg orally twice daily	First line
Amoxicillin–clavulanate	Augmentin®	2000 mg/125 mg orally twice daily	Second line
Doxycycline		100 mg orally twice daily or 200 mg orally once daily	Second line
β-Lactam allergy			
Doxycycline		100 mg orally twice daily or 200 mg orally once daily	
Levofloxacin	Levaquin®	500 mg orally once daily	
Moxifloxacin	Avelox®	400 mg orally once daily	
Risk for antibiotic resistance or failed initial therapy			
Amoxicillin–clavulanate	Augmentin®	2000 mg/125 mg orally twice daily	
Levofloxacin	Levaquin®	500 mg orally once daily	
Moxifloxacin	Avelox®	400 mg orally once daily	
Severe infection requiring hospitalization			
Ampicillin–sulbactam	Unasyn®	1.5–3 g IV every 6 hours	
Levofloxacin	Levaquin®	500 mg orally once daily	
Moxifloxacin	Avelox®	400 mg orally once daily	
Ceftriaxone	Rocephin®	1–2 g IV every 12–24 hours	
Cefotaxime	Claforan®	2 g IV every 4–6 hours	

less than 2 or greater than 65 years, (e) recent hospitalization, (f) antibiotic use within the last month, and (g) immunocompromised persons. Doxycycline is also second line for adults but should be avoided in children.
- The duration of antimicrobial therapy for acute bacterial rhinosinusitis is not well established. Most trials have used 10- to 14-day antibiotic courses for uncomplicated rhinosinusitis. For adults, the recommended duration is 5–7 days.
- If symptoms persist or worsen after 48–72 hours of appropriate antibiotic therapy, then the patient should be reevaluated and alternative antibiotics should be considered.

See Chapter 126, Upper Respiratory Tract Infections, authored by Christopher Frei and Bradi Frei, for a more detailed discussion of this topic.

- The older and more recent definitions of terms related to *sepsis* are given in **Table 46-1**. Sepsis-3 redefined sepsis by combining sepsis and severe sepsis from the Sepsis-2 guideline.

ETIOLOGY AND PATHOPHYSIOLOGY

- Patients at risk for infection who are predisposed to sepsis include advanced or very young age; preexisting conditions including heart failure, diabetes, chronic obstructive pulmonary disease, cirrhosis, alcohol dependence, and end-stage renal disease; and other immunosuppressive diseases such as neoplasm and human immunodeficiency virus (HIV) disease.
- The most common anatomic source of infection that leads to sepsis is the lung (40%–42%), followed by intra-abdominal space (31%–34%) and genitourinary tract (11%–15%). The microorganisms isolated from blood cultures of patients with sepsis or septic shock include gram-negative organisms in 44%–59% of patients, gram-positive bacteria in 37%–52%, anaerobic organisms in 5%, and fungi in 4%–10%.
- *Escherichia coli* is by far the most commonly isolated gram-negative microorganism in sepsis (55%–60%), followed by *Klebsiella* species, *Proteus* species, *Enterobacter* species, and *Pseudomonas aeruginosa*. Mortality increases significantly with increasing severity of sepsis (3.5% for sepsis, 9.9% in severe sepsis, and 29% in septic shock), especially in presence of *P. aeruginosa*. The most common gram-positive organisms are *Staphylococcus aureus*, followed by coagulase-negative *Staphylococci*, *Enterococcus* species, and *Streptococcus pneumoniae*.
- *Candida* species (particularly *Candida albicans*) are common fungal etiologic agents of bloodstream infections. The 30-day mortality rate for sepsis due to candidemia is 54%.
- The pathophysiologic focus of gram-negative sepsis has been on the lipopolysaccharide (endotoxin) component of the gram-negative cell wall membrane. Lipid A is

TABLE 46-1	Comparison of Definitions from Sepsis-2 and Sepsis-3 Guidelines
Sepsis-2 Guideline (2012)	**Sepsis-3 Guideline (2016)**
Systemic inflammatory response syndrome (SIRS) to infectious or noninfectious insults: Two or more of the following: • Temperature >38°C or <36°C • Heart rate >90 beats/minute • Respiratory rate >20 breaths/minute • WBC >12,000/mm³ (12 × 10⁹/L) or <4000 cells/mm³ (4 × 10⁹/L) or >10% (0.10) immature bands	**Sepsis:** Life-threatening organ dysfunction caused by a dysregulated host response to infection • Acute change in total SOFA score ≥2 points **Septic shock:** Sepsis + persistent hypotension requiring vasopressor use and serum lactate >2 mmol/L despite adequate fluid resuscitation
Sepsis: SIRS + probable or documented infection	
Severe sepsis: Sepsis + one or more organ dysfunction or hypoperfusion	
Septic shock: Sepsis + refractory hypotension despite fluid resuscitation (30 mL/kg) or serum lactate >1 mmol/L	

SOFA, sequential organ failure assessment; WBC, white blood cell.

a part of the endotoxin molecule from the gram-negative bacterial cell wall that is highly immunoreactive and is responsible for most of the toxic effects. In gram-positive sepsis, the exotoxin peptidoglycan on the cell wall surface appears to exhibit proinflammatory activity.

- Sepsis involves a complex interaction of proinflammatory (eg, tumor necrosis factor-α [TNF-α]; interleukin [IL]-1, IL-6, IL-12) and anti-inflammatory mediators (eg, IL-1 receptor antagonist, IL-4, and IL-10).

- TNF-α concentrations are elevated early in the inflammatory response during sepsis. TNF-α also stimulates release of cyclooxygenase-derived arachidonic acid metabolites (thromboxane A2 and prostaglandins) that contribute to vascular endothelial damage.

- A primary mechanism of injury with sepsis is through endothelial cells. With inflammation, endothelial cells allow circulating cells (eg, granulocytes) and plasma constituents to enter inflamed tissues, which may result in organ damage.

- A key endogenous substance involved in inflammation of sepsis is activated protein C, which enhances fibrinolysis and inhibits inflammation. Levels of protein C are reduced in patients with sepsis.

- Shock is the most ominous complication associated with gram-negative sepsis and causes death in about one-half of patients. Another complication is disseminated intravascular coagulation (DIC). Simultaneous widespread microvascular thrombosis and profuse bleeding from various sites characterize DIC. DIC can produce acute renal failure, hemorrhagic necrosis of the gastrointestinal (GI) mucosa, liver failure, acute pancreatitis, acute respiratory distress syndrome (ARDS), and pulmonary failure.

- ARDS and acute kidney injury are other common complications of sepsis. ARDS can result in loss of functional alveolar volume, impaired pulmonary compliance, and profound hypoxemia.

- The hallmark of the hemodynamic effect of sepsis is the hyperdynamic state characterized by low systemic vascular resistance (SVR) and high cardiac output with tachycardia and arterial hypotension.

CLINICAL PRESENTATION

- The clinical presentation of sepsis varies significantly depending on the site of the infection (ie, pulmonary versus urinary tract), host response to the infection based on the patient's underlying health status and risk factors, and organ dysfunction. The initial presentations may include general malaise or myalgia and nonspecific signs such as fever (or hypothermia), chills, tachycardia, tachypnea, or change in mental status.

- Progression of uncontrolled sepsis leads to evidence of organ dysfunction, which may include oliguria, hemodynamic instability with hypotension or shock, lactic acidosis, hyperglycemia or hypoglycemia, possibly leukopenia, DIC, thrombocytopenia, ARDS, GI hemorrhage, or coma.

- Sepsis-3 redefined sepsis to "life-threatening organ dysfunction caused by a dysregulated host response to infection." Early recognition using a formal screening tool is critical, such as the SOFA scoring system. SOFA encompasses various organ systems such as pulmonary, hepatic, cardiovascular, renal, and neurological and gives a score ranging from 0 to 4 for each system. A SOFA score of 2 or more is associated with an increased risk of mortality by 10% in hospitalized patients with presumed infection.

TREATMENT

- <u>Goals of Treatment</u>: The primary goals include: timely diagnosis and identification of the pathogen, prompt hemodynamic support, rapid identification of the pathogen and source control either medically and/or surgically, early initiation of appropriate broad-spectrum antimicrobial therapy, and avoidance complications such as organ failure and septic shock.

- Evidence-based treatment recommendations for sepsis and septic shock from the *Surviving Sepsis* campaign are presented in **Table 46-2**.

TABLE 46-2 Evidence-Based Treatment Recommendations and Best Practice Statements

Recommendations	Recommendation Grades
Fluid therapy	
Initial resuscitation from sepsis-associated hypotension with at least 30 mL/kg of IV crystalloid fluid within 1 hour	Strong recommendation, low evidence
Either balanced crystalloids or saline for additional fluids guided by frequent assessment of dynamic variables	Weak recommendation, low evidence
Antimicrobial therapy	
IV broad-spectrum antibiotic within 1 hour of diagnosis of sepsis and septic shock against likely bacterial/fungal pathogens	Strong recommendation, moderate evidence
Reassess antibiotic therapy daily with microbiology and clinical data to narrow coverage (de-escalation)	BPS
Optimize dosing strategies based on pharmacokinetics/pharmacodynamics parameters in patients with sepsis or septic shock	BPS
Empiric combination therapy for patients with multidrug-resistant bacterial pathogens such as *Acinetobacter* and *Pseudomonas* species or septic shock	Weak recommendation, low evidence
Treatment duration of 7–10 days for most serious infections	Weak recommendation, low evidence
Vasopressors	
Initiate vasopressor therapy to maintain MAP ≥65 mm Hg	Strong recommendation, moderate evidence
Norepinephrine as the first-choice vasopressor	Strong recommendation, moderate evidence
Add vasopressin or epinephrine to norepinephrine to maintain adequate blood pressure	Weak recommendation, moderate evidence
Add vasopressin to norepinephrine to decrease norepinephrine dosage	Weak recommendation, moderate evidence
Corticosteroids	
Hydrocortisone 200 mg IV per day for septic shock only when hemodynamically unstable after adequate fluid resuscitation and vasopressors	Weak recommendation, low evidence
Hydrocortisone should be tapered when vasopressors are no longer required	Weak recommendation, low evidence
Glucose control	
Use insulin dosing protocol when two consecutive blood glucose levels are >180 mg/dL (10 mmol/L), targeting an upper blood glucose <180 mg/dL (10 mmol/L)	Strong recommendation, high-level evidence

(Continued)

TABLE 46-2	Evidence-Based Treatment Recommendations and Best Practice Statements (*Continued*)
Recommendations	**Recommendation Grades**
Monitor blood glucose every 1–2 hours until insulin infusion rates are stable, then every 4 hours thereafter	BPS
Venous thomboembolism prophylaxis	
Use daily low-molecular-weight heparin (LMWH) over unfractionated heparin	Strong recommendation, moderate evidence
Combination of LMWH and intermittent pneumatic compression, whenever possible	Weak recommendation, low evidence
If creatinine clearance is <30 mL/min (0.5 mL/ sec), use unfractionated heparin or dalteparin	Weak recommendation, low evidence
Stress ulcer prophylaxis	
Stress ulcer prophylaxis should be given to patients who have bleeding risk factors	Strong recommendation, low evidence
Either proton pump inhibitors or H2 receptor blockers	Weak recommendation, low evidence

BPS, best practice statement; MAP, mean arterial pressure.

ANTIMICROBIAL THERAPY

- Once the source of infection is identified, prompt efforts to eradicate that source should be made as progression of sepsis can occur despite rapid initial resuscitation including fluid and appropriate antimicrobials in the absence of adequate source control.
- The Sepsis-3 guidelines recommend administration of empiric broad-spectrum therapy with one or more IV antimicrobials within 1 hour of recognition of sepsis or septic shock to treat most likely pathogens. Rapid identification of candidemia is critical in prompt initiation of appropriate therapy.
- The regimen selected should be based on the type or anatomic site of infection, the most likely pathogens, acquisition of the organism from the community or healthcare institution, and the usual antibiotic susceptibility and resistance profile of the prevalent pathogens at the institution.
- The antibiotics that may be used for empiric treatment of sepsis based on site of infection are listed in Table 46-3.
- Patients with nosocomial infections are at risk for sepsis with MRSA, and an anti-MRSA agent such as **vancomycin** should be initiated empirically in most cases.
- If *P. aeruginosa* is suspected, or with sepsis from hospital-acquired infections, an antipseudomonal cephalosporin (**ceftazidime** or **cefepime**), antipseudomonal fluoroquinolone (**ciprofloxacin** or **levofloxacin**), or an aminoglycoside should be included in the regimen.
- When *S. aureus* is likely to be methicillin-resistant, **linezolid** may be preferred to vancomycin because of the poor penetration of vancomycin into the lungs, as well as the worldwide emergence of glycopeptide intermediately resistant *S. aureus.*
- The average duration of antimicrobial therapy in a patient with sepsis is 7–10 days in the absence of source control issues, and fungal infections can require 10–14 days. The Surgical Infection Society recommends no more than 4 full days of antimicrobial therapy for patients with adequate source control and no more than 5–7 days in patients in whom a definitive source control was not performed.

TABLE 46-3	Empiric Antimicrobial Regimens in Sepsis		
	Antimicrobial Regimen		
Infection (Site or Type)	**Community-Acquired**	**Hospital-Acquired**	
Urinary tract	Ceftriaxone or ciprofloxacin/ levofloxacin	Ceftriaxone/ceftazidime or ciprofloxacin/levofloxacin	
Respiratory tract	Levofloxacin[a]/ moxifloxacin or ceftriaxone + clarithromycin/ azithromycin	Piperacillin/tazobactam or ceftazidime or cefepime or carbapenem[b] + levofloxacin/ciprofloxacin or aminoglycoside	±Vancomycin or linezolid
Intra-abdominal	Ertapenem or ciprofloxacin/ levofloxacin + metronidazole or ceftriaxone + metronidazole	Carbapenem[b] or piperacillin/ tazobactam or ceftazidime/cefepime + metronidazole	
Skin/Soft tissue	Vancomycin or linezolid or daptomycin	Vancomycin + piperacillin/ tazobactam	
Catheter-related		Vancomycin	
Unknown	Piperacillin/ Tazobactam or carbapenem[b]	Carbapenem[b]	

[a]750 mg once daily.
[b]Imipenem, meropenem, and doripenem.

- Empiric treatment of invasive candidiasis based on clinical assessment of risk factors, surrogate markers such as beta-D-glucan for invasive candidiasis, or culture includes echinocandins, triazoles, or a formulation of **amphotericin B.** The choice depends on the clinical status of the patient, the local susceptibility of the most prevalent *Candida* species, recent exposure to antifungal agents, relative drug toxicity, and the presence of organ dysfunction or shock that would affect drug clearance. Preferred empiric therapy for suspected invasive candidiasis in non-neutropenic patients in the ICU is an echinocandin (**anidulafungin, micafungin, or caspofungin**).
- Triazoles (**fluconazole, voriconazole**) are recommended in hemodynamically stable patients who have not had previous triazole exposure and not known to be colonized with azole-resistant *Candida* species.
- Broad-spectrum-antibiotics should be initiated empirically due to the serious nature of the disease, but the antimicrobial regimen should be reassessed daily based on the microbiological and clinical data.

FLUID AND HEMODYNAMIC SUPPORT

- Early effective fluid resuscitation is crucial for preventing further sepsis-induced tissue hypoperfusion or septic shock. The Sepsis-3 guidelines recommend treating and resuscitating from sepsis-induced hypoperfusion immediately with at least 30 mL/kg of IV crystalloid fluid given judiciously within the first 3 hours. Target MAP is 65 mm Hg (8.6 kPa) to assess the need for vasopressors. Lactate should be normalized in patients with elevated lactate levels as a marker of tissue hypoperfusion.

- Fluid therapy guided by dynamic assessment of fluid responsiveness by examining cardiac output was associated with decreased mortality compared to standard care.
- The Sepsis-3 guidelines recommend a crystalloid product (balanced solution such as lactated Ringers and Plasma-Lyte or normal saline) based on accessibility and cost. Colloid (ie, albumin) can be used in patients who have already received considerable amount of crystalloids and continue to require fluid.
- Hetastarch products should be avoided at all times because they increased the risk of renal failure, need for renal replacement therapy, and death in multiple studies.
- Fluid therapy is based on the four phases of septic shock: ROSE—resuscitation, optimization, stabilization, and evacuation. **R**esuscitation phase occurs within minutes, and the patient will most likely have a positive fluid balance especially after the 30 mL/kg bolus. During the **O**ptimization phase, within hours, the goal is to keep a neutral fluid balance between intake and output. During the **S**tabilization phase, which usually occurs in days, the focus should be on organ support and keeping fluid balance neutral to net negative with maintenance doses (30 mL/kg/day) of fluid only. Lastly, the **E**vacuation phase occurs in days to weeks, and it is suggested to keep fluid balance negative.

INOTROPE AND VASOACTIVE DRUG SUPPORT

- Vasopressors should be used to achieve and maintain MAP goal in fluid-resuscitation refractory shock, and they are titrated up carefully to an end point of adequate organ perfusion. Selection and dosage are based on the pharmacologic properties of various catecholamines and how they influence hemodynamic parameters (**Table 46-4**).
- For septic patients with clinical signs of shock and significant hypotension unresponsive to aggressive fluid therapy, **norepinephrine** is the preferred agent for increasing MAP. In comparison to **dopamine**, it is less arrhythmogenic and was associated with lower risk of mortality. **Epinephrine** is an alternative to norepinephrine for refractory hypotension. **Phenylephrine** is only recommended as a salvage therapy only if tachycardia or arrhythmia makes norepinephrine intolerable.

PERFORMANCE IMPROVEMENT BUNDLE

- The Sepsis-3 guidelines recommend the 3-hour bundle with the use of a 1-hour care, putting the importance of beginning the initial treatment immediately (**Table 46-5**).

ADJUNCTIVE THERAPY

- Recommended blood glucose levels to initiate an insulin protocol are more than 180 mg/dL (>10 mmol/L) with an upper target blood glucose level <180 dL (10 mmol/L) for the majority of critically ill patients to improve the outcome while reducing the risk of hypoglycemia.
- **Hydrocortisone** 200 mg IV per day should be administered only if hemodynamic stability is not achieved after adequate fluid resuscitation and vasopressor therapy, regardless of the state of adrenal insufficiency. Hydrocortisone should be tapered when vasopressors are no longer required because hemodynamic and immunologic rebound effects have been reported with abrupt cessation of corticosteroids.
- Venous thromboembolism (VTE) prophylaxis with daily subcutaneous low-molecular-weight heparin should be initiated in all patients admitted to the ICU with sepsis and septic shock along with mechanical prophylaxis (intermittent pneumatic compression or graduated compression stockings) unless contraindicated.

TABLE 46-4 Mechanism of Action and Hemodynamic Effects of Vasopressors in Septic Shock

Drug	Receptor Affinity				Physiologic Outcome			
	Dopamine	Alpha-1	Beta-1	Beta-2	HR	SV	SVR	CO
Dopamine (0.5–2)[a]	+++	–	+	–	↔↑	↑	↔ or ↑	↑
Dopamine (5–10)[a]	++	+	+++	+	↑	↑	↔ or ↑	↑↑
Dopamine (10–20)[a]	++	+++	++	–	↑	↑	↑↑	↑
Epinephrine	–	++++	++++	+++	↑	↑	↑↑	↑↑
Norepinephrine	–	++++	++	+	↔ or ↑	↕	↑↑	↑
Phenylephrine	–	+++	–	–	↔ or ↓	–	↑↑	↑
Vasopressin	V1 receptor				↔ or ↓	–	↑↑	↔↔ or ↓
Angiotensin II	AT receptor				↑	–	↑	↑

[a]mcg/kg/min.

CO, cardiac output; HR, heart rate; SV, stroke volume; SVR, systemic vascular resistance; V1, vasopressin receptor 1; V2, vasopressin receptor 2.

TABLE 46-5	Sepsis-3 (2016) Performance Improvement Checklist for Bundle-Care Compliance

One-hour bundle
- Measure initial lactate
- Repeat in 2 hours if initial lactate >2 mmol/L
- Obtain cultures (blood, urine, sputum, etc.) prior to administration of antibiotics
- Administer broad-spectrum IV antibiotics within 1 hour
- Initial fluid resuscitation of 30 mL/kg crystalloid for hypotension or lactate $\geq$4 mmol/L
- Vasopressors if MAP <65 mm Hg during or after completion of fluid resuscitation

Outcome measurements
- Length of stay in ICU and hospital
- Rate of organ dysfunction
- Mortality rate

CVP, central venous pressure; MAP, mean arterial pressure; ScvO$_2$, central venous oxygen saturation.

- Stress ulcer prophylaxis should be initiated in all patients with sepsis and septic shock who have risk factors for GI bleeding.

See Chapter 137, Severe Sepsis and Septic Shock, authored by S. Lena Kang-Birken and Sul R. Jung, for a more detailed discussion of this topic.

Sexually Transmitted Diseases 47

- The spectrum of sexually transmitted infections (STIs) includes the classic venereal diseases—gonorrhea, syphilis, chancroid, lymphogranuloma venereum, and granuloma inguinale—as well as a variety of other pathogens known to be spread by sexual contact (Table 47-1). Selected clinical syndromes associated with STIs are listed in Table 47-2. The most current information on epidemiology, diagnosis, and treatment of STIs provided by the Centers for Disease Control and Prevention (CDC) can be found at www.cdc.gov.

TABLE 47-1	Sexually Transmitted Infections
Disease	**Associated Pathogens**
Bacterial	
Gonorrhea	*Neisseria gonorrhoeae*
Syphilis	*Treponema pallidum*
Chancroid	*Haemophilus ducreyi*
Granuloma inguinale	*Calymmatobacterium granulomatis*
Enteric disease	*Salmonella* spp., *Shigella* spp., *Campylobacter* fetus
Campylobacter infection	*Campylobacter jejuni*
Bacterial vaginosis	*Gardnerella vaginalis, Mycoplasma hominis, Bacteroides* spp., *Mobiluncus* spp.
Group B streptococcal infections	Group B *Streptococcus*
Chlamydial	
Nongonococcal urethritis	*Chlamydia trachomatis*
Lymphogranuloma venereum	*C. trachomatis*, type L
Viral	
Acquired immunodeficiency syndrome	Human immunodeficiency virus
Herpes genitalis	Herpes simplex virus, types I and II
Viral hepatitis	Hepatitis A, B, C, and D viruses
Condylomata acuminata	Human papillomavirus
Molluscum contagiosum	Poxvirus
Cytomegalovirus infection	Cytomegalovirus
Mycoplasmal	
Nongonococcal urethritis	*Mycoplasma genitalium*
Protozoal	
Trichomoniasis	*Trichomonas vaginalis*
Amebiasis	*Entamoeba histolytica*
Giardiasis	*Giardia lamblia*
Fungal	
Vaginal candidiasis	*Candida albicans*
Parasitic	
Scabies	*Sarcoptes scabiei*
Pediculosis pubis	*Phthirus pubis*
Enterobiasis	*Enterobius vermicularis*

	TABLE 47-2 Selected Syndromes Associated with Common Sexually Transmitted Pathogens	
Syndrome	**Commonly Implicated Pathogens**	**Common Clinical Manifestations[a]**
Urethritis	*C. trachomatis*, herpes simplex virus, *N. gonorrhoeae*, *Trichomonas vaginalis*, *Ureaplasma urealyticum*, *Mycoplasma genitalium*	Urethral discharge, dysuria
Epididymitis	*C. trachomatis*, *N. gonorrhoeae*	Scrotal pain, inguinal pain, flank pain, urethral discharge
Cervicitis/ Vulvovaginitis	*C. trachomatis*, *Gardnerella vaginalis*, herpes simplex virus, human papillomavirus, *N. gonorrhoeae*, *T. vaginalis*	Abnormal vaginal discharge, vulvar itching/irritation, dysuria, dyspareunia
Genital ulcers (painful)	*Haemophilus ducreyi*, herpes simplex virus	Usually multiple vesicular/pustular (herpes) or papular/pustular (*H. ducreyi*) lesions that can coalesce; painful, tender lymphadenopathy[b]
Genital ulcers (painless)	*Treponema pallidum*	Usually single papular lesion
Genital/Anal warts	Human papillomavirus	Multiple lesions ranging in size from small papular warts to large exophytic condylomas
Pharyngitis	*C. trachomatis*, herpes simplex virus, *N. gonorrhoeae*	Symptoms of acute pharyngitis, cervical lymphadenopathy, fever[c]
Proctitis	*C. trachomatis*, herpes simplex virus, *N. gonorrhoeae*, *T. pallidum*	Constipation, anorectal discomfort, tenesmus, mucopurulent rectal discharge
Salpingitis	*C. trachomatis*, *N. gonorrhoeae*	Lower abdominal pain, purulent cervical or vaginal discharge, adnexal swelling, fever[d]

[a]For some syndromes, clinical manifestations can be minimal or absent.
[b]Recurrent herpes infection can manifest as a single lesion.
[c]Most cases of pharyngeal gonococcal infection are asymptomatic.
[d]Salpingitis increases the risk of subsequent ectopic pregnancy and infertility.

Gonorrhea

- *Neisseria gonorrhoeae* is a gram-negative diplococcus estimated to cause almost 500,000 new infections per year in the United States. Humans are the only known host of this intracellular parasite.

CLINICAL PRESENTATION

- Infected individuals may be symptomatic or asymptomatic, have complicated or uncomplicated infections, and have infections involving several anatomical sites. The majority of women diagnosed with gonorrhea are asymptomatic.
- The most common clinical features of gonococcal infections are presented in **Table 47-3**. Ninety percent of males experience symptoms within 2–6 days following exposure, most commonly mucopurulent penile discharge and dysuria. Approximately 10%–20% of

TABLE 47-3	Presentation of Gonorrhea Infections	
	Males	**Females**
General	Incubation period: 1–14 days	Incubation period: 1–14 days
	Symptom onset in 2–8 days	Symptom onset in 10 days
Site of infection	Most common: urethra	Most common: endocervical canal
	Others: rectum (usually caused by rectal intercourse in MSM), oropharynx, eye	Others: urethra, rectum (usually caused by perineal contamination), oropharynx, eye
Symptoms	Commonly symptomatic, may be asymptomatic	Can be asymptomatic or minimally symptomatic
	Urethral infection: dysuria and urinary frequency	Endocervical infection: usually asymptomatic or mildly symptomatic
	Anorectal infection: asymptomatic to severe rectal pain	Urethral infection: dysuria, urinary frequency
	Pharyngeal infection: asymptomatic to mild pharyngitis	Anorectal and pharyngeal infection; symptoms same as for men
Signs	Purulent urethral or rectal discharge can be scant to profuse. Anorectal: pruritus, mucopurulent discharge, bleeding	Abnormal vaginal discharge or uterine bleeding; purulent urethral or rectal discharge can be scant to profuse
Complications	Rare (epididymitis, prostatitis, inguinal lymphadenopathy, urethral stricture)	Pelvic inflammatory disease and associated complications (ie, ectopic pregnancy, infertility)
	Disseminated gonorrhea	Disseminated gonorrhea (three times more common than in men)

MSM, men who have sex with men.

women with gonorrhea develop pelvic inflammatory disease. Left untreated, pelvic inflammatory disease can be an indirect cause of infertility and ectopic pregnancies.

- In 0.5%–3% of patients with gonorrhea, the gonococci invade the bloodstream and produce disseminated disease. The usual clinical manifestations of disseminated gonococcal infection are tender necrotic skin lesions, tenosynovitis, and monoarticular arthritis.
- Diagnosis of gonococcal infections can be made by gram-stained smears, culture (the most reliable method), or newer methods based on the detection of cellular components of the gonococcus (eg, enzymes, antigens, or DNA) in clinical specimens.
- Nucleic acid amplification techniques (NAATs) have replaced culture in most settings as the primary diagnostic test for gonorrhea infections and when screening for asymptomatic infections.

TREATMENT

- Single-dose intramuscular (IM) **ceftriaxone** remains the only recommended agent for treating gonorrhea as ceftriaxone-based regimens are the only regimens with well-documented efficacy in the treatment of urethral, cervical, rectal, and pharyngeal infections (**Table 47-4**). Ceftriaxone 250 mg should be administered IM

TABLE 47-4	Treatment of Gonorrhea	
Type of Infection	**Recommended Regimens[a]**	**Alternative Regimens[a]**
Uncomplicated infections of the cervix, urethra, and rectum in adults	Ceftriaxone 250 mg IM once *plus* Azithromycin 1 g orally once	Cefixime 400 mg orally once *plus* Azithromycin 1 g orally once, or doxycycline 100 mg PO twice daily for 7 days[b] *or* Gemifloxacin 320 mg orally once or gentamicin 240 mg IM *plus* Azithromycin 2 g orally once
Uncomplicated infections of the pharynx	Ceftriaxone 250 mg IM once *plus* Azithromycin 1 g orally once	Consult with infectious disease expert
Disseminated gonococcal infection in adults (>45 kg)	Ceftriaxone 1–2 g IM or IV every 12–24 hours[c] *plus* Azithromycin 1 g orally once	Cefotaxime 1 g IV every 8 hours[c] or ceftizoxime 1 g IV every 8 hours[c] *plus* Azithromycin 1 g orally once
Uncomplicated infections of the cervix, urethra, pharynx, and rectum in children (<45 kg)	Ceftriaxone 25–50 mg/kg IV or IM once (not to exceed 125 mg)	
Disseminated gonococcal infection in children (<45 kg)	Ceftriaxone 50 mg/kg IV or IM once daily × 7 days (not to exceed 1 g)	
Gonococcal conjunctivitis in adults	Ceftriaxone 1 g IM once[d] *plus* Azithromycin 1 g orally once	
Ophthalmia neonatorum	Ceftriaxone 25–50 mg/kg IV or IM[f] once (not to exceed 125 mg)	
Disseminated gonococcal infection in neonates	Ceftriaxone 25–50 mg/kg/day IV or IM once daily or cefotaxime 25 mg/kg IV or IM twice daily for 7 days, or 10–14 days if meningitis is suspected[f]	

(*Continued*)

TABLE 47-4	Treatment of Gonorrhea (Continued)	
Type of Infection	**Recommended Regimens[a]**	**Alternative Regimens[a]**
Infants born to mothers with gonococcal infection	Prophylaxis: Erythromycin (0.5%) ophthalmic ointment in a single application[e]	
	Treatment:	
	Ceftriaxone 25–50 mg/kg IM or IV once (not to exceed 125 mg)	

[a]Recommendations are those of the CDC.
[b]Tetracyclines are contraindicated during pregnancy. Pregnant women should be treated with recommended cephalosporin-based combination therapy. In severe cephalosporin allergy, consultation with an infectious diseases expert is recommended.
[c]Parenteral treatment duration should be determined in consultation with an infectious diseases expert. Parenteral therapy for meningitis should be continued for at least 10–14 days and at least 4 weeks in endocarditis.
[d]A single lavage of the infected eye with normal saline should be considered; empiric therapy for *C. trachomatis* is recommended.
[e]Efficacy in preventing chlamydial ophthalmia is unclear.
[f]Caution should be taken when administering ceftriaxone to hyperbilirubinemic neonates.
CDC, Centers for Disease Control and Prevention; *C. trachomatis*, *Chlamydia trachomatis*; NAAT, nucleic acid amplification test; *N. gonorrhoeae*, *Neisseria gonorrhoeae*.

in combination with a 1000-mg single dose of oral **azithromycin**. Dual antibiotic therapy with different mechanisms of action is recommended in an effort to delay further development of antimicrobial resistance and increase treatment efficacy. A 400 mg oral dose of **cefixime** may be substituted if ceftriaxone is unavailable.
- Ceftriaxone is the recommended therapy for disseminated gonococcal infection (DGI) including meningitis and endocarditis, and any type of gonococcal infection in children.
- Pregnant women infected with *N. gonorrhoeae* should be treated with ceftriaxone.
- Treatment of gonorrhea during pregnancy is essential to prevent ophthalmia neonatorum. The CDC recommends that **erythromycin (0.5%) ophthalmic ointment** be instilled in each conjunctival sac immediately postpartum to prevent ophthalmia neonatorum.

Syphilis

- The causative organism of syphilis is *Treponema pallidum*, a spirochete.
- Syphilis is usually acquired by sexual contact with infected mucous membranes or cutaneous lesions, although on rare occasions it can be acquired by nonsexual personal contact, accidental inoculation, or blood transfusion.

CLINICAL PRESENTATION AND DIAGNOSIS

- The clinical presentation of syphilis is varied, with progression through multiple stages possible in untreated or inadequately treated patients.

PRIMARY SYPHILIS

- Primary syphilis is characterized by the appearance of a chancre on cutaneous or mucocutaneous tissue exposed to the organism and is highly infectious. Chancres heal within 4–6 weeks, although lymphadenopathy may persist longer.
- Incubation period: 10–90 days (mean, 21 days).
- Site of infection: External genitalia, perianal region, mouth, and throat.
- Signs and symptoms: Single, painless, indurated lesion (chancre) that erodes, ulcerates, and eventually heals (typical); regional lymphadenopathy is common; multiple, painful, purulent lesions possible but uncommon.

SECONDARY SYPHILIS

- The secondary stage of syphilis is characterized by a variety of mucocutaneous eruptions, resulting from widespread hematogenous and lymphatic spread of *T. pallidum*. There is multisystem involvement secondary to hematogenous and lymphatic spread.
- Develops 2–8 weeks after initial infection in untreated or inadequately treated individuals.
- Signs and symptoms of secondary syphilis disappear in 4–10 weeks; however, if untreated, secondary syphilis disappears spontaneously within 1–6 months.
- There is pruritic or nonpruritic rash, mucocutaneous lesions, flu-like symptoms, lymphadenopathy.

LATENT SYPHILIS

- Persons with a positive serologic test for syphilis but with no other evidence of disease have latent syphilis. It develops 4–10 weeks after secondary stage in untreated or inadequately treated individuals.
- There is potentially multisystem involvement (dormant) involving the CNS, heart, eyes, bones, and joints.
- Most untreated patients with late latent syphilis are asymptomatic and have no further sequelae; however, approximately 20% of patients progress either to neurosyphilis or to late syphilis with clinical manifestations other than neurosyphilis.

TERTIARY SYPHILIS AND NEUROSYPHILIS

- Develops in approximately 30% of untreated or inadequately treated individuals 10–30 years after initial infection.
- Tertiary syphilis may include cardiovascular syphilis (aortitis or aortic insufficiency), neurosyphilis (meningitis, general paresis, dementia, tabes dorsalis, eighth cranial nerve deafness, blindness), gummatous lesions involving any organ or tissue.
- If left untreated, syphilis can slowly produce an inflammatory reaction in virtually any organ in the body. Forty percent of patients with primary or secondary syphilis exhibit CNS infection.
- Because *T. pallidum* is difficult to culture in vitro, diagnosis is based primarily on dark-field or direct fluorescent antibody microscopic examination of serous material from a suspected syphilitic lesion or on results from serologic testing.
- Serologic tests are the mainstay in the diagnosis of syphilis and are categorized as nontreponemal or treponemal. Common nontreponemal tests include the venereal disease research laboratory (VDRL) slide test, rapid plasma reagin (RPR) card test, unheated serum reagin (USR) test, and the toluidine red unheated serum test (TRUST).
- Treponemal tests are more sensitive than nontreponemal tests and are used to confirm the diagnosis (ie, the fluorescent treponemal antibody absorption).

TREATMENT

- Treatment recommendations from the CDC for syphilis are presented in **Table 47-5**. Parenteral penicillin G is the treatment of choice for all stages of syphilis. **Benzathine penicillin G** is the only penicillin effective for single-dose therapy. The recommended treatment for syphilis of less than 1 year's duration is benzathine penicillin G 2.4 million units as a single IM dose.
- Alternative regimens recommended for penicillin-allergic patients are **doxycycline** 100 mg orally twice daily or **tetracycline** 500 mg orally four times daily for 2–4 weeks depending on the duration of syphilis infection.
- For pregnant patients, penicillin is the treatment of choice at the dosage recommended for that particular stage of syphilis. To ensure treatment success and prevent

transmission to the fetus, some experts advocate an additional IM dose of benzathine penicillin G, 2.4 million units, 1 week after completion of the recommended regimen.

- Patients treated for primary and secondary syphilis experience the Jarisch–Herxheimer reaction after treatment, characterized by flu-like symptoms such as transient headache, fever, chills, malaise, arthralgia, myalgia, tachypnea, peripheral vasodilation, and aggravation of syphilitic lesions. The Jarisch–Herxheimer reaction should not be confused with penicillin allergy. Most reactions can be managed symptomatically with analgesics, antipyretics, and rest.

- CDC recommendations for serologic follow-up of patients treated for syphilis are given in Table 47-5. Quantitative nontreponemal tests should be performed at 6 and 12 months in all patients treated for primary and secondary syphilis and at 6, 12, and 24 months for early and late latent disease.

- For women treated during pregnancy, monthly, quantitative, nontreponemal tests are recommended in those at high risk of reinfection.

TABLE 47-5	Drug Therapy and Follow-up of Syphilis	
Stage/Type of Syphilis	**Recommended Regimens[a,b]**	**Follow-up Serology**
Primary, secondary, or early latent syphilis (<1 year's duration)	Adults: benzathine penicillin G 2.4 million units IM in a single dose Children: Benzathine penicillin G 50,000 units/kg IM in a single dose, up to 2.4 million units	Quantitative nontreponemal tests at 6 and 12 months for primary and secondary syphilis; at 6, 12, and 24 months for early latent syphilis[c]
Late latent syphilis (>1 year's duration) or latent syphilis of unknown duration or tertiary syphilis or retreatment	Adults: benzathine penicillin G 2.4 million units IM once a week for 3 successive weeks (7.2 million units total) Children: benzathine penicillin G 50,000 units/kg IM once a week for 3 successive weeks, up to 7.2 million units total	Quantitative nontreponemal tests at 6, 12, and 24 months[d,e]
Neurosyphilis	Aqueous crystalline penicillin G 18–24 million units IV (3–4 million units every 4 hours or by continuous infusion) for 10–14 days[f] *or* Aqueous procaine penicillin G 2.4 million units IM daily plus probenecid 500 mg orally four times daily, both for 10–14 days[f]	CSF examination every 6 months until the cell count is normal; if it has not decreased at 6 months or is not normal by 2 years, retreatment should be considered
Congenital syphilis (infants with proven or highly probable disease)	Aqueous crystalline penicillin G 50,000 units/kg/dose IV every 12 hours during the first 7 days of life and every 8 hours thereafter for a total of 10 days *or* Procaine penicillin G 50,000 units/kg IM daily for 10 days	Serologic follow-up only recommended if antimicrobials other than penicillin are used

(Continued)

TABLE 47-5	Drug Therapy and Follow-up of Syphilis (Continued)	
Stage/Type of Syphilis	**Recommended Regimens**[a,b]	**Follow-up Serology**
Penicillin-allergic patients[g]		
Primary, secondary, or early latent syphilis	Doxycycline 100 mg orally two times daily for 14 days[g,h] *or* Tetracycline 500 mg orally four times daily for 14 days[h] or Ceftriaxone 1–2 g IM or IV daily for 10–14 days	Same as for non–penicillin-allergic patients
Late latent syphilis (>1 year's duration) or syphilis of unknown duration	Doxycycline 100 mg orally twice a day for 28 days[h,i] *or* Tetracycline 500 mg orally four times daily for 28 days[h,i]	Same as for non–penicillin-allergic patients

[a]Recommendations are those of the CDC.
[b]The CDC recommends that all patients diagnosed with syphilis be tested for HIV infection.
[c]More frequent follow-up (ie, 3, 6, 9, 12, and 24 months) recommended for HIV-infected patients.
[d]More frequent follow-up (ie, 6, 12, 18, and 24 months) recommended for HIV-infected patients.
[e]No specific recommendations exist for tertiary syphilis because of the lack of available data.
[f]Some experts administer benzathine penicillin G 2.4 million units IM once per week for up to 3 weeks after completion of the neurosyphilis regimens to provide a total duration of therapy comparable to that used for late syphilis in the absence of neurosyphilis.
[g]For nonpregnant patients; pregnant patients should be treated with penicillin after desensitization.
[h]Pregnant patients allergic to penicillin should be desensitized and treated with penicillin.
[i]Limited data suggest that ceftriaxone may be effective, although the optimal dosage and treatment duration are unclear.
CDC, Centers for Disease Control and Prevention; CSF, cerebrospinal fluid; HIV, human immunodeficiency virus.

Chlamydia

- Infections caused by *Chlamydia trachomatis* are believed to be the most common STI in the United States. *C. trachomatis* is an obligate intracellular parasite that has some similarities to viruses and bacteria.

CLINICAL PRESENTATION

- In comparison with gonorrhea, chlamydial genital infections are more frequently asymptomatic, and when present, symptoms tend to be less noticeable. Table 47-6 summarizes the usual clinical presentation of chlamydial infections.
- Similar to gonorrhea, chlamydia may be transmitted to an infant during contact with infected cervicovaginal secretions. Nearly two-thirds of infants acquire chlamydial infection after endocervical exposure, with the primary morbidity associated with seeding of the infant's eyes, nasopharynx, rectum, or vagina.
- Culture of endocervical or urethral epithelial cell scrapings is the most specific method (close to 100%) for detection of chlamydia, but sensitivity is as low as 70%. Between 3 and 7 days are required for results.

TABLE 47-6	Presentation of Chlamydia Infections	
	Males	**Females**
General	Incubation period: 35 days	Incubation period: 7–35 days
	Symptom onset: 7–21 days	Usual symptom onset: 7–21 days
Site of infection	Most common: urethra	Most common: endocervical canal
	Others: rectum (receptive anal intercourse), oropharynx, eye	Others: urethra, rectum (usually caused by perineal contamination), oropharynx, eye
Symptoms	More than 50% of urethral and rectal infections are asymptomatic	More than 66% of cervical infections are asymptomatic
	Urethral infection: mild dysuria, discharge	Urethral infection: usually subclinical; dysuria and frequency uncommon
	Pharyngeal infection: asymptomatic to mild pharyngitis	Rectal and pharyngeal infection: symptoms same as for men
Signs	Scant to profuse, mucoid to purulent urethral or rectal discharge	Abnormal vaginal discharge or uterine bleeding, purulent urethral or rectal discharge can be scant to profuse
	Rectal infection: pain, discharge, bleeding	
Complications	Epididymitis, Reiter's syndrome (rare)	Pelvic inflammatory disease and associated complications (ie, ectopic pregnancy, infertility)
		Reiter's syndrome (rare)

- Tests that allow rapid identification of chlamydial antigens and nucleic acid provide more rapid results, are technically less demanding to perform, less costly, and in some situations have greater sensitivity than culture. Nucleic acid amplification tests (NAATs) are the most sensitive tests for first-catch urine, endocervix and vaginal swab specimens in women, and urethral swab specimens in men, and are therefore the recommended tests for detecting chlamydia infection.

TREATMENT

- **Azithromycin** 1000 mg orally as a single-dose and **doxycycline** 100 mg orally twice daily for 7 days are the regimens of choice for the treatment of uncomplicated urogenital chlamydia infections (Table 47-7).
- Treatment of chlamydial infections with the recommended regimens is highly effective; therefore, posttreatment cultures are not routinely recommended.
- Infants with pneumonitis should receive follow-up testing because **erythromycin** is only 80% effective.
- For infected pregnant women azithromycin is the recommended treatment.

Genital Herpes

- The term *herpes* is used to describe two distinct but antigenically related serotypes of herpes simplex virus (HSV). HSV type 1 (HSV-1) is most commonly associated with oropharyngeal disease; type 2 (HSV-2) is most closely associated with genital disease.

CLINICAL PRESENTATION

- A summary of the clinical presentation of genital herpes is provided in **Table 47-8**.
- Complications from genital herpes infections result from both genital spread and autoinoculation of the virus and occur most commonly with primary first episodes. Lesions at extragenital sites, such as the eye, rectum, pharynx, and fingers, are not uncommon. CNS involvement is seen occasionally and can take several forms, including encephalitis, aseptic meningitis, and transverse myelitis. A major concern is the effect of genital herpes on neonates exposed during pregnancy.
- Tissue culture is the most specific (100%) and sensitive method (80%–90%) of confirming the diagnosis of first-episode genital herpes; however, culture is relatively insensitive in detecting HSV in ulcers in the latter stages of healing and in recurrent infections.

TREATMENT

- <u>Goals of Treatment:</u> To relieve symptoms and to shorten the clinical course, prevent complications and recurrences, and to decrease disease transmission.
- Specific treatment recommendations are given in **Table 47-9**.
- Oral **acyclovir, valacyclovir,** and **famciclovir** are the treatments of choice for outpatients with first-episode genital herpes.

TABLE 47-7	Treatment of Chlamydia Infections	
Infection	**Recommended Regimens[a]**	**Alternative Regimen**
Uncomplicated urethral, endocervical, or rectal infection in adults	Azithromycin 1 g orally once, or doxycycline 100 mg orally twice daily for 7 days	Erythromycin base 500 mg orally four times daily for 7 days, or erythromycin ethylsuccinate 800 mg orally four times daily for 7 days, or levofloxacin 500 mg orally once daily for 7 days, or ofloxacin 300 mg orally twice daily for 7 days
Urogenital infections during pregnancy	Azithromycin 1 g orally as a single dose or amoxicillin 500 mg orally three times daily for 7 days	Amoxicillin 500 mg orally three times daily for 7 days, or erythromycin base 500 mg orally four times daily for 7 days, or erythromycin base 250 mg orally four times daily for 14 days, or erythromycin ethylsuccinate 800 mg orally four times daily for 7 days, or erythromycin ethylsuccinate 400 mg orally four times daily for 14 days
Conjunctivitis of the newborn or pneumonia in infants	Erythromycin base or ethylsuccinate 50 mg/kg/day orally in four divided doses for 14 days[b,c]	Azithromycin suspension 20 mg/kg/day orally once daily for 3 days[c]

[a]Recommendations are those of the CDC.
[b]Topical therapy alone is inadequate for ophthalmia neonatorum and is unnecessary when systemic therapy is administered. Effectiveness of erythromycin treatment is approximately 80%; therefore, a second course of therapy may be required.
[c]An association between oral erythromycin and azithromycin and IHPS has been reported in infants aged <6 weeks. Infants treated with either of these antimicrobials should be followed for signs and symptoms of IHPS.
CDC, Centers for Disease Control and Prevention; IHPS, infantile hypertrophic pyloric stenosis.

TABLE 47-8	Presentation of Genital Herpes Infections
General	Incubation period: 2–14 days (mean, 4 days)
	Can be caused by either HSV-1 or HSV-2
Classification of infection	
First-episode primary	Initial genital infection in individuals lacking antibody to either HSV-1 or HSV-2
First-episode nonprimary	Initial genital infection in individuals with clinical or serologic evidence of prior HSV (usually HSV-1) infection
Recurrent	Appearance of genital lesions at some time following healing of first-episode infection
Signs and symptoms	
First-episode infections	Most primary infections are asymptomatic or minimally symptomatic
	Multiple painful pustular or ulcerative lesions on external genitalia developing over a period of 7–10 days; lesions heal in 2–4 weeks (mean, 21 days)
	Flu-like symptoms (eg, fever, headache, malaise) during first few days after appearance of lesions
	Others—local itching, pain, or discomfort; vaginal or urethral discharge, tender inguinal adenopathy, paresthesias, urinary retention
	Severity of symptoms greater in females than in males
	Symptoms are less severe (eg, fewer lesions, more rapid lesion healing, fewer or milder systemic symptoms) with nonprimary infections
	Symptoms more severe and prolonged in immunocompromised patients
	On average viral shedding lasts approximately 11–12 days for primary infections and 7 days for nonprimary infections
Recurrent	Prodrome seen in approximately 50% of patients prior to appearance of recurrent lesions; mild burning, itching, or tingling are typical prodromal symptoms
	Compared to primary infections, recurrent infections associated with (1) fewer lesions that are more localized, (2) shorter duration of active infection (lesions heal within 7 days), and (3) milder symptoms
	Severity of symptoms greater in females than in males
	Symptoms more severe and prolonged in immunocompromised patients
	On average viral shedding lasts approximately 4 days
	Asymptomatic viral shedding is more frequent during the first year after infection with HSV
Therapeutic implications of HSV-1 vs. HSV-2 genital infection	Primary infections caused by HSV-1 and HSV-2 virtually indistinguishable
	Recurrent infections and subclinical viral shedding are less frequent with HSV-1
	Recurrent infections with HSV-2 tend to be more severe
Complications	Secondary infection of lesions; extragenital infection because of autoinoculation; disseminated infection (primarily in immunocompromised patients); meningitis or encephalitis; neonatal transmission

HSV-1, herpes simplex virus type 1; HSV-2, herpes simplex virus type 2.

- Suppressive with oral antiviral agents reduces the frequency and the severity of recurrences in 70%–80% of patients experiencing frequent recurrences.
- Acyclovir, valacyclovir, and famciclovir have been used to prevent reactivation of infection in patients seropositive for HSV who undergo transplantation procedures or induction chemotherapy for acute leukemia.
- The safety of acyclovir, famciclovir, and valacyclovir therapy during pregnancy is not well established, although experience with both agents in animal studies suggests a low risk of fetal harm.

Trichomoniasis

- Trichomoniasis is caused by *Trichomonas vaginalis,* a flagellated, motile protozoan that is responsible for 3–4 million cases per year in the United States.
- Coinfection with other STIs (eg, gonorrhea) is common in patients diagnosed with trichomoniasis.

CLINICAL PRESENTATION

- The typical presentation of trichomoniasis in men and women is presented in **Table 47-10**.
- *T. vaginalis* produces nonspecific symptoms also consistent with bacterial vaginosis; thus, laboratory diagnosis is required.
- The simplest and most reliable means of diagnosis is a wet-mount examination of the vaginal discharge. Trichomoniasis is confirmed if characteristic pear-shaped, flagellating organisms are observed. Newer diagnostic tests, such as monoclonal antibody or DNA probe techniques, as well as PCR tests that can detect small amounts of trichomonal DNA and are highly sensitive and specific.

TREATMENT

- Recommended and alternative treatment regimens for *T. vaginalis* include either **metronidazole** or **tinidazole**, both of which produce high cure rates.
- Treatment recommendations for *Trichomonas* infections are given in **Table 47-11**.
- GI complaints are more common with the single 2 g dose of either metronidazole or tinidazole and some patients also complain of a bitter metallic taste in the mouth with metronidazole.
- Patients intolerant of the single 2 g dose because of GI adverse effects usually tolerate the alternative metronidazole multidose regimen.
- To achieve maximal cure rates and prevent relapse with the single 2 g dose of metronidazole, simultaneous treatment of infected sexual partners is necessary.
- In patients who fail to respond to an initial course of metronidazole therapy, a second course of therapy with metronidazole 500 mg twice daily for 7 days or a single 2 g dose of tinidazole is recommended.
- Patients taking metronidazole should be instructed to avoid alcohol ingestion during therapy and for 1 or 2 days after completion of therapy because of a possible disulfiram-like effect.
- Because metronidazole is secreted in breast milk, it is recommended that breastfeeding be interrupted for 12–24 hours after maternal ingestion of a single 2 g dose. Metronidazole (pregnancy category B) and tinidazole (pregnancy category C) are contraindicated during the first trimester of pregnancy based on FDA-approved labeling. However, the CDC now recommends that all symptomatic pregnant women, regardless of pregnancy stage, be tested and considered for treatment with metronidazole.

TABLE 47-9	Treatment of Genital Herpes	
Type of Infection	**Recommended Regimens[a,b]**	**Alternative Regimen**
First clinical episode of genital herpes[c]	Acyclovir 400 mg orally three times daily for 7–10 days[d] or Acyclovir 200 mg orally five times daily for 7–10 days[d] or Famciclovir 250 mg orally three times daily for 7–10 days[d] or Valacyclovir 1 g orally twice daily for 7–10 days[d]	Acyclovir 5–10 mg/kg IV every 8 hours for 2–7 days or until clinical improvement occurs, followed by oral therapy to complete at least 10 days of total therapy[e]
Recurrent infection		
Episodic therapy	Acyclovir 400 mg orally three times daily for 5 days[f] or Acyclovir 800 mg orally twice daily for 5 days[f] or Acyclovir 800 mg orally three times daily for 2 days[f] or Famciclovir 125 mg orally twice daily for 5 days[f] or Famciclovir 1 g orally twice daily for 1 day[f] or Famciclovir 500 mg orally once, followed by 250 mg orally twice daily for 2 days[f] or Valacyclovir 500 mg orally twice daily for 3 days[f] or Valacyclovir 1 g orally once daily for 5 days[f]	
Suppressive therapy[g]	Acyclovir 400 mg orally twice daily or Famciclovir 250 mg orally twice daily[h] or Valacyclovir 500 mg or 1000 mg orally once daily[i]	

[a]Recommendations are those of the CDC.
[b]HIV-infected patients can require more aggressive therapy.
[c]Primary or nonprimary first episode.
[d]Treatment duration can be extended if healing is incomplete after 10 days.
[e]Only for patients with severe symptoms or complications that necessitate hospitalization. HSV encephalitis requires 21 days of IV therapy.
[f]Requires initiation of therapy within 24 hours of lesion onset or during the prodrome that precedes some outbreaks.
[g]Consider discontinuation of treatment after 1 year to assess frequency of recurrence.
[h]Famciclovir appears less effective for suppression of viral shedding.
[i]Valacyclovir 500 mg appears less effective than other valacyclovir and acyclovir regimens in patients with 10 or more recurrences per year.
CDC, Centers for Disease Control and Prevention; HIV, human immunodeficiency virus; IV, intravenous.

TABLE 47-10	Presentation of Trichomonas Infections	
	Males	**Females**
General	Incubation period: 3–28 days	Incubation period: 3–28 days
	Organism can be detectable within 48 hours after exposure to infected partner	
Site of infection	Most common: urethra	Most common: endocervical canal
	Others: rectum (usually caused by rectal intercourse in MSM), oropharynx, eye	Others: urethra, rectum (usually caused by perineal contamination), oropharynx, eye
Symptoms	Can be asymptomatic (more common in males than females) or minimally symptomatic	Can be asymptomatic or minimally symptomatic
	Urethral discharge (clear to mucopurulent)	Scant to copious, typically malodorous vaginal discharge (50%–75%) and pruritus (worse during menses)
	Dysuria, pruritus	Dysuria, dyspareunia
Signs	Urethral discharge	Vaginal discharge
		Vaginal pH 4.5–6
		Inflammation/erythema of vulva, vagina, and/or cervix
		Urethritis
Complications	Epididymitis and chronic prostatitis (uncommon)	Pelvic inflammatory disease and associated complications (ie, ectopic pregnancy, infertility)
	Male infertility (decreased sperm motility and viability)	Premature labor, premature rupture of membranes, and low-birth-weight infants (risk of neonatal infections is low)
		Cervical neoplasia

MSM, men who have sex with men.

- Follow-up was previously considered unnecessary in patients who become asymptomatic after treatment with recommended therapy; however, retesting is now recommended for all sexually active women within 3 months following initial treatment due to the high rates of reinfection.
- When patients remain symptomatic, it is important to determine if reinfection has occurred. In these cases, a repeat course of therapy, as well as identification and treatment or retreatment of infected sexual partners, is recommended.

TABLE 47-11	Treatment of Trichomoniasis	
Type	**Recommended Regimens[a]**	**Alternative Regimen**
Symptomatic and asymptomatic infections	Metronidazole 2 g orally in a single dose *or* Tinidazole 2 g orally in a single dose[b]	Metronidazole 500 mg orally two times daily for 7 days[c,d]
Persistent or recurrent infections	Metronidazole 500 mg orally two times daily for 7 days[c]	Metronidazole 2 g orally for 7 days[e] *or* Tinidazole 2 g orally for 7 days[e]
Treatment in pregnancy	Metronidazole 2 g orally in a single dose[e,f]	

[a]Recommendations are those of the CDC.
[b]Randomized controlled trials comparing single 2 g doses of metronidazole and tinidazole suggest that tinidazole is equivalent to, or superior to, metronidazole in achieving parasitologic cure and resolution of symptoms.
[c]Metronidazole labeling approved by the FDA does not include this regimen. Dosage regimens for treatment of trichomoniasis included in the product labeling are the single 2 g dose; 250 mg three times daily for 7 days; and 375 mg twice daily for 7 days. The 250 mg and 375 mg dosage regimens are currently not included in the CDC recommendations.
[d]Recommended treatment regimen for women with HIV coinfection.
[e]For treatment failures with metronidazole 2 g as a single dose and metronidazole 500 mg orally two times daily for 7 days.
[f]Symptomatic pregnant women can be treated with this regimen at any stage of pregnancy.
CDC, Centers for Disease Control and Prevention; HIV, human immunodeficiency virus.

TABLE 47-12	Treatment Regimens for Miscellaneous Sexually Transmitted Infections	
Infection	**Recommended Regimens[a]**	**Alternative Regimen**
Chancroid (*H. ducreyi*)	Azithromycin 1 g orally in a single dose *or* Ceftriaxone 250 mg IM in a single dose *or* Ciprofloxacin 500 mg orally twice daily for 3 days[b] *or* Erythromycin base 500 mg orally four times daily for 7 days	
Lymphogranuloma venereum	Doxycycline 100 mg orally twice daily for 21 days[c]	Erythromycin base 500 mg orally four times daily for 21 days[d]
Nongonococcal urethritis (NGU)	Azithromycin 1 g orally in a single dose *or* Doxycyline 100 mg orally twice daily for 7 days	Erythromycin base 500 mg orally four times daily for 7 days, or erythromycin ethylsuccinate 800 mg orally four times daily for 7 days, or levofloxacin 500 mg orally once daily for 7 days, or ofloxacin 300 mg orally twice daily for 7 days

(Continued)

TABLE 47-12	Treatment Regimens for Miscellaneous Sexually Transmitted Infections *(Continued)*	
Infection	**Recommended Regimens[a]**	**Alternative Regimen**
NGU (persistent or recurrent or due to *Mycoplasma genitalium*)	Azithromycin 1 g orally in a single dose	Fail initial regimen of azithromycin: moxifloxacin 400 mg orally daily for 7 days
HPV infection		
External genital/ Perianal warts	*Provider-administered therapies* Cryotherapy (eg, liquid nitrogen or cryoprobe); repeat weekly as necessary *or* Podophyllin resin 10%–25% in compound tincture of benzoin applied to lesions; repeat weekly as necessary[e,f] *or* TCA 80%–90% *or* BCA 80%–90% applied to warts; repeat weekly as necessary *or* Surgical removal (tangential scissor excision, tangential shave excision, curettage, or electrosurgery) *Patient-applied therapies* Podofilox 0.5% solution or gel applied twice daily for 3 days, followed by 4 days of no therapy; cycle is repeated as necessary for up to four cycles[f] *or* Imiquimod 3.75% or 5% cream applied at bedtime three times weekly for up to 16 weeks[f] *or* Sinecatechins 15% ointment applied three times daily for up to 16 weeks	Intralesional interferon *or* Photodynamic therapy *or* Topical cidofovir
Vaginal and anal warts	Cryotherapy with liquid nitrogen, or TCA or BCA 80%–90% as for external HPV warts; repeat weekly as necessary[g] Surgical removal (not for vaginal or urethral meatus warts)	
Urethral meatus warts	Cryotherapy with liquid nitrogen, or podophyllin resin 10%–25% in compound tincture of benzoin applied at weekly intervals[f,h]	

(Continued)

TABLE 47-12	Treatment Regimens for Miscellaneous Sexually Transmitted Infections *(Continued)*	
Infection	**Recommended Regimens[a]**	**Alternative Regimen**
Prevention (ages 9–14 years)	Gardasil (HPV quadrivalent [types 6, 11, 16, and 18]) recombinant vaccine 0.5 mL IM on day 1; a second dose administered 6–12 months following the first dose[i,j,k]	
	Cervarix (HPV bivalent [types 16 and 18]) recombinant vaccine 0.5 mL IM on day 1; a second dose administered 6–12 months following the first dose[i,j]	
	Gardasil9 (HPV 9-valent [types 6, 11, 16, 18, 31, 33, 45, 52, 58]) recombinant vaccine 0.5 mL IM on day 1; a second dose administered 6–12 months following the first dose[i]	
Prevention (age ≥15 years)	Gardasil (HPV quadrivalent [types 6, 11, 16, and 18]) recombinant vaccine 0.5 mL IM on day 1; a second and third dose are administered 2 and 6 months following the first dose[i,j,k]	
	Cervarix (HPV bivalent [types 16 and 18]) recombinant vaccine 0.5 mL IM on day 1; a second and third dose are administered 1 and 6 months following the first dose[i,j]	
	Gardasil9 (HPV 9-valent [types 6, 11, 16, 18, 31, 33, 45, 52, 58]) recombinant vaccine 0.5 mL IM on day 1; a second and third dose are administered 1 and 6 months following the first dose[i]	

[a]Recommendations are those of the Centers for Disease Control and Prevention (CDC).
[b]Ciprofloxacin is contraindicated for pregnant and lactating women and for persons aged <18 years.
[c]Azithromycin 1 g PO once weekly for 3 weeks can be effective.
[d]Pregnant patients should be treated with erythromycin.
[e]Some experts recommended washing podophyllin off after 1–4 hours to minimize local irritation.
[f]Safety during pregnancy is not established.
[g]Surgical removal of anal warts is also a recommended treatment.
[h]Some specialists recommend the use of podofilox and imiquimod for treating distal meatal warts.
[i]CDC recommendations: vaccination is recommended in girls 11–12 years of age, and in females aged 13–26 years who either were not previously vaccinated, or who did not complete the vaccination series.
[j]FDA-approved labeling for Gardasil: indicated in girls and women 9 through 26 years of age for the prevention of cervical, vulvar, vaginal, and anal cancer caused by HPV types 16 and 18, genital warts (condyloma acuminata) caused by HPV types 6 and 11, and precancerous or dysplastic lesions caused by HPV types 6, 11, 16, and 18.
[k]Vaccination is recommended in males aged 9–26 years to prevent genital warts and anal cancer.
[l]FDA-approved labeling for Cervarix: indicated in females 9 through 25 years of age for the prevention of cervical cancer, cervical intraepithelial neoplasia grade 2 or worse, adenocarcinoma in situ, and cervical intraepithelial neoplasia grade 1 caused by HPV types 16 and 18.
BCA, bichloracetic acid; HPV, human papillomavirus; NGU, nongonococcal urethritis; TCA, trichloroacetic acid.

Other Sexually Transmitted Infections

• Several STIs other than those previously discussed occur with varying frequency in the United States and throughout the world. Although an in-depth discussion of these diseases is beyond the scope of this chapter, recommended treatment regimens are given in **Table 47-12**.

See Chapter 135, Sexually Transmitted Infections, authored by Bryson Duhon, and Yvonne Burnett, for a more detailed discussion of this topic.

- Bacterial infections of the skin can be classified as primary or secondary (Table 48-1). Primary bacterial infections are usually caused by a single bacterial species and involve areas of generally healthy skin (eg, impetigo and erysipelas). Secondary infections develop in areas of previously damaged skin and are frequently polymicrobic.
- The conditions that may predispose a patient to the development of skin and soft-tissue infections (SSTIs) include: (1) a high concentration of bacteria; (2) excessive moisture of the skin; (3) inadequate blood supply; (4) availability of bacterial nutrients; and (5) damage to the corneal layer, allowing for bacterial penetration.
- The majority of SSTIs are caused by gram-positive organisms on the skin surface. *Staphylococcus aureus* and *Streptococcus pyogenes* account for the majority of SSTIs. Other common nosocomial pathogens include *Pseudomonas aeruginosa* (11%), enterococci (9%), and *Escherichia coli* (7%).

Erysipelas

- *Erysipelas* (Saint Anthony's fire) is a distinct form of cellulitis involving the superficial layers of the skin and cutaneous lymphatics. The infection is almost always caused by β-hemolytic streptococci, with *S. pyogenes* (group A streptococci) responsible for most infections.
- The lower extremities are the most common sites for erysipelas. Patients often experience flu-like symptoms (fever, chills, and malaise) prior to the appearance of the lesions. The infected area is painful, often a burning pain. The lesion is intensely erythematous and edematous, often with lymphatic streaking. It has a raised border, which is sharply demarcated from uninfected skin. Leukocytosis is common, and C-reactive protein is generally elevated.
- Mild-to-moderate cases of erysipelas in adults are treated with intramuscular **procaine penicillin G** or **penicillin VK** for 7–10 days. For more serious infections, the patient should be hospitalized and **aqueous penicillin G** administered IV. Penicillin-allergic patients can be treated with **clindamycin**.
- Evidence-based recommendations for treatment of SSTIs are given in **Table 48-2**, and recommended drugs and dosing regimens for outpatient treatment of mild-to-moderate SSTIs are given in **Tables 48-3** and **48-4**.

Impetigo

- *Impetigo* is a superficial skin infection that is seen most commonly in children. It is highly communicable and spreads through close contact. Most cases are caused by *S. pyogenes*, but *S. aureus* either alone or in combination with *S. pyogenes* has emerged as a principal cause of impetigo.

CLINICAL PRESENTATION

- Exposed skin, especially the face, is the most common site for impetigo.
- Pruritus is common, and scratching of the lesions may further spread infection through excoriation of the skin. Other systemic signs of infection are minimal.
- Weakness, fever, and diarrhea are sometimes seen with bullous impetigo.
- Nonbullous impetigo manifests initially as small, fluid-filled vesicles. These lesions rapidly develop into pus-filled blisters that readily rupture. Purulent discharge from the lesions dries to form golden yellow crusts that are characteristic of impetigo.
- In the bullous form of impetigo, the lesions begin as vesicles and turn into bullae containing clear yellow fluid. Bullae soon rupture, forming thin, light brown crusts.
- Regional lymph nodes may be enlarged.

TABLE 48-1	Bacterial Classification of Important Skin and Soft-Tissue Infections
Primary infections	
Erysipelas	Group A streptococci (*Streptococcus pyogenes*)
Impetigo	*Staphylococcus aureus* (including methicillin-resistant strains), group A streptococci
Lymphangitis	Group A streptococci; occasionally *S. aureus*
Cellulitis	Group A streptococci, *S. aureus* (potentially including methicillin-resistant strains); occasionally other gram-positive cocci, gram-negative bacilli, and/or anaerobes
Necrotizing fasciitis	
Type I	Anaerobes (*Bacteroides* spp., *Peptostreptococcus* spp.) and facultative bacteria (streptococci, Enterobacteriaceae)
Type II	Group A streptococci
Type III	*Clostridioides perfringens*
Secondary infections	
Diabetic foot infections	*S. aureus*, streptococci, Enterobacteriaceae, *Bacteroides* spp., *Peptostreptococcus* spp., *Pseudomonas aeruginosa*
Pressure sores	*S. aureus* including methicillin-resistant strains, streptococci, Enterobacteriaceae, *Bacteroides* spp., *Peptostreptococcus* spp., *P. aeruginosa*
Bite wounds	
Animal	*Pasteurella* spp., *S. aureus*, streptococci, *Bacteroides* spp.
Human	*Eikenella corrodens*, *S. aureus*, streptococci, *Corynebacterium* spp., *Bacteroides* spp., *Peptostreptococcus* spp.
Burn wounds	*P. aeruginosa*, Enterobacteriaceae, *S. aureus*, streptococci

TREATMENT

- Although impetigo may resolve spontaneously, antimicrobial treatment is indicated to relieve symptoms, prevent formation of new lesions, and prevent complications such as cellulitis.
- Topical **mupirocin** ointment or **retapamulin** ointment for 5 days is recommended as first-line treatment of mild cases of impetigo not involving multiple lesions or the face.
- Penicillinase-resistant penicillins (eg, **dicloxacillin**) are the systemic agents of choice because of the increased isolation of *S. aureus*. First-generation cephalosporins (eg, **cephalexin**) are also used (see Table 48-3). **Penicillin** may be used for impetigo caused by *S. pyogenes*. It may be administered as either a single intramuscular dose of **benzathine penicillin G** (300,000–600,000 units in children, 1.2 million units in adults) or as oral penicillin VK given for 7 days. Penicillin-allergic patients can be treated with oral **clindamycin, doxycycline, or trimethoprim–sulfamethoxazole**. Recommended doses for antimicrobials are given in **Table 48-4**.

Cellulitis

- Cellulitis is an acute, spreading infectious process that initially affects the epidermis and dermis and may subsequently spread within the superficial fascia. This process is characterized by inflammation but with little or no necrosis or suppuration of soft tissue.

TABLE 48-2 Evidence-Based Recommendations for Treatment of Skin and Soft-Tissue Infections

Recommendations	Recommendation Grade[a]
Folliculitis, furuncles, carbuncles	
Gram stain and culture of pus from carbuncles and abscesses are recommended, but treatment without cultures is reasonable in most patients	Strong, moderate
Carbuncles, abscesses, and large furuncles of mild severity should be treated with incision and drainage	Strong, high
Administration of antibiotics with activity against *Staphylococcus aureus* as an adjunct to incision and drainage should be based on presence or absence of systemic signs of infection	Strong, low
Antibiotics with activity against MRSA are recommended for patients with carbuncles or abscesses of higher severity who have failed initial antibiotic therapy, have severe systemic signs of infection, or are immunocompromised	Strong, low
Erysipelas	
Most infections are caused by *Streptococcus pyogenes*. Penicillin (oral or IV depending on clinical severity) is the drug of choice	A-I
If *S. aureus* is suspected, a penicillinase-resistant penicillin or first-generation cephalosporin should be used	A-I
Impetigo	
Gram stain and culture of pus or exudates should be obtained to help identify causative pathogens	Strong, moderate
Bullous and nonbullous impetigo should be treated with either mupirocin or retapamulin for 5 days	Strong, high
Impetigo should be treated with oral antibiotics active against *S. aureus* unless cultures show streptococci alone. Dicloxacillin or cephalexin is recommended for 7 days. Doxycycline, clindamycin, or sulfamethoxazole-trimethoprim should be used when MRSA is suspected or confirmed	Strong, moderate
Cellulitis	
Cultures of blood or cutaneous aspirates, biopsies, or swabs are not routinely recommended	Strong, moderate
Blood cultures are recommended, and cultures of cutaneous aspirates, biopsies, or swabs should be considered, in patients receiving chemotherapy for malignancies, neutropenia, severe cell-mediated immunodeficiency, immersion injuries, or animal bites	Strong, moderate (blood)
	Weak, moderate (other cultures)

Typical cases of mild nonpurulent cellulitis should be treated with antibiotics active against streptococci	Strong, moderate
Systemic antibiotics are recommended for moderate nonpurulent cellulitis with systemic signs of infection. Use of antibiotics active against methicillin-susceptible *S. aureus* could be considered	Weak, low
Patients with severe nonpurulent cellulitis associated with penetrating trauma, MRSA infection in another location, MRSA nasal colonization, injection drug use, or systemic signs of infection should be treated with vancomycin or other antibiotics active against both MRSA and streptococci	Strong, moderate
Broad-spectrum antibiotic therapy with vancomycin plus either piperacillin–tazobactam, imipenem, or meropenem may be considered for empiric treatment of severe nonpurulent cellulitis in severely immunocompromised patients	Weak, moderate (need for broad-spectrum therapy); strong, moderate (recommended broad-spectrum antibiotic regimen if used)
A treatment duration of 5 days is recommended for cellulitis, but may be extended if lack of clinical response within that time	Strong, high
Elevation of the affected area and treatment of predisposing factors are recommended for cellulitis	Strong, moderate
Systemic corticosteroids for 7 days can be considered for adjunctive treatment of cellulitis in nondiabetic patients	Weak, moderate
Patients with mild nonpurulent cellulitis who do not have systemic signs of infection, altered mental status, or hemodynamic instability should be treated as outpatients	Strong, moderate
Hospitalization is recommended for patients with moderate-to-severe nonpurulent cellulitis who have failed outpatient therapy, have poor adherence to therapy, are immunocompromised, or in whom there is a concern for deeper or necrotizing infection	Strong, moderate
Empiric antibiotics for outpatients with purulent cellulitis should provide activity against community-associated MRSA; coverage of β-hemolytic streptococci is likely not required. Mild-to-moderate infections can generally be treated with oral agents (dicloxacillin, cephalexin, clindamycin) unless resistance is high in the community	A-II
Recommended antibiotics for empiric coverage of MRSA in outpatients include orally administered trimethoprim–sulfamethoxazole, doxycycline, minocycline, clindamycin, and linezolid	A-II for all listed options
If coverage of both β-hemolytic streptococci and community-associated MRSA is desired, empiric antibiotic regimens for outpatient therapy include orally administered clindamycin alone; linezolid alone; or trimethoprim–sulfamethoxazole, doxycycline, or minocycline in combination with amoxicillin	A-II for all listed options

(Continued)

TABLE 48-2 Evidence-Based Recommendations for Treatment of Skin and Soft-Tissue Infections (*Continued*)

Recommendations	Recommendation Grade[a]
Recommendations	
Hospitalized patients with complicated or purulent cellulitis should receive IV antibiotics with activity against MRSA pending culture data. Antibiotic options include vancomycin, linezolid, daptomycin, telavancin, and clindamycin	A-I for all except clindamycin; clindamycin A-III
In the treatment of *S. aureus* infections, trough serum vancomycin concentrations should always be maintained >10 mg/L (7 μmol/L) to avoid development of resistance	B-III
Necrotizing fasciitis	
Patients with severe nonpurulent cellulitis characterized by aggressive infection and associated with signs of systemic toxicity, necrotizing fasciitis, or gas gangrene should have prompt surgical consultation	Strong, low
Early and aggressive surgical debridement of all necrotic tissue is essential	A-III
Necrotizing fasciitis should be empirically treated with broad-spectrum antibiotics such as vancomycin or linezolid plus piperacillin–tazobactam or a carbapenem, or vancomycin or linezolid plus ceftriaxone and metronidazole	Strong, low
Necrotizing fasciitis caused by *S. pyogenes* should be treated with the combination of clindamycin and penicillin	Strong, low
In the treatment of necrotizing fasciitis caused by methicillin-resistant *S. aureus* infections, trough serum vancomycin concentrations of 15–20 mg/L (10–14 μmol/L) are recommended	B-II
Clostridial gas gangrene (myonecrosis) should be treated with clindamycin and penicillin	B-III
Diabetic foot infections	
Clinically uninfected wounds should not be treated with antibiotics	A-III
Empiric antibiotic regimens should be selected based on severity of infection and likely pathogens	A-III
Antibiotic therapy should target only aerobic gram-positive cocci in patients with mild-to-moderate infection who have not received antibiotics within the previous month	C-III
Broad-spectrum empiric antibiotic therapy should be initiated in most patients with severe infections, until culture and susceptibility data are available	A-III

Empiric antibiotics directed against *Pseudomonas aeruginosa* are usually unnecessary except in patients with specific risk factors for infection with this pathogen: patient has been soaking feet, patient has failed previous antibiotic therapy with nonpseudomonal agents, or clinically severe infection	A-III
Empiric antibiotics directed against MRSA should be considered in patients with specific risk factors, including prior history of infection or colonization with MRSA, high local prevalence of MRSA (eg, ≥50% for mild infections, ≥30% for severe infection), or clinically severe infection	C-III
Oral agents with high bioavailability may be used in the treatment of most mild, and many moderate, infections	A-II
Parenteral therapy is initially preferred for all severe, and some moderate, infections. After initial response, step-down therapy to oral agents can be considered	C-III
Definitive therapy should be based on results of appropriately collected cultures and sensitivities, as well as clinical response to empiric antimicrobial agents	A-III
Appropriate wound care, in addition to appropriate antimicrobial therapy, is often necessary for healing of infected wounds	A-III
Antibiotic therapy should only be continued until resolution of signs/symptoms of infection, but not necessarily until the wound is fully healed. The duration of therapy should initially be 1–2 weeks for mild infections and 2–3 weeks for moderate-to-severe infection	C-III
Pressure ulcers	
Optimize the host response by evaluating nutritional status and addressing deficits; stabilizing glycemic control; improving arterial blood flow; and/or reducing immunosuppressant therapy if possible	A-III
Consider the use of topical antiseptics for pressure ulcers that are not expected to heal and are critically colonized/topically infected	B-III
Consider use of silver sulfadiazine in heavily contaminated or infected pressure ulcers until definitive debridement is accomplished	B-III
Consider the use of medical-grade honey in heavily contaminated or infected pressure ulcers until definitive debridement is accomplished	C-III
Limit the use of topical antibiotics on infected pressure ulcers, except in special situations where the benefit to the patient outweighs the risk of antibiotic side effects and resistance	B-III

(Continued)

513

TABLE 48-2 Evidence-Based Recommendations for Treatment of Skin and Soft-Tissue Infections (*Continued*)

Recommendations	Recommendation Grade[a]
Use systemic antibiotics for individuals with clinical evidence of systemic infection, such as positive blood cultures, cellulitis, fasciitis, osteomyelitis, systemic inflammatory response syndrome (SIRS), or sepsis	B-III
Animal bites	
Preemptive early antibiotics should be administered for 3–5 days in patients with any of the following: immunocompromised; asplenic; advanced liver disease; preexisting or resultant edema of the bitten area; moderate-to-severe bite-related injuries, especially to the hands or face; or bite injuries that have penetrated the periosteum or joint capsule	Strong, low
Amoxicillin–clavulanic acid or other antibiotics active against both aerobic and anaerobic bacteria should be used for treatment of infected animal bites	Strong, moderate
Serious infections requiring IV antimicrobial therapy can be treated with a β-lactam/β-lactamase inhibitor combination or second-generation cephalosporin with activity against anaerobes (eg, cefoxitin)	B-II
Penicillinase-resistant penicillins, first-generation cephalosporins, macrolides, and clindamycin should not be used for treatment of infected wounds because of their poor activity against *Pasteurella multocida*	D-III
Human bites	
Antimicrobial therapy should provide coverage against *Eikenella corrodens*, *S. aureus*, and β-lactamase–producing anaerobes	B-III

[a]Qualitative (descriptive) recommendations are from: Stevens DL, Bisno AL, Chambers HF, et al. Practice guidelines for the diagnosis and management of skin and soft-tissue infections: 2014 update by the Infectious Diseases Society of America. Clin Infect Dis. 2014;59:e10–e52.

Strength of recommendation: A, good evidence for use; B, moderate evidence for use; C, poor evidence for use, optional; D, moderate evidence to support not using; E, good evidence to support not using. *Quality of evidence:* I, evidence from ≥1 properly randomized controlled trials; II, evidence from ≥1 well-designed clinical trials without randomization, case–control analytic studies, multiple time series, or dramatic results from uncontrolled experiments; III, evidence from expert opinion, clinical experience, descriptive studies, or reports of expert committees.

Qualitative (descriptive) recommendations: *strong, high:* strong recommendation, high-quality evidence from well-performed randomized controlled trials (RCTs) or exceptionally strong evidence from unbiased observational studies; *strong, moderate:* strong recommendation, moderate quality evidence from RCTs with important limitations or exceptionally strong evidence from unbiased observational studies; *strong, low:* strong recommendation, low-quality evidence for at least one critical outcome from observational studies, RCTs with serious flaws, or indirect evidence; *weak, moderate:* weak recommendation, moderate quality evidence from RCTs with important limitations or exceptionally strong evidence from unbiased observational studies; *weak, low:* weak recommendation, low-quality evidence for at least one critical outcome from observational studies, RCTs with serious flaws, or indirect evidence.

TABLE 48-3	Recommended Oral Drugs for Outpatient Treatment of Mild-to-Moderate Skin and Soft-Tissue Infections	
Infection	**Adults**	**Children**
Folliculitis	None; warm saline compresses usually sufficient	
Furuncles and carbuncles	Trimethoprim–sulfamethoxazole[a,b] Doxycycline[a,b] Minocycline[a,b]	Trimethoprim–sulfamethoxazole[a,b] Clindamycin[a,b]
Erysipelas	Procaine penicillin G Penicillin VK Clindamycin[a] Erythromycin[a]	Penicillin VK Clindamycin[a] Erythromycin[a]
Impetigo	Mupirocin ointment[a] Retapamulin ointment[a] Dicloxacillin Cephalexin Trimethoprim–sulfamethoxazole[a,b] Clindamycin[a,b] Doxycycline[a,b]	Mupirocin ointment[a] Retapamulin ointment[a] Dicloxacillin Cephalexin Trimethoprim–sulfamethoxazole[a] Clindamycin[a]
Lymphangitis	Initial IV therapy, followed by penicillin VK Clindamycin[a]	Initial IV therapy, followed by penicillin VK Clindamycin[a]
Cellulitis	Penicillin VK[c] Cephalexin[c] Dicloxacillin[c] Clindamycin[b,c] Trimethoprim–sulfamethoxazole[b,d] Doxycycline[b,d] Minocycline[b,d] Linezolid[b]	Penicillin VK[c] Cephalexin[c] Dicloxacillin[c] Clindamycin[b,c] Trimethoprim–sulfamethoxazole[b,d] Linezolid[b]
Diabetic foot infections	Dicloxacillin Clindamycin Cephalexin Amoxicillin–clavulanate Levofloxacin ± metronidazole or clindamycin[a,e] Ciprofloxacin ± metronidazole or clindamycin[a,e] Moxifloxacin	

(Continued)

TABLE 48-3	Recommended Oral Drugs for Outpatient Treatment of Mild-to-Moderate Skin and Soft-Tissue Infections (*Continued*)	
Infection	**Adults**	**Children**
Bite wounds (animal or human)	Amoxicillin–clavulanate	Amoxicillin–clavulanate
	Doxycycline[a]	Trimethoprim–sulfamethoxazole + metronidazole or clindamycin[a]
	Moxifloxacin[a]	
	Trimethoprim–sulfamethoxazole + metronidazole or clindamycin[a]	Cefuroxime axetil + metronidazole or clindamycin
	Levofloxacin or ciprofloxacin + metronidazole or clindamycin[a]	Dicloxacillin + penicillin VK
	Cefuroxime axetil + metronidazole or clindamycin	
	Dicloxacillin + penicillin VK	

[a]May be used in patients with penicillin allergy.
[b]Recommended if CA-MRSA is suspected.
[c]For nonpurulent cellulitis when CA-MRSA is not suspected, or purulent cellulitis when CA-MRSA not documented (not penicillin VK).
[d]May be combined with amoxicillin if additional coverage for streptococci is desired.
[e]Fluoroquinolone alone may be suitable for mild infections, while addition of drugs with antianaerobic activity may be recommended for more severe infections.

- Cellulitis is most often caused by *S. pyogenes* or *S. aureus* (see **Table 48-1**).
- Acute cellulitis with mixed aerobic and anaerobic pathogens may occur in diabetics, following traumatic injuries, at sites of surgical incisions to the abdomen or perineum, or where host defenses have been otherwise compromised (vascular insufficiency).

CLINICAL PRESENTATION

- Cellulitis is characterized by erythema and edema of the skin. The lesion, which may be extensive, is painful and nonelevated and has poorly defined margins. Tender lymphadenopathy associated with lymphatic involvement is common. Malaise, fever, and chills are also commonly present. There is usually a history of an antecedent wound from minor trauma, an ulcer, or surgery.
- A Gram stain of a smear obtained by injection and aspiration of 0.5 mL of saline (using a small-gauge needle) into the advancing edge of the erythematous lesion may help in making the microbiologic diagnosis but often yields negative results. Blood cultures are useful, as bacteremia may be present in 30% of cases.

TREATMENT

- <u>Goals of Treatment</u>: Rapid eradication of the infection and prevention of further complications. Antimicrobial therapy of bacterial cellulitis is directed toward the type of bacteria either documented to be present or suspected. Local care of cellulitis includes elevation and immobilization of the involved area to decrease local swelling. Incision and drainage is the primary therapy for infections such as small abscesses and furuncles, and in otherwise uncomplicated patients with mild infections. Systemic antibiotic therapy is often unnecessary in such cases.
- Antibiotic therapy is recommended along with incision and drainage in patients with more complicated abscesses associated with the following: severe or extensive disease involving multiple sites of infection; rapidly progressive infection in the presence of associated cellulitis; signs and symptoms of systemic illness; complicating factors such as extremes of age, comorbidities, or immunosuppression; abscesses in areas

TABLE 48-4 Drug Dosing Table[a]

Drug	Brand Name	Usual Dosing Range	Special Population Dose	Other
Oral agents				
Amoxicillin–clavulanate	Augmentin	875/125 mg orally every 12 hours	Pediatric: 40 mg/kg (of the amoxicillin component) orally in two divided doses	
Cefaclor	Ceclor	500 mg orally every 8 hours	Pediatric: 20–40 mg/kg/day (not to exceed 1 g) orally in three divided doses	
Cefadroxil	Duricef	250–500 mg orally every 12 hours	Pediatric: 30 mg/kg orally in two divided doses	
Cefuroxime axetil	Ceftin	250–500 mg orally every 12 hours	Pediatric: 20–30 mg/kg orally in two divided doses	
Cephalexin	Keflex	250–500 mg orally every 6 hours	Pediatric: 25–50 mg/kg orally in four divided doses	
Ciprofloxacin	Cipro	500–750 mg orally every 12 hours		
Clindamycin	Cleocin	300–600 mg orally every 6–8 hours	Pediatric: 10–30 mg/kg/day orally in three to four divided doses	May be used for oral treatment of MRSA infection
Delafloxacin	Baxdela	450 mg orally every 12 hours		May be used for oral treatment of MRSA infection
Dicloxacillin	Dynapen	250–500 mg orally every 6 hours	Pediatric: 25–50 mg/kg orally in four divided doses	
Doxycycline	Vibramycin	100–200 mg orally every 12 hours		May be used for oral treatment of MRSA infection
Erythromycin	E-Mycin Erythrocin	250–500 mg orally every 6 hours	Pediatric: 30–50 mg/kg orally in four divided doses[a]	

(*Continued*)

TABLE 48-4 Drug Dosing Table[a] (Continued)

Drug	Brand Name	Usual Dosing Range	Special Population Dose	Other
Levofloxacin	Levaquin	500–750 mg orally once daily		
Linezolid	Zyvox	600 mg orally every 12 hours	Pediatric: 20–30 mg/kg/day orally in two to three divided doses	For oral treatment of MRSA infection
Metronidazole	Flagyl	250–500 mg orally every 8 hours	Pediatric: 30 mg/kg orally in three to four divided doses	
Moxifloxacin	Avelox	400 mg orally once daily		
Mupirocin ointment	Bactroban	Apply to affected areas every 8 hours	Pediatric: apply to affected areas every 8 hours	
Penicillin VK	Veetids Pen-V	250–500 mg orally every 6 hours	Pediatric: 25,000–90,000 units/kg orally in four divided doses	
Retapamulin ointment	Altabax	Apply to affected area every 12 hours	Pediatric: apply to affected area every 12 hours	
Tedizolid	Sivextro	200 mg orally once daily		For oral treatment of MRSA infection
Trimethoprim–sulfamethoxazole	Bactrim Septra Cotrimoxazole	160/800 mg orally every 12 hours	Pediatric: 4–6 mg/kg (of the trimethoprim component) orally every 12 hours	Up to double the usual dose may be considered for oral treatment of MRSA infection
Parenteral agents				
Ampicillin	Omnipen Polycillin Principen	1–2 g IV every 6 hours	Pediatric: 200–300 mg/kg/day IV in four to six divided doses	

Generic	Brand	Dose	Comments
Aztreonam	Azactam	1 g IV every 6 hours	Pediatric: 100–150 mg/kg/day IV in four divided doses
Cefazolin	Ancef, Kefzol	1 g IV every 6–8 hours	Pediatric: 75 mg/kg/day IV in three divided doses
Cefepime	Maxipime	1–2 g IV every 12 hours	Pediatric: 100 mg/kg/day IV in two divided doses
Cefotaxime	Claforan	1–2 g IV every 6 hours	150–200 mg/kg/day in three to four divided doses
Cefoxitin	Mefoxin	1–2 g IV every 6 hours	Pediatric: 30–40 mg/kg/day IV in four divided doses
Ceftazidime	Fortaz	1–2 g IV every 8 hours	Pediatric: 150 mg/kg/day IV in three divided doses
Ceftaroline	Teflaro	600 mg IV every 12 hours	For MRSA infection
Ceftriaxone	Rocephin	1 g IV once daily	
Cefuroxime	Zinacef	0.75–1.5 g IV every 8 hours	Pediatric: 150 mg/kg/day IV in three divided doses
Ciprofloxacin	Cipro	400 mg IV every 8–12 hours	
Clindamycin	Cleocin	300–600 mg IV every 6–8 hours; 600–900 mg IV every 6–8 hours for necrotizing fasciitis	Pediatric: 30–50 mg/kg/day IV in three to four divided doses
Dalbavancin	Dalvance	1000 mg IV once on day 1 of therapy, followed by 500 mg IV once on day 8 of therapy; OR 1500 mg IV once with no additional doses	For MRSA infection
Daptomycin	Cubicin	4 mg/kg IV once daily	For MRSA infection
Delafloxacin	Baxdela	300 mg IV every 12 hours	For MRSA infection
Doripenem	Doribax	500 mg IV every 8 hours	For MRSA infection

(Continued)

TABLE 48-4	Drug Dosing Table^a (Continued)			
Drug	Brand Name	Usual Dosing Range	Special Population Dose	Other
Ertapenem	Invanz	1 g IV once daily	Pediatric: 30 mg/kg/day IV in one to two divided doses	
Gentamicin	Garamycin	Traditional: 2 mg/kg loading dose, followed by 1.5 mg/kg IV every 8 hours and guided by measured serum concentrations. Alternative: 5–7 mg/kg IV once daily	Pediatric: 5–7 mg/kg/day IV in three divided doses; doses guided by serum concentrations	
Imipenem–cilastatin	Primaxin	250–500 mg IV every 6–8 hours	Pediatric: 40–80 mg/kg/day IV in four divided doses	
Levofloxacin	Levaquin	500–750 mg IV once daily		
Linezolid	Zyvox	600 mg IV every 12 hours	Pediatric: 20–30 mg/kg/day IV in two to three divided doses	For MRSA infection
Meropenem	Merrem	1 g IV every 8 hours	Pediatric: 60 mg/kg/day IV in three divided doses	
Metronidazole	Flagyl	500 mg IV every 8 hours	Pediatric: 30–50 mg/kg/day IV in three divided doses	
Moxifloxacin	Avelox	400 mg IV once daily		
Nafcillin	Nafcil	1–2 g IV every 4–6 hours	Pediatric: 100–200 mg/kg/day IV in four to six equally divided doses	
Oritavancin	Orbactiv	1200 mg IV once with no additional doses		For MRSA infection

Drug	Brand	Adult Dose	Pediatric Dose	Comment
Penicillin G	Pfizerpen Bicillin Wycillin	1–2 million units IV every 4–6 hours	Pediatric: 100,000–200,000 units/kg/day IV in four divided doses[a]	
Piperacillin–tazobactam	Zosyn	3.375–4.5 g IV every 6 hours	Pediatric: 250–350 mg/kg/day IV in three to four divided doses	
Procaine penicillin G	Bicillin C-R	0.6–1.2 million units IM every 12 hours	Pediatric: 25,000–50,000 units/kg (maximum 1.2 million units) IM once daily	
Tedizolid	Sivextro	200 mg IV once daily		For MRSA infection
Telavancin	Vibativ	10 mg/kg IV once daily		For MRSA infection
Tigecycline	Tigacil	100 mg IV once, and then 50 mg IV every 12 hours		
Tobramycin	Nebcin	Traditional: 2 mg/kg loading dose, followed by 1.5 mg/kg IV every 8 hours and guided by measured serum concentrations. Alternative: 5–7 mg/kg IV once daily	Pediatric: 5–7 mg/kg/day IV in three divided doses; doses guided by serum concentrations	
Vancomycin	Vancocin	30–40 mg/kg/day IV in two divided doses; dosing guided by serum concentrations to achieve trough of 15–20 mg/L (10–14 μmol/L)	Pediatric: 40–60 mg/kg/day IV in three to four divided doses; doses guided by serum concentrations	For MRSA infection

[a]Dosing guidelines in patients with normal renal function.
IM, intramuscularly; MRSA, methicillin-resistant S. aureus.

that are difficult to drain, such as hands, face, and genitalia; or lack of response to previous drainage alone.

- Oral agents recommended for moderate purulent cellulitis include **trimethoprim–sulfamethoxazole** and **doxycycline** (**Figure 48-1**). Oral **linezolid** is also recommended in such cases but is significantly more expensive and apparently no more efficacious than other treatment options.

- Patients with severe purulent cellulitis should be hospitalized for empiric treatment with parenteral antibiotics having activity against MRSA. **Vancomycin, daptomycin, linezolid, televancin,** and **ceftaroline** are all acceptable treatment options with comparable efficacy in adults (**Figure 48-1**). In children, **vancomycin, linezolid,** or **clindamycin** are the preferred treatment options.

- Empiric therapy of nonpurulent cellulitis is directed primarily against group A β-hemolytic streptococci. Recommended empiric therapy of mild nonpurulent cellulitis (ie, no focus of purulence or systemic signs of infection) consists of an orally administered β-lactam such as **penicillin VK, cephalexin,** or **dicloxacillin.**

- Hospitalization and treatment with parenteral antibiotics are also recommended for patients with severe nonpurulent cellulitis as indicated by the presence of systemic findings of infection, failure of previous oral antibiotic therapy, immunocompromised states, or presence of clinical signs of deeper infection such as bullae, skin sloughing, hypotension, or organ dysfunction. Recommended regimens include vancomycin plus **piperacillin–tazobactam,** and **vancomycin** plus **imipenem–cilastatin** or **meropenem.**

Diabetic Foot Infections

- Three key factors are involved in the causation of diabetic foot problems: neuropathy, ischemia, and immunologic defects. Any of these disorders can occur in isolation; however, they frequently occur together.

- There are three major types of diabetic foot infections (DFIs): deep abscesses, cellulitis of the dorsum, and mal perforans ulcers of the sole of the foot. Osteomyelitis may occur in 30%–40% of infections.

- Mild cases of DFIs are often monomicrobial. However, more severe infections are typically polymicrobic; up to 60% of hospitalized patients have polymicrobial infections. Staphylococci and streptococci are the most common pathogens, although gram-negative bacilli and anaerobes occur in 50% of cases.

- Patients with peripheral neuropathy often do not experience pain but seek medical attention for swelling or erythema. Lesions vary in size and clinical features. A foul-smelling odor suggests anaerobic organisms. Temperature may be mildly elevated or normal.

TREATMENT

- <u>Goals of Treatment</u>: (a) Successfully treat infected wounds by using effective nondrug and antibiotic therapy; (b) prevent additional infectious complications; (c) preserve as much normal limb function as possible; (d) avoid unnecessary use of antimicrobials that contribute to increased resistance; and (e) minimize toxicities and cost while increasing patient quality of life.

- Up to 90% of infections can be treated successfully with a comprehensive treatment approach that includes both wound care and antimicrobial therapy. After carefully assessing the extent of the lesion and obtaining necessary cultures, necrotic tissue must be thoroughly debrided, with wound drainage and amputation as required.

- Diabetic glycemic control should be maximized to ensure optimal healing.

- The patient should initially be restricted to bed rest, leg elevation, and control of edema, if present.

- Suggested antibiotic regimens for empiric treatment of DFIs are given in **Table 48-5.** Treatment algorithms for initial management of mild-to-moderate DFI and severe DFI are shown in **Figures 48-2** and **48-3.**

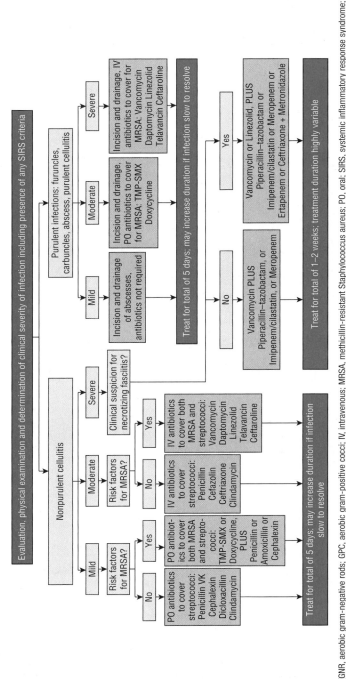

FIGURE 48-1. Recommended treatment algorithm for initial empiric management of selected purulent and nonpurulent skin and soft-tissue infections.

(GNR, aerobic gram-negative rods; GPC, aerobic gram-positive cocci; IV, intravenous; MRSA, methicillin-resistant Staphylococcus aureus; PO, oral; SIRS, systemic inflammatory response syndrome; TMP-SMX, trimethoprim–sulfamethoxazole.)

TABLE 48-5 Suggested Antibiotic Regimens for Empiric Treatment of Diabetic Foot Infections

Severity of Infection	Probable Pathogens	Drug(s)[a]	Duration of Therapy
Mild	*Staphylococcus aureus* (MSSA) *Streptococcus* spp. *S. aureus* (MRSA) • Patients with history of MRSA infection or colonization in past year • Prevalence of MRSA ≥50% in local geographic area • Recent hospitalization	Amoxicillin–clavulanate Cephalexin Dicloxacillin Clindamycin Levofloxacin Moxifloxacin[b]	1–2 weeks; may increase up to 4 weeks if infection slow to resolve
Moderate-to-severe (initially oral or IV antibiotics for moderately severe infections, IV antibiotics for severe infections)	MSSA *Streptococcus* spp. Enterobacteriaceae Obligate anaerobes MRSA • Patients with history of MRSA infection or colonization in past year • Prevalence of MRSA ≥30% in local geographic area	Ampicillin/Sulbactam Cefoxitin Ceftriaxone Imipenem/Cilastatin Ertapenem Levofloxacin Moxifloxacin Tigecycline Levofloxacin or ciprofloxacin + clindamycin Add to one of the above regimens: • Vancomycin • Linezolid • Daptomycin	Moderately severe infection: 1–3 weeks; severe infection: 2–4 weeks

- Recent hospitalization
- Infection severe enough that not empirically covering MRSA poses unacceptable risk of treatment failure

Piperacillin/Tazobactam

Pseudomonas aeruginosa
- Patient has been soaking feet
- Patient has previously failed therapy with nonpseudomonal antibiotic regimen
- Severe infection

Cefepime, ceftazidime, or aztreonam + metronidazole or clindamycin + vancomycin[c]

or

Piperacillin–tazobactam or imipenem–cilastatin or meropenem[b] + vancomycin[c]

Mixed infections potentially including all of the above

[a]Agents not shown in any particular order of preference.
[b]Not specifically recommended in IDSA guidelines but may be appropriate treatment option.
[c]Linezolid or daptomycin may be used in place of vancomycin.
MRSA, methicillin-resistant S. aureus; MSSA, methicillin-susceptible S. aureus.

FIGURE 48-2. Recommended treatment algorithm for initial empiric management of mild-to-moderate diabetic foot infections.

(GNR, aerobic gram-negative rods; GPC, aerobic gram-positive cocci; MRSA, methicillin-resistant *Staphylococcus aureus*; TMP-SMX, trimethoprim–sulfamethoxazole.)

aMay substitute metronidazole in place of clindamycin.

[a]May substitute linezolid or daptomycin for vancomycin.

(GNR, aerobic gram-negative rods; MRSA, methicillin-resistant *Staphylococcus aureus*; MSSA, methicillin-susceptible *S. aureus*.)

FIGURE 48-3. Recommended treatment algorithm for initial empiric management of severe diabetic foot infections.

Infected Pressure Ulcers

- A pressure sore is also called a "decubitus ulcer" or "bed sore." A classification system for pressure sores is presented in **Table 48-6**. Many factors are thought to predispose patients to the formation of pressure ulcers: paralysis, paresis, immobilization, malnutrition, anemia, infection, and advanced age. Factors thought to be most critical to their formation are pressure, shearing forces, friction, and moisture; however, there is still debate as to the exact pathophysiology of pressure sore formation. The areas of highest pressure are generated over the bony prominences.
- Most pressure sores are heavily colonized by microorganisms. A large variety of aerobic gram-positive and gram-negative bacteria, as well as anaerobes, are frequently isolated from wound cultures.

CLINICAL PRESENTATION

- Most pressure sores are in the pelvic region and lower extremities. The most common sites are the sacral and coccygeal areas, ischial tuberosities, and greater trochanter.
- A dark red color on the surface of a pressure sore may indicate local infection. Surrounding erythema, swelling, and heat are commonly present with infection. Purulent discharge, foul odor, and systemic signs (fever and leukocytosis) may be present.
- Pressure sores vary greatly in their severity, ranging from an abrasion to large lesions that can penetrate into the deep fascia involving both bone and muscle.

TABLE 48-6	Pressure Injury Classification
Stage 1	Intact skin with a localized area of nonblanchable erythema. Presence of blanchable erythema or changes in sensation, temperature, or firmness may precede visual changes. Color changes do not include purple or maroon discoloration; these may indicate deep tissue pressure injury.
Stage 2	Partial-thickness loss of skin with exposed dermis. Wound bed is viable, pink or red, moist, and may also present as an intact or ruptured serum-filled blister. Adipose tissue is not visible and deeper tissues are not visible. Granulation tissue, slough, and eschar are not present.
Stage 3[a]	Full-thickness loss of skin, in which adipose tissue is visible in the ulcer and granulation tissue and epibole (rolled wound edges) are often present. Slough and/or eschar may be visible. Depth of tissue damage varies by anatomical location; areas of significant adiposity can develop deep wounds. Undermining and tunneling may occur. Fascia, muscle, tendon, ligament, cartilage, and/or bone are not exposed.
Stage 4[a]	Full-thickness skin and tissue loss with exposed or directly palpable fascia, muscle, tendon, ligament, cartilage, or bone in the ulcer. Slough and/or eschar may be visible. Epibole (rolled edges), undermining, and/or tunneling often occur. Depth varies by anatomical location.
Unstageable[a]	Full-thickness skin and tissue loss in which the extent of tissue damage within the ulcer cannot be confirmed because it is obscured by slough or eschar. If slough or eschar is removed, a stage 3 or stage 4 pressure injury will be revealed.
Deep-tissue pressure injury	Intact or nonintact skin with localized area of persistent nonblanchable deep red, maroon, purple discoloration or epidermal separation revealing a dark wound bed or blood-filled blister. Pain and temperature change often precede skin color changes. This injury results from intense and/or prolonged pressure and shear forces at the bone-muscle interface. The wound may evolve rapidly to reveal the actual extent of tissue injury, or may resolve without tissue loss.

[a]Stage 3, stage 4, and unstageable lesions are unlikely to resolve on their own and often require surgical intervention.

PREVENTION AND TREATMENT

- <u>Goals of Treatment</u>: The primary goal for pressure sores is prevention. Once a pressure sore has developed, the goals of therapy are prevention of complications (ie, infections), preventing sores from growing larger, and preventing the development of sores in other locations.
- Prevention is the single most important aspect in managing pressure sores. Friction and shearing forces can be minimized by proper positioning. Skin care and prevention of soilage are important, with the intent being to keep the surface relatively free from moisture. Relief for a period of only 5 minutes once every 2 hours gives protection against pressure sore formation.
- The goal of therapy is to clean and decontaminate the ulcer in order to permit formation of healthy granulation tissue that promotes wound healing or prepares the wound for an operative procedure. The main factors to be considered for successful wound care are: (1) relief of pressure; (2) debridement of necrotic tissue; (3) wound cleansing; (4) dressing selection; and (5) prevention, diagnosis, and treatment of infection.

- Medical management is generally indicated for lesions that are of moderate size and of relatively shallow depth (stage 1 or 2 lesions) and are not located over a bony prominence.
- Debridement can be accomplished by surgical, mechanical (wet-to-dry dressing changes), or chemical means. Other effective therapies are hydrotherapy, wound irrigation, and dextranomers. Pressure sores should be cleaned with normal saline.
- A short, 2-week trial of topical antibiotic (**silver sulfadiazine** or **triple antibiotic**) is recommended for a clean ulcer that is not healing or is producing a moderate amount of exudate despite appropriate care.

Infected Bite Wounds

- Patients at risk of acquiring an infection after a bite have had a puncture wound, have not sought medical attention within 8 hours of injury, or are older than 50 years.
- An infected dog or cat bite is usually characterized by erythema, and clear or purulent discharge at the wound site. If *Pasteurella multocida* is present, a rapidly progressing cellulitis is observed within 24–48 hours of initial injury.
- Most infections from dog and cat bites are polymicrobial. *Pasteurella* is the most frequent isolate.
- Bite wounds should be irrigated thoroughly with a copious volume of sterile water or saline, and the wound washed vigorously with soap or povidone–iodine in order to reduce the bacterial count in the wound. Surgical debridement and immobilization of the affected area are often required in dog and human bites associated with more extensive tissue injury.
- The role of antimicrobials for non-infected dog bite wounds remains controversial. A 3–5 day antibiotic prophylaxis regimen is recommended in patients with the following factors associated with increased risk for infection: immunocompromised; asplenic; advanced liver disease; preexisting or resultant edema of the affected area; moderate-to-severe bite-related injuries, especially to the hands or face; or bite injuries that have penetrated the periosteum or joint capsule.
- Empiric antibiotics for the treatment of established infection of dog and cat bite wounds should be directed at a variety of aerobic and anaerobic flora. **Amoxicillin–clavulanic** acid is commonly recommended for oral outpatient therapy. Alternative oral agents include **doxycycline** alone, or **trimethoprim–sulfamethoxazole, levofloxacin, ciprofloxacin**, or a second- or third-generation cephalosporin in combination with **metronidazole** or **clindamycin** to provide activity against oropharyngeal anaerobes.
- Treatment options for patients requiring IV therapy include β-lactam–β-lactamase inhibitors (**ampicillin–sulbactam** and **piperacillin–tazobactam**), second-generation cephalosporins with antianaerobic activity (**cefoxitin**), and **ertapenem**. Therapy should generally be continued from 7 to 14 days.
- If the immunization history of a patient with anything other than a clean minor wound is not known, tetanus/diphtheria toxoids (TD) should be administered. Both TD and tetanus immunoglobulin should be administered to patients who have never been immunized.
- If a patient has been exposed to rabies, the treatment objectives consist of thorough irrigation of the wound, tetanus prophylaxis, antibiotic prophylaxis (if indicated), and immunization. Postexposure prophylaxis immunization consists of both passive antibody administration and vaccine administration.

Human Bites

- Infections caused by these injuries are most often caused by the normal oral flora, which includes both aerobic and anaerobic microorganisms. Human bite wounds are notable for potential involvement of *Eikenella corrodens* in approximately 30% of infections.

- Management of bite wounds consists of aggressive irrigation and topical wound dressing, surgical debridement, and immobilization of the affected area. Primary closure for human bites is not generally recommended. Tetanus toxoid and antitoxin may be indicated.
- All patients with human bite injuries should receive prophylactic antibiotic therapy ("early preemptive therapy") for 3–5 days due to high infection risk.
- **Amoxicillin–clavulanic** acid (500 mg every 8 hours) is commonly recommended. Alternatives for penicillin-allergic patients include fluoroquinolones or **trimethoprim–sulfamethoxazole** in combination with **clindamycin** or **metronidazole**.
- Patients with serious injuries or clenched-fist injuries should be started on IV antibiotics. Treatment options for patients requiring IV therapy include β-lactam–β-lactamase inhibitor combinations (**ampicillin–sulbactam, piperacillin–tazobactam**), second-generation cephalosporins with antianaerobic activity (eg, **cefoxitin**), and **ertapenem**.

See Chapter 128, Skin and Soft-Tissue Infections, authored by Douglas N. Fish, for a more detailed discussion of this topic.

CHAPTER 49

Surgical Prophylaxis

- Antibiotics administered prior to the contamination of previously sterile tissues or fluids are considered prophylactic. The goal of prophylactic antibiotics is to prevent an infection from developing.
- Presumptive antibiotic therapy is administered when an infection is suspected but not yet proven. Therapeutic antibiotics are required for established infection.
- *Surgical-site infections* (SSIs) are classified as either incisional (eg, cellulitis of the incision site) or involving an organ or space (eg, with meningitis). Incisional SSIs may be superficial (skin or subcutaneous tissue) or deep (fascial and muscle layers). Both types, by definition, occur by postoperative day 30. This period extends to 1 year from the date of surgery in the case of prosthesis implantation involvement with a deep incisional or organ/space infection

RISK FACTORS FOR SURGICAL WOUND INFECTION

- The traditional classification system developed by the National Research Council (NRC) stratifying surgical procedures by infection risk is reproduced in **Table 49-1**. The NRC wound classification for a specific procedure is determined intraoperatively and is the primary determinant of whether antibiotic prophylaxis is warranted.
- The Study on the Efficacy of Nosocomial Infection Control (SENIC) analyzed more than 100,000 surgery cases and identified abdominal operations, operations lasting more than 2 hours, contaminated or dirty procedures, and more than three underlying medical diagnoses as factors associated with an increased incidence of SSI. When the NRC classification described in **Table 49-1** was stratified by the number of SENIC risk factors present, the infection rates varied by as much as a factor of 15 within the same operative category.
- The SENIC risk assessment technique has been modified to include the American Society of Anesthesiologists preoperative assessment score (**Table 49-2**). An American Society of Anesthesiologists score greater than or equal to three was a strong predictor for the development of an SSI.

BACTERIOLOGY

- Bacteria involved in SSI are acquired either from the patient's normal flora (endogenous) or from contamination during the surgical procedure (exogenous).
- The loss of normal flora through the use of broad-spectrum antibiotics can destabilize homeostasis, allowing pathogenic bacteria to proliferate and infection to occur.
- Normal flora can become pathogenic when translocated to a normally sterile tissue site or fluid during surgical procedures.
- The five most common pathogens encountered in surgical wounds are *Staphylococcus aureus*, coagulase-negative staphylococci, Enterococci, *Escherichia coli*, and *Pseudomonas aeruginosa*.
- Impaired host defenses, vascular occlusive states, traumatized tissues, and the presence of a foreign body greatly decrease the number of bacteria required to cause an SSI.

| TABLE 49-1 | National Research Council Wound Classification, Risk of Surgical Site Infection, and Indication for Antibiotics |

| | SSI Rate (%) | | | |
Classification	**Preoperative Antibiotics**	**No Preoperative Antibiotics**	**Criteria**	**Antibiotics**
Clean	0.8	5.1	No acute inflammation or transection of GI, oropharyngeal, genitourinary, biliary, or respiratory tracts; elective case, no technique break	Not indicated unless high-risk procedure[a]
Clean–contaminated	1.3	10.1	Controlled opening of aforementioned tracts with minimal spillage/minor technique break; clean procedures performed emergently or with major technique breaks	Prophylactic antibiotics indicated
Contaminated	10.2	21.9	Acute, nonpurulent inflammation present; major spillage/technique break during clean–contaminated procedure	Prophylactic antibiotics indicated
Dirty	N/A	N/A	Obvious preexisting infection present (abscess, pus, or necrotic tissue present)	Therapeutic antibiotics required

[a]High-risk procedures include implantation of prosthetic materials and other procedures where surgical site infection is associated with high morbidity (see the text).
N/A, not applicable; SSI, surgical site infection.

ANTIBIOTIC ISSUES

SCHEDULING ANTIBIOTIC ADMINISTRATION

- The following principles must be considered when providing antimicrobial surgical prophylaxis:
  - ✓ Antimicrobials should be delivered to the surgical site prior to the initial incision. They should be administered within 60 minutes prior to the initial incision, preferably at the time of anesthetic induction. Antibiotics should not be prescribed to be given "on-call to the OR (operating room)."
  - ✓ Bactericidal antibiotic tissue concentrations should be maintained throughout the surgical procedure.
- Strategies to ensure appropriate antimicrobial prophylaxis use are described in Table 49-3.

TABLE 49-2	Surgical Site Infection Incidence (%) Stratified by NRC Wound Classification and SENIC Risk Factors[a]			
Number of SENIC Risk Factors	**Clean**	**Clean–Contaminated**	**Contaminated**	**Dirty**
0	1.1	0.6	N/A	N/A
1	3.9	2.8	4.5	6.7
2	8.4	8.4	8.3	10.9
3	15.8	17.7	11.0	18.8
4	N/A	N/A	23.9	27.4

[a]Study on the Efficacy of Nosocomial Infection Control (SENIC) risk factors include abdominal operation, operations lasting >2 hours, contaminated or dirty procedures by National Research Council (NRC) classification, and more than three underlying medical diagnoses.
N/A, not applicable; NRC, National Research Council; SENIC, Study on the Efficacy of Nosocomial Infection Control.
Reproduced, with permission, from Wilson AP, Hodgson B, Liu M, et al. Reduction in wound infection rates by wound surveillance with postdischarge follow-up and feedback. Br J Surg. 2006;93:630-638.

TABLE 49-3	Strategies for Implementing an Institutional Program to Ensure Appropriate Use of Antimicrobial Prophylaxis in Surgery

1. **Educate:** Develop an educational program that enforces the importance and rationale of timely antimicrobial prophylaxis. Make this educational program available to all healthcare practitioners involved in the patient's care.

2. **Standardize the ordering process:** Establish a protocol (eg, a preprinted order sheet) that standardizes antibiotic choice according to current published evidence, formulary availability, institutional resistance patterns, and cost.

3. **Standardize the delivery and administration process**: Use system that ensures antibiotics are prepared and delivered to the holding area in a timely fashion. Standardize the administration time to <1 hour preoperatively. Designate responsibility and accountability for antibiotic administration. Provide visible reminders to prescribe/administer prophylactic antibiotics (eg, checklists). Develop a system to remind surgeons/nurses to readminister antibiotics intraoperatively during long procedures.

4. **Provide feedback**: Follow up with regular reports of compliance and infection rates.

ANTIMICROBIAL SELECTION

- The choice of the prophylactic antimicrobial depends on the type of surgical procedure, most likely pathogenic organisms, safety and efficacy of the antimicrobial, current literature evidence supporting its use, and cost.
- Typically, gram-positive coverage is included in the choice of surgical prophylaxis because organisms such as *S. aureus* and *S. epidermidis* are common skin flora.
- Parenteral antibiotic administration is favored because of its reliability in achieving suitable tissue concentrations.
- First-generation cephalosporins (particularly **cefazolin**) are the preferred choice, particularly for clean surgical procedures. Antianaerobic cephalosporins (eg, **cefoxitin** or **cefotetan**) are appropriate choices when broad-spectrum anaerobic and gram-negative coverage are desired.
- Although third-generation cephalosporins (eg, **ceftriaxone**) have been advocated for prophylaxis because of their increased gram-negative coverage and prolonged half-lives, their inferior gram-positive and anaerobic activity and high cost have discouraged the widespread use of these agents.

- **Vancomycin** may be considered for prophylactic therapy in surgical procedures involving implantation of a prosthetic device in which the rate of methicillin-resistant *S. aureus* (MRSA) is high. If the risk of MRSA is low and a β-lactam hypersensitivity exists, **clindamycin** can be used instead of cefazolin in order to limit vancomycin use.

RECOMMENDATIONS FOR SPECIFIC TYPES OF SURGERIES

- Specific recommendations are summarized in **Table 49-4**.

GASTRODUODENAL SURGERY

- The risk of infection rises with conditions that increase gastric pH and subsequent bacterial overgrowth, such as obstruction, hemorrhage, malignancy, and acid-suppression therapy (clean-contaminated).
- A single dose of intravenous (IV) **cefazolin** will provide adequate prophylaxis for most cases. Oral **ciprofloxacin** may be used for patients with β-lactam hypersensitivity.
- Postoperative therapeutic antibiotics may be indicated if perforation is detected during surgery, depending on whether an established infection is present.

HEPATOBILIARY SURGERY

- Antibiotic prophylaxis has been proven beneficial for surgery involving the biliary tract.
- Most frequently encountered organisms include *E. coli, Klebsiella*, and Enterococci. Single-dose prophylaxis with **cefazolin** is currently recommended. **Ciprofloxacin** and **levofloxacin** are alternatives for patients with β-lactam hypersensitivity.
- For patients undergoing elective laparoscopic cholecystectomy, antibiotic prophylaxis has traditionally not been recommended but newer trials and systematic reviews are conflicting and assessments of current practice are reflective of this.
- Ciprofloxacin and levofloxacin are effective alternatives for β-lactam-allergic patients undergoing open cholecystectomy.
- Detection of an active infection during surgery (gangrenous gallbladder or suppurative cholangitis) is an indication for therapeutic postoperative antibiotics.

COLORECTAL SURGERY

- Anaerobes and gram-negative aerobes predominate in SSIs (see **Table 49-4**), although gram-positive aerobes are also important. Therefore, the risk of an SSI in the absence of an adequate prophylactic regimen is substantial.
- Risk factors for SSIs include age over 60 years, hypoalbuminemia, poor preoperative bowel preparation, corticosteroid therapy, malignancy, and operations lasting longer than 3.5 hours.
- Reducing bacteria load with a thorough bowel preparation regimen (4 L of polyethylene glycol solution or 90 mL of sodium phosphate solution administered orally the day before surgery) is controversial, even though it is used by most surgeons.
- While oral or parenteral antimicrobials have been used, combination therapy (oral and IV) was superior to oral regimens alone and IV regimens alone. The combination of 1 g of **neomycin** and 1 g of **erythromycin base** given orally 19, 18, and 9 hours preoperatively is the most commonly used oral regimen in the United States. **Cefoxitin** and **cefotetan** are the IV agents used most commonly, but other second- and some third-generation cephalosporins also are effective.
- Postoperative antibiotics are unnecessary in the absence of any untoward events or findings during surgery.

APPENDECTOMY

- Preoperative antimicrobials are effective at reducing the risk of infection after appendectomy and should be administered in all cases.

TABLE 49-4 Most Likely Pathogens and Specific Recommendations for Surgical Prophylaxis

Type of Operation	Likely Pathogens	Recommended Prophylaxis Regimen[a]	Comments	Grade of Recommendation[b]
GI surgery				
Gastroduodenal	Enteric gram-negative bacilli, gram-positive cocci, oral anaerobes	Cefazolin 1 g × 1	High-risk patients only (obstruction, hemorrhage, malignancy, acid suppression therapy, morbid obesity)	IA
Bariatric Surgery	Enteric gram-negative bacilli, gram-positive cocci, oral anaerobes	Cefazolin 2 g × 1	Intraoperative redosing required for procedures longer than 4 hours	IB
Cholecystectomy	Enteric gram-negative bacilli, anaerobes	Cefazolin 1 g × 1 for high-risk patients; laparoscopic: controversial	High-risk patients only (open biliary tract procedures, acute cholecystitis, common duct stones, previous biliary surgery, jaundice, age >60 years, obesity, diabetes mellitus)	IA
Transjugular intrahepatic portosystemic shunt (TIPS)	Enteric gram-negative bacilli, anaerobes	Ceftriaxone 1 g × 1	Longer-acting cephalosporins preferred	IA
Appendectomy	Enteric gram-negative bacilli, anaerobes	Cefoxitin or cefotetan 1 g × 1 or cefazolin 1 g plus metronidazole 1 g × 1	Second intraoperative dose of cefoxitin may be required if procedure lasts longer than 3 hours	IA
Colorectal	Enteric gram-negative bacilli, anaerobes	Orally: neomycin 1 g + erythromycin base 1 g at 1, 2, and 11 pm 1 day preoperatively plus mechanical bowel preparation IV: cefoxitin or cefotetan 1 g × 1	Role of mechanical bowel preparation is controversial. It is widely used despite evidence suggesting it may have no effect on SSI or other clinical outcomes	IA

(Continued)

TABLE 49-4 Most Likely Pathogens and Specific Recommendations for Surgical Prophylaxis *(Continued)*

Type of Operation	Likely Pathogens	Recommended Prophylaxis Regimen[a]	Comments	Grade of Recommendation[b]
GI endoscopy	Variable, depending on procedure, but typically enteric gram-negative bacilli, gram-positive cocci, oral anaerobes	Orally: amoxicillin 2 g × 1 IV: ampicillin 2 g × 1 or cefazolin 1 g × 1	Recommended only for high-risk patients undergoing high-risk procedures (see the text)	IA
Urologic surgery				
Prostate resection, shock-wave lithotripsy, ureteroscopy	*E. coli*	Ciprofloxacin 500 mg orally or Trimethoprim–sulfamethoxazole 1 DS tablet	All patients with positive preoperative urine cultures should receive a course of antibiotic treatment	IA–IB
Removal of external urinary catheters, cystography, urodynamic studies, simple cystourethroscopy	*E. coli*	Ciprofloxacin 500 mg orally or Trimethoprim–sulfamethoxazole 1 DS tablet	Should be considered only in patients with risk factors (see the text)	IB
Gynecological surgery				
Cesarean section	Enteric gram-negative bacilli, anaerobes, group B streptococci, enterococci	Cefazolin 2 g × 1 and azithromycin 500 mg IV × 1	Antimicrobial administration should be prior to the initial incision as opposed to after umbilical cord clamping	IA
Hysterectomy	Enteric gram-negative bacilli, anaerobes, group B streptococci, enterococci	Vaginal: cefazolin 1 g × 1 Abdominal: cefotetan 1 g × 1 or cefazolin 1 g × 1	Metronidazole 1 g IV × 1 is recommended alternative for penicillin allergy	IA

Head and neck surgery

Maxillofacial surgery	*Staphylococcus aureus,* streptococci spp, oral anerobes	Cefazolin 2 g or clindamycin 600 mg	Repeat intraoperative dose for operations longer than 4 hours	IA
Head and neck cancer resection	*S. aureus,* streptococci spp, oral anerobes	Clindamycin 600 mg at induction and every 8 hours × 2 more doses	Add gentamicin for clean–contaminated procedures	IA

Cardiothoracic surgery

Cardiac surgery	*S. aureus, S. epidermidis, Corynebacterium*	Cefazolin 1 g every 8 hours × 48 hours Intranasal mupirocin twice daily for 5 days preoperatively for patients colonized with *S. aureus*	Patients >80 kg (>176 lb) should receive 2 g of cefazolin instead; in areas with high prevalence of *S. aureus* resistance, vancomycin should be considered	IA
Thoracic surgery	*S. aureus, S. epidermidis, Corynebacterium,* enteric gram-negative bacilli	Cefuroxime 750 mg IV every 8 hours × 48 hours	First-generation cephalosporins are deemed inadequate, and shorter durations of prophylaxis have not been adequately studied	IA

Vascular surgery

Abdominal aorta and lower extremity vascular surgery	*S. aureus, S. epidermidis,* enteric gram-negative bacilli	Cefazolin 1 g at induction and every 8 hours × 2 more doses	Although complications from infections may be infrequent, graft infections are associated with significant morbidity	IB

Orthopedic surgery

Joint replacement	*S. aureus, S. epidermidis*	Cefazolin 1 g × 1 preoperatively, then every 8 hours × 2 more doses Intranasal mupirocin twice daily for 5 days preoperatively for patients colonized with *S. aureus*	Vancomycin reserved for penicillin-allergic patients or where institutional prevalence of methicillin-resistant *S. aureus* warrants use	IA

(Continued)

TABLE 49-4 Most Likely Pathogens and Specific Recommendations for Surgical Prophylaxis *(Continued)*

Type of Operation	Likely Pathogens	Recommended Prophylaxis Regimen[a]	Comments	Grade of Recommendation[b]
Hip fracture repair	*S. aureus, S. epidermidis*	Cefazolin 1 g × 1 preoperatively, then every 8 hours for 48 hours	Compound fractures are treated as if infection is presumed	IA
Open/Compound fractures	*S. aureus, S. epidermidis*; gram-negative bacilli, polymicrobial	Cefazolin 1 g × 1 preoperatively, then every 8 hours for a course of presumed infection	Gram-negative coverage (ie, gentamicin) often indicated for severe open fractures	IA
Neurosurgery				
CSF shunt procedures	*S. aureus, S. epidermidis*	Cefazolin 1 g every 8 hours × 3 doses or ceftriaxone 2 g × 1	No agents have been shown to be better than cefazolin in randomized comparative trials	IA
Spinal surgery	*S. aureus, S. epidermidis*	Cefazolin 1 g × 1	Limited number of clinical trials comparing different treatment regimens	IB
CSF shunt procedures	*S. aureus, S. epidermidis*	Cefazolin 1 g every 8 hours × 3 doses or ceftriaxone 2 g × 1	No agents have been shown to be better than cefazolin in randomized comparative trials	IA
Craniotomy	*S. aureus, S. epidermidis*	Cefazolin 1 g × 1 or cefotaxime 1 g × 1	Vancomycin 1 g IV × 1 can be substituted for patients with penicillin allergy	IA

[a]One-time doses are optimally infused at induction of anesthesia except as noted. Repeat doses may be required for long procedures. See the text for references.
[b]Strength of recommendations: Category IA: Strongly recommended and supported by well-designed experimental, clinical, or epidemiologic studies. Category IB: Strongly recommended and supported by some experimental, clinical, or epidemiologic studies and strong theoretical rationale. Category II: Suggested and supported by suggestive clinical or epidemiologic studies or theoretical rationale.
CSF, cerebrospinal fluid; DS, double strength.

- A cephalosporin with antianaerobic activity, such as **cefoxitin** or **cefotetan**, is recommended as first-line therapy; however, cefotetan may be superior for longer operations because of its longer duration of action.
- Single-dose therapy with cefotetan is adequate. Intraoperative dosing of cefoxitin may be required if the procedure extends beyond 3 hours.

UROLOGIC PROCEDURES

- As long as the urine is sterile preoperatively, the risk of SSI after urologic procedures is low, and the benefit of prophylactic antibiotics in this setting is controversial. *E. coli* is the most frequently encountered organism.
- Antibiotic prophylaxis is warranted for all patients undergoing transurethral resection of the prostate or bladder tumors, shock wave lithotripsy, percutaneous renal surgery, or ureteroscopy.
- Specific recommendations are listed in **Table 49-4.**
- Urologic procedures requiring an abdominal approach such as a nephrectomy or cystectomy require prophylaxis appropriate for a clean-contaminated abdominal procedure.

CESAREAN SECTION

- Antibiotics are efficacious to prevent SSIs for all women undergoing cesarean section regardless of underlying risk factors.
- **Cefazolin**, 2 g IV, remains the drug of choice. For patients with a β-lactam allergy, preoperative **metronidazole** is an acceptable alternative.
- Antimicrobial administration should occur at the time of the initial incision instead of at the time of umbilical cord clamping.

HYSTERECTOMY

- Vaginal hysterectomies are associated with a high rate of postoperative infection when performed without the benefit of prophylactic antibiotics.
- A single preoperative dose of **cefazolin** or **cefoxitin** is recommended for vaginal hysterectomy. For patients with β-lactam hypersensitivity, a single preoperative dose of **metronidazole** or **doxycycline** is effective.
- Abdominal hysterectomy SSI rates are correspondingly lower than vaginal hysterectomy rates. However, prophylactic antibiotics are still recommended regardless of underlying risk factors.
- First-, second-, or third-generation cephalosporins can be used for prophylaxis.

HEAD AND NECK SURGERY

- Use of prophylactic antibiotics during head and neck surgery depends on the procedure type. Clean procedures, such as thyroidectomy or a simple tooth extraction, are associated with low rates of SSI and antimicrobial prophylaxis is not recommended. Head and neck procedures involving an incision through a mucosal layer carry a high risk of SSI.
- Specific recommendations for prophylaxis are listed in **Table 49-4.**
- Although typical doses of **cefazolin** are ineffective for anaerobic infections, the recommended 2 g dose produces concentrations high enough to be inhibitory to these organisms. A 24-hour duration has been used in most studies, but single-dose therapy may also be effective.
- A single dose of **clindamycin** is adequate for prophylaxis in maxillofacial surgery unless the procedure lasts longer than 4 hours, when a second dose should be administered intraoperatively. For most head and neck cancer resection surgeries, including free-flap reconstruction, 24 hours of clindamycin is appropriate,

CARDIAC SURGERY

- Although most cardiac surgeries are technically clean procedures, prophylactic antibiotics have been shown to lower rates of SSI.

- The usual pathogens are skin flora (see Table 49-4) and, rarely, gram-negative enteric organisms.
- Risk factors for developing an SSI after cardiac surgery include obesity, renal insufficiency, connective tissue disease, reexploration for bleeding, and poorly timed administration of antibiotics.
- **Cefazolin** has been extensively studied and is currently considered the drug of choice. Patients weighing more than 80 kg should receive 2 g cefazolin rather than 1 g. Doses should be administered no earlier than 60 minutes before the first incision and no later than the beginning of induction of anesthesia.
- Extending antibiotic administration beyond 48 hours does not lower SSI rates.
- **Vancomycin** use may be justified in hospitals with a high incidence of SSI with MRSA or when sternal wounds are to be explored for possible mediastinitis.

NONCARDIAC VASCULAR SURGERY

- Prophylactic antibiotics are beneficial, especially in procedures involving the abdominal aorta and the lower extremities.
- Twenty-four hours of prophylaxis with IV **cefazolin** is adequate. For patients with β-lactam allergy, 24 hours of oral **ciprofloxacin** is effective.

ORTHOPEDIC SURGERY

- Prophylactic antibiotics are beneficial in cases involving implantation of prosthetic material (pins, plates, and artificial joints).
- The most likely pathogens mirror those of other clean procedures and include staphylococci and, infrequently, gram-negative aerobes.
- **Cefazolin** is the drug of choice. For hip fracture repairs and joint replacements, it should be administered for 24 hours. **Vancomycin** is not recommended unless a patient has a history of β-lactam hypersensitivity or the propensity for MRSA infection at the institution necessitates its use.

NEUROSURGERY

- The use of prophylactic antibiotics in neurosurgery is controversial.
- Single doses of **cefazolin** appear to lower SSI risk after craniotomy.

See Chapter 141, Antimicrobial Prophylaxis in Surgery, authored by Salmaan Kanji, for a more detailed discussion of this topic.

50   Tuberculosis

- *Tuberculosis* (TB) is a communicable infectious disease caused by *Mycobacterium tuberculosis*. It can produce silent, latent infection, as well as progressive, active disease. Globally, 2 billion people are infected and roughly 1.5 million people die from TB each year.

PATHOPHYSIOLOGY AND ETIOLOGY

- *M. tuberculosis* is transmitted from person to person by coughing or other activities that cause the organism to be aerosolized. Close contacts of TB patients are most likely to become infected.
- Human immunodeficiency virus (HIV) is the most important risk factor for progressing to active TB, especially among people 25–44 years of age. An HIV-infected individual with TB infection is over 100-fold more likely to develop active disease than an HIV-seronegative patient.
- Approximately 90% of patients who experience primary disease have no further clinical manifestations other than a positive skin test either alone or in combination with radiographic evidence of stable granulomas. Tissue necrosis and calcification of the originally infected site and regional lymph nodes may occur, resulting in the formation of a radiodense area referred to as a *Ghon complex.*
- Approximately 5% of patients (usually children, the elderly, or the immunocompromised) experience progressive primary disease at the site of the primary infection (usually the lower lobes) and frequently by dissemination, leading to meningitis and often to involvement of the upper lobes of the lung as well.
- Approximately 10% of patients develop reactivation disease, which arises subsequent to the hematogenous spread of the organism. In the United States, most cases of TB are believed to result from reactivation.
- Occasionally, a massive inoculum of organisms may be introduced into the bloodstream, causing widely disseminated disease and granuloma formation known as *miliary TB.*

CLINICAL PRESENTATION AND DIAGNOSIS

- Patients with TB typically present with cough, weight loss, fatigue, fever, and night sweats. Symptom onset may be gradual.
- Frank hemoptysis usually occurs late in the course of disease but may present earlier.
- On physical examination, the patient is usually thin with evidence or recent weight loss. Dullness to chest percussion, rales, and increased vocal fremitus are often present, but a normal lung examination is common compared to the degree of radiological lung involvement.
- The white blood cell (WBC) count is usually moderately elevated with lymphocyte predominance. A high platelet count (thrombocytosis) and mild-to-moderate anemia are common.
- Sputum smear is done to detect mycobacteria. A fiber-optic bronchoscopy is performed if sputum tests are inconclusive and suspicion is high.
- Chest radiograph shows patchy or nodular infiltrates in the apical areas of the upper lobes or the superior segment of the lower lobes. There may be cavitation that shows air–fluid levels as the infection progresses.
- Clinical features associated with extrapulmonary TB vary depending on the organ system(s) involved but typically consist of slowly progressive decline of organ function with low-grade fever and other constitutional symptoms.
- Patients with HIV may have atypical presentation. HIV-positive patients are less likely to have positive skin tests, cavitary lesions, or fever. They have a higher incidence of extrapulmonary TB and are more likely to present with progressive primary disease.

- TB in older persons is easily confused with other respiratory diseases. It is far less likely to present with positive skin tests, fevers, night sweats, sputum production, or hemoptysis. TB in children may present as typical bacterial pneumonia and is called *progressive primary TB*.
- The most widely used screening method for tuberculous infection is the tuberculin skin test, which uses purified protein derivative (PPD). Populations most likely to benefit from skin testing are listed in **Table 50-1**. Testing for latent TB is summarized in **Figure 50-1**.
- The Mantoux method of PPD administration consists of the intracutaneous injection of PPD containing five tuberculin units. The test is read 48–72 hours after injection by measuring the diameter of the zone of induration.
- Some patients may exhibit a positive test 1 week after an initial negative test; this is referred to as a *booster effect*.
- Confirmatory diagnosis of a clinical suspicion of TB must be made via chest radiograph and microbiologic examination of sputum or other infected material to rule out active disease.
- When active TB is suspected, attempts should be made to isolate *M. tuberculosis* from the infected site. Daily sputum collection over 3 consecutive days is recommended.
- Tests to measure release of interferon-γ in the patient's blood in response to TB antigens may provide quick and specific results for identifying *M. tuberculosis*.

TREATMENT

- <u>Goals of Treatment</u>: (1) Rapid identification of a new TB case; (2) Initiation of specific anti-TB treatment; (3) Eradicating *M. tuberculosis* infection; (4) Achievement of a noninfectious state in the patient, thus ending isolation; (5) Preventing the development of resistance; (6) Adherence to the treatment regimen by the patient; and (7) Cure of the patient as quickly as possible (generally at least 6 months of treatment).
- Drug treatment is the cornerstone of TB management. A minimum of two drugs, and generally three or four drugs, must be used simultaneously. Directly observed therapy (DOT) by a healthcare worker is a cost-effective way to ensure completion of treatment and is considered the standard of care.
- Drug treatment is continued for at least 6 months, and 18–24 months for cases of multidrug-resistant TB (MDR-TB).
- Debilitated patients may require therapy for other medical conditions, including substance abuse and HIV infection, and some may need nutritional support.
- Surgery may be needed to remove destroyed lung tissue, space-occupying lesions, and some extrapulmonary lesions.

PHARMACOLOGIC THERAPY

Latent Infection

- As described in **Table 50-2**, chemoprophylaxis should be initiated in patients to reduce the risk of progression to active disease.
- **Isoniazid**, 300 mg (5–10 mg/kg of body weight) daily in adults, is the preferred treatment for latent TB in the United States, generally given for 9 months.
- **Rifampin**, 600 mg daily for 4 months, can be used when isoniazid resistance is suspected or when the patient cannot tolerate isoniazid. **Rifabutin**, 300 mg daily, may be substituted for rifampin for patients at high risk of drug interactions.
- The CDC recommends the 12-week **isoniazid/rifapentine** regimen as an equal alternative to 9 months of daily isoniazid for treating latent tuberculosis infection (LTBI) in otherwise healthy patients aged 12 years or older who have a predictive factor for greater likelihood of TB developing, which included recent exposure to contagious TB, conversion from negative to positive on an indirect test for infection (ie, interferon-gamma release assays [IGRA] or tuberculin skin test), and radiographic findings of healed pulmonary TB.

TABLE 50-1   Criteria for Tuberculosis Positivity

Reaction ≥5 mm of induration	Reaction ≥10 mm of induration	Reaction ≥15 mm of induration
HIV-infected persons	Recent immigrants (ie, within the last 5 years) from high-prevalence countries	Persons with no risk factors for TB
A recent contact of a person with TB disease	Injection drug users	
Fibrotic changes on chest radiograph consistent with prior TB	Residents and employees[a] of the following high-risk congregate settings: prisons and jails, nursing homes and other long-term facilities for the elderly, hospitals and other healthcare facilities, residential facilities for patients with AIDS, and homeless shelters	
Patients with organ transplants and other immunosuppressed patients (receiving the equivalent of 15 mg/day or more of prednisone for 1 month or longer, taking TNF-α antagonists)[b]	Mycobacteriology laboratory personnel, persons with the following clinical conditions that place them at high risk: silicosis, diabetes mellitus, chronic renal failure, some hematologic disorders, other specific malignancies, gastrectomy, and jejunoileal bypass	
	Children younger than 5 years of age or infants, children, and adolescents exposed to adults at high risk	

Interpretation of Interferon Gamma Release Assay (IGRA) Results

The interpretation of IGRAs is based on the amount of IFN-γ, in T-SPOT®.TB. An IGRA is recommended over a tuberculin skin test (TST) in persons at least 5 years of age who are likely to have *M. tuberculosis* infection; who are at low or moderate risk of the disease progressing; in whom it has been determined that latent tuberculosis infection (LTBI) testing is necessary; and who have been vaccinated against Calmette-Guerin or are not likely to return for follow up after a TST. The TST is a viable second option in certain circumstances, such as if an IGRA is unavailable. Laboratories should provide both the qualitative and quantitative results.

Qualitative results are reported positive, negative, indeterminate, or borderline.

Quantitative results are reported as numerical values that include a response to the TB antigen and two controls, nil and mitogen.

Quantitative results may be useful for clinical decision making in individual cases, in combination with risk factors.

[a]For persons who are otherwise at low risk and who are tested at the start of employment, a reaction of ≥15 mm induration is considered positive.
[b]Risk of TB for patients treated with corticosteroids increases with higher dose and longer duration.
AIDS, acquired immunodeficiency syndrome; HIV, human immunodeficiency virus; TB, tuberculosis.
Source: Centers for Disease Control and Prevention. Screening for tuberculosis and tuberculosis infection in high-risk populations: recommendations of the Advisory Council for the Elimination of Tuberculosis. M.M.W.R. 1995;44(No. RR-11):19–34.

Group	Testing Strategy	Considerations
Likely to be Infected **High** Risk of Progression (TST ≥ 5 mM)	**Adults** **Acceptable:** IGRA OR TST Consider dual testing where a positive result from either result would be considered **positive** **Children ≤ 5 years of age** **Acceptable:** TST **Acceptable:** IGRA OR TST Consider dual testing where a positive result from either result would be considered **positive**[1]	Prevalence of BCG vaccination Expertise of staff and/or laboratory Test availability Patient perceptions Staff perceptions Programmatic concerns
Likely to be Infected **Low** to **Intermediate** Risk of Progression (TST ≥ 10 mM)	**Preferred:** IGRA where available **Acceptable:** IGRA OR TST	

Unlikely to be Infected
(TST > 15 mM)
	Testing for LTBI is not recommended
	If necessary:
	    Preferred: IGRA where available.
	    Acceptable: Either IGRA OR TST
	For serial testing:
	    Acceptable: Either IGRA OR TST
	
	Consider repeat or dual testing where a negative result from either would be considered **negative**[2]	

Performing A Second Diagnostic Test When The Initial Test Is A Negative Is A Strategy To Increase Sensitivity. This May Reduce Specificity, But The Panel Decided That This Is An Acceptable Trade Off In Situations In Which The Consequences Of Missing Ltbi Exceed The Consequences Of Inappropriate Therapy. 2Performing A Confirmatory Test Following An Initial Positive Result Is Based Upon Both The Evidence That False-Positive Results Are Common Among Individuals Who Are Unlikely To Be Infected With Mycobacterium Tuberculosis And The Committee's Presumption That Performing A Second Test On Those Patients Whose Initial Test Was Positive Will Help Identify Initial False-Positive Results.

(Adapted from Jamil SM, et al. Diagnosis of tuberculosis in adults and children. Ann Am Thorac. 2017;14(2):275–278.)

FIGURE 50-1. Summary of recommendations for testing for latent tuberculosis infection (LTBI).

TABLE 50-2 Choosing the Most Effective Treatment of LTBI

Drug	Duration	Dose	Frequency	Comments
Isoniazid	9 months	Adult: 5 mg/kg Children: 10–20 mg/kg[a]	Daily	In HIV-infected patients, isoniazid may be administered concurrently with nucleoside reverse transcriptase inhibitors (NRTIs), protease inhibitors, or non-NRTIs (NNRTIs) Preferred regimen in children 2–11 years
	9 months	Adult: 15 mg/kg Children: 20–40 mg/kg[a]	Twice weekly[c]	Directly observed treatment (DOT) must be used with twice-weekly dosing
	6 months	Adult: 5 mg/kg Children: Not recommended	Daily	Treatment for LTBI for 6 months rather than 9 months may be more cost-effective and result in greater adherence by patients
	6 months	Adult: 15 mg/kg Children: Not recommended	Twice weekly[c]	Directly observed treatment (DOT) must be used with twice-weekly dosing
Isoniazid and rifapentine	3 months	Rifapentine 10.0–14.0 kg: 300 mg 14.1–25.0 kg: 450 mg 25.1–32.0 kg: 600 mg 32.1–49.9 kg: 750 mg ≥50.0 kg: 900 mg	Once weekly[c]	Equal alternative to 9 months of daily isoniazid for otherwise healthy patients age >12 years DOT is recommended Not recommended for children <2 years; HIV-infected patients taking antiretroviral therapy, presumed resistance, pregnant women or women expecting to become pregnant during the treatment period DOT must be used
Rifampin	4 months	Adult: 10 mg/kg Children: 15–20 mg/kg[b]	Daily	For persons who are contacts of patients with isoniazid-resistant rifampin-susceptible Can be considered for persons who cannot tolerate isoniazid or who have been exposed to isoniazid-resistant TB Rifampin should not be used to treat HIV-infected person taking some combinations of ART

[a]The American Academy of Pediatrics recommends an INH dosage of 10–15 mg/kg for the daily regiment and 20–30 mg/kg for twice-weekly regimen.

[b]In the United States, the recommended regimen for the treatment of LTBI in children is a 9-month course of isoniazid. For the treatment of LTBI in infants, children, and adolescents when isoniazid could not be tolerated or the child has had contact with a case patient infected with an isoniazid resistant but rifamycin susceptible organism, the American Academy of Pediatrics recommends 6 months of daily rifampin (180 doses) at a dosage of 10 mg/kg.

[c]Intermittent regimens must be provided via directly observed therapy (DOT), that is, healthcare worker observes the ingestion of medication.

Source: Adapted from Latent tuberculosis infection: A guide for primary health care providers. US Department of Health and Human Services/CDC. Atlanta, GA, 2013.

- Pregnant women, alcoholics, and patients with poor diets who are treated with isoniazid should receive pyridoxine, 10–50 mg daily, to reduce the incidence of central nervous system (CNS) effects or peripheral neuropathies.

Treating Active Disease

- Table 50-3 lists options for treatment of culture-positive pulmonary TB caused by drug-susceptible organisms. Doses of antituberculosis drugs are given in Table 50-4. Other sources should be consulted for treatment recommendations when TB is concurrent with HIV infection. The standard TB treatment regimen is **isoniazid, rifampin, pyrazinamide, and ethambutol** for 2 months, followed by isoniazid and rifampin for 4 months. Ethambutol can be stopped if susceptibility to isoniazid, rifampin, and pyrazinamide is shown.
- Appropriate samples should be sent for culture and susceptibility testing prior to initiating therapy for all patients with active TB. The data should guide the initial drug selection for the new patient. If susceptibility data are not available, the drug resistance pattern in the area where the patient likely acquired TB should be used.
- If the patient is being evaluated for the retreatment of TB, it is imperative to know what drugs were used previously and for how long.
- The standard TB treatment regimen is isoniazid, rifampin, pyrazinamide, and ethambutol for 2 months, followed by isoniazid and rifampin for 4 months, a total of 6 months of treatment.
- Patients who are slow to respond, those who remain culture positive at 2 months of treatment, those with cavitary lesions on chest radiograph, and HIV-positive patients should be treated for 9 months and for at least 6 months from the time they convert to smear and culture negativity.

Drug Resistance

- If the organism is drug resistant, the aim is to introduce two or more active agents that the patient has not received previously. With MDR-TB, no standard regimen can be proposed. It is critical to avoid monotherapy or adding only a single drug to a failing regimen.
- Drug resistance should be suspected in the following situations:
  - ✓ Patients who have received prior therapy for TB
  - ✓ Patients from geographic areas with a high prevalence of resistance (South Africa, Mexico, Southeast Asia, the Baltic countries, and the former Soviet states)
  - ✓ Patients who are homeless, institutionalized, IV drug abusers, and/or infected with HIV
  - ✓ Patients who still have acid-fast bacilli–positive sputum smears after 2 months of therapy
  - ✓ Patients who still have positive cultures after 2–4 months of therapy
  - ✓ Patients who fail therapy or relapse after retreatment
  - ✓ Patients known to be exposed to MDR-TB cases

Special Populations

Tuberculous Meningitis and Extrapulmonary Disease

- In general, **isoniazid, pyrazinamide, ethionamide**, and **cycloserine** penetrate the cerebrospinal fluid readily. Patients with CNS TB are often treated for longer periods (9–12 months). Extrapulmonary TB of the soft tissues can be treated with conventional regimens. TB of the bone is typically treated for 9 months, occasionally with surgical debridement.

Children

- TB in children may be treated with regimens similar to those used in adults, although some physicians still prefer to extend treatment to 9 months. Pediatric doses of drugs should be used.

TABLE 50-3 Drug Regimens for Microbiologically Confirmed Pulmonary Tuberculosis Caused by Drug Susceptible Organisms

		Initial Phase		Continuation Phase	
Regimen	Drugs[a]	Interval and Doses[b] (Minimal Duration)	Drugs	Interval and Doses[c] (Minimal Duration)	Comments[c,e]
1	Isoniazid Rifampin Pyrazinamide Ethambutol	7 days/week for 56 doses (8 weeks) or 5 days/week for 40 doses (8 weeks)[c]	Isoniazid/ Rifampin	7 days/week for 126 doses (18 weeks) or 5 days/week for 90 doses (18 weeks)[c]	This is preferred regimen for patient with newly diagnosed pulmonary tuberculosis.
2	Isoniazid Rifampin Pyrazinamide Ethambutol	7 days/week for 56 doses or 5 days/week for 40 doses (8 weeks)	Isoniazid/ Rifampin	Three times weekly for 54 doses (18 weeks)[d]	Preferred alternative regimen in situations in which more frequent DOT during continuation phase is difficult to achieve.
3	Isoniazid Rifampin Pyrazinamide Ethambutol	3 times weekly for 24 doses (8 weeks)	Isoniazid/ Rifampin	Three times weekly for 54 doses (18 weeks)	Use regimen with caution in patients with HIV and/or cavitary disease. Missed doses can lead to treatment failure, relapse, and acquired drug resistance.

(Continued)

TABLE 50-3 Drug Regimens for Microbiologically Confirmed Pulmonary Tuberculosis Caused by Drug Susceptible Organisms *(Continued)*

		Initial Phase		Continuation Phase	
Regimen	Drugs[a]	Interval and Doses[b] (Minimal Duration)	Drugs	Interval and Doses[c] (Minimal Duration)	Comments[c,e]
4	Isoniazid Rifampin Ethambutol Pyrazinamide	7 days/week for 14 doses, then twice weekly for 12 doses[e]	Isoniazid/ Rifampin	Twice weekly for 36 doses (18 weeks)	Do not use twice weekly regimens in HIV-infected patients or patients with smear positive and/or cavitary disease. If doses are missed, then therapy is equivalent to once weekly, which is inferior.

[a]Other combinations may be appropriate in certain circumstances.

[b]When DOT is used, drugs may be given 5 days/week and the necessary number of doses adjusted accordingly. Although there are no studies that compare 5 with 7 daily doses, extensive experience indicates this would be an effective practice. DOT should be used when drugs are administered <7 days/week.

[c]Based on expert opinion, patients with cavitation on initial chest radiograph and positive cultures at completion of 2 months of therapy should receive a 7-month (31-week) continuation phase.

[d]Pyridoxine (vitamin B₆), 25–50 mg/day, is given with INH to all persons at risk of neuropathy (eg, pregnant women; breastfeeding infants; persons with HIV; patients with diabetes, alcoholism, malnutrition, or chronic renal failure; or patients with advanced age). For patients with peripheral neuropathy, experts recommend increasing pyridoxine dose to 100 mg/day.

[e]Alternatively, some US tuberculosis control programs have administered intensive-phase regimens 5 days/week for 15 doses (3 weeks), then twice weekly for 12 doses.

DOT, directly observed therapy; EMB, ethambutol; HIV, human immunodeficiency virus; INH, isoniazid; PZA, pyrazinamide; RIF, rifampin.

Source: Reprinted, with permission, from Nahid P, et al. Executive Summary: Official American Thoracic Society/Centers for Disease Control and Prevention/Infectious Diseases Society of America Clinical Practice Guidelines: Treatment of Drug-Susceptible Tuberculosis, Clinical Infectious Diseases, Volume 63, Issue 7, 1 October 2016, pp. 853–867.

TABLE 50-4 Antituberculosis Drugs for Adults and Children

Drug	Preparation	Adults/Children	Typical Doses[a]			
			Daily	1× Per Week	2× Per Week	3× Per Week
First-line drugs						
Isoniazid	Tablets (50, 100, 300 mg); elixir (50 mg/5 mL); aqueous solution (100 mg/mL) for IV or intramuscular injection	Adults	5 mg/kg	15 mg/kg	15 mg/kg	15 mg/kg
		Children	10–15 mg/kg		20–30 mg/kg	—
Rifampin[h]	Capsule (150, 300 mg); powder may be suspended for oral administration; aqueous solution for IV injection	Adults[b]	10 mg/kg	—	10 mg/kg	10 mg/kg
		Children	10–20 mg/kg	—	10–20 mg/kg	—
Rifabutin	Capsule (150 mg)	Adults[b]	5 mg/kg	—		5 mg/kg
		Children	Appropriate dosing for children is unknown			
Rifapentine[h]	Tablet (150 mg, film coated)	Adults	—	10–20 mg/kg (continuation phase)	—	—
		Children	The drug is not approved for use in children <12 years old			
Pyrazinamide	Tablet (500 mg, scored)	Adults	40–55 kg: 1000 mg 56–75 kg: 1500 mg 76–90 kg: 2000 mg	—	40–55 kg: 2000 mg 56–75 kg: 3000 mg 76–90 kg: 4000 mg	40–55 kg: 1500 mg 56–75 kg: 2500 mg 76–90 kg: 3000 mg
		Children	30–40 mg/kg	—	50 mg/kg	—

(Continued)

TABLE 50-4 Antituberculosis Drugs for Adults and Children (Continued)

Drug	Preparation	Adults/Children	Typical Doses[a] Daily	1× Per Week	2× Per Week	3× Per Week
Ethambutol	Tablet (100, 400 mg)	Adults	40–55 kg: 800 mg 56–75 kg: 1200 mg 76–90 kg: 1600 mg	— — —	40–55 kg: 2000 mg 56–75 kg: 2800 mg 76–90 kg: 4000 mg	40–55 kg: 1200 mg 56–75 kg: 2000 mg 76–90 kg: 2400 mg
		Children[b]	30–40 mg/kg	—	—	50 mg/kg
Second-line drugs						
Cycloserine	Capsule (250 mg)	Adults	10–15 mg/kg/day, usually 500–750 mg/day in two doses[c]	No data	No data	No data
		Children	10–15 mg/kg/day	—	—	—
Ethionamide	Tablet (250 mg)	Adults[d]	15–20 mg/kg/day, usually 500–750 mg/day in a single daily dose or two divided doses[f]	No data	No data	No data
		Children	15–20 mg/kg/day	No data	No data	No data
Streptomycin	Aqueous solution (1-g vials) for IV or intramuscular administration	Adults	15 mg/kg/day[e]	—	—	—
		Children[i]	15–20 mg/kg/day	—	25–30 mg/kg	25 mg/kg

Amikacin/Kanamycin	Aqueous solution (500-mg and 1-g vials) for IV or intramuscular administration	Adults	15 mg/kg/day^e	—	—	25 mg/kg
		Children^i	15–20 mg/kg/day IV or intramuscular as a single daily dose	—	25–30 mg/kg	—
Capreomycin	Aqueous solution (1-g vials) for IV or intramuscular administration	Adults	15 mg/kg/day^g	e	25–30 mg/kg	25 mg/kg
		Children^i	15–20 mg/kg/day as a single daily dose	—		25–30 mg/kg
p-Aminosalicylic acid (PAS)	Granules (4-g packets) can be mixed with food; tablets (500 mg) are still available in some countries, but not in the United States; a solution for IV administration is available in Europe	Adults	8–12 g/day in two or three doses	No data	No data	No data
		Children	200–300 mg/kg/day in two to four divided doses	No data	No data	No data
Levofloxacin	Tablets (250, 500, 750 mg); aqueous solution (500-mg vials) for IV injection	Adults	500–1000 mg daily	No data	No data	No data
		Children	f	f	f	f
Moxifloxacin	Tablets (400 mg); aqueous solution (400 mg/250 mL) for IV injection	Adults	400 mg daily	No data	No data	No data
		Children	g	g	g	g

(Continued)

TABLE 50-4 Antituberculosis Drugs for Adults and Children (*Continued*)

Drug	Preparation	Adults/Children	Typical Doses[a]			
			Daily	1× Per Week	2× Per Week	3× Per Week
Bedaquiline		Adults	Weeks 1–2: 400 mg daily. Weeks 3–24: 200 mg three times weekly.	No data	No data	No data
		Children	The drug is not approved for use in children			

[a]The authors of this chapter do not agree with the use of maximum doses, since this arbitrarily caps doses for patients who otherwise might need larger doses. These maximum doses were not based on prospective studies in large or overweight individuals, and do not consider patients with documented malabsorption of their medications. Clinical judgment should be used in such circumstances.

[b]The drug can likely be used safely in older children but should be used with caution in children younger than 5 years, in whom visual acuity cannot be monitored. In younger children, ethambutol at the dose of 15 mg/kg/day can be used if there is suspected or proven resistance to isoniazid or rifampin.

[c]Although this is the dose recommended generally, most clinicians with experience using cycloserine indicate that it is unusual for patients to be able to tolerate this amount. Serum concentration measurements are often useful in determining the optimal dose for a given patient.

[d]The single daily dose can be given at bedtime or with the main meal to reduce nausea.

[e]Dose: 15 mg/kg/day (1 g), and 10 mg/kg in persons older than 59 years (750 mg). Usual dose: 750–1000 mg administered intramuscularly or IV, given as a single dose 5–7 days/week and reduced to two or three times per week after the first 2–4 months or after culture conversion, depending on the efficacy of the other drugs in the regimen.

[f]The long-term (more than several weeks) use of levofloxacin in children and adolescents has not been approved because of concerns about effects on bone and cartilage growth. However, most experts agree that the drug should be considered for children with tuberculosis caused by organisms resistant to both isoniazid and rifampin. The optimal dose is not known.

[g]The long-term (more than several weeks) use of moxifloxacin in children and adolescents has not been approved because of concerns about effects on bone and cartilage growth. The optimal dose is not known.

[h]Higher doses of rifampin and rifapentine are being studied. Rifabutin dose may need to be adjusted when there is concomitant use of protease inhibitors or non-nucleoside reverse transcriptase inhibitors.

[i]Larger total body water content and faster clearance of injectable drugs in most children. Dosing can be guided by serum concentrations.

For purposes of this document, adult dosing begins at age 15 years.

Source: Reprinted, with permission, from Nahid P, et al. Executive Summary: Official American Thoracic Society/Centers for Disease Control and Prevention/Infectious Diseases Society of America Clinical Practice Guidelines: *Treatment of Drug-Susceptible Tuberculosis, Clinical Infectious Diseases, Volume 63, Issue 7, 1 October 2016, pp. 853–867.*

TABLE 50-5	Dosing Recommendations for Adults with Reduced Renal Function and for Adults Receiving Hemodialysis	
Drug	**Change in Frequency?**	**Recommended Dose and Frequency for Patients with Creatinine Clearance <30 mL/min (0.50 mL/sec) or for Patients Receiving Hemodialysis[a,b,c,d]**
Isoniazid	No change	300 mg once daily, or 900 mg three times per week
Rifampin	No change	600 mg once daily, or 600 mg three times per week
Pyrazinamide	Yes	25–35 mg/kg per dose three times per week (not daily)
Ethambutol	Yes	15–25 mg/kg per dose three times per week (not daily)
Levofloxacin	Yes	750–1000 mg per dose three times per week (not daily)
Cycloserine	Yes	250 mg once daily, or 500 mg/dose three times per week[e]
Ethionamide	No change	250–500 mg/dose daily
p-Aminosalicylic acid	No change	4 g/dose, twice daily
Streptomycin	Yes	12–15 mg/kg per dose two or three times per week (not daily)
Capreomycin	Yes	12–15 mg/kg per dose two or three times per week (not daily)
Kanamycin	Yes	12–15 mg/kg per dose two or three times per week (not daily)
Amikacin	Yes	12–15 mg/kg per dose two or three times per week (not daily)

[a]Standard doses are given unless there is intolerance.
[b]The medications should be given after hemodialysis on the day of hemodialysis.
[c]Monitoring of serum drug concentrations should be considered to ensure adequate drug absorption, without excessive accumulation, and to assist in avoiding toxicity.
[d]Data currently are not available for patients receiving peritoneal dialysis. Until data become available, begin with doses recommended for patients receiving hemodialysis and verify adequacy of dosing, using serum concentration monitoring.
[e]The appropriateness of 250-mg daily doses has not been established. There should be careful monitoring for evidence of neurotoxicity.

Source: Reprinted, with permission, from Nahid P, et al. Executive Summary: Official American Thoracic Society/Centers for Disease Control and Prevention/Infectious Diseases Society of America Clinical Practice Guidelines: Treatment of Drug-Susceptible Tuberculosis, Clinical Infectious Diseases, Volume 63, Issue 7, 1 October 2016, pp. 853–867.

Pregnant Women

- The usual treatment of pregnant women is **isoniazid, rifampin, and ethambutol** for 9 months.
- Women with TB should be cautioned against becoming pregnant, as the disease poses a risk to the fetus as well as to the mother. Isoniazid or ethambutol is relatively safe when used during pregnancy. Supplementation with B vitamins is particularly important during pregnancy. **Rifampin** has been rarely associated with birth defects, but those

TABLE 50-6 Recommended Regimens for the Concomitant Treatment of TB and HIV Infection in Adults

Combined Regimen for Treatment of HIV and TB	Pharmacokinetic Effect of the Rifamycin	Tolerability/Toxicity	Antiviral Activity when Used with Rifamycin	Recommendations (Comments)
Efavirenz-based antiretroviral therapy[a] with rifampin-based TB treatment	Well-characterized, modest decrease in concentrations in some patients	Low rates of discontinuation	Excellent	Preferred (efavirenz should not be used during the first trimester of pregnancy)
PI-based antiretroviral therapy[a] with rifabutin-based TB treatment	Little effect of rifabutin on PI concentrations, but marked increases in rifabutin concentrations	Low rates of discontinuation (if rifabutin is appropriately dose-reduced)	Favorable, although published clinical experience is not extensive	Preferred for patients unable to take efavirenz[b] (caution to ensure patients who discontinue PI not to continue to receive reduced rifabutin dose)
Nevirapine-based antiretroviral therapy with rifampin-based TB treatment	Moderate decrease in concentrations	Concern about hepatotoxicity when used with isoniazid, rifampin, and pyrazinamide	Suboptimal when nevirapine is initiated using once-daily dosing largely favorable when nevirapine is given twice daily throughout cotreatment	Alternative for patients who cannot take efavirenz, though efavirenz is preferred (nevirapine should not be initiated among women with CD4 >250 [0.25 × 10^9/L] or men with CD4 >400 cells/μL [0.40 × 10^9/L])
Raltegravir-based antiretroviral therapy with rifampin-based TB treatment	Significant decrease in concentrations with standard dosing	Limited experience	Limited published clinical experience	Alternative at higher doses for patients who cannot take efavirenz and who have baseline viral load <100,000 copies/mL (100 × 10^6/L)

(Continued)

TABLE 50-6 Recommended Regimens for the Concomitant Treatment of TB and HIV Infection in Adults (*Continued*)

Combined Regimen for Treatment of HIV and TB	Pharmacokinetic Effect of the Rifamycin	Tolerability/Toxicity	Antiviral Activity when Used with Rifamycin	Recommendations (Comments)
Dolutegravir-based antiretroviral therapy with rifampin-based TB-treatment	Coadministration with rifampicin results in decreases in dolutegravir plasma exposure requiring increased dose of dolutegravir	Limited experience	Limited published clinical experience	Alternative for patients who cannot take efavirenz
Zidovudine/Lamivudine/Abacavir/Tenofovir with rifampin-based TB treatment	50% decrease in zidovudine, possible effect on abacavir not evaluated	Anemia	No published clinical experience, but this regimen is less effective than efavirenz- or aatazanavir-based regimens in person not taking rifampin	Alternative for patients who cannot take efavirenz or nevirapine and if rifabutin not available
Zidovudine/Lamivudine/Tenofovir with rifampin-based TB treatment	50% decrease in zidovudine, no other effects predicted	Anemia	Favorable, but not evaluated in a randomized trial	Alternative for patients who cannot take efavirenz and abacavir and if rifabutin not available
Zidovudine/Lamivudine/Abacavir with rifampin-based TB treatment	50% decrease in zidovudine, possible effect on abacavir not evaluated	Anemia	Early favorable experience, but this combination is less effective than efavirenz- or nevirapine-based regimens in persons not taking rifampin	Alternative for patients who cannot take efavirenz and tenofovir and if rifabutin not available

TABLE 50-6 Recommended Regimens for the Concomitant Treatment of TB and HIV Infection in Adults (*Continued*)

Combined Regimen for Treatment of HIV and TB	Pharmacokinetic Effect of the Rifamycin	Tolerability/Toxicity	Antiviral Activity when Used with Rifamycin	Recommendations (Comments)
Superboosted[c] lopinavir-based antiretroviral therapy or double dose lopinavir/ritonavir-based therapy with rifampin-based TB treatment	Moderate decrease in concentrations	Hepatitis	Early favorable experience of superboosting among young children and double dose among adults already on antiretroviral drugs at the time of rifampin initiation	Alternative if rifabutin not available; double dose an option among adults already taking lopinavir-based antiretroviral therapy and virologically suppressed at the time of tuberculosis treatment initiation; superboosting has not been adequately tested in adults but may be effective

[a]With two nucleoside analogues.

[b]Includes patients with NNRTI-resistant HIV, those unable to tolerate efavirenz, and women during the first one to two trimesters of pregnancy.

[c]Superboosting of lopinavir is achieved by giving lopinavir 400 mg together with 400 mg ritonavir twice daily. Double dose lopinavir/ritonavir is lopinavir 800 mg plus ritonavir 200 mg twice daily.

ART, antiretroviral therapy; HIV, human immunodeficiency virus; TB, tuberculosis.

Source: CDC. *Managing Drug Interactions in the Treatment of HIV-Related Tuberculosis [online], 2013. Available at: http://www.cdc.gov/tb/TB_HIV_Drugs/default.htm.*

seen are occasionally severe, including limb reduction and CNS lesions. **Pyrazinamide** has not been studied in a large number of pregnant women, but anecdotal information suggests that it may be safe. **Ethionamide** may be associated with premature delivery, congenital deformities, and Down syndrome when used during pregnancy, so it cannot be recommended in pregnancy. **Streptomycin** has been associated with hearing impairment in the newborn, including complete deafness and must be reserved for critical situations where alternatives do not exist. **Cycloserine** is not recommended during pregnancy. Fluoroquinolones should be avoided in pregnancy and during nursing.

Renal Failure

- In nearly all patients, isoniazid and rifampin do not require dose modifications in renal failure. Pyrazinamide and ethambutol typically require a reduction in dosing frequency from daily to three times weekly (**Table 50-5**).

EVALUATION OF THERAPEUTIC OUTCOMES AND PATIENT MONITORIG

- The most serious problem with TB therapy is nonadherence to the prescribed regimen. The most effective way to ensure adherence is with DOT.
- Patients who are AFB smear positive should have sputum samples sent for acid-fast bacilli stains every 1–2 weeks until two consecutive smears are negative. Once on maintenance therapy, patients should have sputum cultures performed monthly until negative, which generally occurs over 2–3 months. If sputum cultures continue to be positive after 2 months, drug susceptibility testing should be repeated, and serum drug concentrations should be checked.
- Patients should have blood urea nitrogen, serum creatinine, aspartate transaminase or alanine transaminase, and a complete blood count determined at baseline and periodically, depending on the presence of other factors that may increase the likelihood of toxicity (advanced age, alcohol abuse, and possibly pregnancy). Hepatotoxicity should be suspected in patients whose transaminases exceed five times the upper limit of normal or whose total bilirubin exceeds 3 mg/dL (51.3 μmol/L). At this point, the offending agent(s) should be discontinued and alternatives selected.
- See **Table 50-6** for drug monitoring recommendations.

See Chapter 130, Tuberculosis, authored by Rocsanna Namdar and Charles A. Peloquin, for a more detailed discussion of this topic.

51 Urinary Tract Infections and Prostatitis

- Infections of the urinary tract represent a wide variety of clinical syndromes including urethritis, cystitis, prostatitis, and pyelonephritis.
- A *urinary tract infection* (UTI) is defined as the presence of microorganisms in the urine that cannot be accounted for by contamination. The organisms have the potential to invade the tissues of the urinary tract and adjacent structures.
- Lower tract infections include cystitis (bladder), urethritis (urethra), prostatitis (prostate gland), and epididymitis. Upper tract infections involve the kidney and are referred to as *pyelonephritis*.
- *Uncomplicated UTIs* are not associated with structural or functional abnormalities that may interfere with the normal flow of urine or the voiding mechanism. *Complicated UTIs* are the result of a predisposing lesion of the urinary tract, such as a congenital abnormality or distortion of the urinary tract, stone, indwelling catheter, prostatic hypertrophy, obstruction, or neurologic deficit that interferes with the normal flow of urine and urinary tract defenses.
- *Recurrent UTIs,* two or more UTIs occurring within 6 months or three or more within 1 year, are characterized by multiple symptomatic episodes with asymptomatic periods occurring between these episodes. These infections are due to reinfection or to relapse. Reinfections are caused by a different organism and account for the majority of recurrent UTIs. Relapse represents the development of repeated infections caused by the same initial organism.

PATHOPHYSIOLOGY

- The bacteria causing UTIs usually originate from bowel flora of the host. Organisms typically gain entry into the urinary tract via three routes: the ascending, hematogenous (descending), and lymphatic pathways.
- The most common cause of uncomplicated UTIs is *E. coli*, accounting for more than 80%–90% of community-acquired infections. Additional causative organisms are *Staphylococcus saprophyticus, Klebsiella pneumoniae, Proteus* spp., *Pseudomonas aeruginosa,* and *Enterococcus* spp.
- The urinary pathogens in complicated or nosocomial infections may include *E. coli*, which accounts for less than 50% of these infections, *Proteus* spp., *K. pneumoniae, Enterobacter* spp., *P. aeruginosa,* staphylococci, and enterococci. Enterococci represent the second most frequently isolated organisms in hospitalized patients.
- Most UTIs are caused by a single organism; however, in patients with stones, indwelling urinary catheters, or chronic renal abscesses, multiple organisms may be isolated.
- Vancomycin-resistant *E. faecalis* and *E. faecium* (vancomycin-resistant enterococci) have become more widespread, especially in patients with long-term hospitalizations or underlying malignancies.

CLINICAL PRESENTATION

- The typical signs and symptoms of urinary tract infections are:
  ✓ Lower UTI: Dysuria, urgency, frequency, nocturia, and suprapubic heaviness, gross hematuria, and costovertebral tenderness.
  ✓ Upper UTI: Flank pain, fever, nausea, vomiting, and malaise.
- Symptoms alone are unreliable for the diagnosis of bacterial UTIs. The key to the diagnosis of a UTI is the ability to demonstrate significant numbers of microorganisms present in an appropriate urine specimen to distinguish contamination from infection.

- Older patients frequently do not experience specific urinary symptoms, but they will present with altered mental status, change in eating habits, or gastrointestinal (GI) symptoms.
- A standard urinalysis should be obtained in the initial assessment of a patient. Microscopic examination of the urine should be performed by preparation of a Gram stain of unspun or centrifuged urine. The presence of at least one organism per oil-immersion field in a properly collected uncentrifuged specimen correlates with greater than 100,000 colony-forming units (CFU)/mL (10^5 CFU/mL [$>10^8$ CFU/L]) of urine.
- A quantitative count of 10^5 CFU/mL (10^8 CFU/L) or more is considered indicative of a UTI; however, up to 50% of women will present with clinical symptoms of a UTI with lower counts (10^3 CFU/mL [10^6CFU/L]).
- The presence of pyuria (>10 white blood cells/mm^3 [10×10^6/L]) in a symptomatic patient correlates with significant bacteriuria. A count of 5–10 WBC/mm^3 (5×10^6–10×10^6/L) is accepted as the upper limit of normal.
- The nitrite test can be used to detect the presence of nitrate-reducing bacteria in the urine (eg, *E. coli*). The leukocyte esterase test is a rapid dipstick test to detect pyuria.
- The most reliable method of diagnosing UTIs is by quantitative urine culture. Patients with infection usually have more than 10^5 bacteria/mL (10^8/L) of urine, although as many as one-third of women with symptomatic infection have less than 10^5 bacteria/mL (10^8/L).

TREATMENT

- <u>Goals of Treatment</u>: Eradicate the invading organisms, prevent or treat systemic consequences of infection, prevent recurrence of infection, and decrease the potential for collateral damage with excessively broad antimicrobial therapy.
- The management of a patient with a UTI includes initial evaluation, selection of an antibacterial agent and duration of therapy, and follow-up evaluation.
- The initial selection of an antimicrobial agent for the treatment of UTI is primarily based on the severity of the presenting signs and symptoms, the site of infection, and whether the infection is determined to be complicated or uncomplicated. Other considerations include antibiotic susceptibility, side-effect potential, cost, current antimicrobial exposure, and the comparative inconvenience of different therapies.

PHARMACOLOGIC TREATMENT

- Eradication of bacteria from the urinary tract is directly related to the sensitivity of the organism and the achievable concentration of the antimicrobial agent in the urine.
- Management of UTIs is best accomplished by first categorizing the type of infection: acute uncomplicated cystitis, symptomatic abacteriuria, asymptomatic bacteriuria, complicated UTIs, recurrent infections, or prostatitis.
- Most *E. coli* remain susceptible to **trimethoprim–sulfamethoxazole**, although resistance is increasing. In light of rising resistance and in order to decrease the overuse of broad-spectrum antimicrobials, agents such as **nitrofurantoin** and **fosfomycin** are now considered first-line treatments along with trimethoprim–sulfamethoxazole in acute uncomplicated cystitis.
- **Table 51-1** lists the most common agents used to treat lower UTIs in adults, along with comments concerning their general use.
- **Table 51-2** presents an overview of various therapeutic options for outpatient therapy for UTI.
- **Table 51-3** describes empiric treatment regimens for specific clinical situations.

Acute Uncomplicated Cystitis

- These infections are predominantly caused by *E. coli,* and antimicrobial therapy should be directed against this organism initially. Because the causative organisms

TABLE 51-1	Commonly Used Antimicrobial Agents in the Treatment of UTIs		
Drug	**Adverse Drug Reactions**	**Monitoring Parameters**	**Comments**
Oral therapy			
Trimethoprim–sulfamethoxazole	Rash, Stevens–Johnson syndrome, renal failure, photosensitivity, hematologic (neutropenia, anemia, etc.)	Serum creatinine, BUN, electrolytes, signs of rash, and CBC	Highly effective against most aerobic enteric bacteria except *P. aeruginosa*. High urinary tract tissue concentrations and urine concentrations are achieved, which may be important in complicated infection treatment. Also effective as prophylaxis for recurrent infections
Nitrofurantoin	GI intolerance, neuropathies, and pulmonary reactions	Baseline serum creatinine and BUN	Effective as both a therapeutic and prophylactic agent in patients with recurrent UTIs. Main advantage is the lack of resistance even after long courses of therapy
Fosfomycin trometamol	Diarrhea, headache, and angioedema	No routine tests recommended	Single-dose therapy for uncomplicated infections, low levels of resistance, use with caution in patients with hepatic dysfunction
Fluoroquinolones			
Ciprofloxacin Levofloxacin	Hypersensitivity, photosensitivity, GI symptoms, dizziness, confusion, and tendonitis (black box warning)	CBC, baseline serum creatinine, and BUN	Greater spectrum of activity, including *P. aeruginosa*. Effective for pyelonephritis and prostatitis. Avoid in pregnancy and children. Moxifloxacin should not be used owing to inadequate urinary concentrations
Penicillins			
Amoxicillin–clavulanate	Hypersensitivity (rash, anaphylaxis), diarrhea, superinfections, and seizures	CBC, signs of rash, or hypersensitivity	Due to increasing *E. coli* resistance, amoxicillin–clavulanate is the preferred penicillin for uncomplicated cystitis

(Continued)

| | **TABLE 51-1** | Commonly Used Antimicrobial Agents in the Treatment of UTIs *(Continued)* |

Drug	Adverse Drug Reactions	Monitoring Parameters	Comments
Cephalosporins			
Cefaclor	Hypersensitivity (rash, anaphylaxis), diarrhea, superinfections, and seizures	CBC, signs of rash, or hypersensitivity	No major advantages over other agents for treating UTIs, and they are more expensive. Not active against enterococci
Cefpodoxime-proxetil			
Parenteral therapy			
Aminoglycosides			
Gentamicin	Ototoxicity, nephrotoxicity	Serum creatinine and BUN, serum drug concentrations, and individual pharmacokinetic monitoring	Renally excreted and achieve good concentrations in the urine. Amikacin generally is reserved for multidrug-resistant bacteria
Tobramycin			
Amikacin			
Penicillins			
Ampicillin–sulbactam	Hypersensitivity (rash, anaphylaxis), diarrhea, superinfections, and seizures	CBC, signs of rash, or hypersensitivity	Generally are equally effective for susceptible bacteria. The extended-spectrum penicillins are more active against *P. aeruginosa* and enterococci and often are preferred over cephalosporins. They are very useful in renally impaired patients or when an aminoglycoside is to be avoided
Piperacillin–tazobactam			
Cephalosporins			
Ceftriaxone	Hypersensitivity (rash, anaphylaxis), diarrhea, superinfections, and seizures	CBC, signs of rash, or hypersensitivity	Second- and third-generation cephalosporins have a broad spectrum of activity against gram-negative bacteria, but are not active against enterococci and have limited activity against *P. aeruginosa*. Ceftazidime and cefepime are active against *P. aeruginosa*. They are useful for nosocomial infections and urosepsis due to susceptible pathogens
Ceftazidime			
Cefepime			
Ceftozolane/Tazobactam			
Ceftazidime/Avabactam			

(Continued)

TABLE 51-1	Commonly Used Antimicrobial Agents in the Treatment of UTIs (Continued)		
Drug	**Adverse Drug Reactions**	**Monitoring Parameters**	**Comments**
Carbapenems/ Monobactams			
Imipenem– cilistatin Meropenem Meropenem/ Vaborbactam Doripenem Ertapenem Aztreonam	Hypersensitivity (rash, anaphylaxis), diarrhea, superinfections, and seizures	CBC, signs of rash, or hypersensitivity	Carbapenems have a broad spectrum of activity, including gram-positive, gram-negative, and anaerobic bacteria. Imipenem, meropenem, and doripenem are active against *P. aeruginosa* and enterococci, but ertapenem is not. Aztreonam is a monobactam that is only active against gram-negative bacteria, including some strains of *P. aeruginosa*. Generally useful for nosocomial infections when aminoglycosides are to be avoided and in penicillin-sensitive patients
Fluoroquinolones			
Ciprofloxacin Levofloxacin	Hypersensitivity, photosensitivity, GI symptoms, dizziness, confusion, and tendonitis (black box warning)	CBC, baseline serum creatinine, and BUN	Broad-spectrum activity against both gram-negative and gram-positive bacteria. They provide urine and high-tissue concentrations and are actively secreted in reduced renal function

BUN, blood urea nitrogen; CBC, complete blood count; GI, gastrointestinal; UTIs, urinary tract infections.

and their susceptibilities are generally known, a cost-effective approach to management is recommended that includes a urinalysis and initiation of empiric therapy without a urine culture (**Figure 51-1**).

- Short-course therapy (3-day therapy) with **trimethoprim–sulfamethoxazole** or a **fluoroquinolone** (eg, **ciprofloxacin** or **levofloxacin**, but not moxifloxacin) is superior to single-dose therapy for uncomplicated infection. Fluoroquinolones should be reserved for patients with suspected or possible pyelonephritis due to the collateral damage risk. Instead, a 3-day course of trimethoprim–sulfamethoxazole, a 5-day course of nitrofurantoin, or a one-time dose of **fosfomycin** should be considered

TABLE 51-2	Overview of Outpatient Antimicrobial Therapy for Lower Tract Infections in Adults			
Indications	**Antibiotic**	**Oral Dose**	**Interval**[a]	**Duration**
Lower tract infections				
Uncomplicated	Trimethoprim–sulfamethoxazole	1 DS tablet	Twice a day	3 days
	Nitrofurantoin monohydrate	100 mg	Twice a day	5 days
	Fosfomycin trometamol	3 g	Single dose	1 day
	Ciprofloxacin	250 mg	Twice a day	3 days
	Levofloxacin	250 mg	Once a day	3 days
	Amoxicillin–clavulanate	500 mg	Every 8 hours	5–7 days
	Pivmecillinam	400 mg	Twice a day	3 days
Complicated	Trimethoprim–sulfamethoxazole	1 DS tablet	Twice a day	7–10 days
	Ciprofloxacin	250–500 mg	Twice a day	7–10 days
	Levofloxacin	250 mg	Once a day	10 days
		750 mg	Once a day	5 days
	Amoxicillin–clavulanate	500 mg	Every 8 hours	7–10 days
Recurrent infections	Nitrofurantoin	50 mg	Once a day	6 months
	Trimethoprim–sulfamethoxazole	1/2 SS tablet	Once a day	6 months
Acute pyelonephritis	Trimethoprim–sulfamethoxazole	1 DS tablet	Twice a day	14 days
	Ciprofloxacin	500 mg	Twice a day	14 days
		1000 mg ER	Once a day	7 days
	Levofloxacin	250 mg	Once a day	10 days
		750 mg	Once a day	5 days
	Amoxicillin–clavulanate	500 mg	Every 8 hours	14 days

[a]Dosing intervals for normal renal function.
DS, double strength; SS, single strength.

as first-line therapy. In areas where there is more than 20% resistance of *E. coli* to trimethoprim–sulfamethoxazole, nitrofurantoin or fosfomycin should be utilized. Amoxicillin or ampicillin is not recommended because of the high incidence of resistant *E. coli*. Follow-up urine cultures are not necessary in patients who respond.

Complicated Urinary Tract Infections

Acute Pyelonephritis

- The presentation of high-grade fever (>38.3°C [100.9°F]) and severe flank pain should be treated as acute pyelonephritis, and aggressive management is warranted. Severely ill patients with pyelonephritis should be hospitalized and IV drugs administered initially. Milder cases may be managed with oral antibiotics in an outpatient setting.

TABLE 51-3 Evidence-Based Empirical Treatment of UTIs and Prostatitis

Diagnosis	Pathogens	Treatment Recommendation	Comments
Acute uncomplicated cystitis	Escherichia coli, Staphylococcus saprophyticus	1. Nitrofurantoin × 5 days (A,I)[a] 2. Trimethoprim–sulfamethoxazole × 3 days (A,I)[a] 3. Fosfomycin trometamol × 1 dose (A,I)[a] 4. Fluoroquinolone × 3 days (A,I)[a] 5. β-Lactams × 3–7 days (B,I)[a] 6. Pivmecillinam × 3–7 days (A,I)	Short-course therapy more effective than single dose Reserve fluoroquinolones as alternatives to development of resistance (A-III)[a] β-Lactams as a group are not as effective in acute cystitis than trimethoprim–sulfamethoxazole or the fluoroquinolones; do not use amoxicillin or ampicillin[a] Pivmecillinam not available in the United States
Pregnancy	As above	1. Amoxicillin–clavulanate × 7 days 2. Cephalosporin × 7 days 3. Trimethoprim–sulfamethoxazole × 7 days	Avoid trimethoprim–sulfamethoxazole during the third trimester
Acute pyelonephritis			
Uncomplicated	E. coli	1. Fluoroquinolone × 7 days (A,I)[a] 2. Trimethoprim–sulfamethoxazole (if susceptible) × 14 days (A,I)[a]	Can be managed as outpatient
	Gram-positive bacteria	1. Amoxicillin or amoxicillin–clavulanic acid × 14 days	
Complicated	E. coli P. mirabilis K. pneumoniae P. aeruginosa Enterococcus faecalis	1. Quinolone × 14 days 2. Extended-spectrum penicillin plus aminoglycoside	Severity of illness will determine duration of IV therapy; culture results should direct therapy Oral therapy may complete 14 days of therapy
Prostatitis	E. coli K. pneumoniae Proteus spp. P. aeruginosa	1. Trimethoprim–sulfamethoxazole × 4–6 weeks 2. Fluoroquinolone 4–6 weeks	Acute prostatitis may require IV therapy initially Chronic prostatitis may require longer treatment periods or surgery

[a]Strength of recommendations: A, good evidence for; B, moderate evidence for; C, poor evidence for and against; D, moderate against; E, good evidence against. Quality of evidence: I, at least one proper randomized, controlled study; II, one well-designed clinical trial; III, evidence from opinions, clinical experience, and expert committees.

UTI, urinary tract infection.

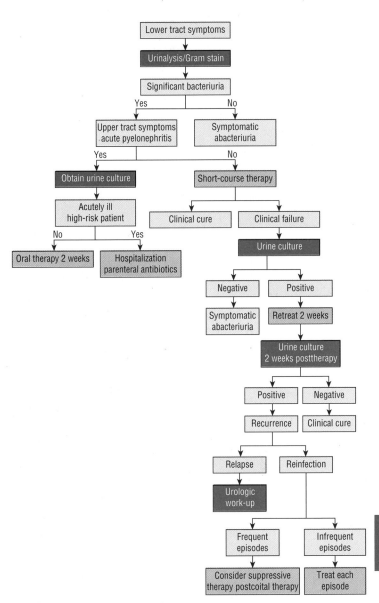

FIGURE 51-1. Management of urinary tract infections in women.

- At the time of presentation, a Gram stain of the urine should be performed, along with urinalysis, culture, and sensitivities.
- In the mild to moderately symptomatic patient for whom oral therapy is considered, an effective agent should be administered for 7–14 days, depending on the agent used. Fluoroquinolones (**ciprofloxacin** or **levofloxacin**) orally for 7–10 days are the first-line choice in mild-to-moderate pyelonephritis. Other options include

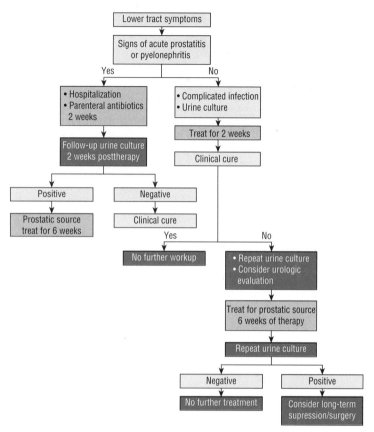

FIGURE 51-2. Management of urinary tract infections in men.

trimethoprim–sulfamethoxazole for 14 days. If a Gram stain reveals gram-positive cocci, *Streptococcus faecalis* should be considered and treatment directed against this pathogen (**ampicillin**).

- In the seriously ill patient, the traditional initial therapy is an IV fluoroquinolone, an aminoglycoside with or without ampicillin, or an extended-spectrum cephalosporin with or without an aminoglycoside.
- If the patient has been hospitalized in the last 6 months, has a urinary catheter, or is in a nursing home, the possibility of *P. aeruginosa* and enterococci infection, as well as multiple-resistant organisms, should be considered. In this setting, **ceftazidime, ticarcillin–clavulanic acid, piperacillin, aztreonam, meropenem**, or **imipenem**, in combination with an aminoglycoside, is recommended. If the patient responds to initial combination therapy, the aminoglycoside may be discontinued after 3 days.
- Follow-up urine cultures should be obtained 2 weeks after the completion of therapy to ensure a satisfactory response and to detect possible relapse.

Urinary Tract Infections in Men

- Therapy in men requires prolonged treatment (**Figure 51-2**).
- A urine culture should be obtained before treatment, because the cause of infection in men is not as predictable as in women.

- If gram-negative bacteria are presumed, trimethoprim–sulfamethoxazole or a fluoroquinolone is a preferred agent. Initial therapy is for 10–14 days. For recurrent infections in men, cure rates are much higher with a 6-week regimen of trimethoprim–sulfamethoxazole.

Recurrent Infections

- Recurrent episodes of UTI (reinfections and relapses) account for a significant portion of all UTIs. These patients are most commonly women and can be divided into two groups: those with fewer than two or three episodes per year and those who develop more frequent infections.
- In patients with infrequent infections (ie, fewer than three infections per year), each episode should be treated as a separately occurring infection. Short-course therapy should be used in symptomatic female patients with lower tract infection.
- In patients who have frequent symptomatic infections, long-term prophylactic antimicrobial therapy may be instituted (see Table 51-2). Therapy is generally given for 6 months, with urine cultures followed monthly.
- In women who experience symptomatic reinfections in association with sexual activity, voiding after intercourse may help prevent infection. Also, self-administered, single-dose prophylactic therapy with **trimethoprim–sulfamethoxazole** taken after intercourse significantly reduces the incidence of recurrent infection in these patients.
- Women who relapse after short-course therapy should receive a 2-week course of therapy. In patients who relapse after 2 weeks, therapy should be continued for another 2–4 weeks. If relapse occurs after 6 weeks of treatment, urologic examination should be performed, and therapy for 6 months or even longer may be considered.

SPECIAL CONDITIONS

URINARY TRACT INFECTION IN PREGNANCY

- In patients with significant bacteriuria, symptomatic or asymptomatic treatment is recommended to avoid possible complications during the pregnancy. Therapy should consist of an agent with a relatively low adverse-effect potential (**cephalexin, amoxicillin**, or **amoxicillin/clavulanate**) administered for 7 days.
- Tetracyclines should be avoided because of teratogenic effects and sulfonamides should not be administered during the third trimester because of the possible development of kernicterus and hyperbilirubinemia. Also, the fluoroquinolones should not be given because of their potential to inhibit cartilage and bone development in the newborn.

CATHETERIZED PATIENTS

- When bacteriuria occurs in asymptomatic, short-term catheterized patients (<30 days), the use of systemic antibiotic therapy should be withheld and the catheter removed as soon as possible. If the patient becomes symptomatic, the catheter should again be removed, and treatment as described for complicated infections should be started.
- The use of prophylactic systemic antibiotics in patients with short-term catheterization reduces the incidence of infection over the first 4–7 days. In long-term catheterized patients, however, antibiotics only postpone the development of bacteriuria and lead to emergence of resistant organisms.

See Chapter 134, Urinary Tract Infections and Prostatitis, authored by Julianna M. Fernandez and Elizabeth A. Coyle, for a more detailed discussion of this topic.

52 Vaccines, Toxoids, and Other Immunobiologics

- *Vaccines* are substances administered to generate a protective immune response. They can be live attenuated or killed.
- *Toxoids* are inactivated bacterial toxins. They retain the ability to stimulate the formation of antitoxins, which are antibodies directed against the bacterial toxin.
- *Adjuvants* are inert substances, such as aluminum salts (ie, alum), which enhance vaccine antigenicity by prolonging antigen absorption.
- *Immune sera* are sterile solutions containing antibody derived from human (immunoglobulin [Ig]) or equine (antitoxin) sources.

VACCINE AND TOXOID RECOMMENDATIONS

- The childhood, adolescent, and adult immunization schedules are updated frequently and published annually. Recommendations for the use of influenza vaccine are issued annually. Healthcare providers involved in primary care and immunization delivery must keep themselves abreast of these changes in a systematic way. Electronic newsletters and browsing reliable websites are efficient methods for obtaining information (Table 52-1).
- In general, killed vaccines can be administered simultaneously at separate sites. Killed and live-attenuated vaccines may be administered simultaneously at separate sites. If they cannot be administered simultaneously, they can be administered at any interval between doses with the exception of cholera (killed) and yellow fever (live) vaccines, which should be given at least 3 weeks apart. If live vaccines are not administered simultaneously, their administration should be separated by at least 4 weeks.

TABLE 52-1	Web Resources for Vaccine Information
Recommended Internet sites for vaccine information	
http://www.cdc.gov/vaccines/	Vaccines and Immunizations Centers for Disease Control and Prevention
www.immunize.org	Immunization Action Coalition
www.nfid.org/	National Foundation for Infectious Diseases
www.cdc.gov/mmwr/	Morbidity and Mortality Weekly Report
http://www.nationalacademies.org/hmd/	The National Academies of Sciences, Engineering, and Medicine. Health and Medicine Division
http://www.hrsa.gov/vaccinecompensation/	Vaccine Injury Compensation Program
http://www.chop.edu/centers-programs/vaccine-education-center/	Vaccine Education Center Children's Hospital of Philadelphia
https://vaers.hhs.gov/index.html	Vaccine Adverse Event Reporting System
Recommended electronic newsletters	
www.immunize.org/express	The Immunization Action Coalition's newsletter
www.cdc.gov/mmwr/	Morbidity and Mortality Weekly Report

- Administration of live vaccines, such as rubella or varicella, are deferred until postpartum and are routinely recommended for new mothers who do not have evidence of immunity prior to hospital discharge. These live vaccines can be administered without regard to administration of Rho(D) Ig (RDIg) in the postpartum period. Pregnant women should receive Tdap during the late second trimester or third trimester of pregnancy. Additionally, Tdap is recommended for all new mothers who have not received a Tdap before because household contacts are frequently implicated as the source of pertussis infection in a young infant.
- In general, severely immunocompromised individuals should not receive live vaccines.
- Patients with chronic conditions that cause limited immunodeficiency (eg, renal disease, diabetes, liver disease, and asplenia) and who are not receiving immunosuppressants may receive live-attenuated and killed vaccines, as well as toxoids.
- Patients with active malignant disease may receive killed vaccines or toxoids but should not be given live vaccines. Live virus vaccines may be administered to persons with leukemia who have not received chemotherapy for at least 3 months.
- If a person has been receiving high-dose corticosteroids or has had a course lasting longer than 2 weeks, then at least 1 month should pass before immunization with live virus vaccines.
- Responses to live and killed vaccines generally are suboptimal for human immune deficiency virus (HIV)–infected patients and decrease as the disease progresses.
- Whenever possible, transplant patients should be immunized before transplantation. Live vaccines generally are not given after transplantation.

DIPHTHERIA TOXOID ADSORBED AND DIPHTHERIA ANTITOXIN

- Two strengths of diphtheria toxoid are available: pediatric strength (D) and adult strength (d), which contain less antigen. Primary immunization with D is indicated for children older than 6 weeks. Generally, D is given along with tetanus and acellular pertussis (DTaP) vaccines at 2, 4, and 6 months of age, and then at 15–18 months and 4–6 years of age.
- For nonimmunized adults, a complete three-dose series of diphtheria toxoid should be administered, with the first two doses given at least 4 weeks apart and the third dose 6–12 months after the second. One dose in the series should be Tdap. The combined preparation, tetanus–diphtheria (Td), is recommended in adults because it contains less diphtheria toxoid than DTaP, with fewer reactions seen from the diphtheria preparation. Booster doses are given every 10 years.
- Adverse effects to diphtheria toxoid include mild to moderate tenderness, erythema, and induration at the injection site.

TETANUS TOXOID, TETANUS TOXOID ADSORBED, AND TETANUS IMMUNOGLOBULIN

- In children, primary immunization against tetanus is usually done in conjunction with diphtheria and pertussis vaccination using DTaP or a combination vaccine that includes other antigens. A 0.5-mL dose is recommended at 2, 4, 6, and 15–18 months of age.
- In children 7 years and older and in adults who have not been previously immunized, a series of three 0.5-mL doses of Td is administered intramuscularly (IM) initially. The first two doses are given 1–2 months apart and the third dose 6–12 months later. Boosters are recommended every 10 years.
- Tetanus toxoid may be given to immunosuppressed patients if indicated.
- Tetanus Ig (TIg) is used to provide passive tetanus immunization after the occurrence of traumatic wounds in nonimmunized or suboptimally immunized persons (**Table 52-2**). A dose of 250–500 units is administered IM. When administered with tetanus toxoid, separate sites for administration should be used.
- TIg is also used for the treatment of tetanus. In this setting, a single dose of 3000–6000 units is administered IM.

TABLE 52-2	Tetanus Prophylaxis			
Vaccination History	**Clean, Minor Wounds**		**All Other Wounds**	
	Td[a]	TIG	Td[a]	TIG
Unknown or fewer than three doses	Yes	No	Yes	Yes
Three or more doses	No[a,b]	No	No[a,c]	No

[a]A single dose of Tdap should be used for the next dose of tetanus–diphtheria toxoid for individuals aged >10 years.
[b]Yes, if more than 10 years since last dose.
[c]Yes, if more than 5 years since last dose.

HAEMOPHILUS INFLUENZAE TYPE B VACCINES

- *Haemophilus influenzae* type b (Hib) vaccines currently in use are conjugate products, consisting of either a polysaccharide or oligosaccharide of polyribosylribitol phosphate (PRP) covalently linked to a protein carrier.
- Hib conjugate vaccines are indicated for routine use in all infants and children younger than 5 years.
- The primary series of Hib vaccination consists of 0.5-mL IM doses at 2, 4, and 6 months of age. If PRP-OMP (PRP conjugated to an outer membrane protein) is used, it should be given at ages 2 and 4 months. A booster dose is recommended at age 12–15 months.
- For infants 7–11 months of age who have not been vaccinated, three doses of Hib vaccine should be given: two doses spaced 4 weeks apart and then a booster dose at age 12–15 months (but at least 8 weeks since the second dose). For unvaccinated children ages 12–14 months, two doses should be given, with an interval of 2 months between doses. In a child older than 15 months, a single dose of any of the four conjugate vaccines is indicated.

HEPATITIS VACCINES

- Information on hepatitis vaccines can be found in Chapter 25.

HUMAN PAPILLOMAVIRUS VACCINE

- ACIP recommends HPV vaccine for the prevention of HPV-related disease in individuals aged 9–26 years. Individuals who start the HPV series between the ages of 9 and 14 years should receive two doses separated by 6 months. This vaccine is administered as a three-dose series using a schedule of 0, 1–2, and 6 months for individuals who start the series at age 15 years or older. The vaccines are recommended for adolescents aged 11–12 years and catch-up immunization for individuals aged 13–26 years.
- The ACIP recommended shared clinical decision-making for HPV vaccine for individuals aged 27–45 years. The vaccine is administered as a three-dose series (0, 1–2, and 6 months).
- The vaccine is well tolerated, with injection site reactions and headache and fatigue occurring as commonly as in placebo groups.

INFLUENZA VIRUS VACCINE

- See Chapter 41 for information regarding influenza vaccination.

MEASLES VACCINE

- Measles vaccine is a live-attenuated vaccine that is administered for primary immunization to persons 12–15 months of age or older, usually as a combination of measles, mumps, and rubella (MMR). A second dose is recommended at 4–6 years of age.

- Measles-containing vaccine should not be given to pregnant women or immunosuppressed patients. An exception is HIV-infected patients, who are at very high risk for severe complications if they develop measles.
- The vaccine should not be given within 1 month of any other live vaccine unless the vaccine is given on the same day (as with the MMR vaccine).
- Measles vaccine is indicated in all persons born after 1956 or in those who lack documentation of wild virus infection by either history or antibody titers.

MENINGOCOCCAL VACCINES

- There are two meningococcal conjugate vaccines: Menactra is licensed for individuals 9 months–55 years old and Menveo for those 2 months–55 years old. They are recommended for all children 11–12 years old with a second dose at 16 years of age.
- The vaccine is indicated in high-risk populations such as those exposed to the disease, those in the midst of uncontrolled outbreaks, travelers to an area with epidemic hyperendemic meningococcal disease, and individuals who have terminal complement deficiencies or asplenia. Reimmunization at 5-year intervals is recommended for individuals who are at high risk. The polysaccharide vaccine should be reserved for those older than 55 years who require immunization.
- Also, there are two meningococcal serogroup B vaccines (Trumenba and Bexsero), and are licensed for individuals 10–25 years of age. Either vaccine is recommended for individuals at high risk for invasive meningococcal disease.

MUMPS VACCINE

- The vaccine (usually given in conjunction with measles and rubella, MMR) is given beginning at age 12–15 months, with a second dose prior to entry into elementary school.
- Two doses of mumps vaccine are recommended for school-age children, international travelers, college students, and healthcare workers born after 1956.
- Postexposure vaccination is of no benefit.
- Mumps vaccine should not be given to pregnant women or immunosuppressed patients. The vaccine should not be given within 6 weeks (preferably 3 months) of administration of Ig.

PERTUSSIS VACCINE

- Acellular pertussis vaccine is usually administered in combination with diphtheria and tetanus toxoids (as DTaP).
- The primary immunization series for pertussis vaccine consists of four doses given at ages 2, 4, 6, and 15–18 months. A booster dose is recommended at age 4–6 years. Pertussis vaccine is administered in combination with diphtheria and tetanus (DTaP). Administration of an acellular pertussis-containing vaccine is also recommended for adolescents once between ages 11 and 18 years and a single dose of Tdap should be administered to all adults.
- Tdap should be administered to females in their late second or third trimester of pregnancy. Tdap should also be administered to all close contacts, including household contacts and out of home care providers.
- Systemic reactions, such as moderate fever, occur in 3%–5% of those receiving vaccines. Very rarely, high fever, febrile seizures, persistent crying spells, and hypotonic hyporesponsive episodes occur after vaccination.
- There are only two contraindications to pertussis administration: (1) an immediate anaphylactic reaction to a previous dose and (2) encephalopathy within 7 days of a previous dose, with no evidence of other cause.

PNEUMOCOCCAL VACCINES

- Pneumococcal polysaccharide vaccine is a mixture of capsular polysaccharides from 23 of the most prevalent types of *Streptococcus pneumoniae* seen in the United States (PPV23). The vaccine is administered IM or subcutaneously as a single 0.5 mL dose.
- Pneumococcal vaccine (PPV23) is recommended for the following immunocompetent persons:
  - ✓ Persons 65 years or older. If an individual received vaccine more than 5 years earlier and was younger than 65 at the time of administration, revaccination should be given.
  - ✓ Persons ages 2–64 years with chronic illness.
  - ✓ Persons ages 2–64 years with functional or anatomical asplenia. When splenectomy is planned, pneumococcal vaccine should be given at least 2 weeks before surgery. A single revaccination is recommended at 5 years in subjects older than 10 years and at 3 years in subjects younger than 10 years).
  - ✓ Persons aged 19–64 years who smoke cigarettes or have asthma.
  - ✓ Persons with cochlear implants.
- Pneumococcal vaccination (PPV23) is recommended for immunocompromised persons 2 years of age or older with:
  - ✓ HIV infection
  - ✓ Leukemia, lymphoma, Hodgkin disease, or multiple myeloma
  - ✓ Generalized malignancy
  - ✓ Chronic renal failure of nephritic syndrome
  - ✓ Patients receiving immunosuppressive therapy
  - ✓ Organ or bone marrow transplant recipients
- Because children younger than 2 years do not respond adequately to the pneumococcal polysaccharide vaccine, a pneumococcal conjugate vaccine was created (PCV13).
- PCV 13 valent (Prevnar-13) is administered as a 0.5-mL IM injection at 2, 4, and 6 months of age and between 12 and 15 months of age. A single dose of PCV13 should be administered to children aged 6–18 years with sickle cell disease or splenic dysfunction, HIV infection, immunocompromising conditions, cochlear implant, or cerebral spinal fluid leak should be immunized. It is also licensed for individuals aged 50 years and older.

POLIOVIRUS VACCINES

- Two types of trivalent poliovirus vaccines are currently licensed for distribution in the United States: an enhanced inactivated poliovirus vaccine (IPV) and a live-attenuated, oral poliovirus vaccine (OPV). IPV is the recommended vaccine for the primary series and booster dose for children in the United States, whereas OPV is recommended in areas of the world that have circulating poliovirus.
- IPV is given to children ages 2, 4, and 6–18 months and 4–6 years. Primary poliomyelitis immunization is recommended for all children and young adults up to age 18 years. Allergies to any component of IPV, including streptomycin, polymyxin B, and neomycin, are contraindications to vaccine use.
- The routine use of OPV in the United States has been discontinued.

RUBELLA VACCINE

- The vaccine is given with measles and mumps vaccines (MMR) at 12–15 months of age, then at 4–6 years.
- The vaccine should not be given to immunosuppressed individuals, although MMR vaccine should be administered to young children with HIV without severe immunosuppression as soon as possible after their first birthday. The vaccine should not be given to individuals with anaphylactic reaction to neomycin.

- Although the vaccine has not been associated with congenital rubella syndrome, its use in pregnancy is contraindicated. Women should be counseled not to become pregnant for 4 weeks after vaccination.

VARICELLA VACCINE

- Varicella virus vaccine is recommended for all children 12–18 months of age, with a second dose prior to entering school between 4 and 6 years of age. It is also recommended for persons above this age if they have not had chickenpox. Persons ages 13 years and older should receive two doses separated by 4–8 weeks.
  ✓ The vaccine is contraindicated in immunosuppressed or pregnant patients.
  ✓ Children with asymptomatic or mildly symptomatic HIV should receive two doses of varicella vaccine 3 months apart.

ZOSTER VACCINE

- Two vaccines for the prevention of zoster are available, a live-attenuated vaccine (Zostavax) and a recombinant zoster vaccine (Shingrix). The recombinant zoster vaccine is 91% effective for preventing zoster and is currently the preferred product for use as recommended by the ACIP for use in immunocompetent individuals aged 50 years and older as a two-dose series at 0 and 2–6 months.
- Almost 80% of those who receive the recombinant vaccine report injection site pain with 9% of those reporting injection site reactions that interfere with their normal activities.

IMMUNOGLOBULIN

- Ig is available as both IM (IGIM) and IV (IGIV) preparations.
- Table 52-3 lists the suggested dosages for IGIM in various disease states.
- The uses for IGIV are as follows:
  ✓ Primary immunodeficiency states, including both antibody deficiencies and combined deficiencies
  ✓ Idiopathic thrombocytopenia
  ✓ Chronic lymphocytic leukemia in patients who have had a serious bacterial infection
  ✓ Kawasaki disease (mucocutaneous lymph node syndrome)
  ✓ Pediatric HIV infection
  ✓ Allogeneic bone marrow transplant
  ✓ Chronic inflammatory demyelinating polyneuropathy and multifocal motor neuropathy
  ✓ Multifocal motor neuropathy
  ✓ Kidney transplantation involving a recipient with high antibody concentrations or an ABO incompatible donor

TABLE 52-3	Indications and Dosage of Intramuscular Immunoglobulin in Infectious Diseases
Primary immunodeficiency states	1.2 mL/kg IM then 0.6 mL/kg every 2–4 weeks
Hepatitis A exposure	0.02 mL/kg IM within 2 weeks if <1 year or >39 years of age
Hepatitis A prophylaxis	0.02 mL/kg IM for exposure <3 months' duration
	0.06 mL/kg IM for exposure up to 5 months' duration
Hepatitis B exposure	0.06 mL/kg (HBIG preferred in known exposures)
Measles exposure	0.5 mL/kg (maximum dose 15 mL) as soon as possible

RHO(D) IMMUNOGLOBULIN

- Rho(D) Ig (RDIg) suppresses the antibody response and formation of anti-Rho(D) in Rho(D)-negative, D^u-negative women exposed to Rho(D)-positive blood and prevents the future chance of erythroblastosis fetalis in subsequent pregnancies with a Rho(D)-positive fetus.
- RDIg, when administered IM within 72 hours of delivery of a full-term infant, reduces active antibody formation from 1% to 0.2%.
- RDIg is also used in the case of a premenopausal woman who is Rho(D) negative and has inadvertently received Rho(D)-positive blood or blood products.
- RDIg may be used after abortion, miscarriage, amniocentesis, or abdominal trauma.

See Chapter 142, Vaccines, Toxoids, and Other Immunobiologics, authored by Mary S. Hayney, for a more detailed discussion of this topic.

CHAPTER

53 | Alzheimer Disease

- *Alzheimer disease* (AD) affects ~7.5 million Americans of all ages and is a progressive illness of unknown cause characterized by loss of cognitive and physical functioning, commonly with behavior symptoms.

PATHOPHYSIOLOGY

- Dominantly inherited forms of AD are fewer than 1% of cases. More than half of young-onset, dominantly inherited cases are attributed to chromosomal alterations that affect processing of the amyloid precursor protein. Genetic susceptibility to late-onset AD is primarily linked to the apolipoprotein E (*APOE*) genotype, but an interaction of multiple genes with the environment may be at play.
- AD risk factors include age, decreased reserve capacity of the brain, head injury, Down syndrome, depression, mild cognitive impairment, and risk factors for vascular disease, including hypertension, elevated homocysteine, elevated low-density lipoprotein cholesterol, low high-density lipoprotein cholesterol, obesity, metabolic syndrome, and diabetes.
- Signature findings include intracellular neurofibrillary tangles (NFTs), extracellular amyloid plaques in the cortex and medial temporal lobe, degeneration of neurons and synapses, and cortical atrophy. AD-affected individuals appear to have a higher burden of plaques and NFTs in their younger years compared to age-matched controls.
- Proposed mechanisms for these changes include: (1) β-amyloid protein aggregation, leading to formation of plaques; (2) hyperphosphorylation of tau protein, leading to NFTs; (3) synaptic failure and depletion of neurotrophin and neurotransmitters; (4) mitochondrial dysfunction; and (5) oxidative stress. The amyloid cascade hypothesis states that there is an imbalance between production and clearance of β-amyloid, with aggregation and accumulation of β-amyloid leading to AD. Whether this is the primary pathology in most forms of AD remains to be shown.
- Of neurotransmitter deficits, loss of cholinergic activity is most prominent, and it correlates with AD severity. Cholinergic cell loss seems to be a consequence of AD pathology, not the cause of it.
- Other neurotransmitter considerations include: (1) serotonergic neurons of the raphe nuclei and noradrenergic cells of the locus ceruleus are lost; (2) monoamine oxidase type B activity is increased; (3) glutamate pathways of the cortex and limbic structures are abnormal; and (4) excitatory neurotransmitters, including glutamate, may be neurotoxic.

CLINICAL PRESENTATION

- Cognitive decline is gradual and includes memory loss, aphasia, apraxia, agnosia, disorientation, and impaired executive function. Other non-cognitive symptoms include depression, psychotic symptoms, aggression, motor hyperactivity, uncooperativeness, wandering, and combativeness. Patients become increasingly unable to care for themselves. Table 53-1 shows the stages of AD.

TABLE 53-1	Stages of Alzheimer Disease
Mild (MMSE score 26–21)	Patient has difficulty remembering recent events. Ability to manage finances, prepare food, and carry out other household activities declines. May get lost while driving. Begins to withdraw from difficult tasks and to give up hobbies. May deny memory problems.
Moderate (MMSE score 20–10)	Patient requires assistance with activities of daily living. Frequently disoriented with regard to time (date, year, and season). Recall of recent events is severely impaired. May forget some details of past life events and names of family and friends. Functioning may fluctuate from day to day. Patient generally denies problems. May become suspicious or tearful. Loses ability to drive safely. Agitation, paranoia, and delusions are common.
Severe (MMSE score 9–0)	Patient loses ability to speak, walk, and feed self. Incontinent of urine and feces. Requires care 24 hours a day, 7 days a week.

MMSE, Mini-Mental State Examination.

DIAGNOSIS

- The National Institute on Aging and the Alzheimer's Association view AD as a spectrum beginning with an asymptomatic preclinical phase progressing to the symptomatic preclinical phase and then to the dementia phase. AD is a clinical diagnosis, based largely on identified symptoms and difficulty with activities of daily living revealed by patient and caregiver interviews.
- Patients with suspected AD should have a history and physical examination with appropriate laboratory tests (serum B_{12}, folate, thyroid panel, blood cell counts, serum electrolytes, and liver function tests), and computed tomography (CT) or magnetic resonance imaging (MRI) may aid diagnosis.
- International guidelines recommend structural imaging (ie, noncontrast enhanced CT or MRI) be performed when evaluating people with suspected dementia to identify structural abnormalities consistent with AD or other pathology, such as brain atrophy, vascular damage, or tumors. To exclude other diagnoses, cerebrospinal fluid analysis or an electroencephalogram can occasionally be justified.
- Obtain information on medication use; alcohol or other substance use; family medical history; and history of trauma, depression, or head injury. Rule out medication use (eg, anticholinergics, sedatives, hypnotics, opioids, antipsychotics, and anticonvulsants) as contributors to dementia symptoms. Rule out medications that could contribute to delirium (eg, digoxin, nonsteroidal anti-inflammatory drugs [NSAIDs], histamine-2 [H_2] receptor antagonists, amiodarone, antihypertensives, and corticosteroids).
- The Folstein Mini-Mental State Examination (MMSE) can help establish a history of deficits in two or more areas of cognition at baseline against which to evaluate change in severity over time. The average expected decline in an untreated patient is 2–4 points per year (Table 53-1). Other scales for assessment are also available.
- In the future, improved brain imaging and validated biomarkers of disease will enable a more accurate diagnosis with identified cognitive strengths and weaknesses and neuroanatomic localization of deficits.

TREATMENT

- <u>Goals of Treatment</u>: The goal of treatment in AD is to maintain cognitive functioning and activities of daily living as long as possible, with a secondary goal to treat the psychiatric and behavioral symptoms.

NONPHARMACOLOGIC THERAPY

- The general approach to nonpharmacologic strategies for cognitive and non-cognitive symptoms of AD is to identify the symptom and causative factors, and adapt the caregiving environment to remedy the situation.
- Sleep disturbances, wandering, urinary incontinence, agitation, and aggression should be managed with behavioral and environmental interventions whenever possible, for example, redirecting the patient's attention and removing stressors and triggers.
- On initial diagnosis, the patient and caregiver should be educated on the course of illness, available treatments, legal decisions, changes in lifestyle that will become necessary, and other quality-of-life issues.
- Primary prevention of AD may include smoking cessation, increasing physical activity, and reducing midlife obesity, hypertension, and diabetes. Also adherence to the Mediterranean Diet or Dietary Approaches to Stop Hypertension (DASH) Diet may reduce the risk of cognitive impairment or decline.

PHARMACOLOGIC THERAPY OF COGNITIVE SYMPTOMS

- Cholinesterase inhibitors and NMDA-receptor antagonists are indicated for treatment of AD. Current guidelines do not have a specific preference for cholinesterase inhibitor initiation.
- Reasonable expectations of treatment may be a slowed decline in abilities and delayed long-term care placement.
- Dosing regimens should be simplified and patient and caregiver preferences considered in an effort to improve medication adherence and persistence.
- Gaps in treatment may be associated with a loss of benefits when medication is stopped but this is controversial.

Cholinesterase Inhibitors

- **Table 53-2** summarizes dosing of the cholinesterase inhibitors and memantine.
- No comparative trials have assessed the effectiveness of one agent over another. **Donepezil**, **rivastigmine**, and **galantamine** are indicated in mild-to-moderate AD; donepezil is also indicated for severe AD.
- MMSE is practical to use in the clinical setting to measure changes in cognitive function. Successful treatment would show a decline in MMSE sco re of less than 2 points per year.
- The three cholinesterase inhibitors have similar efficacy in mild-to-moderate AD, and duration of benefit lasts 3–24 months. Because of their short half-lives, if rivastigmine or galantamine treatment is interrupted for several days or longer, retitrate starting at the lowest dose. Gradual dose titration over several months improves tolerability. When switching from one agent to another, a washout period is recommended.
- **Table 53-3** lists common side effects and monitoring parameters for the cholinesterase inhibitors. Abrupt discontinuation can cause worsening of cognition and behavior in some patients.

N-Methyl-D-Aspartate (NMDA) Receptor Antagonist

- **Memantine** (Namenda) blocks glutamatergic neurotransmission by antagonizing NMDA receptors, which may prevent excitotoxic reactions. It is used as monotherapy and in combination with a cholinesterase inhibitor. It is indicated for treatment of moderate to severe AD, but not for mild AD. It is not metabolized by the liver and is primarily excreted unchanged in the urine. Dosing must be adjusted in patients with renal impairment. It is usually well tolerated; side effects include constipation, confusion, dizziness, and headache (**Table 53-3**).
- Combination therapy with cholinesterase inhibitors and memantine, individually or as **Namzaric**, is generally prescribed for people with moderate-to-severe AD and has been shown to slow cognitive and functional decline to a statistically

TABLE 53-2	Dosing of Drugs Used for Cognitive Symptoms				
Drug	Brand Name	Initial Dose	Usual Range	Special Population Dose	Other
Cholinesterase inhibitors					
Donepezil	Aricept, Aricept ODT	5 mg daily in the evening	5–10 mg daily in mild to moderate AD 10–23 mg daily in moderate to severe AD	No dosage adjustments recommended	Available as: tablet, ODT, oral solution Can be taken with or without food Weight loss associated with 23 mg daily dose
Rivastigmine	Exelon	1.5 mg twice daily (capsule, oral solution) 4.6 mg/day (transdermal patch)	3–6 mg twice a day (capsule, oral solution) 9.5–13.3 mg/day (transdermal patch)	Capsule/oral solution: renal impairment, hepatic impairment, or low body weight (<50 kg [<110 lb]): patients may be able to only tolerate lower doses Transdermal patch: mild to moderate hepatic impairment or low body weight: consider maximum daily dose of 4.6 mg every 24 hours	Available as: capsule, oral solution, transdermal patch Take with meals Also indicated for Parkinson disease dementia Application of multiple transdermal patches at same time associated with hospitalization and death
Galantamine	Razadyne, Razadyne ER	4 mg twice daily (tablet, oral solution) 8 mg daily in the morning (extended-release capsule)	8–12 mg twice a day (tablet, oral solution) 16–24 mg (extended-release capsule)	Moderate renal or hepatic impairment: maximum daily dose of 16 mg Severe renal or hepatic impairment: not recommended	Available as: tablet, oral solution, extended-release capsule Take with meals

N-methyl-D-aspartate (NMDA) receptor antagonist

Memantine	Namenda, Namenda XR	5 mg daily (tablet, oral solution) 7 mg daily (extended-release capsule)	10 mg twice daily 28 mg daily (extended-release capsule)	Severe renal impairment: recommended maintenance dose of 5 mg twice daily (tablet, oral solution) or 14 mg daily (extended-release capsule) Severe hepatic impairment: administer with caution	Available as: tablet, oral solution, extended-release capsule Can be taken with or without food Can open capsule and sprinkle contents on applesauce for ease of administration

Cholinesterase inhibitor + NMDA receptor antagonist

Memantine + donepezil	Namzaric	7 mg/10 mg (if patient is stabilized on donepezil and not currently on memantine) 28 mg/10 mg (if patient is stabilized on memantine and donepezil)	28 mg/10 mg daily	Severe renal impairment: 14 mg/10 mg daily	Available as: memantine extended-release and donepezil capsule Can be taken with or without food Can open capsule and sprinkle contents on applesauce for ease of administration

ODT, orally disintegrating tablet.

TABLE 53-3	Monitoring Drug Therapy for Cognitive Symptoms		
Drug	**Adverse Drug Reaction**	**Monitoring Parameters**	**Comments**
Galantamine	Serious skin reactions (Stevens–Johnson syndrome and acute generalized exanthematous pustulosis)	Appearance of skin rash	Discontinue galantamine at first sign of skin rash, unless clearly not drug related
			If signs/symptoms are suggestive of a serious reaction, consider alternative treatment and do not rechallenge
Rivastigmine	Allergic dermatitis	Application site reaction spread beyond patch size, evidence of a more intense local reaction (increasing erythema, edema, papules, vesicles), and persistence of symptoms for more than 48 hours after patch removal	Discontinue rivastigmine if evidence of disseminated allergic dermatitis appears
			Patients sensitized by exposure to the transdermal patch may not be able to take rivastigmine by mouth either; allergy testing and close medical supervision recommended
Cholinesterase inhibitors	Dizziness, syncope, bradycardia, atrial arrhythmias, sinoatrial and atrioventricular block, myocardial infarction	Report of dizziness or falls, pulse, blood pressure, and postural blood pressure change	Dizziness is usually mild, transient, and not related to cardiovascular problems
			Routine pulse checks at baseline, monthly during titration, and every 6 months thereafter
	Nausea, vomiting, diarrhea, anorexia, weight loss	Weight and GI complaints	Take with food to decrease GI upset
			Usually transient, dose-related GI adverse effects seen with drug initiation, dosage titration, or drug switch
			Debilitated patients or those weighing <55 kg (<121 lb) may be more likely to experience GI adverse effects and significant weight loss, particularly when rivastigmine is prescribed or when titrating to donepezil 23 mg
			GI adverse effects less prominent with transdermal versus oral rivastigmine

(Continued)

	Adverse Drug	Monitoring	
Drug	**Reaction**	**Parameters**	**Comments**
Cholinesterase inhibitors (con't)	Peptic ulcer disease, GI bleeding	Signs or symptoms of active or occult GI bleeding	Of particular concern for patients at increased risk of developing ulcers, such as those with a history of ulcer disease or concurrently taking NSAIDs
	Insomnia, vivid/ abnormal dreams, nightmares	Complaints of sleep disturbances, daytime drowsiness	Donepezil can be taken in the morning to decrease risk of sleep disturbances
Memantine	Headache, confusion, dizziness, hallucinations	Report of dizziness or falls, hallucinations	Confusion may be observed during dose titration and is usually transient
	Constipation	GI complaints	Memantine may mitigate GI adverse effects associated with cholinesterase inhibitor therapy

TABLE 53-3 Monitoring Drug Therapy for Cognitive Symptoms *(Continued)*

GI, gastrointestinal; NSAIDs, nonsteroidal anti-inflammatory drugs.

significant degree compared to cholinesterase inhibitor monotherapy or no treatment. Memantine may help mitigate some of the GI adverse effects seen with cholinesterase inhibitors.

Other Drugs

- Use of estrogen, NSAIDS, prednisone, statins, or ginkgo biloba is not recommended to prevent or treat dementia.
- Vitamin E is under investigation for prevention of AD and is not recommended for treatment of AD.
- Do not use ginkgo biloba in individuals taking anticoagulants or antiplatelet drugs, and use cautiously in those taking NSAIDs.
- There is currently insufficient evidence to recommend medical foods such as Axona, Souvenaid, and Cerefolin NAC for treatment of AD.

PHARMACOLOGIC THERAPY OF NONCOGNITIVE SYMPTOMS

- No drug is FDA approved for the treatment of AD behavioral and psychological symptoms such as psychotic symptoms, inappropriate or disruptive behavior, and depression.
- General guidelines include: (1) starting with reduced doses and titrating slowly; (2) monitoring closely; (3) periodically attempting to taper and discontinue medication; and (4) careful documentation.
- Some evidence supports that cholinesterase inhibitors and memantine may be beneficial in treating non-cognitive symptoms, but they do not reduce acute agitation. Avoid anticholinergic psychotropic medications as they may worsen cognition.

Antidepressants

- Depression and dementia share many symptoms, and the diagnosis of depression can be difficult, especially later in the course of AD.

- A **selective serotonin reuptake inhibitor** (SSRI) is usually given to depressed patients with AD, and the best evidence is for **sertraline** and **citalopram**. **Tricyclic antidepressants** are usually avoided.
  ✓ Common side effects seen with SSRIs can be found in Chapter 68.

Antipsychotics

- Antipsychotic medications have traditionally been used for disruptive behaviors and neuropsychiatric symptoms, but the risks and benefits must be carefully weighed.
- Atypical antipsychotics (ie, **aripiprazole, risperidone, olanzapine**, and **quetiapine**) have been shown to be more effective compared to placebo; however, the higher risk of adverse effects and mortality offset this benefit. Antipsychotics in AD should be restricted to patients with severe symptoms that have not responded to other measures, and treatment should be tapered as early as possible and rarely used beyond 12 weeks.
  ✓ Common adverse events include somnolence, extrapyramidal symptoms, abnormal gait, worsening cognition, cerebrovascular events, and increased risk of death (see black-box warning). See Chapter 70 for more information.

Miscellaneous Therapies

- Evidence for benzodiazepine use is lacking and not advised due to significant adverse effects.
- Use of antiepileptic medication (ie, carbamazepine and gabapentin) may be alternatives for agitation, but evidence is conflicting. Use of valproic acid is no longer recommended due to severe adverse effects.

EVALUATION OF THERAPEUTIC OUTCOMES

- At baseline interview both patient and caregiver to identify target symptoms; define therapeutic goals; and document cognitive status, physical status, functional performance, mood, thought processes, and behavior.
- Use the MMSE for cognition, Bristol Activities of Daily Living Scale for activities of daily living, and Neuropsychiatric Inventory Questionnaire for assessment of behavioral disturbances to quantify changes in symptoms and functioning.
- Observe the patient carefully for potential side effects. The specific side effects to be monitored and the method and frequency of monitoring should be documented.
- Assess for drug effectiveness, side effects, adherence to regimen, and need for dosage adjustment or change in treatment at 2–4 weeks, and 8–12 weeks after initiation, followed by every 3–6 months thereafter. Several months to 1 year of treatment may be required to determine whether medications for cognition are beneficial.
- Drug deprescribing for people with AD is aided by the availability of deprescribing guidelines. When to stop treatment due to lack of efficacy, if ever, is controversial.

See Chapter 71, Alzheimer Disease, authored by Emily P. Peron, Kristin M. Zimmerman, Ericka L Crouse, Patricia W. Slattum, and Sarah E. Hobgood, for a more detailed discussion of this topic.

54 Epilepsy and Status Epilepticus

- *Epilepsy* is a common neurologic condition in which a person is prone to recurrent epileptic seizures. Epilepsies are characterized by different seizure types, ranging in severity and etiologies often with neurobiological, cognitive, psychological, and social consequences. *Status epilepticus* (SE) is a neurologic emergency associated with brain damage and death with generalized convulsive status epilepticus (GCSE) being the most common and severe form. It occurs when the length of the continuous seizure activity extends past 5 minutes or time of ongoing seizure activity extends past 30 minutes, after which there is a risk of long-term consequences.

PATHOPHYSIOLOGY

- Seizures result from excessive excitation or disordered inhibition of neurons, resulting in changes in electrical activity as measured by the electroencephalogram (EEG). Initially, a small number of neurons fire abnormally. Normal membrane conductances and inhibitory synaptic currents then break down, and excitability spreads locally (focal seizure) or more widely (generalized seizure). Epileptic seizures result only when there is also synchronization of excessive neuronal firing.
- Seizure initiation is likely caused by an imbalance between excitatory (eg, glutamate, calcium, sodium, substance P, and neurokinin B) and inhibitory (γ-aminobutyric acid [GABA], adenosine, potassium, neuropeptide Y, opioid peptides, and galanin) neurotransmission.
- GCSE is largely caused by glutamate acting on postsynaptic *N*-methyl-D-aspartate (NMDA) and α-amino-3-hydroxy-5-methylisoxazole-4-propionate (AMPA)/kainate receptors. Sustained depolarization can result in neuronal death.
- GABA$_A$ receptors may become less responsive to endogenous GABA and GABA agonists.
- Epilepsy etiologies can be classified into six categories: (1) genetic; (2) structural; (3) infectious; (4) metabolic; (5) immune; and (6) unknown.

CLINICAL PRESENTATION

EPILEPSY

- **Figure 54-1** shows the International League Against Epilepsy (ILAE) framework for the classification of seizure types.
- Many patients, particularly those with focal onset seizures with dyscognitive features or generalized tonic–clonic (GTC) seizures, are amnestic to the actual seizure event.
- Symptoms depend on seizure type and where the abnormal firing occurs. Although seizures can vary between patients, they tend to be stereotyped within an individual.
- Focal seizures (ie, partial seizures) begin in one hemisphere of the brain, and unless they become secondarily generalized (ie, evolve to a bilateral convulsive seizure), result in an asymmetric seizure. Focal seizures manifest as alterations in motor functions (eg, twitching or shaking), sensory (eg, numbness or tingling) or somatosensory symptoms, aberrations in behavior, or automatisms. Focal seizures without dyscognitive features (formerly called simple partial seizures) are associated with no impairment of consciousness. In focal seizures with dyscognitive features (formerly called complex partial seizures), there is impairment of consciousness and awareness and no memory of the event.
- Absence seizures generally occur in young children or adolescents and exhibit a sudden onset, interruption of ongoing activities, a blank stare, and possibly a brief upward rotation of the eyes. There is only a very brief (seconds) period of altered consciousness. Absence seizures have a characteristic two to four cycles per second spike and slow-wave EEG pattern.

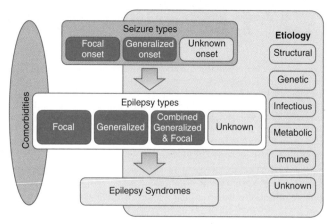

FIGURE 54-1. ILAE 2017 Classification of seizure types—expanded version.

- GTC seizures are major convulsive episodes and are always associated with a loss of consciousness. Motor symptoms are bilateral. GTC seizures may be preceded by premonitory symptoms (ie, an aura). A tonic–clonic seizure that is preceded by an aura is likely a focal seizure that is secondarily generalized. Tonic–clonic seizures begin with a short tonic contraction of muscles followed by a period of rigidity and clonic movements. The patient may lose sphincter control, bite the tongue, or become cyanotic. The episode is frequently followed by a deep sleep.
- Interictally (between seizure episodes), there are typically no objective, pathognomonic signs of epilepsy.
- Myoclonic seizures are brief shock-like muscular contractions (jerks) of the face, trunk, and extremities. They may be isolated events or rapidly repetitive. There is no alteration of consciousness.
- In atonic seizures (the hallmark of Lennox–Gastaut syndrome), there is a sudden loss of muscle tone that may be described as a head drop, dropping of a limb, or slumping to the ground.

STATUS EPILEPTICUS

- The four stages of GCSE are (1) stablization, (2) initial therapy, (3) secondary therapy, and (4) third therapy as indicated in **Table 54-1**.
  - ✓ During first therapy phase of GCSE, each seizure produces marked increases in plasma epinephrine, norepinephrine, and steroid concentrations that may cause hypertension, tachycardia, and cardiac arrhythmias. Muscle contractions and hypoxia can cause acidosis, hypotension, shock, rhabdomyolysis, and secondary hyperkalemia, and acute tubular necrosis may ensue.
  - ✓ In second therapy phase, beginning 30 minutes into the seizure, the patient begins to decompensate and may become hypotensive with compromised cerebral blood flow. Serum glucose may be normal or decreased, and hyperthermia, respiratory deterioration, hypoxia, and ventilatory failure may develop.
  - ✓ The third therapy phase consists of refractory and supra-refractory GCSE where motor activity may cease, but electrical seizures may persist.
- Younger children, older persons, and those with preexisting epilepsy have a higher propensity for sequelae.
- Overall worldwide case fatality rate of 14.9%, with the highest rate in those >60 years of age (24.9%) and in those with refractory GCSE (33.3%).

TABLE 54-1	Generalized Convulsive Status Epilepticus		
Phase	**Time**	**Stage**	**Definition**
Stabilization phase	0–5 minutes		An acute condition characterized by convulsive seizures. This may include pre-hospitalization or emergency room care
Initial-therapy phase (5–20 minutes)	0–20 minutes	Impending GCSE	
Second-therapy phase (20–40 minutes)	20–40 minutes	Established GCSE	An acute condition characterized by continuous or intermittent seizures without full recovery of consciousness between events for at least 20 minutes
Third-therapy phase	40–60 minutes	Refractory GCSE	An acute condition characterized by continuous seizures despite initial treatment with 2 ASDs
	>24 hours	Supra-refractory	An acute condition characterized by seizures that continue 24 hours or longer after the administration of anesthesia, including cases in which SE recurs on reduction or withdrawal of anesthesia

ASD, antiseizure drug; GCSE, generalized convulsive status epilepticus; SE, status epilepticus.

- Variables affecting outcome are (1) the time between onset of GCSE and the initiation of treatment and (2) the duration of the seizure. The mortality rate is 2.6%, 19%, and 32% for those with seizures lasting 10–29 minutes, longer than 30 minutes, and longer than 60 minutes, respectively.

DIAGNOSIS

- Ask the patient and family to characterize the seizure for signs/symptoms, triggers, frequency, duration, precipitating factors, time of occurrence, presence of an aura, impairment of consciousness, ictal activity, and postictal state.
- Physical, neurologic, and laboratory examination may identify an etiology.
- A person is considered to have epilepsy if they have (1) at least 2 unprovoked (or reflex) seizures occurring greater than 24 hours apart; (2) 1 unprovoked (or reflex) seizure and a probability of further seizures of at least 60% after 2 unprovoked seizures, occurring over the next 10 years; or (3) a diagnosis of an epilepsy syndrome.
- In some cases, particularly following GTC seizures, serum prolactin levels may be transiently elevated. A serum prolactin level obtained within 10–20 minutes of a tonic–clonic seizure can help differentiate seizure activity from pseudoseizure activity but not from syncope.
- Laboratory tests may rule out treatable causes of seizures (hypoglycemia, altered serum electrolyte concentrations, infections, etc.) that are not epilepsy.
- EEG is very useful in the diagnosis of various seizure disorders, but epileptiform activity is found in only about 50% of patients with epilepsy.
- Brain imaging with either a computerized tomography (CT) scan or magnetic resonance imaging (MRI) can detect structural lesions that can aid in the diagnosis of seizures and epilepsy types.

TREATMENT

EPILEPSY

- <u>Goals of Treatment</u>: Control or reduce the frequency and severity of seizures, minimize side effects, and ensure compliance, allowing the patient to live as normal a life as possible. Complete suppression of seizures must be balanced against tolerability of side effects, and the patient should be involved in defining the balance. Side effects and comorbidities (eg, anxiety and depression) as well as social issues (eg, driving, job security, relationships, and social stigma) have significant impact on quality of life.

STATUS EPILEPTICUS

- <u>Goals of Treatment</u>: (1) Identify GCSE subtype and precipitating factors; (2) terminate clinical and electrical seizure activity as soon as possible, and preserve cardiorespiratory function; (3) minimize side effects; (4) prevent recurrent seizures; and (5) avoid pharmacoresistant epilepsy and/or neurologic sequelae.

NONPHARMACOLOGIC THERAPY

Epilepsy

- Nonpharmacologic therapies are available for drug-resistant patients with epilepsy as well as for drug-responsive patients in which the benefits of nonpharmacologic therapies outweigh its risk (ie, ketogenic diet, vagus nerve stimulation [VNS], and surgery among other modalities).

Status Epilepticus

- Therapy starts with the stabilization phase where the time of seizure onset should be noted, vital signs should be assessed, a protected airway should be established, ventilation should be maintained, and oxygen should be administered. Intravenous access should be established and hyperthermia, if present, should be aggressively treated (eg, rectal or IV acetaminophen and cooling blanket).
- Laboratory values should be drawn, including anticonvulsant serum concentrations.
- Continuous EEG monitoring may need to occur for patients with persistent GCSE and frequent arterial blood gas determinations are necessary to assess for metabolic acidosis.

PHARMACOLOGIC THERAPY

Epilepsy

- Drug selection depends on the seizure type and epilepsy classification as well as patient-specific characteristics including age, gender, susceptibility to adverse effects, comorbid medical conditions, interactions with other medications, ability to comply with a prescribed regimen, and cost of therapy/insurance coverage. Figure 54-2 is a suggested algorithm for treatment of epilepsy.
- Most anti-seizure drugs (ASDs) affection channel (sodium and Ca) kinetics, augmentation of inhibitory neurotransmission (increasing CNS GABA), and modulation of excitatory neurotransmission (decreasing or antagonizing glutamate and aspartate). ASDs effective against GTC and focal seizures probably work by delaying recovery of sodium channels from activation. Drugs that reduce corticothalamic T-type Ca currents are effective against generalized absence seizures.
- Begin with monotherapy. About 65% of patients can be maintained on one ASD, although not necessarily seizure free.
- Up to 60% of patients with epilepsy are nonadherent, commonly leading to treatment failure.
- Patients who have had two or more seizures should generally be started on ASDs; however, some providers start after one seizure.
- Provide the patient with a seizure and side-effect diary.
- ASD dosing is shown in Table 54-2.

- Many newer ASDs have been tested only as adjunctive therapy, but many providers will use them off-label as monotherapy.
- Evidence for comparable effectiveness is mostly available for older agents and for a few newer ones. In general, the newer ASDs appear to have comparable efficacy to the older drugs, and some may be better tolerated.
- **Carbamazepine, ethosuximide, gabapentin, levetiracetam, oxcarbazepine, phenytoin valproic acid,** and **zonisamide** have strong enough evidence to be labeled efficacious or effective or as probably efficacious or effective as initial monotherapy in certain seizure types.
- Some ASDs may possibly precipitate or aggravate certain seizure types, and it is suggested that they be used with caution in those patients. Examples are **carbamazepine, gabapentin, oxcarbazepine, phenytoin, tiagabine,** and **vigabatrin** in children with absence or juvenile myoclonic epilepsy.
- Initiate ASD with a low dose (ie, one-fourth to one-third of the anticipated maintenance dose), and titrated gradually over 3–4 weeks to a moderate dose. If seizures continue, titrate to a maximum dose. If the first ASD is ineffective or causes intolerable side effects, add a second ASD (preferably with a different mechanism of action), and then taper and discontinue the ineffective or intolerable drug. If the second ASD is ineffective, then polytherapy may be indicated.
- Clinicians should determine the optimal serum concentration for each patient as seizure control may occur before the "minimum" of the therapeutic serum range is reached, and some patients may need serum concentrations beyond the "maximum."
- The therapeutic range for ASDs may be different for different seizure types (eg, higher for focal seizures with dyscognitive features than for GTC seizures).
- Serum concentration determinations can be useful to document lack of or loss of efficacy, establish noncompliance, and guide therapy in patients with renal and/or hepatic disease and patients taking multiple drugs, as well as in women who are pregnant or taking oral contraceptives.
- Lower doses of ASDs are often required in older individuals due to compromised renal or hepatic function and some patients have increased receptor sensitivity to CNS drugs, making the accepted therapeutic range invalid. Older persons often take many medications, and thus are more prone to experience neurocognitive effects and drug–drug interactions involving ASDs that affect the CPY450 system (eg, carbamazepine, phenytoin, valproic acid, and phenobarbital). Hypoalbuminemia is common in older populations, and highly bound ASDs (eg, valproic acid) can be problematic. They also experience body mass changes which can affect elimination half-life and volume of distribution. **Lamotrigine** is often considered a drug of choice for older patients with focal onset seizures because of effectiveness and tolerability.
- After 12 months of treatment, the percentage who are seizure free is highest for those with only GTC seizures (48%–55%), lowest for those who have only focal seizures (23%–26%), and intermediate for those with mixed seizure types (25%–32%).
- ASD withdrawal can be considered in a patient meeting the following profile: seizure free for 2–5 years, a history of a single type of focal seizure or primary generalized seizures, a normal neurologic exam and normal IQ, and an EEG that has normalized with treatment. Factors favoring an unsuccessful withdrawal of ASDs include a history of a high frequency of seizures, repeated episodes of SE, a combination of seizure types, and development of abnormal mental functioning. Always withdraw ASDs gradually.
- Drug resistance is defined as failure of adequate trials of two tolerated and appropriately chosen and used ASD schedules (whether as monotherapies or in combination) to achieve sustained seizure freedom.
- For populations known to have altered plasma protein binding, measure free rather than total serum concentrations if the ASD is highly protein bound. Conditions altering ASD protein binding include chronic renal failure, liver disease, hypoalbuminemia, burns, pregnancy, malnutrition, displacing drugs, and age (neonates and older persons). Unbound concentration monitoring is especially useful for phenytoin.

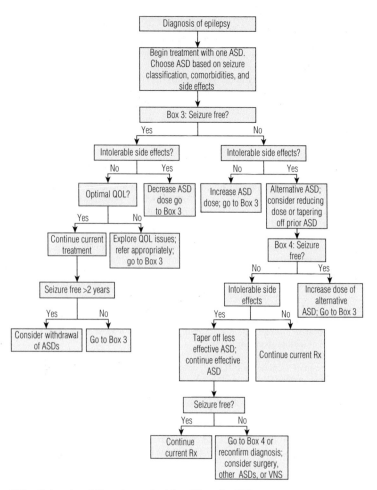

(ASD, antiseizure drug; VNS, vagal nerve stimulation; QOL, quality of life)

FIGURE 54-2. An algorithm for ASD therapy.

- Neonates and infants display decreased efficiency in renal elimination and may metabolize drugs more slowly, but by age 2 or 3 years children may metabolize drugs more rapidly than adults. Thus, neonates and infants require lower doses of ASD, but children require higher doses of many ASDs than adults.
- ASD side effects and monitoring are shown in **Table 54-3**. Concentration-dependent side effects can often be alleviated by decreasing the dose or avoided by increasing the dose very slowly.
- CNS side effects are frequent and include sedation, dizziness, blurred vision, poor concentration, and ataxia.
- Barbiturates can cause more cognitive impairment than other ASDs, but in children, they can cause paradoxical excitement. In general, the newer agents have less effect on cognition, except topiramate.

TABLE 54-2	Antiseizure Drug Dosing and Target Serum Concentration Ranges			
Drug	Brand Name	Initial or Starting Dose	Usual Range or Maximum Dose	Comments Target Serum Concentration Range
First generation				
Carbamazepine	Tegretol Tegretol XR	400 mg/day	400–1600 mg	4–12 mcg/mL[a] (17–51 μmol/L)
Clonazepam	Klonopin	1.5 mg/day	20 mg	20–70 ng/mL (67–233 pmol/L)
Ethosuximide	Zarontin	500 mg/day	500–1500 mg	40–100 mcg/mL (282–708 μmol/L)
Phenobarbital	Various	1–3 mg/kg/day (10– 20 mg/kg LD)	180–300 mg	10–40 mcg/mL[a] (43–172 μmol/L)
Phenytoin	Dilantin	3–5 mg/kg (200–400 mg) (15–20 mg/kg LD)	300–600 mg	Total: 10–20 mcg/mL (40–79 μmol/L) Unbound: 0.5–3 mcg/mL (2–12 μmol/L)
Primidone	Mysoline	100–125 mg/day	750–2000 mg	5–10 mcg/mL (23–46 μmol/L)
Valproic acid	Depakene Depakote DR/ER Depacon	15 mg/kg (500–1000 mg)	60 mg/kg (3000–5000 mg)	50–100 mcg/mL (347–693 μmol/L)
Second generation				
Felbamate	Felbatol	1200 mg/day	3600 mg	30–60 mcg/mL (126–252 μmol/L)
Gabapentin	Neurontin	300–900 mg/day	4800 mg	2–20 mcg/mL (12–117 μmol/L)
Lamotrigine	Lamictal Lamictal XR	25 mg every other day if on VPA; 25–50 mg/day if not on VPA	100–200 mg if on VPA; 300–500 mg if not on VPA	4–20 mcg/mL (16–78 μmol/L)

(Continued)

TABLE 54-2 Antiseizure Drug Dosing and Target Serum Concentration Ranges *(Continued)*

Drug	Brand Name	Initial or Starting Dose	Usual Range or Maximum Dose	Comments Target Serum Concentration Range
Second generation (con't)				
Levetiracetam	Keppra Keppra XR	500–1000 mg/day	3000 mg	12–46 mcg/mL (70–270 µmol/L)
Oxcarbazepine	Trileptal Oxtellar XR	300–600 mg/day	1200–2400 mg	3–35 mcg/mL (MHD) (12–139 µmol/L)
Tiagabine	Gabitril	4 mg/day	56 mg	0.02–0.2 mcg/mL (0.05–0.5 µmol/L)
Topiramate	Topamax Trokendi XR	25–50 mg/day	200–400 mg	5–20 mcg/mL (15–59 µmol/L)
Zonisamide	Zonegran	100 mg/day	600 mg	10–40 mcg/mL (47–188 µmol/L)
Third generation				
Brivaracetam	Briviact	100 mg/day	200 mg/day	Not defined
Cannabadiol	Epidiolex	5 mg/kg/day	10–20 mg/kg/day	Not defined
Clobazam	Onfi	≤30 kg: 5 mg/day; >30 kg: 10 mg/day	≤30 kg up to 20 mg; >30 kg up to 40 mg	0.03–0.3 mcg/mL (0.1–1.0 µmol/L)
Eslicarbazepine	Aptiom	400 mg/day	800–1600 mg	Not defined
Lacosamide	Vimpat	100 mg/day	400 mg	Not defined
Perampanel	Fycompa	2 mg/day	8–12 mg	Not defined
Pregabalin	Lyrica	150 mg/day	600 mg	Not defined
Rufinamide	Banzel	400–800 mg/day	3200 mg	Not defined
Vigabatrin	Sabril	1000 mg/day	3000 mg	0.8–36 mcg/mL (6–279 µmol/L)

aUnits mcg/mL and mg/L are numerically equivalent, and units ng/mL and mcg/L are numerically equivalent.
LD, loading dose; MHD, 10-monohydroxycarbazepine derivative.

- The most widely recognized idiosyncratic reactions are ASD-induced drug rashes, which can progress to Stevens–Johnson syndrome/toxic epidermal necrolysis. Variants of the HLA-B gene, HLA-B*1502, have been associated with increased risk of developing Stevens–Johnson syndrome as well as toxic epidermal necrolysis with carbamazepine (and possibly phenytoin, lamotrigine, and oxcarbazepine). This variant is found in up to 15% of individuals of Asian, southeast Asian, and south Asian origin. Patients with this variant should generally avoid these drugs. Also, the HLA genotype HLA-A*3101 is associated with carbamazepine-induced skin reactions in individuals of Chinese, Japanese, and European populations.
- Others reactions include hepatitis and blood dyscrasias. When acute organ failure occurs, it usually happens within the first 6 months of ASD therapy. Any patient taking ASDs who complains of lethargy, vomiting, fever, or rash should have a laboratory assessment, including white blood cell counts and liver function tests.
- A side effect of long-term use of ASDs is osteomalacia or osteoporosis. It is hypothesized that phenytoin, phenobarbital, carbamazepine, oxcarbazepine, felbamate, and valproic acid may interfere with vitamin D metabolism. Patients taking these drugs should receive vitamin D supplementation and calcium and bone mineral density testing if other risk factors for osteoporosis are present. Laboratory tests may reveal elevated bone-specific alkaline phosphatase and decreased serum Ca and 25-OH vitamin D, as well as intact parathyroid hormone.
- **Table 54-4** shows ASD elimination pathways and major effects on hepatic enzymes. Use caution when ASDs are added to or discontinued from a drug regimen. Pharmacokinetic interactions are common complicating factor in ASD selection.
- Phenobarbital, phenytoin, primidone, and carbamazepine are potent inducers of cytochrome P450 (CYP450), epoxide hydrolase, and uridine diphosphate glucuronosyltransferase enzyme systems. Valproic acid inhibits many hepatic enzyme systems and displaces some drugs from plasma albumin.
- Felbamate and topiramate can act as inducers with some isoforms and inhibitors with others.

First-Generation ASDs

Carbamazepine

- Food, especially fat, may enhance the bioavailability of carbamazepine.
- Controlled- and sustained-release preparations dosed every 12 hours are bioequivalent to immediate-release preparations dosed every 6 hours. The sustained-release capsule can be opened and sprinkled on food.
- Carbamazepine may be continued unless the white blood cell count drops to less than 2500/mm^3 (2.5×10^9/L) and the absolute neutrophil count drops to less than 1000/mm^3 (1×10^9/L).
- Carbamazepine may interact with other drugs by inducing their metabolism. The interaction of erythromycin and clarithromycin (CYP3A4 inhibition) with carbamazepine is particularly significant. Autoinduction of its own metabolism starts 3–5 days after initiating and is complete in 21–28 days. Reversal of autoinduction is rapid after discontinuation.

Ethosuximide

- Titration over 1–2 weeks to maintenance doses of 20 mg/kg/day usually produces therapeutic serum concentrations. It is usually given in two equal doses daily.
- There is some evidence for nonlinear metabolism at higher serum concentrations.

Phenobarbital

- Phenobarbital, a potent enzyme inducer, interacts with many drugs.

Phenytoin

- Phenytoin is a first-line ASD for many seizure types (see **Table 54-3**).
- Absorption may be saturable at higher doses (above 400 mg). Do not change brands without careful monitoring. The IM route is best avoided, as absorption is erratic. Fosphenytoin can safely be administered IV and intramuscularly (IM). Equations are available to normalize the phenytoin concentration in patients with hypoalbuminemia or renal failure.

TABLE 54-3	Antiseizure Drugs (ASDs)		
ASD and Available Formulations	**Advantages**	**Disadvantages**	**DDI: Effect of Drug on Concomitant ASD**
First-generation ASDs			
Carbamazepine Chewable tablet, ER tablet, liquid suspension	Useful in comorbid bipolar disorder and trigeminal neuralgia	Worsens other seizure types in patients with absence epilepsy; avoid if prior rash with other ASDs due to possible cross-reaction; increased risk of SJS/TEN in HLA-B*1502 and HLA-A*3101 allele in Asians; auto-inducer; active metabolite carbamazepine 10,11 epoxide contributes to idiosyncratic side effects; can cause fetal harm	Potent inducer of CYP3A4, CYP1A2, CYP2B6, CYP2C9/19; decreases levels of brivaracetam, clonazepam, eslicarbazepine, ethosuximide, lamotrigine, oxcarbazepine, perampanel, phenytoin, tiagabine, topiramate, valproate
Clonazepam (Schedule IV) Tablet, ODT	Useful in patients with panic disorder, myoclonic seizures, and subcortical myoclonus	May increase TC seizures when used in mixed seizure types; tolerance and dependence may occur; use with other CNS depressant may produce additive effects; may cause respiratory depression; contraindicated in acute narrow angle glaucoma and severe liver impairment; withdrawal symptoms may occur after discontinuation; no adequate data in pregnancy—may cause fetal harm	May affect levels of phenytoin
Ethosuximide Capsule, liquid solution	Drug of choice for absence seizures	Worsens generalized TC seizures and other seizure types; contraindicated in those with allergies to succinimides; may cause fetal harm; use with caution in hepatic/renal dysfunction	May affect levels of phenytoin, carbamazepine, phenobarbital, phenytoin, primidone, valproate
Phenobarbital (Schedule III) Tablet, elixir, injectable solution		Tolerance and dependence may occur; slow taper needed when discontinuing after prolonged use; use with other CNS depressants may produce additive CNS effects; may cause respiratory depression; can cause fetal harm	May decrease levels of carbamazepine, eslicarbazepine, ethosuximide, lamotrigine, oxcarbazepine, perampanel, phenytoin, rufinamide, tiagabine, topiramate, valproate

DDIs: Effect of Concomitant ASDs on Drug	Common and Dose-Related Adverse Effects	Rare and Serious Adverse Effects[a]	Long-Term Adverse Effects
Phenobarbital, phenytoin, primidone decrease levels; valproate increases carbamazepine-10,11 epoxide	CNS effects including diplopia, dizziness, drowsiness, unsteadiness, lethargy	Boxed warning: Increased risk of SJS/TEN and HLA-B*1502 allele; aplastic anemia and agranulocytosis Other blood dycrasias including thrombocytopenia, leukopenia; DRESS; hyponatremia; increased intraocular pressure; cardiovascular effects including second- and third-degree AV heart block; hepatotoxicity; genitourinary effect; nephrotoxicity	Hyponatremia (periodically monitor sodium); metabolic bone disease including osteoporosis, osteopenia, osteomalacia
May be affected by enzyme-inducing or enzyme-inhibiting ASDs	CNS effects including sedation, ataxia; paradoxical reactions such as agitation, irritability, aggression, anxiety, anger, nightmares, hallucinations and psychoses	Boxed warning: Concomitant use with opioids may result in profound sedation, respiratory depression, coma, and death Blood dyscrasias including leukopenia, thrombocytopenia, eosinophilia; rash; cardiovascular or respiratory depression; hepatotoxicity; muscle weakness	Physiologic dependence; loss of effect; hair loss; hirsutism; ankle and facial edema
Valproate may increase or decrease levels	GI distress including nausea/vomiting, cramps diarrhea; anorexia and weight loss; CNS effects including drowsiness, dizziness, hiccoughs	Blood dyscrasias including leukopenia, agranulocytosis, pancytopenia; rash including SJS; DRESS; hepatic/renal dysfunction; lupus erythematosus	Behavioral changes
Valproate increases levels; phenytoin increases or decreases levels	CNS effects including residual sedation, drowsiness, lethargy, confusion, ataxia, vertigo; paroxysmal excitement, irritability and hyperactivity in older persons and children; GI effects including nausea, vomiting	Respiratory depression and apnea; rash (SJS, TEN); cardiac effects including bradycardia, hypotension, syncope; hepatotoxicity	Behavioral changes; connective tissue disorder; intellectual blunting; metabolic bone disease (osteoporosis, osteopenia, osteomalacia); folate deficiency (with megaloblastic anemia)

(Continued)

TABLE 54-3	Antiseizure Drugs (ASDs) (Continued)		
ASD and Available Formulations	**Advantages**	**Disadvantages**	**DDI: Effect of Drug on Concomitant ASD**
First-generation ASDs (con't)			
Phenytoin ER capsule; liquid suspension; injectable; chewable tablet (Fosphenytoin, a prodrug desterified by esterases in the blood to phenytoin, also available as injectable solution only)	Useful in nonadherence as dosed once daily	May aggravate seizures in patients with absence seizures; can increase blood sugar levels in diabetes; HLA-B*1502 may be a risk factor for the development of SJS/TEN in patients of Asian ancestry; monitoring of free phenytoin levels required in pregnancy, older persons or low albumin; compromised absorption with concomitant tube feeds	May decrease levels of brivaracetam, carbamazepine, clonazepam, eslicarbazepine, ethosuximide, felbamate, lamotrigine, oxcarbazepine, perampanel, tiagabine, topiramate, valproate
Primidone Tablet	Useful in essential tremor	Contraindicated in patients with porphyria	May decrease levels of carbamazepine, eslicarbazepine, ethosuximide, lamotrigine, oxcarbazepine, perampanel, phenytoin, rufinamide, tiagabine, topiramate, valproate
Valproate Divalproex DR sprinkle capsule, Divalproex DR tablet, Divalproex ER 24-hour tablet, valproic acid IR capsule, valproate sodium injectable solution	Useful in comorbid bipolar disorder and migraine	Contraindicated in significant hepatic dysfunction, mitochondrial disorders caused by DNA polymerase γ (POLG) mutations, urea cycle disorders; use with caution in pancreatitis, bleeding and other hematopoietic disorders; hyperammonemia with and without encephalopathy associated with concomitant topiramate use; pregnancy category D—contraindicated in women of childbearing potential and pregnancy category X for pregnant patients treated for migraine prophylaxis	May increase levels of eslicarbazepine, ethosuximide, felbamate, lamotrigine, oxcarbazepine, phenytoin, phenobarbital, rufinamide, topiramate

DDIs: Effect of Concomitant ASDs on Drug	Common and Dose-Related Adverse Effects	Rare and Serious Adverse Effects[a]	Long-Term Adverse Effects
Ethosuximide, felbamate, oxcarbazepine, methsuximide, topiramate may increase levels; carbamazepine, vigabatrin may decrease levels; phenobarbital, valproate may increase or decrease levels	CNS effects including ataxia, nystagums, slurred speech, decreased coordination, mental confusion, dizziness, insomnia, transient nervousness, headaches	Blood dyscrasias including thrombocytopenia, leukopenia, granulocytopenia, agranulocytosis, pancytopenia; rash (SJS/TEN); DRESS; hepatotoxicity, cardiac effects; purple glove syndrome with IV administration	Connective tissue changes including skin thickening, gingival hyperplasia, coarsening of facial features, enlargement of lips; hirsutism; metabolic bone disease (osteoporosis, osteopenia, osteomalacia); peripheral neuropathy; cerebellar atrophy; folate deficiency (with megaloblastic anemia)
Valproate may increase levels; phenytoin may increase or decrease levels	CNS effects including ataxia, vertigo, nystagmus, diplopia, drowsiness, fatigue; GI effect including nausea/vomiting, anorexia, fatigue; emotional disturbances including hyperirritability	Blood dyscrasias including granulocytopenia, agranulocytosis; rash (SJS, TEN); liver dysfunction	Behavioral changes; intellectual blunting; connective tissue disorder; metabolic bone disease (rickets, osteomalacia); folate deficiency (with megaloblastic anemia)
Carbamazepine, phenobarbital, phenytoin, primidone decrease levels; felbamate can increase levels; estrogen OCPs may affect levels	GI effects including abdominal pain/GI upset (worse with IR), constipation, diarrhea, anorexia, increased appetite, weight gain, nausea/vomiting; CNS effects including blurred vision, ataxia, dizziness, headache, insomnia, nystagmus, somnolence, thinking abnormal, tremor; dose dependent thrombocytopenia (associated with valproate concentrations >100 mg/mL; 693 umol/L).	Boxed warning: hepatotoxicity especially for children <2 years of age and with mitochondrial disorders; fetal risk including neural tube defects, other major malformations, and decreased IQ; pancreatitis including fatal hemorrhagic pancreatitis Hyperammonemia with and without encephalopathy; hypothermia with and without hyperammonemia; DRESS; bleeding and other hematopoietic disorders	Hair and nail changes including alopecia, hirsutism, hair texture and color changes, nail and nail bed disorders; irregular menses and polycystic ovary-like syndrome; weight gain; cerebral pseudoatrophy; osteoporosis and osteopenia

(Continued)

TABLE 54-3	Antiseizure Drugs (ASDs) (Continued)		
ASD and Available Formulations	**Advantages**	**Disadvantages**	**DDI: Effect of Drug on Concomitant ASD**
Second-generation ASDs			
Gabapentin Tablet, capsule, oral solution	Useful in postherpetic neuralgia, chronic pain, and neuropathy; few drug–drug interactions	Considered weakly efficacious; potential abuse when taken with opioids; withdrawal reaction characterized by anxiety, insomnia, nausea, sweating, and increased pain; absorption may be impaired for doses >1,200 mg; no adequate data in pregnancy—may cause fetal harm	
Lamotrigine Tablet, chewable tablet[a], ODT[a], XR tablet[a]	Useful in bipolar disease; XR useful in nonadherence as dosed once daily	Slow titration required to avoid rash including SJS; increased risk if patient with prior rash to other ASD and concomitant use of valproic acid; rash incidence higher in children; may exacerbate myoclonus; dosage adjustment required in patients with moderate and severe liver impairment; no adequate data in pregnancy—may cause fetal harm	Does not inhibit liver enzymes
Levetiracetam Tablet, XR tablet[a], injectable solution	Minimal drug–drug interactions; XR useful in nonadherence as dosed once daily	May worsen depression, PTSD, anxiety, thought disorders; dose adjustment in dialysis/renal failure is necessary; pregnancy category C	
Oxcarbazepine Tablet, tablet ER[a], liquid suspension[a]	Useful in bipolar disorder; ER useful in nonadherence as dosed once daily	Higher incidence of hyponatremia (as high as 25%); must check HLA-B*1502 in Asians to predict SJS or TEN; active MHD metabolite may decrease in pregnancy; no adequate data in pregnant women—may cause fetal harm	Inhibitor of CYP2C19 and inducer of CYP3A4/5; increases phenytoin levels; decreases lamotrigine levels through UGT induction; decreases estrogen OCP levels

DDIs: Effect of Concomitant ASDs on Drug	Common and Dose-Related Adverse Effects	Rare and Serious Adverse Effects[a]	Long-Term Adverse Effects
Valproate increases lamotrigine levels by 2x; carbamazepine, phenytoin, phenobarbital, primidone decrease levels by 40%; estrogen OCPs decrease lamotrigine by 50%	CNS effects including dizziness, headache, diplopia, ataxia, blurred vision, somnolence, tremor; GI effects including nausea/vomiting, abdominal pain, diarrhea; other effects including rhinitis, pharyngitis, infection, fever; rash	Boxed warning: Rash including SJS, TEN with increased risk if given with valproate, exceeding recommended initial dose or dose escalation DRESS; blood dyscrasias; hemophagocytic lymphohistiocytosis (HLH)	Rash usually appears after 3–4 weeks of therapy and is typically generalized, erythematous, and morbilliform but can progress to SJS
	CNS effects including somnolence, fatigue; behavior effects including aggression, agitation, anger, anxiety, apathy, depersonalization, depression, emotional lability, hostility, irritability	Psychosis, hallucinations	
Carbamazepine, phenytoin and phenobarbital decreases active metabolite levels	CNS effects including dizziness, somnolence, diplopia, fatigue, ataxia, abnormal vision, headache, nystagmus, tremor; GI effects including nausea, vomiting	Hyponatremia; rash (SJS, TEN); DRESS; blood dyscrasias	Hyponatremia

(Continued)

TABLE 54-3	Antiseizure Drugs (ASDs) (*Continued*)		
ASD and Available Formulations	**Advantages**	**Disadvantages**	**DDI: Effect of Drug on Concomitant ASD**
Second-generation ASDs (con't)			
Tiagabine Tablet		Has been associated with new-onset seizure, status epilepticus, and exacerbation of EEG abnormalities in those with existing epilepsy; dosage reduction may be necessary in patients with liver disease; pregnancy category C	
Topiramate Sprinkle capsule, tablet, XR tablet, capsule, capsule ER	Useful in comorbid migraine and obesity; XR useful in nonadherence as dosed once daily	Avoid in patients with preexisting cognitive issues; renally dose adjust with CrCl <70 mL/min; can cause fetal harm	Weak inhibitor of CYP2C19 and inducer of CYP3A4; decreases estrogen OCP levels
Zonisamide Capsule	Useful in tremor; useful in nonadherence as dosed once daily	Contraindicated in those with sulfa allergy; dose efficacy may plateau at 400 mg; should not be used in renal failure due to increases in SCr and BUN and possible effects on GFR; pregnancy category C	
Third-generation ASDs			
Brivaracetam (Schedule V) Tablet, oral solution, injection solution	Consider converting well-controlled patients from levetiracetam if intolerable psychiatric side effects	Dosage adjustments required in hepatic impairment; no adequate data in pregnancy—may cause fetal harm	Increases carbamazepine metabolite; increases phenytoin levels
Cannabidiol (Schedule V) Oral solution	Useful for refractory seizures in LGS and Dravet syndrome	Avoid in patients with hypersensitivity reactions to cannabis, THC; liver function and bilirubin monitoring before and at 1, 3, and 6 months of treatment specially if given with valproate; no adequate data in pregnant woman—may cause fetal harm	Increases lamotrigine levels; increase levels of clobazam active metabolite by 3 times

DDIs: Effect of Concomitant ASDs on Drug	Common and Dose-Related Adverse Effects	Rare and Serious Adverse Effects[a]	Long-Term Adverse Effects
Carbamazepine, phenytoin, primidone, phenobarbital decrease levels; valproate increases levels by 40%	CNS effects including dizziness, lightheadedness, somnolence, thinking abnormal; behavior effects including asthenia, lack of energy, nervousness, irritability, difficulty with concentration or attention; GI effects including abdominal pain and nausea	Increase in generalized seizures and nonconvulsive SE in patients with refractory epilepsy; occurrence of seizures and SE in patients without epilepsy; moderately severe to incapacitating generalized weakness; exacerbation of EEG abnormalities; rash including SJS	Possibility of long-term ophthalmologic effects
Phenytoin carbamazepine decreases levels	CNS effects including fatigue, difficulty concentrating, confusion, language problems, tremor paresthesias; behavioral effects including nervousness, anxiety	Renal stones; glaucoma; oligohidrosis and hyperthermia; metabolic acidosis; rash (SJS, TEN); hypothermia and hyperammonemia with and without encephalopathy when used with valproate	Weight loss, renal stones, metabolic acidosis
CYP3A4 inhibitors or inducers may alter levels; carbamazepine, phenobarbital, phenytoin, valproate decrease levels	CNS effects including sedation, ataxia, confusion, depression, difficulty concentrating, word-finding difficulties	Oligohidrosis and hyperthermia; renal stones; metabolic acidosis; rash (SJS, TEN); DRESS; fulminant hepatic necrosis; blood dyscrasias	Weight loss, renal stones, metabolic acidosis
CYP2C19 inhibitors may alter levels	CNS effects including sedation, fatigue, ataxia, nystagums; behavioral effects including irritability, aggressive behavior, anxiety; GI effects including nausea, vomiting	Angioedema; bronchospasm; decreased neutrophils; psychosis	
CYP3A4 and CYP2C19 inhibitors will increase levels; CYP3A4 and CYP2C19 inducers will decrease levels	CNS effects including somnolence, fatigue, malaise, asthenia; sleep disorders including insomnia, poor quality sleep; GI effects including decreased appetite; diarrhea; transaminase elevations	Hepatotoxicity; hypoxia; respiratory failure	

(Continued)

TABLE 54-3	Antiseizure Drugs (ASDs) (Continued)		
ASD and Available Formulations	Advantages	Disadvantages	DDI: Effect of Drug on Concomitant ASD
Third-generation ASDs (con't)			
Clobazam (Schedule IV) Tablet, oral suspension		Monitor patients with history of substance abuse; use with other CNS depressant may produce additive CNS effects; may cause respiratory depression, coma, and death; no adequate data in pregnant women—may cause fetal harm	Inhibitor of CYP2C9 and inducer of CYP3A4; affects levels of CYP2C9, CYP3A4 substrates; decreases estrogen OCP levels
Eslicarbazepine Tablet	Useful in nonadherence as dosed once daily	Avoid in severe hepatic impairment; dose adjustment in renal failure; avoid concomitant use with carbamazepine and oxcarbazepine; no adequate data in pregnancy—may cause fetal harm	Inhibitor of CYP2C19; affects carbamazepine, phenytoin, phenobarbital, primidone levels; decreases estrogen OCP levels
Lacosamide (Schedule V) Tablet, oral solution, Injectable solution	Minimal drug–drug interactions	Avoid in third-degree heart block; use with caution in patients with underlying proarrhythmic conditions or on concomitant medications that affect cardiac conduction; no adequate data in pregnancy—may cause fetal harm	Substrate of CYP3A4, CYP2C9, and CYP2C19; carbamazepine, phenytoin, phenobarbital, primdone, decrease levels by 15%–20%
Perampanel (Schedule III) Tablet, oral suspension	Useful in mixed seizure types; useful in nonadherence as dosed once daily	Avoid in active psychosis or unstable recurrent affective disorders with significant hostility or aggressive behavior; avoid in severe hepatic/renal impairment or hemodialysis; no adequate data in pregnancy—may cause fetal harm	Modest enzyme inducer at high doses; carbamazepine, eslicarbazepine, oxcarbazepine, phenobarbital, phenytoin, primidone, topiramate decrease levels; valproate has no effect on levels; decreases estrogen OCP levels
Pregabalin (Schedule V) Capsule, tablet CR, oral solution	Useful in patients with diabetic peripheral neuropathy, postherpetic neuralgia, fibromyalgia, neuropathic pain with spinal cord injury; minimal DDIs due to renal excretion	Preexisting cognitive disorders; no adequate data in pregnancy—may cause fetal harm	

DDIs: Effect of Concomitant ASDs on Drug	Common and Dose-Related Adverse Effects	Rare and Serious Adverse Effects[a]	Long-Term Adverse Effects
Carbamazepine, felbamate, phenobarbital, phenytoin, primidone decrease levels	CNS effects including somnolence, sedation, lethargy; pyrexia; constipation; drooling	Boxed warning: Concomitant use with opioids increases risk of death Rash (SJS, TEN); anemia; liver enzyme elevations; respiratory depression	
Carbamazepine, phenobarbital, primidone, and phenytoin decrease levels	CNS effects including dizziness, somnolence, nausea, headache, diplopia, fatigue, vertigo, ataxia, blurred vision, tremor	Hyponatremia; rash (SJS); anaphylaxis, angioedema, DRESS; cardiac effects including prolonged PR interval, AV block; hepatotoxicity; blood dyscrasias	Hyponatremia
CYP2C19 inhibitor but no clinically significant effects	CNS effects including ataxia, dizziness, diplopia, headache, tremor; GI effects including nausea, vomiting	Cardiac effects including AV conduction abnormalities, prolonged PR interval, atrial arrhythmias, syncope (especially in patients with diabetes)	
	CNS effects including dizziness, somnolence, fatigue, falls, vertigo, ataxia, headache, confusion; GI effects including nausea, weight gain, vomiting, abdominal pain; behavioral effects including irritability anxiety	Boxed warning: Aggression, hostility, irritability, anger, and homicidal ideation	Weight gain
	CNS effects including dizziness, somnolence, blurred vision, difficulty with concentration and attention; dry mouth; edema and weight gain	Potential for abuse when taken with opiates	Weight gain

(Continued)

TABLE 54-3	Antiseizure Drugs (ASDs) (Continued)		
ASD and Available Formulations	**Advantages**	**Disadvantages**	**DDI: Effect of Drug on Concomitant ASD**
Third-generation ASDs (con't)			
Rufinamide Tablet, oral suspension		Contraindicated in severe liver impairment or in familial short QT syndrome; use caution with other drugs that shorten QT interval; no adequate data in pregnancy—may cause fetal harm	Weak inhibitor of CYP2E1; weak inducer of CYP3A4; modestly decreases levels of carbamazepine, lamotrigine; increases levels of phenobarbital, phenytoin; decreases estrogen OCP levels
Vigabatrin Tablet, powder packet	Useful in infantile spasms for whom potential benefit outweighs risk of vision loss	Permanent vision loss in most patients after a certain duration of exposure requiring eye exams Q3 months; requires REMS program registration; no adequate data in pregnancy—may cause fetal harm	Inducer of CYP2C9; decreases levels of phenytoin by 20%; possibly increases levels of carbamazepine by 10%; increases C_{max} of clonazepam

[a]All ASDs may increase the risk of suicidal thoughts or behavior and patients treated with an ASD should be monitored for the emergence or worsening of depression, suicidal thoughts or behavior, or any unusual changes in mood or behavior.

AMPA, A-amino-3-hydroxy-5-methyl-4-isoxazolepropionic acid; ASD, antiseizure drug; AV, atrioventricular; BUN, blood urea nitrogen; C_{max}, maximum concentration; CNS, central nervous system; CR, controlled-release; CrCl, creatinine clearance; CYP, cytochrome p450 isoenzyme system; DDI, drug–drug interaction; DR, delayed-release; DRESS, drug rash with eosinophilia and systemic symptoms;

- Zero-order kinetics occurs within the usual therapeutic range, so any change in dose may produce disproportional changes in serum concentrations.
- Most adult patients can be maintained on a single-daily dose, but children often require more frequent administration. Only extended-release preparations should be used for single-daily dosing.
- For phenytoin serum concentration less than 7 mcg/mL (28 μmol/L), the daily dose should be increased by 100 mg; if the concentration is 7–12 mcg/mL (28–48 μmol/L), the daily dose can be increased by 50 mg; and if the concentration is greater than 12 mcg/mL (48 μmol/L), the daily dose can be increased by 30 mg or less. At concentrations greater than 50 mcg/mL (200 μmol/L), phenytoin can exacerbate seizures.
- If protein-binding interactions are suspected, free rather than total phenytoin serum concentrations are a better therapeutic guide.
- Folic acid replacement enhances phenytoin clearance and can result in loss of efficacy. Phenytoin tablets and suspension contain phenytoin acid, whereas the capsules and parenteral solution are phenytoin sodium. Ninety-two milligrams of phenytoin acid is approximately equal to 100 mg of phenytoin sodium.

DDIs: Effect of Concomitant ASDs on Drug	Common and Dose-Related Adverse Effects	Rare and Serious Adverse Effects[a]	Long-Term Adverse Effects
Carbamazepine, phenobarbital, phenytoin decrease levels by 19%–46%; valproate increases levels up to 70%	CNS effects including somnolence, fatigue, coordination abnormalities, dizziness, gait disturbances, ataxia; GI effects including nausea	DRESS; rash (SJS); status epilepticus; leukopenia; QT interval shortening	
	CNS effects including fatigue, somnolence, nystagmus, tremor, blurred vision, memory impairment, abnormal coordination, confusion; weight gain; edema; peripheral neuropathy In pediatric patients: aggression; infection including upper respiratory tract infection, bronchitis, ear infection, and acute otitis media	Boxed warning: Progressive and permanent bilateral peripheral visual constriction including tunnel vision; reduced visual acuity Seizure exacerbation, particularly absence and myoclonic seizures in patients with generalized epilepsies; anemia	Onset of vision loss is unpredictable with risk increasing in a dose-related and life exposure-related manner; abnormal MRI signal changes in infants treated for infantile spasms strongly suggestive of intramyelinic edema in select brain areas

EEG, electroencephalogram; FDA, Food and Drug Administration; ER, extended release; GABA, gamma-aminobutyric acid; GAT1, GABA transporter type 1; GI, gastrointestinal; GFR, glomerular filtration rate; HLA, human leukocyte antigen; IQ, intelligence quotient; IR, immediate release; IV, intravenous; LGS, Lennox–Gastaut syndrome; OCP, oral contraceptives; ODT, orally dissolving tablet; PTSD, posttraumatic stress disorder; SJS, Steven–Johnson syndrome; TEN, toxic epidermal necrolysis; TBI, traumatic brain injury; TC, tonic–clonic; UGT, UDP-glucuronosyltransferase; XR, extended-release.

Valproic acid and divalproex sodium

- The free fraction may increase as the total serum concentration increases, and monitoring free concentrations may be more useful than total concentrations, especially at higher serum concentrations and in patients with hypoalbuminemia.
- At least 10 metabolites have been identified, and some may be active.
- It is first-line therapy for primary generalized seizures, such as absence, myoclonic, and atonic seizures, and is approved for adjunctive and monotherapy treatment of focal onset seizures. It can also be useful in mixed seizure disorders.
- GI complaints may be minimized with the enteric-coated formulation or by giving with food.
- Although carnitine supplementation may partially ameliorate hyperammonemia, it is expensive and is not generally supported.
- Valproic acid is an enzyme inhibitor. Carbapenems and combination oral contraceptives may lower serum levels of valproic acid.
- Once-daily dosing is possible with the extended-release divalproex, but more frequent dosing is the norm due to reports of breakthrough seizures.

TABLE 54-4 Antiseizure Drug Elimination Pathways and Major Effects on Hepatic Enzymes

Antiepileptic Drugs	Major Hepatic Enzymes	Renal Elimination (%)	Induces	Inhibits
First generation				
Carbamazepine	CYP3A4	3	CYP1A2; CYP2B6; CYP2C9/19; CYP3A; GT	None
Clonazepam	CYP3A	2	None	None
Ethosuximide	CYP3A4; CYP2E1	10–20	None	None
Phenobarbital	CYP2C9; CYP2C19	25	CYP 3A4/2C9/2C19/1A2; GT	None
Phenytoin	CYP2C9; CYP2C19	Unknown	CYP3A; CYP2C; GT	None
Primidone		<1		
Valproate	GT; β-oxidation	<3	None	CYP2C9; GT epoxide hydrolase
Second generation				
Felbamate	CYP3A4; CYP2E1; other	50	CYP3A4	CYP2C19; β-oxidation
Gabapentin	None	Almost completely	None	None
Lamotrigine	GT	10	GT	None
Levetiracetam	None (undergoes nonhepatic hydrolysis)	66	None	None
Oxcarbazepine (MHD is active oxcarbazepine metabolite)	Cytosolic system	<1 (27 as MHD)	CYP3A4; CYP3A5; GT	CYP2C19
Tiagabine	CYP3A4; CYP1A2; CYP2D6; CYP2C19	2	None	None
Topiramate	Not known	70	CYP3A (dose dependent)	CYP2C19
Zonisamide	CYP3A4	35	None	None

Third generation

Brivaracetam	CYP2C19	<10	None	CYP2C19 (weak), GT epoxide hydrolase
Cannabidiol	CYP2C19; CYP3A4; GT	Minor	CYP1A2; CYP2B6; GT	CYP2C8/9 and 19
Clobazam	CYP3A4; CYP2C19; CYP2B6	2	CYP3A4 (weak)	CYP2C9
Eslicarbazepine	Undergoes hydrolysis	67	GT (mild)	CYP2C19
Lacosamide	CYP2C9/19; CYP3A4	40	None	CYP2C19
Perampanel	CYP3A4/5; CYP1A2; CYP2B6	Undefined	CYP3A4/5; CYP2B6; GT	CYPA3A4/5; CYP2C8; GT
Pregabalin	None	100	None	None
Rufinamide	Hydrolysis	2	CYP3A4 (weak)	CYP2E1 (weak)
Vigabatrin	None	Almost completely	CYP2C9	None

CYP, cytochrome P450 isoenzyme system; GT, glucuronyltransferase.

- The enteric-coated tablet divalproex sodium causes fewer GI side effects. It is metabolized in the gut to valproic acid. When switching from Depakote to Depakote-ER, the dose should be increased by 14%–20%.

Second-Generation ASDs

Felbamate
- Felbamate is approved as adjunctive treatment for seizures of Lennox–Gastaut syndrome and is effective as monotherapy or adjunctive therapy for focal onset seizures as well. Because of reports of aplastic anemia (1 in 3000 patients) and hepatitis (1 in 10,000 patients), felbamate is recommended only for patients refractory to other ASDs. Risk factors for aplastic anemia may include a history of cytopenia, ASD allergy or toxicity, viral infection, and/or immunologic problems.

Gabapentin
- Gabapentin is a second-line agent for patients with focal onset seizures.
- Binding is saturable, causing dose-dependent bioavailability. It is eliminated exclusively renally, and dosage adjustment is necessary in patients with impaired renal function.
- Dosing is initiated at 300 mg at bedtime and increased to 300 mg twice daily on the second day and 300 mg three times daily on the third day. Further titrations are then made. When the total daily dose is 3600 mg/day or greater, divide the daily dose into at least four doses.

Lamotrigine
- Lamotrigine is useful as both adjunctive therapy and monotherapy for partial seizures and can be considered first- or second-line therapy. It is also approved for primary GTC seizures, and for primary generalized seizure of Lennox–Gastaut syndrome.

Levetiracetam
- Renal elimination of unchanged drug accounts for 66% of levetiracetam clearance, and the dose should be adjusted for impaired renal function. It is metabolized in blood by nonhepatic enzymatic hydrolysis.
- It is effective in the adjunctive treatment of focal onset seizures in patients 1 month of age and older, myoclonic seizures in patients 12 years and older, and primary GTC seizures in patients 6 years and older.
- The recommended initial adult dose is 500 mg orally twice daily. In some intractable seizure patients, the oral dose has been titrated rapidly over 3 days up to 3000 mg/day (1500 mg twice daily). It can be loaded orally or intravenously.

Oxcarbazepine
- The relationship between dose and serum concentration is linear. It does not autoinduce its own metabolism.
- It is indicated for use as adjunctive therapy for partial seizures in patients 6 years and older.
- Concurrent use of oxcarbazepine with ethinyl estradiol and levonorgestrel-containing contraceptives may render these agents less effective.
- In patients converted from carbamazepine, the typical maintenance doses of oxcarbazepine are 1.5 times the carbamazepine dose or less if patients are on larger carbamazepine doses. See manufacturer's recommendations for dosing by weight.

Tiagabine
- Tiagabine is adjunctive therapy for patients 12 years and older with focal onset seizures who have failed initial therapy.
- Tiagabine is displaced from protein by naproxen, salicylates, and valproate.

Topiramate
- Topiramate is a first-line ASD for patients with partial seizures as an adjunct or for monotherapy. It is also approved for tonic–clonic seizures in primary generalized epilepsy and for generalized seizures in Lennox–Gastaut syndrome.

- The dose should be adjusted in renally impaired patients.
- It increases the clearance of ethinyl estradiol.
- Dose increments may occur every 1 or 2 weeks. For patients on other ASDs, doses greater than 400 mg/day do not appear to lead to improved efficacy and may increase side effects.

Zonisamide
- Zonisamide, a broad-spectrum sulfonamide ASD, is approved as adjunctive therapy for partial seizures in adults.
- Start dosing in adults at 100 mg/day and increase by 100 mg/day every 2 weeks. It is suitable for once- or twice-daily dosing, but once-daily dosing may cause more side effects.

Third-Generation ASDs

Brivaracetam
- Dosage adjustment is required in all stages of hepatic impairment.

Cannabadiol
- Cannabadiol is a purified drug derived from marijuana whose exact antiseizure mechanism is unknown.
- It is FDA approved for Dravet syndrome and LGS.

Clobazam
- Abrupt discontinuation can cause a withdrawal syndrome (eg, behavioral disorder, tremor, anxiety, dysphoria, insomnia, convulsions, and psychosis).
- As an inducer of CYP3A4, clobazam may lower serum levels of some oral contraceptives. It is an inhibitor of CYP2D6. In older persons and poor metabolizers of CYP2C19, initiate dosing as in patients weighing less than 30 kg.
- It is more effective than clonazepam for Lennox–Gastaut syndrome but less effective than clonazepam for myoclonic jerks and absence seizures. It is adjunctive treatment for seizures of Lennox–Gastaut syndrome.

Eslicarbazepine
- Eslicarbazepine acetate is a prodrug that undergoes hydrolysis to S-licarbazepine, the major active metabolite of oxcarbazepine. It is FDA approved for monotherapy or adjunctive therapy of focal onset seizures.
- It is mostly renally excreted, and dosage adjustment is needed when creatinine clearance is less than 50 mL/min (0.8 mL/sec). It may increase the PR interval on the ECG. It causes less hyponatremia than oxcarbazepine.

Ezogabine
- Ezogabine is approved for adjunctive treatment of focal onset seizures, and is recommended only after several alternative drugs have been tried.
- Lower doses are recommended in older persons.
- It can cause urinary retention and QT prolongation.
- Alcohol may increase systemic exposure to ezogabine with an increase in side effects. It can increase lamotrigine clearance and reduce digoxin clearance.
- It may cause falsely elevated results on urine and serum bilirubin laboratory tests.
- It must be taken three times daily.

Lacosamide
- Lacosamide is approved as adjunctive therapy in patients 17 years old or greater with focal onset seizures.
- There is a linear relationship between daily doses and serum concentrations up to 800 mg/day. Moderate hepatic and renal impairment both increase systemic drug exposure by up to 40%.
- The starting dose is 100 mg/day in two divided doses, with dose increase by 100 mg/day every week until a daily dose of 200–400 mg has been reached.

Perampanel
- Perampanel has a half-life of approximately 100 hours, and its clearance in increased two- to threefold by enzyme-inducing ASDs.
- It is FDA approved for adjunctive therapy of focal onset seizures in patients 12 years and older and as adjunctive therapy for primary GTC in patients 12 years and older.

Pregabalin
- Pregabalin is FDA approved as adjunctive therapy for adults with focal onset seizures. It is considered a second-line agent for those who have failed initial treatment.
- It is eliminated unchanged primarily by renal excretion; dosage adjustment is required in patients with significant renal dysfunction.

Rufinamide
- Rufinamide is an adjunctive agent used for seizures of LGS in patients 1 year and older and in adults. Reserve rufinamide for patients who have failed other ASDs.
- Children may have a higher clearance of rufinamide than adults.
- It is dosed twice daily because of slow absorption and a short half-life. Drug interactions are common.
- Multiorgan hypersensitivity has occurred within 4 weeks of dose initiation in children younger than 12 years.

Vigabatrin
- Vigabatrin is monotherapy for infantile spasms in infants 1 month–2 years of age, and a third-line adjunctive agent for refractory complex partial seizures in patients 10 years and older.
- It is excreted unchanged in the urine. Dosage adjustment is necessary in pediatric and renally impaired patients.
- Access to vigabatrin is restricted as all providers must be certified in the Vigabatrin Risk Evaluation and Mitigation Strategy (REMS) Program.

Special Considerations in Patients of Reproductive Age
- Estrogen has a seizure-activating effect, and progesterone has a seizure-protective effect. Enzyme-inducing ASDs (eg, phenobarbital, phenytoin, carbamazepine, topiramate, oxcarbazepine, and perhaps rufinamide, lamotrigine, clobazam, and felbamate) may cause oral contraceptive failures; supplemental birth control is advised if breakthrough bleeding occurs. Women taking these ASDs should take twice the usual dose of emergency contraception.
- For catamenial epilepsy (seizures just before or during menses) or seizures that occurring during ovulation, conventional ASDs should be tried first, but intermittent supplementation with higher-dose ASDs or benzodiazepines should be considered. Acetazolamide has been used with limited success. Progestational agents may also be effective.
- Seizures often improve in frequency at menopause.
- Women with epilepsy who are seizure free for 9–12 months before becoming pregnant, have an 84%–92% chance of being seizure free during pregnancy. Fluctuations in ASD serum concentrations during pregnancy may be due to reduced gastric motility, nausea and vomiting, increased drug distribution, increased renal elimination, altered hepatic enzyme activity, or changes in protein binding.
- ASD monotherapy is preferred in pregnancy. Clearance of phenytoin, carbamazepine, lamotrigine, oxcarbazepine, and levetiracetam increases during pregnancy, and protein binding may be reduced. Serum concentrations of phenobarbital, primidone, ethosuximide, and valproic acid may also fluctuate during pregnancy. Serum concentrations of ASDs should be monitored closely durng pregnancy. There is a higher incidence of adverse pregnancy outcomes in women taking ASDs, including an increased risk of major congenital malformations (MCMs).
- Valproic acid is associated with a risk of MCMs 3.5–4 times that of offspring of nonepileptic women. There is also an increased risk of neurodevelopmental effects including effects on cognition in children. **Valproic** acid should not be used in pregnancy, but when it is used, doses should not exceed 500–600 mg/day.

- Topiramate use during pregnancy has been associated with cleft palate and possibly low birth weight and hypospadias.
- Teratogenic effects may possibly be prevented by adequate folate intake, although strong evidence is lacking. Prenatal vitamins with folic acid (0.4–5 mg/day) are recommended for women of childbearing potential taking ASDs. Higher folate doses should be used in women who have previously delivered a child with a neural tube defect and women who are taking valproic acid.
- ASDs with low protein binding will accumulate in breast milk.
- Other adverse outcomes of maternal seizures are growth, psychomotor, and mental retardation. Vitamin K, 10 mg/day orally, given to the woman during the last month of pregnancy may prevent neonatal hemorrhagic disorder. Alternatively, parenteral vitamin K can be given to the newborn at delivery.
- Data suggest that men with epilepsy have reduced fertility, and that carbamazepine, oxcarbazepine, and valproic acid are associated with sperm abnormalities. Valproic acid seems to cause testicular atrophy resulting in reduced testosterone volume, whereas levetiracetam appears to slightly increase serum testosterone.

STATUS EPILEPTICUS

- For any tonic–clonic seizure that does not stop automatically or when doubt exists regarding the diagnosis, treatment of GCSE should begin during the diagnostic workup. **Figure 54-3** is an algorithm for treatment of GCSE. **Table 54-5** includes doses of medication for GCSE, and **Table 54-6** has adverse drug reactions and monitoring of parameters.

Stabilization Phase

- Thiamine (100 mg IV) should be given prior to IV glucose (see **Figure 54-3**).

Initial Therapy Phase (5–20 Minutes)

- Benzodiazepines are effective initial therapy in most patients. Benzodiazepine preference is based on pharmacokinetics, route of administration, pharmacoeconomics, adverse-effect profile, and current availability. Evidence-based guidelines recommend the initial use of IM midazolam, IV lorazepam, or IV diazepam (see **Figure 54-3**) in adults and the use of IV lorazepam or IV diazepam in children.
- IV **diazepam** is extremely lipophilic and quickly distributed into the brain, but it redistributes rapidly into body fat, causing a very short duration of effect (<0.5 hour). Therefore, give a longer-acting anticonvulsant (eg, phenytoin or phenobarbital) immediately after the diazepam.
- IV **lorazepam** is currently considered the benzodiazepine of choice by most practitioners. It takes longer to reach peak brain levels than diazepam but has a longer duration of action (12–24 hours).
- IV **midazolam** is water soluble and diffuses rapidly into the CNS but has a very short half-life. Maintenance doses must be given by continuous infusion. Midazolam has a more reliable IM absorption than either diazepam or lorazepam. There is increasing interest in giving it buccally, IM, and intranasally when IV access cannot be obtained readily. Buccal midazolam may be more effective than rectal diazepam in children.
- Guidelines also recommend the use of IV phenobarbital as an alternative first-line agent in adults during the initial therapy stage.
  - ✓ If the initial loading dose does not stop the seizures within 20–30 minutes, an additional dose (10–20 mg/kg) can be given, before moving to anesthetic agents. When necessary, larger loading doses (eg, 30 mg/kg) have been used in neonates.
- Once GCSE is controlled, the maintenance dose should be started within 12–24 hours.

Second-Therapy Phase: Established GCSE (20–40 Minutes)

- Phenytoin is second-line for GCSE unresponsive to the benzodiazepines or in seizures that recur after successful benzodiazepine treatment.

PREHOSPITAL CARE
- Monitor Vital signs (HR, RR)
- PR diazepam (0.2-0.5 mg/kg)
- Consider IN midazolam (0.15-0.3 mg/kg) or IM midazolam (0.2 mg/kg up to 10 mg)
- Transport to hospital if seizures persist

INITIAL HOSPITAL CARE
- Time from seizure onset
- Assess and control airway and cardiac function; pulse oximetry
- 100% oxygen
- Place IV catheter; Intraosseous if unable to place IV and patient is younger than 6 years
- Begin IV fluids; blood pressure support as needed
- Thiamine 100 mg (adult)
- Pyridoxine 50-100 mg (infant)
- Glucose (adult: 50 mL of 50%; children: 1 mL/kg of 10%) if serum glucose is <60 mg/dL (<3.3 mmol/L)
- Naloxone 0.1 mg/kg for suspected narcotic overdose
- Antibiotics if infection suspected
- Treat hyperthermia

LABORATORY STUDIES
- CBC with differential
- Serum chemistry profile (eg, electrolytes, glucose, renal/hepatic function, calcium, magnesium)
- Arterial blood gas
- Blood cultures
- Serum anticonvulsant concentration
- Urine drug/alcohol screen
- EEG as needed

IMPENDING GSCE (0-30 minutes)
- IV lorazepam (0.1 mg/kg over 30-60 seconds up to 6 mg) may repeat in 5 minutes if no response or IN midazolam (0.15-0.3 mg/kg up to 10 mg) or IM midazolam (0.2 mg/kg up to 10 mg)
- Additional therapies may not be required if seizure stops

ESTABLISHED GSCE (30-60 minutes)
First-line
Phenytoin (IV): 18-20 mg/kg over 20 minutes (<1 mg/kg/min; max 50 mg/min); may give an additional 5 mg/kg as needed or Fosphenytoin (IV or IM): 18-20 mg PE/kg (<3 mg PE/kg/min; max <150 mg PE/min)
Second-line
Phenobarbital (IV): 15-20 mg/kg over 20 minutes (<100 mg/min)
Valproate (IV): 25-30 mg/kg over 5-15 minutes (<3 mg/kg/min up to 200 mg/min) followed by an infusion of 1-mg/kg/h
Third-line
Lacosamide (IV): 50-400 mg; 200 mg given over 15 minutes
Levetiracetam (IV): 40-60 mg/kg, maximum 3,000 mg (administer 2-5 mg/kg/min)

REFRACTORY GSCE (>120 minutes)
Implement continuous EEG monitoring
Assure patient is normovolemic
Assure cerebral perfusion pressure is >70 mm Hg (>9.3 kPa)
Administer volume as stated above and then begin vasopressors to achieve adequate mean arterial pressure (>120 mm Hg [>16.0 kPa]) Continuous ECG monitoring if on propofol
First-line
- Midazolam: 0.2-0.4 mg/kg bolus at a rate of 2 mg/min followed by 0.05-2 mg/kg/h
- Pentobarbital: 10-20 mg/kg bolus at a rate of ≤50 mg/min followed by 1-5 mg/kg/h
- Propofol: 1-2 mg/kg bolus followed by <4 mg/kg/h in children; larger dose may be used in adults

SUPER-REFRACTORY GSCE (>24 hours)
Implement continuous EEG monitoring
Assure patient is normovolemic
Assure cerebral perfusion pressure is >70 mm Hg (>9.3 kPa)
Administer volume as stated above and then begin vasopressors to achieve adequate mean arterial pressure (>120 mm Hg [>16.0 kPa])

- Ketamine
- Hypothermia
- Lidocaine
- Topiramate
- Inhaled Anesthetics
- Immunomodulating therapies
- Ketogenic diet
- Vagus Nerve Stimulator

ªBecause variability exists in dosing, monitor serum concentration
(BP, blood pressure; CBC, complete blood count; CI, continuous infusion; D12.5W, 12.5% dextrose in water; D25W, 25% dextrose in water; D50W, 50% dextrose in water; EEG, electroencephalogram; GCSE, generalized convulsive status epilepticus; HR, heart rate; IN, intranasal; PE, phenytoin equivalents; PR, per rectum; RR, respiratory rate.)

FIGURE 54-3. Algorithm for the treatment of GCSE.

TABLE 54-5	Dosing of Medications Used in the Initial and Established Treatment of GCSE		
Drug (Route)	**Brand Name**	**Initial Dose (Maximum Dose)**	**Maintenance Dose**
Diazepam (IV)	Valium plus generic		
Adult		0.25 mg/kg[a,b,c] (20 mg)	Not used
Pediatric		0.25–0.5 mg/kg[a,c] (20 mg)	Not used
Fosphenytoin (IV)	Cerebyx plus generic		
Adult		20–25 mg PE/kg	4–5 mg PE/kg/day
Pediatric		20–25 mg PE/kg	5–10 mg PE/kg/day
Levetiracetam (IV)	Keppra plus generics		
Adult		2000–3000 mg	1000 mg thrice a day
Pediatric		40–60 mg/kg (3000 mg)	40–60 mg/kg/day, given twice or thrice a day
Lorazepam (IV)	Ativan plus generic		
Adult		4 mg[b,c] (6 mg)	Not used
Pediatric		0.1 mg/kg[a,c] (6 mg)	Not used
Midazolam (IV, IM)	Versed plus generic		
Adult		200 mcg/kg[a,d] (10 mg)	50–500 mcg/kg/hr[e]
Pediatric		150 mcg/kg[a,d] (10 mg)	60–120 mcg/kg/hr[e]
Phenobarbital (IV)	Generic		
Adult		10–20 mg/kg[e]	1–4 mg/kg/day[e]
Pediatric		15–20 mg/kg[e]	3–5 mg/kg/day[e]
Phenytoin (IV)	Dilantin plus generic		
Adult		20–25 mg/kg[f]	4–5 mg/kg/day[e]
Pediatric		20–25 mg/kg[f]	5–10 mg/kg/day[e]
Valproate (IV)	Depacon plus generic		
Adult		15–30 mg/kg (3000 mg)	1–4 mg/kg/hr[e]
Pediatric		20–25 mg/kg (3000 mg)	1–4 mg/kg/hr[e], or give every 4–6 hours

[a]Doses can be repeated every 10–15 minutes until the maximum dosage is given.
[b]Initial doses in the older persons are 2–5 mg.
[c]Larger doses can be required if patients chronically on a benzodiazepine (eg, clonazepam).
[d]Can be given by the intramuscular, rectal, or buccal routes.
[e]Titrate dose as needed.
[f]Administer additional loading dose based on serum concentration.
[g]The rate should not exceed 25 mg/min in older patients and those with known atherosclerotic cardiovascular disease.
GCSE, generalized convulsive status epilepticus; PE, phenytoin equivalents.

- Phenytoin has a 20–36 hour half-life, but it cannot be delivered fast enough to be a first-line agent.
- Phenytoin should be diluted to 5 mg/mL or greater in normal saline. Maintenance doses should be started within 12–24 hours of the loading dose.
- In determining a loading dose, consider whether the patient was taking phenytoin prior to admission and the phenytoin serum concentration if known. A larger loading dose is required in obese patients.

TABLE 54-6	Adverse Drug Reactions and Monitoring of Patients Receiving Drugs for GCSE		

Drug	Adverse Drug Reaction	Monitoring Parameters	Comments
Diazepam	Hypotension and cardiac arrhythmias	Vital signs and ECG during administration	Propylene glycol causes hypotension and cardiac arrhythmias when administered too rapidly; hypotension may occur with large doses
Fosphenytoin	Hypotension and cardiac arrhythmias; paresthesia, pruritus	Vital signs and ECG during administration	Hypotension is less than phenytoin, as product does not contain propylene glycol; pruritus generally involves the face and groin areas, is dose and rate related, and subsides 5–10 minutes after infusion
Lidocaine	Fasciculations, visual disturbances, tinnitus, seizures		Occur at serum concentrations between 6 and 8 mg/L (25.6–34.1 μmol/L); seizures >8 mg/L (34.1 μmol/L)
Lorazepam	Apnea, hypotension, bradycardia, cardiac arrest, respiratory depression, metabolic acidosis, and renal toxicity	Vital signs and ECG during administration; HCO_3 and serum creatinine; cumulative dose of propylene glycol	Accumulation of propylene glycol during prolong continuous infusions may cause acidosis
Pentobarbital	Hypotension	Vital signs and ECG during administration	Rate of infusion should be slower or dopamine should be added if hypotension occurs
Phenytoin	Hypotension and cardiac arrhythmia; nystagmus	Vital signs and ECG during administration	Contains propylene glycol. Large loading doses are generally not given to older individuals with preexisting cardiac disease or in critically ill patients with marginal blood pressure. The infusion rate should be slowed if the QT interval widens or if hypotension or arrhythmias develop; horizontal nystagmus suggests toxicity
Phenobarbital	Hypotension, respiratory, and CNS depression	Vital signs and mental status; EEG if used in anesthesia doses	Contains propylene glycol; if hypotension occurs, slow the rate of administration or begin dopamine; apnea and hypopnea can be more profound in patients treated initially with benzodiazepines

(Continued)

TABLE 54-6	Adverse Drug Reactions and Monitoring of Patients Receiving Drugs for GCSE (Continued)		
Drug	**Adverse Drug Reaction**	**Monitoring Parameters**	**Comments**
Propofol	Progressive metabolic acidosis, hemodynamic instability, and bradyarrhythmias	Vital signs, ECG, osmolar gap; EEG if used in anesthesia doses	Referred to as propofol-related infusion syndrome, which can be fatal
Topiramate	Metabolic acidosis	Acid base status (serum bicarbonate)	Extremely rare

CNS, central nervous system; ECG, electrocardiogram; EEG, electroencephalogram.

- Fosphenytoin, the water-soluble phosphate ester of phenytoin, is a phenytoin prodrug.
- Do not give the loading dose IM unless IV access is impossible.
- Serum phenytoin concentrations should not be obtained for at least 2 hours after IV and 4 hours after IM administration.
- IV valproate or levetiracetam are acceptable first-line agents if a benzodiazepine fails to control seizures after 20 minutes, or if seizures recur following a benzodiazepine and/or a hydantoin. Dosing for these agents is outlined in Table 54-5.

Third-Phase Therapies: Refractory GCSE (40–60 Minutes)

- When adequate doses of a benzodiazepine, and a single dose of a second anticonvulsant (hydantoin, valproate, levetiracetam, and/ or barbiturate) have failed, the condition is termed refractory. Approximately 10%–15% of patients will develop refractory GCSE. Doses of agents used to treat refractory GCSE are given in Table 54-7.
- There is no consensus regarding the agent of choice, sequencing of therapy, or treatment of refractory GCSE.
  ✓ Some clinicians recommend anesthetic doses of midazolam as the first-line treatment for refractory GCSE (see Table 54-7) in combination with another drugs that are mechanistically different. Most patients respond within an hour.
  ✓ Successful benzodiazepine discontinuation is enhanced by serum phenytoin concentrations >20 mg/L (79 μmol/L) and phenobarbital concentrations >40 mg/L (172 μmol/L).
- A short-acting barbiturate (eg, pentobarbital or thiopental) (see Figure 54-3) may require intubation and respiratory support as well as continuous EEG and monitoring of vital signs.
  ✓ Give a loading dose of pentobarbital to provide serum concentration (40 mg/L; 177 μmol/L) sufficient to induce an isoelectric EEG. Usual duration of coma is 2–3 days, aiming to discontinue use as soon as possible.
- Propofol is very lipid soluble and has a large volume of distribution and a rapid onset of action. It has comparable efficacy to midazolam for refractory GCSE. Adverse effects and monitoring are shown in Table 54-6 and dosing is shown in Table 54-7. Once EEG burst suppression is achieved, the dose should be reduced.
- Topiramate tablets can be crushed, dissolved in a small amount of water, and given orally or nasogastrically. Response tends to be delayed hours to days. If metabolic acidosis occurs, it can be treated with citrates, with a goal of maintaining a serum bicarbonate level of at least 20 mEq/L (mmol/L).

Super-Refractory GCSE (>24 Hours)

- **Ketamine** appears to be a reasonable option to consider in refractory GCSE that has failed inhaled analgesics (Figure 54-3). Advantages include maintenance of

TABLE 54-7 Dosing of Medications Used to Treat Refractory or Super-Refractory GCSE

Drug (Brand Name)	Initial Dose (Maximum Dose)	Maintenance Dose	Comments
Ketamine (generics)			
Adult	1–4 mg	1–5 mg/kg/hr	
Pediatric	0.5–2 mg/kg	1–10 mg/kg/hr	
Lacosamide (Vimpat)			
Adult	200–400 mg	200 mg bid	Administer IV over 15 minutes, monitor serum concentrations
Pediatric	6–10 mg/kg (400 mg)	6–12 mg/kg/day, given twice a day	
Lidocaine (generics)			
Adult	50–100 mg	1.5–3.5 mg/kg/hr	Administer IV in ≤2 minutes
Pediatric	1 mg/kg (maximum 3–5 mg/kg in the first hour)	1.2–3 mg/kg/hr	
Midazolam (Versed plus generic)			
Adult	200 mcg/kg[a]	50–500 mcg/kg/hr[b]	Initial dose may be given IM; administer IV over 0.5–1 mg/min; continuous-infusion rate should be increased every 15 minutes in those who do not respond and should be guided by EEG response; development of tachyphylaxis can require frequent increases in dose; decrease dose by 1 mcg/kg/min every 2 hours once GCSE is controlled
pediatric	150 mcg/kg[a]	60–120 mcg/kg/hr[b]	

Pentobarbital (generics)			
Adult	10–20 mg/kg	1–5 mg/kg/hr[b]	Over 1–2 hours, the rate of infusion should be slowed or dopamine should be added if hypotension occurs; gradually titrate dose upward until there is evidence of burst suppression on EEG (ie, isoelectric EEG) or prohibitive adverse effects occur. Twelve hours after a burst suppression is obtained, the rate should be titrated downward every 2–4 hours
Pediatric	15–20 mg/kg	1–5 mg/kg/hr[b]	
Propofol (Diprivan plus generic)			
Adult	2 mg/kg	5–10 mg/kg/hr[b]	Over 10 seconds in adults and 20–30 seconds in pediatric patients
Pediatric	3 mg/kg	2–4 mg/kg/hr[c]	
Topiramate (Topamax plus generic)			
Adult	300–500 mg	400–1600 mg/day	Given orally in divided dose every 12 hours. Doses as large as 25 mg/kg/day for 2–5 days have been used in children. Monitor serum bicarbonate levels and serum concentrations
Pediatric	5–15 mg/kg (400 mg)	5–10 mg/kg/day, given thrice a day	

[a]Doses can be repeated twice at 10–15 minute intervals until the maximum dosage is given.
[b]Titrate dose as needed.
[c]Generally recommended not to exceed a dose of 4 mg/kg/hr and a duration of 48 hours.
EEG, electroencephalogram; GCSE, generalized convulsive status epilepticus; IM, intramuscular; IV, intravenous.

arterial blood pressure, pulse, and cardiac output, but it may cause hallucinations upon awakening, increased salivation, and increased intraocular and intracranial pressures.

- IV **lidocaine** is not recommended unless other agents have failed. Serum concentrations should be monitored to avoid drug accumulation and toxicity (**Table 54-6**).
- Inhaled anesthetics are used once other approaches fail. **Halothane, isoflurane**, are difficult to administer outside the operating room, and an anesthesiologist is required. They have no proven advantages over traditional anticonvulsants, and they can increase intracranial pressure.
- In the absence of contraindications, a trial of large doses of steroids (eg, 1 g/day of IV **prednisolone** for 3 days, followed by 1 mg/kg/day in four divided doses) should be used in patients with unidentified etiology for super-refractory GCSE. Responders should continue long-term steroids, IV immunoglobulins, and other immunomodulatory agents, such as **cyclophosphamide** or **rituximab**.

EVALUATION OF THERAPEUTIC OUTCOMES

- The goal therapeutic outcome for all ASDs is seizure freedom or reduction in seizure frequency, while minimizing adverse effects.
- Monitor long term for seizure control, side effects, social adjustment including quality of life, drug interactions, compliance, and side effects. Clinical response is more important than serum drug concentrations.
- Screen periodically for psychiatric disorders (eg, anxiety and depression).
- Ask patients and caregivers to record severity and frequency of seizures. Medication adherence should be assessed continually.
- The morbidity and mortality associated with GCSE can be minimized by the rapid implementation of a rational therapeutic plan.
- An EEG is an extremely important tool used to determine when abnormal electrical activity has been aborted, but also can assist in determining which anticonvulsant was effective.

See Chapter 73, Epilepsy, authored by Viet-Huong V. Nguyen, Sunita Dergalust, and Edward Chang and Chapter 74, Status Epilepticus, authored by Stephanie J. Phelps and James W. Wheless, for a more detailed discussion of these topics.

CHAPTER 55

Headache: Migraine and Tension-Type

Migraine Headache

- *Migraine*, a common, recurrent, primary headache of moderate-to-severe intensity, interferes with normal functioning and is associated with gastrointestinal (GI), neurologic, and autonomic symptoms. In migraine with aura, focal neurologic symptoms precede or accompany the attack.

PATHOPHYSIOLOGY

- Activation of trigeminal sensory nerves triggers the release of vasoactive neuropeptides, including calcitonin gene-related peptide (CGRP), neurokinin A, and substance P from perivascular axons. Vasodilation of dural blood vessels may occur with extravasation of dural plasma resulting in inflammation.
- Twin studies suggest 50% heritability of migraine, with a multifactorial polygenic basis. Migraine triggers may be modulators of the genetic set point that predisposes to migraine headache.
- Specific populations of serotonin (5-HT) receptors appear to be involved in the pathophysiology and treatment of migraine headache.

CLINICAL PRESENTATION

- Migraine headache is characterized by recurring episodes of throbbing head pain, frequently unilateral.
- Up to 79% of patients with migraines have premonitory symptoms (not to be confused with aura) in the hours or days before headache onset. Neurologic symptoms (phonophobia, photophobia, hyperosmia, and difficulty concentrating) are most common, but psychological (anxiety, depression, euphoria, irritability, drowsiness, hyperactivity, and restlessness), autonomic (eg, polyuria, diarrhea, and constipation), and constitutional (eg, stiff neck, yawning, thirst, food cravings, and anorexia) symptoms may also occur.
- A migraine aura is experienced by approximately 25% of patients with migraines. Aura evolves over 5–20 minutes and lasts less than 60 minutes. Headache usually occurs within 60 minutes of the end of the aura. Visual auras can include both positive features (eg, scintillations, photopsia, teichopsia, and fortification spectrum) and negative features (eg, scotoma and hemianopsia). Sensory symptoms such as paresthesias or numbness of the arms and face, dysphasia or aphasia, weakness, and hemiparesis may also occur.
- Migraine headache may occur at any time but usually occurs in the early morning. Pain is usually gradual in onset, peaking in intensity over minutes to hours and lasting 4–72 hours. Pain is typically in the frontotemporal region and is moderate to severe. Headache is usually unilateral and throbbing with GI symptoms (eg, nausea and vomiting) almost invariably accompanying the headache. Other systemic symptoms include anorexia, constipation, diarrhea, abdominal cramps, nasal stuffiness, blurred vision, diaphoresis, facial pallor, and localized facial, scalp, or periorbital edema. Sensory hyperacuity (photophobia, phonophobia, or osmophobia) is frequent. Many patients seek a dark, quiet place.
- Once the headache pain wanes, a resolution phase characterized by exhaustion, malaise, and irritability ensues.

DIAGNOSIS

- The International Headache Society (IHS) has published diagnostic criteria for classic migraine variants and other migraine subtypes

- A comprehensive headache history is essential and includes age at onset; frequency, timing, and duration of attacks; possible triggers; ameliorating factors; description and characteristics of symptoms; associated signs and symptoms; treatment history; and family and social history.
- Neuroimaging should be considered in patients with unexplained abnormal neurologic examination or atypical headache history.
- Onset of migraine headaches after age 50 suggests an organic etiology, such as a mass lesion, cerebrovascular disease, or temporal arteritis.

TREATMENT

- <u>Goals of Treatment</u>: The goal is to achieve consistent, rapid headache relief with minimal adverse effects and symptom recurrence, and minimal disability and emotional distress, enabling the patient to resume normal activities. Ideally, patients should be able to manage their headaches without emergency department or physician office visits.

NONPHARMACOLOGIC TREATMENT

- Apply ice to the head and recommend periods of rest or sleep, usually in a dark, quiet environment.
- Identify and avoid triggers of migraine attacks (Table 55-1).
- Behavioral interventions (relaxation therapy, biofeedback, and cognitive therapy) may help patients who prefer nondrug therapy or when drug therapy is ineffective or not tolerated.

PHARMACOLOGIC TREATMENT

- Administer acute migraine therapies at the onset of migraine (Table 55-2 and Figure 55-1).

Antiemetic Pretreatment

- Pretreatment with an antiemetic (eg, **metoclopramide**, **chlorpromazine**, or **prochlorperazine**) 15–30 minutes before oral or nonoral migraine treatments (rectal suppositories, nasal spray, or injections) may be advisable when nausea and vomiting are severe. In addition to its antiemetic effects, metoclopramide helps reverse gastroparesis and enhances absorption of oral medications.
- **Prochlorperazine** (IM, IV, or rectal), **metoclopramide** (IV), as well as parenteral chlorpromazine and **droperidol** have been used for refractory migraine.
- Frequent or excessive use of acute migraine medications can result in increasing headache frequency and drug consumption known as medication-overuse headache. This occurs commonly with overuse of simple or combination analgesics, **opioids ergotamine tartrate**, and **triptans**. Limit use of acute migraine therapies to 2 or 3 days per week or 10 days per month.

Analgesics and Nonsteroidal Anti-Inflammatory Drugs

- Simple analgesics and nonsteroidal anti-inflammatory drugs (NSAIDs) are first-line treatments for mild to moderate migraine attacks; some severe attacks are also responsive. **Aspirin, diclofenac, ibuprofen, naproxen sodium**, and the combination of **acetaminophen plus aspirin and caffeine** are effective. Evidence is limited with **ketorolac** and **flurbiprofen**.
- NSAIDs appear to prevent neurogenically mediated inflammation in the trigemino-vascular system by inhibiting prostaglandin synthesis.
- Rectal analgesic preparations are options for patients with severe nausea and vomiting.
- The combination of acetaminophen, aspirin, and caffeine is approved in the United States for relieving migraine pain.
- Aspirin and acetaminophen are also available by prescription in combination with a short-acting barbiturate (**butalbital**). Use of these analgesics or narcotics should be limited because of concerns about overuse, medication-overuse headache, and withdrawal

TABLE 55-1	Commonly Reported Triggers of Migraine

Food triggers

Alcohol

Caffeine/Caffeine withdrawal

Chocolate

Fermented and pickled foods

Monosodium glutamate (eg, in Chinese food, seasoned salt, and instant foods)

Nitrate-containing foods (eg, processed meats)

Saccharin/Aspartame (eg, diet foods or diet sodas)

Tyramine-containing foods

Environmental triggers	**Behavioral–physiologic triggers**
Glare or flickering lights	Excess or insufficient sleep
High altitude	Fatigue
Loud noises	Menstruation, menopause
Strong smells and fumes	Sexual activity
Tobacco smoke	Skipped meals
Weather changes	Strenuous physical activity (eg, prolonged overexertion)
	Stress or poststress

Ergot Alkaloids and Derivatives

- Ergot alkaloids are useful for moderate to severe migraine attacks. They are nonselective $5HT_1$ receptor agonists that constrict intracranial blood vessels and inhibit the development of neurogenic inflammation in the trigeminovascular system. Venous and arterial constriction occurs.
- **Ergotamine tartrate** is available for oral, sublingual, and rectal administration. Oral and rectal preparations contain caffeine to enhance absorption and potentiate analgesia.
- **Dihydroergotamine (DHE)** is available for intranasal and parenteral (IM, IV, or subcutaneous [SC]) administration. Patients can self-administer IM or SC DHE. The nasal spray formulation of DHE has been shown to be effective.
- Nausea and vomiting are common with ergotamine derivatives, so consider antiemetic pretreatment and titrate to a dose that is not nauseating. Other common side effects include abdominal pain, weakness, fatigue, paresthesias, muscle pain, diarrhea, and chest tightness. Symptoms of severe peripheral ischemia (ergotism) include cold, numb, painful extremities; continuous paresthesias; diminished peripheral pulses; and claudication. Gangrenous extremities, myocardial infarction (MI), hepatic necrosis, and bowel and brain ischemia have occurred rarely with ergotamine. Do not use ergotamine derivatives and triptans within 24 hours of each other.
- Contraindications to use of ergot derivatives include renal and hepatic failure; coronary, cerebral, or peripheral vascular disease; uncontrolled hypertension; sepsis; and women who are pregnant or nursing.
- DHE does not appear to cause rebound headache, but dosage restrictions for ergotamine tartrate should be strictly observed to prevent this complication.

TABLE 55-2	Dosing of Acute Migraine Therapies[a]	
Drug	**Dose**	**Usual Range/Comments**
Analgesics		
Acetaminophen[a] (Tylenol)	1000 mg at onset; repeat every 4–6 hours as needed	Maximum daily dose is 4 g
Acetaminophen 250 mg/aspirin 250 mg/ caffeine 65 mg[a] (Excedrin Migraine)	2 tablets at onset and every 6 hours	Available over-the-counter as Excedrin Migraine
Nonsteroidal anti-inflammatory drugs		
Aspirin[a]	500–1000 mg every 4–6 hours	Maximum daily dose is 4 g
Ibuprofen[a] (Motrin)	200–800 mg every 6 hours	Avoid doses >2.4 g/day
Naproxen sodium[a] (Aleve, Anaprox)	550–825 mg at onset; can repeat 220 mg in 3–4 hours	Avoid doses >1.375 g/day
Diclofenac[a] (Cataflam, Voltaren)	50–100 mg at onset; can repeat 50 mg in 8 hours	Avoid doses >150 mg/day
Ergotamine tartrate		
Oral tablet (1 mg) with caffeine 100 mg[b] (Cafergot)	2 mg at onset; then 1–2 mg every 30 minutes as needed	Maximum dose is 6 mg/day or 10 mg/week; consider pretreatment with an antiemetic
Rectal suppository (2 mg) with caffeine 100 mg[b] (Cafergot, Migergot)	Insert 1/2–1 suppository at onset; repeat after 1 hour as needed	Maximum dose is 4 mg/day or 10 mg/week; consider pretreatment with an antiemetic
Dihydroergotamine		
Injection 1 mg/mL (D.H.E. 45)[b]	0.25–1 mg at onset IM, IV or subcutaneous; repeat every hour as needed	Maximum dose is 3 mg/day or 6 mg/week
Nasal spray 4 mg/mL[a] (Migranal)	One spray (0.5 mg) in each nostril at onset; repeat sequence 15 minutes later (total dose is 2 mg or 4 sprays)	Maximum dose is 3 mg/day; prime sprayer 4 times before using; do not tilt head back or inhale through nose while spraying; discard open ampules after 8 hours
Serotonin agonists (triptans)		
Sumatriptan[a] (Imitrex) Injection	6 mg subcutaneous at onset; can repeat after 1 hour if needed	Maximum daily dose is 12 mg
Oral tablets	25, 50, 85, or 100 mg at onset; can repeat after 2 hours if needed	Optimal dose is 50–100 mg; maximum daily dose is 200 mg; combination product with naproxen, 85/500 mg

(Continued)

TABLE 55-2	**Dosing of Acute Migraine Therapies[a] (Continued)**	
Drug	**Dose**	**Usual Range/Comments**
Serotonin agonists (triptans) (con't)		
Nasal spray	5, 10, or 20 mg at onset; can repeat after 2 hours if needed	Optimal dose is 20 mg; maximum daily dose is 40 mg; single-dose device delivering 5 or 20 mg; administer one spray in one nostril
Zolmitriptan[a] (Zomig, Zomig-ZMT)		
Oral tablets	2.5 or 5 mg at onset as regular or orally disintegrating tablet; can repeat after 2 hours if needed	Optimal dose is 2.5 mg; maximum dose is 10 mg/day
		Do not divide ODT dosage form
Nasal spray	5 mg (one spray) at onset; can repeat after 2 hours if needed	Maximum daily dose is 10 mg/day
Naratriptan[a] (Amerge)	1 or 2.5 mg at onset; can repeat after 4 hours if needed	Optimal dose is 2.5 mg; maximum daily dose is 5 mg
Rizatriptan[a] (Maxalt, Maxalt-MLT)	5 or 10 mg at onset as regular or orally disintegrating tablet; can repeat after 2 hours if needed	Optimal dose is 10 mg; maximum daily dose is 30 mg; onset of effect is similar with standard and orally disintegrating tablets; use 5-mg dose (15 mg/day maximum) in patients receiving propranolol
Almotriptan[a] (Axert)	6.25 or 12.5 mg at onset; can repeat after 2 hours if needed	Optimal dose is 12.5 mg; maximum daily dose is 25 mg
Frovatriptan[a] (Frova)	2.5 or 5 mg at onset; can repeat in 2 hours if needed	Optimal dose 2.5–5 mg; maximum daily dose is 7.5 mg (3 tablets)
Eletriptan[a] (Relpax)	20 or 40 mg at onset; can repeat after 2 hours if needed	Maximum single dose is 40 mg; maximum daily dose is 80 mg
Miscellaneous		
Metoclopramide[b] (Reglan)	10 mg IV at onset	Useful for acute relief in the office or emergency department setting
Prochlorperazine[b] (Compazine)	10 mg IV or IM, 25 mg rectally at onset	Useful for acute relief in the office or emergency department setting

[a]Limit use of symptomatic medications to fewer than 10 days/month when possible to avoid medication-overuse headache. Level A—established efficacy (≥2 Class I studies).
[b]Level B—probably effective (1 Class I or 2 Class II studies).
ODT, orally disintegrating tablet.

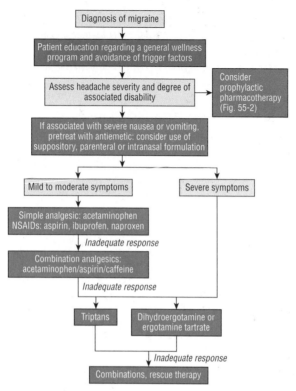

FIGURE 55-1. Treatment algorithm for migraine headaches.

Serotonin Receptor Agonists (Triptans)

- The triptans (**Table 55-3**) are appropriate first-line therapies for patients with mild-to-severe migraine or as rescue therapy when nonspecific medications are ineffective.
- They are selective agonists of the $5HT_{1B}$ and $5HT_{1D}$ receptors. Relief of migraine headache results from: (1) normalization of dilated intracranial arteries, (2) inhibition of vasoactive peptide release, and (3) inhibition of transmission through second-order neurons ascending to the thalamus.
- **Sumatriptan** SC injection is packaged as an autoinjector device for self-administration. Compared with the oral formulation, SC administration offers enhanced efficacy and more rapid onset of action. Intranasal sumatriptan also has a faster onset of effect than the oral formulation and produces similar rates of response.
- Second-generation triptans (all except sumatriptan) have higher oral bioavailability and longer half-lives than oral sumatriptan, which could theoretically reduce headache recurrence. However, comparative clinical trials are necessary to determine their relative efficacy. **Frovatriptan** and **naratriptan** have the longest half-lives, slowest onset of action, and less headache recurrence.
- Pharmacokinetic characteristics of the triptans are shown in **Table 55-3**.
- Lack of response to one triptan does not preclude effective therapy with another triptan.

TABLE 55-3	Pharmacokinetic Characteristics of Triptans			
Drug	**Half-Life (Hours)**	**Time to Maximal Concentration (t_{max})**	**Bioavailability (%)**	**Elimination**
Almotriptan	3–4	1.4–3.8 hours	80	MAO-A, CYP3A4, CYP2D6
Eletriptan	4–5	1–2 hours	50	CYP3A4
Frovatriptan	25	2–4 hours	24–30	Mostly unchanged, CYP1A2
Naratriptan	5–6	2–3 hours	63–74	Largely unchanged, CYP450 (various isoenzymes)
Rizatriptan	2–3		45	MAO-A
Oral tablets		1–1.2 hours		
Disintegrating		1.6–2.5 hours		
Sumatriptan	2			MAO-A
SC injection		12–15 minutes	97	
Oral tablets		2.5 hours	14	
Nasal spray		1–2.5 hours	17	
Zolmitriptan	3		40–48	CYP1A2, MAO-A
Oral		2 hours		
Disintegrating		3.3 hours		
Nasal		4 hours		

CYP, cytochrome P450; MAO-A, monoamine oxidase type A.

- Side effects of triptans include paresthesias, fatigue, dizziness, flushing, warm sensations, and somnolence. Minor injection site reactions are reported with SC use, and taste perversion and nasal discomfort may occur with intranasal administration.
- Up to 25% of patients report chest tightness; pressure; heaviness; or pain in the chest, neck, or throat. The mechanism of these symptoms is unknown, but a cardiac source is unlikely in most patients. Isolated cases of MI and coronary vasospasm with ischemia have been reported. Use triptans cautiously in patients at risk for unrecognized coronary artery disease. Do a cardiovascular assessment before giving triptans to postmenopausal women, men over 40 years of age, and patients with uncontrolled risk factors, and administer the first dose under medical supervision. Ischemic heart disease, uncontrolled hypertension, cerebrovascular disease, hemiplegic and basilar migraine, and pregnancy are contraindications to their use.
- Do not give triptans within 24 hours of ergotamine derivative administration or within 2 weeks of therapy with monoamine oxidase inhibitors. Concomitant use of triptans with selective serotonin reuptake inhibitors or serotonin–norepinephrine reuptake inhibitors can cause serotonin syndrome, a potentially life-threatening condition.

Opioids

- There is inadequate evidence for opioids and derivatives (eg, **meperidine, butorphanol, oxycodone,** and **hydromorphone**) for the treatment of migraines. Combinations of either oral **codeine** or **tramadol** and acetaminophen are probably effective, and **butorphanol** nasal spray has established efficacy.

- Reserve these for patients with moderate to severe infrequent headaches in whom conventional therapies are contraindicated or as rescue medication after failure to respond to conventional therapies. Closely supervise opioid therapy.

Prophylactic Therapy

- Prophylactic therapies (Table 55-4 and Figure 55-2) are administered daily to reduce the frequency, severity, and duration of attacks, and to increase responsiveness to acute therapies.
- Consider prophylaxis in the setting of recurring migraines that produce significant disability; frequent attacks requiring symptomatic medication more than twice per week; symptomatic therapies that are ineffective, contraindicated, or produce serious side effects; uncommon migraine variants that cause profound disruption or risk of neurologic injury; and patient preference to limit the number of attacks.
- Preventive therapy may also be given intermittently when headaches recur in a predictable pattern (eg, exercise-induced or menstrual migraine).
- Because efficacy of various prophylactic agents appears to be similar, drug selection is based on side-effect profiles and comorbid conditions. Response to an agent is unpredictable, and a 2- to 3-month trial is necessary to achieve clinical benefit.
- Only **propranolol**, **timolol**, **divalproex sodium**, **topiramate**, **erenumab-aooe**, **fremanezumab-vfrm**, and **galcanezumab-gnlm** are Food and Drug Administration (FDA) approved for migraine prevention. Other established agents also have probable efficacy.
- Initiate prophylaxis with low doses, and advance slowly until a therapeutic effect is achieved or side effects become intolerable. Continue prophylaxis for at least 6–12 months after headache frequency and severity have diminished, and then gradual tapering or discontinuation may be reasonable.

B-Adrenergic Antagonists

- **Propranolol**, **timolol**, and **metoprolol** reduce the frequency of migraine attacks by 50% in more than 50% of patients. **Atenolol** and **nadolol** are probably also effective.
- Side effects include drowsiness, fatigue, sleep disturbances, vivid dreams, memory disturbance, depression, sexual dysfunction, bradycardia, and hypotension.
- Use with caution in patients with heart failure, peripheral vascular disease, atrioventricular conduction disturbances, asthma, depression, and diabetes.

Antidepressants

- The tricyclic antidepressants (TCAs) **amitriptyline** and **venlafaxine** are probably effective for migraine prophylaxis. There are insufficient data to support or refute the efficacy of other antidepressants.
- Their beneficial effects in migraine prophylaxis are independent of antidepressant activity and may be related to downregulation of central $5HT_2$ receptors, increased synaptic norepinephrine, and enhanced opioid receptor actions.
- TCAs are usually well tolerated at the doses used for migraine prophylaxis, but anticholinergic effects may limit use, especially in elderly patients or those with benign prostatic hyperplasia or glaucoma. Evening doses are preferred because of sedation. Increased appetite and weight gain can occur. Orthostatic hypotension and slowed atrioventricular conduction are occasionally reported.

Anticonvulsants

- **Valproic acid**, **divalproex sodium** (a 1:1 molar combination of valproate sodium and valproic acid), and **topiramate** can reduce the frequency, severity, and duration of headaches. **Carbamazepine** is possibly effective.
- Side effects of valproic acid and divalproex sodium include nausea (less common with divalproex sodium and gradual dosing titration), tremor, somnolence, weight

TABLE 55-4	Dosing of Prophylactic Migraine Therapies		
Drug	**Initial Dose**	**Usual Range**	**Comments**
β-Adrenergic antagonists			
Atenolol[a] (Tenormin)	50 mg/day	50–200 mg/day	
Metoprolol[b] (Toprol, Toprol XL)	100 mg/day in divided doses	100–200 mg/day in divided doses	Dose short-acting 4 times a day and long-acting 2 times a day; available as extended release
Nadolol[a] (Corgard)	40–80 mg/day	80–240 mg/day	
Propranolol[b] (Inderal, Inderal LA)	40 mg/day in divided doses	40–160 mg/day in divided doses	Dose short-acting 2–3 times a day and long-acting 1–2 times a day; available as extended release
Timolol[b] (Blocadren)	20 mg/day in divided doses	20–60 mg/day in divided doses	
Antidepressants			
Amitriptyline[a] (Elavil)	10 mg at bedtime	20–50 mg at bedtime	
Venlafaxine[a] (Effexor, Effexor-XR)	37.5 mg/day	75–150 mg/day	Available as extended release; increase dose after 1 week
Anticonvulsants			
Topiramate[b] (Topamax)	25 mg/day	50–200 mg/day in divided doses	As effective as amitriptyline, propranolol, or valproate; increase by 25 mg/week
Valproic acid/ Divalproex sodium[b] (Depakene, Depakote, Depakote ER)	250–500 mg/day in divided doses, or daily for extended release	500–1500 mg/day in divided doses, or daily for extended release	Monitor levels if compliance is an issue
Nonsteroidal anti-inflammatory drugs			
Ibuprofen[a] (Motrin)	400–1200 mg/day in divided doses	Same as initial dose	Use intermittently, such as for menstrual migraine prevention; daily or prolonged use may lead to medication-overuse headache and is limited by potential toxicity
Ketoprofen[a] (Orudis)	150 mg/day in divided doses	Same as initial dose	
Naproxen sodium[a] (Aleve, Anaprox)	550–1100 mg/day in divided doses	Same as initial dose	

(Continued)

TABLE 55-4	Dosing of Prophylactic Migraine Therapies (*Continued*)		
Drug	**Initial Dose**	**Usual Range**	**Comments**
Serotonin agonists (triptans)			
Frovatriptan[b] (Frova)	2.5 mg/day or 5 mg/day in divided doses	Same as initial dose	Taken in the perimenstrual period to prevent menstrual migraine
Naratriptan[a] (Amerge)	2 mg/day in divided doses	Same as initial dose	
Zolmitriptan[a] (Zomig)	5–7.5 mg/day in divided doses	Same as initial dose	
Miscellaneous			
Magnesium[a]	400 mg/day	800 mg/day in divided doses	May be more helpful in migraine with aura and menstrual migraine
MIG-99[a] (feverfew)	10–100 mg/day in divided doses	Same as initial dose	Withdrawal may be associated with increased headaches
Petasites[b]	100–150 mg/day in divided doses	150 mg/day in divided doses	Use only commercial preparations, plant is carcinogenic
Riboflavin[a]	400 mg/day in divided doses	400 mg/day in divided doses	Benefit only after 3 months

[a]Level B—probably effective (1 Class I or 2 Class II studies).
[b]Level A—established efficacy (≥2 Class I studies).

gain, hair loss, and hepatotoxicity (the risk of hepatotoxicity appears to be low in patients older than 10 years on monotherapy). Obtain baseline liver function tests. The extended-release formulation of divalproex sodium is administered once daily and is better tolerated than the enteric-coated formulation. Valproate is contraindicated in pregnancy and patients with a history of pancreatitis or chronic liver disease.
• Paresthesias (~50% of patients) and weight loss (9%–12% of patients) are common side effects of topiramate. Other side effects include fatigue, anorexia, diarrhea, difficulty with memory, language problems, taste perversions, and nausea. Use topiramate cautiously or avoid in those with a history of kidney stones or cognitive impairment.

Nonsteroidal Anti-Inflammatory Drugs

• NSAIDs are modestly effective for reducing the frequency, severity, and duration of migraine attacks. For migraine prevention, evidence for efficacy is strongest for naproxen and weakest for aspirin.
• They may be used intermittently to prevent headaches that recur in a predictable pattern (eg, menstrual migraine). Initiate up to 1 week before the time of headache vulnerability, and continue until vulnerability is passed.
• Potential GI and renal toxicity limit daily or prolonged use.

Calcitonin Gene-Related Peptide Antagonists

• Several anti-CGRP receptor monoclonal antibodies (**erenumab-aooe, fremanezumab-vfrm, and galcanezumab-gnlm**) have demonstrated efficacy in the prevention of episodic and chronic migraines (with or without aura). Concerns regarding their adverse effects were not substantiated in clinical trials. Data regarding long-term safety and efficacy are still needed. Cost and access may limit their use.

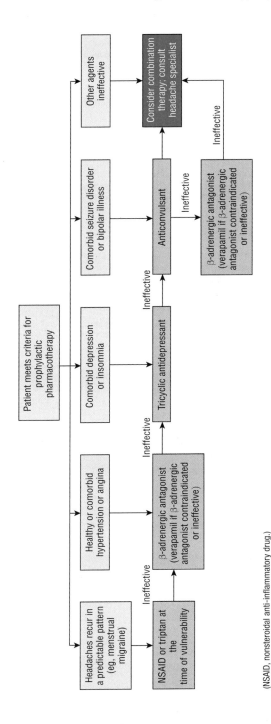

(NSAID, nonsteroidal anti-inflammatory drug.)

FIGURE 55-2. Treatment algorithm for prophylactic management of migraine headaches.

Other Drugs

- **Verapamil** has been widely used, but evidence for efficacy is inadequate.
- **Frovatriptan** is effective for prophylaxis of menstrual migraine, and **naratriptan** and **zolmitriptan** are probably effective.
- Other medications that may be effective include petasites, riboflavin (vitamin B_2), extract of feverfew, magnesium, subcutaneous histamine, lisinopril, candesartan, clonidine, guanfacine, and coenzyme Q10, but additional research is needed to confirm efficacy.

EVALUATION OF THERAPEUTIC OUTCOMES

- Monitor patients taking abortive therapy for frequency of use of prescription and nonprescription medications and for side effects.
- Document patterns of abortive medication used to establish the need for prophylactic therapy. Monitor prophylactic therapies closely for adverse reactions, abortive therapy needs, adequate dosing, and compliance.

Tension-Type Headache

- *Tension-type headache*, the most common type of primary headaches, is more common in women than men. Pain is usually mild to moderate and nonpulsatile. Episodic headaches may become chronic in some patients.

PATHOPHYSIOLOGY

- Pain is thought to originate from myofascial factors and peripheral sensitization of nociceptors. Central mechanisms are also involved. Mental stress, nonphysiologic motor stress, a local myofascial release of irritants, or a combination of these may be the initiating stimulus.

CLINICAL PRESENTATION

- Premonitory symptoms and aura are absent, and pain is usually mild to moderate, bilateral (having a hatband pattern), and nonpulsatile.
- Mild photophobia or phonophobia may occur. Pericranial or cervical muscles may have tender spots or localized nodules in some patients.

DIAGNOSIS

- The IHS has published diagnostic criteria for primary headache disorder.
- A comprehensive headache history is essential and includes age at onset; frequency, timing, and duration of attacks; possible triggers; ameliorating factors; description and characteristics of symptoms; associated signs and symptoms; treatment history; and family and social history.

TREATMENT

- <u>Goals of Treatment</u>: Pain relief and prevention of further headaches are the main desired outcomes of treatment.

NONPHARMACOLOGIC THERAPY

- Nonpharmacologic therapies include reassurance and counseling, stress management, relaxation training, and biofeedback. Evidence supporting physical therapeutic options (eg, heat or cold packs, ultrasound, electrical nerve stimulation, massage, acupuncture, trigger point injections, and occipital nerve blocks) has been inconsistent.

PHARMACOLOGIC THERAPY

Acute Treatment

- Simple analgesics (alone or in combination with caffeine) and NSAIDs are the mainstay of acute therapy. **Acetaminophen, aspirin, diclofenac, ibuprofen, naproxen, ketoprofen,** and **ketorolac** are effective.
- The combination of aspirin or acetaminophen with **butalbital**, or rarely, **codeine** are effective options, but avoid the use of butalbital and codeine combinations when possible. There is no evidence to support the efficacy of muscle relaxants.
- Give acute medication for episodic headache no more often than 3 days (butalbital-containing), 9 days (combination analgesics), or 15 days (NSAIDs) per month to prevent the development of chronic tension-type headache.

Prophylactic Therapy

- Consider preventive treatment if headache frequency is more than two per week, duration is longer than 3–4 hours, or severity results in medication overuse or substantial disability.
- The TCAs are used most often for prophylaxis of tension headache, but **venlafaxine, mirtazapine, gabapentin, topiramate,** and **tizanidine** may also be effective. Limited data suggest that trigger point injections of lidocaine may reduce headache frequency.

EVALUATION OF THERAPEUTIC OUTCOMES

- Monitor for frequency, intensity, and duration of headaches and for any change in the headache pattern. Encourage patients to keep a headache diary to document frequency, duration, and severity of headaches, headache response, and potential triggers of migraine headaches.

See Chapter 78, Headache Disorders, authored by T. Kristopher Harrell and Deborah S. Minor, for a more detailed discussion of this topic.

- *Pain* is a subjective, unpleasant, sensory, and emotional experience associated with actual or potential tissue damage or abnormal functioning of nerves. It may be classified as acute, chronic, or cancer pain.

PATHOPHYSIOLOGY

ADAPTIVE (PHYSIOLOGIC) PAIN

- Nociceptive (eg, from touching something too hot, too cold, or sharp) and inflammatory pain (eg, trauma or surgery) are both adaptive and protective.
- The steps in processing pain are:
  ✓ Transduction—Stimulation of nociceptors.
    o Nociceptors, found in both somatic and visceral structures, are activated by mechanical, thermal, and chemical stimuli. Noxious stimuli may cause release of cytokines and chemokines that sensitize and/or activate nociceptors.
  ✓ Conduction—Receptor activation leads to action potentials that continue along afferent fibers to the spinal cord. Stimulation of large-diameter, sparsely myelinated fibers evokes sharp, well-localized pain. Stimulation of small-diameter, unmyelinated fibers produces aching, poorly localized pain.
  ✓ Transmission—Afferent nociceptive fibers synapse in the spinal cord's dorsal horn, releasing excitatory neurotransmitters (eg, glutamate and substance P). The spinothalamic tract and other pathways bring the signal to the brain's higher cortical structures.
  ✓ Perception—The experience of pain occurs when signals reach higher cortical structures. Relaxation, meditation, and distraction can lessen pain, and anxiety and depression can worsen pain.
  ✓ Modulation—Possible modulating factors include glutamate, substance P, endogenous opioids, γ-aminobutyric acid (GABA), norepinephrine, and serotonin.
- The interface between neurons and immune cells in the central nervous system (CNS) may facilitate maintenance of chronic pain.

MALADAPTIVE (PATHOLOGIC) PAIN

- Pathophysiologic pain (eg, postherpetic neuralgia, diabetic neuropathy, fibromyalgia, irritable bowel syndrome, chronic headaches) is often described as chronic pain. It results from damage or abnormal functioning of nerves in the CNS or peripheral nervous system (PNS). Pain circuits sometimes rewire themselves anatomically and biochemically, resulting in chronic pain, hyperalgesia, or allodynia.

CLINICAL PRESENTATION

ACUTE PAIN

Symptoms

- Acute pain can be sharp or dull, burning, shock-like, tingling, shooting, radiating, fluctuating in intensity, varying in location, and occurring in a temporal relationship with an obvious noxious stimulus. Infants and older individuals may present differently.

Signs

- Hypertension, tachycardia, diaphoresis, mydriasis, and pallor. In some cases there are not obvious physical signs. There are no laboratory tests for pain.

CHRONIC PAIN

Symptoms

- Symptoms can be very similar to acute pain, and may change over time (ie, sharp to dull). Attention must also be given to emotional factors that alter the pain threshold.

Signs

- In most cases there are no obvious signs. Depression, sleep disturbances, and anxiety are often present. No laboratory tests are diagnostic, but may identify etiology.

DIAGNOSIS

- Pain is always subjective and best diagnosed based on patient description, history, and physical examination. A baseline description of pain can be obtained using a symptom assessment mnemonic (ie, OLDCARTS or SOCRATES). Ongoing assessment should include a consistent and validated scale.

TREATMENT

- Goals of Treatment:
  - ✓ Acute pain: pain relief that allows for attainment of defined functional goals.
  - ✓ Chronic or noncancer pain: improve level of functioning, decrease pain, reduce medication use if possible, and improve quality of life.
  - ✓ Cancer pain: pain relief that enables patients to tolerate diagnostic and therapeutic manipulations and preserves function as much as possible while minimizing adverse effects.
- **Figures 56-1** and **56-2** are algorithms for management of acute pain and pain in oncology patients, respectively.

GENERAL APPROACH

- Multimodal therapy, with concomitant use of different nonpharmacologic and pharmacologic interventions to obtain additive therapeutic effects, should be employed to optimize management.
- Use of pharmacogenomic testing results may be beneficial in making therapeutic decisions among agents, because genetic variability in the CYP450 isoenzymes and opioid receptors may affect response and side effects.

NONPHARMACOLOGIC THERAPY

- The use of nonpharmacologic therapies should always be considered first-line therapy, either alone or in combination with appropriate analgesics.
- Physical therapy, exercise programs, weight loss, and electroanalgesia as well as complementary and integrative approaches (ie, acupuncture, Tai chi, yoga, mindfulness, meditation, relaxation, and biofeedback).

PHARMACOLOGIC THERAPY

Nonopioid Agents

Acetaminophen and Nonsteroidal Anti-Inflammatory Drugs

- Initiate treatment with the most effective analgesic with the fewest side effects. See **Table 56-1** for adult dosages of Food and Drug Administration (FDA)–approved nonopioid analgesics.
- **Acetaminophen** and **nonsteroidal anti-inflammatory drugs** (NSAIDS) are often preferred over opioids for mild to moderate pain. The NSAIDs reduce prostaglandins, decreasing the number of pain impulses received by the CNS.
- NSAIDs may be particularly useful for cancer-related bone pain and chronic low back pain. An adequate trial of an NSAID is about 1 month in duration. Chronic use may cause gastrointestinal (GI), cardiac, and renal toxicities.
- Topical NSAIDs may have similar efficacy as oral NSAIDs with improved safety when treating small or superficial joint arthritis.

FIGURE 56-1. Algorithm for acute pain.

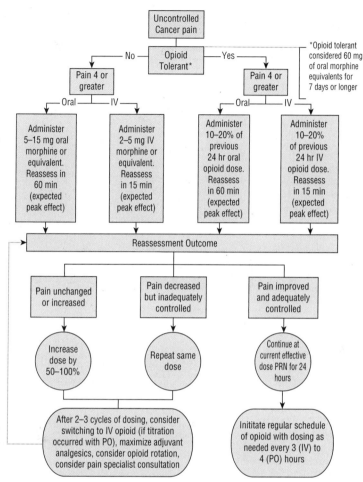

* Other daily oral opioid doses for consideration of tolerance includes codeine 150 mg, fentanyl transdermal 25 mcg, hydromorphone 8 mg, methadone 20 mg, oxycodone 30 mg, oxymorphone 20 mg

Table adapted from reference 31

FIGURE 56-2. Algorithm for cancer pain crisis.

Anticonvulsants

- Anticonvulsants **carbamazepine** and **oxcarbazepine** block voltage-gated sodium channels and potentiate the effects of GABA and are considered the drugs of choice for trigeminal neuralgia (**Table 56-2**).
  ✓ Common side effects during initiation include dizziness, drowsiness, unsteadiness, nausea, and vomiting and can be avoided with low starting doses.
  ✓ Serious dermatologic reactions can occur, including toxic epidermal necrolysis and Stevens–Johnson syndrome (SJS). The risk of dermatological adverse effects

TABLE 56-1	Nonopioid Analgesics		
Class and Generic Name (Brand Name)	**Approximate Half-Life (hr)**	**Usual Dosage Range (mg)**	**Maximal Dose (mg/day)**
Salicylates			
Acetylsalicylic acid[a]—aspirin (various)	0.25	325–1000 every 4-6 hr	4000
Choline and magnesium trisalicylate (various)	9–17	1000–1500 every 12 hr 750 every 8 hr (elderly)	3000
Diflunisal (Dolobid, various)	8–12	500–1000 initial, 250–500 every 8–12 hr	1500
Salsalate (various)	1	1000 every 12 hr or 500 every 6 hr	3000
Para-aminophenol			
Acetaminophen[a] (oral: Tylenol, various; parenteral: Ofirmev)	2–3	325–1000 every 4–6 hr	4000[b] Dosing for peds lower based on weight
Fenamates			
Meclofenamate (various)	0.8–3.3	50–100 every 4–6 hr	400
Mefenamic acid (Ponstel)	2	Initial 500, 250 every 6 hr (max. 7 days)	1000[c]
Pyranocarboxylic acid			
Etodolac (various) (immediate release)	7.3	200–400 every 6–8 hr	1000 (1200 with extended-release product)
Acetic acid			
Diclofenac potassium (Cataflam, various, Flector [patch] Voltaren Gel, Pennsaid [solution])	1.9	In some patients, initial 100, 50 three times per day Patch available: to be applied twice daily to painful area (intact skin only), gel and solution dosing joint specific	150[d]
Propionic acids			
Ibuprofen[a] (Motrin, Caldolor, various)	2–2.5	200–400 every 4–6 hr injectable, 400–800 every 6 hr (infused over 30 min)	3200[e], 2400[e], 1200[f]
Fenoprofen (Nalfon, various)	3	200 every 4–6 hr	3200

(Continued)

TABLE 56-1 Nonopioid Analgesics (*Continued*)

Class and Generic Name (Brand Name)	Approximate Half-Life (hr)	Usual Dosage Range (mg)	Maximal Dose (mg/day)
Propionic acids (continued)			
Ketoprofen (various)	2	25–50 every 6–8 hr	300 (200 with extended-release product)
Naproxen (Naprosyn, Anaprox, various)	12–17	500 initial 500 every 12 hr or 250 every 6–8 hr	1000[c]
Naproxen sodium[a] (Aleve, various, combined with esomeprazole [Vimovo])	12–17	In some patients, 440 initial[f], 220 every 8–12 hr[f]	660[f]
Pyrrolizine carboxylic acid			
Ketorolac–parenteral (Toradol, various)	5–6	30[g]–60 (single IM dose only) 15[g]–30 (single IV dose only) 10[g]–30 every 6 hr (IV dose) (max. 5 days)	30[g]–60 15[g]–30 60[g]–120
Ketorolac—oral, indicated for continuation with parenteral only (various)	5–6	10 every 4–6 hr (max. 5 days, which includes parenteral doses) In non-elderly patients, initial oral dose of 20	40 126
Ketorolac—nasal spray, indicated for acute, moderate to moderately severe pain		1 spray (15.75 mg) in each nostril every 6–8 hr in adults <65 years and weight ≥50 kg	
Pyrazols			
Celecoxib (Celebrex)	11	Initial 400 followed by another 200 on first day, then 200 twice daily (note some recommend maintenance doses of 200 mg/day due to cardiovascular concerns)	400

[a]Available both as an over-the-counter preparation and as a prescription drug.
[b]Food and Drug Administration maximum dose. OTC maximum dose 3000 mg daily. Lower with weight-based dosing in pediatric patients.
[c]Up to 1250 mg on the first day.
[d]Up to 200 mg on the first day.
[e]Some individuals may respond better to 3200 mg as opposed to 2400 mg, although well-controlled trials show no better response; consider risk versus benefits when using 3200 mg/day.
[f]Over-the-counter dose.
[g]Dose for elderly and those under 50 kg (110 lb).
FDA, Food and Drug Administration; hr, hours; IM, intramuscular; IV, intravenous; ND, no data.

TABLE 56-2	Co-analgesics: Oral Anticonvulsants	
Medication	**Dosing**	**Notes**
Carbamazepine and carbamazepine XR	Initial dose: 100 mg twice daily	Significant drug–drug interactions
	Titrate dose by 100 mg twice daily	Monitor CBC, LFTs, sodium level
	Target dose: 300–900 mg/day	Recommended testing HLA-B^{a}1502 in patients with Asian ancestry
	Maximum dose: 1200 mg/day	Therapeutic drug levels only indicated for high-dose therapy to avoid toxicity. No correlation between analgesia and serum drug concentration
Gabapentin	100–300 mg steps	Median dose for response 1600–2400 mg/day
	Increase every 3–5 days as tolerated by 100–300 mg increments	Risk of misuse/abuse
		Requires renal dose adjustment
Gabapentin (Gralise)	Take once daily with evening meal	Refer to gabapentin
	Day 1: 300 mg	
	Day 2: 600 mg	
	Day 3–6: 900 mg	
	Days 7–10: 1200 mg	
	Days 11–14: 1500 mg	
	Day 15: 1800 mg	
	Maximum dose: 1800 mg/day	
Gabapentin enacarbil	Initial dose: 600 mg every morning × 3 days	Refer to gabapentin
	Titrate dose: 600 mg twice daily	
	Maximum dose: 1200 mg/day	
Lamotrigine	Initial 25 mg daily	Stevens–Johnson syndrome
	Titrate every 2 weeks to 50 mg/day, 100 mg/day, and 200 mg/day	
	Maximum dose: 400 mg/day	
Oxcarbazepine	Initial: 150 mg BID	Improved tolerability and less drug–drug interactions compared to CBZ
	Titrate by 300 mg every 3 days	
	Target dose: 300–600 mg twice daily	
	Max dose: 1800 mg/day	
Oxcarbamazepine XR	Initial dose: 600 mg daily	Refer to oxcarbazepine
	Titrate by 600 mg/day weekly	
	Maximum: 2400 mg/day	
Pregabalin	Initial dose: 150 mg/day in 2 or 3 divided doses	Refer to gabapentin
	Titrate dose by 300 mg/day at 1 week	
	Maximum dose: varies by indication. Overall 600 mg/day	*(Continued)*

TABLE 56-2	Co-analgesics: Oral Anticonvulsants (*Continued*)	
Medication	**Dosing**	**Notes**
Pregabalin CR	Initial dose: 165 mg daily	Refer to gabapentin
	Maximum dose: 330 mg/day (DPN) or 330–660 mg/day (PHN)	
Topiramate and Topiramate XR	Initial dose: 25 mg daily × 1 week	Monitor serum bicarbonate and renal function
	Titrate by 25–50 mg week	Increase risk for kidney stones
	Target dose: 50 mg twice daily (migraine) or 200–400 mg/day neuropathic pain	Weight loss
		Decreased sweating/hyperthermia
		Hyperammonemia

ªFDA-approved indication.
DPN, diabetic peripheral neuropathy; PHN, postherpetic neuralgia.
All anticonvulsants associated with increased risk for suicidal thoughts and behaviors.

is higher in patients who come from Asian descent with an inherited variant, HLA-B*1502, so in at-risk ethnicities, patients should be tested for this allele before initiation of carbamazepine.
✓ Cardiovascular effects include hyper/hypotension, congestive heart failure, edema, arrhythmias, atrioventricular block. Elevation in hepatic enzymes should be monitored periodically during treatment.
✓ The primary metabolic pathway for carbamazepine is CYP3A4. Additionally, carbamazepine autoinduces its own metabolism, making titration difficult also resulting in many drug–drug interactions through induction of CYP3A4, CYP1A2, CYP2B6, CYP2C9, and CYP2C19.
✓ Oxcarbazepine is the keto-derivative of carbamazepine which has similar adverse reactions.
- Gabapentinoids, including **gabapentin** and **pregabalin**, are commonly used for treating neuropathic pain. Pharmacologically they decrease release of excitatory neurotransmitters glutamate, norepinephrine, and substance P.
  ✓ Common adverse effects, namely dizziness and sedation, can be mitigated with slow dose titration.
  ✓ All anticonvulsants are associated with increased risk for suicidal thoughts and behavior. Recent reports of misuse and abuse, resulted in them being controlled substances.
- **Lamotrigine** is a fourth-line agent for use in a specialist setting due to risk of life-threatening rash requiring increased monitoring and careful dose titration (Table 56-2).
  ✓ Additional side effects include dizziness, nausea, headache, insomnia, somnolence, fatigue, rhinitis, abdominal pain diplopia, ataxia, and blurred vision.
- **Topirmate** is also listed as a fourth-line agent for migraines and low back pain.

Antidepressants

- **Tricyclic antidepressants** (TCAs) are often used for the treatment of neuropathic pain (Table 56-3) and some guidelines list them as first line.
- **Duloxetine, venlafaxine**, and **milnacipran** are serotonin norepinephrine reuptake inhibitors (SNRIs) that have evidence to support their use in various chronic pain syndromes.

Skeletal Muscle Relaxants

- Skeletal muscle relaxants (SMRs) include antispasmodic and antispasticity medications (Table 56-4).

- Medications used for spasticity include **baclofen, dantrolene, diazepam**, and **tizanidine**.
- Antispasmodics include **carisoprodol, chlorzoxazone, cyclobenzaprine, diazepam, metaxalone, methocarbamol, orphenadrine**, and **tizanidine**.

Topicals

- Topicals address local symptoms while minimizing systemic exposure and risk for adverse effects (Table 56-5) and guidelines suggest use of topical NSAIDS before oral treatment for knee or hand osteoarthritis.
- **Capsaicin** is recommended for peripheral neuropathic pain. Capsaicin is more effective if used on a schedule basis, and the burning that may occur with initial application also decreases over time with repeated, scheduled use.
- **Lidocaine** may also be applied topically and may be the treatment of choice when CNS adverse effects are a concern.
- For managing cancer pain, radiopharmaceuticals (eg, **strontium-89** or **samarium**), **corticosteroids, denosumab**, and certain bisphosphonates are useful co-analgesics in treating bone pain.

Emerging Agents

- **Cannabis** has been primarily studied in the treatment of neuropathic pain; however, the route of administration, dose, and monitoring recommendations are still unclear.
- Guidelines for the use of **ketamine** for treating maladaptive pain syndrome are available, but appropriate dose, duration, and patient selection for chronic pain are still unclear.

Opioid Agents

- Limited data support the safety and efficacy of opioids for chronic noncancer pain. If used it should follow a complete assessment of the pain complaint, the patient's functionality goals, and risk factors for opioid misuse, abuse, diversion, or overdose.
- For definitions of physical dependence, substance abuse, substance dependence, tolerance, and withdrawal, see Chapters 69 and 72.
- The onset of action of oral opioids is about 45 minutes, and peak effect usually is seen in about 1–2 hours.
- Equianalgesic doses, dosing guidelines, and major adverse effects are shown in Tables 56-6, 56-7, and 56-8. Equianalgesic doses are only a guide, and doses must be individualized.
- Combining opioid analgesics with alcohol or other CNS depressants amplifies CNS depression and is potentially lethal.
- Partial agonists and antagonists (eg, **nalbuphine**) compete with agonists for opioid receptor sites and exhibit mixed agonist–antagonist activity. They may produce analgesia with fewer side effects.
- Initially give analgesics around-the-clock for acute pain. As pain subsides, as-needed schedules can be used. Around-the-clock administration is also useful for management of chronic pain.
- Patients with severe pain may receive high doses of opioids with no unwanted side effects, but as pain subsides, patients may not tolerate even low doses.
- Most opioid-related itching or rash is due to histamine release from cutaneous mast cells, and is not a true allergic response. When opioid allergies occur, an opioid from a different structural class may be cautiously tried. For these purposes, the mixed agonist–antagonist class behaves most like the morphine-like agonists.
- With patient-controlled analgesia (PCA), patients self-administer preset amounts of IV opioids via a syringe pump electronically interfaced with a timing device. PCA provides better pain control, improved patient satisfaction, and relatively few differences in side effects compared to traditional as needed administration.
- Administration of opioids directly into the CNS (see Table 56-9) (eg, epidural and intrathecal/subarachnoid routes) is commonly used by anesthesiology pain consult services for acute pain, chronic noncancer pain, and cancer pain. These methods require very careful monitoring as marked sedation, respiratory depression, pruritus,

TABLE 56-3	Co-analgesics: Antidepressants		
Medication	**Role**	**Dosing**	**Notes**
Tricyclic antidepressants (TCAs)			
Amitriptyline Desipramine Imipramine Nortriptyline	Fibromyalgia Low back pain Migraine prophylaxis Neuropathic pain	Initial: 10–25 mg at bedimte Titrate by 10–25 mg every 3–7 days Maximum: 150 mg	Secondary amines (desipramine, nortriptyline) less anticholinergic activity = less ADE Multiple cardiac ADE (including QTc prolongation, orthostatic hypotension, arrhythmias, tachycardia) Doses >100 mg/day associated with sudden cardiac death Lowers seizure threshold
Serotonin norepinephrine reuptake inhibitors (SNRIs)			
Duloxetine	Chronic musculoskeletal pain (low back pain [LBP], osteoarthritis)[a] Diabetic peripheral neuropathy (DPN)[a] Fibromyalgia[a] Chemotherapy-induced neuropathic pain (CINP)	Initial: 30 mg daily × 1 week (2 weeks if elderly) Target dose: 60 mg daily Maximum dose: 120 mg/day though limited evidence for doses >60 mg providing additional benefit in pain	Avoid CrCl <30 mL/min (0.50 mL/sec) Avoid chronic liver disease or cirrhosis Hypertension Hyponatremia Increased risk of bleeding (GI and CNS)
Milnacipran	Fibromyalgia[a]	Day 1: 12.5 mg daily Days 2–3: 12.5 mg BID Days 4–7: 25 mg BID Then increase to 50 mg BID Target dose: 100 mg/day Maximum dose: 200 mg/day	Avoid CrCl <30 mL/min (0.50 mL/sec) Caution with severe hepatic impairment Increase risk for bleeding

(Continued)

639

TABLE 56-3	Co-analgesics: Antidepressants (*Continued*)		
Medication	**Role**	**Dosing**	**Notes**
Serotonin norepinephrine reuptake inhibitors (SNRIs) (continued)			
Venlafaxine	CINP DPN Fibromyalgia LBP Migraine prophylaxis Painful polyneuropathy Tension-type headache	Initial: venlafaxine SA 37.5 mg daily Titrate: by no more than 75 mg/day every 4 days Maximum dose: 225 mg/day	Higher doses needed to achieve SNRI effect Dose adjustments with renal/hepatic impairment Hypertension Hyponatremia QTc prolongation Increased bleeding risk

^aFDA-approved indication(s).
ADE, adverse drug event; GI, gastrointestinal; and CNS central nervous system.

TABLE 56-4	Skeletal Muscle Relaxants (*Continued*)	
Medication	**Dosing**	**Notes**
Baclofen	Initial: 5 mg 3 times daily Titrate: every 3 days to effect Maximum: 80 mg/day	Withdrawal syndrome (hallucinations, seizures) Respiratory depression Requires renal dose adjustment
Carisoprodol	250–300 mg 4 times daily	Meprobamate (a barbiturate) is primary metabolite and has abuse potential Schedule IV controlled substance Withdrawal syndrome Respiratory depression with opioids, benzodiazepines, or barbiturates Metabolized by CYP2C19 which has genetic variabilities
Chlorzoxazone	Initial: 250–500 mg 3–4 times daily Maximum dose: 750 mg 3–4 times daily	Rare hepatotoxicity Urine discoloration Respiratory depression when combined with opioids, benzodiazepines, or barbiturates
Cyclobenzaprine	Initial: 5 mg 3 times daily Titrate: increase to 7.5–10 mg 3 times daily × 2–3 weeks Elderly: 5 mg dose with less frequent doses	Anticholinergic effects Avoid in elderly Caution in patients with cardiac conduction/arrhythmias Avoid closed angle glaucoma Hepatic dose adjustments

(*Continued*)

TABLE 56-4	Skeletal Muscle Relaxants (*Continued*)	
Medication	**Dosing**	**Notes**
Dantrolene	Initial: 25 mg PO daily × 1 week	Black box warning—hepatitis (dose-dependent)
	Titrate dose:	Discontinue at 45 days if no benefit
	25 mg 3 times daily × 7 days	
	50 mg 3 times daily × 7 days	
	100 mg three times daily	
	Maximum dose: 400 mg/day	
Diazepam	Adults: 2–10 mg 3–4 times daily	Long half-life
		Avoid in elderly and renal/hepatic impairment
		Withdrawal with abrupt discontinuation
Methocarbamol	Initial: 1500 mg 4 times daily × 2–3 days	Urine discoloration
	Then: 750–1000 mg 4 times daily	Respiratory depression with opioids, benzodiazepines, or barbiturates
Metaxalone	800 mg 3–4 times daily	Respiratory depression when used with opioids, benzodiazepines, or barbiturates
		Contraindicated in severe liver/renal impairment
Orphenadrine	100 mg twice daily	Anticholinergic effects
		Rare aplastic anemia
Tizanidine	Initial: 4 mg	Hypotension
	Titrate by 2–4 mg every 6–8 hours	Hepatotoxicity
	Maximum: 36 mg/day	Tablets and capsules not bioequivalent
		Withdrawal syndrome with abrupt discontinuation

vomiting, urinary retention, and hypotension can occur. All agents administered directly into the CNS should be preservative-free.

- **Naloxone** is used to reverse respiratory depression, but continuous infusion may be required. Monitor respiratory function for at least 24 hours after a single dose of intrathecal or epidural morphine with standing orders for naloxone if needed.

Morphine and Congeners (Phenanthrenes)

- Many clinicians consider **morphine** the first-line agent for moderate-to-severe pain. It may be used for pain associated with myocardial infarction, as it decreases myocardial oxygen demand, but this is controversial.
  - ✓ Tidal exchange and minute volume can be affected by opioids. Patients with underlying pulmonary dysfunction are at increased risk for respiratory depression, which can be reversed by **naloxone**.
  - ✓ Morphine-induced respiratory depression can increase intracranial pressure and cloud the neurologic examination results.
  - ✓ Hypovolemic patients are at risk for morphine-induced orthostatic hypotension.

TABLE 56-5 Topical Analgesics

Medication	Uses	Mechanism of Action	Dosing	Notes
Capsaicin cream (various)	Temporary relief of minor aches and pains of muscles and joints Localized neuropathic pain	Transient receptor potential vanilloid 1 (TRPV1) receptor agonist	Apply 3–4 times daily	Continue scheduled use for 2–4 weeks for best results
Capsaicin 8% patch (Qutenza)	PHN	Transient receptor potential vanilloid 1 (TRPV1) receptor agonist	Apply 1–4 patches to affected area for 60 min Repeat no more frequently than every 3 months Max: 4 patches	Administer under supervision of physician Specific administration directions in packaging information Apply topical anesthetic before applying Monitor blood pressure due to transient increase in blood pressure during application
Diclofenac 1% gel (Voltaren)	Pain of osteoarthritis of joints amenable to topical treatment (knees, hands)	Nonsteroid anti-inflammatory drugs (NSAIDs)	Lower extremities: 4 g four times daily, max. 16 g/day Upper extremities: 2 g 4 times daily, max. 8 g/day Total dose maximum: 32 g/day	Same black box warnings as PO NSAIDs despite low systemic bioavailability (6% of systemic exposure from oral diclofenac) Use dosing card to measure amount
Diclofenac epolamine 1.3% patch (Flector)	Topical treatment of acute pain due to minor strains, sprains, and contusions	NSAIDs	1 patch to most painful area twice daily	Systemic effects were <1% after 4 days of repeated dosing

Diclofenac topical solution (Pennsaid)	Pain from osteoarthritis of the knee	NSAIDs	1.5%: 40 drops to each affected knee 4 times daily. Apply 10 drops at a time 2%: 2 pumps (40 mg) on each painful knee twice daily	Same black box warnings as PO NSAIDs
Lidocaine gel/Ointment/Patch (various)	Neuropathic pain	Sodium channel blocker	Cream/Ointment: Apply to affected area 3 times daily Patch: apply 1 patch to affected area up to 12 hr	Apply to intact skin only
Lidocaine 5% patch (Lidoderm)	PHN	Sodium channel blocker	Apply 1–3 patches to site of pain for 12 hr Maximum: 3 patches	May cut lidocaine patches Apply to intact skin only Severe hepatic impairment increases risk of side effects
Menthol/Methyl salicylate (various)	Minor aches and pains of muscles and joints (simple backache, arthritis, strains, bruises, sprains)	Rubefacient	Apply topically 3–4 times a day to affected area	Do not apply to damaged skin
Trolamine salicylate cream 10% (various)	Aches and pains of muscles and joints (arthritis, simple backache, bruises, sprains, strains)	Rubefacient	Apply topically 3–4 times a day to affected area	Do not apply to damaged skin

TABLE 56-6　Opioid Analgesics

Class and Generic Name (Brand Name)	Chemical Source	Metabolic Pathway/Metabolites	Route[a]	Equianalgesic Dose in Adults (mg)	Approximate Onset (min)/ Half-Life (hr)[b]
Phenanthrenes (morphine-like agonists)					
Morphine (Embeda, Arymo ER, MorphaBond)	Naturally occurring	Phase II via glucuronidation/M3G (inactive) and M6G[i] (active)	IM/IV	10	10–20/2
			PO	25–30	
Hydromorphone (Dilaudid, Exalgo, various)	Semisynthetic	Phase II via glucuronidation/H3G (active)[m], H6G[n]	IM/IV	7.5	10–20/2–3
			PO		
Oxymorphone (Numorphan, Opana)	Semisynthetic	Phase II via glucuronidation/O3G (inactive)[o]	IM/IV[a]	1	10–20/2–3
			PO	10	
Levorphanol (various)	Semisynthetic	Phase II via glucuronidation/Levorphanol-3-glucuronide (inactive)	PO	Variable	10–20/12–16
Codeine (various)	Naturally occurring	CYP2D6/Morphine (active), Phase II glucuronidation/codeine-6-glucuronide (unknown), CYP3A4/norcodeine (inactive)	PO	15–30[c]	10–30/3
Hydrocodone (available as combination, single entity extended release—Hysingla ER, Zohydro ER)	Semisynthetic	CYP3A4/Norhydrocodone (inactive); CYP2D6/hydromorphone (active)	PO	5–10[c]	30–60/4
Oxycodone (OxyContin, Xtampza, RoxyBond/Troxyco ER [oxycodone and acetaminophen])	Semisynthetic	CYP3A4/Noroxycodone (active), CYP2D6/oxymorphone (active)	PO	15–30[d]	30–60/2–3
Phenylpiperidines (meperidine-like agonists)					
Meperidine (Demerol, various)	Synthetic	Phase II hydrolysis/Meperidinic acid, CYP2B6, CYP3A4, and CYP2C19/normeperidine	IM / IV	75	10–20/3–5
			PO	300[d]; not recommended	

Drug	Source	Metabolism/Metabolite	Route	Dose	
Fentanyl (Sublimaze, Duragesic, Lazanda, Abstral, Fentora, Subsys, OTFC, various)	Synthetic	CYP3A4/Norfentanyl (inactive)	IM/IV	0.125[e]	7–15/3–4
			Transdermal, buccal, transmucosal, sublingual, nasal, nebulized	Variable[f]	
				Variable[f]	
Diphenylheptanes (methadone-like agonists)					
Methadone (Dolophine, various)	Synthetic	CYP3A4, CYP2B6, CYP2C19, CYP2C9, CYP2D6/ EDDP (inactive)[p]	IM/IV	Variable[g] (acute)	
			PO	Variable[g] (acute)	30–60/12–190
Phenylpropanolamines					
Tramadol (Ultram, Rybix, Ryzolt, ConZip, various)	Synthetic	CYP3A4/Nortramadol (inactive), CYP2D6/O-desmethyltramadol (active)	PO	50–100[c,h,i]	<60/5–7
Tapentadol (Nucynta)	Synthetic	Phase II glucuronidation/ tapentadol-o-glucuronide (inactive), CYP2C9 and CYP2C19/N-desmethyltapentadol (inactive), CYP2D6/hydroxytapentadol	PO	50–10[c,h,i]	Within 60/4
Agonist–antagonist derivatives					
Pentazocine (Talwin, various)	Synthetic	Liver/Alcoholic and carboxylic acid derivatives (inactive), pentazocine glucuronide (inactive)	IM	Not recommended	
			PO	50[c]	15–30/2–3
Butorphanol (Stadol, various)	Synthetic	CYP3A4/Hydroxybutorphanol (active), norbutorphanol (inactive)	IM/IV	2	10–20/3–4
			Intranasal	1[c] (one spray)	

(Continued)

TABLE 56-6 Opioid Analgesics (*Continued*)

Class and Generic Name (Brand Name)	Chemical Source	Metabolic Pathway/Metabolites	Route[a]	Equianalgesic Dose in Adults (mg)	Approximate Onset (min)/ Half-Life (hr)[b]
Agonist–antagonist derivatives (continued)					
Nalbuphine (Nubain, various)	Synthetic	CYP3A4 CYP2C19/Nornalbuphine, 6-ketonalbuphine	IM/IV	10	<15/5
Buprenorphine (Buprenex, Butrans, Suboxone, Belbuca, Subutex, various)	Synthetic	CYP3A4/Norbuprenorphine (active)	IM/IV	0.3	10–20/2–3
			Transdermal Sublingual	Variable	

[a]The IM route should be avoided whenever possible—produces significant pain with administration and rate and extent of absorption is highly variable. If IV route is unavailable then administer subcutaneously (SC).
[b]ER/LA formulations may vary greatly in terms of onset and duration of analgesia. The reader should consult individual prescribing labels.
[c]Starting dose only (equianalgesia not shown).
[d]Starting doses lower (oxycodone 5–10 mg, meperidine 50–150 mg).
[e]Equivalent PO morphine dose = variable.
[f]For breakthrough pain only. Equianalgesic dose conversion should be avoided for Transmucosal Immediate Release Fentanyl (TIRF) products.
[g]The equianalgesic dose of methadone when compared with other opioids will decrease progressively the higher the previous opioid dose. Caution should be exercised when initiating in opioid naive patients.
[h]First day of dosing may administer second dose 1 hour after first dose.
[i]Onset of action may differ for long-acting formulations. Ceiling dose recommendations exist and may differ from immediate release dosing recommendations.
[j]FDA approved as abuse-deterrent formulation.
[k]Morphine-3-glucuronide (accumulates in renal failure).
[l]Morphine-6-glucuronide (accumulates in renal failure).
[m]Hydromorphone-3-glucuronide (accumulates in renal failure).
[n]Hydromorphone-6-glucuronide.
[o]Oxymorphone-3-glucuronide.
[p]2-ethylidene-1,5-dimethyl-3,3-diphenylpyrrolidene (EDDP).
[q]Oral transmucosal fentanyl citrate (OTFC).
IM, intramuscular; IV, intravenous; PO, oral.

✓ Most clinicians avoid morphine in patients with creatinine clearance less than or equal to 30ml/min [0.5 ml/sec] due to accumulation of active metabolites.

- Counsel patients to take the extended-release **oxymorphone** without food, as high-fat meals can greatly increase absorption, increasing risk of toxicity.
- **Hydromorphone** may have fewer side effects, especially pruritus, compared with other opioids and **levorphanol** has an extended half-life and purported NMDA glutamate receptor activity.
- **Codeine**, alone or combined with other analgesics (eg, acetaminophen), is commonly used for mild-to-moderate pain. **Oxycodone** is useful for moderate-to-severe pain, especially when combined with nonopioids.

Meperidine and Congeners (Phenylpiperidines)

- **Meperidine** is less potent and has a shorter duration of action than morphine.
  - ✓ With high doses or in patients with renal failure, the metabolite normeperidine accumulates, causing tremor, muscle twitching, and possibly seizures. In most settings, meperidine offers no advantages over morphine.
  - ✓ Do not combine meperidine with monoamine oxidase inhibitors because severe respiratory depression or serotonin syndrome may occur.
- **Fentanyl**, often used as an adjunct to general anesthesia, is more potent and faster acting than meperidine.

Methadone and Congeners (Diphenylheptanes)

- **Methadone** has extended duration of action. Studies show a growing number of methadone-related deaths. High doses cause cardiac arrhythmias. Do not titrate more frequently than every 5–7 days. Although effective for acute pain, it is used for chronic cancer pain.
- There is a growing number of methadone-related deaths. The equianalgesic dose of methadone may decrease with higher doses of the previous opioid.

Opioid Agonist–Antagonist Derivatives

- This analgesic class may cause less respiratory depression than opioids and may have lower abuse potential than morphine. However, psychotomimetic responses (eg, hallucinations and dysphoria), a limited analgesic effect, and the propensity to initiate withdrawal in opioid-dependent patients have limited their use.
- Buprenorphine is a pharmacologically complex opioid. When used with or without naloxone, for opioid use disorder, a special DEA license is required by the prescriber.

Centrally Acting Opioids

- **Tramadol** and **tapentadol** are indicated for relief of moderate to moderately severe pain.
  - ✓ Their side effects are similar to other opioids, although the seizure risk with tramadol may be higher.

Opioid Antagonists

- **Naloxone**, a pure opioid antagonist that binds competitively to opioid receptors, does not produce analgesia or opioid side effects. It reverses the toxic effects of agonist and agonist–antagonist opioids. In some states in the United States, pharmacists are assuming greater roles in administering or dispensing naloxone for patients who have experienced opioid overdoses.
- Opioid antagonists may act centrally (eg, naloxone or **naltrexone**) or be limited to peripheral action only (eg, **naloxegol, methylnaltrexone, or naldemedine**).
- **Table 56-10** lists dosing for central and peripheral opioid antagonists.

TABLE 56-7 Dosing Guidelines

Agent(s)	Doses (Use Lowest Effective Dose, Titrate Up or Down Based on Patient Response, Opioid-Tolerant Patients May Need Dose Modification)	Notes
NSAIDs/Acetaminophen/Aspirin	Use lowest effective dose for the shortest duration possible	Used in mild-to-moderate pain
		May use in conjunction with opioid agents to decrease doses of each
		Regular alcohol use and of acetaminophen may result in liver toxicity
		Care must be exercised to avoid overdose when combination products containing these agents are used
		Underlying renal impairment, hypovolemia, and CHF may predispose to nephrotoxicity
Morphine	PO 5–30 mg every 4 hr[a]	Drug of choice in severe pain
	IM 5–20 mg every 4 hr[a]	Use immediate-release product with SR product to control breakthrough pain in cancer patients
	IV 5–15 mg every 4 hr[a]	Typical patient controlled analgesia IV dose is 1 mg with a 10-min lock-out interval
	SR 15–30 mg every 12 hr (may need to be every 8 hr in some patients)	Every 24-hr products available
	Rectal 10–20 mg every 4 hr[a]	
Hydromorphone	PO 2–4 mg every 4–6 hr[a]	Use in severe pain
	XR 8 mg to 64 mg every 24 hr	More potent than morphine; otherwise, no advantages

	IM 1–2 mg every 4–6 hr[a]	
	IV 0.5–2 mg every 4 hr[a]	Typical patient-controlled analgesia IV dose is 0.2 mg with a 10-min lock-out interval
Oxymorphone	Rectal 3 mg every 6–8 hr[a]	Every 24-hr product (Exalgo) available
	IM 1–1.5 mg every 4–6 hr[a]	Use in severe pain
	IV 0.5 mg every 4–6 hr[a]	No advantages over morphine
	PO immediate-release 5–10 mg every 4–6 hr[a]	Use immediate-release product with controlled-release product to control breakthrough pain in cancer or chronic pain patients
	PO extended-release 5–10 mg every 12 hr[a]	Manufacturer recommends 5 mg every 12 hr in opioid-naïve patients
		Take ER on empty stomach
Levorphanol	PO 2–3 mg every 6–8 hr[a] (Levo-Dromoran)	Use in severe pain
	PO 2 mg every 3–6 hr[a] (Levorphanol Tartrate)	Extended half-life useful in cancer patients
	IM 1–2 mg every 6–8 hr[a]	In chronic pain, wait 3 days between dosage adjustments
	IV 1 mg every 3–6 hr[a]	
Codeine	PO 15–60 mg every 4–6 hr[a]	Use in mild-to-moderate pain
	IM 15–60 mg every 4–6 hr[a]	Weak analgesic; analgesic prodrug
Hydrocodone	PO 5–10 mg every 4–6 hr[a]	Use in moderate/severe pain
Oxycodone	PO 5–15 mg every 4–6 hr[a]	Use in moderate/severe pain
	Controlled release 10–20 mg every 12 hr	Use immediate-release product with controlled-release product to control breakthrough pain in cancer or chronic pain patients
		CR reformulated to deter abuse

(Continued)

TABLE 56-7 Dosing Guidelines (Continued)

Agent(s)	Doses (Use Lowest Effective Dose, Titrate Up or Down Based on Patient Response, Opioid-Tolerant Patients May Need Dose Modification)	Notes
Meperidine	IM 50–150 mg every 3–4 hr[a]	Use in severe pain
	IV 5–10 mg every 5 min prn[a]	Oral not recommended
		Do not use in renal failure
		May precipitate tremors, myoclonus, and seizures
		Monoamine oxidase inhibitors can induce hyperpyrexia and/or seizures or opioid overdose symptoms
Fentanyl	IV 25–50 mcg/hr	Used in severe pain
	IM 50–100 mcg every 1–2 hr[a]	**Do not use transdermal in acute pain**
	Transdermal 25 mcg/h every 72 hr	Transmucosal for breakthrough cancer pain in patients already receiving or tolerant to opioids
	Transmucosal (Actiq/OTFC Lozenge and Onsolis buccal film) 200 mcg may repeat × 1, 30 min after first dose is started, then titrate	**Always start with lowest dose despite daily opioid intake; product-specific titration recommendations exist**
	Transmucosal (Fentora Buccal Tablet) 100 mcg, may repeat × 1, 30 min after first dose is started, then titrate	
	Intranasal (Lazanda Spray) 100 mcg (one spray) in one nostril. Wait 2 hr prior to redosing	
	Sublingual (Subsys Spray) 100 mcg (1 spray). Wait 4 hr rprior to redosing	
	Sublingual (Abstral Tablet) 100 mcg tablets placed sublingually. Must wait 2 hr prior to redosing	

Drug	Dosing	Comments
Methadone[g]	PO 2.5–10 mg every 8–12 hr[a] IM 2.5–10 mg every 8–12 hr[a]	Effective in severe chronic pain Some chronic pain patients can be dosed every 12 hr Equianalgesic dose of methadone when compared with other opioids will decrease progressively the higher the previous opioid dose. Avoid dose titrations more frequently than weekly in chronic pain maintenance
Pentazocine	PO 50–100 mg every 3–4 hr[b] (max. 600 mg daily, for those 50 mg tablet containing 0.5 mg of naloxone) PO 25 mg every 4 hr[b] (max. 150 mg daily, for those 25 mg tablet containing 325 mg of acetaminophen)	Second-line agent for moderate-to-severe pain; may precipitate withdrawal in opiate-dependent patients; parenteral doses not recommended
Butorphanol	IM 1–4 mg every 3–4 hr[b] IV 0.5–2 mg every 3–4 hr[b] Intranasal 1 mg (1 spray) every 3–4 hr[b] If inadequate relief after initial spray, may repeat in other nostril × 1 in 60–90 min Max. 2 sprays (one per nostril) every 3–4 hr[b]	Second-line agent for moderate-to-severe pain May precipitate withdrawal in opiate-dependent patients
Nalbuphine	IM/IV 10 mg every 3–6 hr[b] (max. 20 mg dose, 160 mg daily)	Second-line agent for moderate-to-severe pain; may precipitate withdrawal in opiate-dependent patients Used frequently in low doses to treat/prevent opioid-induced pruritus
Buprenorphine	IM 0.3 mg every 6 hr[b]	Second-line agent for moderate-to-severe pain

(Continued)

651

TABLE 56-7 Dosing Guidelines *(Continued)*

Agent(s)	Doses (Use Lowest Effective Dose, Titrate Up or Down Based on Patient Response, Opioid-Tolerant Patients May Need Dose Modification)	Notes
Buprenorphine (continued)	Slow IV 0.3 mg every 6 hr[b]	May precipitate withdrawal in opiate-dependent patients
		Transdermal delivery systems (5, 7.5, 10, 15, 20 micrograms/h) available for every 7 day administration. Detailed manufacturer dosing conversion recommendations exist
Naloxone	May repeat × 1, 30–60 min after initial dose	Naloxone may not be effective in reversing respiratory depression
	IV/IM 0.4–2 mg	When reversing opiate side effects in patients needing analgesia, dilute and titrate (0.1–0.2 mg every 2–3 min) so as not to reverse analgesia
Tramadol	PO 50–100 mg every 4–6 hr[a]	Maximum dose for nonextended-release, 400 mg/24 hr maximum for extended release, 300 mg/24 hr
	If rapid onset not required, start 25 mg/day and titrate over several days	Decrease dose in patient with renal impairment and in the elderly
	Extended release PO 100 mg every 24 hr	
Tapentadol	PO 50–100 mg every 4–6 hr[a]	First day of therapy may administer second dose after the first within 1 hr, maximum dose first day 700 mg, max. dose thereafter 600 mg (maximum dose for CR 500 mg)

[a]May start with an around-the-clock regimen and switch to prn if/when the painful signal subsides or is episodic.
[b]May reach a ceiling analgesic effect.
CR, controlled release; HCL, hydrochloride; IM, intramuscular; IV, intravenous;; mcg, microgram; mg, milligram; NSAID, nonsteroidal anti-inflammatory drug; OTFC, Oral transmucosal fentanyl citrate; PO, oral; prn, as needed; SR, sustained release; XR, extended release.

TABLE 56-8	Major Adverse Effects of the Opioid Analgesics
Effect	**Manifestation**
Mood changes	Dysphoria, euphoria
Somnolence	Sedation, inability to concentrate
Stimulation of chemoreceptor trigger zone	Nausea, vomiting
Respiratory depression	Decreased respiratory rate, periodic breathing, oxygen desaturation
Decreased gastrointestinal motility	Constipation
Increase in sphincter tone	Biliary spasm, urinary retention (varies among agents)
Histamine release	Urticaria, pruritus, rarely exacerbation of asthma due to bronchospasm (varies among agents)
Tolerance	Larger doses for same effect
Dependence	Withdrawal symptoms upon abrupt discontinuation
Addiction	Genetic predisposition leads to loss of control of drug use, continued use despite harm, compulsion to use, cravings
Hypogonadism	Fatigue, depression, loss of analgesia, sexual dysfunction, amenorrhea (women)
Sleep	Disrupts sleep–wake cycle, causes dose-dependent rapid eye movement (REM) suppression

TABLE 56-9	Intraspinal Opioids			
Agent	**Single Dose (mg)**	**Onset of Pain Relief (min)**	**Duration of Pain Relief (hr)**	**Continual Infusion Dose (mg/hr)**
Epidural route				
Morphine	1–6	30	6–24	0.1–1
Hydromorphone	0.8–1.5	5–8	4–8	0.1–0.3
Fentanyl	0.025–0.1	5	2–8	0.025–0.1
Sufentanil	0.01–0.06	5	2–4	0.01–0.05
Subarachnoid route				
Morphine	0.1–0.3	15	8–34	–
Fentanyl	0.005–0.025	5	3–6	–

Doses above should not be interpreted as equianalgesic doses for conversion to or from the specific opioid or route of administration.

REGIONAL ANALGESIA

- Regional analgesia with local anesthetics (Table 56-11) is useful for both acute and chronic pain. Anesthetics can be positioned by injection (eg, in the joints, epidural or intrathecal space, nerve plexus, or along nerve roots), or applied topically.
- High plasma concentrations of local anesthetics can cause dizziness, tinnitus, drowsiness, seizures, and respiratory arrest. Cardiovascular effects include myocardial depression, heart block, hypotension, bradycardia, and cardiac arrest. Skillful application, frequent administration, and specialized follow-up are required.

TABLE 56-10 Central and Peripheral Opioid Antagonists

Generic Name (Brand Name)	Activity	Role	Route	Dose in Adults (mg)	Special Considerations
Naldemedine (Symproic)	Peripheral	CNMP[a], OIC[b]	PO	0.2 mg qday	Avoid with severe hepatic impairment
Naloxone (Narcan, various)	Systemic	Opioid reversal	IV, IM, IN	0.4–2 mg[e]	Onset 1–2 (IV) minutes, 2–5 (IM) minutes Half-life 0.5–1.3 hr
Methylnaltrexone (Relistor)	Peripheral	Cancer and CNMP OIC[b]	SC (both), PO (CNMP)	Variable	Renal dose adjustments
Naltrexone (ReVia, Vivitrol)	Systemic	AUD,[c] OUD[d]	PO, IM	12 mg Qday–Q12 (PO) 380 mg q4weeks (IM)	Opioid free for 7–10 days before initiation
Alvimopan (Entereg)	Peripheral	Postoperative ileus	PO	12 mg PO 30 min–5 hr before surgery then 12 mg PO BID starting day after surgery for maximum of 7 days	Limited to 15 doses
Naloxegol (Movantik)	Peripheral	CNMP[a], OIC[b]	PO	12.5–25 mg qday 1 hour before, 2 hours after a meal	Renal dose adjustments Avoid with moderate 3A4 inhibitors

[a]Chronic nonmalignant pain.
[b]Opioid-induced constipation.
[c]Alcohol use disorder.
[d]Opioid use disorder.
[e]Starting doses to be used in cases of opioid overdose.
Data from individual package inserts.

TABLE 56-11	Local Anesthetics[a]	
Agent (Brand Name)	**Onset (min)**	**Duration (hr)**
Esters		
Procaine (Novocain, various)	2–5	0.25–1
Chloroprocaine (Nesacaine, various)	6–12	0.5
Tetracaine (Pontocaine)	≤15	2–3
Amides		
Mepivacaine (Polocaine, various)	3–5	0.75–1.5
Bupivacaine (Marcaine, various)	5	2–4
Bupivacaine liposomal (Exparel— wound infiltration only)	variable	24 local 96 systemic
Lidocaine (Xylocaine, various)	<2	0.5–1
Prilocaine (Citanest)	<2	1–2
Ropivacaine[b] (Naropin)	10–30	0.5–6

[a]Unless otherwise indicated, values are for infiltrative anesthesia.
[b]Epidural administration.

SPECIAL POPULATIONS

- The elderly and young are at higher risk of undertreatment. In these populations, it is important to monitor signs (eg, heart rate) and to talk with parents or caregivers.
- Those with chronic, debilitating, and life-threatening illnesses need specialized pain control and palliative care.
- Pharmacologic therapy of cancer pain (see **Figure 56-2**) should be coupled with psychological, surgical, and supportive therapies using an interdisciplinary approach. Continuous assessment of pain response, side effects, and behavior are required.

EVALUATION OF THERAPEUTIC OUTCOMES

- Pain intensity, pain relief, and medication side effects must be assessed regularly. The frequency of assessment depends on the type of pain, analgesic used, route of administration, and concomitant medications. Postoperative pain and acute exacerbations of cancer pain may require hourly assessment. Chronic nonmalignant pain may need only daily (or less frequent) monitoring. Quality of life must be assessed regularly.
- The four A's (eg, *a*nalgesia, *a*ctivity, *a*berrant drug behavior, and *a*dverse effects) are key assessment measures for patients with chronic pain.
- Patients taking opioids should be counseled on proper intake of fluids and fiber, and a stimulant laxative should be added with chronic opioid use. Peripherally acting mu-opioid receptor antagonists (PAMORAs) are available for treating opioid-induced constipation.
- Concomitant use of CNS depressants should be avoided with opioid analgesics.

See Chapter 77, Pain Management, authored by Chris M. Herndon, James B. Ray, and Courtney M. Kominek, for a more detailed discussion of this topic.

Parkinson Disease 57

- *Parkinson disease* (PD) has highly characteristic neuropathologic findings and a clinical presentation, including motor deficits and, in some cases, mental deterioration.

PATHOPHYSIOLOGY

- The true etiology of PD is unknown.
- Two hallmark features in the substantia nigra pars compacta are loss of neurons and presence of Lewy bodies. The degree of nigrostriatal dopamine loss correlates positively with severity of motor symptoms.
- Reduced activation of dopamine$_1$ and dopamine$_2$ receptors results in greater inhibition of the thalamus and reduced activation of the motor cortex. Clinical improvement may be tied to restoring activity more at the dopamine$_2$ receptor than at the dopamine$_1$ receptor.

CLINICAL PRESENTATION

- PD develops insidiously and progresses slowly over many years.

GENERAL FEATURES

- The patient exhibits bradykinesia and at least one of the following: resting tremor, rigidity, or postural instability. Asymmetry of motor features is supportive.

MOTOR SYMPTOMS

- Only two-thirds of patients with PD have tremor on diagnosis, and some never develop this sign. Tremor in PD is present most commonly in the hands, sometimes with a characteristic pill-rolling motion.
- The patient experiences hypokinetic movements, decreased manual dexterity, difficulty arising from a seated position, diminished arm swing during ambulation, dysarthria (slurred speech), dysphagia (difficulty with swallowing), festinating gait (tendency to pass from a slow to a quickened pace), flexed posture, "freezing" at initiation of movement, hypomimia (reduced facial animation), hypophonia (reduced voice volume), and micrographia.

AUTONOMIC AND SENSORY SYMPTOMS

- The patient experiences bladder dysfunction, constipation, diaphoresis, fatigue, olfactory impairment, orthostatic intolerance, pain, paresthesia, paroxysmal vascular flushing, seborrhea, sexual dysfunction, and sialorrhea (drooling).

MENTAL STATUS CHANGES

- The patient experiences anxiety, apathy, bradyphrenia (slowness of thought processes), cognitive impairment, depression, and hallucinosis/psychosis.

SLEEP DISTURBANCES

- The patient experiences excessive daytime sleepiness, insomnia, obstructive sleep apnea, and rapid eye movement (REM) sleep behavior disorder.

DIAGNOSIS

- The clinical diagnosis of PD is based on the presence of bradykinesia and at least one of the three other features: muscular rigidity, resting tremor, and postural instability (Table 57-1).
- There are no laboratory tests available to diagnose PD, including genetic testing.
- Neuroimaging may be useful for excluding other diagnoses.
- Medication history should be obtained to rule out drug-induced parkinsonism.

TABLE 57-1	Diagnostic Criteria and Differential Diagnosis for Parkinson Disease

Parkinson disease
- Step 1: Presence of bradykinesia and at least one of the following: resting tremor, rigidity, or postural instability
- Step 2: Exclude other types of parkinsonism or tremor disorders (see "Differential Diagnosis")
- Step 3: Presence of at least three supportive positive criteria:
  - Asymmetry of motor signs/symptoms
  - Unilateral onset
  - Progressive disorder
  - Resting tremor
  - Excellent response to carbidopa/levodopa
  - levodopa response for 5 years or longer
  - Presence of levodopa dyskinesias

Differential diagnosis
- Essential tremor
- Pharmacotoxicity (drug-induced)
  - Antiemetics (eg, metoclopramide, prochlorperazine)
  - Antipsychotics (eg, chlorpromazine, fluphenazine, haloperidol, olanzapine, risperidone, thioridazine)
  - Other drugs (α-methyldopa, cinnarizine, flunarizine, tetrabenazine)
- Environmental toxicity (eg, manganese, organophosphates)
- Infections (eg, human immunodeficiency virus, subacute sclerosing panencephalitis)
- Metabolic disorder (eg, hypothyroidism, parathyroid abnormalities)
- Neoplasms, strokes, traumatic lesions involving the nigrostriatal pathways
- Normal-pressure hydrocephalus
- Parkinsonism with other neuronal system degenerations
  - Corticobasal ganglionic degeneration
- Multiple-system atrophies
- Progressive supranuclear palsy
- Familial (hereditary) parkinsonism
  - Autosomal dominant
  - α-Synuclein gene mutation (*PARK1* and *PARK4*)
  - L-responsive dystonia
  - Leucine-rich repeat kinase 2 (LRRK2) mutation
  - Rapid-onset dystonia parkinsonism (DYT12)
  - Spinocerebellar ataxias (SCA2, SCA3)
- Autosomal recessive
  - Wilson disease
  - Young-onset parkinsonism (DJ-1, parkin, PINK1)
- X-linked recessive
  - Fragile X tremor/ataxia syndrome (FXTAS)
  - Lubag (DYT3 or Filipino dystonia parkinsonism)

TREATMENT

- <u>Goals of Treatment</u>: The goals of treatment are to minimize symptoms, disability, and side effects while maintaining quality of life. Education of patients and caregivers, exercise, and proper nutrition are essential.
- To date, no treatments have been shown to effectively change the course of PD by slowing or halting its progression (disease modification).

NONPHARMACOLOGIC THERAPY

- Surgery should be considered an adjunct to pharmacotherapy when patients are experiencing frequent motor fluctuations or disabling dyskinesia or tremor despite an optimized medical regimen

- Other biotherapies, such as stem cell and gene-based approaches, are currently under investigation and remain highly experimental.

PHARMACOLOGIC THERAPY

General Approach

- An algorithm for management of early to advanced PD is shown in **Figure 57-1**. **Table 57-2** is a summary of available antiparkinson medications and their dosing, and **Table 57-3** shows side effect monitoring.

Age is not the sole determinant for drug choice. Other factors such as cognitive function and overall tolerability of drug (especially in older patients) should be considered.

FIGURE 57-1. General approach to the management of early to advanced Parkinson disease.

		Starting Dose[b] (mg/day)	Maintenance Dose[b] (mg/day)	Dosage Forms (mg)
TABLE 57-2	Dosing of Drugs Used in Parkinson Disease[a]			
Generic Name	Trade Name			
Anticholinergic drugs				
Benztropine	Cogentin	0.5–1	1–6	0.5, 1, 2
Trihexyphenidyl	Artane	1–2	6–15	2, 5, 2/5 mL
Carbidopa/Levodopa products				
Carbidopa/ levodopa	Sinemet	300[c]	300–2000[c]	10/100, 25/100, 25/250
Carbidopa/ levodopa ODT	Parcopa	300[c]	300–2000[c]	10/100, 25/100, 25/250
Carbidopa/ levodopa CR	Sinemet CR	400[c]	400–2000[c]	25/100, 50/200
Carbidopa/ levodopa IR/ER	Rytary	435[c]	435–2450[c]	23.75/95, 36.25/145, 48.75/195, 61.25/245[d]
Carbidopa/ levodopa enteral suspension	Duopa	1000[c]	1000–2000[c]	4.63/20 per mL
Carbidopa/ levodopa/ entacapone	Stalevo	600[e]	600–1600[e]	12.5/50/200, 18.75/75/200, 25/100/200, 31.25/125/200, 37.5/150/200, 50/200/200
Carbidopa	Lodosyn	25	25–75	25
Levodopa	Inbrija	84	84–420	42[f]
Dopamine agonists				
Apomorphine	Apokyn	1–3	3–12	30/3 mL[g]
Bromocriptine	Parlodel	2.5–5	15–40	2.5, 5
Pramipexole	Mirapex	0.125	1.5–4.5	0.125, 0.25, 0.5, 1, 1.5
Pramipexole ER	Mirapex ER	0.375	1.5–4.5	0.375, 0.75, 1.5, 3, 4.5
Ropinirole	Requip	0.75	9–24	0.25, 0.5, 1, 2, 3, 4, 5
Ropinirole XL	Requip XL	2	8–24	2, 4, 6, 8, 12
Rotigotine	Neupro	2	2–8	1, 2, 3, 4, 6, 8
COMT inhibitors				
Entacapone	Comtan	200–600	200–1600	200
Tolcapone	Tasmar	300	300–600	100, 200
MAO-B inhibitors				
Rasagiline	Azilect	0.5–1	0.5–1	0.5, 1
Safinamide	Xadago	50	50–100	50, 100
Selegiline	Eldepryl	5–10	5–10	5
Selegiline ODT	Zelapar	1.25	1.25–2.5	1.25, 2.5

(Continued)

TABLE 57-2   Dosing of Drugs Used in Parkinson Disease[a] (Continued)

Generic Name	Trade Name	Starting Dose[b] (mg/day)	Maintenance Dose[b] (mg/day)	Dosage Forms (mg)
Miscellaneous				
Amantadine	Symmetrel	100	200–300	100, 50/5 mL
Amantadine ER	Gocovri	137	274	68.5, 137
Amantadine ER	Osmolex	129	129–258	129, 193, 258

[a]Marketed in the United States for Parkinson disease.
[b]Dosages may vary.
[c]Dosages expressed as levodopa component.
[d]Dosages of Rytary were developed to avoid confusion with other oral carbidopa/levodopa products that contain levodopa in multiples of 50 mg.
[e]Dosages expressed as entacapone component.
[f]Capsule containing levodopa dry powder for inhalation
[g]Sterile solution of subcutaneous injection with supplied pen injector.
COMT, catechol-*O*-methyltransferase; CR, controlled-release; IR, immediate-release; ER, extended-release; MAO, monoamine oxidase; ODT, orally disintegrating tablet.

TABLE 57-3   Monitoring of Potential Adverse Reactions to Drug Therapy for Parkinson Disease

Generic Name	Adverse Drug Reaction	Monitoring Parameter	Comments
Amantadine	Confusion	Mental status; renal function	Reduce dosage; adjust dose for renal impairment
	Livedo reticularis	Lower extremity examination; ankle edema	Reversible upon drug discontinuation
Benztropine and Trihexyphenidyl	Anticholinergic effects, confusion, drowsiness	Dry mouth, mental status, constipation, urinary retention, vision	Reduce dosage; avoid in elderly and in those with a history of constipation, memory impairment, urinary retention
Carbidopa/ levodopa	Drowsiness	Mental status	Reduce dose
	Dyskinesias	Abnormal involuntary movements	Reduce dose; add amantadine
	Nausea		
		Nausea	Take with food (eg, nonprotein snack)
COMT inhibitors			
Entacapone	Augmentation of levodopa side effects; also diarrhea	See carbidopa/ levodopa; also bowel movements	Reduce dose of levodopa; antidiarrheal agents
Tolcapone	See entacapone; also liver toxicity	See carbidopa/ levodopa; also ALT/AST	See carbidopa/levodopa; also at start of therapy and for every dose increase, ALT and AST levels at baseline and every 2–4 weeks for the first 6 months of therapy; afterward monitor based on clinical judgment.

(Continued)

TABLE 57-3	Monitoring of Potential Adverse Reactions to Drug Therapy for Parkinson Disease *(Continued)*		
Generic Name	**Adverse Drug Reaction**	**Monitoring Parameter**	**Comments**
Dopamine agonists			
Apomorphine	Drowsiness	Mental status	Reduce dose
	Nausea	Nausea	Premedicate with trimethobenzamide
	Orthostatic hypotension	Blood pressure, dizziness upon standing	Reduce dose
Bromocriptine	See pramipexole; also pulmonary fibrosis	Mental status; also chest radiograph	Reduce dose; chest radiograph at baseline and once yearly
Pramipexole and Ropinirole	Confusion	Mental status	Reduce dose
	Drowsiness	Mental status	Reduce dose
	Edema	Lower extremity swelling	Reduce dose or discontinue medication
	Hallucinations/ delusions	Behavior, mental status	Reduce dose or discontinue medication
	Impulsivity	Behavior	Discontinue medication
	Nausea	Nausea	Titrate dose upward slowly; take with food
	Orthostatic hypotension	Blood pressure, dizziness upon standing	Reduce dose
Rotigotine	See pramipexole; also skin irritation at site of patch application	See pramipexole; also skin examination	See pramipexole; rotate patch application site
MAO-B inhibitors			
Rasagiline	Nausea	Nausea	Take with food
Selegiline	Agitation/ Confusion	Mental status	Reduce dose
	Insomnia	Sleep	Administer dose earlier in day
	Hallucinations	Behavior, mental status	Reduce dose
	Orthostatic hypotension	Blood pressure, dizziness upon standing	Reduce dose

ALT, alanine aminotransferase; AST, aspartate aminotransferase; COMT, catechol-*O*-methyltransferase; MAO, monoamine oxidase.

- Initial monotherapy usually begins with a monoamine oxidase-B (MAO-B) inhibitor.
- Ultimately, all patients will require the use of **carbidopa/levodopa** either as monotherapy or in combination with other agents.
- With the development of motor fluctuations, patients should administer carbidopa/levodopa more frequently or addition of a COMT inhibitor, MAO-B inhibitor, or dopamine agonist to the carbidopa/levodopa regimen should be considered.
- For management of carbidopa/levodopa–induced peak-dose dyskinesias, a reduction in levodopa dose and/or addition of amantadine should be considered.

Anticholinergic Medications

- Anticholinergic drugs can improve tremor and sometimes dystonic features in some patients, but they rarely substantially improve bradykinesia or other disabilities. They can be used as monotherapy or in conjunction with other antiparkinson drugs.
- Anticholinergic side effects include dry mouth, blurred vision, constipation, and urinary retention. More serious reactions include forgetfulness, confusion, sedation, depression, and anxiety (see Table 57-3). Patients with preexisting cognitive deficits and the elderly are at greater risk for central anticholinergic side effects.

Amantadine

- Amantadine often provides modest benefit for tremor, rigidity, and bradykinesia, but is most often used for levodopa-induced dyskinesia.
- Doses should be reduced in patients with renal dysfunction (100 mg/day with creatinine clearances of 30–50 mL/min [0.50–0.84 mL/sec], 100 mg every other day for creatinine clearances of 15–29 mL/min [0.25–0.49 mL/sec], and 200 mg every 7 days for creatinine clearances less than 15 mL/min [0.25 mL/sec]) and those on hemodialysis.
- Adverse effects include sedation, dry mouth, hallucinations, dizziness, and confusion. Livedo reticularis (a diffuse mottling of the skin in the upper or lower extremities) is a common but reversible side effect.

Levodopa and Carbidopa/Levodopa

- **Levodopa** is the immediate precursor of dopamine and, in combination with a peripherally acting L-amino acid decarboxylase (L-AAD) inhibitor (carbidopa or benserazide), remains the most effective drug for the symptomatic treatment of PD.
- In the central nervous system (CNS) and peripherally, levodopa is converted by L-AAD to dopamine. In the periphery, carbidopa or benserazide can block L-AAD, thus increasing CNS penetration of administered levodopa and decreasing dopamine adverse effects (eg, nausea, cardiac arrhythmias, postural hypotension, and vivid dreams). Benserazide is unavailable in the United States.
- The usual maximal dose of levodopa tolerated is approximately 1000 to 1500 mg/day.
- About 75 mg of carbidopa is required to effectively block peripheral L-AAD, but some patients need more. Carbidopa/levodopa 25/100 mg tablet three times daily is the usual initial maintenance dose. Also available are the 25/250 mg and 10/100 mg dosage forms. Controlled-release preparations of carbidopa/levodopa are also available (Table 57-2). For patients with difficulty swallowing, an orally disintegrating tablet is available, and a capsule containing beads is available which can be sprinkled on food (Rytary).
- After oral levodopa administration, time to peak plasma concentrations varies intra- and intersubject. Meals delay gastric emptying, but antacids promote gastric emptying. Levodopa is absorbed primarily in the proximal duodenum via a saturable large neutral amino acid transport system, thus high-protein meals can interfere with bioavailability.
- Levodopa is not bound to plasma proteins, and the elimination half-life is approximately 1 hour. Adding carbidopa or benserazide can extend the half-life to 1.5 hours, and adding a COMT inhibitor (eg, **entacapone**) can extend it to approximately 2–2.5 hours.
- Sinemet CR and Rytary are 70% and 75% bioavailable compared to the standard immediate release carbidopa/levodopa formulation.
  - ✓ Long-term, levodopa-associated motor complications can be disabling. The most common of these are "end-of-dose wearing off" and "peak-dose dyskinesias." The risk of developing motor fluctuations or dyskinesias is approximately 10% per year of levodopa therapy. However, motor complications can occur 5–6 months after starting levodopa, especially when excessive doses are used initially. Table 57-4 shows these motor complications and suggests management strategies.

TABLE 57-4	Common Motor Complications and Possible Initial Treatments
Effects	**Possible Treatments**
End-of-dose "wearing off" (motor fluctuation)	Increase frequency of carbidopa/levodopa doses; add either COMT inhibitor or MAO-B inhibitor or dopamine agonist; add or switch to extended-release carbidopa/levodopa (ie, Rytary); use levodopa inhalation
"Delayed on" or "no on" response	Give carbidopa/levodopa on empty stomach; use carbidopa/levodopa ODT; avoid carbidopa/levodopa SR; use apomorphine subcutaneous or levodopa inhalation
Start hesitation ("freezing")	Increase carbidopa/levodopa dose; add a dopamine agonist or MAO-B inhibitor; utilize physical therapy along with assistive walking devices or sensory cues (eg, rhythmic commands, stepping over objects)
Peak-dose dyskinesia	Provide smaller doses of carbidopa/levodopa; reduce dose of adjunctive dopamine agonist; add amantadine

COMT, catechol-*O*-methyltransferase; MAO, monoamine oxidase; ODT, orally disintegrating tablet; SR, sustained release.

✓ End-of-dose "wearing off" is related to the increasing loss of neuronal dopamine storage capability and the short half-life of levodopa. Bedtime administration of a dopamine agonist or a drug formulation that provides sustained drug levels overnight (eg, carbidopa/levodopa CR or IR/ER, ropinirole XL, pramipexole ER, rotigotine transdermal patch) can help reduce nocturnal off episodes and improve functioning upon awakening. Administration of Rytary may also be useful, as therapeutic levels of levodopa are rapidly achieved and maintained for 4–5 hours (see Table 57-4).

✓ "Delayed-on" or "no-on" can result from delayed gastric emptying or decreased absorption in the duodenum. Chewing or crushing carbidopa/levodopa tablets and taking with a glass of water or using the orally disintegrating tablet on an empty stomach may help. Subcutaneous **apomorphine** may be used as rescue therapy.

✓ "Freezing," an episodic inhibition of lower extremity motor function, may be worsened by anxiety and may increase falls.

✓ Dyskinesias, involuntary choreiform movements usually involving the neck, trunk, and extremities, are usually associated with peak striatal dopamine levels. Less commonly, dyskinesias can develop during the rise and fall of levodopa effects (the dyskinesias-improvement-dyskinesias or diphasic pattern of response).

✓ "Off-period" dystonia muscle contractions occur most commonly in distal lower extremities (eg, feet or toes), often in the early morning. Consider bedtime administration of sustained-release products, use of **baclofen**, or selective denervation with **botulinum toxin**. If dystonia occurs as part of an levodopa peak dose effect, management is similar to that of dyskinesias.

Monoamine Oxidase B Inhibitors

• Three selective MAO-B inhibitors (**rasagiline, safinamide, selegiline**) are available for management of PD.

• Rasagiline and selegiline contain a propargylamine moiety, which is essential for conferring irreversible ("suicide") inhibition of MAO-B, in contrast to safinamide, which is a reversible MAO-B inhibitor. At therapeutic doses, all three agents preferentially inhibit MAO-B over MAO-A.

• Concomitant use of MAO-B inhibitors with meperidine and other selected opioid analgesics is contraindicated due to the small risk of serotonin syndrome. However, drugs with serotonergic antidepressants can be used concomitantly when clinically warranted.

- As monotherapy in early PD, both selegiline and rasagiline provide modest improvements in motor function.
- As add-on therapy, all three MAO-B inhibitors can provide up to 1 hour of extra "on" time for patients
- Selegiline also increases the peak effects of levodopa and can worsen preexisting dyskinesias or psychiatric symptoms, such as delusions. Metabolites of selegiline are L-methamphetamine and L-amphetamine. The oral disintegrating tablet may provide improved response and fewer side effects than the conventional formulation.
- Both rasagiline and safinamide are well tolerated with minimal GI or neuropsychiatric side effects

Catechol-*O*-Methyltransferase Inhibitors

- **Tolcapone** and **entacapone** are used in conjunction with carbidopa/levodopa to prevent the peripheral conversion of levodopa to dopamine (increasing the area under the curve of levodopa by approximately 35%). Thus, "on" time is increased by approximately 1–2 hours, and dosage requirements of levodopa are decreased. Avoid concomitant use of nonselective MAO inhibitors to prevent inhibition of the pathways for normal catecholamine metabolism.
- Tolcapone's use is limited by the potential for fatal liver toxicity, requiring strict monitoring of liver function. Reserve tolcapone for patients with fluctuations unresponsive to other therapies.
- Because entacapone has a shorter half-life, 200 mg is given with each dose of carbidopa/levodopa up to eight times a day.
- Dopaminergic adverse effects may occur and are managed by reducing the carbidopa/levodopa dose. Brownish orange urine discoloration may occur (as with tolcapone), but hepatotoxicity is not reported with entacapone.

Dopamine Agonists

- The ergot derivative **bromocriptine** and the nonergots **pramipexole**, **rotigotine**, and **ropinirole** are beneficial adjuncts in patients experiencing fluctuation in response to levodopa. They decrease the frequency of "off" periods and provide an levodopa-sparing effect.
- Titrate the dose of dopamine agonists slowly to enhance tolerability, and find the least dose that provides optimal benefit (see Table 57-2).
- The nonergots are safer and are effective as monotherapy in mild-to-moderate PD and as adjuncts to levodopa in patients with motor fluctuations.
- There is less risk of developing motor complications from monotherapy with dopamine agonists than from levodopa. Because younger patients are more likely to develop motor fluctuations, dopamine agonists are preferred in this population. Older patients are more likely to experience psychosis and orthostatic hypotension from dopamine agonists; therefore, carbidopa/levodopa may be the best initial medication in elderly patients. For patients with cognitive problems or dementia, dopamine agonists are best avoided.
- Common side effects of dopamine agonists are shown in Table 57-3. Other side effects include vivid dreams and sleep attacks. When added to levodopa, dopamine agonists may worsen dyskinesias. Hallucinations or delusions should be managed by dosage reduction or discontinuation and if needed addition of an atypical antipsychotic, such as clozapine, quetiapine, or pimavanserin (FDA approved for psychosis in PD).
- **Bromocriptine** is not commonly used because of its safety profile, which includes a risk of pulmonary fibrosis.
- **Pramipexole** is primarily renally excreted, and the initial dose must be adjusted in renal insufficiency. A once-daily extended-release formulation is available.
- **Ropinirole** is metabolized by cytochrome P4501A2; fluoroquinolones and smoking may alter ropinirole clearance. A once-daily formulation is available.
- **Rotigotine** patch provides continuous release over 24 hours, and disposition is not affected by hepatic or renal impairment.

- **Apomorphine** is a nonergot dopamine agonist given as a subcutaneous "rescue" injection. For patients with advanced PD with intermittent "off" episodes despite optimized therapy, subcutaneous apomorphine triggers an "on" response within 20 minutes, and duration of effect is up to 100 minutes. Most patients require 0.06 mg/kg. Prior to injection, patients should be premedicated with the antiemetic **trimethobenzamide**. It is contraindicated with the serotonin-3-receptor blockers (eg, ondansetron).

TABLE 57-5	Monitoring Parkinson Disease Therapy

1. Monitor medication administration times. Educate the patient that immediate-release carbidopa/levodopa is absorbed best on an empty stomach but is commonly taken with food (preferably nonprotein snack) to minimize nausea. Avoid administration of conventional selegiline in the late afternoon or evening to minimize insomnia.

2. Monitor to ensure that the patient and/or caregivers understand the prescribed medication regimen. For example, they should understand that catechol-*O*-methyltransferase inhibitors work by enhancing the effect of levodopa and that the patient should not discontinue medication without notifying the clinician.

3. Monitor and inquire specifically about dose-by-dose effects of medication, including response to doses of medication and the presence of dyskinesias, "wearing-off" effects, dizziness, nausea, orthostasis, or visual hallucinations. Offer suggestions to help alleviate these, or encourage the patient to discuss them with the clinician.

4. Monitor caregiver involvement and facilitation for early detection of abnormal behaviors, dyskinesias, falls, hallucinations, impulsivity, memory problems, mood changes, and sleep disorders.

5. Monitor for nonadherence and, if present, inquire for possible reasons (eg, dosing convenience, financial issues, and adverse effects) and offer suggestions.

6. Monitor for presence of drugs that can exacerbate idiopathic Parkinson disease motor features (eg, D_2-receptor blockers).

7. Monitor for presence of drugs that can exacerbate nonmotor symptoms. Evaluate whether the presence of an anticholinergic agent is causing confusion or cognitive impairment.

EVALUATION OF THERAPEUTIC OUTCOMES

- Comprehensive monitoring is essential to achieve desired outcomes (**Table 57-5**). Educate patients and caregivers about recording medication doses and administration times and duration of "on" and "off" periods.
- Monitor symptoms, side effects, and activities of daily living, and individualize therapy. Concomitant medications that may worsen motor symptoms, memory, falls, or behavioral symptoms should be discontinued if possible.

See Chapter 76, Parkinson Disease, authored by Jack J. Chen and Khashayar Dashtipour, for a more detailed discussion of this topic.

CHAPTER

58   **Obesity**

- *Obesity* occurs when there is an imbalance between energy intake and energy expenditure over time, resulting in increased energy storage.

PATHOPHYSIOLOGY

- The etiology of obesity is usually unknown, but it is likely multifactorial and related to varying contributions from genetic, environmental, and physiologic factors.
- Genetic factors appear to be the primary determinants of obesity in some individuals, determining both obesity and distribution of fat, whereas environmental factors are more important in others. The total number and identity of contributing genes are still being determined.
- Environmental factors include reduced physical activity or work, abundant food supply, relatively sedentary lifestyles, increased availability of high-fat foods, and cultural factors and religious beliefs.
- Medical conditions including Cushing disease, growth hormone deficiency, insulinoma, leptin deficiency, and psychiatric disorders such as depression, binge-eating disorder, and schizophrenia and genetic syndromes such as Prader–Willi syndrome can be associated with weight gain.
- Medications associated with unintended weight gain include insulin, corticosteroids, some antidepressants, conventional antipsychotics, and several anticonvulsants.
- Many neurotransmitters and neuropeptides stimulate or depress the brain's appetite network, impacting total calorie intake.
- The degree of obesity is determined by the net balance of energy ingested relative to energy expended over time. The single largest determinant of energy expenditure is metabolic rate, which is expressed as *resting energy expenditure* or *basal metabolic rate*. Physical activity is the other major factor that affects total energy expenditure and is the most variable component.
- Major types of adipose tissue are: (1) white adipose tissue, which manufactures, stores, and releases lipid; and (2) brown adipose tissue, which dissipates energy via uncoupled mitochondrial respiration. Adrenergic stimulation activates lipolysis in fat cells and increases energy expenditure in adipose tissue and skeletal muscle.

CLINICAL PRESENTATION

- Obesity is associated with serious health risks and increased risk of all-cause mortality. Central obesity reflects high levels of intra-abdominal or visceral fat that is associated with the development of hypertension, dyslipidemia, type 2 diabetes, and cardiovascular disease (sometimes referred to as the "metabolic syndrome").
- Body mass index (BMI) and waist circumference (WC) are recognized, acceptable markers of excess body fat that independently predict disease risk (**Table 58-1**).
- BMI is calculated as weight (kg) divided by the square of the height (m²).
- WC, the most practical method of characterizing central adiposity, is the narrowest circumference between the last rib and the top of the iliac crest.

TABLE 58-1	Classification of Overweight and Obesity by Body Mass Index, Comorbidity Risk, Waist Circumference, and Associated Disease Risk

				Disease Risk[a] (Relative to Normal Weight and Waist Circumference)	
				Men	
				≤40 in. (102 cm)	**>40 in. (102 cm)**
				Women	
	BMI (kg/m²)	**Obesity Class**	**Comorbidity Risk**	**≤35 in. (89 cm)**	**>35 in. (89 cm)**
Underweight	<18.5		Low but other problems	—	—
Normal weight[b]	18.5–24.9		Average	—	High
Overweight	25.0–29.9		Increased	Increased	High
Obesity	30.0–34.9	I	Moderate	High	Very high
	35.0–39.9	II	Severe	Very high	Very high
Extreme obesity	≥40	III	Very severe	Extremely high	Extremely high

[a]Disease risk for type 2 diabetes, hypertension, and cardiovascular disease.
[b]Increased waist circumference can also be a marker for increased risk even in persons of normal weight.
BMI, body mass index.
Adapted from Preventing and Managing the Global Epidemic of Obesity. Report of the World Health Organization Consultation on Obesity. Geneva: World Health Organization, 1997. Reprinted with permission from National Institutes of Health, National Heart, Lung, and Blood Institutes. 1997, http://www.nhlbi.nih.gov/guidelines/obesity/ob_home.htm.

TREATMENT

- Goals of Treatment: Current clinical practice guidelines recommend a "complication-centric approach" to assess for the presence and severity of weight-related complications to determine appropriate treatment and intensity of weight loss therapy in individuals with overweight and obesity. The primary goal is to ameliorate weight-related complications and ultimately improve health and quality of life rather than a preset decrease in body weight.

GENERAL APPROACH

- Nonpharmacologic therapy, including reduced caloric intake, increased physical activity, and behavior modification, is the mainstay of obesity management. Set goals based on factors including initial body weight, patient motivation and desire, presence of obesity-related comorbid conditions, and age.
- Current adult practice guidelines recommend reduced caloric intake through adherence to a low-calorie diet. Adherence to this type of diet with increased exercise, and in-person behavioral counseling sessions have been reported to result in an average weight loss of 8 kg (17.6 lb) over 6 months.
- Bariatric surgery, which reduces the stomach volume or absorptive surface of the alimentary tract, remains the most effective intervention for obesity. Surgery should

be reserved for those with extreme obesity (BMI $\geq$40 kg/m²) or BMI >35 kg/m² with significant comorbidities such as hypertension, type 2 diabetes, or obstructive sleep apnea.

- Implantable medical devices are an option for individuals who do not qualify for bariatric surgery or choose to not undergo the procedure. These devices are designed to work in conjunction with prescribed diet and exercise programs.

PHARMACOLOGIC THERAPY

- Pharmacotherapy is an adjunct to comprehensive lifestyle intervention in adults who are motivated to lose weight, have failed to achieve or sustain weight loss with lifestyle change alone, and have a BMI $\geq$30 kg/m² or BMI $\geq$27 kg/m² with at least one weight-related comorbidity (Table 58-2).
- Long-term pharmacotherapy may have a role for patients who have no contraindications to approved drug therapy (Table 58-3).
- **Orlistat** (180 or 360 mg in three divided doses/day) is a lipase inhibitor that induces weight loss by lowering dietary fat absorption; it also improves lipid profiles, glucose control, and other metabolic markers. Soft stools, abdominal pain or colic, flatulence, fecal urgency, and/or incontinence occur in 80% of individuals using prescription strength, are mild to moderate in severity, and improve after 1–2 months of therapy. Orlistat is approved for long-term use. It interferes with the absorption of fat-soluble vitamins, cyclosporine, levothyroxine, and oral contraceptives. A nonprescription formulation is also available.
- **Phentermine** in combination with **topiramate extended release** is indicated for chronic weight management. Doses are gradually titrated from phentermine 3.75 to 15 mg and topiramate 23–92 mg over 4 months, but the drug should be stopped after 12 weeks if 5% weight loss is not achieved. Common adverse effects include constipation, dry mouth, paraesthesia, dysgeusia, and insomnia.
- **Naltrexone** in combination with **bupropion extended release** is indicated for chronic weight management. Doses are gradually increased over 4 weeks, starting with one tablet daily (8 mg naltrexone/90 mg bupropion) to a maintenance dose of two tablets twice daily. Patients should avoid taking their dose with a high-fat meal. Common adverse effects include nausea, constipation, headache, vomiting, dizziness, insomnia, dry mouth, and diarrhea. Discontinue treatment if 5% weight loss is not achieved after 12 weeks.
- **Liraglutide** is a glucagon-like peptide-1 receptor agonist indicated for chronic weight management at a dose of 3 mg daily. It is administered subcutaneously and is available in prefilled, multidose pens. A 5-week dose escalation schedule is recommended to improve tolerability of GI adverse events, beginning with 0.6 mg daily and increasing weekly by 0.6 mg increments to a maintenance dose of 3 mg daily. Common adverse effects include nausea, diarrhea, constipation, vomiting, dyspepsia, hypoglycemia, and abdominal pain. Discontinue liraglutide if weight loss of at least 4% is not achieved after 16 weeks of therapy.
- **Amphetamines** should generally be avoided because of their powerful stimulant effects and addictive potential.
- **Lorcaserin** is a selective serotonin receptor agonist (5-HT_{2C}) that was removed from the market in February 2020.
- Many complementary and alternative therapy products are promoted for weight loss. Regulation of dietary supplements is less rigorous than that of prescription and over-the-counter drug products; manufacturers do not have to prove safety and effectiveness prior to marketing.

EVALUATION OF THERAPEUTIC OUTCOMES

- Assess progress once or twice monthly for 1–2 months, then monthly. Each encounter should document weight, WC, BMI, blood pressure, medical history, and patient assessment of tolerability of drug therapy.

TABLE 58-2 FDA-Approved Pharmacotherapeutic Agents for Weight Loss

Drug	Brand Name	Initial Dose	Usual Range	Special Population Dose	Comment
Gastrointestinal lipase inhibitor					
Orlistat	Xenical	120 mg three times daily with each main meal containing fat	120 mg three times daily with each main meal containing fat		Approved for long-term use Take during or up to 1 hour after the meal Omit dose if meal is occasionally missed or contains no fat
Orlistat	Alli[a]	60 mg three times daily with each main meal containing fat	60 mg three times daily with each main meal containing fat		Same as Xenical
Phentermine–topiramate combination					
Phentermine and topiramate extended-release	Qsymia	3.75 mg of phentermine and 23 mg of topiramate once daily for 14 days; then increase to 7.5 mg of phentermine and 46 mg of topiramate once daily	7.5 mg of phentermine and 46 mg of topiramate once daily to a maximum dose of phentermine 15 mg and topiramate 92 mg once daily	Maximum dose for patients with moderate or severe renal impairment or patients with moderate hepatic impairment is 7.5 mg of phentermine and 46 mg of topiramate	Approved for long-term use Take dose in the morning to avoid insomnia Controlled substance: C–IV

Naltrexone–bupropion combination

Bupropion and naltrexone extended-release	Contrave	8 mg naltrexone/90 mg bupropion (1 tablet) once daily in the morning for 1 week; then 8 mg naltrexone/90 mg bupropion twice daily (morning and evening) for 1 week; then 16 mg naltrexone/180 mg bupropion in the morning and 8 mg naltrexone/90 mg bupropion in the evening for 1 week; then 16 mg naltrexone/180 mg bupropion twice daily (morning and evening)	16 mg naltrexone and 180 mg bupropion (2 tablets) twice daily	Maximum dose for patients with moderate or severe renal impairment is 8 mg naltrexone/90 mg bupropion (1 tablet) twice daily Maximum dose for patients with hepatic impairment is 8 mg naltrexone/90 mg bupropion (1 tablet) once daily in the morning	Approved for long-term use Do not take dose with high-fat meal

Glucagon-like peptide-1 agonist

Liraglutide	Saxenda	0.6 mg once daily for 1 week 1.2 mg once daily for 1 week 1.8 mg once daily for 1 week 2.4 mg once daily for 1 week 3.0 mg once daily for 1 week[a] administered by subcutaneous injection	3 mg once daily	Use with caution in mild, moderate, and severe renal and hepatic impairment	Approved for long-term use Inject subcutaneously in the abdomen, thigh, or upper arm Administer at any time of day without regard to the timing of meals

Noradrenergic agents

Phendimetrazine	Bontril PDM; Bontril slow-release	Conventional tablet: start at 17.5 mg two or three times daily, given 1 hour before meals Extended-release capsule: 105 mg once daily 30–60 minutes before morning meal	70–105 mg/day	Use caution in patients with renal impairment	Approved for short-term monotherapy Controlled substance: C–III Prescriptions should be written for the smallest quantity to minimize possibility of overdose

(Continued)

TABLE 58-2 FDA-Approved Pharmacotherapeutic Agents for Weight Loss (Continued)

Drug	Brand Name	Initial Dose	Usual Range	Special Population Dose	Comment
Phentermine	Lomaira Adipex-P	8 mg three times daily, given half hour before meal Orally disintegrating tablet: 15 or 30 mg once every morning Phentermine hydrochloride: 15–37.5 mg/day given in one or two divided doses; administer before breakfast or 1–2 hours after breakfast	8 mg three times daily, given half hour before meal Orally disintegrating tablet: 15 or 30 mg once every morning Phentermine hydrochloride: 15–37.5 mg/day given in one or two divided doses; administer before breakfast or 1–2 hours after breakfast	Use with caution in patients with renal impairment	Approved for short-term monotherapy Controlled substance: C–IV Prescriptions should be written for the smallest quantity to minimize possibility of overdose Individualize to achieve adequate response with lowest effective dose
Diethylpropion	Tenuate, Tenuate Dospan	Immediate release: 25 mg three times daily administered 1 hour before meals Controlled release: 75 mg once daily administered at midmorning	75 mg/day	Use with caution in patients with renal impairment	Approved for short-term monotherapy Dose should not be administered in the evening or at bedtime Controlled substance: C–IV

aAvailable without a prescription.

TABLE 58-3	Clinical and Economic Considerations for Long-Term Pharmacotherapy Options			
Drug	**Brand Name**	**Weight Loss Above Diet and Exercise Alone (1 year)**	**Cost for 30 days of Therapy[a]**	**Comments**
Orlistat	Xenical	2.9–3.4 kg (6.5–7.5 lb)	$685.81	Use may be limited by GI intolerance
Phentermine and topiramate extended-release	Qsymia	6.6–8.6 kg (14.5–18.9 lb)	$186.00, 7.5–46 mg $199.50, 15–92 mg	Limited distribution under FDA Risk Evaluation Mitigation Strategy (REMS)
Bupropion and naltrexone extended-release	Contrave	4.9 kg (10.8 lb)	$277.99	Lowers seizure threshold (bupropion) Rare reports of hepatotoxicity (naltrexone) Drug interactions with opioids, CYP2B6 inducers, and CYP2D6 substrates
Liraglutide	Saxenda	5.8 kg (12.8 lb)	$1242.00	Injectable Reduces A1C and fasting glucose Risk of medullary thyroid carcinoma and multiple endocrine neoplasia syndrome type 2 Rare reports of pancreatitis, gall bladder disease, and suicidal ideation

[a]Cost of therapy based on maintenance dose using wholesaler acquisition cost (WAC) as of January 9, 2018.

- Discontinue medication therapy after 3 months if the patient has failed to demonstrate weight loss or maintenance of prior weight.
- Diabetic patients require more intense medical monitoring and self-monitoring of blood glucose. Weekly healthcare visits for 1–2 months may be necessary until the effects of diet, exercise, and weight loss medication become more predictable.
- Monitor patients with hyperlipidemia or hypertension to assess effects of weight loss on appropriate end points.

See Chapter 161, Obesity, authored by Amy Heck Sheehan, Judy T. Chen, and Jack A. Yanovski, for a more detailed discussion of this topic.

Nutrition Assessment and Support

- Malnutrition is a consequence of nutrient imbalance resulting from inadequate intake, absorption, or utilization of protein and energy. Undernutrition can result in changes in subcellular, cellular, or organ function that increase the individual's risks of morbidity and mortality.
- For information on overnutrition or obesity, see Chapter 58.
- Nutrition screening provides a systematic way to identify individuals in any care environment with preexisting malnutrition or those at risk for malnutrition for whom a detailed nutrition assessment is warranted.
- Nutrition assessment is the first step in developing a nutrition care plan. Goals of nutrition assessment are to identify the presence of factors associated with an increased risk of developing undernutrition and complications, estimate nutrition needs, and establish baseline parameters for assessing the outcome of therapy.
- This assessment should include a comprehensive medical, surgical, and dietary history and a nutrition-focused physical exam (NFPE) including anthropometrics and laboratory measurements.
- The NFPE uses a system-based approach to assess for abnormal nutrition-related clinical and physical findings in each region of the body.

NUTRITION ASSESSMENT

ANTHROPOMETRIC MEASUREMENTS

- Anthropometric measurements are physical measurements of the size, weight, and proportions of the human body used to compare an individual with normative population standards. Common measurements are weight, stature, head circumference (for children younger than 3 years of age) and waist circumference. Measurements of limb size (eg, skinfold thickness and mid-arm muscle and wrist circumferences), along with bioelectrical impedance analysis (BIA), may be useful in selected individuals.
- Interpretation of actual body weight (ABW) should consider ideal weight (IBW) for height, usual body weight (UBW), fluid status, and age. Change over time can be calculated as the percentage of UBW. Unintentional weight loss, especially rapid weight loss (5% of UBW in 1 month or 10% of UBW in 6 months), increases risk of nutrition-related poor clinical outcomes in adults.
- The best indicator of adequate nutrition in children is appropriate growth. Weight, stature, head circumference (until 3 years), and body mass index (BMI) (after 2 years) should be plotted on the appropriate growth curve. Average weight gain for newborns is 10–20 g/kg/day (24–35 g/day for term infants and 10–25 g/day for preterm infants depending on gestational age).
- BMI is another index of weight-for-height. Interpretation of BMI should include consideration of gender, frame size, race/ethnicity, and age. BMI values greater than 25 kg/m^2 are indicative of overweight, and values less than 18.5 kg/m^2 are indicative of undernutrition. BMI is calculated as follows:

  Body weight (kg)/[height (m)]^2 **or** [Body weight (lb) $\times$ 703]/[height (in.)]^2

- Measurements of skinfold thickness estimate subcutaneous fat, mid-arm muscle circumference estimates skeletal muscle mass, and waist circumference estimates abdominal (visceral) fat content.
- BIA is a simple, noninvasive, and relatively inexpensive way to assess LBM, total body water (TBW), and water distribution. It is based on differences between fat tissue and lean tissue's resistance to conductivity. Hydration status should be considered in interpretation of BIA results.

BIOCHEMICAL AND IMMUNE FUNCTION STUDIES

- LBM can be assessed by measuring serum visceral proteins (Table 59-1). They are of greatest value for assessing uncomplicated starvation and recovery, and less useful for assessing status during acute stress. Interpret visceral proteins relative to overall clinical status because they are affected by many factors other than nutrition.
- Nutrition affects immune status both directly and indirectly. Total lymphocyte count and delayed cutaneous hypersensitivity reactions are immune function tests useful in nutrition assessment, but their lack of specificity limits their usefulness as nutrition status markers.
- Delayed cutaneous hypersensitivity is commonly assessed using antigens to which the patient was likely previously sensitized. The recall antigens used most frequently are mumps and *Candida albicans*. Anergy is associated with severe malnutrition; immune response can be restored with nutrition repletion.

SPECIFIC NUTRIENT DEFICIENCIES

- Biochemical assessment of trace element, vitamin, and essential fatty acid deficiencies should be based on the nutrient's function, but few practical methods are available. Therefore, most assays measure serum concentrations of the individual nutrient.
- Clinical syndromes are associated with deficiencies of the following trace elements: zinc, copper, manganese, selenium, chromium, iodine, fluoride, molybdenum, and iron.
- Single vitamin deficiencies are uncommon; multiple vitamin deficiencies more commonly occur with malnutrition. For information on iron deficiency and other anemias, see Chapter 33.

TABLE 59-1	Serum Proteins Used for Assessment of Lean Body Mass			
Serum Protein	**Half-Life (Days)**	**Function**	**Factors Resulting in Increased Values**	**Factors Resulting in Decreased Values**
Albumin	18–20	Maintains plasma oncotic pressure; transports small molecules	Dehydration, anabolic steroids, insulin, infection	Fluid overload; edema; kidney dysfunction; nephrotic syndrome; poor dietary intake; impaired digestion; burns; heart failure; cirrhosis; thyroid, adrenal, or pituitary hormones; trauma; sepsis
Transferrin	8–9	Binds Fe in plasma; transports Fe to bone	Fe deficiency, pregnancy, hypoxia, chronic blood loss, estrogens	Chronic infection, cirrhosis, burns, enteropathies, nephrotic syndrome, cortisone, testosterone
Prealbumin (transthyretin)	2–3	Binds T_3 and, to a lesser extent, T_4; retinol-binding protein carrier	Impaired kidney function	Cirrhosis, hepatitis, stress, surgery, inflammation, hyperthyroidism, cystic fibrosis, burns, zinc deficiency

Fe, iron; T_3, triiodothyronine; T_4, thyroxine.

- Essential fatty acid deficiency is rare but can occur with prolonged lipid-free parenteral nutrition (PN), very low-fat enteral formulations or diets, severe fat malabsorption, or severe malnutrition. The body can synthesize all fatty acids except for linoleic and α-linolenic acid.
- Carnitine can be synthesized from lysine and methionine, but hepatic synthesis is decreased in premature infants. Low carnitine levels can occur in premature infants receiving PN or carnitine-free diets.

ASSESSMENT OF NUTRIENT REQUIREMENTS

- Assessment of nutrient requirements must be made in the context of patient-specific factors (eg, age, gender, size, disease state, clinical condition, nutrition status, and physical activity).
- Adults should consume 45%–65% of total calories from carbohydrates, 20%–35% from fat, and 10%–35% from protein. Recommendations are similar for children, except that infants should consume 40%–50% of total calories from fat.

Energy Requirements

- Energy requirements of individuals can be estimated using validated predictive equations or directly measured, depending on factors including severity of illness and resources available. The simplest method is to use population estimates of calories required per kilogram of body weight.
- Healthy adults with normal nutrition status and minimal illness severity require an estimated 20–25 kcal ABW/kg/day (84–105 kJ ABW/kg/day). Daily energy requirements for children are approximately 150% of basal metabolic rate with additional calories to support activity and growth. Consult references for equations used to estimate energy expenditure in adults and children.
- Energy requirements for all ages increase with fever, sepsis, major surgery, trauma, burns, long-term growth failure, and chronic conditions (eg, bronchopulmonary dysplasia, congenital heart disease, and cystic fibrosis).

Protein, Fluid, and Micronutrient Requirements

Protein

- Protein requirements are based on age, gender, nutrition status, disease state, and clinical condition. The usual recommended daily protein allowances are 0.8 g/kg for adults, 1.5 g/kg for adults over 60 years of age, 1.5–2 g/kg for patients with metabolic stress (eg, infection, trauma, and surgery), and 2.5–3 g/kg for patients with burns.

Fluid

- Daily adult fluid requirements are approximately 30–40 mL/kg.
- Fluid requirements for children and preterm infants who weigh less than 10 kg are at least 100 mL/kg/day. An additional 50 mL/kg should be provided for each kilogram of body weight between 11 and 20 kg, and 20 mL/kg for each kilogram greater than 20 kg.
- Factors that may result in increased fluid requirements include but are not limited to gastrointestinal (GI) losses, fever, sweating, and increased metabolism, whereas kidney or heart failure and hypoalbuminemia with starvation are examples of factors that may result in decreased fluid requirements.
- Assess fluid status by monitoring urine output and specific gravity, serum electrolytes, and weight changes. An hourly urine output of at least 1 mL/kg for children and 40–50 mL for adults is needed to ensure tissue perfusion.

Micronutrients

- Requirements for micronutrients (ie, electrolytes, minerals, trace elements, and vitamins) vary with age, sex, route of ingestion, and underlying clinical conditions.

- Sodium, potassium, magnesium, and phosphorus requirements are typically decreased in patients with kidney failure, whereas calcium requirements are increased (see Chapters 74 and 75).

Drug–Nutrient Interactions

- Concomitant drug therapy can alter serum concentrations of vitamins (Table 59-2), minerals, and electrolytes.
- Some drug delivery vehicles contain nutrients. For example, the vehicle for propofol is 10% lipid emulsion, and most IV therapies include dextrose or sodium.

TABLE 59-2	Drug and Nutrient Interactions
Drug	**Effect**
Angiotensin-converting enzyme inhibitors	Increased urinary zinc losses
Angiotensin receptor blockers	Increased urinary zinc losses
Antacids	Thiamine deficiency
Antibiotics	Vitamin K deficiency
Aspirin	Folic acid deficiency; increased vitamin C excretion
Cathartics	Increased requirements for vitamins D, C, and B_6
Cholestyramine	Vitamins A, D, E, and K and β-carotene malabsorption
Colestipol	Vitamins A, D, E, and K and β-carotene malabsorption
Corticosteroids	Decreased vitamins A, D, and C
Diuretics (loop)	Thiamine deficiency
Diuretics (thiazides)	Increased urinary zinc losses
Efavirenz	Vitamin D deficiency caused by increased metabolism of 25(OH)D and 1,25(OH)$_2$D
Histamine$_2$ antagonists	Vitamin B_{12} malabsorption (reduced acid results in impaired release of B_{12} from food)
Isoniazid	Vitamin B_6 and niacin deficiency
Isotretinoin	Vitamin A increases toxicity
Mercaptopurine	Niacin deficiency
Methotrexate	Folic acid inhibits effect
Orlistat	Vitamins A, D, E, and K malabsorption caused by fat malabsorption
Pentamidine	Folic acid deficiency
Phenobarbital	Increased vitamin D metabolism
Phenytoin	Increased vitamin D metabolism; decreased folic acid concentrations
Primidone	Folic acid deficiency
Protease inhibitors	Vitamin D deficiency (impaired renal hydroxylation)
Proton pump inhibitors	Decreased iron and vitamin B_{12} absorption (reduced acid results in impaired release of B_{12} from food)
Sulfasalazine	Folic acid malabsorption
Trimethoprim	Folic acid depletion
Warfarin	Vitamin K inhibits effect; vitamins A, C, and E may increase effect
Valproic acid	Zinc
Zidovudine	Folic acid and B_{12} deficiencies increase myelosuppression

NUTRITION SUPPORT

- The primary objective of nutrition support therapy is to promote positive clinical outcomes of an illness and improve quality of life.

ENTERAL NUTRITION

- Enteral nutrition (EN) delivers nutrients by tube or mouth into the GI tract; we will focus on delivery through a feeding tube. The goal of EN is to provide calories, macronutrients, and micronutrients to those who are unable to achieve these requirements from an oral diet.
- EN is indicated for the patient who cannot or will not eat enough to meet nutritional requirements and who has a functioning GI tract and a method of enteral access. Potential indications include neoplastic disease, organ dysfunction, hypermetabolic states, GI disease, and neurologic impairment.
- Distal mechanical intestinal obstruction, bowel ischemia, and necrotizing enterocolitis are contraindications to EN. Contraindications to tube placement include active peritonitis and uncorrectable coagulopathy. Conditions that challenge the success of EN include severe diarrhea, protracted vomiting, enteric fistulas, severe GI hemorrhage, hemodynamic instability, and intestinal dysmotility.
- EN has replaced PN as the preferred method for the feeding of critically ill patients requiring specialized nutrition support. Advantages of EN over PN include maintaining GI tract structure and function; fewer metabolic, infectious, and technical complications; and lower costs.
- The timing of initiation of EN in the critically ill patients is of clinical significance. Initiation within 24–48 hours of admission to an intensive care unit appears to attenuate the stress response and reduce infectious complications and mortality. If patients are only mildly to moderately stressed and well nourished, EN initiation can be delayed until oral intake is inadequate for 5–7 days.

Access

- EN can be administered through four routes, which have different indications, tube placement options, advantages, and disadvantages (Table 59-3). The choice depends on the anticipated duration of use and the feeding site (ie, stomach vs. small bowel).
- The stomach is generally the least expensive and least labor-intensive access site; however, patients who have impaired gastric emptying are at risk for aspiration and pneumonia.
- Long-term access with gastrostomy and jejunostomy tubes should be considered when EN is anticipated for more than 4–6 weeks.

Administration Methods

- EN can be administered by continuous, cyclic, bolus, and intermittent methods. The choice depends on the location of the feeding tube tip, patient's clinical condition, intestinal function, and tolerance to tube feeding.
- Continuous EN is preferred for initiating therapy and has the advantage of being well tolerated. Disadvantages include cost and inconvenience associated with pump and administration sets.
- Cyclic EN has the advantage of allowing breaks from the infusion system, thereby increasing mobility, especially if EN is administered nocturnally.
- Bolus EN is most commonly used in patients in the home or long-term care setting who have a gastrostomy. Advantages include short administration time (eg, 5–10 minutes) and minimal equipment (eg, a syringe). Bolus EN has the potential disadvantages of causing cramping, nausea, vomiting, aspiration, and diarrhea.
- Intermittent EN is similar to bolus EN except that the feeding is administered over 20–60 minutes, which improves tolerability but requires more equipment (eg, reservoir bag and infusion pump). Like bolus EN, intermittent EN mimics normal eating patterns.

TABLE 59-3	Options and Considerations in the Selection of Enteral Access			
Access	EN Duration/Patient Characteristics	Tube Placement Options	Advantages	Disadvantages
Nasogastric or orogastric	Short term Intact gag reflex Normal gastric emptying	Manually at bedside	Ease of placement Allows for all methods of administration Inexpensive Multiple commercially available tubes and sizes	Potential tube displacement Potential increased aspiration risk
Nasojejunal	Short term Impaired gastric motility or emptying High risk of GER or aspiration	Manually at bedside Fluoroscopically Endoscopically	Potential reduced aspiration risk Allows for early postinjury or postoperative feeding Multiple commercially available tubes and sizes	Manual transpyloric passage requires greater skill Potential tube displacement or clogging Bolus or intermittent feeding not tolerated
Gastrostomy	Long term Normal gastric emptying	Surgically Endoscopically Radiologically Laparoscopically	Allows for all methods of administration Low-profile buttons available Large-bore tubes less likely to clog Multiple commercially available tubes and sizes	Attendant risks associated with each type of procedure Potential increased aspiration risk Risk of stoma site complications
Jejunostomy	Long term Impaired gastric motility or gastric emptying High risk of GER or aspiration	Surgically Endoscopically Radiologically Laparoscopically	Allows for early postinjury or postoperative feeding Potential reduced aspiration risk Multiple commercially available tubes and sizes Low-profile buttons available	Attendant risks associated with each type of procedure Bolus or intermittent feeding not tolerated Risk of stoma site complications

EN, enteral nutrition; GER, gastroesophageal reflux.

- Protocols outlining initiation and advancement criteria are a useful strategy to optimize achievement of nutrient goals based on GI tolerance. Clinical signs of intolerance include abdominal distention or cramping, high gastric residual volumes, aspiration, and diarrhea.
- Continuous EN feedings are typically started in adults at 20–50 mL/hr and advanced by 10–25 mL/hr every 4–8 hours until the goal is achieved. Intermittent EN feedings are started at 120 mL every 4 hours and advanced by 30–60 mL every 8–12 hours.

Formulations

- Historically, EN formulations were created to provide essential nutrients, including macronutrients (eg, carbohydrates, fats, and proteins) and micronutrients (eg, electrolytes, trace elements, vitamins, and water).
- Over time, formulations have been enhanced to improve tolerance and meet specific patient needs. For example, immunonutrients or pharmaconutrients are added to modify the disease process or improve clinical outcome; however, these health claims are not regulated by the FDA.
- The molecular form of the protein source determines the amount of digestion required for absorption within the small bowel. The carbohydrate component usually provides the major source of calories; polymeric entities are preferred over elemental sugars. Vegetable oils rich in polyunsaturated fatty acids are the most common sources of fat in EN formulations.
- Soluble and insoluble fiber has been added to several EN formulations. Potential benefits of soluble fiber include trophic effects on colonic mucosa, promotion of sodium and water absorption, and regulation of bowel function.
- Osmolality is a function of the size and quantity of ionic and molecular particles primarily related to protein, carbohydrate, electrolyte, and mineral content. The osmolality of EN formulations for adults ranges from 280 to 875 mOsm/kg (mmol/kg). Osmolality is commonly thought to affect GI tolerability, but there is a lack of supporting evidence.

Classification of Enteral Feeding Formulations

- EN formulations are classified by their composition and intended patient population (Table 59-4). Formularies should focus on clinically significant characteristics of available products, avoid duplicate formulations, and include only specialty formulations with evidence-based indications.

Complications and Monitoring

- Monitor patients for metabolic, GI, and mechanical complications of EN (Table 59-5).
- Metabolic complications associated with EN are similar to those of PN, but the incidence is lower.
- GI complications include nausea, vomiting, abdominal distention, cramping, aspiration, diarrhea, and constipation. Gastric residual volume is thought to increase the risk of vomiting and aspiration.
- Mechanical complications include tube occlusion or malposition and inadvertent nasopulmonary intubation. Techniques for clearing occluded tubes include pancreatic enzymes in sodium bicarbonate and using a declogging device. Techniques for maintaining patency include flushing with at least 15–30 mL of water before and after medication administration and intermittent feedings and at least every 8 hours during continuous feeding.

Drug Delivery Via Feeding Tube

- Administering drugs via tube feeding is a common practice. If the drug is a solid that can be crushed (eg, *not* a sublingual, sustained-release, or enteric-coated formulation) or is a capsule, mix with 15–30 mL of water or other appropriate solvent and administer. Otherwise, a liquid dosage preparation should be used. Administer multiple medications separately, each followed by flushing the tube with 5–15 mL of water.

TABLE 59-4	Adult Enteral Feeding Formulation Classification System	
Category	**Features**	**Indications**
Standard polymeric	Isotonic 1–1.2 kcal/mL (4.2–5 kJ/mL) NPC:N 125:1–150:1 May contain fiber	Designed to meet the needs of the majority of patients Patients with functional GI tract Not suitable for oral use
High protein	NPC:N <125:1 May contain fiber	Patients with protein requirements >1.5 g/kg/day, such as trauma patients and those with burns, pressure sores, or wounds Patients receiving propofol
High caloric density	1.5–2 kcal/mL (6.3–8.4 kJ/mL) Lower electrolyte content per calorie Hypertonic	Patients requiring fluid and/or electrolyte restriction, such as kidney insufficiency
Elemental	High proportion of free amino acids Low in fat	Patients who require low fat Use has generally been replaced by peptide-based formulations
Peptide-based	Contains dipeptides and tripeptides Contains MCTs	Indications/benefits not clearly established Trial may be warranted in patients who do not tolerate intact protein due to malabsorption
Disease specific		
Kidney	Caloric dense Protein content varies Low-electrolyte content	Alternative to high-caloric density formulations, but generally more expensive
Liver	Increased branched-chain and decreased aromatic amino acids	Patients with hepatic encephalopathy
Lung	High fat, low carbohydrate Anti-inflammatory lipid profile and antioxidants	Patients with ARDS and severe ALI
Diabetes mellitus	High fat, low carbohydrate	Alternative to standard, fiber-containing formulation in patients with uncontrolled hyperglycemia
Immune-modulating	Supplemented with glutamine, arginine, nucleotides, and/or omega-3 fatty acids	Patients undergoing major elective GI surgery, trauma, burns, head and neck cancer, and critically ill patients on mechanical ventilation Use with caution in patients with sepsis Select nutrients may be beneficial or harmful in subgroups of critically ill patients
Oral supplement	Sweetened for taste Hypertonic	Patients who require supplementation to an oral diet

ALI, acute lung injury; ARDS, acute respiratory distress syndrome; MCT, medium-chain triglyceride; NPC:N, nonprotein calorie-to-nitrogen ratio.

	TABLE 59-5	Suggested Monitoring for Adult Patients on Enteral Nutrition

Parameter	During Initiation of EN Therapy	During Stable EN Therapy
Vital signs	Every 4–6 hours	As needed with suspected change (ie, fever)
Clinical assessment		
Weight	Daily	Weekly
Total intake/Output	Daily	As needed with suspected change in intake/output
Tube-feeding intake	Daily	Daily
Enterostomy tube site assessment	Daily	Daily
GI tolerance		
Stool frequency/Volume	Daily	Daily
Abdomen assessment	Daily	Daily
Nausea or vomiting	Daily	Daily
Gastric residual volumes	Every 4–8 hours (varies)	As needed when delayed gastric emptying suspected
Tube placement	Prior to starting, then ongoing	Ongoing
Laboratory		
Electrolytes, blood urea nitrogen/serum creatinine, glucose	Daily until stable, then 2–3 times/week	Every 1–3 months
Calcium, magnesium, phosphorus	Daily until stable, then 2–3 times/week	Every 1–3 months
Liver function tests	Weekly	Every 1–3 months
Trace elements, vitamins	If deficiency/toxicity suspected	If deficiency/toxicity suspected

EN, enteral nutrition.

- Mixing of liquid medications with EN formulations can cause physical incompatibilities that inhibit drug absorption and clog small-bore feeding tubes. Incompatibility is more common with formulations containing intact (vs. hydrolyzed) protein and medications formulated as acidic syrups. Mixing of liquid medications and EN formulations should be avoided whenever possible.
- The most significant drug–nutrient interactions result in reduced bioavailability and suboptimal pharmacologic effect (Table 59-6). Continuous feeding requires interruption for drug administration, and medications should be spaced between bolus feedings.

PARENTERAL NUTRITION

- PN provides macro- and micronutrients by central or peripheral venous access to meet specific nutritional requirements of the patient.
- PN should be considered when a patient cannot meet nutritional requirements enterally for an extended time period.

Components of Parenteral Nutrition

- Macronutrients (ie, water, protein, dextrose, and lipid) are used for energy (dextrose and lipid) and as structural substrates (protein and lipid).
- Protein is provided as crystalline amino acids (CAAs). When oxidized, 1 g of protein yields 4 calories (~17 J). Including the caloric contribution from protein in calorie calculations is controversial; therefore, PN calories can be calculated as either total or nonprotein calories.
- Standard CAA products contain a balanced profile of essential, semi-essential, and nonessential L-amino acids and are designed for patients with "normal" organ

TABLE 59-6	Select Medications with Special Considerations for Enteral Feeding Tube Administration	
Drug	**Interaction**	**Comments**
Phenytoin	Reduced bioavailability in the presence of tube feedings	To minimize interaction, holding tube feedings 1–2 hours before and after phenytoin has been suggested
	Possible phenytoin binding to calcium caseinates or protein hydrolysates in enteral feeding	Adjust tube-feeding rate to account for time held for phenytoin administration
		Monitor phenytoin serum concentration and clinical response closely
		Consider switching to IV phenytoin or an alternative-treatment option if unable to reach therapeutic serum concentration
Fluoroquinolones Tetracyclines	Potential for reduced bioavailability because of complexation of drug with divalent and trivalent cations found in enteral feeding	Consider holding tube feeding 1 hour before and after administration
		Avoid jejunal administration of ciprofloxacin
		Monitor clinical response
Warfarin	Decreased absorption of warfarin because of enteral feeding; therapeutic effect antagonized by vitamin K in enteral formulations	Adjust warfarin dose based on INR
		Anticipate need to increase warfarin dose when enteral feedings are started and decrease dose when enteral feedings are stopped
		Consider holding tube feeding 1 hour before and after administration
Omeprazole Lansoprazole	Administration via feeding tube complicated by acid-labile medication within delayed-release, base-labile granules	Granules become sticky when moistened with water and may occlude small-bore tubes
		Granules should be mixed with acidic liquid when given via a gastric feeding tube
		An oral liquid suspension can be extemporaneously prepared for administration via a feeding tube

INR, International normalized ratio.

function and nutritional requirements. Standard CAA products differ in protein concentration, total nitrogen, and electrolyte content but have similar effects on protein markers.

- The primary energy source in PN solutions is carbohydrate, usually as dextrose monohydrate, which is available in concentrations ranging from 5% to 70%. When oxidized, 1 g of hydrated dextrose provides 3.4 kcal (14.2 kJ).
- Commercially available intravenous lipid emulsions (IVLE) provide calories and essential fatty acids. These products differ in triglyceride source, fatty acid content, and essential fatty acid concentration.
- When oxidized, 1 g of fat yields 9 kcal (38 kJ). Because of the caloric contribution from egg phospholipid and glycerol, caloric content of IVLE is 1.1 kcal/mL (4.6 kJ/mL) for the 10%, 2 kcal/mL (8.4 kJ/mL) for the 20%, and 3 kcal/mL (12.6 kJ/mL) for the 30% emulsions.
- Essential fatty acid deficiency can be prevented by giving IVLE, 0.5–1 g/kg/day for neonates and infants and 100 g/wk for adults.

- IVLE 10% and 20% products can be administered by a central or peripheral vein, added directly to PN solution as a total nutrient admixture (TNA) or three-in-one system (lipids, protein, glucose, and additives), or co-infused with a CAA and dextrose solution, commonly referred to as a two-in-one solution. IVLE 30% is approved only for TNA preparation.
- Micronutrients (ie, vitamins, trace elements, and electrolytes) support metabolic activities for cellular homeostasis such as enzyme reactions, fluid balance, and regulation of electrophysiologic processes.
- Multivitamin products have been formulated to comply with guidelines for adults, children, and infants. These products contain 13 essential vitamins, including vitamin K.
- Requirements for trace elements depend on the patient's age and clinical condition.
- Chromium, copper, manganese, selenium, and zinc are considered essential and available as single- or multiple-entity products for addition to PN solutions.
- Sodium, potassium, calcium, magnesium, phosphorus, chloride, and acetate are necessary components of PN for maintenance of numerous cellular functions.
- Electrolyte requirements depend on the patient's age, disease state, organ function, previous and current drug therapy, nutrition status, and extrarenal losses.

Specifics of Parenteral Nutrition

- The patient's clinical condition determines whether PN is administered through a peripheral or central vein.
- Peripheral parenteral nutrition (PPN) candidates do not have large nutritional requirements, are not fluid restricted, and are expected to regain GI tract function within 10–14 days. Solutions for PPN have lower final concentrations of amino acid (3%–5%), dextrose (5%–10%), and micronutrients as compared with central parenteral nutrition (CPN).
- Primary advantages of PPN include a lower risk of infectious and technical complications.
- CPN is useful in patients who require PN for more than 7–14 days and who have large nutrient requirements, poor peripheral venous access, or fluctuating fluid requirements.
- CPN solutions are highly concentrated hypertonic solutions that must be administered through a large central vein. The choice of venous access site depends on factors including patient age and anatomy. Peripherally inserted central catheters (PICCs) are often used for both short- and long-term central venous access in acute or home care settings.
- Disadvantages include risks associated with catheter insertion, use, and care. Central venous access has a greater potential for infection.
- PN regimens for adults can be ordered on traditional paper order forms or by using standardized electronic order forms. Standardized order forms are popular because they help educate practitioners and foster cost-efficient nutrition support by minimizing errors in ordering, compounding, and administering.
- Pediatric PN regimens typically require an individualized approach because practice guidelines often recommend nutrient intake based on weight. Labeling should reflect "amount per kilogram per day."

EVALUATION OF THERAPEUTIC OUTCOMES

- Assessing the outcome of EN includes monitoring objective measures of body composition, protein and energy balance, and subjective outcome for physiologic muscle function and wound healing.
- Measures of disease-related morbidity include length of hospital stay, infectious complications, and patient's sense of well-being. Ultimately, the successful use of EN avoids the need for PN.
- Outcomes with PN are determined through routine assessment of the clinical condition of the patient, with a focus on nutritional and metabolic effects of the PN regimen.
- Biochemical and clinical parameters should be monitored routinely in patients receiving PN (**Figure 59-1**).

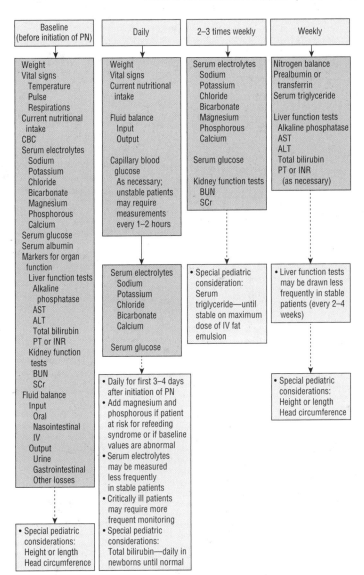

Baseline (before initiation of PN)	Daily	2–3 times weekly	Weekly

Weight
Vital signs
  Temperature
  Pulse
  Respirations
Current nutritional
  intake
CBC
Serum electrolytes
  Sodium
  Potassium
  Chloride
  Bicarbonate
  Magnesium
  Phosphorous
  Calcium
Serum glucose
Serum albumin
Markers for organ
  function
  Liver function tests
    Alkaline
      phosphatase
    AST
    ALT
    Total bilirubin
    PT or INR
  Kidney function
    tests
    BUN
    SCr
Fluid balance
  Input
    Oral
    Nasointestinal
    IV
  Output
    Urine
    Gastrointestinal
    Other losses
	Weight
	Vital signs
	Current nutritional
	  intake
	
	Fluid balance
	  Input
	  Output
	
	Capillary blood
	  glucose
	    As necessary;
	    unstable patients
	    may require
	    measurements
	    every 1–2 hours
		Serum electrolytes
		  Sodium
		  Potassium
		  Chloride
		  Bicarbonate
		  Magnesium
		  Phosphorous
		  Calcium
		
		Serum glucose
		
		Kidney function tests
		  BUN
		  SCr
			Nitrogen balance
			Prealbumin or
			  transferrin
			Serum triglyceride
			
			Liver function tests
			  Alkaline phosphatase
			  AST
			  ALT
			  Total bilirubin
			  PT or INR
			  (as necessary)

Serum electrolytes
  Sodium
  Potassium
  Chloride
  Bicarbonate
  Calcium

Serum glucose

• Special pediatric
  consideration:
  Serum
  triglyceride—until
  stable on maximum
  dose of IV fat
  emulsion

• Liver function tests
  may be drawn less
  frequently in stable
  patients (every 2–4
  weeks)

• Daily for first 3–4 days
  after initiation of PN
• Add magnesium and
  phosphorous if patient
  at risk for refeeding
  syndrome or if baseline
  values are abnormal
• Serum electrolytes
  may be measured
  less frequently
  in stable patients
• Critically ill patients
  may require more
  frequent monitoring
• Special pediatric
  considerations:
  Total bilirubin—daily in
  newborns until normal

• Special pediatric
  considerations:
  Height or length
  Head circumference

• Special pediatric
  considerations:
  Height or length
  Head circumference

(ALT, alanine aminotransferase; AST, aspartate aminotransferase; BUN, blood urea nitrogen;
CBC, complete blood cell count; INR, international normalized ratio; PN, parenteral nutrition;
PT, prothrombin time; SCr, serum creatinine)

FIGURE 59-1. Monitoring strategy for patients receiving parenteral nutrition (PN).

See Chapter 158, Assessment of Nutrition Status and Nutrition Requirements, authored by Katherine Hammond Chessman and Vanessa J. Kumpf; Chapter 159, Parenteral Nutrition, authored by Todd W. Mattox and Catherine M. Crill; and Chapter 160, Enteral Nutrition, authored by Vanessa J. Kumpf and Diana W. Mulherin, for a more detailed discussion of this topic.

CHAPTER

60

Breast Cancer

- *Breast cancer* is a malignancy originating from breast tissue. Disease confined to a localized breast lesion is referred to as *early, primary, localized,* or *curable.* Disease detected clinically or radiologically in sites distant from the breast is referred to as *advanced* or *metastatic breast cancer* (MBC), which is usually incurable.

EPIDEMIOLOGY

- Two variables most strongly associated with occurrence of breast cancer are gender and age. Additional risk factors include endocrine factors (eg, early menarche, nulliparity, late age at first birth, and hormone replacement therapy), genetic factors (eg, personal and family history, mutations of tumor suppresser genes [*BRCA1* and *BRCA2*]), and environmental and lifestyle factors (eg, radiation exposure, weight, height, and alcohol use).
- Breast cancer cells often spread undetected by contiguity, lymph channels, and through the blood early in the course of the disease, resulting in metastatic disease after local therapy. The most common metastatic sites are lymph nodes, skin, bone, liver, lungs, and brain.

PREVENTION OF BREAST CANCER

- Selective estrogen receptor modulators (SERMs) and aromatase inhibitors (AIs) are being studied for pharmacologic risk reduction of breast cancer.
- The most clinical information is available for the SERMs, **tamoxifen** and **raloxifene**, which reduce the rates of invasive breast cancer in women at high risk for developing the disease. Tamoxifen increased incidence of endometrial cancer and both agents increased thromboembolic events.
- **Exemestane** and **anastrozole** taken for 5 years significantly reduced the rates of invasive breast cancers in postmenopausal women with tolerable adverse events.
- Risk reduction strategies include mastectomy, oophorectomy, and pharmacologic agents. Clinical guidelines recommend the use of tamoxifen, raloxifene, anastrozole, or exemestane for postmenopausal women at high risk.

CLINICAL PRESENTATION

- A painless, palpable lump is the initial sign of breast cancer in most women. The typical malignant mass is solitary, unilateral, solid, hard, irregular, and nonmobile. Nipple changes are less commonly seen. More advanced cases present with prominent skin edema, redness, warmth, and induration.
- Symptoms of MBC depend on the site of metastases but may include bone pain, difficulty breathing, abdominal pain or enlargement, jaundice, and mental status changes.
- Many women first detect some breast abnormalities themselves, but it is increasingly common for breast cancer to be detected during routine screening mammography in asymptomatic women.

DIAGNOSIS

- Initial workup should include a careful history, physical examination of the breast, three-dimensional mammography, and, possibly, other breast imaging techniques, such as ultrasound and magnetic resonance imaging (MRI).
- Breast biopsy is indicated for a mammographic abnormality that suggests malignancy or for a palpable mass on physical examination.

STAGING

- Stage (anatomical extent of disease) is based on primary tumor extent and size (T_{1-4}), presence and extent of lymph node involvement (N_{1-3}), and presence or absence of distant metastases (M_{0-1}). The staging system determines prognosis and assists with treatment decisions. Simplistically stated, these stages may be represented as follows:
  - ✓ *Early breast cancer*
    - ❖ Stage 0: Carcinoma in situ or disease that has not invaded the basement membrane
    - ❖ Stage I: Small primary invasive tumor without lymph node involvement
    - ❖ Stage II: Involvement of regional lymph nodes
  - ✓ *Locally advanced breast cancer*
    - ❖ Stage III: Usually a large tumor with extensive nodal involvement in which the node or tumor is fixed to the chest wall
  - ✓ *Advanced or metastatic breast cancer*
    - ❖ Stage IV: Metastases in organs distant from the primary tumor
- Staging for breast cancer is separated into clinical and pathologic staging. Clinical stage is assigned before surgery and is based on physical examination (assessment of tumor size and presence of axillary lymph nodes), imaging (eg, mammography, ultrasonography), and pathologic examination of tissues (eg, biopsy results). Pathologic staging occurs after surgery and adds data from surgical exploration and resection.

PATHOLOGIC EVALUATION

- Development of malignancy is a multistep process involving preinvasive (or noninvasive) and invasive phases. The goal of treatment for noninvasive carcinomas is to prevent the development of invasive disease.
- Pathologic evaluation of breast lesions establishes the histologic diagnosis and confirms the presence or absence of prognostic factors.
- Most breast carcinomas are adenocarcinomas and are classified as ductal or lobular.

PROGNOSTIC FACTORS

- The ability to predict prognosis is used to design personalized treatment recommendations.
- Age at diagnosis and ethnicity can affect prognosis.
- Tumor size and presence and number of involved axillary lymph nodes are independent factors that influence the risk for breast cancer recurrence and subsequent metastatic disease. Other disease characteristics that provide prognostic information are histologic subtype, nuclear or histologic grade, lymphatic and vascular invasion, and proliferation indices.
- Hormone receptors (estrogen [ER] and progesterone [PR]) are not strong prognostic markers but are used clinically to predict response to endocrine therapy.
- *HER2* overexpression occurs in about 20%–30% of breast cancers and is associated with increased tumor aggressiveness, increased rates of recurrence, and increased rates of mortality.
- Genetic profiling tools provide additional prognostic information to aid in treatment decisions for subgroups of patients with otherwise favorable prognostic features.

TREATMENT

- <u>Goals of Treatment</u>: Adjuvant therapy for early and locally advanced breast cancer is administered with curative intent. Neoadjuvant therapy is given to eradicate micrometastatic disease, determine prognosis, and potentially conserve breast tissue for a better cosmetic result. Palliation is the desired therapeutic outcome in the treatment of MBC.
- Treatment is rapidly evolving. Specific information regarding the most promising interventions can be found only in the primary literature.
- Treatment can cause substantial toxicity, which differs depending on the individual agent, administration method, and combination regimen. A comprehensive review of toxicities is beyond the scope of this chapter; consult appropriate references.

EARLY BREAST CANCER (STAGE I AND II)

Local-Regional Therapy

- Surgery alone can cure most patients with in situ cancers, 70%–80% of stage I cancers, and approximately one-half of those with stage II cancers.
- Breast-conserving therapy (BCT) is an appropriate primary therapy for most women with stages I and II disease and is preferable because it provides survival rates equivalent to modified radical mastectomy. BCT includes removal of part of the breast, surgical evaluation of axillary lymph nodes, and radiation therapy (RT) to prevent local recurrence.
- RT is administered to the entire breast over 3–5 weeks to eradicate residual disease after BCT. Reddening and erythema of the breast tissue with subsequent shrinkage of total breast mass are minor complications associated with RT.
- Multiple sites of cancer within the breast and the inability to attain negative pathologic margins on the excised breast specimen are indications for mastectomy.
- Axillary lymph nodes should be sampled for staging and prognostic information. Lymphatic mapping with sentinel lymph node biopsy is a less invasive alternative to axillary dissection.

Systemic Adjuvant Therapy

- Systemic adjuvant therapy is the administration of systemic therapy following definitive local therapy (surgery, radiation, or both) when there is no evidence of metastatic disease but a high likelihood of disease recurrence. The goal of such therapy is cure.
- Administration of chemotherapy, endocrine therapy, targeted therapy, or some combination of these agents results in improved disease-free survival (DFS) and/or overall survival (OS) for high-risk patients in specific prognostic subgroups.
- The National Comprehensive Cancer Network (NCCN) practice guidelines are updated at least annually and should be consulted for treatment recommendations.
- Several multigene expression assays are commercially available as decision-support tools for adjuvant chemotherapy.

Adjuvant Chemotherapy

- Early administration of effective combination chemotherapy at a time of low tumor burden should increase the likelihood of cure and minimize emergence of drug-resistant tumor cell clones. Combination regimens have historically been more effective than single-agent chemotherapy (**Table 60-1**).
- Anthracycline-containing regimens (eg, **doxorubicin** and **epirubicin**) reduce the rate of recurrence and death as compared with regimens that contain **cyclophosphamide**, **methotrexate**, and **fluorouracil**.
- The addition of taxanes, **docetaxel** and **paclitaxel**, to adjuvant regimens comprised of the drugs listed above resulted in reduced risk of distant recurrence, any recurrence, and breast cancer mortality compared with a nontaxane regimen in node-positive breast cancer patients. The use of taxane-containing regimens in node-negative patients remains controversial.

TABLE 60-1	Selected Neo/Adjuvant Chemotherapy Regimens for Breast Cancer
Dose-Dense AC → Paclitaxel[a]	**AC → Paclitaxel**
Doxorubicin 60 mg/m^2 IV bolus, day 1	Doxorubicin 60 mg/m^2 IV, day 1
Cyclophosphamide 600 mg/m^2 IV, day 1	Cyclophosphamide 600 mg/m^2 IV, day 1
Repeat cycles every 14 days for 4 cycles (must be given with growth factor support)	Repeat cycles every 21 days for 4 cycles
Followed by paclitaxel 80 mg/m^2 IV weekly	Followed by paclitaxel 80 mg/m^2 IV weekly
Repeat cycles every 7 days for 12 cycles	Repeat cycles every 7 days for 12 cycles
TC[a]	**TAC**
Docetaxel 75 mg/m^2 IV, day 1	Docetaxel 75 mg/m^2 IV, day 1
Cyclophosphamide 600 mg/m^2 IV, day 1	Doxorubicin 50 mg/m^2 IV bolus, day 1
Repeat cycles every 21 days for 4 cycles	Cyclophosphamide 500 mg/m^2 IV, day 1 (doxorubicin should be given first)
Dose-Dense AC → Dose-Dense Paclitaxel[a]	Repeat cycles every 21 days for 6 cycles (must be given with growth factor support)
Doxorubicin 60 mg/m^2 IV bolus, day 1	
Cyclophosphamide 600 mg/m^2 IV, day 1	**CMF**
Repeat cycles every 14 days for 4 cycles (must be given with growth factor support)	Cyclophosphamide 100 mg/m^2 per day orally, days 1–14
Followed by paclitaxel 175 mg/m^2 IV over 3 hours	Methotrexate 40 mg/m^2 IV, days 1 and 8
Repeat cycles every 14 days for 4 cycles (must be given with growth factor support)	5-fluorouracil 600 mg/m^2 IV, days 1 and 8
	Repeat cycles every 28 days for 6 cycles

[a]Designated as a preferred regimen in the NCCN Breast Cancer Guidelines.
AC, Adriamycin (doxorubicin), Cytoxan (cyclophosphamide); CMF, cyclophosphamide, methotrexate, 5-fluorouracil; TAC, Taxotere (docetaxel), Adriamycin (doxorubicin), cyclophosphamide; TC, Taxotere (docetaxel), cyclophosphamide.

- Initiate chemotherapy within 12 weeks of surgical removal of the primary tumor. Optimal duration of adjuvant treatment is unknown but appears to be 12–24 weeks, depending on the regimen used.
- *Dose intensity* refers to the amount of drug administered per unit of time, which can be achieved by increasing dose, decreasing time between doses, or both. *Dose density* is one way of achieving dose intensity by decreasing time between treatment cycles.
- Dose-dense adjuvant regimens for node-positive breast cancer resulted in prolonged DFS and OS. No benefit in DFS or OS was shown for sequential versus concurrent chemotherapy, but sequential therapy appears to be less toxic.
- Concomitant or sequential administration of a taxane with an anthracycline-based regimen is standard of care in node-positive breast cancer.
- Dose increases in standard regimens appear to not be beneficial and may be harmful.
- Avoid dose reductions in standard regimens unless necessitated by severe toxicity.
- Short-term toxicities of adjuvant chemotherapy are generally well tolerated, especially with the availability of serotonin-antagonist and substance P/neurokinin 1–antagonist antiemetics and myeloid growth factors.
- Survival benefit for adjuvant chemotherapy in stage I and II breast cancer is modest. The absolute reduction in mortality at 10 years is 5% in node-negative and 10% in node-positive disease.

Adjuvant Biologic or Targeted Therapy

- **Trastuzumab** in combination with or sequentially after adjuvant chemotherapy is indicated in patients with early stage, *HER2*-positive breast cancer. The risk of recurrence was reduced up to 50% in clinical trials.

- Unanswered questions with the use of adjuvant trastuzumab include optimal concurrent chemotherapy, optimal dose, schedule and duration of therapy, and use of other concurrent therapeutic modalities.

Adjuvant Endocrine Therapy

- Tamoxifen, **toremifene**, oophorectomy, ovarian irradiation, luteinizing hormone–releasing hormone (LHRH) agonists, and AIs are hormonal therapies used in the treatment of primary or early-stage breast cancer. Tamoxifen was the gold standard adjuvant hormonal therapy for three decades and is generally considered the adjuvant hormonal therapy of choice for premenopausal women. It has both estrogenic and antiestrogenic properties, depending on the tissue and gene in question.
- Tamoxifen 20 mg daily, beginning soon after completing chemotherapy and continuing for 5 years, reduces the risk of recurrence and mortality. It is usually well tolerated; however, symptoms of estrogen withdrawal (hot flashes and vaginal bleeding) may occur but decrease in frequency and intensity over time. Tamoxifen reduces the risk of hip radius and spine fractures. It increases the risks of stroke, pulmonary embolism, deep vein thrombosis, and endometrial cancer, particularly in women age 50 years or older. Administration of tamoxifen for 10 years in patients with a higher risk of recurrence is supported by recent studies.
- Premenopausal women benefit from ovarian ablation with LHRH agonists (eg, **goserelin**) in the adjuvant setting, either with or without concurrent tamoxifen. Trials are ongoing to further define the role of LHRH agonists.
- Guidelines recommend incorporation of AIs into adjuvant hormonal therapy for postmenopausal, hormone-sensitive breast cancer. Experts believe that **anastrozole**, **letrozole**, and **exemestane** have similar antitumor efficacy and toxicity profiles. Adverse effects with AIs include bone loss/osteoporosis, hot flashes, myalgia/arthralgia, vaginal dryness/atrophy, mild headaches, and diarrhea.
- The optimal drug, dose, sequence, and duration of administration of AIs in the adjuvant setting are not known.

LOCALLY ADVANCED BREAST CANCER (STAGE III)

- Neoadjuvant or primary chemotherapy is the initial treatment of choice. Benefits include rendering inoperable tumors resectable and increasing the rate of BCT.
- Primary chemotherapy with an anthracycline- and taxane-containing regimen is recommended. The use of trastuzumab and **pertuzumab** with chemotherapy is appropriate for patients with *HER2*-positive tumors.
- Surgery followed by chemotherapy and adjuvant RT should be administered to minimize local recurrence.
- Cure is the primary goal of therapy for most patients with stage III disease.

METASTATIC BREAST CANCER (STAGE IV)

- Treatment of MBC with cytotoxic, endocrine, or targeted therapy often results in regression of disease, improvements in quality of life, and improved OS with the addition of some biologic or targeted therapies.
- The choice of therapy for MBC is based on the extent of disease involvement and the presence or absence of certain tumor or patient characteristics, as described below.
- The most important predictive factors are the presence of *HER2*, ER, and PR receptors in the primary or metastatic tumor tissue.
- Consider adding bone-modifying agents (eg, **pamidronate**, **zoledronic acid**, or **denosumab**) to treat breast cancer patients with metastases to the bone to decrease rates of skeletal-related events, such as fractures, spinal cord compression, and pain, and the need for radiation to the bones or surgery.

Biologic or Targeted Therapy

- Fifteen percent to 20% of patients with MBC overexpress *HER2*. Five anti-*HER2* agents are available in the United States: trastuzumab, **lapatinib**, **pertuzumab**, **ado-trastuzumab emtansine**, and **neratinib**.

- First-line therapy with a pertuzumab-trastuzumab-taxane combination is the preferred option for *HER2*-overexpressing MBC in patients who have not received pertuzumab in the neoadjuvant or adjuvant setting. Second-line *HER2*-targeted therapy for MBC depends on the specific agent given as first-line therapy. Subsequent therapy (third-line) for *HER2*-positive MBC is controversial.
- Consider combination endocrine plus *HER2*-directed therapy when chemotherapy is not tolerated or after achieving maximal response with chemotherapy-*HER2* therapy approach.
- All *HER2*-targeted therapies are cardiotoxic with the type of toxicity differing among agents. The incidence of heart failure is ~5% with single-agent trastuzumab and unacceptably high in combination with an anthracycline.
- *HER2*-targeted regimens for MBC are summarized in **Table 60-2**.

TABLE 60-2 Selected Regimens for *HER2*-Positive Metastatic Breast Cancer

Select Chemotherapy/Biologic Therapy Regimens

Docetaxel + Trastuzumab + Pertuzumab	**Ado-Trastuzumab Emtansine (T-DM1)**
Docetaxel 75 mg/m^2 IV day 1	Ado-Trastuzumab Emtansine 3.6 mg/kg IV day 1
Trastuzumab 8 mg/kg IV day 1 followed 21 days later by 6 mg/kg IV	Repeat cycle every 21 days
Pertuzumab 840 mg IV day 1 followed 21 days later by 420 mg IV	**Trastuzumab + Chemotherapy**
Repeat cycle every 21 days	Trastuzumab 8 mg/kg IV day 1 followed 21 days later by 6 mg/kg IV day 1
Paclitaxel + Trastuzumab + Pertuzumab	Repeat cycle every 21 days (for every 21 day chemotherapy)
Paclitaxel 80 mg/m^2 IV days 1, 8, 15	**OR**
Trastuzumab 8 mg/kg IV day 1 followed 21 days later by 6 mg/kg IV	Trastuzumab 4 mg/kg IV day 1 followed 7 days later by 2 mg/kg IV day 1
Pertuzumab 840 mg IV day 1 followed 21 days later by 420 mg IV	Repeat cycle weekly (for weekly chemotherapy)
Repeat cycle every 21 days	Chemotherapy may include any one of the following:
	Paclitaxel, docetaxel, protein-bound paclitaxel, capecitabine, vinorelbine, gemcitabine

Select Endocrine Therapy/Biologic Therapy Regimens

Trastuzumab + Lapatinib (± Aromatase Inhibitor)	**Trastuzumab (± Aromatase Inhibitor or Fulvestrant or Tamoxifen)**
Lapatinib 1000 mg orally daily continuously	Trastuzumab 8 mg/kg IV day 1 followed 21 days later by 6 mg/kg IV day 1
Trastuzumab 8 mg/kg IV day 1 followed 21 days later by 6 mg/kg IV	Repeat cycle every 21 days
Repeat cycle every 21 days	*(aromatase inhibitor, fulvestrant, and tamoxifen dosed per Table 60-3)*
(aromatase inhibitor dosed per Table 60-3)	
Lapatinib + Capecitabine	**Lapatinib + Aromatase Inhibitor**
Lapatinib 1250 mg orally daily continuously	Lapatinib 1500 mg orally daily continuously
Capecitabine 1000 mg/m^2 twice daily × 14 days	*(aromatase inhibitor dosed daily continuously per Table 60-3)*
Repeat cycle every 21 days	

- Other targeted agents including mTOR inhibitors (eg, **everolimus**) and cyclin-dependent kinases (CDK) (eg, **abemaciclib**, **palbociclib**, and **ribociclib**) are used in combination with endocrine agents to improve outcomes. To date, CDK inhibitors have improved progression-free survival in combination with AIs (as first-line therapy), fulvestrant (as first- and second-line therapy), and tamoxifen (as first-line therapy) (see Table 60-3).

Endocrine Therapy

- Consider endocrine therapy in combination with a targeted agent when feasible although this increases the risk of adverse events that require supportive management strategies. The choice of endocrine therapy is based on the menopausal status of the patient, prior therapies and previous response, duration of response, or disease-free interval.
- Endocrine therapy is the treatment of choice for patients who have hormone receptor-positive metastases in soft tissue, bone, pleura, or, if asymptomatic, viscera. Compared with chemotherapy, endocrine therapy has an equal probability of response and a better safety profile.
- Patients are sequentially treated with endocrine therapy until their tumors cease to respond, at which time chemotherapy can be given.
- No one endocrine therapy has clearly superior survival benefit. Choice of agent is based primarily on mechanism of action, toxicity, and patient preference (Table 60-3).
- AIs are generally first-line therapy in postmenopausal women. AIs reduce circulating and target organ estrogens by blocking peripheral conversion from an androgenic precursor, the primary source of estrogens in postmenopausal women. The third-generation AIs anastrozole, letrozole, and exemestane are more selective and have an improved toxicity profile. When compared with tamoxifen, patients receiving AIs had similar response rates as well as lower incidence of thromboembolic events and vaginal bleeding.
- Tamoxifen, an estrogen agonist/antagonist, is the preferred initial agent when metastases are present in premenopausal women except when metastases occur within 1 year of adjuvant tamoxifen. In addition to the side effects described for adjuvant therapy, tumor flare or hypercalcemia occurs in approximately 5% of patients with MBC.
- **Toremifene**, also an estrogen agonist/antagonist, has similar efficacy and tolerability as tamoxifen and is an alternative to tamoxifen in postmenopausal patients. **Fulvestrant** is a second-line intramuscular agent with similar efficacy and safety when compared with anastrozole or exemestane in patients who progressed on tamoxifen.
- Surgical or chemical ovarian ablation is considered by some experts to be the endocrine therapy of choice in premenopausal women and produces similar overall response rates as tamoxifen. Medical castration with an LHRH analogue (**goserelin**, **leuprolide**, or **triptorelin**) is a reversible alternative to surgery.
- Progestins are generally reserved for third-line therapy. They cause weight gain, fluid retention, and thromboembolic events.

Chemotherapy

- Chemotherapy is used as initial therapy for women with hormone receptor-negative tumors, with triple negative tumors, and after failure of endocrine/targeted therapy regimens.
- Chemotherapy is chosen based on overall efficacy, the risk of toxicity, performance status and presence of comorbidities in the patient, aggressiveness of disease (eg, indolent vs. visceral crisis), and patient preferences related to chemotherapy schedules, dosing route (eg, oral vs. intravenous), and frequency (eg, weekly vs. every 3 weeks).

TABLE 60-3	Therapies Used for Hormone Receptor–Positive Metastatic Breast Cancer				
Drug	Brand Name	Initial Dose	Usual Range	Special Population Dose	Comments
Aromatase Inhibitors: Nonsteroidal					
Anastrozole	Arimidex, generic	1 mg orally daily			
Letrozole	Femara, generic	2.5 mg orally daily		Caution in severe liver impairment[a]	
Aromatas Inhibitor: Steroidal					
Exemestane	Aromasin, generic	25 mg orally daily			Take after meals
Estrogen Agonists/Antagonists					
Tamoxifen	Nolvadex, generic	20 mg orally daily		See text regarding *CYP2D6*	
Toremifene	Fareston	60 mg orally daily			
Antiestrogen: SERD					
Fulvestrant	Faslodex	500 mg IM every 28 days (after loading days 1, 15, 29)	250–500 mg (see text for details)	Moderate liver impairment[a] administer 250 mg IM every 28 days (after loading days 1, 15, 29)	
LHRH Agonists					
Goserelin	Zoladex	3.6 mg SC every 28 days		Premenopausal women only	
Leuprolide	Lupron (IM), generic	3.75 mg IM every 28 days	Other formulations and doses are not used for breast cancer	Premenopausal women only	Not FDA approved for breast cancer; other formulations are administered differently
Triptorelin	Trelstar	3.75 mg IM every 28 days		Premenopausal women only	Not FDA-approved for breast cancer

Progestins

Megestrol acetate	Megace, generic	40 mg orally 4 times a day	80 mg twice daily also appropriate	Absorption may be increased when taken with food
Medroxyprogesterone	DepoProvera, generic	400 mg IM every week	400–1000 mg IM every week	May need to decrease dose in severe liver impairment[a]

Androgens

Fluoxymesterone	Androxy, generic	10 mg orally twice a day	10–20/day in divided doses	Avoid in severe renal or liver impairment[a]

Estrogens

Ethinyl estradiol	Multiple generics	1 mg orally 3 times a day	Lower doses not effective	Avoid in jaundice or "marked" liver disease	Take with food
Conjugated estrogens	Premarin	2.5 mg orally 3 times a day	Lower doses not effective	Avoid in jaundice or "marked" liver disease	Take with food

Biologic/Targeted Therapies

Abemaciclib (± Letrozole or Fulvestrant)	Verzenio	Single agent 200 mg orally twice a day continuously OR Combination 150 mg orally twice a day continuously	50–200 mg twice a day	Adjust dose for diarrhea, myelosuppression, and/or severe hepatic impairment. Monitor for hepatotoxicity and thromboembolism. Avoid concomitant strong inhibitors of CYP3A4 and moderate/strong inducers of CYP3A4	Do not split tablets

(Continued)

TABLE 60-3 Therapies Used for Hormone Receptor–Positive Metastatic Breast Cancer (*Continued*)

Drug	Brand Name	Initial Dose	Usual Range	Special Population Dose	Comments
Palbociclib (+ Letrozole or Fulvestrant)	Ibrance	125 mg orally daily × 21 days, followed by 7 days off, repeated every 28 days	75–125 mg daily	Adjust dose for myelosuppression and severe hepatic impairment. Monitor for nausea, diarrhea, and hepatotoxicity. Avoid concomitant strong inhibitors of *CYP3A4* and moderate/strong inducers of *CYP3A4*	Do not open capsules
Ribociclib (+ Letrozole or Fulvestrant)	Kisqali	600 mg orally daily × 21 days, followed by 7 days off, repeated every 28 days	200–600 mg daily	Adjust dose for myelosuppression and/or severe hepatic or renal impairment. Monitor for hepatotoxicity and QT prolongation. Avoid concomitant strong inhibitors of *CYP3A4* and moderate/strong inducers of *CYP3A4*	Do not split tablets
Everolimus (+ Exemestane or Fulvestrant or Tamoxifen)	Afinitor	10 mg orally daily	2.5–10 mg daily	Adjust dose in mild, moderate, and severe liver impairment; also monitor for myelosuppression, hyperglycemia, dyslipidemia, renal dysfunction. May need to adjust dose with concomitant *CYP3A4* inhibitors/inducers	Do not split tablets

aSevere liver impairment: Child–Pugh class C; moderate liver impairment: Child–Pugh class B; minor liver impairment: Child–Pugh class A.
IM, intramuscular; LHRH, luteinizing hormone-releasing hormone; SC, subcutaneous; SERD, selective estrogen receptor downregulator.

- Response rates are high with combination chemotherapy, but sequential use of single agents is an effective strategy and may be preferred due to decreased rates of adverse events. In the palliative setting, when efficacy is similar, the least toxic approach is preferred (Table 60-4).

TABLE 60-4	Select Chemotherapy Regimens for *HER2*-Negative Metastatic Breast Cancer

Single-Agent Chemotherapy

Paclitaxel	**Vinorelbine**
Paclitaxel 175 mg/m^2 IV over 3 hours	Vinorelbine 25 mg/m^2/week IV
Repeat cycles every 21 days	Repeat cycles every 7 days (adjust dose based on absolute neutrophil count; see product information)
or	
Paclitaxel 80 mg/m^2/week IV over 1 hour	
Repeat dose every 7 days	
Docetaxel	**Gemcitabine**
Docetaxel 60–100 mg/m^2 IV over 1 hour	Gemcitabine 800–1200 mg/m^2/week IV, days 1, 8, and 15
Repeat cycles every 21 days	Repeat cycles every 28 days (may need to hold day 15 dose based on blood counts)
Protein-Bound Paclitaxel	**Ixabepilone**
Protein-Bound Paclitaxel 260 mg/m^2 IV over 30 minutes	Ixabepilone 40 mg/m^2 IV over 3 hours
Repeat cycles every 21 days	Repeat cycles every 21 days
or	**Eribulin**
Protein-Bound Paclitaxel 100–125 mg/m^2 IV over 30 minutes on days 1, 8, and 15	Eribulin 1.4 mg/m^2/dose IV over 2–5 minutes on days 1 and 8
Repeat cycle every 28 days	Repeat dose every 21 days
Capecitabine	**Liposomal Doxorubicin**
Capecitabine 1000–1250 mg/m^2 orally twice daily for 14 days	Liposomal Doxorubicin 50 mg/m^2 IV over variable duration
Repeat cycles every 21 days	Repeat cycles every 28 days
Olaparib	**Talazoparib**
Olaparib tablet 300 mg orally twice daily	Talazoparib tablet 1 mg orally daily
Repeat cycles every 28 days	Repeat cycles every 28 days

Combination Chemotherapy Regimens

Gemcitabine + Carboplatin	**Paclitaxel + Gemcitabine**
Gemcitabine 1000 mg/m^2 IV, days 1 and 8	Paclitaxel 175 mg/m^2 IV over 3 hours, day 1
Carboplatin AUC 2 IV, days 1 and 8	Gemcitabine 1250 mg/m^2 IV days 1 and 8
Repeat cycles every 21 days	Repeat cycles every 21 days
Docetaxel + Capecitabine	**Paclitaxel + Bevacizumab**
Docetaxel 75 mg/m^2 IV over 1 hour, day 1	Paclitaxel 90 mg/m^2 IV over 1 hour, days 1, 8, and 15
Capecitabine 950 mg/m^2 orally twice daily for 14 days	Bevacizumab 10 mg/kg IV over 30–90 minutes, days 1 and 15
Repeat cycles every 21 days	Repeat cycles every 28 days

Adapted from NCCN Clinical Practice Guidelines in Oncology (NCCN Guidelines®). Breast Cancer V.3.2019. National Comprehensive Cancer Network, Inc. Accessed September 20, 2019.

- Treatment with sequential single agents is recommended over combination regimens unless the patient has rapidly progressive disease, life-threatening visceral disease, or the need for rapid symptom control.
- Most patients experience partial responses to chemotherapy, but complete disappearance of disease occurs in less than 10% of patients. The median duration of response is highly variable, ranging from 5–18 months; the median OS is 14–33 months. A specific chemotherapy regimen is continued until there is unequivocal evidence of progressive disease or intolerable side effects.
- **Anthracyclines** and **taxanes** produce response rates of 50% to 60% when used as first-line therapy for MBC. Single-agent **capecitabine**, **vinorelbine**, and **gemcitabine** have response rates of 20% to 25% when used after an anthracycline and a taxane.
- **Ixabepilone**, a microtubule stabilizing agent, is indicated as monotherapy or in combination with capecitabine. **Eribulin** is a second antimicrotubule agent approved as monotherapy in patients who have received at least two prior chemotherapy regimens for MBC.

Radiation Therapy

- Commonly used to treat painful bone metastases or other localized sites of disease, including brain and spinal cord lesions. Pain relief is seen in approximately 90% of patients who receive RT for painful bone metastases.

EVALUATION OF THERAPEUTIC OUTCOMES

EARLY BREAST CANCER

- The goal of adjuvant therapy, chemotherapy, biologic or targeted therapy, and endocrine therapy, in early-stage disease is cure. Adjuvant therapy is intended to eradicate micrometastases and thus cure the patient of breast cancer, which cannot be fully evaluated for years after initial diagnosis and treatment. In addition, because disease cannot be detected at the time adjuvant therapy is started, an assessment of disease response is not possible.
- Adjuvant chemotherapy can cause significant toxicity. Optimize supportive care measures such as antiemetics and growth factors to maintain dose intensity.

LOCALLY ADVANCED BREAST CANCER

- The goal of neoadjuvant chemotherapy in locally advanced breast cancer is cure. Complete pathologic response, determined at the time of surgery, is the desired end point.

METASTATIC BREAST CANCER

- Palliation is the therapeutic end point in the treatment of MBC. Optimizing quality of life is an important therapeutic end point. Valid and reliable tools are available for objective assessment of quality of life in patients with breast cancer.
- The least toxic therapies are used initially, with increasingly aggressive therapies applied in a sequential manner that does not significantly compromise quality of life.
- Tumor response is measured by changes in laboratory tests, diagnostic imaging, or physical signs or symptoms.

See Chapter 145, Breast Cancer, authored by Bonnie Lin Boster, Neelam K. Patel, and Laura Boehnke Michaud, for a more detailed discussion of this topic.

- *Colorectal cancer* (CRC) is a malignant neoplasm involving the colon, rectum, and anal canal.

PATHOPHYSIOLOGY

- Development of a colorectal neoplasm is a multistep process of genetic and phenotypic alterations of normal bowel epithelium structure and function leading to dysregulated cell growth, proliferation, and tumor development.
- Features of colorectal tumorigenesis include genomic instability, activation of oncogene pathways, mutational inactivation or silencing of tumor-suppressor genes, DNA mismatch repairs, and activation of growth factor pathways.
- Adenocarcinomas account for about 92% of tumors of the large intestine.

PREVENTION AND SCREENING

- *Primary prevention* is aimed at preventing CRC in an at-risk population. Trials with celecoxib in people with familial adenomatous polyposis (FAP) showed reduction in size and number of polyps after 6–9 months of treatment, but there is a lack of long-term benefit.
- *Secondary prevention* is aimed at preventing malignancy in a population that has already manifested an initial disease process. Secondary prevention includes procedures ranging from colonoscopic removal of precancerous polyps detected during screening colonoscopy to total colectomy for high-risk individuals (eg, FAP).
- Current US guidelines for average-risk individuals include annual occult fecal blood testing starting at age 50 years and examination of the colon every 5 or 10 years, depending on the procedure.

CLINICAL MANIFESTATIONS

- Signs and symptoms of CRC can be extremely varied, subtle, and nonspecific. Early-stage CRC is often asymptomatic and detected by screening procedures.
- Blood in the stool is the most common sign; however, any change in bowel habits, vague abdominal discomfort, or abdominal distention may be a warning sign. Less common signs and symptoms include nausea, vomiting, and, if anemia is severe, fatigue.
- Twenty percent of patients present with metastatic disease most commonly in the liver, lung, and bones.

DIAGNOSIS

- Perform a physical examination and obtain a careful personal and family history. Evaluate entire large bowel by colonoscopy.
- Obtain baseline laboratory tests: complete blood cell count, international normalized ratio (INR), activated partial thromboplastin time, liver and renal function tests, and serum carcinoembryonic antigen (CEA). Serum CEA serves as a marker for monitoring CRC response to treatment, but it is too insensitive and nonspecific to be used as a screening test for early-stage CRC.
- Radiographic imaging studies may include chest radiographs, bone scan, chest and abdominal computed tomography scans, positron emission tomography, ultrasonography, and magnetic resonance imaging.
- Determine CRC stage at diagnosis to predict prognosis and develop treatment options. Stage is based on size of the primary tumor (T_{1-4}), presence and extent of lymph node involvement (N_{0-2}), and presence or absence of distant metastases (M).

✓ Stage I disease involves tumor invasion of the submucosa (T_1) or muscularis propria (T_2) and negative lymph nodes.

✓ Stage II disease involves tumor invasion through the muscularis propria into pericolorectal tissues (T_3), or penetration to the surface of the visceral peritoneum (T_{4a}), or directly invades or is adherent to other organs or structures (T_{4b}), and negative lymph nodes.

✓ Stage III disease includes T_{1-4} and positive regional lymph nodes.

✓ Stage IV disease includes any T, any N, and distant metastasis.

PROGNOSIS

- Stage at diagnosis is the most important independent prognostic factor for survival and disease recurrence. Five-year relative survival is approximately 90% for those with localized tumor as compared with 14% for those with metastatic disease at diagnosis.
- Poor prognostic clinical factors at diagnosis include bowel obstruction or perforation, high preoperative CEA level, distant metastases, and location of the primary tumor in the rectum or rectosigmoid area.
- Molecular markers, particularly MSI, 18q/*DCC* mutation or LOH, *BRAF V600E* mutation, and *RAS* mutations are also associated with CRC prognosis.

TREATMENT

- <u>Goals of Treatment</u>: The goals include cure for stages I, II, and III; the intent is to eradicate micrometastatic disease after surgical resection. Most stage IV disease is incurable; palliative treatment is given to reduce symptoms, avoid disease-related complications, and prolong survival. Twenty to 30% of patients with metastatic disease may be cured if their metastases are resectable.
- Treatment modalities are surgery, radiation therapy (RT), chemotherapy, and biomodulators.

OPERABLE DISEASE

Surgery

- Complete surgical resection of the primary tumor with regional lymphadenectomy is a curative approach for patients with operable CRC.
- The preferred surgical procedure for rectal cancer is a total excision of the mesorectum that includes tissue containing perirectal fat and draining lymph nodes.
- Common complications of colorectal surgery include infection, anastomotic leakage, obstruction, adhesions, sexual dysfunction, and malabsorption syndromes.

Adjuvant Radiation Therapy

- Adjuvant RT has a limited role in colon cancer because most recurrences are extrapelvic and occur in the abdomen.

Adjuvant Chemotherapy for Colon Cancer

- Adjuvant therapy is administered after complete tumor resection to eliminate residual micrometastatic disease. Adjuvant therapy is not indicated for stage I CRC because more than 90% of patients are cured by surgical resection alone.
- Results of adjuvant chemotherapy studies in patients with stage II disease are conflicting. Despite a lack of consensus among practitioners, the approach to treatment of high-risk stages II and III disease is similar.
- Adjuvant chemotherapy is the standard of care for stage III colon cancer.
- Standard adjuvant regimens include a fluoropyrimidine (**fluorouracil** [with **leucovorin**] or **capecitabine**) as a single agent or in combination with **oxaliplatin**. Leucovorin enhances cytotoxic activity of fluorouracil.

- Administration method affects clinical activity and toxicity. In most common combination regimens, fluorouracil is administered by both IV bolus injection and by continuous IV infusion. No one treatment schedule is superior for overall patient survival.
- Continuous IV infusion of fluorouracil is generally well tolerated but is associated with palmar-plantar erythrodysesthesia (hand–foot syndrome) and stomatitis. IV bolus administration is associated with leukopenia, which is dose limiting and can be life threatening. Both administration methods are associated with a similar incidence of mucositis, diarrhea, nausea and vomiting, and alopecia.
- In rare cases, patients deficient in dihydropyrimidine dehydrogenase, responsible for the catabolism of fluorouracil, develop severe toxicity, including death, after fluorouracil administration.
- National guidelines recommend oxaliplatin-based regimens as the first-line option for patients with stage III colon cancer who can tolerate combination therapy. It is commonly administered with fluorouracil/leucovorin. Oxaliplatin is associated with both acute and persistent neuropathies, including rare, acute pharyngolaryngeal dysesthesia, neutropenia, and gastrointestinal (GI) toxicity.
- Selection of an adjuvant regimen (Table 61-1) is based on patient-specific factors, including performance status, comorbid conditions, and patient preference based on lifestyle factors. Age should also be considered as subset analysis of large clinical trials has shown that patients older than 70 years may not benefit from adjuvant oxaliplatin.
- Fluorouracil/leucovorin regimens currently have limited use but are acceptable options in patients who cannot receive oxaliplatin and are unable to tolerate oral capecitabine.

Adjuvant Therapy for Rectal Cancer

- Rectal cancer is more difficult to resect with wide margins, so local recurrences are more frequent than with colon cancer. Adjuvant RT plus chemotherapy is considered the standard of care for stages II and III rectal cancer.
- RT reduces the risk of local tumor recurrence in patients undergoing surgery for rectal cancer. RT is given prior to surgery to decrease tumor size, making it more resectable.
- Preoperative (neoadjuvant) chemoradiation shrinks rectal tumors prior to surgical resection, improving sphincter preservation. Preoperative infusional fluorouracil-based regimens or oral capecitabine plus RT are recommended. Patients should receive adjuvant chemotherapy following surgery to total 6 months of chemotherapy.

METASTATIC DISEASE

- Patients with metastatic colorectal cancer (MCRC) are considered to have resectable, potentially resectable, or unresectable metastatic disease. Surgery and RT are used to manage isolated sites of tumor. Chemotherapy is used for disseminated disease and is the primary treatment modality for unresectable MCRC.
- Tumor RAS (KRAS exon 2 and nonexon 2 and NRAS) and BRAF genotyping for mutation status and determination of tumor methylation or mismatch repair (MMR) or microsatellite instability (MSI) status (if not previously done) are recommended when metastatic disease is diagnosed to identify appropriate treatment options.

Resectable or Potentially Resectable MCRC

- Surgical resection of metastases with curative intent is the primary goal.
- Neoadjuvant or conversional chemotherapy is administered to increase complete resection rates with resectable and potentially resectable liver or lung lesions

TABLE 61-1	Chemotherapy Regimens for the Adjuvant Treatment of Colorectal Cancer	
Regimen	**Agents**	**Comments**
FOLFOX	Oxaliplatin 85 mg/m^2 IV on day 1 Leucovorin 400 mg/m^2 IV on day 1 Fluorouracil 400 mg/m^2 IV bolus, after leucovorin on day 1, then 1200 mg/m^2/day × 2 days CIV (total 2400 mg/m^2 over 46–48 hours) Repeat every 2 weeks × 24 weeks[a]	Preferred regimen for stage III colon and rectal cancers; common toxicities: sensory neuropathy, neutropenia.
CapeOx	Oxaliplatin 130 mg/m^2 IV day 1 Capecitabine 1000 mg/m^2 twice daily orally days 1 through 14 Each cycle lasts 3 weeks × 24 weeks[b]	Improved DFS in patients with stage III colon cancer compared to capecitabine alone or Roswell Park Regimen; common dose-limiting toxicities: neuropathies and hand–foot syndrome. A preferred regimen for adjuvant rectal therapy.
Capecitabine	Capecitabine 1000 mg/m^2–1250 mg/m^2 PO twice daily on days 1 through 14 Each cycle lasts 14 days and is repeated every 3 weeks × 24 weeks	Equivalent DFS as compared with the Mayo Clinic regimen with improved tolerability; hand–foot syndrome common, useful for patients without vascular access or who have difficulties with travel to infusion center
Roswell Park Regimen	Leucovorin 500 mg/m^2 IV day 1 over 2 hours Fluorouracil 500 mg/m^2 IV bolus 1 hour after leucovorin Repeat weekly for 6 of 8 weeks × 4 cycles	Leukopenia common dose-limiting toxicity; diarrhea, and stomatitis common
Simplified Biweekly	Leucovorin 400 mg/m^2 per day IV Fluorouracil 400 mg IV bolus, after leucovorin, then 1200 mg/m^2/day days 1 and 2 (total 2400 mg/m^2 over 46–48 hours) for 2 consecutive days Repeat every 2 weeks × 12 cycles	Hand–foot syndrome common

[a]Known as mFOLFOX6; survival benefit has not been demonstrated for patients 70 years and older.
[b]In patients with low-risk stage III (T1-3, any N), 3 months of CapeOX is noninferior to 6 months of CapeOX for DFS but this has not been proven for FOLFOX. In patients with high-risk stage III disease (T4, N1-2, or any T, N2), 3 months of FOLFOX is inferior to 6 months of FOLFOX for DFS, but this has not been proven with CapeOX. Grade 3 neuropathy is lower with 3 months of CapeOX or FOLFOX.
CIV, continuous intravenous infusion; DFS, disease-free survival; OS, overall survival; PO, by mouth.

(**Table 61-2**). Chemotherapy with or without biologic agents is given over 2–3 months pre-op. Adjuvant (postoperative) chemotherapy is administered to complete a total of 6 months of chemotherapy.

- Consider hepatic-directed therapy in addition to or as an alternative to surgical resection in patients with liver-only or liver-predominant MCRC. Hepatic artery infusion (HAI) delivers chemotherapy (eg, **floxuridine** and fluorouracil) through the hepatic artery directly into the liver. Tumor ablation uses radiofrequency ablation or micro-wave energy to generate heat to destroy tumor cells. Cryoablation is also used. These strategies are less successful than surgical interventions.

Unresectable MCRC

- Systemic chemotherapy palliates symptoms and improves survival in patients with unresectable disease. RT may control localized symptoms. Most MCRCs are incur-able; however, randomized trials confirm that chemotherapy prolongs life and improves quality of life.
- Consider goals of therapy, history of prior chemotherapy, tumor *RAS* and MMR/MSI mutation status, performance status/comorbidities, and risk of drug-related toxicities to determine a management strategy. Regimens are the same for metastatic cancer of the colon and rectum.
- Accepted initial chemotherapy regimens incorporate a fluoropyrimidine. Addition of **irinotecan** or oxaliplatin significantly improves response rates, progression-free survival, and median survival. Addition of the targeted anti-angiogenesis agent **bevacizumab** further improves response rate and survival (see **Table 61-2**).
- **Capecitabine** monotherapy is suitable for first-line therapy in patients not likely to tolerate IV chemotherapy. Available for oral administration, it is converted to fluoro-uracil and is a suitable replacement for infusional fluorouracil in combination with oxaliplatin (CapeOx).
- Bevacizumab is a humanized monoclonal antibody directed against vascular endo-thelial growth factor (VEGF). Addition of bevacizumab to fluorouracil-based regi-mens modestly increases PFS and OS as compared to chemotherapy alone.
  - ✓ Hypertension is common with bevacizumab and easily managed with oral antihy-pertensive agents. Other safety concerns include bleeding, thrombocytopenia, and proteinuria. GI perforation is a rare but potentially fatal complication necessitating prompt evaluation of abdominal pain associated with vomiting or constipation. Bevacizumab can interfere with wound healing; schedule surgery at least 6 weeks after the last dose of bevacizumab and wait at least 6–8 weeks after surgery to restart.
- **Cetuximab** and **panitumumab** are EGFR inhibitors used in patients with wild-type *RAS* and wild-type *BRAF* tumors in combination with FOLFOX or FOLFIRI or administered alone (**Table 61-2**). Patients with left-sided primary tumors have improved overall survival when treated with EGFR inhibitors while those with right-sided tumors (cecum to hepatic flexure) do not. Severe infusion reactions, including anaphylaxis, can occur with cetuximab (3%) and panitumumab (1%). Skin toxicity is also commonly seen and is not part of the infusion reaction. The presence of papulo-pustular skin rash has been shown to correlate with response and survival and most commonly occurs within 2 to 4 weeks of therapy initiation.
- Patients may receive consecutive regimens; the sequence of drugs appears less impor-tant than exposure to all active agents in the course of chemotherapy treatments.

METASTATIC DISEASE: SECOND-LINE AND SUBSEQUENT THERAPY

- The selection of second-line chemotherapy is primarily based on the type of and response to prior therapy received, site and extent of disease, and patient factors and treatment preferences. The optimal sequence of regimens has not been established (**Table 61-3**).
- Patients with wild-type *RAS* and wild-type *BRAF* tumors who experience progression on therapies that do not contain an EGFR inhibitor may benefit from the combina-tion of cetuximab or panitumumab and irinotecan or FOLFIRI.
- Patients with *BRAF V600E* mutations may benefit from a regimen containing iri-notecan and cetuximab with or without **vemurafenib** (a second-generation, select BRAF inhibitor) or a second regimen containing **dabrafenib** (a BRAF inhibitor), **trametinib** (a MEK inhibitor), and panitumumab (an EGFR inhibitor).
- Angiogenesis inhibitors including VEGF inhibitors bevacizumab, **ramucircumab**, and **ziv-aflibercept** and the oral multikinase inhibitor **regorafenib** may be used in patients with progressive disease.

TABLE 61-2 Initial Chemotherapeutic Regimens for Metastatic Colorectal Cancer[a]

Regimen	Agents	Major Dose-Limiting Toxicities	Comments
Patients Appropriate for Intensive Therapy with *RAS* Mutations			
FOLFOX ± bevacizumab	Oxaliplatin 85 mg/m² IV day 1 Leucovorin 400 mg/m² IV day 1 Fluorouracil 400 mg/m² IV bolus, after leucovorin day 1, then 1200 mg/m²/day × 2 days CIV (total 2400 mg/m² over 46–48 hours) Repeat every 2 weeks ± Bevacizumab 5 mg/kg IV day 1 before FOLFOX Repeat cycle every 2 weeks	FOLFOX: sensory neuropathy, neutropenia Bevacizumab: hypertension, thrombosis, proteinuria	Most commonly used first-line regimen
CapeOx ± bevacizumab	Oxaliplatin 130 mg/m² IV day 1 Capecitabine 1000 mg/m² orally twice a day, days 1–14 Repeat cycle every 3 weeks ± Bevacizumab 7.5 mg/kg IV day 1 Repeat cycle every 3 weeks	CapeOx: diarrhea, hand–foot syndrome, neuropathies Bevacizumab: hypertension, thrombosis, proteinuria	Reduced capecitabine dose better tolerated; patient must be able to be adherent and report side effects in a timely fashion
FOLFIRI ± bevacizumab	Irinotecan 180 mg/m² IV day 1 Leucovorin 400 mg/m² IV day 1 Fluorouracil 400 mg/m² IV bolus, after leucovorin day 1, then 1200 mg/m²/day × 2 days CIV (total 2400 mg/m² over 46–48 hours) ± Bevacizumab 5 mg/kg IV day prior to FOLFIRI Repeat cycle every 2 weeks	FOLFIRI: diarrhea, mucositis, neutropenia Bevacizumab: hypertension, thrombosis, proteinuria	May be preferred in patients who have preexisting neuropathy or those in which neuropathy may be debilitating to their line of work (eg, musician)

Regimen	Dosing	Side Effects	Comments
Fluorouracil/Leucovorin ± bevacizumab	See Table 61-1 for fluorouracil/leucovorin regimen options ± Bevacizumab 5 mg/kg IV day prior to fluorouracil and leucovorin Repeat cycle every 2 weeks	Fluorouracil/Leucovorin: diarrhea, hand–foot syndrome, mucositis, neutropenia Bevacizumab: hypertension, thrombosis, proteinuria	Infusional fluorouracil/leucovorin regimen preferred to bolus fluorouracil regimen. Infusional regimens tend to have more hand–foot syndrome and stomatitis and bolus regimens more neutropenia; weekly or bimonthly schedule of leucovorin plus fluorouracil (either bolus or continuous infusion) may be more convenient for the patient in terms of fewer scheduled clinic appointments, less interference with work schedules, and ease of dose adjustments based on toxicity
Capecitabine ± bevacizumab	Capecitabine 850–1250 mg/m² orally twice a day, days 1–14 ± Bevacizumab 7.5 mg/kg IV day 1 Repeat cycle every 3 weeks	Capecitabine: hand–foot syndrome, diarrhea, hyperbilirubinemia Bevacizumab: hypertension, thrombosis, proteinuria	May be preferred in those without a port or limited venous access; patient must be able to be adherent and report side effects in a timely fashion
FOLFOXIRI ± bevacizumab	Irinotecan 165 mg/m² IV day 1 prior to oxaliplatin Oxaliplatin 85 mg/m² IV day 1 prior to leucovorin day 1 Leucovorin 400 mg/m² IV day 1 prior to fluorouracil Fluorouracil 1200 mg/m²/day × 2 days CIV (total 2400 mg/m² over 48 hours)[b] Repeat cycle every 2 weeks ± Bevacizumab 5 mg/kg IV day 1 before FOLFOXIRI Repeat cycle every 2 weeks	FOLFOXIRI: neutropenia, diarrhea, stomatitis, peripheral neurotoxicity, thrombocytopenia Bevacizumab: hypertension, thrombosis, proteinuria	More neutropenia and peripheral neurotoxicity compared to FOLFIRI; often used in medically fit individuals with diffuse aggressive disease to palliate symptoms and as potential conversion therapy

(Continued)

TABLE 61-2 Initial Chemotherapeutic Regimens for Metastatic Colorectal Cancer[a] (*Continued*)

Regimen	Agents	Major Dose-Limiting Toxicities	Comments
Patients Appropriate for Intensive Therapy with *RAS* or *BRAF* Wild-Type and Left-Sided Tumors			
FOLFOX + cetuximab or panitumumab	FOLFOX regimen + cetuximab (400 mg/m² IV loading dose, then cetuximab 250 mg/m² IV weekly thereafter OR cetuximab 500 mg/m² IV every 2 weeks) IV before FOLFOX OR FOLFOX regimen + panitumumab 6 mg/kg IV day 1 before FOLFOX Repeat cycle every 2 weeks	FOLFOX: sensory neuropathy, neutropenia Cetuximab: papulopustular and follicular rash, asthenia, constipation, diarrhea, allergic reactions, hypomagnesemia Panitumumab: rash, diarrhea, hypomagnesemia	Only *RAS* wild-type tumor
FOLFIRI + cetuximab or panitumumab	FOLFIRI + cetuximab (400 mg/m² IV loading dose, then cetuximab 250 mg/m² IV weekly thereafter OR cetuximab 500 mg/m² IV every 2 weeks) IV before FOLFIRI OR FOLFIRI + panitumumab 6 mg/kg IV day 1 before FOLFIRI Repeat cycle every 2 weeks	FOLFIRI: diarrhea, mucositis, neutropenia Cetuximab: papulopustular and follicular rash, asthenia, constipation, diarrhea, allergic reactions, hypomagnesemia Panitumumab: rash, diarrhea, hypomagnesemia	Only *RAS* wild-type tumor; preferred for patients with preexisting neuropathy or those in which neuropathy may be debilitating to their line of work (eg, musician)

Patients NOT Appropriate for Intensive Therapy with *RAS* Mutations

Infusional fluorouracil + leucovorin ± bevacizumab	Fluorouracil 400 mg/m² IV bolus, after leucovorin on day 1, then 1200 mg/m²/day × 2 days CIV (total 2400 mg/m² over 46–48 hours) Repeat cycle every 2 weeks ± Bevacizumab 5 mg/kg IV day 1 prior to fluorouracil and leucovorin Repeat cycle every 2 weeks	Infusional fluorouracil/leucovorin: neutropenia, diarrhea Bevacizumab: hypertension, bleeding, proteinuria	Infusional fluorouracil/leucovorin regimen preferred to bolus fluorouracil regimen
Capecitabine ± bevacizumab	Capecitabine 850–1250 mg/m² orally twice a day, days 1–14 ± Bevacizumab 7.5 mg/kg IV day 1 Repeat cycle every 3 weeks	Capecitabine: hand–foot syndrome, diarrhea, hyperbilirubinemia Bevacizumab: hypertension, thrombosis, proteinuria	

Patients NOT Appropriate for Intensive Therapy with *RAS* or *BRAF* Wild-Type and Left-Sided Tumors

Cetuximab^c	Cetuximab 400 mg/m² IV loading dose, then cetuximab 250 mg/m² IV weekly thereafter OR Cetuximab 500 mg/m² IV every 2 weeks	Papulopustular and follicular rash, asthenia, constipation, diarrhea, allergic reactions, hypomagnesemia	Only *RAS* wild-type tumor
Panitumumab^c	6 mg/kg IV over 60 minutes every 2 weeks	Rash, hypomagnesemia, rare allergic reactions	Only *RAS* wild-type tumor

Patients NOT Appropriate for Intensive Therapy with dMMR or MSI-H

Nivolumab	3 mg/kg IV every 2 weeks or 240 mg IV every 2 weeks^d	Immune-mediated side effects (most common: skin, liver, kidney, gastrointestinal tract, lung, and endocrine systems)	Only in dMMR or MSI-H tumors. Patients should be closely monitored for side effects and report any side effects immediately as interruption of treatment or initiation of corticosteroids may be needed

(Continued)

TABLE 61-2 Initial Chemotherapeutic Regimens for Metastatic Colorectal Cancer[a] (*Continued*)

Regimen	Agents	Major Dose-Limiting Toxicities	Comments
Pembrolizumab	2 mg/kg IV every 2 weeks or 200 mg IV every 3 weeks[d]	Immune-mediated side effects (most common: skin, liver, kidney, gastrointestinal tract, lung, and endocrine systems)	Only in dMMR or MSI-H tumors. Patients should be closely monitored for side effects and report any side effects immediately as interruption of treatment or initiation of corticosteroids may be needed
Nivolumab + ipilimumab[c]	Nivolumab 3 mg/kg IV over 30 minutes and ipilimumab 1 mg/kg IV over 30 minutes every 3 weeks × 4 doses, then nivolumab 3 mg/kg IV or nivolumab 240 mg IV every 2 weeks[d]	Immune-mediated side effects (most common: skin, liver, kidney, gastrointestinal tract, lung, and endocrine systems)	Only in dMMR or MSI-H tumors. Patients should be closely monitored for side effects and report any side effects immediately as interruption of treatment or initiation of corticosteroids may be needed

[a]National Comprehensive Cancer Network (NCCN) Guideline recommendations for initial therapy. All recommendations are Category 2A unless otherwise noted. Category 2A: based upon lower-evidence, there is uniform NCCN consensus that the intervention is appropriate.

[b]Original dosing was 1600 mg/m²/day but it is recommended that US patients use this dose as they don't tolerate fluorouracil as well.

[c]NCCN Category 2B: based upon lower-evidence, there is NCCN consensus that the intervention is appropriate.

[d]Flat dosing is preferred.

TABLE 61-3	Second-line and Salvage Chemotherapy Regimens for Metastatic Colorectal Cancer[a]
Disease Progression with First-Line Regimen	**Comments**
First-Line Therapy: Oxaliplatin-Based Regimen +/- Bevacizumab (ie, FOLFOX, CapeOX)	
Second-line options	
1. FOLFIRI or irinotecan	Use with caution in patients with elevated bilirubin
2. FOLFIRI + bevacizumab or ziv-aflibercept or ramucirumab	Use with caution in patients with elevated bilirubin; bevacizumab is preferred antiangiogenic agent based on toxicity and cost
3. Irinotecan + bevacizumab or ziv-aflibercept or ramucirumab	Use with caution in patients with elevated bilirubin; bevacizumab is preferred antiangiogenic agent based on toxicity and cost
4. FOLFIRI + cetuximab or panitumumab	Only if *RAS* wild-type and *BRAF* wild-type; if neither previously given; use with caution in patients with elevated bilirubin
5. Irinotecan ± cetuximab or panitumumab	Only if *RAS* wild-type and *BRAF* wild-type; if neither previously given; use with caution in patients with elevated bilirubin
6. Irinotecan ± (cetuximab or panitumumab) + vemurafenib	Only if *RAS* wild-type and *BRAF V600E* mutation positive; use with caution in patients with elevated bilirubin
7. Dabrafenib + trametinib + (cetuximab or panitumumab)	Only if *BRAF V600E* mutation positive
8. Encorafenib + binimetinib + (cetuximab or panitumumab)	Only if *BRAF V600E* mutation positive
9. Nivolumab ± ipilimumab	Only if dMMR/MSI-H
10. Pembrolizumab	Only if dMMR/MSI-H
11. Trastuzumab + (pertuzumab or lapatinib)	Only if *HER2*-amplified and *RAS* wild-type
First-Line Therapy: Irinotecan-Based Regimen +/- Bevacizumab (ie, FOLFIRI)	
Second-line options	
1. FOLFOX or CapeOx ± bevacizumab	Bevacizumab FDA-approved to continue with second-line options
2. FOLFOX + cetuximab or panitumumab	Only if *RAS* wild-type and *BRAF* wild-type
3. Irinotecan + cetuximab or panitumumab	Only if *RAS* wild-type and *BRAF* wild-type; if neither previously given; use with caution in patients with elevated bilirubin
4. Irinotecan + (cetuximab or panitumumab) + vemurafenib	Only if *RAS* wild-type and *BRAF V600E* mutation positive; use with caution in patients with elevated bilirubin
5. Dabrafenib + trametinib + (cetuximab or panitumumab)	Only if *BRAF V600E* mutation positive
6. Encorafenib + binimetinib + (cetuximab or panitumumab)	Only if *BRAF V600E* mutation positive
7. Nivolumab ± ipilimumab	Only if dMMR/MSI-H
8. Pembrolizumab	Only if dMMR/MSI-H

(Continued)

TABLE 61-3	Second-line and Salvage Chemotherapy Regimens for Metastatic Colorectal Cancer[a] (Continued)
Disease Progression with First-Line Regimen	**Comments**
9. Trastuzumab + (pertuzumab or lapatinib)	Only if *HER2*-amplified and *RAS* wild-type
First-Line Therapy: Fluorouracil-Based Regimen +/- Bevacizumab (ie, Fluorouracil/ Leucovorin, Capecitabine)	
Second-line options	
1. FOLFOX or CapeOx ± bevacizumab	
2. FOLFIRI or irinotecan ± bevacizumab or ziv-aflibercept or ramucirumab	Bevacizumab has least toxicity and lower cost of antiangiogenic agents
3. Irinotecan + oxaliplatin (IROX) ± bevacizumab	Use with caution in patients with elevated bilirubin
4. Nivolumab ± ipilimumab	Only if dMMR/MSI-H
5. Pembrolizumab	Only if dMMR/MSI-H
6. Trastuzumab + (pertuzumab or lapatinib)	Only if *HER2*-amplified and *RAS* wild-type
Therapy After Second Progression or Third Progression	
1. Regorafenib	Used after progressed through all available regimens
2. Irinotecan ± cetuximab or panitumumab	Only if *RAS* wild-type and neither previously given; use with caution in patients with elevated bilirubin
3. Trifluridine/Tipiracil	Used after progressed through all available regimens
4. Nivolumab ± ipilimumab	Only if dMMR/MSI-H and not previously given
5. Pembrolizumab	Only if dMMR/MSI-H and not previously given
6. Trastuzumab + (pertuzumab or lapatinib)	Only if *HER2*-amplified and *RAS* wild-type
7. Clinical trial	If available and only if patient eligible
8. Best supportive care	Appropriate for patients who do not want to pursue treatment or quality of life is expected to decrease

[a]National Comprehensive Cancer Network (NCCN) Guideline recommendations for initial therapy. All recommendations are Category 2A unless otherwise noted. Category 2A: based upon lower-evidence, there is uniform NCCN consensus that the intervention is appropriate.
CapeOx, capecitabine plus oxaliplatin; dMMR, DNA mismatch repair deficiency; FOLFIRI, fluorouracil plus leucovorin plus irinotecan; FOLFOX, fluorouracil plus leucovorin plus oxaliplatin; MSI-H, high microsatellite instability.

- *HER2*, a member of the same kinase family as EGFR, is rarely overexpressed in CRC; however, it is more common in those with *RAS* and *BRAF* wild-type tumors. *HER2* inhibitor therapy can be an option for those with *HER2* overexpression when other options have failed.
- **Pembrolizumab**, a humanized, IgG4 monoclonal antibody that binds to PD-L1 with high affinity, is effective in MCRC patients with dMMR who have progressed through 2–4 other regimens. **Nivolumab**, another humanized IgG4 monoclonal antibody PD-1 inhibitor, has also been evaluated with or without **ipilimumab** in patients with MCRC who have dMMR/MSI-H tumors.

EVALUATION OF THERAPEUTIC OUTCOMES

- Goals of monitoring are to evaluate benefit of treatment and detect recurrence.
- Patients who undergo curative surgical resection, with or without adjuvant therapy, require routine follow-up. Consult practice guidelines for specifics.
- Evaluate patients for anticipated side effects such as loose stools or diarrhea, nausea or vomiting, mouth sores, fatigue, and fever.
- Patients should be closely monitored for side effects that require prompt intervention, such as irinotecan-induced diarrhea, bevacizumab-induced GI perforation, hypertension and proteinuria, oxaliplatin-induced neuropathy, and cetuximab- and panitumumab-induced skin rash.
- Less than one-half of patients develop symptoms of recurrence, such as pain syndromes, changes in bowel habits, rectal or vaginal bleeding, pelvic masses, anorexia, and weight loss. Recurrences in asymptomatic patients can be detected because of increased serum CEA levels.
- Monitor quality-of-life indices, especially in patients with metastatic disease.

See Chapter 147, Colorectal Cancer, authored by Lisa M. Holle, Jessica M. Clement, and Lisa E. Davis, for a more detailed discussion of this topic.

62 Lung Cancer

- *Lung cancer* is a solid tumor originating from the bronchial epithelial cells. This chapter distinguishes between nonsmall cell lung cancer (NSCLC) and small cell lung cancer (SCLC) because they have different natural histories and responses to therapy.

PATHOPHYSIOLOGY

- Lung carcinomas arise from normal bronchial epithelial cells that have acquired multiple genetic lesions and are capable of expressing a variety of phenotypes.
- Activation of proto-oncogenes, inhibition or mutation of tumor suppressor genes, and production of autocrine (self-stimulatory) growth factors contribute to cellular proliferation and malignant transformation. Molecular changes, such as overexpression of c-KIT in SCLC and epidermal growth factor receptor (EGFR) in NSCLC, also affect disease prognosis and response to therapy.
- Smoking is responsible for approximately 80% of lung cancer cases. Other risk factors are exposure to environmental respiratory carcinogens (eg, asbestos, benzene, and arsenic), genetic risk factors, and history of other lung diseases (eg, chronic obstructive pulmonary disease [COPD] and asthma).
- The major cell types are SCLC (~15% of all lung cancers), adenocarcinoma (~50%), squamous cell carcinoma (<30%), and large cell carcinoma. The last three types are grouped together and referred to as NSCLC.

CLINICAL PRESENTATION

- The most common initial signs and symptoms are cough, dyspnea, chest pain, or discomfort, with or without hemoptysis. Many patients also exhibit systemic symptoms such as anorexia, weight loss, and fatigue.
- Disseminated disease can cause neurologic deficits from CNS metastases, bone pain, or pathologic fractures secondary to bone metastases, or liver dysfunction from hepatic involvement.
- Paraneoplastic syndromes are signs and symptoms that occur at sites away from the primary tumor or its metastases and are not associated with direct tumor involvement. They occur more frequently with lung cancer than any other tumor, and more frequently with SCLC than with NSCLC.

DIAGNOSIS

- Chest radiographs, endobronchial ultrasound, computed tomography (CT) scan, and positron emission tomography (PET) scan are the most valuable diagnostic tests. Integrated CT–PET technology appears to improve diagnostic accuracy in staging NSCLC over CT or PET alone.
- Pathologic confirmation is established by examination of sputum cytology and/or tumor biopsy by bronchoscopy, mediastinoscopy, percutaneous needle biopsy, or open-lung biopsy.
- All patients must have a thorough history and physical examination to detect signs and symptoms of the primary tumor, regional spread of the tumor, distant metastases, paraneoplastic syndromes, and ability to withstand aggressive surgery or chemotherapy.

STAGING

- The World Health Organization has established a TNM staging classification for NSCLC based on primary tumor size and extent (T), regional lymph node involvement (N), and presence or absence of distant metastases (M).
- A simpler system is commonly used to compare therapeutic modalities. Stage I includes tumors confined to the lung without lymphatic spread, stage II includes large tumors with ipsilateral peribronchial or hilar lymph node involvement, stage III includes other lymph node and regional involvement, and stage IV includes any tumor with distant metastases.
- A two-stage classification is widely used for SCLC. Limited disease is confined to one hemithorax and can be encompassed by a single radiation port. All other disease is classified as extensive.

TREATMENT

NONSMALL CELL LUNG CANCER

- <u>Goals of Treatment</u>: Definitive cure is the desired outcome with early-stage disease. Prolongation of survival is desired in patients with advanced-stage disease.
- The stage of NSCLC and the patient's comorbidities and performance status (ie, the ability to perform activities of daily living) determine which treatment modalities will be used. The intent of treatment—curative or palliative—influences the aggressiveness of therapy.

Recommendations for Chemotherapy, Radiation Therapy, and Surgery

- Genetic testing of tumors should be performed at the time of diagnosis in all patients, including those with localized disease.
- Local disease (stages IA and IB) is associated with a favorable prognosis. Surgery is the mainstay of treatment and may be used alone or in some situations with radiation therapy (RT) and/or chemotherapy.
- Stage IIA and IIB diseases are primarily treated with surgery followed by adjuvant chemotherapy (Table 62-1). Platinum-based regimens are preferred and should be given concurrently rather than sequentially with RT. Chemoradiotherapy is recommended for medically inoperable patients who can tolerate combined modality therapy.
- Optimal outcomes for stage III disease are achieved with multimodality therapy. Patients with operable disease should be considered for surgery preceded or followed by systemic chemotherapy. Current recommendations for patients with resectable stage IIIA disease include chemotherapy followed by surgery or radiation, depending on individual patient and tumor features.
- Patients with stage IIIA disease who are not surgical candidates or have a tumor that cannot be resected, and nearly all stage IIIB patients, are typically treated with both an active platinum-containing regimen and concurrent radiotherapy. Patients who respond to chemotherapy should then receive maintenance therapy with **durvalumab**, a programmed death ligand-1 (PD-L1) inhibitor that significantly improves 2-year survival and median progression-free survival (PFS).
- Patients with stage III disease who are not candidates for radiation are treated like those with stage IV disease. Chemotherapy is administered to palliate symptoms, improve quality of life, and increase duration of survival. Therapy depends on patient-specific factors (performance status is most important) and tumor characteristics.
- Three pathways have been identified for advanced NSCLC: (1) immune sensitive (PD-L1+), (2) targetable genetic mutation-driven, which is further divided based on the mutation (EGFR, ALK, BRAF, NTRK, and ROS1), and (3) nonbiomarker-driven therapy treatment, which is further classified as squamous histology or nonsquamous histology due to drug toxicity and efficacy. Select regimens for each group are outlined in Table 62-2.

TABLE 62-1	Common Chemotherapy Regimens Used in the Adjuvant Treatment of Nonsmall Cell Lung Cancer	
Regimen	**Drugs and Doses**	**Frequency and Number of Cycles**
Cisplatin/ Etoposide	Cisplatin 100 mg/m² IV day 1	Every 28 days for 4 cycles
	Etoposide 100 mg/m² IV daily on days 1, 2, and 3	
Cisplatin/ Vinorelbine	Cisplatin 50 mg/m² IV days 1 and 8	Every 28 days for 4 cycles
	Vinorelbine 25 mg/m² IV days 1, 8, 15, and 22	
	Cisplatin 100 mg/m² IV day 1	Every 28 days for 4 cycles
	Vinorelbine 30 mg/m² IV days 1, 8, 15, and 22	
Carboplatin/ Paclitaxel	Carboplatin AUC 6 IV day 1	Every 21 days for 4 cycles
	Paclitaxel 200 mg/m² IV day 1	
Cisplatin/ Pemetrexed	Cisplatin 75 mg/m² IV day 1	Every 21 days for 4 cycles (for nonsquamous histology only)
	Pemetrexed 500 mg/m² IV day 1	

- First-line therapy for patients with NSCLC with PD-L1+ tumors is **pembrolizumab**, an immune checkpoint inhibitor that binds to the programmed death-1 (PD-1) receptor on T cells. As compared with a platinum doublet chemotherapy regimen, pembrolizumab demonstrated increased median PFS. Use chemotherapy as second-line therapy after failing pembrolizumab.
- Treatment options for patients with advanced lung cancer and a targetable genetic driver mutation include:
  (1) Patients with a tumor that harbors a *mutation in the EGFR receptor* should receive first-line EGFR tyrosine kinase inhibitor therapy with **osimertinib**. Osimertinib, a third-generation EGFR tyrosine kinase inhibitor, shows the most impressive activity in patients with EGFR-positive tumors. In addition to significantly longer PFS, osimertinib has improved CNS penetration resulting in improved CNS response rates and less CNS disease as the cause of progression. First- and second-generation EGFR tyrosine kinase inhibitors include **afatinib**, **erlotinib**, or **gefitinib**. A meta-analysis suggests that these three agents have similar PFS results and response rates about two times higher than chemotherapy. Subsequent therapy after progression during treatment with an EGFR inhibitor depends on initial treatment and further genetic evaluation of the tumor. Most patients will proceed to a platinum doublet chemotherapy with or without an immunotherapy agent.
  (2) Patients with a tumor with an *ALK rearrangement* should receive initial treatment with an ALK inhibitor, with a preference for **alectinib**. Other ALK inhibitors approved for first-line therapy are **ceritinib** and **crizotinib**. **Lorlatinib** was recently approved as second-line therapy after failure on a first-line ALK inhibitor.
  (3) Patients with a tumor with a *mutation in ROS1* should be treated with **crizotinib**. Patients should receive lorlatinib as second-line therapy.
  (4) Patients with a tumor with the *BRAF V600E mutation* should receive combination therapy with two kinase inhibitors, **trametinib** and **dabrafenib**.
  (5) Patients with a tumor with a *neurotrophic receptor kinases (NTRK) gene fusion* should receive **larotrectinib**.
- Combination chemotherapy is the preferred option for patients with metastatic NSCLC who are not candidates for targeted therapies or have progressed despite

TABLE 62-2 Selected Regimens Used to Treat Advanced-Stage Nonsmall cell Lung Cancer

| | Nonbiomarker Driven | | | | EGFR Mutation Positive | | ALK Rearrangement Positive | |
| | Nonsquamous | | Squamous Cell | | | | | |
Place in Therapy	Regimen	Drugs, Doses, Frequency	Regimen	Drugs, Doses, Frequency	Regimen	Drugs, Doses, Frequency	Regimen	Drugs, Doses, Frequency
First line	Carboplatin/ Paclitaxel/ Bevacizumab	Carboplatin AUC 6 IV on day 1 Paclitaxel 200 mg/m² IV on day 1 Bevacizumab 15 mg/kg IV on day 1 Repeat cycle every 3 weeks × 6 cycles—bevacizumab maintenance until progression	Gemcitabine/ Cisplatin	Gemcitabine 1250 mg/m² IV on days 1 and 8 Cisplatin 75 mg/m² IV on day 1 Repeat cycle every 21 days × 6 cycles	Erlotinib	Erlotinib 150 mg (one 150 mg capsule) daily on an empty stomach	Crizotinib	Crizotinib 250 mg (one 250 mg capsule) twice daily without regard to meals
	Carboplatin/ Pemetrexed	Carboplatin AUC 5 IV on day 1 Pemetrexed 500 mg/m² IV on day 1 Repeat cycle every 3 weeks	Carboplatin/ Paclitaxel/ Pembrolizumab	Carboplatin AUC 6 IV on day 1 Paclitaxel 200 mg/m² IV on day 1 or nab-paclitaxel 100 mg/m² IV on days 1, 8, 15 Pembrolizumab 200 mg IV on day 1	Afatinib	Afatinib 40 mg (one 40 mg tablet) daily on an empty stomach	Alectinib	Alectinib 600 mg (four 150 mg capsules) twice daily with food

(Continued)

TABLE 62-2 Selected Regimens Used to Treat Advanced-Stage Nonsmall Cell Lung Cancer *(Continued)*

| Place in Therapy | Nonbiomarker Driven | | | | EGFR Mutation Positive | | ALK Rearrangement Positive | |
| | Nonsquamous | | Squamous Cell | | | | | |
	Regimen	Drugs, Doses, Frequency	Regimen	Drugs, Doses, Frequency	Regimen	Drugs, Doses, Frequency	Regimen	Drugs, Doses, Frequency
				Repeat cycle every 3 weeks × 4 cycles—pembrolizumab maintenance up to 31 additional doses or until progression	Osimertinib	Osimertinib 80 mg (one 80 mg tablet) daily without regard to meals		
	Platinum/ Pemetrexed/ Pembrolizumab	Cisplatin 75 mg/m² or carboplatin AUC 5 IV on day 1 Pemetrexed 500 mg/m² IV on day 1 Pembrolizumab 200 mg IV on day 1 Repeat cycle every 3 weeks × 4 cycles—pembrolizumab maintenance up to 31 additional doses or until progression						

(Continued)

Carboplatin/ Paclitaxel/ Bevacizumab/ Atezolizumab	Carboplatin AUC 6 IV on day 1 Paclitaxel 200 mg/m² IV on day 1 Bevacizumab 15 mg/kg IV on day 1 Atezolizumab 1200 mg IV on day 1 Repeat cycle every 3 weeks × 4 or 6 cycles—atezolizumab and bevacizumab maintenance until progression				
Second line	Docetaxel/ Ramucirumab	Docetaxel 75 mg/m² IV day 1 Ramucirumab 10 mg/kg IV day 1 Repeat every 21 days	Osimertinib (if patient has not previously received)	Osimertinib 80 mg (one 80 mg tablet) daily without regard to meals	
	Nivolumab	Nivolumab 3 mg/kg IV day 1 Repeat every 2 weeks	Docetaxel/ Ramucirumab	Docetaxel 75 mg/ m² IV day 1 Ramucirumab 10 mg/kg IV day 1 Repeat every 21 days	
	Pembrolizumab	Pembrolizumab 2 mg/kg IV day 1 Repeat every 3 weeks	Nivolumab	Nivolumab 3 mg/kg IV day 1 Repeat every 2 weeks	
			Pembrolizumab	Pembrolizumab 2 mg/kg IV day 1 Repeat every 3 weeks	
			Brigatinib	Brigatinib 90 mg (one 90 mg tablet) daily for 7 days, then 180 mg (one 180 mg tablet) daily. Take without regards to meals	

targeted therapies and are candidates for further therapy. Platinum-based chemotherapy doublets consisting of **cisplatin** or **carboplatin** combined with **paclitaxel** (or **nab-paclitaxel**), **docetaxel**, **gemcitabine**, **pemetrexed**, or **vinorelbine** are considered standard care and equally effective in nonsquamous NSCLC.

- Guidelines recommend adding **bevacizumab**, a recombinant, humanized monoclonal antibody that neutralizes vascular endothelial growth factor (VEGF) to chemotherapy for patients with advanced NSCLC of nonsquamous cell histology, no history of recent significant hemoptysis, no CNS metastasis, and not receiving therapeutic anticoagulation.

- The most recent treatment advance for metastatic NSCLC is the addition of PD-1 (nivolumab, pembrolizumab) or PD-L1 (**atezolizumab**) inhibitors, regardless of the level of PD-L1 expression. Clinical guidelines recommend the combination of PD-1 or PD-L1 directed therapy and chemotherapy as first-line therapy for patients with nonbiomarker-driven NSCLC.

- Maintenance therapy is the ongoing use of one or more agents after a positive tumor response to four to six cycles of an initial chemotherapy regimen until disease progression. Continuation or switch maintenance therapy improves survival of NSCLC patients with nonsquamous histology. In continuation maintenance therapy, patients receive ongoing treatment with at least one of the agents used in the initial chemotherapy regimen. Alternatively, switch maintenance therapy starts a new agent not included in the initial regimen. Pemetrexed is the most established maintenance chemotherapy option.

- Monotherapy with nivolumab, pembrolizumab, atezolizumab, docetaxel, or pemetrexed is the most commonly considered option for second-line therapy in patients with a good performance status who progress during or after first-line chemotherapy. Nivolumab, pembrolizumab, and atezolizumab are options in the second-line setting for patients who have not previously received one of the drugs in the class.

- The efficacy of docetaxel has recently been improved with the addition of **ramucirumab** which binds to VEGF. Guidelines list nivolumab, pembrolizumab, or atezolizumab as preferred second-line regimens but docetaxel with or without ramucirumab has emerged as a standard second-line option because immunotherapy and pemetrexed are commonly used as first-line and maintenance therapy.

SMALL CELL LUNG CANCER

- <u>Goals of Treatment</u>: The goals include cure or prolonged survival, which requires aggressive combination chemotherapy.

Limited Disease

- Use of surgery in SCLC is limited to solitary nodules without evidence of metastasis to lymph nodes.
- SCLC is very radiosensitive; radiation is preferred for treatment of local disease over surgery. Radiation is given concurrently with chemotherapy, and the regimen of choice is **etoposide** and cisplatin (EP regimen; see **Table 62-3**).
- Radiotherapy is used to prevent and treat brain metastases, a frequent occurrence with SCLC. Prophylactic cranial irradiation (PCI) is used in patients with limited or extensive disease to reduce the risk of brain metastases.

Extensive Disease

- The EP regimen is the regimen of choice to treat extensive-stage SCLC, with **irinotecan** and cisplatin as an acceptable alternative. The addition of the PD-L1 inhibitor atezolizumab to carboplatin/etoposide improved median PFS and overall survival and is the first significant improvement over standard platinum plus etoposide chemotherapy.
- Concurrent radiotherapy is not routinely used in extensive disease.

TABLE 62-3 Chemotherapy Regimens Used in the Treatment of SCLC

	Regimen	Drugs and Doses
First line	Etoposide/Cisplatin (EP)	Cisplatin 75 mg/m² IV on day 1
		Etoposide 100 mg/m² IV on days 1–3; repeat cycle every 3 weeks for 4–6 cycles
		or
		Cisplatin 60 mg/m² IV on day 1
		Etoposide 120 mg/m² IV on days 1–3; repeat cycle every 3 weeks for 4–6 cycles
	Etoposide/Carboplatin (EC)	Carboplatin AUC 5–6 IV on day 1
		Etoposide 120 mg/m² IV on days 1–3; repeat cycle every 3 weeks for 4–6 cycles
	Cisplatin/Irinotecan (IP)	Cisplatin 60 mg/m² IV on day 1
		Irinotecan 60 mg/m² IV on days 1, 8, 15; repeat cycle every 4 weeks for 4–6 cycles
		or
		Cisplatin 30 mg/m² IV on day 1
		Irinotecan 65 mg/m² IV on days 1 and 8; repeat cycle every 3 weeks for 4–6 cycles
	EC + atezolizumab[a]	Carboplatin AUC 5 IV on day 1
		Etoposide 100 mg/m² IV on days 1–3
		Atezolizumab 1200 mg IV on day 1; repeat cycle every 3 weeks for 4 cycles followed by
		Atezolizumab 1200 mg every 3 weeks as maintenance
Second line	Topotecan	Topotecan 1.5 mg/m²/day IV days 1–5; repeat every 3 weeks
	Nivolumab	Nivolumab 3 mg/kg IV; repeat every 2 weeks

[a]Extensive stage only.

Relapsed Disease

- Relapsed SCLC is usually less sensitive to chemotherapy. **Topotecan** (IV and oral) is considered the second-line treatment of choice, but other agents should be considered because of its modest efficacy. If relapse occurs more than 3 months after first-line chemotherapy, national guidelines recommend single-agent topotecan, gemcitabine, irinotecan, paclitaxel, docetaxel, oral etoposide, **temozolomide**, and vinorelbine; CAV regimen (**cyclophosphamide, doxorubicin,** and **vincristine**); and participation in a clinical trial.
- Nivolumab was recently approved for relapsed SCLC.
- SCLC that recurs within 3 months of first-line chemotherapy is considered refractory to chemotherapy and unlikely to respond to a second-line regimen. Patients should receive best supportive care or be enrolled in a clinical trial.

EVALUATION OF THERAPEUTIC OUTCOMES

- Evaluate tumor response to chemotherapy for NSCLC at the end of the second or third cycle and at the end of every second cycle thereafter. Patients with stable disease, objective response, or measurable decrease in tumor size should continue treatment until four to six cycles have been administered. Consider maintenance therapy with pemetrexed in responding patients with nonsquamous histology.

- Evaluate efficacy of first-line therapy for SCLC after two or three cycles of chemotherapy. If there is no response or progressive disease, therapy can be discontinued or changed to a non–cross-resistant regimen. If responsive to chemotherapy, the induction regimen should be administered for four to six cycles. Responding patients benefit from the addition of PCI following initial therapy.
- Intensive therapeutic monitoring is required for all patients with lung cancer to avoid drug-related and radiotherapy-related toxicities. These patients frequently have numerous concurrent medical problems requiring close attention.
- References should be consulted for management of common toxicities associated with the aggressive chemotherapy regimens used for lung cancer.

See Chapter 146, Lung Cancer, authored by Val R. Adams and Keith A. Hecht, for a more detailed discussion of this topic.

Lymphomas

- *Lymphomas* are a heterogeneous group of malignancies that arise from malignant transformation of immune cells residing predominantly in lymphoid tissues. Differences in histology have led to the classification of Hodgkin and non-Hodgkin lymphoma (HL and NHL, respectively), which are addressed separately in this chapter.

Hodgkin Lymphoma

PATHOPHYSIOLOGY

- B-cell transcriptional processes are disrupted during malignant transformation, preventing expression of B-cell surface markers and production of immunoglobulin messenger RNA. Alterations in the normal apoptotic pathways favor cell survival and proliferation.
- Malignant Reed–Sternberg cells overexpress nuclear factor-κB, which is associated with cell proliferation and antiapoptotic signals. Infections with viral and bacterial pathogens upregulate nuclear factor-κB. Epstein–Barr virus is found in many, but not all, HL tumors.

CLINICAL PRESENTATION

- Most patients with HL present with a painless, rubbery, enlarged lymph node in the supradiaphragmatic area and commonly have mediastinal nodal involvement. Asymptomatic adenopathy of the inguinal and axillary regions may also be present.
- Constitutional, or "B," symptoms (eg, fever, drenching night sweats, and weight loss) are present at diagnosis in approximately 25% of patients with HL.

DIAGNOSIS AND STAGING

- Diagnosis requires the presence of Reed–Sternberg cells in the lymph node biopsy.
- Staging is performed to provide prognostic information and to guide therapy. Clinical staging is based on noninvasive procedures such as history, physical examination, laboratory tests, and radiography, including positron emission tomography (PET). Pathologic staging is based on biopsy findings of strategic sites (eg, bone marrow, spleen, and abdominal nodes) using an invasive procedure (eg, laparoscopy).
- At diagnosis, approximately half of patients have localized disease (stages I, II, and II$_E$) and the others have advanced disease, of which 10%–15% is stage IV.
- Prognosis predominantly depends on age and amount of disease; patients older than 65–70 years have a lower cure rate than younger patients. Patients with limited stage disease (stages I and II) have a 90%–95% cure rate, whereas those with advanced disease (stages III and IV) have a 60%–80% cure rate.

TREATMENT

- <u>Goals of Treatment</u>: The goal is to maximize curability while minimizing short- and long-term treatment-related complications.
- Treatment options include radiation therapy (RT), chemotherapy, or both (combined-modality therapy). The therapeutic role of surgery is limited, regardless of stage.
- RT is an integral part of treatment and can be used alone for select patients with early-stage disease, although most patients will receive chemotherapy and radiation.
- Long-term complications of RT, chemotherapy, and chemoradiotherapy include gonadal dysfunction, secondary malignancies (eg, lung, breast, and GI tract, as well as leukemia), and cardiac disease.

INITIAL CHEMOTHERAPY

- Treat all stages and risk-groups of HL with 8–12 weeks of chemotherapy and then obtain a restaging PET-CT (Table 63-1). Most patients with unfavorable disease will require RT.

SALVAGE CHEMOTHERAPY

- Response to salvage therapy depends on the extent and site of recurrence, previous therapy, and duration of first remission. Choice of salvage therapy should be guided by response to initial therapy and a patient's ability to tolerate therapy.
- Patients who relapse after an initial complete response can be treated with the same regimen, a non–cross-resistant regimen, RT, or high-dose chemotherapy and autologous hematopoietic stem cell transplantation (HSCT).
- Lack of complete remission after initial therapy or relapse within 1 year after completing initial therapy is associated with a poor prognosis. Patients with these prognostic factors are candidates for high-dose chemotherapy and HSCT.
- Immune checkpoint inhibitors, specifically PD-1 (programmed death 1 pathway) inhibitors (eg, **nivolumab** and **pembrolizumab**), are approved for relapsed HL.

Non-Hodgkin Lymphoma

PATHOPHYSIOLOGY

- NHLs are derived from monoclonal proliferation of malignant B or T lymphocytes and their precursors. Current classification schemes characterize NHLs according to cell of origin, clinical features, and morphologic features.
- The World Health Organization (WHO) classification uses *grade* to refer to histologic parameters such as cell and nuclear size, density of chromatin, and proliferation fraction, and *aggressiveness* to denote clinical behavior of a tumor.

CLINICAL PRESENTATION

- Patients present with a variety of symptoms, which depend on site of involvement and whether it is nodal or extranodal.
- Adenopathy can be localized or generalized. Involved nodes are painless, rubbery, and discrete and usually located in the cervical and supraclavicular regions. Mesenteric or GI involvement can cause nausea, vomiting, obstruction, abdominal pain, palpable abdominal mass, or GI bleeding. Bone marrow involvement can cause symptoms related to anemia, neutropenia, or thrombocytopenia.
- Forty percent of patients with NHL present with B symptoms—fever, drenching night sweats, and weight loss.

DIAGNOSIS AND STAGING

- Diagnosis is established by biopsy of an involved lymph node. Diagnostic workup of NHL is generally similar to that of HL.
- NHL classification systems continue to evolve. Slow-growing or indolent lymphomas are favorable (untreated survival measured in years), whereas rapid-growing or aggressive lymphomas are unfavorable (untreated survival measured in weeks to months).
- Prognosis depends on histologic subtype and clinical risk factors (eg, age >60 years, performance status of two or more, abnormal lactate dehydrogenase, extranodal involvement, and stage III or IV disease). These risk factors are used to calculate the International Prognostic Index (IPI) that is most useful in patients with aggressive lymphomas.
- A newer prognostic index for patients with indolent (follicular) lymphomas uses similar risk factors except that poor performance status is replaced with low hemoglobin (<12 g/dL [120 g/L; 7.45 mmol/L]). Current research is focused on prognostic importance of phenotypic and molecular characteristics of NHL.

TABLE 63-1	Combination Chemotherapy Regimens for Hodgkin Lymphoma		
Drug	**Dosage (mg/m²)**	**Route**	**Days**
MOPP			
Mechlorethamine	6	IV	1, 8
Vincristine	1.4	IV	1, 8
Procarbazine	100	Oral	1–14
Prednisone	40	Oral	1–14
Repeat every 21 days			
ABVD			
Doxorubicin (Adriamycin)	25	IV	1, 15
Bleomycin	10	IV	1, 15
Vinblastine	6	IV	1, 15
Dacarbazine	375	IV	1, 15
Repeat every 28 days			
MOPP/ABVD			
Alternating months of MOPP and ABVD			
MOPP/ABV hybrid			
Mechlorethamine	6	IV	1
Vincristine	1.4	IV	1
Procarbazine	100	Oral	1–7
Prednisone	40	Oral	1–14
Doxorubicin	35	IV	8
Bleomycin	10	IV	8
Vinblastine	6	IV	8
Repeat every 28 days			
Stanford V			
Doxorubicin	25	IV	Weeks 1, 3, 5, 7, 9, 11
Vinblastine	6	IV	Weeks 1, 3, 5, 7, 9, 11
Mechlorethamine	6	IV	Weeks 1, 5, 9
Etoposide	60	IV	Weeks 3, 7, 11
Vincristine	1.4	IV	Weeks 2, 4, 6, 8, 10, 12
Bleomycin	5	IV	Weeks 2, 4, 6, 8
Prednisone	40	Oral	Every other day for 12 weeks; begin tapering at week 10
One course (12 weeks)			

(Continued)

TABLE 63-1	Combination Chemotherapy Regimens for Hodgkin Lymphoma (*Continued*)		
Drug	**Dosage (mg/m²)**	**Route**	**Days**
BEACOPP (standard-dose)			
Bleomycin	10	IV	8
Etoposide	100	IV	1–3
Adriamycin (doxorubicin)	25	IV	1
Cyclophosphamide	650	IV	1
Oncovin (vincristine)	1.4[a]	IV	8
Procarbazine	100	Oral	1–7
Prednisone	40	Oral	1–14
Repeat every 21 days			
BEACOPP (escalated-dose)			
Bleomycin	10	IV	8
Etoposide	200	IV	1–3
Adriamycin (doxorubicin)	35	IV	1
Cyclophosphamide	1250	IV	1
Oncovin (vincristine)	1.4[a]	IV	8
Procarbazine	100	Oral	1–7
Prednisone	40	Oral	1–14
Granulocyte colony-stimulating factor		Subcutaneously	8+
Repeat every 21 days			
A-AVD			
Brentuximab vedotin	1.2 mg/kg	IV	1, 15
Doxorubicin	25	IV	1, 15
Vinblastine	6	IV	1, 15
Dacarbazine	375	IV	1, 15

[a]Vincristine dose capped at 2 mg.

TREATMENT

- Goals of Treatment: The goals are to relieve symptoms and, whenever possible, cure the patient of disease while minimizing the risk of serious toxicity.

GENERAL PRINCIPLES

- Appropriate therapy for NHL depends on many factors, including patient age, histologic type, stage and site of disease, presence of adverse prognostic factors, and patient preference.
- Treatment is divided into two categories: limited disease (eg, localized disease; Ann Arbor stages I and II) and advanced disease (eg, Ann Arbor stage III or IV and stage II patients with poor prognostic features).
- Treatment options include RT, chemotherapy, and biologic agents. RT is used for remission induction with early stage, localized disease and, more commonly, as a palliative measure in advanced disease.
- Effective chemotherapy ranges from single-agent therapy for indolent (follicular) lymphomas to aggressive, complex combination regimens for aggressive disease.

FOLLICULAR LYMPHOMAS

- Follicular lymphomas occur in older adults, with a majority having advanced disease that includes the chromosomal translocation t(14;18). Clinical course is generally indolent, with median survival of 8–10 years. The natural history of follicular lymphoma is unpredictable, with spontaneous regression of objective disease seen in 20%–30% of patients.

Localized Follicular Lymphoma

- Options for stages I and II follicular lymphoma include locoregional RT and immunotherapy (ie, **rituximab**) with or without chemotherapy or RT.
- RT is the standard treatment and is usually curative. Chemotherapy is not recommended, unless the patient has high-risk, stage II disease.

Advanced Follicular Lymphoma

- Management of stages II bulky, III, and IV indolent lymphoma is controversial because standard approaches are not curative. Median time to relapse is only 18–36 months. After relapse, response can be reinduced; however, response rates and durations decrease with each retreatment.
- Therapeutic options are diverse and include watchful waiting, RT, single-agent chemotherapy, combination chemotherapy, biologic therapy, radioimmunotherapy, and combined-modality therapy. Immediate aggressive therapy does not improve survival compared with conservative therapy (ie, watchful waiting followed by single-agent chemotherapy, rituximab, or RT, when treatment is needed).
- Oral alkylating agents **chlorambucil** or **cyclophosphamide**, used alone or in combination with **prednisone**, are the mainstay of treatment. These single agents are as effective as combination regimens and produce minimal toxicity, but secondary acute leukemia is a concern. **Bendamustine** is an IV alkylating agent approved for relapsed or refractory indolent NHL.
- **Fludarabine** is an adenosine analogue that produces high response rates in previously untreated and relapsed advanced follicular lymphoma. Fludarabine is associated with prolonged myelosuppression and profound immunosuppression, increasing the risk of opportunistic infections, such as fungal infections.
- Rituximab, a chimeric monoclonal antibody directed at the CD20 molecule on B cells, is one of the most widely used therapies for follicular lymphoma. It is approved for first-line therapy either alone or combined with chemotherapy and as maintenance therapy for patients with stable disease or with partial or complete response following induction chemotherapy.
  - ✓ The most common chemotherapy regimen used with rituximab is the CHOP regimen (Table 63-2). Practice guidelines list rituximab maintenance for up to 2 years as an option in both first- and second-line therapy.
  - ✓ Rituximab adverse effects are usually infusion related, especially after the first infusion, and consist of fever, chills, respiratory symptoms, fatigue, headache,

TABLE 63-2	CHOP Regimen		
Drug	**Dose**	**Route**	**Treatment Days**
Cyclophosphamide	750 mg/m^2	IV	1
Doxorubicin	50 mg/m^2	IV	1
Vincristine[a]	1.4 mg/m^2	IV	1
Prednisone	100 mg	Oral	1–5
One cycle is 21 days			

[a]Vincristine dose is typically capped at 2 mg.
Another name for doxorubicin is hydroxydaunorubicin.

pruritus, and angioedema. Pretreatment with oral acetaminophen, 650 mg, and diphenhydramine, 50 mg, 30 minutes before the infusion is recommended.

- A second anti-CD20 monoclonal antibody, **obinutuzumab**, is approved in combination with chemotherapy, as first-line, second-line, and subsequent therapy options for treatment of follicular lymphoma.

- ^{90}Y-**ibritumomab tiuxetan** is an anti-CD20 radioimmunoconjugate, linking mouse antibodies to radioisotopes. Radiation is selectively delivered to tumor cells expressing the CD20 antigen and to adjacent tumor cells that do not express it.
  - ✓ Radioimmunotherapy is generally well tolerated. Toxicities include infusion-related reactions, myelosuppression, and possibly myelodysplastic syndrome or acute myelogenous leukemia.

- Phosphatidylinositol-3-kinase (PI3K) inhibitors, **idealisib** and **copanlisib**, reduce a messenger that affects malignant B lymphocyte proliferation and survival. They are treatment options for second-line therapy with relapsed or refractory follicular lymphoma. Both agents are associated with serious adverse reactions including severe neutropenia, diarrhea, infection, and pneumonia.

- High-dose chemotherapy followed by HSCT is an option for relapsed follicular lymphoma. The recurrence rate is lower after allogeneic than after autologous HSCT, but the benefit is offset by increased treatment-related mortality.

AGGRESSIVE LYMPHOMAS

- Diffuse large B-cell lymphomas (DLBCLs) are the most common lymphoma in patients of all ages but most commonly seen in the seventh decade. Extranodal disease is present at diagnosis in 30%–40% of patients. IPI score correlates with prognosis. Diffuse aggressive lymphomas are sensitive to chemotherapy, with cure achieved in some patients.

Treatment of Localized Disease

- Stage I and nonbulky stage II should be treated with three or four cycles of rituximab and CHOP (R-CHOP) followed by locoregional RT or six to eight cycles of R-CHOP with no RT.

- Patients with at least one adverse risk factor should receive six cycles of R-CHOP followed by locoregional RT.

Treatment of Advanced Disease

- Bulky stage II and stages III and IV lymphoma should be treated with R-CHOP or rituximab and CHOP-like chemotherapy until achieving complete response (usually 4–6 cycles). Maintenance therapy following a complete response does not improve survival.

- Consider high-dose chemotherapy with autologous HSCT in high-risk patients who respond to standard chemotherapy and meet HSCT criteria.

- Although historically elderly adults have lower complete response and survival rates than younger patients, full-dose R-CHOP is recommended as initial treatment for aggressive lymphoma in the elderly.

Treatment of Refractory or Relapsed Disease

- Approximately one-third of patients with aggressive lymphoma will require salvage therapy at some point. Salvage therapy is more likely to induce response if the response to initial chemotherapy was complete (chemosensitivity) than if it was primarily or partially resistant to chemotherapy.

- High-dose chemotherapy with autologous HSCT is the therapy of choice for younger patients with chemosensitive relapse.

- Salvage regimens incorporate drugs not used as initial therapy. Commonly used regimens include DHAP (**dexamethasone**, **cytarabine**, and **cisplatin**), ESHAP (**etoposide**, **methylprednisolone**, cytarabine, and cisplatin), and MINE (**mesna, ifosfamide, mitoxantrone,** and **etoposide**). None is clearly superior to the others.

- Rituximab is being evaluated in combination with many salvage regimens.

NON-HODGKIN LYMPHOMA IN ACQUIRED IMMUNODEFICIENCY SYNDROME

- Patients with AIDS have more than a 100-fold increased risk of developing NHL, which is usually aggressive (eg, Burkitt or DLBCL).
- Treatment of AIDS-related lymphoma is difficult because underlying immunodeficiency increases the risk of treatment-related myelosuppression.
- Standard combination regimens (eg, CHOP) yield disappointing results. Newer approaches, including dose-adjusted EPOCH (etoposide, prednisone, vincristine, cyclophosphamide, and doxorubicin), appear promising. The role of rituximab in the treatment of AIDS-related DLBCL is not clear.
- Prophylactic antibiotics should be continued during chemotherapy, but the optimal timing for highly active antiretroviral therapy (HAART) is not clear in patients with AIDS-related lymphoma.

EVALUATION OF THERAPEUTIC OUTCOMES

- The primary outcome to be identified is tumor response, which is based on physical examination, radiologic evidence, PET/computed tomography (CT) scanning, and other baseline findings.

See Chapter 149, Lymphomas, authored by Alexandre Chan, Chia Jie Tan, and Jolynn Sessions, for a more detailed discussion of this topic.

- *Prostate cancer* is a malignant neoplasm that arises from the prostate gland. Prostate cancer has an indolent course; localized prostate cancer is curable by surgery or radiation therapy, but advanced prostate cancer is not yet curable.

PATHOPHYSIOLOGY

- The normal prostate is composed of acinar secretory cells that are altered when invaded by cancer. The major pathologic cell type is adenocarcinoma (>95% of cases).
- Prostate cancer can be graded. Well-differentiated tumors grow slowly, whereas poorly differentiated tumors grow rapidly and have a poor prognosis.
- Metastatic spread can occur by local extension, lymphatic drainage, or hematogenous dissemination. Skeletal metastases from hematogenous spread are the most common sites of distant spread. The lung, liver, brain, and adrenal glands are the most common sites of visceral involvement, but these organs are not usually involved initially.
- Hormonal regulation of androgen synthesis is mediated through a series of biochemical interactions between the hypothalamus, pituitary, adrenal glands, and testes (**Figure 64-1**).
- The testes and the adrenal glands are the major sources of androgens, specifically dihydrotestosterone (DHT).
- Luteinizing hormone–releasing hormone (LHRH) from the hypothalamus stimulates the release of luteinizing hormone (LH) and follicle-stimulating hormone (FSH) from the anterior pituitary gland.
- LH complexes with receptors on the Leydig cell testicular membrane, stimulating the production of testosterone and small amounts of estrogen.
- FSH acts on testicular Sertoli cells to promote maturation of LH receptors and produce an androgen-binding protein.
- Circulating testosterone and estradiol influence the synthesis of LHRH, LH, and FSH by a negative-feedback loop at the hypothalamic and pituitary level.

CHEMOPREVENTION

- The use of 5-α-reductase inhibitors, **finasteride** and **dutasteride**, to prevent prostate cancer has been debated for more than a decade. Current guidelines do not recommend the use of these agents for prostate cancer chemoprevention.

SCREENING

- Screening recommendations for prostate cancer have changed, and digital rectal examination (DRE) and prostate-specific antigen (PSA) are no longer recommended for patients without a discussion with their clinician about risks versus benefits. The American Urologic Association does not recommend routine screening in men between the ages of 40 and 54 years of average risk. They recommend that men aged 55–69 years discuss the risks and benefits of prostate cancer screening. Men who elect to have screening should do so no more than every 2 years; a recent study suggests that screening every 5 years may be adequate.
- PSA is a glycoprotein produced and secreted by prostate epithelial cells. Acute urinary retention, acute prostatitis, and BPH influence PSA, thereby limiting the usefulness of PSA alone for early detection, but it is a useful marker for monitoring response to therapy.

(ACTH, adrenocorticotropic hormone; DHT, dihydrotestosterone; FSH, follicle-stimulating hormone; GH, growth hormone; LH, luteinizing hormone; LHRH, luteinizing hormone–releasing hormone; mRNA, messenger RNA; PROL, prolactin; R, receptor.)

FIGURE 64-1. Hormonal regulation of the prostate gland.

CLINICAL PRESENTATION

- Localized prostate cancer is usually asymptomatic.
- Locally invasive prostate cancer is associated with ureteral dysfunction or impingement, such as alterations in micturition (eg, urinary frequency, hesitancy, and dribbling), and impotence.
- Advanced disease commonly presents with back pain and stiffness due to osseous metastases. Untreated spinal cord lesions can lead to cord compression. Lower extremity edema can occur as a result of lymphatic obstruction. Anemia and weight loss are nonspecific signs of advanced disease.

TREATMENT

- <u>Goals of Treatment</u>: In early-stage prostate cancer, the goal is to minimize morbidity and mortality. Surgery and radiation therapy are curative but also associated with significant morbidity and mortality. In advanced prostate cancer, treatment focuses on providing symptom relief and maintaining quality of life.

GENERAL APPROACH

- Initial treatment depends on disease stage, Gleason score, presence of symptoms, and patient's life expectancy. The most appropriate therapy for early-stage prostate cancer is unknown. See **Table 64-1** for management recommendations based on risk of recurrence.
- Initial treatment modality for advanced prostate cancer is androgen ablation (eg, orchiectomy or LHRH agonists with or without antiandrogens). After disease progression, secondary hormonal manipulations, cytotoxic chemotherapy, and supportive care are used.

NONPHARMACOLOGIC THERAPY

Observation

- Observation or watchful waiting involves monitoring the course of disease and initiating treatment if the cancer progresses. PSA and DRE are performed every 6 months.
- Advantages include avoiding adverse effects of definitive therapies and minimizing risk of unnecessary therapies. The major disadvantage is the risk of cancer progression requiring more intense therapy.

Surgery and Radiation Therapy

- Bilateral orchiectomy rapidly reduces circulating androgens to castrate levels. Many patients are not surgical candidates due to advanced age, and other patients find this procedure psychologically unacceptable. Orchiectomy is the preferred initial treatment for patients with impending spinal cord compression or ureteral obstruction.
- Radical prostatectomy and radiation therapy are potentially curative therapies but are associated with complications that must be weighed against expected benefit. Consequently, many patients postpone therapy until symptoms develop.
- Complications of radical prostatectomy include blood loss, stricture formation, incontinence, lymphocele, fistula formation, anesthetic risk, and impotence. Nerve-sparing techniques facilitate return of sexual potency after prostatectomy.
- Acute complications of radiation therapy include cystitis, proctitis, hematuria, urinary retention, penoscrotal edema, and impotence.
- Chronic complications of radiation therapy include proctitis, diarrhea, cystitis, enteritis, impotence, urethral stricture, and incontinence.

PHARMACOLOGIC THERAPY

Drug Treatments of First Choice

Luteinizing Hormone–Releasing Hormone Agonists

- LHRH agonists are a reversible method of androgen ablation and are as effective as orchiectomy.
- There are no comparative trials of LHRH agonists, so the choice is usually based on cost and patient and physician preference for a dosing schedule (**Table 64-2**). **Leuprolide acetate, leuprolide depot, leuprolide implant, triptorelin depot, triptorelin implant,** and **goserelin acetate implant** are currently available. Dosing intervals range from once monthly to every 6 months. Leuprolide implant is a mini-osmotic pump that delivers daily doses for 1 year. Testosterone castration levels are achieved in 28 days with leuprolide.
- The most common adverse effects of LHRH agonists include disease flare-up during the first week of therapy (eg, increased bone pain or urinary symptoms), hot flashes, erectile impotence, decreased libido, and injection-site reactions. Use of an antiandrogen (eg, **flutamide, bicalutamide,** or **nilutamide**) prior to initiation of LHRH therapy and for 2–4 weeks after is a strategy to minimize initial tumor flare.

TABLE 64-1	\multicolumn{2}{l}{Initial Management of Prostate Cancer Based on Expected Survival and Recurrence Risk}

Recurrence Risk	Expected Survival (Years)	Initial Therapy
Very low		
T_{1c}, Gleason score less than 6 and PSA less than 10 ng/mL (mcg/L)	<20	Observation
T_{1c}, Gleason score less than 6 and PSA less than 10 ng/mL (mcg/L)	20 or more	Observation or Radical prostatectomy with or without pelvic lymph node dissection or Radiation therapy
Low		
T_1–T_{2a} and Gleason and PSA less than 10 ng/mL (mcg/L) and <5% tumor in the specimen	10 or more	Observation or Radical prostatectomy with or without pelvic lymph node dissection or radiation therapy
	<10	Observation
Intermediate		
T_{2b}–T_{2c} or Gleason 7 or PSA 10–20 ng/mL (mcg/L)	10 or more	Observation or Radical prostatectomy with pelvic lymph node dissection or Radiation therapy with or without 4–6 months of neoadjuvant ADT with or without brachytherapy
T_{2b}–T_{2c} or Gleason 7 or PSA 10–20 ng/mL (mcg/L)	10 or more	Radical prostatectomy with pelvic lymph node dissection or Radiation therapy with or without 4–6 months of neoadjuvant ADT with or without brachytherapy
High		
T_{3a}, Gleason 8–10, PSA >20 ng/mL (mcg/L)	5 years or more	Radiation therapy and ADT[a] (2–3 years) with or without brachytherapy or Radical prostatectomy and pelvic lymph node dissection

(Continued)

	Expected Survival (Years)	
TABLE 64-1		Initial Management of Prostate Cancer Based on Expected Survival and Recurrence Risk *(Continued)*
Recurrence Risk		**Initial Therapy**
Very high		
T_{3b}–T_4 or Gleason pattern 5 or >4 cores with Gleason score 8–10		Radiation therapy and ADT (2–3 years) with or without brachytherapy
		or
		Radical prostatectomy and pelvic lymph node dissection
		or
		ADT
Very high		
Any T, N_1		ADT (2–3 years) with or without abiraterone and prednisone
		or
		Radiation therapy and ADT (2–3 years) with or without abiraterone and prednisone (or methylprednisolone)
Any T, Any N, M_1		Orchiectomy
		or
		LHRH agonist[b] with or without an antiandrogen
		or
		LHRH antagonist
		or
		Observation

[a]Androgen deprivation therapy to achieve serum testosterone levels <50 ng/dL (1.7 nmol/L).
[b]LHRH agonist, medical castration, or surgical castration is equivalent.
ADT, androgen-deprivation therapy; LHRH, luteinizing hormone–releasing hormone; PSA, prostate-specific antigen.

- Decreases in bone mineral density complicate androgen deprivation therapy (ADT), resulting in increased risk of osteoporosis, osteopenia, and skeletal fractures. Calcium and vitamin D supplements and a baseline bone mineral density are recommended. Consider administering an antiresorptive agent (eg, **denosumab** or **zoledronic acid**) to reduce the risk of skeletal-related events.
- Screen patients receiving ADT for cardiovascular disease and diabetes due to increased risk of metabolic effects.

Gonadotropin-Releasing Hormone Antagonists

- The gonadotropin-releasing hormone (GnRH) antagonist **degarelix** binds reversibly to GnRH receptors in the pituitary gland, reducing the production of testosterone to castrate levels in 7 days or less. A major advantage of degarelix over LHRH agonists is the lack of tumor flare.
- Degarelix is administered as a subcutaneous injection every 28 days. Injection site reactions are the most frequently reported adverse effects and include pain,

TABLE 64-2 Hormonal Therapies for Prostate Cancer

Drug (Brand Name)	Usual Dose	Toxicities	Hepatic/Renal Adjustments	Monitoring Parameters	Drug Interactions	Administration
First-Generation Antiandrogens						
Flutamide (Eulexin)	750 mg/day	Gynecomastia Hot flashes GI disturbances (diarrhea) Loss of libido LFT abnormalities Breast tenderness Methemoglobinemia	Contraindicated in patients with hepatic impairment No dosage adjustment necessary in chronic renal impairment	Monitor serum transaminases prior to start of therapy and monthly for the first 4 months, then periodically thereafter Monitor for tumor reduction, testosterone/estrogen, and alkaline phosphatase serum levels	Substrate of CYP1A2 and CYP3A4	Administered orally in three divided doses; capsule may be opened into applesauce, pudding, or other soft foods
Bicalutamide (Casodex)	50 mg/day (up to 150 mg/day—unlabeled use)	Gynecomastia Hot flashes GI disturbances (diarrhea) Decreased libido LFT abnormalities Breast tenderness	Discontinue if ALT >2 times upper limit of normal or patient develops jaundice	Monitor serum transaminases prior to start of therapy and monthly for the first 4 months, then periodically thereafter Periodic monitoring of CBC, EKG, echocardiograms, serum testosterone, luteinizing hormone, and PSA	Inhibits CYP3A4 May increase the concentration of vitamin K antagonists	May be taken with or without food

(Continued)

TABLE 64-2 Hormonal Therapies for Prostate Cancer (Continued)

Drug (Brand Name)	Usual Dose	Toxicities	Hepatic/Renal Adjustments	Monitoring Parameters	Drug Interactions	Administration
Nilutamide (Nilandron)	300 mg/day for first month then 150 mg/day	Gynecomastia Hot flashes GI disturbances (constipation) LFT abnormalities Breast tenderness Visual disturbances (impaired dark adaptation) Alcohol intolerance Interstitial pneumonitis	Contraindicated in patients with hepatic impairment Discontinue if ALT >2 times upper limit of normal or patient develops jaundice	Monitor serum transaminases prior to start of therapy and monthly for the first 4 months, then periodically thereafter Chest x-ray at baseline and consider pulmonary function testing (at baseline)	Substrate of CYP2C19 and weak inhibitor of CYP2C19	May be taken with or without food
Second-Generation Antiandrogens						
Apalutamide (Erleada)	240 mg/day	GI disturbances (diarrhea, nausea) Hot flashes Fatigue Hypertension Rash Decreased weight Falls and fractures Peripheral edema Seizures	No adjustment necessary for renal or hepatic impairment	CBC baseline and periodically LFTs baseline and periodically	Strong inducer of CYP3A4 and CYP2C19, and a weak inducer of CYP2C9	May be taken with or without food

Drug	Dose	Adverse Effects	Monitoring	Drug Interactions	Administration
Enzalutamide (Xtandi)	160 mg/day	GI disturbances (diarrhea) Musculoskeletal disorders (back pain, arthralgias, muscle pain, weakness) Asthenia Peripheral edema CNS (headache, dizziness) Seizures LFT abnormalities	No adjustment necessary for renal or hepatic impairment	CBC baseline and periodically LFTs baseline and periodically	Strong CYP3A4 and moderate CYP2C9 and CYP2C19 inducer; avoid CYP3A4, CYP2C9, and CYP2C19 sensitive substrates. CYP2C8 substrate, avoid strong inducers and inhibitors of CYP2C8. If vitamin K antagonists are necessary, conduct additional INR monitoring
Darolutamide (Nubeqa)	1200 mg/day	Fatigue GI disturbances (diarrhea, constipation, nausea) Rash Musculoskeletal disorders (back pain, arthralgias, pain in an extremity) Falls, including accidents/bone fractures Hypertension Seizures	For moderate hepatic impairment or severe renal impairment (not on dialysis): reduce dose to 600 mg/day	CBC baseline and periodically LFTs baseline and periodically	Breast cancer resistance protein (BCRP) transporter Inhibitor Darolutamide inhibits OATP1B1 and OATP1B3

Note: the column order in the image (reading the rotated table left to right) places the rightmost handwritten column as "Administration":

- Enzalutamide: May be taken with or without food
- Darolutamide: Take with food

(Continued)

TABLE 64-2 Hormonal Therapies for Prostate Cancer *(Continued)*

Drug (Brand Name)	Usual Dose	Toxicities	Hepatic/Renal Adjustments	Monitoring Parameters	Drug Interactions	Administration
Androgen Synthesis Inhibitor						
Abiraterone acetate (Zytiga)	1000 mg/day + prednisone 5 mg BID	GI disturbances (diarrhea) Edema Hypokalemia Hypophosphatemia LFT abnormalities Hypertriglyceridemia	250 mg daily for Child–Pugh Class B; avoid use in Child–Pugh Class C Withhold treatment if LFTs >5 times the ULN or bilirubin >3 ULN	Monitor serum transaminases prior to start of therapy, every 2 weeks for 3 months, then monthly thereafter Monitor for signs and symptoms of adrenocorticoid insufficiency; monthly for hypertension, hypokalemia, and fluid retention	Substrate of CYP3A4. Use with caution with CYP3A4 inhibitors and inducers Inhibits CYP1A2, CYP2C19, CYP2C8, CYP2C9, CYP2D6, CYP3A4, and P-glycoprotein Use sensitive substrates with caution	Take on an empty stomach, at least 1 hour before or 2 hours after food
Luteinizing-Hormone Agonists						
Leuprolide (Lupron)	7.5 mg IM every month 22.5 mg IM every 3 months 30 mg IM every 4 months 45 mg IM every 6 months	Hot flashes Decreased libido Gynecomastia Osteoporosis Fatigue Weight gain	No adjustment necessary for renal or hepatic impairment	Serum testosterone ~4 weeks after initiation, PSA, blood glucose, and A1C prior to initiation and periodically thereafter	May diminish the effects of antidiabetic agents	Vary injection site

Drug	Dose	Renal/Hepatic Adjustment	Adverse Effects	Monitoring	Drug Interactions	Administration
Goserelin (Zoladex)	3.6 mg SQ implant every month 10.8 mg SQ implant every 3 months	No adjustment necessary for renal or hepatic impairment	Hot flashes Decreased libido Gynecomastia Osteoporosis Fatigue Weight gain	Monitor bone mineral density, serum calcium, and cholesterol/lipids	May diminish the effects of antidiabetic agents	Vary injection site
Triptorelin (Trelstar)	3.75 mg IM every month 11.25 mg IM every 3 months 22.5 mg IM every 6 months	No adjustment necessary for renal or hepatic impairment	Hot flashes Decreased libido Gynecomastia Osteoporosis Fatigue Weight gain	Monitor serum testosterone levels and PSA	May diminish the effects of antidiabetic agents	Vary injection site
Gonadotropin-Releasing Hormone Antagonists						
Degarelix (Firmagon)	240 mg SQ loading dose 80 mg SQ every 28 days (following 28 days after loading dose)	Use with caution with CL_{cr} <50 mL/min (0.83 mL/sec) Do not use in patients with severe hepatic impairment	Hot flashes Decreased libido Gynecomastia Osteoporosis Fatigue Weight gain	PSA periodically, serum testosterone monthly until castration achieved then every other month, LFTs at baseline in addition to serum electrolytes and bone mineral density	Use with caution with agents that may increase QTc interval	Vary injection site

ALT, alanine aminotransferase; BID, twice daily; CBC, complete blood count; CL_{cr}, creatinine clearance; CNS, central nervous system; CYP, cytochrome P450; EKG, electrocardiogram; GI, gastrointestinal; IM, intramuscular injection; INR, international normalized ratio; LFT, liver function test; PSA, prostate-specific antigen; SQ, subcutaneous injection; ULN, upper limit of normal.

erythema, swelling, induration, and nodules. Osteoporosis may develop, and calcium and vitamin D supplementation should be considered.

Antiandrogens

- Monotherapy with flutamide, bicalutamide, and nilutamide is no longer recommended due to decreased efficacy as compared with patients treated with LHRH agonist therapy. Antiandrogens are indicated for advanced prostate cancer only when combined with an LHRH agonist (flutamide and bicalutamide]) or orchiectomy (nilutamide). In combination, antiandrogens can reduce the LHRH agonist–induced flare.
- **Apalutamide**, **enzalutamide**, and **darolutamide** are second-generation antiandrogens. Apalalutamide was initially approved in the nonmetastatic castration naive patient population but has since been approved for castrate-resistant prostate cancer (CRPC). Enzalutamide may be used in the first-line setting to delay the initiation of chemotherapy in both nonmetastatic and metastatic disease
- Adverse effects of antiandrogens are summarized in **Table 64-2**.

Combined Androgen Blockade

- The role of combined androgen blockade (CAB), also referred to as *maximal androgen deprivation* or *total androgen blockade*, continues to be evaluated. The combination of LHRH agonists or orchiectomy with antiandrogens is the CAB approach most extensively studied.
- Some clinicians consider CAB to be the initial hormone therapy of choice for newly diagnosed patients because the major benefit is seen in patients with minimal disease. Some argue that treatment should not be delayed because combined androgen deprivation trials demonstrate a survival advantage for young patients with good performance status and minimal disease who were initially treated with hormone therapy.

Alternative Drug Treatments

- Selection of salvage therapy depends on what was used as initial therapy. Radiotherapy can be used after failed radical prostatectomy. Androgen ablation can be used after progression of disease after radiation therapy or radical prostatectomy.
- An antiandrogen or orchiectomy may be indicated if testosterone levels are not suppressed (ie, >20 ng/dL [0.7 nmol/L]) after initial LHRH agonist therapy. If testosterone levels are suppressed, the disease is considered androgen-independent and palliative androgen-independent salvage therapy can be used.
- Androgen withdrawal should be attempted if initial therapy consists of CAB with an LHRH agonist and antiandrogen. Mutations of the androgen receptor may allow antiandrogens to become agonists. Androgen withdrawal produces responses lasting 3–14 months in up to 35% of patients.
- Androgen synthesis inhibitors provide symptomatic but brief relief in approximately 50% of patients. **Aminoglutethimide** causes adverse effects in 50% of patients, such as lethargy, ataxia, dizziness, and self-limiting rash. The adverse effects of **ketoconazole** include GI intolerance, transient increases in liver and renal function tests, and hypoadrenalism. **Abiraterone** targets CYP17A1, resulting in decreased circulating levels of testosterone (**Table 64-2**). Review medication profiles for potential drug interactions because abiraterone is an inhibitor of CYP2D6.

Chemotherapy

- **Docetaxel**, 75 mg/m^2 every 3 weeks, combined with **prednisone**, 5 mg twice daily, improves survival in CRPC. The most common adverse events include nausea, alopecia, and myelosuppression (**Table 64-3**).
- **Cabazitaxel** 25 mg/m^2 every 3 weeks with prednisone 10 mg daily significantly improves progression-free and overall survival in patients previously treated with docetaxel and prednisone. Neutropenia, febrile neutropenia, neuropathy, and diarrhea are the most significant toxicities.

TABLE 64-3 Chemotherapy and Immunotherapy for Prostate Cancer

Drug (Brand Name)	Usual Dose	Toxicities	Hepatic/Renal Adjustments	Monitoring Parameters	Drug Interactions	Administration
Antimicrotubule Agents						
Docetaxel (Taxotere)	75 mg/m^2 IV every 3 weeks	Fluid retention, alopecia, mucositis, myelosuppression, hypersensitivity	Do not administer if AST/ALT >1.5 times the upper limit of normal and alkaline phosphatase >2.5 times the upper limit of normal	CBC with differential, LFTs, bilirubin, alkaline phosphatase, renal function. Monitor for hypersensitivity reactions	Avoid concomitant use of CYP3A4 inhibitors	Administer IV infusion over 1 hour. Premedication with corticosteroids for 3 days beginning the day before
Cabazitaxel (Jevtana)	25 mg/m^2 IV every 3 weeks	Fluid retention, constipation, mucositis, myelosuppression, hypersensitivity	Discontinue if ALT >2 times upper limit of normal or patient develops jaundice	CBC weekly during the first cycle, then prior to each treatment. Monitor for hypersensitivity	Avoid concomitant use of CYP3A4 inducers and inhibitors	Administer IV infusion over 1 hour
Immunotherapy						
Sipuleucel-T (Provenge)	Each injection contains >50 million autologous CD54+ cells (obtained through leukapheresis) activated with PAP-GM-CSF. Dose is given ~ every 2 weeks for 3 total doses	Hypersensitivity, chills, fatigue, fever, headache, myalgias	No dosage adjustment necessary for renal or hepatic dysfunction	No specific laboratory monitoring recommended	Immunosuppressants may decrease the therapeutic effects of sipuleucel-T	Administer IV infusion over 1 hour. Observe the patient for 30 minutes after completion of the infusion. Premedicate with acetaminophen and an antihistamine 30 minutes prior to administration

ALT, alanine aminotransferase; AST, aspartate aminotransferase; CBC, complete blood count; CYP, cytochrome P450; LFT, liver function test; PAP-GM-CSF, prostatic acid phosphatase granulocyte-macrophage colony-stimulating factor.

Immunotherapy

- **Sipuleucel-T** is a novel autologous cellular immunotherapy indicated for asymptomatic or minimally symptomatic metastatic CRPC. Use is controversial because trials have not been done to compare it to standard second-line hormonal interventions.

Nuclear Medicine

- Radium-223, an alpha emitter, can be used in first-, second-, or third-line therapy in patients with metastatic CRPC with symptomatic primary bone metastases. It has not been approved for use with concomitant chemotherapy.
- Radium-223 improved survival, pain-related outcomes, quality of life and decreased opioid needs. The most common adverse effects include nausea, diarrhea, vomiting, peripheral edema, and bone marrow suppression.

EVALUATION OF THERAPEUTIC OUTCOMES

- Monitor primary tumor size, involved lymph nodes, and tumor marker response such as PSA with definitive, curative therapy. PSA level is checked every 6 months for the first 5 years, then annually.
- With metastatic disease, clinical benefit can be documented by evaluating performance status, weight, quality of life, analgesic requirements, and PSA or DRE at 3-month intervals.

See Chapter 148, Prostate Cancer, authored by LeAnn B. Norris, for a more detailed discussion of this topic.

CHAPTER 65

Glaucoma

- *Glaucomas* are ocular disorders that lead to an optic neuropathy characterized by changes in the optic nerve head (optic disc) that is associated with loss of visual sensitivity and field.

PATHOPHYSIOLOGY

- There are two major types of glaucoma: *primary open-angle glaucoma* (POAG) or ocular hypertension, which accounts for most cases and is therefore the focus of this chapter, and *primary angle closure glaucoma* (PACG). Either type can be a primary inherited disorder, congenital, or secondary to disease, trauma, or drugs.
- In POAG, the specific cause of optic nerve damage is unknown. Increased intraocular pressure (IOP) was historically considered to be the sole cause. Additional contributing factors include increased susceptibility of the optic nerve to ischemia, excitotoxicity, autoimmune reactions, and other abnormal physiologic processes.
- Although IOP is a poor predictor of which patients will have visual field loss, the risk of visual field loss increases with increasing IOP. IOP is not constant; it changes with pulse, blood pressure, forced expiration or coughing, neck compression, and posture. IOP demonstrates diurnal variation with a minimum pressure around 6 PM and a maximum pressure upon awakening.
- The balance between the inflow and outflow of aqueous humor determines IOP. Inflow is increased by β-adrenergic agents and decreased by α_2- and β-adrenergic blockers, dopamine blockers, carbonic anhydrase inhibitors (CAIs), meltatonin-1 agonists, and adenylate cyclase stimulators. Outflow is increased by cholinergic agents (eg, pilocarpine), which contract the ciliary muscle and open the trabecular meshwork, and by prostaglandin analogues and β- and α_2-adrenergic agonists, which affect uveoscleral outflow.
- Secondary OAG has many causes, including exfoliation syndrome, pigmentary glaucoma, systemic diseases, trauma, surgery, ocular inflammatory diseases, and drugs. Secondary glaucoma can be classified as pretrabecular (normal meshwork is covered and prevents outflow of aqueous humor), trabecular (meshwork is altered or material accumulates in the intertrabecular spaces), or posttrabecular (episcleral venous blood pressure is increased).
- Many drugs can increase IOP (Table 65-1). The potential to induce or worsen glaucoma depends on the type of glaucoma and on whether it is adequately controlled.
- PACG occurs when there is a physical blockage of the trabecular meshwork, resulting in increased IOP.

CLINICAL PRESENTATION

- POAG is bilateral, often asymmetric, progresses slowly, and is usually asymptomatic until onset of substantial visual field loss. Central visual acuity is maintained, even in late stages.
- Patients with PACG typically experience intermittent prodromal symptoms (eg, blurred or hazy vision with halos around lights and, occasionally, headache). Acute episodes produce symptoms associated with a cloudy, edematous cornea; ocular pain; nausea, vomiting, and abdominal pain; and diaphoresis.

TABLE 65-1	Drugs That May Induce or Potentiate Increased Intraocular Pressure

Open-angle glaucoma

Ophthalmic corticosteroids (high risk)

Systemic corticosteroids

Nasal/Inhaled corticosteroids

Fenoldopam

Ophthalmic anticholinergics

Succinylcholine

Vasodilators (low risk)

Cimetidine (low risk)

Closed-angle glaucoma

Topical anticholinergics

Topical sympathomimetics

Systemic anticholinergics

Heterocyclic antidepressants

Low-potency phenothiazines

Antihistamines

Ipratropium

Benzodiazepines (low risk)

Theophylline (low risk)

Vasodilators (low risk)

Systemic sympathomimetics (low risk)

CNS stimulants (low risk)

Serotonin-selective reuptake inhibitors

Imipramine

Venlafaxine

Topiramate

Tetracyclines (low risk)

Carbonic anhydrase inhibitors (low risk)

Monoamine oxidase inhibitors (low risk)

Topical cholinergics (low risk)

DIAGNOSIS

- POAG is confirmed by the presence of characteristic optic disc changes and visual field loss, with or without increased IOP. *Normal tension glaucoma* refers to disc changes, visual field loss, and IOP less than 21 mm Hg (2.8 kPa). *Ocular hypertension* refers to IOP greater than 21 mm Hg (2.8 kPa) without disc changes or visual field loss.
- PACG is usually visualized by gonioscopy. IOP is generally markedly elevated (eg, 40–90 mm Hg [5.3–12 kPa]) when symptoms are present. Additional signs include hyperemic conjunctiva, cloudy cornea, shallow anterior chamber, and occasionally edematous and hyperemic optic disc.

TREATMENT OF OCULAR HYPERTENSION AND OPEN-ANGLE GLAUCOMA

- <u>Goal of Treatment</u>: The goal is to preserve visual function by reducing IOP to a level at which no further optic nerve damage occurs.
- Treat ocular hypertension if the patient has a significant risk factor such as IOP greater than 25 mm Hg (3.3 kPa), vertical cup:disc ratio greater than 0.5, or central corneal thickness less than 555 μm. Additional risk factors to be considered include family history of glaucoma, black, Latino/Hispanic ethnicity, severe myopia, and presence of only one eye. The goal of therapy is to lower IOP by 20%–30% from baseline to decrease the risk of optic nerve damage.
- Treat all patients with elevated IOP and characteristic optic disc changes or visual field defects. An initial target IOP reduction of 25%–30% is desired in patients with POAG.
- Initiate drug therapy in a stepwise manner (**Figure 65-1**), starting with lower concentrations of a single well-tolerated topical agent (**Table 65-2**). Historically, β-blockers (eg, **timolol**) were the treatment of choice provided no contraindications existed.
- Newer agents are also suitable for first-line therapy. Prostaglandin analogs (eg, **latanoprost, bimatoprost,** and **travoprost**) offer once-daily dosing, better IOP reduction, good tolerance, and availability of lower-cost generics. **Brimonidine** and topical CAIs are also suitable for first-line therapy.
- If more than one agent is needed, fixed combination products reduce the number of daily doses, which might improve adherence and prevent washout effect seen when a second medication is administered too soon after the initial medication. They also reduce exposure to ophthalmic preservatives.
- **Pilocarpine** is used as third-line therapy because of adverse events or reduced efficacy as compared with newer agents.
- **Carbachol, dipivefrin,** topical cholinesterase inhibitors, and oral CAIs (eg, **acetazolamide**) are used as last-resort options after failure of less toxic combination options.
- **Netarsudil** is the first approved Rho kinase inhibitor. Efficacy appears to be similar to that of β-blockers. It may be used in combination therapy.
- Surgical procedures such as laser trabeculoplasty or surgical trabeculectomy can be considered when drug therapy fails, is not tolerated, or is excessively complicated. Antiproliferative agents such as **fluorouracil** and **mitomycin C** are used to modify the healing process and maintain patency.

TREATMENT OF CLOSED-ANGLE GLAUCOMA

- Acute angle-closure crisis (AACC) with high IOP requires rapid reduction in IOP. Iridectomy is the definitive treatment producing a hole in the iris that permits aqueous humor flow to move directly from the posterior to the anterior chamber.
- Drug therapy of an acute attack typically consists of a miotic (eg, pilocarpine), secretory inhibitor (eg, β-blocker, α_2-agonist, latanoprost, or CAI), or prostaglandin agonist.
- Osmotic agents are used to rapidly decrease IOP. Examples include oral **glycerin**, 1–2 g/kg, and **mannitol**, 1–2 g/kg IV.
- Topical corticosteroids can be used to reduce ocular inflammation and synechiae.

EVALUATION OF THERAPEUTIC OUTCOMES

- Successful outcomes require identifying an effective, well-tolerated regimen; closely monitoring therapy; and patient adherence. Whenever possible, therapy for open-angle glaucoma should be started as a single agent in one eye to facilitate evaluation of drug efficacy and tolerance. Many drugs or combinations may need to be tried before the optimal regimen is identified.

^aFourth-line agents are not commonly used any longer or are commercially unavailable.
^bMost clinicians believe the laser procedure should be performed earlier (eg, after three-drug maximum or with a poorly adherent patient).
(CAI, carbonic anhydrase inhibitor.)

FIGURE 65-1. Algorithm for the pharmacotherapy of open-angle glaucoma.

TABLE 65-2 Topical Drugs Used in the Treatment of Open-Angle Glaucoma

Drug	Pharmacologic Properties	Common Brand Names/Generic	Dose Form	Strength (%)	Usual Dose[a]	Mechanism of Action
β-Adrenergic blocking agents						
Betaxolol	Relative β$_1$ selective	Generic	Solution	0.5	One drop twice a day	All reduce aqueous production of ciliary body
Carteolol	Nonselective, intrinsic sympathomimetic activity	Betoptic-S	Suspension	0.25	One drop twice a day	
		Generic	Solution	1	One drop twice a day	
Levobunolol	Nonselective	Betagan/Generic	Solution	0.25, 0.5	One drop twice a day	
Metipranolol	Nonselective	OptiPranol	Solution	0.3	One drop twice a day	
Timolol	Nonselective	Timoptic, Betimol, Istalol/Generic	Solution	0.25, 0.5	One drop every day—one to two times a day	
		Timoptic-XE/Generic	Gelling solution	0.25, 0.5	One drop every day[a]	
Adrenergic agonists						
α$_2$-Adrenergic agonists						
Apraclonidine	Specific α$_2$-agonists	Iopidine	Solution	0.5, 1	One drop two to three times a day	Both reduce aqueous humor production; brimonidine known to also increase uveoscleral outflow; only brimonidine has primary indication

(*Continued*)

TABLE 65-2	Topical Drugs Used in the Treatment of Open-Angle Glaucoma (Continued)					
Drug	Pharmacologic Properties	Common Brand Names/Generic	Dose Form	Strength (%)	Usual Dose[a]	Mechanism of Action
Brimonidine		Alphagan P 0.1/Generic 0.2, 0.15	Solution	0.2, 0.15, 0.1	One drop two to three times a day	All increase aqueous humor outflow through trabecular meshwork
Cholinergic agonists direct acting						
Carbachol	Direct and indirect acting	Carboptic, Isopto Carbachol	Solution	1.5, 3	One drop two to three times a day[a]	
Pilocarpine	Direct acting	Isopto Carpine, Pilocar/ Generic	Solution	1, 2, 4	One drop two to three times a day[a] One drop four times a day	
Cholinesterase inhibitor						
Echothiophate	Indirect acting cholinesterase inhibitor	Phospholine Iodide	Solution	0.125	Once or twice a day	
Carbonic anhydrase inhibitors						
Topical						
Brinzolamide	Carbonic anhydrase type II inhibition	Azopt	Suspension	1	Two to three times a day	All reduce aqueous humor production of ciliary body
Dorzolamide		Trusopt/Generic	Solution	2	Two to three times a day	
Systemic						
Acetazolamide		Generic	Tablet	125 mg, 250 mg	125–250 mg two to four times a day	
		Injection	500 mg/vial			
		Diamox Sequels	Capsule	250–500 mg 500 mg	500 mg twice a day	

		Generic	Tablet	25 mg, 50 mg	25–50 mg two to three times a day	Increases aqueous uveoscleral outflow and to a lesser extent trabecular outflow
Methazolamide			Tablet	25 mg, 50 mg	25–50 mg two to three times a day	
Prostaglandin analogs						
Latanoprost	Prostanoid agonist	Xalatan/Generic	Solution	0.005	One drop every night	Increases aqueous uveoscleral outflow and to a lesser extent trabecular outflow
Latanoprostene Bunod	Prostanoid agonist	Vyzulta	Solution	0.024	One drop every night	
Bimatoprost	Prostamide agonist	Lumigan 0.01/ Generic 0.03	Solution	0.01, 0.03	One drop every night	
Travoprost	Prostanoid agonist	Travatan Z/ GenericTravoprost	Solution	0.004	One drop every night	
Tafluprost	Prostanoid agonist	Zioptan	Preservative free solution	0.0015	One drop every night	
Rho kinase inhibitor						
Netarsudil	Rho kinase inhibitor	Rhopressa	Solution	0.02	One drop every night	
Combinations						
Timolol—dorzolamide		Cosopt Generic	Solution	Timolol 0.5/ Dorzolamide 2	One drop twice daily	
Timolol—brimonidine		Combigan	Solution	Timolol 0.5/ Brimonidine 0.2	One drop twice daily	
Brinzolamide—brimonidine		Simbrinza	Suspension	Brinzolamide 1/ Brimonidine 0.2	One drop three times daily	
Netarsudil-latanoprost		Rocklatan	Solution	Netarsudil 0.02/ Latanoprost 0.005	One drop every night	

aUse of nasolacrimal occlusion will increase the number of patients successfully treated with longer dosage intervals.

- Monitoring therapy for POAG should be individualized. Assess IOP response every 4–6 weeks initially, every 3–4 months after IOPs become acceptable, and more frequently if therapy is changed. Visual field and disc changes are monitored annually, unless glaucoma is unstable or worsening.
- There is no specific target IOP because the correlation between IOP and optic nerve damage is poor. Typically, a reduction of 25%–30% is desired.
- The target IOP also depends on disease severity and is generally less than 21 mm Hg (2.8 kPa) for early visual field loss or optic disc changes, with progressively lower targets for greater levels of glaucomatous damage. Targets as low as less than 10 mm Hg (1.3 kPa) are desired for very advanced disease, continued damage at higher IOPs, normal-tension glaucoma, and pretreatment pressures in the low to middle teens.
- Monitor medication adherence because it is commonly inadequate and a cause of therapy failure.

See Chapter 110, Glaucoma, authored by Richard G. Fiscella, Timothy S. Lesar, Ohoud A. Owaidhah, and Deepak P. Edward, for a more detailed discussion of this topic.

CHAPTER 66 | Anxiety Disorders

- *Anxiety disorders* (eg, generalized anxiety disorder [GAD] and panic disorder [PD]) have prominent features of anxiety and avoidance that are irrational or that impair functioning. In posttraumatic stress disorder (PTSD), there is previous exposure to trauma and intrusive, avoidant, and hyperarousal symptoms.

ETIOLOGY

- Evaluation of anxiety requires a physical and mental status examination; complete psychiatric diagnostic exam; appropriate laboratory tests.
- Anxiety symptoms may be associated with medical illnesses (**Table 66-1**) or medications (**Table 66-2**), and they may be present in several major psychiatric illnesses (eg, mood disorders, schizophrenia, organic mental syndromes, and substance withdrawal).

PATHOPHYSIOLOGY

- *Noradrenergic model.* The autonomic nervous system of anxious patients is hypersensitive and overreacts to various stimuli. The locus ceruleus (LC) may have a role in regulating anxiety, because it activates norepinephrine release and stimulates the sympathetic and parasympathetic nervous systems. Chronic noradrenergic overactivity downregulates α_2-adrenoreceptors in patients with GAD and PTSD, while this receptor is hypersensitive in PD. Drugs with anxiolytic or antipanic effects (eg, benzodiazepines and antidepressants) inhibit LC firing, decrease noradrenergic activity, and block the effects of anxiogenic drugs.
- *γ-Aminobutyric acid (GABA) receptor model.* GABA is the major inhibitory neurotransmitter in the central nervous system (CNS). Benzodiazepines enhance the inhibitory effects of GABA, which regulates or inhibits serotonin (5-hydroxytryptamine; 5-HT), norepinephrine, and dopamine activity. The number of $GABA_A$ receptors can change with alterations in the environment, and GABA receptor subunit expression can be altered by hormonal changes. Abnormal functioning of several neurotransmitter systems, including norepinephrine, GABA, glutamate, dopamine, and 5-HT, may affect manifestations of anxiety disorders.
- *5-HT model.* Abnormalities in serotonergic functioning may play a role. Preclinical models suggest that greater 5-HT function facilitates avoidance behavior; but primate studies show that reducing 5-HT increases aggression. GAD symptoms may reflect excessive 5-HT transmission or overactivity of the stimulatory 5-HT pathways. The selective serotonin reuptake inhibitors (SSRIs) increase 5-HT levels at the synapse and are effective in blocking manifestations of panic and anxiety.
- Cortisol reduces the stress response by tempering the sympathetic reaction. Patients with PTSD hypersecrete corticotropin-releasing factor but have subnormal levels of cortisol at the time of trauma and chronically. Dysregulation of the hypothalamic–pituitary–adrenal axis may be a risk factor for eventual development of PTSD.
- Neuroimaging studies support the role of the amygdala, anterior cingulate cortex, and insula in the pathophysiology of anxiety. In GAD, there is an abnormal increase in the brain's fear circuitry and increased activity in the prefrontal cortex. Patients with PD have abnormalities of midbrain structures. In PTSD, the amygdala plays a role in the persistence of traumatic memory. Hypofunctioning in the ventromedial

TABLE 66-1	Common Medical Illnesses Associated with Anxiety Symptoms

Cardiovascular: Angina, arrhythmias, cardiomyopathy, congestive heart failure, hypertension, ischemic heart disease, mitral valve prolapse, myocardial infarction

Endocrine and metabolic: Cushing disease, diabetes, hyperparathyroidism, hyperthyroidism, hypothyroidism, hypoglycemia, hyponatremia, hyperkalemia, pheochromocytoma, vitamin B_{12} or folate deficiencies

Gastrointestinal: Crohn disease, irritable bowel syndrome, ulcerative colitis, peptic ulcer disease

Neurologic: Migraine, seizures, stroke, neoplasms, poor pain control

Respiratory system: Asthma, chronic obstructive pulmonary disease, pulmonary embolism, pneumonia

Others: Anemias, cancer, systemic lupus erythematosus, vestibular dysfunction

TABLE 66-2	Drugs Associated with Anxiety Symptoms

Anticonvulsants: carbamazepine, phenytoin

Antidepressants: bupropion, selective serotonin reuptake inhibitors, serotonin–norepinephrine reuptake inhibitors

Antihypertensives: clonidine, felodipine

Antibiotics: quinolones, isoniazid

Bronchodilators: albuterol, theophylline

Corticosteroids: prednisone

Dopamine agonists: amantadine, levodopa

Herbals: ma huang, ginseng, ephedra

Illicit substances: ecstasy, marijuana

Nonsteroidal anti-inflammatory drugs: ibuprofen, indomethacin

Stimulants: amphetamines, caffeine, cocaine, methylphenidate, nicotine

Sympathomimetics: pseudoephedrine, phenylephrine

Thyroid hormones: levothyroxine

Toxicity: anticholinergics, antihistamines, digoxin

prefrontal cortex is theorized to prevent extinction in patients with PTSD and is inversely correlated with severity of symptoms.

- Glutamate signaling abnormalities may distort amygdala-dependent emotional processing under stress, which may contribute to the dissociative and hypervigilant symptoms in PTSD.

Generalized Anxiety Disorder

CLINICAL PRESENTATION AND DIAGNOSIS

- Psychological and cognitive symptoms of GAD include excessive anxiety, worries that are difficult to control, feeling keyed up or on edge, and trouble concentrating or mind going blank.

- Physical symptoms include restlessness, fatigue, muscle tension, sleep disturbance, and irritability.
- The diagnosis of GAD requires excessive anxiety and worry most days for at least 6 months with at least three physical symptoms present. Significant distress or impairment in functioning is present, and the disturbance is not caused by a substance or another medical condition.
- Women are twice as likely as men to have GAD. The illness has a gradual onset at an average age of 21 years. The course is chronic, with multiple exacerbations and remissions.

TREATMENT

- <u>Goals of Treatment</u>: The goals are to reduce severity, duration, and frequency of symptoms and improve functioning. The long-term goal is minimal or no anxiety symptoms, no functional impairment, prevention of recurrence, and improved quality of life.

NONPHARMACOLOGIC THERAPY

- Nonpharmacologic modalities include psychotherapy, short-term counseling, stress management, psychoeducation, meditation, and exercise. Ideally, patients with GAD should have psychological therapy, alone or in combination with antianxiety drugs. Cognitive behavioral therapy (CBT), though not widely available, is the most effective psychological therapy. Patients should avoid caffeine, nicotine, stimulants, excessive alcohol, and diet pills.
- A treatment algorithm from the International Psychopharmacology Algorithm Project (IMAP) is shown in **Figure 66-1**.

PHARMACOLOGIC THERAPY

- Drug choices for GAD and PD are shown in **Table 66-3**, and non-benzodiazepine antianxiety agents for GAD and their dosing are shown in **Table 66-4**.

Antidepressants

- Antidepressants are effective for acute and long-term management of GAD (Table 66-4). They are the treatment of choice for long-term management of chronic anxiety, especially in the presence of depressive symptoms. **Venlafaxine extended-release, duloxetine, paroxetine**, and **escitalopram** are FDA-approved for GAD, and **imipramine** is considered a second-line agent. Antianxiety response requires 2–4 weeks or longer. See Chapter 68 for additional information on antidepressants.
- Selective serotonin reuptake inhibitors (SSRIs), extended-release venlafaxine, and duloxetine are effective in acute therapy (response rates of 60%–68%). In a meta-analysis, **fluoxetine** was most likely to achieve remission of GAD symptoms; sertraline was best tolerated.
- Common side effects and monitoring parameters for patients taking medications used for anxiety disorders are shown in **Table 66-5**.
- Some patients require small initial doses of antidepressants for the first week to limit the development of transient increased anxiety, also known as jitteriness syndrome.
- All antidepressants carry a black box warning regarding suicidality (suicidal thinking and behaviors) in children, adolescents, and young adults less than 25 years and recommends specific monitoring parameters (consult the FDA-approved labeling or the FDA website).
- Clinical practice guidelines recommend use of fluoxetine, sertraline, or citalopram for pregnant women; however, jitteriness, myoclonus, and irritability in the neonate and premature infant have been reported and paroxetine should be avoided due to cardiovascular malformation risk.

Benzodiazepines

- All benzodiazepines possess anxiolytic properties, although only 7 marketed agents have FDA approval for the treatment of GAD, as the other agents have different FDA-approved indications.

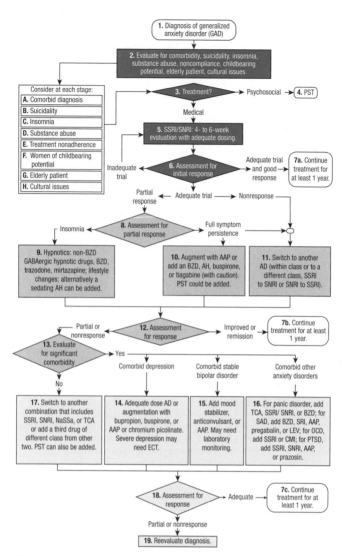

Dark blue, first-line treatment (nodes 2, 3, 5, 6); medium blue, second-line treatment (nodes 8–12); light blue, third-line treatment, no comorbidity (nodes 13, 17, 18, 19); gray, third-line treatment, with comorbidity (nodes 14–16). Levels of evidence used in development of the flowchart were: 1, more than one placebo-controlled trial with sample sizes over 30; 2, one placebo-controlled trial (or active vs. active drug comparison) with sample size of 30 or greater; 3, one or small ($n < 30$) placebo-controlled trial; 4, case reports or open-label trials; and 5, expert consensus without published evidence. (Used by permission of the International Psychopharmacology Algorithm Project. IPAP—Generalized Anxiety Disorder Algorithm. http://www.ipap.org./gad/index.php, accessed December 22, 2015.)

(AAP, atypical antipsychotic; AD, antidepressant; AH, antihistamine; BZD, benzodiazepine; CMI, clomipramine; ECT, electroconvulsive therapy; GAD, generalized anxiety disorder; LEV, levetiracetam; NaSSa, noradrenergic and selective serotonergic antidepressant; PST, psychosocial treatment; SAD, social anxiety disorder; SNRI, serotonin-norepinephrine reuptake inhibitor; SRI, serotonin reuptake inhibitor; SSRI, selective serotonin reuptake inhibitor; TCA, tricyclic antidepressant.)

FIGURE 66-1. International Psychopharmacology Algorithm Project (IPAP) generalized anxiety disorder (GAD) algorithm flowchart.

TABLE 66-3	Drug Choices for Anxiety Disorders		
Anxiety Disorder	**First-Line Drugs**	**Second-Line Drugs**	**Alternatives**
Generalized anxiety disorder	Duloxetine	Benzodiazepines	Hydroxyzine
	Escitalopram	Buspirone	Quetiapine
	Paroxetine	Imipramine	
	Sertraline	Pregabalin	
	Venlafaxine XR		
Panic disorder	SSRIs	Alprazolam	Phenelzine
	Venlafaxine XR	Citalopram	
		Clomipramine	
		Clonazepam	
		Imipramine	

SSRI, selective serotonin reuptake inhibitor; XR, extended-release.

TABLE 66-4	Nonbenzodiazepine Antianxiety Agents for Generalized Anxiety Disorder			
Drug	**Brand Name**	**Initial Dose**	**Usual Range (mg/day)**[a]	**Comments**
Antidepressants				
Duloxetine	Cymbalta	30 or 60 mg/day	60–120	FDA-approved
Escitalopram	Lexapro	10 mg/day	10–20	FDA-approved, available generically
Imipramine	Tofranil	50 mg/day	75–200	Available generically
Paroxetine	Paxil Pexeva	20 mg/day	20–50	FDA-approved, available generically, avoid in pregnancy
Sertraline	Zoloft	50 mg/day	50–200	Available generically
Venlafaxine XR	Effexor XR	37.5 or 75 mg/day	75–225[b]	FDA-approved, available generically
Vilazodone	Viibryd	10 mg/day	20–40[b]	During concomitant use of a strong CYP3A4 inhibitor (eg, itraconazole, clarithromycin, voriconazole), dose should not exceed 20 mg once daily
Vortioxetine	Brintellix	5 mg/day	5–20	(Continued)

TABLE 66-4	Nonbenzodiazepine Antianxiety Agents for Generalized Anxiety Disorder (*Continued*)			
Drug	**Brand Name**	**Initial Dose**	**Usual Range (mg/day)**[a]	**Comments**
Azapirone				
Buspirone	BuSpar	7.5 mg twice daily	15–60[b]	FDA-approved, available generically
Diphenylmethane				
Hydroxyzine	Vistaril	25 or 50 mg four times daily (adult)	200–400	FDA-approved, available generically, also approved for children with anxiety and tension
Anticonvulsant				
Pregabalin	Lyrica	50 mg three times daily	150–600	Dosage adjustment required in renal impairment
Atypical antipsychotic				
Quetiapine XR	Seroquel XR	50 mg at bedtime	150–300	

[a]Older patients are usually treated with approximately one-half of the dose listed.
[b]No dosage adjustment is required in older patients.
XR, extended-release.

- Benzodiazepines are the most effective and frequently prescribed drugs for the treatment of acute anxiety (**Table 66-6**). About 65%–75% of patients with GAD have a marked to moderate response, and most of the improvement occurs in the first 2 weeks of therapy. They are more effective for somatic and autonomic symptoms of GAD, whereas antidepressants are more effective for the psychic symptoms (eg, apprehension and worry).
- The dose must be individualized. Older patients are more sensitive to benzodiazepines and may experience falls when taking them.
- The most common side effect of benzodiazepines is CNS depression. Tolerance usually develops to this effect. Other side effects are disorientation, psychomotor impairment, confusion, aggression, excitement, ataxia, and anterograde amnesia (see Table 66-5).
- Start with low doses, and adjust weekly (see Table 66-6). Benzodiazepines should be used with a regular dosing regimen and not on an as-needed basis when used for the treatment of an anxiety disorder
- Treatment of acute anxiety generally should be 2–4 weeks. Manage persistent symptoms with antidepressants.
- Long half-life benzodiazepines may be dosed once daily at bedtime, providing nighttime hypnotic and next day anxiolytic effects.
- Use low doses of short-elimination half-life agents in older patients.
- **Diazepam** and **clorazepate** have high lipophilicity and are rapidly absorbed and distributed into the CNS. They have rapid antianxiety effects, but a shorter duration of effect after a single dose than would be predicted based on half-life, as they are rapidly distributed to the periphery.

TABLE 66-5 Monitoring of Adverse Effects Associated with Medications Used for Anxiety Disorders

Medication Class/Drug	Adverse Drug Reaction	Monitoring Parameter	Comments
SSRIs	Jitteriness syndrome	Patient interview	
	Suicidality	Patient interview	Monitor weekly in first few weeks in patients with comorbid depression and patients under age 25
	Nausea, diarrhea	Patient interview	Typically transient
	Headache	Patient interview	Typically transient
	Weight gain	Body weight, BMI, waist circumference	Paroxetine may be more likely to cause weight gain
	Sexual dysfunction	Patient interview	Significant reason for nonadherence
	Hyponatremia	Basic metabolic panel	Monitor at baseline and periodically thereafter. More frequent monitoring required in high-risk groups, especially patients >65 years
	Thrombocytopenia	Complete blood count	Reported with citalopram
	Teratogenicity	Pregnancy test at baseline	Avoid paroxetine in pregnancy; Pregnancy Category D
	QT prolongation	ECG	Before starting citalopram, consider ECG and measurement of QT interval in patients with cardiac disease
	Discontinuation syndrome	Patient interview	Avoid abrupt discontinuation in all but fluoxetine
SNRIs	Jitteriness syndrome	Patient interview	
	Suicidality	Patient interview	Monitor weekly in first few weeks in patients with comorbid depression and patients under age 25
	Nausea, diarrhea	Patient interview	Typically transient
	Headache	Patient interview	Typically transient
	Elevated blood pressure	Blood pressure	Monitor blood pressure on initiation and regularly during treatment
	Sexual dysfunction	Patient interview	Significant reason for nonadherence
	Discontinuation syndrome	Patient interview	Avoid abrupt discontinuation

(Continued)

TABLE 66-5 Monitoring of Adverse Effects Associated with Medications Used for Anxiety Disorders (*Continued*)

Medication Class/Drug	Adverse Drug Reaction	Monitoring Parameter	Comments
TCAs	Jitteriness syndrome	Patient interview	
	Suicidality	Patient interview	Monitor weekly in first few weeks in patients with comorbid depression and patients under age 25
	Anticholinergic effects	Patient interview	Contraindicated with narrow-angle glaucoma, prostatic hypertrophy, and urinary retention
	Weight gain	Body weight, BMI, waist circumference	Significant reason for nonadherence
	Sexual dysfunction	Patient interview	Administer dosage at bedtime when feasible
	Sedation	Patient interview	At baseline and periodically in children and patients >40 years of age
	Arrhythmia	ECG	
	Orthostatic hypotension	Blood pressure with position changes	
	Cholinergic rebound	Patient interview	Avoid abrupt discontinuation; taper doses
Benzodiazepines	Drowsiness, fatigue	Patient interview	Avoid operating large machinery; tolerance to sedation develops after repeated dosing
	Anterograde amnesia and memory impairment	Patient interview	Risk of anterograde amnesia is worsened with concomitant intake of alcohol
	Dependence	Patient interview; Prescription Monitoring Program	Monitor for early refills or escalation of dosage
	Withdrawal symptoms	Physical examination; patient interview	Taper doses on discontinuation
	Respiratory depression	Respiratory rate	Avoid administering with other CNS depressants (ie, opioids, alcohol)
	Psychomotor impairment	Physical examination	Increased risk of falls
	Paradoxical disinhibition	Physical examination; family report	Increase in anxiety, irritability, or agitation may be seen in older patients or children

Other drugs

Drug	Adverse effect	Monitoring parameter	Comments
Buspirone	Nausea, abdominal pain	Patient interview	Typically transient
	Drowsiness, dizziness	Patient interview	Typically transient
Phenelzine	Jitteriness syndrome	Patient interview	
	Suicidality	Patient interview	Monitor weekly in first few weeks in patients with comorbid depression and patients under age 25
	Hypertensive crisis	Blood pressure	Tyramine-free diet and avoidance of drug interactions required
Pregabalin	Orthostatic hypotension	Blood pressure with position changes	Fasting labs at baseline and then periodically
	Dizziness, somnolence	Patient interview	
	Peripheral edema	Physical examination	
Quetiapine	Thrombocytopenia	Complete blood count	
	Weight gain	Body weight	
	Sedation	Patient interview	
	Metabolic syndrome	Body weight, BMI, waist circumference, fasting lipids and glucose	Fasting labs at baseline and then periodically
	Akathisia	Patient interview	
	Tardive dyskinesia	Abnormal Involuntary Movement Scale	
	Orthostatic hypotension	Blood pressure with position changes	

BMI, body mass index; ECG, electrocardiogram; SNRI, serotonin–norepinephrine reuptake inhibitor; SSRIs, selective serotonin reuptake inhibitors; TCAs, tricyclic antidepressants.

		Approved Dosage Range (mg/day)	Maximum Dosage for Older Patients (mg/day)	Approximate Equivalent Dose (mg)	
TABLE 66-6	**Benzodiazepine Antianxiety Agents**				
Drug	**Brand Name**				**Comments**
Alprazolam[a]	Niravam[b], Xanax	0.75–4	2	0.5	Associated with interdose rebound anxiety
	Xanax XR	1–10[c]			
Chlordiazepoxide[a]	Librium	25–400	40	10	
Clonazepam[a]	Klonopin	1–4[c]	3	0.25–0.5	
	Klonopin Wafer[b]				
Clorazepate[a]	Tranxene	7.5–60	30	7.5	
Diazepam[a]	Valium	2–40	20	5	
Lorazepam[a]	Ativan	0.5–10	3	1	Preferred in elderly
Oxazepam[a]	Serax	30–120	60	30	Preferred in elderly

[a]Available generically.
[b]Orally disintegrating formulation.
[c]Panic disorder dose.
XR, extended-release.

- **Lorazepam** and **oxazepam** are less lipophilic, have a slower onset, but a longer duration of action. They are not recommended for immediate relief of anxiety.
- **Avoid intramuscular (IM) diazepam** and **IM chlordiazepoxide** because of variability in rate and extent of absorption. **IM lorazepam** provides rapid and complete absorption.
- Several benzodiazepines are converted to desmethyldiazepam, which has a long half-life and can accumulate. Intermediate- or short-acting benzodiazepines are preferred for chronic use in older patients and those with liver disorders because of minimal accumulation and achievement of steady state within 1–3 days.
- Combining benzodiazepines with alcohol or other CNS depressants may be fatal.
- Addition of nefazodone, ritonavir, or ketoconazole (CYP3A4 inhibitors) can increase the blood levels of alprazolam and diazepam. Drugs that induce cytochrome CYP3A4 (eg, carbamazepine, St. John's wort) can reduce benzodiazepine levels. Drugs that inhibit or induce CYP2C19 (eg, fluoxetine, fluvoxamine, omeprazole) or *N*-acetyltransferase 2 activity can alter diazepam and clonazepam metabolism, respectively.
- Consult the drug interaction literature for more information on benzodiazepine drug interactions.
- Benzodiazepine use in pregnant women has been associated with teratogenic effects (ie, cleft lip and palate, "floppy baby syndrome," and neonatal withdrawal. Antidepressants are preferred. If a benzodiazepine must be used, diazepam and chlordiazepoxide may be preferred but may cause sedation, lethargy, and weight loss in breastfed infants.

Benzodiazepine Discontinuation

- After benzodiazepines are abruptly discontinued, three events can occur: (1) rebound symptoms are an immediate but transient return of original symptoms with an increased intensity compared with baseline; (2) recurrence or relapse is the return of original symptoms at the same intensity as before treatment; or (3) withdrawal is the emergence of new symptoms and a worsening of preexisting symptoms.
- The onset of withdrawal symptoms is within 24–48 hours after discontinuation of short-elimination half-life benzodiazepines and 3–8 days after discontinuation of long-elimination half-life drugs.
- Discontinuation strategies include:
  - ✓ A 25% per week reduction in dosage until 50% of the dose is reached, and then reduce by one eighth every 4–7 days. If therapy duration exceeds 8 weeks, a taper over 2–3 weeks is recommended, but if duration of treatment is 6 months, a taper over 4–8 weeks is reasonable. Longer durations of treatment may require a 2- to 4-month taper.
- Adjunctive use of **pregabalin** can help to reduce withdrawal symptoms during the benzodiazepine taper.

Abuse, Dependence, Withdrawal, and Tolerance

- Benzodiazepine dependence is defined by appearance of a withdrawal syndrome (ie, anxiety, insomnia, agitation, muscle tension, irritability, nausea, diaphoresis, nightmares, depression, hyperreflexia, tinnitus, delusions, hallucinations, and seizures) upon abrupt discontinuation.
- Those with a history of drug abuse should not receive benzodiazepines. Those with GAD and PD are at high risk for dependence because of the chronicity of the illnesses.

Buspirone

- **Buspirone** is a 5-HT$_{1A}$ partial agonist that lacks anticonvulsant, muscle relaxant, sedative-hypnotic, motor impairment, and dependence-producing properties.
- It is a second-line agent for GAD because of inconsistent reports of long-term efficacy, and delayed onset of effect. It is an option for patients who fail other anxiolytic therapies or patients with a history of alcohol or substance abuse. It does not provide rapid or "as needed" antianxiety effects.
- Buspirone can be titrated in increments of 5 mg/day every 2 or 3 days as needed.
- The onset of anxiolytic effects requires 2 weeks or more; maximum benefit may require 4–6 weeks. Improvement in psychic symptoms precedes improvement in somatic symptoms.
- It may be less effective in patients who have previously taken benzodiazepines.
- It has a mean $t_{1/2}$ of 2.5 hours, and it is dosed two to three times daily (see Table 66-4).
- Buspirone may elevate blood pressure in patients taking a monoamine oxidase inhibitor (MAOI).
- Verapamil, itraconazole, and fluvoxamine can increase buspirone levels through CYP3A4 inhibition, and rifampin reduces buspirone blood levels 10-fold.

Alternative Pharmacotherapy

- **Hydroxyzine**, often used in primary care, is considered a second-line agent.
- **Pregabalin** produced anxiolytic effects similar to lorazepam, alprazolam, and venlafaxine in acute trials. Sedation and dizziness were the most common adverse effects.
- **Quetiapine** extended release, 150 mg/day, was superior to placebo and as effective as **paroxetine** 20 mg/day and **escitalopram** 10 mg/day, but with earlier onset of action. Quetiapine is not FDA-approved for GAD and the long-term risks are unknown.

EVALUATION OF THERAPEUTIC OUTCOMES

- Initially, monitor anxious patients every 2 weeks for reduction in anxiety symptoms, improvement in functioning, and side effects. The Hamilton Rating Scale for Anxiety or the Sheehan Disability Scale can help measure drug response.
- Treatment resistance may be diagnosed after poor, partial, or lack of response is seen with at least two antidepressants from different classes. For those who do not achieve an appropriate response with a first-line agent the dose may be increased, changed to a different agent in the same class or different class, or augmented. If treatment fails, the clinician should assess for (a) symptoms (eg, psychotic symptoms) that need additional medications or (b) treatment nonadherence. Patients should also be assessed for concurrent substance use disorder, concurrent illnesses, and suicidal thoughts.

Panic Disorder

CLINICAL PRESENTATION

- Psychological symptoms include depersonalization (feeling detached from oneself); derealization (feelings of being detached from one's environment); and fear of losing control, going crazy, or dying.
- Physical symptoms include abdominal distress, chest pain or discomfort, chills, dizziness or lightheadedness, feeling of choking, heart sensations, nausea, palpitations, paresthesias, sensation of shortness or breath or smothering, sweating, tachycardia, and trembling or shaking.
- Recurrent unexpected panic attacks. At least one attack has been followed by at least 1 month of either or both (1) persistent worry about having another panic attack or their consequences or (2) maladaptive change in behavior related to the attacks.
- During an attack, there must be at least four symptoms in addition to intense fear or discomfort. Symptoms reach a peak within 10 minutes and usually last no more than 20 or 30 minutes.
- Up to 50% of Panic Disorder (PD) patients develop agoraphobia, which is marked fear or anxiety about being in at least 2 situations where escape could be difficult or help unavailable (eg, being in crowded places or crossing bridges). Patients may become homebound.

TREATMENT

- <u>Goals of Treatment</u>: Complete resolution of panic attacks, marked reduction in anticipatory anxiety, elimination of phobic avoidance, and no functional impairment.

NONPHARMACOLOGIC THERAPY

- Cognitive Behavioral Therapy (CBT) is associated with short-term improvement in 80%–90% of patients and 6-month improvement in 75% of patients. Adding psychosocial treatment to pharmacotherapy may reduce likelihood of relapse when drug therapy is stopped.
- Educate patient to avoid caffeine, nicotine, alcohol, drugs of abuse, and stimulants. Aerobic exercise may benefit patients with PD.

PHARMACOLOGIC THERAPY

- SSRIs or **venlafaxine XR** are first-line agents for PD (**Table 66-7**), but benzodiazepines (second line agents) are the most commonly used drugs. **Imipramine** is considered second line. An algorithm for drug therapy of PD is shown in **Figure 66-2**.
- If pharmacotherapy is used, antidepressants, especially the SSRIs, are preferred in older patients and youth. The benzodiazepines are second line in these patients because of potential problems with disinhibition.

TABLE 66-7	Drugs Used in the Treatment of Panic Disorder		
Class/Generic Name	**Brand Name**	**Starting Dose**	**Antipanic Dosage Range (mg)**
SSRIs			
Citalopram	Celexa	10 mg/day	20–40
Escitalopram	Lexapro	5 mg/day	10–20
Fluoxetine	Prozac	5 mg/day	10–30
Fluvoxamine	Luvox	25 mg/day	100–300
Paroxetine	Paxil	10 mg/day	20–60
	Pexeva		
	Paxil CR	12.5 mg/day	25–75
Sertraline	Zoloft	25 mg/day	50–200
SNRI			
Venlafaxine XR	Effexor XR	37.5 mg/day	75–225
Benzodiazepines			
Alprazolam	Xanax	0.5 mg three times a day	4–10
	Xanax XR	0.5–1 mg/day	3–10
Clonazepam	Klonopin	0.25 mg once or twice daily	1–4
Diazepam	Valium	2–5 mg three times a day	5–20
Lorazepam	Ativan	0.5–1 mg three times a day	2–8
TCA			
Imipramine	Tofranil	10 mg/day	75–250
MAOI			
Phenelzine	Nardil	15 mg/day	45–90

CR, controlled release; MAOI, monoamine oxidase inhibitor; SNRI, serotonin–norepinephrine reuptake inhibitor; SSRIs, selective serotonin reuptake inhibitors; TCA, tricyclic antidepressant; XR, extended release.

- The acute phase of treatment usually lasts 1–3 months with SSRIs. Therapy should be altered if there is no response after 6–8 weeks of an adequate dose. With benzodiazepines the acute phase lasts approximately 1 month.
- Usually patients are treated for 12–24 months before discontinuation is attempted over 4–6 months. Many patients require long-term therapy.

Antidepressants

- **Citalopram** use is limited by QT prolongation.
- Stimulatory side effects (eg, anxiety, insomnia, and jitteriness) that can occur in tricyclic antidepressant (TCA) and SSRI-treated patients may hinder adherence and dose escalation. Low initial doses and gradual dose titration may eliminate these effects (see Table 66-7).
- Imipramine blocks panic attacks within 4 weeks in 75% of patients, but reducing anticipatory anxiety and phobic avoidance requires 8–12 weeks.
- Twenty-five percent of PD patients discontinue TCAs because of side effects.
- SSRIs eliminate panic attacks in 60%–80% of patients within about 4 weeks, but some patients require 8–12 weeks.
- Venlafaxine extended release is superior to placebo and similar in efficacy to **paroxetine** in relieving panic attacks, anticipatory anxiety, fear, and avoidance.

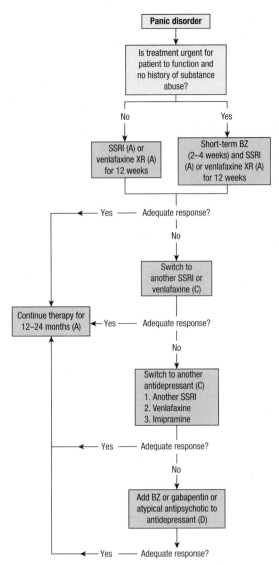

Strength of recommendations: A, directly based on category I evidence (ie, meta-analysis of randomized controlled trials [RCT] or at least one RCT); B, directly based on category II evidence (ie, at least one controlled study without randomization or one other type of quasi-experimental study); C, directly based on category III evidence (ie, nonexperimental descriptive studies); D, directly based on category IV evidence (ie, expert committee reports or opinions and/or clinical experience of respected authorities).

(BZ, benzodiazepine; SSRI, selective serotonin reuptake inhibitor.)

FIGURE 66-2. Algorithm for the pharmacotherapy of panic disorder.

Benzodiazepines

- Benzodiazepines are second-line agents for PD except when rapid response is essential. Avoid benzodiazepine monotherapy in patients with PD who are depressed, have a history of depression, or a history of alcohol or drug abuse. They are often used concomitantly with antidepressants in the first 4–6 weeks to achieve a more rapid antipanic response.
- Relapse rates of 50% or higher are common despite slow drug tapering.
- **Alprazolam** and **clonazepam** are the preferred benzodiazepines for PD. Therapeutic response typically occurs within 1–2 weeks. The use of extended-release alprazolam or clonazepam avoids breakthrough symptoms between doses.
  - ✓ A regular dosing schedule is preferred as the goal is to prevent panic attacks rather than reduce symptoms once an attack has already occurred
  - ✓ The starting dose of clonazepam is 0.25 mg once or twice daily, with a dose increase of 0.25–0.5 mg every 3 days to 4 mg/day if needed.
  - ✓ The starting dose of alprazolam is 0.25 three times daily (or 0.5 mg once daily of extended-release alprazolam), slowly increasing over several weeks as needed. Most patients require 3–6 mg/day.

EVALUATION OF THERAPEUTIC OUTCOMES

- Evaluate patients with PD every 1–2 weeks during the first few weeks to fine-tune dosing and to monitor side effects. Once stabilized, they can be seen every 2 months. The Panic Disorder Severity Scale (with a remission goal of three or less with no or mild agoraphobic avoidance, anxiety, disability, or depressive symptoms) and the Sheehan Disability Scale (with a goal of less than or equal to one on each item) can be used to measure disability. During drug discontinuation, the frequency of appointments should be increased.

Posttraumatic Stress Disorder

CLINICAL PRESENTATION

- In adults and children older than 6, there is exposure to actual or threatened death, serious injury, or sexual violence, either directly, or by witnessing the event(s) happening to others, learning about the event(s) happening to someone close, or experiencing repeated or extreme exposure to details of the event(s).
- Duration of intrusive, avoidance, alterations in thinking and mood, and hyperarousal symptoms (**Table 66-8**) must be present longer than 1 month and cause significant distress or impairment. There must be at least one intrusive symptom, one symptom of avoidance of stimuli associated with the trauma, at least two symptoms of negative alterations in thinking and mood, and at least two symptoms of increased arousal. PTSD co-occurs with mood, anxiety, and substance use disorders.

TREATMENT

- <u>Goals of Treatment</u>: Reduction in core symptoms, disability, comorbidity and improved quality of life.
- Immediately after the trauma, patients should receive treatment individualized to their presenting symptoms (eg, nonbenzodiazepine hypnotic or short courses of trauma-focused cognitive behavioral therapy [CBT]). Brief courses of CBT in close proximity to the trauma can help prevent PTSD.
- If symptoms persist for 3–4 weeks, and there is social or occupational impairment, patients can receive pharmacotherapy or psychotherapy, or both.

TABLE 66-8	Clinical Presentation of Posttraumatic Stress Disorder

Intrusion symptoms
- Recurrent, intrusive distressing memories of the trauma
- Recurrent, disturbing dreams of the event
- Feeling that the traumatic event is recurring (eg, dissociative flashbacks)
- Physiologic reaction to or psychological distress from reminders of the trauma

Avoidance symptoms
- Avoidance of conversations, thoughts, or feelings about the trauma
- Avoidance of people, places, or activities that are reminders of the event

Persistent negative alterations in thinking and mood
- Inability to recall an important aspect of the trauma
- Anhedonia
- Estrangement from others
- Restricted affect
- Negative beliefs about oneself
- Distorted beliefs causing one to blame others or themselves for the trauma
- Negative mood state

Hyperarousal symptoms
- Decreased concentration
- Easily startled
- Self-destructive behavior
- Hypervigilance
- Insomnia
- Irritability or anger outbursts

Specifiers
- Dissociative symptoms: depersonalization or derealization
- With delayed expression: full criteria are not met until at least 6 months posttrauma

NONPHARMACOLOGIC THERAPY

- Psychotherapies include stress management, eye movement desensitization and reprocessing (EMDR), and psychoeducation. Trauma-focused CBT and EMDR are more effective than stress management or group therapy to reduce PTSD symptoms.

PHARMACOLOGIC THERAPY

- **Figure 66-3** shows an algorithm for the pharmacotherapy of PTSD.
- The SSRIs and venlafaxine are first-line pharmacotherapy for PTSD (**Table 66-9**). The TCAs and MAOIs also can be effective, but side effects can be problematic.
- **Sertraline** and **paroxetine** are approved for acute treatment of PTSD, and sertraline is approved for long-term management.
- Antiadrenergics and atypical antipsychotics can be used as augmenting agents.
- Large prospective studies document the effectiveness of sertraline and paroxetine in acute management of PTSD. Long-term use of SSRIs (9–12 months) was effective in preventing relapse.
- In a 12-week trial comparing **venlafaxine XR** and sertraline, venlafaxine XR was effective in reducing the avoidance/numbing and hyperarousal cluster, whereas sertraline improved all PTSD symptom clusters.
- **Mirtazapine,** amitriptyline and imipramine are second line drugs. **Phenelzine** is considered a third-line drug.
- If there is no improvement in the acute stress response 3–4 weeks following trauma, SSRIs should be started in a low dose with slow titration upward toward antidepressant doses. Eight to 12 weeks is an adequate duration of treatment to determine response.
- Responders to drug therapy should continue treatment for at least 12 months. When discontinued, drug therapy should be tapered slowly over 1 month or more to reduce the likelihood of relapse.

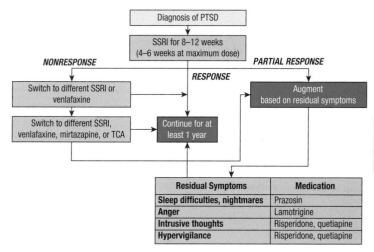

FIGURE 66-3. Algorithm for the pharmacotherapy of posttraumatic stress disorder (PTSD).

Residual Symptoms	Medication
Sleep difficulties, nightmares	Prazosin
Anger	Lamotrigine
Intrusive thoughts	Risperidone, quetiapine
Hypervigilance	Risperidone, quetiapine

TABLE 66-9	Dosing of Antidepressants in the Treatment of PTSD		
Drug	**Brand Name**	**Initial Dose**	**Usual Range (mg/day)**
SSRIs			
Fluoxetine[a]	Prozac	10 mg/day	10–40[b]
Paroxetine[a]	Paxil, Pexeva	10–20 mg/day	20–40; max 50 mg/day[c]
Sertraline[a]	Zoloft	25 mg/day	50–100; max 200 mg/day[c]
Other agents			
Amitriptyline[a]	Elavil	25 or 50 mg/day	75–200[b]
Imipramine[a]	Tofranil	25 or 50 mg/day	75–200[b]
Mirtazapine[a]	Remeron	15 mg/night	30–60[b]
Phenelzine[a]	Nardil	15 or 30 mg every night	45–90[b]
Venlafaxine extended-release[a]	Effexor XR	37.5 mg/day	75–225[b]

[a]Available generically.
[b]Dosage used in clinical trials but not FDA approved.
[c]Dosage is FDA approved.
PTSD, posttraumatic stress disorder; SSRIs, selective serotonin reuptake inhibitors.

- **Prazosin**, in daily doses of 1–4 mg, can be useful in some patients with PTSD. It may be particularly helpful for nightmares and insomnia.
- **Risperidone, quetiapine,** α_1-adrenergic antagonists, antidepressants, mood stabilizers, and anticonvulsants may be used as augmenting agents in partial responders.

EVALUATION OF THERAPEUTIC OUTCOMES

• See patients frequently for the first 3 months, then monthly for 3 months. In months 6–12, patients can be seen every 2 months. Those who respond to pharmacotherapy should continue treatment for at least 12 months.
• Monitor for symptom response, suicidal ideation, disability, side effects, and treatment adherence. The Clinician-Administered PTSD Scale (CAPS) can be useful to assess symptom severity.

See Chapter 87, Anxiety Disorders: Generalized Anxiety, Panic, and Social Anxiety Disorders, authored by Sarah T. Melton and Cynthia K. Kirkwood, and Chapter 88, Posttraumatic Stress Disorder and Obsessive-Compulsive Disorder, authored by Kristen N. Gardner, Jolene R. Bostwick, and Ericka L. Crouse, for a more detailed discussion of this topic.

- *Bipolar disorder* is a common, lifelong, often severe cyclic mood disorder characterized by recurrent fluctuations in mood, energy, and behavior. The mania or hypomania is not substance-related or caused by other medical or psychiatric disorders.

PATHOPHYSIOLOGY

- **Table 67-1** lists medical conditions, medications, and treatments that may induce mania.
- Bipolar disorder is influenced by developmental, genetic, neurobiological, and psychological factors. Multiple gene loci are likely involved in the heredity of mood disorders.

CLINICAL PRESENTATION

- Different types of episodes may occur sequentially with or without a period of normal mood (euthymia) between them. There can be mood fluctuations that continue for months or after one episode, and there can be years without recurrence of any type of mood episode.

DIAGNOSIS

- The *Diagnostic and Statistical Manual of Mental Disorders*, 5th edition classifies bipolar disorders into five subtypes:
  (1) Bipolar I disorder: At least one manic episode, which may have been preceded by and may be followed by hypomanic or major depressive episode(s).
  (2) Bipolar II disorder: At least one hypomanic episode and a current or past major depressive episode.
  (3) Cyclothymic disorder: Chronic fluctuations between subsyndromal depressive and hypomanic episodes.
  (4) Other specified bipolar and related disorder.
  (5) Unspecified bipolar and related disorder.
- See **Table 67-2** for diagnostic criteria for major depressive episode, manic episode, and hypomanic episode.
- A medical, psychiatric, and medication history; physical examination; and laboratory testing are necessary to rule out organic causes of mania or depression.
- Delusions, hallucinations, and suicide attempts are more common in bipolar depression than in unipolar depression.
- Acute mania usually begins abruptly, and symptoms increase over several days. Bizarre behavior, hallucinations, and paranoid or grandiose delusions may occur. There is marked impairment in functioning. Manic episodes may be precipitated by stressors, sleep deprivation, antidepressants, central nervous system (CNS) stimulants, or bright light.
- In hypomanic episodes, there is no marked impairment in social or occupational functioning, no delusions, and no hallucinations. Some patients may be more productive than usual, but 5%–15% of patients may rapidly switch to a manic episode.

COURSE OF ILLNESS

- Childhood onset is associated with more mood episodes, rapid cycling, and comorbid psychiatric conditions.

TABLE 67-1	**Secondary Causes of Mania**

Medical conditions that induce mania
- CNS disorders (brain tumor, strokes, head injuries, subdural hematoma, multiple sclerosis, systemic lupus erythematosus, temporal lobe seizures, Huntington disease)
- Infections (encephalitis, neurosyphilis, sepsis, human immunodeficiency virus)
- Electrolyte or metabolic abnormalities (calcium or sodium fluctuations, hyperglycemia or hypoglycemia)
- Endocrine or hormonal dysregulation (Addison disease, Cushing disease, hyperthyroidism or hypothyroidism, menstrual-related or pregnancy-related or perimenopausal mood disorders)

Medications or drugs that induce mania
- Alcohol intoxication
- Drug withdrawal states (alcohol, α_2-adrenergic agonists, antidepressants, barbiturates, benzodiazepines, opiates)
- Antidepressants (MAOIs, TCAs, 5-HT and/or NE and/or DA reuptake inhibitors, 5-HT antagonists)
- DA-augmenting agents (CNS stimulants: amphetamines, cocaine, sympathomimetics; DA agonists, releasers, and reuptake inhibitors)
- Hallucinogens (LSD, PCP)
- Marijuana intoxication precipitates psychosis, paranoid thoughts, anxiety, and restlessness
- NE-augmenting agents (α_2-adrenergic antagonists, β-agonists, NE reuptake inhibitors)
- Steroids (anabolic, adrenocorticotropic hormone, corticosteroids)
- Thyroid preparations
- Xanthines (caffeine, theophylline)
- Nonprescription weight loss agents and decongestants (ephedra, pseudoephedrine)
- Herbal products (St. John's wort)

Somatic therapies that induce mania
- Bright light therapy
- Deep brain stimulation
- Sleep deprivation

CNS, central nervous system; DA, dopamine; 5-HT, serotonin; LSD, lysergic acid diethylamide; MAOI, monoamine oxidase inhibitor; NE, norepinephrine; PCP, phencyclidine; TCA, tricyclic antidepressant.

- Rapid cyclers, 20% of patients with bipolar disorder, have four or more episodes per year (major depressive, manic, or hypomanic). Rapid cycling is associated with frequent and severe episodes of depression and a poorer long-term prognosis.
- Women are more likely to have depressive symptoms, older age of onset, better adherence, and thyroid abnormalities. Men may have more manic episodes and substance use.
- Suicide attempts occur in up to 50% of patients with bipolar disorder, and ~10%–19% of individuals with bipolar I disorder commit suicide. Patients with bipolar II disorder may have a higher rate of suicide attempts than bipolar I patients.

TREATMENT

- <u>Goals of Treatment</u>: (1) Eliminate mood episode with complete remission of symptoms (ie, acute treatment); (2) prevent recurrences or relapses of mood episodes (ie, continuation phase treatment); (3) return to baseline psychosocial functioning; (4) maximize adherence with therapy; (5) minimize adverse effects; (6) use medications with the best tolerability and fewest drug interactions; (7) minimize polypharmacy when possible; (8) treat comorbid substance use and abuse; (9) eliminate alcohol, marijuana, cocaine, amphetamines, and hallucinogens; (10) minimize nicotine use and stop caffeine intake at least 8 hours prior to bedtime; and (11) avoid stressors or substances that precipitate an acute episode.

TABLE 67-2	Evaluation and Diagnosis of Mood Episodes	
Diagnosis Episode	**Impairment of Functioning or Need for Hospitalization**[a]	**DSM-5 Criteria**[b]
Major depressive	Yes	At least 2-week period of either depressed mood or loss of interest or pleasure in normal activities, associated with at least five of the following symptoms: • Depressed, sad mood (adults); can be irritable mood in children • Decreased interest and pleasure in normal activities • Decreased or increased appetite, weight loss or weight gain • Insomnia or hypersomnia • Psychomotor retardation or agitation • Decreased energy or fatigue • Feelings of excessive guilt or worthlessness • Impaired concentration or indecisiveness • Recurrent thoughts of death, suicidal thoughts or attempts
Manic	Yes	At least 1-week period of abnormally and persistently elevated mood (expansive or irritable) and energy, associated with at least three of the following symptoms (four if the mood is only irritable): • Inflated self-esteem (grandiosity) • Decreased need for sleep • Increased talking (pressure of speech) • Racing thoughts (flight of ideas) • Distractibility (poor attention) • Increased goal-directed activity (socially, at work, or sexually) or psychomotor agitation • Excessive involvement in activities that are pleasurable but have a high risk for serious consequences (buying sprees, sexual indiscretions, poor judgment in business ventures)
Hypomanic	No	At least 4 days of abnormally and persistently elevated mood (expansive or irritable) and energy, associated with at least three of the following symptoms (four if the mood is only irritable): • Inflated self-esteem (grandiosity) • Decreased need for sleep • Increased talking (pressure of speech) • Racing thoughts (flight of ideas) • Distractibility (poor attention) • Increased goal-directed activity (socially, at work, or sexually) or psychomotor agitation • Excessive involvement in activities that are pleasurable but have a high risk for serious consequences (buying sprees, sexual indiscretions, poor judgment in business ventures)

[a]Impairment in social or occupational functioning; may include need for hospitalization because of potential self-harm, harm to others, or psychotic symptoms.

[b]The disorder is not caused by a medical condition (eg, hypothyroidism) or substance-induced disorder (eg, antidepressant treatment, medications, drugs of abuse). Numerous specifiers are available to further characterize episodes (eg, with mixed features, with anxious distress, with rapid cycling, with melancholic features).

GENERAL APPROACH

- Table 67-3 shows an algorithmic approach to treating acute episodes including refractory episodes in adults.
- Treatment must be individualized because the clinical presentation, severity, and frequency of episodes vary widely among patients. Adherence to treatment is the most important factor in achieving goals.
- During acute episodes, medications can be added and then tapered once the patient is stabilized and euthymic.
- Patients with bipolar disorder should remain on a mood stabilizer (eg, lithium, valproate, or a second-generation antipsychotic [SGA]) lifelong.

NONPHARMACOLOGIC THERAPY

- Patients and family members should be educated about bipolar disorder (eg, symptoms, causes, and course) and treatment options.
- Nonpharmacologic approaches should address adequate nutrition, sleep, exercise, and stress reduction.
- Psychological interventions include cognitive behavioral therapy (CBT), interpersonal and social rhythm therapy, group psychoeducation, family focused therapy, and enhanced relapse prevention/individual psychoeducation.

PHARMACOLOGIC THERAPY

- See Table 67-4 for product and dosing information on medications for bipolar disorder.
- **Lithium, divalproex sodium (valproate), extended-release carbamazepine, aripiprazole, asenapine, cariprazine, olanzapine, quetiapine, risperidone**, and **ziprasidone** are currently approved by the U.S. Food and Drug administration (FDA) for treatment of acute mania. Lithium, aripiprazole, olanzapine, intramuscular (IM) risperidone, and lamotrigine are approved for maintenance treatment.
- **Quetiapine** and **lurasidone** are the only FDA-approved monotherapy antipsychotics for bipolar depression.
- Combination therapies (see Table 67-3) can provide better acute response and long-term prevention of relapse and recurrence than monotherapy in some bipolar patients.
- Sources of useful guidelines include the Canadian Network for Mood and Anxiety Treatments (CANMAT), International Society for Bipolar Disorders (ISBD), and International Task Force of the World Federation of Societies of Biological Psychiatry (WFSBP).

Lithium

- Lithium is a first-line agent for acute mania, acute bipolar depression, and maintenance treatment of bipolar I and II disorders.
- Lithium is rapidly absorbed, neither protein bound nor metabolized, and excreted unchanged in the urine and other body fluids.
- It may require 6–8 weeks to show antidepressant efficacy. It produces a prophylactic response in up to two-thirds of patients and reduces suicide risk.
- Abrupt discontinuation or noncompliance with lithium therapy can increase the risk of relapse.
- Initial GI and CNS side effects are often dose related and are worse at peak serum concentrations (1–2 hours postdose). Lowering the dose, taking doses with food, using extended-release products, and once-daily dosing at bedtime may help. Diarrhea can sometimes be improved by switching to a liquid formulation.
- A benign fine hand tremor occurs in many patients whereas a coarse hand tremor may be a sign of toxicity. The fine tremor may be treated by switching to a long-acting preparation, lowering the dose, or adding propranolol, 20–120 mg/day.

TABLE 67-3	Algorithm and Guidelines for the Acute Treatment of Mood Episodes in Patients with Bipolar I Disorder

Acute Manic or Mixed Episode	Acute Depressive Episode
General Guidelines	**General Guidelines**
Assess for secondary causes of mania or mixed states (eg, alcohol or drug use)	Assess for secondary causes of depression (eg, alcohol or drug use)
Discontinue antidepressants	Taper off antipsychotics, benzodiazepines, or sedative–hypnotic agents if possible
Taper off stimulants and caffeine if possible	
Treat substance abuse	Treat substance abuse
Encourage good nutrition (with regular protein and essential fatty acid intake), exercise, adequate sleep, stress reduction, and psychosocial therapy	Encourage good nutrition (with regular protein and essential fatty acid intake), exercise, adequate sleep, stress reduction, and psychosocial therapy

Hypomania	Mania	Mild-to-Moderate Depressive Episode	Severe Depressive Episode
First, optimize current mood stabilizer if noncompliance is suspected OR initiate mood-stabilizing medication: lithium[a], valproate[a], carbamazepine[a], or SGAs	**First,** optimize previously prescribed mood stabilizer or medication regimen if noncompliance suspected OR initiate new mood-stabilizing two- or three-drug combinations (lithium[a], valproate[a], or SGA) **plus** a benzodiazepine (lorazepam or clonazepam) and/or antipsychotic for short-term adjunctive treatment of agitation or insomnia; lorazepam is recommended for catatonia	**First,** initiate and/or optimize mood-stabilizing medication: lithium[a], quetiapine, lurasidone	**First,** optimize current mood stabilizer if noncompliance is suspected OR initiate a new mood-stabilizing medication: lithium[a] or quetiapine or lurasidone
Consider adding a benzodiazepine (lorazepam or clonazepam) for short-term adjunctive treatment of agitation or insomnia if needed		Alternative anticonvulsants: lamotrigine[c], valproate[a]; antipsychotics: fluoxetine/olanzapine combination	Alternative fluoxetine/olanzapine combination
Alternative medication treatment options: oxcarbazepine	Do not combine antipsychotics		If psychosis is present, initiate an antipsychotic in combination with above
	Alternative medication treatment options: carbamazepine[a]; if patient does not respond or tolerate, consider oxcarbazepine		Do not combine antipsychotics
			Alternative anticonvulsants: lamotrigine[c], valproate[a]

(Continued)

TABLE 67-3	Algorithm and Guidelines for the Acute Treatment of Mood Episodes in Patients with Bipolar I Disorder (*Continued*)		
Acute Manic or Mixed Episode		**Acute Depressive Episode**	
Hypomania	Mania	Mild-to-Moderate Depressive Episode	Severe Depressive Episode
Second, if response is inadequate, consider a two-drug combination: Lithium[a] **plus** an anticonvulsant or an SGA Anticonvulsant **plus** an anticonvulsant or SGA	**Second**, if response is inadequate, consider a three-drug combination: Lithium[a] **plus** an anticonvulsant **plus** an antipsychotic Anticonvulsant **plus** an anticonvulsant **plus** an antipsychotic **Third**, if response is inadequate, consider ECT for mania with psychosis or catatonia[b], or add clozapine for treatment-refractory illness		**Second,** if response is inadequate, consider carbamazepine[a] or adding antidepressant[d] **Third**, if response is inadequate, consider a three-drug combination: Lithium **plus** lamotrigine[c] **plus** an antidepressant[d] Lithium **plus** quetiapine **plus** antidepressant[d] **Fourth**, if response is inadequate, consider ECT for treatment-refractory illness and depression with psychosis or catatonia[b]

[a]Use standard therapeutic serum concentration ranges if clinically indicated; if partial response or breakthrough episode, adjust dose to achieve higher serum concentrations without causing intolerable adverse effects; valproate is preferred over lithium for mixed episodes and rapid cycling; lithium and/or lamotrigine is preferred over valproate for bipolar depression.

[b]ECT is used for severe mania or depression during pregnancy and for mixed episodes; prior to treatment, anticonvulsants, lithium, and benzodiazepines should be tapered off to maximize therapy and minimize adverse effects.

[c]Lamotrigine is not approved for the acute treatment of depression, and the dose must be started low and slowly titrated up to decrease adverse effects if used for maintenance therapy of bipolar I disorder. Lamotrigine may be initiated during acute treatment with plans to transition to this medication for long-term maintenance. A drug interaction and a severe dermatologic rash can occur when lamotrigine is combined with valproate (ie, lamotrigine doses must be halved from standard dosing titration).

[d]Controversy exists concerning the use of antidepressants, and they are often considered third line in treating acute bipolar depression, except in patients with no recent history of severe acute mania or potentially in bipolar II patients.

ECT, electroconvulsive therapy; SGA, second-generation antipsychotic.

- Polydipsia with polyuria with or without nephrogenic diabetes insipidus (DI) can occur. About 30%–50% of patients develop nephrogenic DI soon after initiating lithium, and it persists in about 10%–25% of patients. It is typically reversible with discontinuation of lithium. Nocturia is common and is managed by changing to once-daily dosing at bedtime.
- Lithium reduces the kidneys' ability to concentrate urine and may cause a nephrogenic DI with low urine-specific gravity and low osmolality polyuria (urine volume >3 L/day). This may be treated with loop or thiazide diuretics. If a thiazide diuretic is used, lithium doses should be decreased by 50% and lithium and potassium levels monitored. Amiloride has weaker natriuretic effects and seems to have little effect on lithium clearance.
- Hypothyroidism can occur in lithium-treated patients (more common in women) and does not require discontinuation of lithium. Exogenous thyroid hormone (ie, levothyroxine) can be added to the regimen. If lithium is discontinued, the need for the levothyroxine should be reassessed because hypothyroidism can be reversible.
- Lithium may cause cardiac effects including T-wave flattening or inversion (up to 30% of patients), atrioventricular block, and bradycardia. In patients with significant cardiac disease, an ECG and consultation with a cardiologist are recommended at baseline and periodically during therapy.
- Other late-appearing lithium side effects are benign reversible leukocytosis, acne, folliculitis, and weight gain.
- Lithium toxicity can occur with serum levels greater than 1.5 mEq/L (mmol/L), but older persons may have toxic symptoms at lower levels. Severe toxic symptoms (eg, vomiting, diarrhea, incontinence, incoordination, impaired cognition, arrhythmias, seizures, permanent neurologic impairment, and kidney damage) may occur with serum concentrations above 2 mEq/L (mmol/L).
  - ✓ Factors predisposing to lithium toxicity include sodium restriction, dehydration, vomiting, diarrhea, age greater than 50 years, heart failure, cirrhosis, drug interactions that decrease lithium clearance, heavy exercise, sauna baths, hot weather, and fever. Tell patients to maintain adequate sodium and fluid intake and to avoid excessive use of alcohol and caffeine-containing beverages.
  - ✓ If lithium toxicity is suspected, discontinue lithium and send the patient immediately to the emergency department.
  - ✓ Consider intermittent hemodialysis in these situations:
    - o In lithium-naive patients, when lithium serum concentrations are at least 4 mEq/L (mmol/L).
    - o In patients previously taking lithium, when lithium serum concentrations are 2.5 mEq/L (mmol/L) or greater and moderate-to-severe neurologic toxicity is present or as clinically indicated.
    - o Continue hemodialysis until serum lithium concentration is below 1 mEq/L (mmol/L) when drawn 8 hours after the last dialysis.
  - ✓ Thiazide diuretics, nonsteroidal anti-inflammatory drugs, angiotensin-converting enzyme inhibitors, and salt-restricted diets can elevate lithium levels. Neurotoxicity can occur when lithium is combined with antipsychotics, methyldopa, metronidazole, phenytoin, and verapamil. Combining lithium with calcium channel blockers is not recommended because of reports of neurotoxicity. Acetaminophen or aspirin and loop diuretics are less likely to interfere with lithium clearance. Caffeine and theophylline can enhance renal elimination of lithium.
- Lithium is usually initiated with 600 mg/day for prophylaxis and 900–1200 mg/day for acute mania. Give immediate-release preparations two or three times daily and extended-release products once or twice daily. After patients are stabilized, many patients can switch to once-daily dosing.
- In general, lithium serum concentrations should be maintained between 0.6 and 1.0 mEq/L (mmol/L). Lithium levels are considered to be at steady state after approximately 5 days with samples drawn 12 hours postdose. Initially, check serum lithium

concentrations once or twice weekly. After a desired serum concentration is achieved, check levels in 2 weeks, and when stable, check them every 3–6 months.

- Lithium clearance increases by 50%–100% during pregnancy. Monitor serum levels monthly during pregnancy and weekly the month before delivery. At delivery, reduce dose to prepregnancy levels and maintain hydration.
- A reasonable therapeutic trial in outpatients is at least 4–6 weeks with lithium serum concentrations of 0.6–1.2 mEq/L (mmol/L). Although serum concentrations less than 0.6 mEq/L (mmol/L) may be associated with higher relapse rates, some patients can do well at 0.4–0.7 mEq/L (mmol/L). Acutely manic patients can require serum concentrations of 1–1.2 mEq/L (mmol/L), and some need up to 1.5 mEq/L (mmol/L). For bipolar prophylaxis in older patients, serum concentrations of 0.4–0.6 mEq/L (mmol/L) are recommended.

Anticonvulsants

- For more in-depth information on the side effects, pharmacokinetics, and drug interactions of anticonvulsants, refers to Chapter 54.

Valproate Sodium and Valproic Acid

- Divalproex sodium (sodium valproate), FDA-approved for acute manic or mixed episodes, is the most prescribed mood stabilizer in the United States. It is as effective as lithium and olanzapine for pure mania, and it can be more effective than lithium for rapid cycling, mixed states, and bipolar disorder with substance abuse. It reduces the frequency of (or prevents) recurrent manic, depressive, and mixed episodes.
- Lithium, carbamazepine, antipsychotics, or benzodiazepines can augment the antimanic effects of valproate. Valproate can be added to lithium to achieve synergistic effects in patients who are treatment refractory and are rapid cyclers or have mixed features, and the combination is effective as maintenance therapy of bipolar I disorder. The potential for drug interactions necessitate blood level monitoring of both agents. SGAs can be added to valproate for breakthrough mania, but they can increase the risk of sedation and weight gain. Combining valproate with lamotrigine increases the risk of rashes, ataxia, tremor, sedation, and fatigue.
- The most frequent dose-related side effects of valproate are GI complaints, fine tremor, and sedation. Giving it with food, reducing the initial dose and making gradual increases, or switching to the extended-release formulation can help alleviate the GI complaints. Reducing the dose or adding a β-blocker may alleviate tremors. Giving the total dose at bedtime can minimize daytime sedation. Other side effects are ataxia, lethargy, alopecia, pruritus, prolonged bleeding, transient increases in liver enzymes, weight gain, and hyperammonemia. Thrombocytopenia can occur at higher doses; lowering the valproate dose may normalize platelet counts. Fatal necrotizing hepatitis is rare and idiosyncratic, occurring in children on multiple anticonvulsants. Life-threatening pancreatitis has been reported.
- For healthy inpatient adults with acute mania, the initial starting dose of valproate is typically 20 mg/kg/day given in divided doses over 12 hours. The daily dose is adjusted by 250–500 mg every 1–3 days based on response and tolerability. The maximum dose is 60 mg/kg/day (see Table 67-4).
  - ✓ For outpatients who are hypomanic or euthymic, or for older patients, the initial dose is generally lower (5–10 mg/kg/day in divided doses) and gradually titrated to avoid side effects.
  - ✓ After establishing the optimal dose, the dose can be given twice daily or at bedtime if tolerated.
  - ✓ Extended-release divalproex can be given once daily, but bioavailability can be 15% lower than that of immediate release products.
- Most clinicians seek a serum concentration range of 50–125 mcg/mL (347–866 μmol/L) measured 12 hours after the last dose. Patients with cyclothymia or bipolar II disorder respond at lower blood levels, while patients with more severe forms may require up to 150 mcg/mL (1040 μmol/L). Serum levels are most useful when assessing for adherence or toxicity.

TABLE 67-4	Products, Dosage and Administration, and Clinical Use of Agents Used in the Treatment of Bipolar Disorder		
Drug (Brand Name)	**Initial Dosing**	**Usual Dosing; Special Population Dosing**	**Comments**
Lithium salts			
Lithium carbonate (Eskalith[a,b]) (Eskalith CR) (Lithobid) Lithium citrate (Cibalith-S[a,b])	300 mg twice daily	900–2400 mg/day in two to four divided doses, preferably with meals Renal impairment: lower doses required with frequent serum monitoring There is wide variation in the dosage needed to achieve therapeutic response and trough serum lithium concentration (ie, 0.6–1.2 mEq/L [mmol/L] for maintenance therapy and 0.8–1.2 mEq/L [mmol/L] for acute mood episodes taken 12 hours after the last dose)	Use alone or in combination with other medications (eg, valproate, carbamazepine, antipsychotics) for acute treatment of mania and for maintenance treatment
Anticonvulsants			
Divalproex sodium (Depakote[a]) (Depakote ER) Valproic acid[a] (Depakene) Valproate sodium (Depacon)	250–500 mg twice daily Loading dose of divalproex (20–30 mg/kg/day) can be given	750–3000 mg/day (20–60 mg/kg/day) given once daily or in divided doses Titrate to clinical response Dose adjustment needed with hepatic impairment	Use alone or in combination with other medications (eg, lithium, carbamazepine, antipsychotics) for acute treatment of mania and for maintenance treatment Use caution when combining with lamotrigine because of potential drug interaction
Lamotrigine (Lamictal[b])	25 mg daily	50–400 mg/day in divided doses. Increase dosage slowly (eg, 25 mg/day for 2 weeks, then 50 mg/day for weeks 3 and 4, and then 50 mg/day increments at weekly intervals up to 200 mg/day) Dose adjustment needed with hepatic impairment	Use alone or in combination with other medications (eg, lithium, carbamazepine) for long-term maintenance treatment for bipolar I disorder

(Continued)

TABLE 67-4 Products, Dosage and Administration, and Clinical Use of Agents Used in the Treatment of Bipolar Disorder *(Continued)*

Drug (Brand Name)	Initial Dosing	Usual Dosing; Special Population Dosing	Comments
Carbamazepine (Equetro[a]) (Tegretol) (Epitol) (Tegretol-XR) (Carbatrol)	200 mg twice daily	200–1800 mg/day in two to four divided doses Titrate to clinical response Dose adjustment needed with hepatic impairment	Use alone or in combination with other medications (eg, lithium, valproate, antipsychotics) for the acute and long-term maintenance treatment of mania or mixed episodes for bipolar I disorder. APA guidelines recommend reserving it for patients unable to tolerate or who have inadequate response to lithium or valproate Extended-release tablets should be swallowed whole and not be broken or chewed Carbitrol capsules can be opened and contents sprinkled over food
Oxcarbazepine (Trileptal)	300 mg twice daily	300–1200 mg/day in two divided doses Titrate dosage based on clinical response Dose adjustment required with severe renal impairment	Use after patients have failed treatment with carbamazepine or have intolerable side effects May have fewer adverse effects and be better tolerated than carbamazepine
Atypical antipsychotics			
Aripiprazole (Abilify[a,b]) (Abilify Maintena[b])	10–15 mg daily	10–30 mg/day once daily	
Asenapine (Saphris[a])	5–10 mg twice daily sublingually	5–10 mg twice daily sublingually	

(Continued)

TABLE 67-4	Products, Dosage and Administration, and Clinical Use of Agents Used in the Treatment of Bipolar Disorder (Continued)		
Drug (Brand Name)	**Initial Dosing**	**Usual Dosing; Special Population Dosing**	**Comments**
Cariprazine (Vraylar[a])	1.5 mg daily	3–6 mg daily	
Lurasidone (Latuda[c])	20 mg daily	20–120 mg daily with food	
Olanzapine (Zyprexa[a,b]) (Zyprexa Zydis)	2.5–5 mg twice daily	5–20 mg/day once daily or in divided doses	
Olanzapine and fluoxetine (Symbyax[c])	6 mg olanzapine and 25 mg fluoxetine daily	6–12 mg olanzapine and 25–50 mg fluoxetine daily	
Quetiapine (Seroquel[a,b])	50 mg twice daily	50–800 mg/day in divided doses or once daily when stabilized	
Risperidone (Risperdal[a]) (Risperdal M-Tab) (Risperdal Consta[b])	0.5–1 mg twice daily	0.5–6 mg/day once daily or in divided doses	
Ziprasidone (Geodon[a])	40–60 mg twice daily	40–160 mg/day in divided doses	
Benzodiazepines			
Various	Dosage should be slowly adjusted up and down according to response and adverse effects	Use in combination with other medications (eg, antipsychotics, lithium, valproate) for acute treatment of mania or mixed episodes Use as a short-term adjunctive sedative–hypnotic agent	

[a]FDA-approved for acute mania.
[b]FDA-approved for maintenance.
[c]FDA-approved for acute bipolar depression.
FDA-approved agents may be used as monotherapy in various phases of the illness as noted in the table footnotes.

Carbamazepine

- Because of drug interactions, carbamazepine is usually reserved for use after treatment failure with lithium or divalproex sodium.
- It has acute antimanic effects, but its long-term effectiveness is less clear. It may be less effective than lithium for maintenance therapy and for bipolar depression.
- The combination of carbamazepine with lithium, valproate, and antipsychotics is often used for manic episodes in treatment-resistant patients.
- Adverse effects of carbamazepine are summarized in Chapter 54.

- Carbamazepine induces the hepatic metabolism of antidepressants, anticonvulsants, antipsychotics, and many other medications. Women taking oral contraceptives who receive carbamazepine should be counseled to use a nonhormonal method of contraception.

- Certain medications that inhibit CYP3A4 (eg, cimetidine, diltiazem, erythromycin, fluoxetine, fluvoxamine, itraconazole, ketoconazole, nefazodone, and verapamil) added to carbamazepine therapy may cause carbamazepine toxicity. When carbamazepine is combined with valproate, reduce the carbamazepine dose, as its free levels can be increased. Do not combine clozapine and carbamazepine because of possible additive bone marrow suppression.

- For inpatients in an acute manic episode, doses can be started at 400–600 mg/day in divided doses with meals and increased by 200 mg/day every 2–4 days up to 10–15 mg/kg/day. Outpatients should be started at lower doses and titrated upward more slowly to avoid side effects. Many patients tolerate once-daily dosing after stabilization.

- During the first month of therapy, serum concentrations may decrease because of autoinduction of cytochrome P450 3A4 enzymes, requiring a dose increase.

- Carbamazepine serum levels are usually obtained every 1 or 2 weeks during the first 2 months, then every 3–6 months during maintenance. Serum samples are drawn 10–12 hours postdose and at least 4–7 days after dosage initiation or change. Most clinicians attempt to maintain levels between 6–10 mcg/mL (25–42 μmol/L), but some patients may require 12–14 mcg/mL (51–59 μmol/L).

- Use of carbamazepine in patients of Asian ancestry requires genetic testing for human leukocyte antigen (HLA) allele, HLA-B 1502, to help detect a higher risk of Stevens–Johnson syndrome and toxic epidermal necrolysis.

Oxcarbazepine

- Oxcarbazepine is not FDA-approved for treatment of bipolar disorder in the United States. Guidelines typically recommend it as a third-line option for mania, a third- or fourth-line option for maintenance treatment, and it is not recommended for treatment of bipolar depression.

- Initial dosing is usually 150–300 mg twice daily, which can be increased by 300–600 mg every 3–6 days up to 1200 mg/day in divided doses (with or without food).

- Discontinue oxcarbazepine at the first sign of a skin reaction, as severe dermatologic reactions have been reported (eg, Stevens–Johnson syndrome). Other adverse effects may include impaired cognitive or psychomotor performance, somnolence, fatigue, incoordination, and hyponatremia. Severe hyponatremia is more common with oxcarbazepine than with carbamazepine.

- Oxcarbazepine is a CYP 2C19 inhibitor and a 3A3/4 inducer. It induces the metabolism of oral contraceptives, necessitating use of alternative contraception measures. Oxcarbazepine does not autoinduce its own metabolism.

Lamotrigine

- Lamotrigine has both antidepressant and mood-stabilizing effects. It may have augmenting properties when combined with lithium or valproate. It has a low rate of switching patients to mania. Although it is less effective for acute mania compared with lithium and valproate, it may be beneficial for the maintenance therapy of treatment-resistant bipolar I and II disorders. It seems most effective for prevention of bipolar depression.

- Common adverse effects include headache, nausea, dizziness, ataxia, diplopia, drowsiness, tremor, maculopapular rash, and pruritus. Although most rashes resolve with continued therapy, some progress to life-threatening Stevens–Johnson syndrome. Discontinue lamotrigine if the rash is diffuse, involves mucous membranes, and is accompanied by fever or sore throat. The incidence of rash is greatest with concomitant administration of valproate, rapid dose escalation of lamotrigine, and higher than recommended lamotrigine initial doses.

- In patients taking valproate, dose lamotrigine at about one-half the standard doses, and titrate upward more slowly than usual.
- For maintenance treatment of bipolar disorder, the usual dosage range of lamotrigine is 50–300 mg/day. The target dose is generally 200 mg/day (100 mg/day when combined with valproate and 400 mg/day when combined with carbamazepine). For patients not taking medications that affect lamotrigine's clearance, the dose is 25 mg/day for the first 2 weeks, then 50 mg/day for weeks 3 and 4, 100 mg/day for the next week, then 200 mg/day. Patients who stop dosing for more than a few days should restart the dose escalation schedule.

Antipsychotics

- First-generation (eg, fluphenazine, haloperidol) and second-generation (eg, aripiprazole, asenapine, clozapine, lurasidone, quetiapine, risperidone, ziprasidone) antipsychotics are effective as monotherapy or as add-on therapy for acute mania. Long-term antipsychotics can be needed for some patients, but the risks versus benefits must be weighed in view of long-term side effects (eg, obesity, type 2 diabetes, hyperlipidemia, hyperprolactinemia, and tardive dyskinesia).
- Both first- and second-generation antipsychotics are effective in ~70% of patients with acute mania associated with agitation, aggression, and psychosis.
- Clinical trials support the use of quetiapine and lurasidone as monotherapy and adjunctive treatment for bipolar depression. Data also support use of combined fluoxetine/olanzapine for bipolar depression.
- Oral aripiprazole, olanzapine, and long-acting risperidone are effective monotherapy options for maintenance treatment in bipolar disorder. First-generation depot antipsychotics (eg, haloperidol decanoate, fluphenazine decanoate) can be useful for maintenance treatment in patients who are noncompliant or treatment-resistant.
- Controlled studies in acute mania suggest that lithium or valproate plus an antipsychotic is more effective than any of these agents alone.
- Clozapine monotherapy has acute and long-term mood stabilizing effects in refractory bipolar disorder but requires regular white blood cell monitoring for agranulocytosis.
- Higher initial antipsychotic doses (eg, olanzapine 20 mg/day) may be required for acute mania. After mania is controlled (usually 7–28 days), the antipsychotic can be gradually tapered and discontinued, and the patient maintained on mood stabilizer monotherapy.
- For more information on the side effects, pharmacokinetics, and drug interactions of specific antipsychotics, refer to Chapter 70.

Alternative Medications

- High-potency benzodiazepines (eg, clonazepam and lorazepam) are common alternatives (or adjuncts) to antipsychotics for acute mania, agitation, anxiety, panic, and insomnia, or in patients who cannot take mood stabilizers. IM lorazepam may be used for acute agitation. When no longer required, benzodiazepines should be gradually tapered and discontinued to avoid withdrawal symptoms. A relative contraindication for long-term use is a history of drug or alcohol abuse or dependency.
- Many clinicians consider adjunctive antidepressants third-line for acute bipolar depression, except in those with no history of severe and/or recent mania or potentially in bipolar II patients. The rate of mood switching from depression to mania with tricyclic antidepressants and venlafaxine is higher than the rate associated with use of selective serotonin reuptake inhibitors. Before initiating an antidepressant, be sure the patient has a therapeutic dose or blood level of a primary mood stabilizer. Be cautious in using antidepressants in those with a history of mania after a depressive episode, and those with frequent cycling. Generally, the antidepressant should be withdrawn 2–6 months after remission.

TABLE 67-5 Guidelines for Baseline and Routine Laboratory Tests and Monitoring for Patients with Bipolar Disorder Taking Mood Stabilizers

	Baseline: Physical Examination and General Chemistry[a]	Hematologic Tests[b]		Metabolic Tests[c]		Liver Function Tests[d]		Renal Function Tests[e]		Thyroid Function Tests[f]		Serum Electrolytes[g]		Dermatologic[h]	
	Baseline	Baseline	6–12 months	Baseline	6–12 months	Baseline	6–12 months	Baseline	6–12 months	Baseline	6–12 months	Baseline	6–12 months	Baseline	6–12 months
SGAs[i]	X			X	X										
Carbamazepine[j]	X	X	X			X	X	X					X	X	X
Lamotrigine[k]	X													X	X
Lithium[l]	X	X		X				X	X	X	X	X	X	X	X
Oxcarbazepine[m]	X	X										X			
Valproate[n]	X	X	X	X		X	X							X	X

[a]Screen for drug abuse and serum pregnancy.
[b]Complete blood cell count (CBC) with differential and platelets.
[c]Fasting glucose, serum lipids, and weight.
[d]Lactate dehydrogenase, aspartate aminotransferase, alanine aminotransferase, total bilirubin, and alkaline phosphatase.
[e]Serum creatinine, blood urea nitrogen, urinalysis, urine osmolality, and specific gravity.
[f]Triiodothyronine, total thyroxine, thyroxine uptake, and thyroid-stimulating hormone.
[g]Serum sodium.
[h]Rashes, hair thinning, and alopecia.
[i]Second-generation antipsychotics: Monitor for increased appetite with weight gain (primarily in patients with initial low or normal body mass index); monitor closely if rapid or significant weight gain occurs during early therapy; cases of hyperlipidemia and diabetes reported.

^{k}Carbamazepine: Manufacturer recommends CBC and platelets (and possibly reticulocyte counts and serum iron) at baseline, and that subsequent monitoring be individualized by the clinician (eg, CBC, platelet counts, and liver function tests every 2 weeks during the first 2 months of treatment, and then every 3 months if normal). Monitor more closely if patient exhibits hematologic or hepatic abnormalities or if the patient is receiving a myelotoxic drug; discontinue if platelets are <100,000/mm³ (<100 × 10⁹/L), if white blood cell (WBC) count is <3000/mm³ (<3 × 10⁹/L), or if there is evidence of bone marrow suppression or liver dysfunction. Serum electrolyte levels should be monitored in the elderly or those at risk for hyponatremia. Carbamazepine interferes with some pregnancy tests.

^{k}Lamotrigine: If renal or hepatic impairment, monitor closely and adjust dosage according to manufacturer's guidelines. Serious dermatologic reactions have occurred within 2–8 weeks of initiating treatment and are more likely to occur in patients receiving concomitant valproate, with rapid dosage escalation, or using doses exceeding the recommended titration schedule.

^{l}Lithium: Obtain baseline electrocardiogram for patients older than 40 years or if preexisting cardiac disease (benign, reversible T-wave depression can occur). Renal function tests should be obtained every 2–3 months during the first 6 months, and then every 6–12 months; if impaired renal function, monitor 24-hour urine volume and creatinine every 3 months; if urine volume >3 L/day, monitor urinalysis, osmolality, and specific gravity every 3 months. Thyroid function tests should be obtained once or twice during the first 6 months, and then every 6–12 months; monitor for signs and symptoms of hypothyroidism; if supplemental thyroid therapy is required, monitor thyroid function tests and adjust thyroid dose every 1–2 months until thyroid function indices are within normal range, and then monitor every 3–6 months.

^{m}Oxcarbazepine: Hyponatremia (serum sodium concentrations <125 mEq/L [mmol/L]) has been reported and occurs more frequently during the first 3 months of therapy; serum sodium concentrations should be monitored in patients receiving drugs that lower serum sodium concentrations (eg, diuretics or drugs that cause inappropriate antidiuretic hormone secretion) or in patients with symptoms of hyponatremia (eg, confusion, headache, lethargy, and malaise). Hypersensitivity reactions have occurred in approximately 25%–30% of patients with a history of carbamazepine hypersensitivity and require immediate discontinuation.

^{n}Valproate: Weight gain reported in patients with low or normal body mass index. Monitor platelets and liver function during first 3–6 months if evidence of increased bruising or bleeding. Monitor closely if patients exhibit hematologic or hepatic abnormalities or in patients receiving drugs that affect coagulation, such as aspirin or warfarin; discontinue if platelets are <100,000/mm³/L (<100 × 10⁹/L) or if prolonged bleeding time. Pancreatitis, hyperammonemic encephalopathy, polycystic ovary syndrome, increased testosterone, and menstrual irregularities have been reported; not recommended during first trimester of pregnancy due to risk of neural tube defects.

SGAs, second-generation antipsychotics.

Special Populations

- The occurrence of Epstein anomaly in infants exposed to lithium during the first trimester is estimated to be between 1 and 10.78:1000, and the risk of neural tube defects is 13.4:1000.
- When lithium is used during pregnancy, use the lowest effective dose to prevent relapse, thus lessening the risk of "floppy" infant syndrome, hypothyroidism, and nontoxic goiter in the infant. Monitor closely and adjust dose as appropriate.
- Breastfeeding is usually discouraged for women taking lithium.
- When valproate, carbamazepine, and lamotrigine are taken during the first trimester, the risk of neural tube defects is ~4%, ~3%, and ~2%, respectively. Administration of folic acid can reduce the risk of neural tube defects.
- Women taking valproate may breastfeed, but mother and infant should have identical laboratory monitoring.
- First-generation antipsychotics seem to have little teratogenic risk when used during pregnancy. Data on the SGAs are more limited. Risk to benefit ratio must be considered before using antipsychotics during pregnancy.
- Lithium, valproic acid, and carbamazepine are used in pediatric bipolar disorder, but data are limited. Aripiprazole and risperidone are FDA-approved for bipolar mania in adolescents 13–17 years. Quetiapine is approved as monotherapy or adjunctive therapy to lithium or divalproex in manic patients aged 10–17 years. Olanzapine is approved for manic or mixed episodes in patients aged 13–17 years.
- Lithium is FDA-approved as a mood stabilizer for children older than 12 years.
- A guideline for treatment of children and adolescents with bipolar disorder is *Practice Parameters for the Assessment and Treatment of Children and Adolescents with Bipolar Disorder.*
- The elimination half-life of lithium and valproate increases with age. Older patients can have many medical comorbidities and increased sensitivity to side effects of mood stabilizers and antipsychotics.

EVALUATION OF THERAPEUTIC OUTCOMES

- Mood episodes: Document symptoms on a daily mood chart (document life stressors, type of episode, length of episode, and treatment outcome); monthly and yearly life charts are valuable for documenting patterns of mood cycles.
- See **Table 67-5** for guidelines for laboratory monitoring of patients on mood stabilizers.
- Assess medication adherence; missing medication doses is a primary reason for nonresponse and recurrence of episodes.
- Ask patients about adverse effects, especially sedation and weight gain; manage side effects rapidly and vigorously to avoid nonadherence.
- Be aware of suicidal ideation or attempts. Suicide completion rates with bipolar I disorder are 10%–15%; suicide attempts are primarily associated with depressive episodes, mixed episodes with severe depression, or presence of psychosis.
- Assess patients with partial treatment response or nonresponse for accurate diagnosis, concomitant medical or psychiatric conditions, medication adherence, and use of medications or substances that exacerbate mood symptoms.
- Involve patients and family members in treatment to monitor target symptom response and side effects and to enhance adherence and reduce stressors. Standardized rating scales may be useful in monitoring for response.

See Chapter 86, Bipolar Disorder, authored by Shannon J. Drayton and Christopher S. Fields, for a more detailed discussion of this topic.

CHAPTER 68

Depressive Disorders

- The essential feature of *major depressive disorder* (MDD) is a clinical course characterized by one or more major depressive episodes without a history of manic or hypomanic episodes.
- Refer to guidelines published by the American Psychiatric Association, the British Association of Psychopharmacology, and the Canadian Network for Mood and Anxiety Treatments (CANMAT) because they have similarities in their recommendations.

PATHOPHYSIOLOGY

- *Monoamine hypothesis:* Decreased brain levels of the neurotransmitters norepinephrine (NE), serotonin (5-HT), and dopamine (DA) may cause depression.
- *Postsynaptic changes in receptor sensitivity:* Studies have demonstrated that desensitization or downregulation of NE or 5-HT$_{1A}$ receptors may relate to onset of antidepressant effects.
- *Dysregulation hypothesis:* Failure of homeostatic neurotransmitter regulation, rather than absolute increases or decreases in their activities.
- *Inflammatory hypothesis:* Chronic stress and inflammation may alter glutamatergic and GABA transmission. Brain-derived neurotrophic factor (BDNF) is a primary mediator of neuronal changes as well as synaptogenesis whose expression is reduced due to stress and may be associated with depression.
- Neuroactive steroids are a growing area of research for depression.

CLINICAL PRESENTATION

- *Emotional symptoms:* Diminished ability to experience pleasure, loss of interest in usual activities, sadness, pessimism, crying, hopelessness, anxiety, feelings of worthlessness or guilt, and psychotic features (eg, auditory hallucinations and delusions). Recurrent thoughts of death, suicidal ideation without a specific plan, suicide attempt, or a plan for committing suicide.
- *Physical symptoms:* Weight gain or loss, fatigue, pain (especially headache), sleep disturbance, decreased or increased appetite, loss of sexual interest, and gastrointestinal (GI) and cardiovascular complaints (especially palpitations).
- *Cognitive symptoms:* Decreased ability to concentrate, poor memory for recent events, confusion, and indecisiveness.
- *Psychomotor disturbances:* Psychomotor retardation (slowed physical movements, thought processes, and speech) or psychomotor agitation.

DIAGNOSIS

- MDD is characterized by one or more major depressive episodes, as defined by the *Diagnostic and Statistical Manual of Mental Disorders*, 5th ed. Five or more of the above symptoms must have been present nearly every day during the same 2-week period and cause significant distress or impairment. Depressed mood or loss of interest or pleasure must be present in adults (or irritable mood in children and adolescents). **Table 68-1** outlines a common acronym for MDD diagnostic criteria.
- The depressive episode must not be attributable to physiological effects of a substance or medical condition.
- There must not be a history of manic-like or hypomanic-like episodes unless they were induced by a substance or medical condition.

TABLE 68-1	Diagnostic Criteria for Major Depressive Episode
S	Suicidal ideation with or without plan, suicide attempt; recurrent thoughts of death
I	Interest—loss of interest or pleasure in activities; anhedonia
G	Guilt—inappropriate or excessive in nature; feelings of worthlessness
E	Energy decreased
C	Concentration decreased; difficulty making decisions
A	Appetite changes; typically decreased; resulting in 5% change in weight from baseline
P	Psychomotor agitation or retardation
S	Sleep impairment; typically insomnia but may be hypersomnia

- At least five symptoms must be consistently present over a 2-week period.
- Symptoms must include depressed mood or anhedonia.
- Symptoms must cause substantial distress or impairment in functioning.
- Other medical conditions or substance use do not account for symptoms.

- Diagnosis requires a medication review, physical examination, mental status examination, a complete blood count with differential, thyroid function tests, and electrolyte determination.
- Many chronic illnesses (eg, stroke, Parkinson disease, traumatic brain injury, hypothyroidism) and substance abuse and dependence disorders are associated with depression. Medications associated with depressive symptoms include many antihypertensives, oral contraceptives, isotretinoin, interferon-β_{1a}, and many others.
- Standardized rating scale should be used to diagnose depression and evaluate treatment.

TREATMENT

- <u>Goals of Treatment</u>: Resolution of current symptoms (ie, remission), prevention of further episodes of depression (ie, relapse or recurrence), and prevention of suicide.

NONPHARMACOLOGIC TREATMENT

- Psychotherapy (eg, cognitive therapy, behavioral therapy, or interpersonal psychotherapy) is recommended as primary treatment for mild to moderately severe major depressive episode. For severe depression, it may be used in combination with medications as its effect is considered additive. Psychotherapy alone is not recommended for acute treatment of severe and/or psychotic MDD.
- Electroconvulsive therapy (ECT) may be considered when a rapid response is needed, risks of other treatments outweigh potential benefits, there is history of a poor response to drugs, and the patient prefers ECT. A rapid therapeutic response (10–14 days) has been reported.
- Repetitive transcranial magnetic stimulation has demonstrated efficacy and does not require anesthesia as does ECT.
- Recent data suggest the benefit of physical activity in patients with MDD, and the American Psychiatry Association has endorsed inclusion of exercise into MDD treatment plans.

PHARMACOLOGIC THERAPY

General Approach

- **Figure 68-1** shows an algorithm for treatment of uncomplicated MDD. **Table 68-2** guides adult dosing of antidepressants.

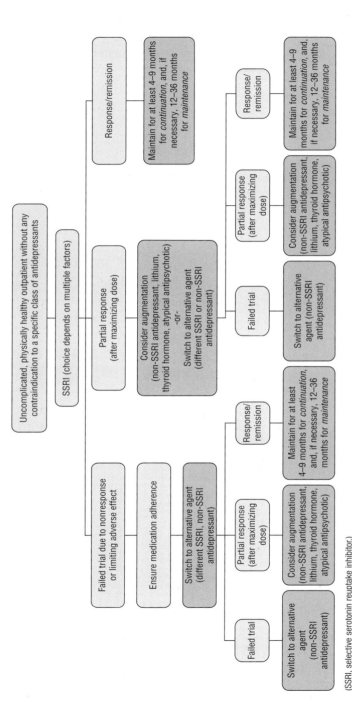

(SSRI, selective serotonin reuptake inhibitor.)

FIGURE 68-1. Algorithm for treatment of uncomplicated MDD. Note: Both the BAP guidelines and the STAR*D trial suggest that switching and augmentation strategies are supported by stronger evidence compared to dose increases (among poor antidepressant responders).

TABLE 68-2 Adult Dosing Guidance for Currently Available Antidepressant Medications

Drug (Brand Name)	Initial Dose (mg/day)	Usual Dosage Range (mg/day)	Comments (eg, Maximum Daily Dosage, Suggested Therapeutic Plasma Concentration)[a]
Selective serotonin reuptake inhibitors (SSRIs)			
Citalopram (Celexa)	20	20–40	Doses >40 mg/day not recommended due to QT prolongation risk; maximum 20 mg/day for CYP2C19 poor metabolizers or coadministration with CYP2C19 inhibitors; 20 mg/day recommended for patients older than 60 years of age
Escitalopram (Lexapro)	10	10–20	Maximum 20 mg/day; dose may be increased to maximum daily dose after at least 1 week if needed; 5 mg tablet available for unique circumstances
Fluoxetine (Prozac)	20	20–60	Maximum 80 mg/day; dose may be increased in 20 mg increments; doses of 5 or 10 mg/day have been used as initial therapy; doses >20 mg/day may be given in a single daily dose or divided twice daily
Fluvoxamine (Luvox)	50	50–300	Maximum 300 mg/day; daily doses >100 mg total dose should be divided twice daily, with the larger dose given at night
Paroxetine (Paxil)	20	20–50	Maximum 300 mg/day (ER formulation)
			Maximum 50 mg/day (IR formulation); titrate 10 mg/day increments weekly
			Maximum 62.5 mg/day (CR formulation); titrate 12.5 mg/day increments weekly
Sertraline (Zoloft)	50	50–200	Maximum 200 mg/day; titrate 25 mg/day increments weekly
Serotonin–norepinephrine reuptake inhibitors (SNRIs)			
Newer-generation SNRIs			
Desvenlafaxine (Pristiq)	50	50	Doses up to 400 mg/day have been studied; however, AEs are increased and no additional benefit has been shown at doses exceeding 50 mg/day. Dose reductions or discontinuation may be required if sustained hypertension occurs
Duloxetine (Cymbalta)	30	30–90	Maximum 120 mg/day (given once or twice daily); doses exceeding 60 mg/day not shown to provide increased efficacy for the treatment of MDD

Venlafaxine (Effexor)	37.5–75	75–225	Maximum 375 mg/day (IR); maximum 225 mg/day (ER); may increase in increments up to 75 mg/day at a minimum of every 4 days. Dose reductions or discontinuation may be required if sustained hypertension occurs
Levomilnacipran (Fetzima)	20	40–120	Initial dose (20 mg) for 2 days before dose increases is recommended at intervals of 2 or more days. Dose adjustment or discontinuation may be required if sustained elevated heart rate or hypertension occurs
Tricyclic antidepressants (TCAs)			
Amitriptyline (Elavil)	25	100–200	Maximum 300 mg/day for MDD; depending on the total dose, it may be given as a single daily dose at bedtime or in divided doses throughout the day; therapeutic serum level 100–250 ng/mL (mcg/L; 370–925 nmol/L); parent drug plus metabolite (nortriptyline)
Desipramine (Norpramin)	25	100–200	Maximum 300 mg/day; suggested therapeutic concentration range for combined imipramine + desipramine: 150–300 ng/mL (mcg/L; 550–1100 nmol/L)
Doxepin (Sinequan)	25	100–200	Maximum 300 mg/day; may be given in a single daily dose at bedtime (if tolerated) or in divided doses throughout the day; a single dose should not exceed 150 mg
Imipramine (Tofranil)	25	100–200	Maximum 300 mg/day; may be given in a single daily dose at bedtime (if tolerated) or in divided doses throughout the day; suggested therapeutic concentration range for combined imipramine + desipramine: 150–300 ng/mL (mcg/L; 550–1100 nmol/L)
Nortriptyline (Pamelor)	25	50–150	Maximum 150 mg/day; total daily may be given as a single daily dose (if tolerated) or 25 mg doses given three to four times daily; therapeutic serum level 50–150 ng/mL (mcg/L; 190–570 nmol/L)
Norepinephrine and dopamine reuptake inhibitor (NDRI)			
Bupropion (Wellbutrin)	150 (75 mg given twice daily)	150–450	Maximum 450 mg/day (IR, ER), 400 mg/day (SR); ER dosed once daily; SR dosed once or twice daily; IR may be dosed up to three times daily. Adhering to labeled maximum daily and maximum single doses minimizes effect on seizure threshold
Mixed serotonergic effects (mixed 5-HT)			
Nefazodone (Serzone)	100	200–400	Maximum 600 mg/day; daily doses should be divided twice daily

(Continued)

787

TABLE 68-2 Adult Dosing Guidance for Currently Available Antidepressant Medications (*Continued*)

Drug (Brand Name)	Initial Dose (mg/day)	Usual Dosage Range (mg/day)	Comments (eg, Maximum Daily Dosage, Suggested Therapeutic Plasma Concentration)[a]
Trazodone (Desyrel; Oleptro)	50	150–300	Maximum 600 mg/day; IR daily dose should be divided three times daily and may increase by 50 mg/day increments every 3–7 days; ER dose titration initiated at 150 mg at bedtime and can be increased 75 mg/day every 3 days
Vilazodone (Viibryd)	10	20–40	Target dose 20–40 mg/day unless coadministered with CYP3A4 inhibitor (dose not to exceed 20 mg/day). Dose titration: 10 mg/day for 7 days, 20 mg/day for 7 days, and then may increase to 40 mg/day. Dose must be taken with food to ensure adequate drug absorption and bioavailability
Vortioxetine (Brintellix)	10	20	Maximum 20 mg/day; minimal difference in efficacy and side effects in clinical trials between 10 and 20 mg
Serotonin and α₂-adrenergic antagonist			
Mirtazapine (Remeron)	15	15–45	Maximum 45 mg/day; dose adjustment may be required for renal impairment
Monoamine oxidase inhibitors (MAOIs)			
Phenelzine (Nardil)	15	30–90	Divided dosing 2–3 times daily; dosing may be increased to 90 mg/day based on tolerance and response
Selegiline (transdermal) (Emsam)	6	6–12	Not to exceed 12 mg/24 hours; dose may be increased by 3 mg/day increments every 2 weeks; site of application should be rotated
Tranylcypromine (Parnate)	10	20–40	Maximum 60 mg/day; divided dosing; increase by 10 mg at 1- to 3-week intervals
Isocarboxazid (Marplan)	10–20	30–60	Maximum 60 mg/day; divided dosing

Second-generation antipsychotics (SGA) as augmentation (5HT$_{2A}$ and D$_2$ modulators)

Aripiprazole (Abilify)	2	2–15	FDA-approved for augmentation; CANMAT Level 1 evidence, 1st line
Brexpiprazole (Rexulti)	1	1–3	Not FDA-approved for augmentation; CANMAT Level 1 evidence, 2nd line
Olanzapine (Zyprexa)	2.5	2.5–10	Not FDA-approved for augmentation; CANMAT Level 1 evidence, 2nd line
Quetiapine (Seroquel)	50	150–300	FDA-approved for augmentation; CANMAT Level 1 evidence, 1st line
Risperidone (Risperdal)	1	1–3	Not FDA-approved for augmentation; CANMAT Level 1 evidence, 1st line
Alternative augmentation agents (not FDA-approved for antidepressant augmentation)			
Buspirone (Buspar)	10	10–60	Divided dosing 2–3 times daily. 5HT1A partial agonist
Lithium	300	600–1200	Dose based on therapeutic levels (target 0.6–1 mEq/L [mmol/L]). Mechanism in depression not fully understood
Triiodothyronine (Cytomel)	0.025	0.025–0.05	Once daily dosing; monitor free T3 levels

[a]SI conversion for cases where reference ranges are for a mixture of parent drug and active metabolite is calculated based on a 1:1 ratio.
AE, adverse effects; CR, continuous release; ER, extended release; IR, immediate release; MDD, major depressive disorder; SR, sustained release; CANMAT, Canadian Network for Mood and Anxiety Treatments.

- Antidepressants are equal in efficacy when administered in comparable doses, and they are often classified by chemical structure and/or presumed mechanism.
- The initial choice of antidepressant is often made empirically and influenced by the patient's or family member's history of response, concurrent medical conditions, medications the patient is taking, presenting symptoms, potential for drug–drug interactions, side effect profiles, patient preference, and drug cost.
- An individual's pharmacogenomics may be useful when choosing therapy as a way to better predict antidepressant side effects or response. Dosing recommendations to aid in the interpretation of results are available through the Clinical Pharmacogenomics Implementation Consortium (CPIC) as well as the FDA-approved package inserts.
- 50%–60% of patients with varying types of depression improve with drug therapy.
- At least a 6-week trial of an antidepressant at maximum dosage is considered an adequate trial of that medication.
- The acute phase of treatment lasts 6–12 weeks, and the goal is remission (ie, absence of symptoms). The continuation phase (4–9 months after remission) seeks to eliminate residual symptoms or prevent relapse. The maintenance phase (12–36 months or more) seeks to prevent recurrence of a new episode of depression.
- Give older patients one-half of the initial dose given to younger adults, and increase the dose more slowly. Older patients may require 6–12 weeks of treatment to achieve the desired antidepressant response.
- Early in treatment, all antidepressants can increase suicidal thinking and behavior in children, adolescents, and young adults less than 25 years of age. Suicide risk may also be elevated in the 30 days after discontinuation.
- Some clinicians recommend lifelong therapy for persons younger than 40 years with two or more prior episodes and for all persons with three or more prior episodes.
- Educate patients and their support systems about the delay in antidepressant response (typically 2–4 weeks) and the importance of adherence before starting therapy and throughout treatment.
- Occurrence of a withdrawal syndrome with some antidepressants may be reduced with a slow taper over weeks or months when the medication is being discontinued.
- Table 68-3 shows antidepressant potency and relative selectivity for inhibition of various receptors. Specific adverse effects seen with select antidepressants are given in Table 68-4.
- The ability of any antidepressant to inhibit or induce the CYP450 enzymes can be a significant factor determining its capability to cause a pharmacokinetic drug–drug interaction.

Selective Serotonin Reuptake Inhibitors

- The SSRIs inhibit the reuptake of 5-HT into the presynaptic neuron. They are generally chosen as first-line antidepressants because of their relative safety in overdose and improved tolerability compared with earlier agents (Figure 68-1).
- The SSRIs, with the possible exceptions of **citalopram** and **sertraline**, may have a nonlinear pattern of drug accumulation with chronic dosing. Hepatic impairment, renal impairment, and age can influence the pharmacokinetics of SSRIs. The pharmacokinetics of the antidepressants is summarized in Table 68-5.
- Any antidepressant that enhances serotonergic activity can be associated with serotonin syndrome characterized by mental status changes, autonomic instability, and neuromuscular abnormalities. Combining an SSRI with another 5-HT augmenting agent is also a risk.
- The primary adverse effects for SSRIs are nausea, vomiting, diarrhea, headache, insomnia, fatigue, and sexual dysfunction and have a reduced incidence of sedative, anticholinergic, and cardiovascular adverse effects or weight gain.
- A few patients have anxiety symptoms early in treatment which may be reduced by starting with lower doses and slowly titrating up.

TABLE 68-3	Relative Potencies of Norepinephrine and Serotonin Reuptake Blockade and Selected Receptor Antagonism Profile of Antidepressants

	Reuptake Antagonism				
	NE	5-HT	M1	H1	α1
Selective serotonin reuptake inhibitors (SSRIs)					
Citalopram	0	++++	0	+	0
Escitalopram	0	++++	0	0	0
Fluoxetine	+	++++	0	0	0
Fluvoxamine	0	++++	0	+	0
Paroxetine	++	++++	+	+	0
Sertraline	0	++++	0	0	0
Serotonin–norepinephrine reuptake inhibitors (SNRIs)					
Duloxetine	+++	++++	+	0	+
Levomilnacipran	++++	+++	+	0	0
Venlafaxine[a] and desvenlafaxine	+++	++++	+	+	0
Tricyclic antidepressants (TCAs)					
Amitriptyline	++	++++	++++	++++	+++
Desipramine	++++	++	++	++	++
Doxepin	++	++	+++	++++	++
Imipramine	++	++++	+++	+++	++++
Nortriptyline	++++	++	++	++	+
Mixed serotonergic (mixed 5-HT)					
Nefazodone	0	++	0	+++	+++
Trazodone	0	++	0	++++	+++
Vilazodone	0	++++	0	+	0
Vortioxetine	0	++++	0	+	0
Norepinephrine and dopamine reuptake inhibitor (NDRI)					
Bupropion[b]	+	0	+	0	0
Serotonin and α₂-receptor antagonist					
Mirtazapine	0	0	0	++	++

[a]Venlafaxine: primarily 5-HT at lower doses, NE at higher doses, and DA at very high doses.
[b]Bupropion: also blocks dopamine reuptake.
α1, antiadrenergic, hypotension; H1, antihistamine, sedation; M1, antimuscarinic/anticholinergic side effects.
++++, high; +++, moderate; ++, low; +, very low; 0, absent or not adequately studied.

- Citalopram and escitalopram may to an increase in QT interval at doses above 40 mg/day.
- Potentially fatal reactions may occur when any SSRI and MAOI are coadministered. A 5-week washout after fluoxetine discontinuation is critical before starting an MAOI.
- If an SSRI is added to a regimen which includes drugs known to interact with SSRIs, the SSRI starting dose should be low and slowly titrated.
- Table 68-6 compares second- and third-generation antidepressants for their effects on CYP450 enzymes. CYP2D6 and 3A4 are responsible for the metabolism of more than 80% of currently marketed drugs. Consult the drug interaction literature for detailed information concerning any real or potential psychotherapeutic drug interactions.

TABLE 68-4 Adverse Drug Reactions and Monitoring Parameters Associated with Select Antidepressants

Drug	ADR(s)	Monitoring	Comments
Antidepressants from each pharmacologic class			
Common to all antidepressants	Suicidality	Behavioral changes Mental status	(US black box warning) for all antidepressants; caregivers should be alerted to monitor for acute changes in behavior (especially early in treatment)
Selective serotonin reuptake inhibitors (SSRIs)			
Common to all SSRIs	Anxiety or nervousness	Assess severity and impact on patient functioning and quality of life	Most prominent on initial treatment; lower initial doses recommended in patients with prominent anxiety
	Hyponatremia	Serum sodium	More likely in older females; sodium may decrease within 72 hours of initiating antidepressant
	Nausea	Frequency and severity	May improve with slower dose titration
	Sleep changes (insomnia and somnolence)	Sleep patterns	Among SSRI class: fluoxetine may be more activating; fluvoxamine and paroxetine may be more sedating
	Sexual dysfunction	Assess severity and impact on patient functioning and quality of life	Spontaneous self-reporting may be low; clinician should assess symptoms; reversible on drug discontinuation
SSRI-specific			
Citalopram (possibly escitalopram)	QTc interval prolongation	Electrocardiogram; electrolytes (eg, potassium, magnesium)	Caution use in "at-risk" patients (eg, electrolyte disturbance); discontinue if QTc persistently >500 msec or increased >5 msec over baseline
Fluoxetine	Anorexia	Weight (over time)	SSRIs are generally considered weight neutral
Paroxetine	Anticholinergic effects	Symptoms: dry mouth, constipation, urinary retention, mental status	Paroxetine possesses relatively more anticholinergic effects than other SSRIs

Serotonin–norepinephrine reuptake inhibitors (SNRIs)

Common to all SNRIs

Cardiovascular changes	Increases in blood pressure; heart rate	Possibly less likely with duloxetine; may need to lower/discontinue dose
Insomnia	Sleep patterns	Possibly less likely with duloxetine
Nausea	Frequency and severity	May improve with slower dose titration
Sexual dysfunction	Assess severity and impact on patient functioning and quality of life	Spontaneous self-reporting may be low; clinicians should assess symptoms; reversible on drug discontinuation
Sweating	Frequency and severity	May require change in therapy

SNRI-specific

Desvenlafaxine	Dose-related hyperlipidemia	Lipid profile	Elevations in total cholesterol, low-density lipoproteins, and triglycerides
Duloxetine	Liver toxicity	Liver function tests	May be transient upon initiation or sustained

Mixed serotonergic effects (mixed 5-HT)

Nefazodone	Liver toxicity	Liver function tests	Nefazodone black box warning in the United States for hepatotoxicity
Trazodone	Orthostatic hypotension	Blood pressure, pulse	May be more severe as compared with other antidepressants; rate-limiting side effect
	Priapism	Patient report of sexual side effects, especially painful erection	Patient should seek medical attention for prolonged erection (ie, >4 hours)
Vilazodone and vortioxetine	Nausea	Frequency and severity	Most common dose-limiting side effect

Serotonin and α_2-adrenergic antagonist

Mirtazapine	Weight gain	Body weight	Frequently occurring and significant (>7% over baseline) weight gain among adults; diet mediated

Norepinephrine and dopamine reuptake inhibitor (NDRI)

Bupropion	Seizure activity	Electroencephalogram if indicated	See Table 68-2 for proper dosing, which can help decrease seizure risk; caution use in patients with eating disorders or alcohol use disorders

TABLE 68-5	Pharmacokinetic Properties of Antidepressants		
Generic Name	**Elimination Half-Life**[a]	**Plasma Protein Binding (%)**	**Clinically Important Metabolites**
Selective serotonin reuptake inhibitors (SSRIs)			
Citalopram	33 hours	80	None
Escitalopram	27–32 hours	56	None
Fluoxetine	4–6 days[b]	94	Norfluoxetine[c]
Fluvoxamine	15–26 hours	77	None
Paroxetine	24–31 hours	95	None
Sertraline	27 hours	99[d]	None
Serotonin–norepinephrine reuptake inhibitors (SNRIs)			
Desvenlafaxine	11 hours	30	None
Duloxetine	12 hours	90	None
Levomilnacipran	12 hours	22	None
Venlafaxine	5 hours	27–30	O-Desmethyl-venlafaxine
Tricyclic Antidepressants (TCAs)			
Amitriptyline	9–46 hours	90–97	Nortriptyline
Desipramine	11–46 hours	73–92	2-Hydroxy-desipramine
Doxepin	8–36 hours	68–82	Desmethyl-doxepin
Imipramine	6–34 hours	63–96	Desipramine
Nortriptyline	16–88 hours	87–95	10-Hydroxy-nortriptyline
Mixed serotonergic (mixed 5-HT)			
Nefazodone	2–4 hours	99	meta-Chlorophenyl-piperazine
Trazodone	6–11 hours	92	meta-Chlorophenyl-piperazine
Vilazodone	25 hours	>95	
Vortioxetine	66 hours	98	
Norepinephrine/Dopamine reuptake inhibitor (NDRI)			
Bupropion	10–21 hours	82–88	Hydroxy-bupropion
			Threohydro-bupropion
			Erythrohydro-bupropion
Serotonin and α_2—adrenergic antagonists			
Mirtazapine	20–40 hours	85	None

[a]Biologic half-life in slowest phase of elimination.
[b]Four to 6 days with chronic dosing; norfluoxetine, 4–16 days.
[c]Take with food to increase area under the curve concentrations by greater than 60%.
[d]Increases 30%–40% when taken with food.

TABLE 68-6	Second- and Third-Generation Antidepressants and Cytochrome (CYP) P450 Enzyme Inhibitory Potential			
	CYP Enzyme			
Drug	**1A2**	**2C**	**2D6**	**3A4**
Bupropion	0	0	+++	0
Citalopram	0	0	+	NA
Duloxetine	0	0	+++	0
Escitalopram	0	0	+	0
Fluoxetine	0	++	++++	++
Fluvoxamine	++++	++	0	+++
Mirtazapine	0	0	0	0
Nefazodone	0	0	0	++++
Paroxetine	0	0	++++	0
Sertraline	0	++	+	+
(des)-Venlafaxine	0	0	0/+	0

++++, high; +++, moderate; ++, low; +, very low; 0, absent.

Serotonin–Norepinephrine Reuptake Inhibitors and Antidepressants with Mixed Serotonin Effects

- The serotonin–norepinephrine reuptake inhibitors include **venlafaxine, desvenlafaxine, duloxetine**, and **levomilnacipran**. Some studies suggest a slight efficacy advantage for venlafaxine compared to other antidepressants.
- Common side effects for these medications may be dose-related and include nausea, sexual dysfunction, activation, and hyperhidrosis.
- Venlafaxine may cause a dose-related increase in diastolic blood pressure. Dosage reduction or discontinuation may be necessary if sustained hypertension occurs. Nausea and vomiting may be worse with venlafaxine and there may be higher side effect-related discontinuation rates with venlafaxine and duloxetine than with the SSRIs.
- The most common side effects of duloxetine are nausea, dry mouth, constipation, decreased appetite, insomnia, and increased sweating.
- Mirtazapine enhances central noradrenergic and serotonergic activity by antagonizing central presynaptic α_2-adrenergic autoreceptors and heteroreceptors. It also antagonizes 5-HT$_2$ and 5-HT$_3$ receptors and blocks histamine receptors. It may be an option for patients who experience sexual dysfunction taking other antidepressants. Mirtazapine's most common adverse effects are somnolence, weight gain, dry mouth, and constipation.
- Levomilnacipran is a single-isomer, extended-release form of milnacipran which is FDA-approved to treat fibromyalgia which pharmacologically inhibits NE reuptake more than 5HT reuptake. This agent may increase blood pressure and heart rate and its place in therapy for MDD is unknown.
- Trazodone and nefazodone antagonize the 5-HT$_2$ receptor and inhibit the reuptake of 5-HT. They can also enhance 5-HT$_{1A}$ neurotransmission. Trazodone blocks α_1-adrenergic and histaminergic receptors increasing dizziness and sedation.
  - ✓ Trazodone cause minimal anticholinergic effects. Sedation, dizziness, and cognitive slowing are the most frequent dose-limiting side effects with trazodone. Common side effects with nefazodone are dizziness, orthostatic hypotension, and somnolence.
  - ✓ Priapism occurs rarely with trazodone (1 in 6000 male patients). Surgical intervention may be required, and impotence may result.
  - ✓ Nefazodone carries a black box warning for life-threatening liver failure. Do not initiate nefazodone in individuals with active liver disease or elevated serum transaminases.

- Vilazodone and vortioxetine are other antidepressants with mixed serotonin effects that are a combination SSRI and 5-HT$_{1A}$ presynaptic receptor partial agonists. Vilazodone may be particularly useful for depressed patients with anxiety, and vortioxetine may be helpful for depressed patients with cognitive difficulties.
  - ✓ Vilazodone is associated with nausea, diarrhea, dizziness, insomnia, and decreased libido, especially in men.
  - ✓ Vortioxetine causes nausea and constipation and sexual dysfunction in men at the highest dose (20 mg/day).

Bupropion

- **Bupropion** inhibits both the NE and DA reuptake that makes it one of the most activating antidepressants.
  - ✓ The occurrence of seizures with bupropion is dose related and may be increased by predisposing factors (eg, history of head trauma or central nervous system [CNS] tumor). At the ceiling dose (450 mg/day), the incidence of seizures is 0.4%.
  - ✓ Other side effects are nausea, vomiting, tremor, insomnia, dry mouth, and skin reactions. It is contraindicated in patients with bulimia or anorexia nervosa, as these patients have a higher risk for seizures. It causes less sexual dysfunction than SSRIs.

Tricyclic Antidepressants

- Tricyclic antidepressant (TCA) use has diminished because of the availability of equally effective therapies that are safer on overdose and better tolerated. They inhibit the reuptake of NE and 5-HT and have affinity for adrenergic, cholinergic, and histaminergic receptors.
- TCAs cause anticholinergic side effects (eg, dry mouth, blurred vision, constipation, urinary retention, tachycardia, memory impairment, and delirium) and sedation. Additional adverse effects include weight gain, orthostatic hypotension, cardiac conduction delay, and sexual dysfunction.
- **Desipramine** carries an increased risk of death in patients with a family history of sudden cardiac death, cardiac dysrhythmias, or cardiac conduction disturbances.
- Abrupt withdrawal of TCAs (especially high doses) may result in cholinergic rebound (eg, dizziness, nausea, diarrhea, insomnia, and restlessness).
- **Maprotiline**, a tetracyclic drug, causes seizures at a higher incidence than do standard TCAs and is contraindicated in patients with a history of seizure disorder.
- Metabolism of the TCAs appears to be linear within the usual dosage range. Dose-related kinetics cannot be ruled out in older patients. Factors reported to influence TCA plasma concentrations include renal or hepatic dysfunction, genetics, age, cigarette smoking, and concurrent drug administration.
- In acutely depressed patients, there is a correlation between antidepressant effect and plasma concentrations for some TCAs (eg, **amitriptyline, nortriptyline, imipramine**, and **desipramine**). The best-established therapeutic range is for **nortriptyline**, and data suggest a therapeutic window (Table 68-2).
- Some indications for TCA plasma level monitoring include inadequate response; relapse; serious or persistent adverse effects; use of higher than standard doses; suspected non-adherence, toxicity, pharmacokinetic interactions; elderly, pediatric, and adolescent patients; pregnant patients; patients of African or Asian descent (because of slower metabolism); cardiac disease; and changing brands. Plasma concentrations should be obtained at steady state, usually after a minimum of 1 week at constant dosage, during the elimination phase, and usually in the morning 12 hours after the last dose.
- TCAs may interact with other drugs that modify hepatic cytochrome P450 (CYP450) enzyme activity or hepatic blood flow. TCAs also are involved in interactions through displacement from protein-binding sites.
- Increased plasma concentrations of TCAs and symptoms of toxicity may occur when fluoxetine or paroxetine (both inhibitors of CYP2D6) are added.

Monoamine Oxidase Inhibitors

- **Isocarboxazide**, **phenelzine**, and **tranylcypromine** increase the concentrations of NE, 5-HT, and DA within the neuronal synapse through inhibition of monoamine oxidase (MAO). They are nonselective inhibitors of MAO-A and MAO-B. **Selegiline**, available as a transdermal patch for treatment of major depression, inhibits brain MAO-A and MAO-B but has reduced effects on MAO-A in the gut.
- Table 68-7 shows dietary and medication restrictions for patients taking phenelzine or tranylcypromine.
- The most common adverse effect of MAOIs is postural hypotension (more likely with phenelzine than tranylcypromine), which can be minimized by divided dosing.
- Phenelzine is mildly to moderately sedating, but tranylcypromine is often stimulating, and the last dose of the day is administered in the early afternoon. Sexual dysfunction in both genders is common. Phenelzine has been associated with hepatocellular damage and weight gain.
- Hypertensive crisis is a potentially fatal reaction that can occur when MAOIs are taken concurrently with certain foods, especially those high in tyramine, and with certain drugs (see Table 68-7). Symptoms of hypertensive crisis include occipital headache, stiff neck, nausea, vomiting, sweating, and sharply elevated blood pressure. Hypertensive crisis may be treated with agents such as captopril. Education of patients taking MAOIs regarding dietary and medication restrictions is critical. Patients taking transdermal selegiline patch doses greater than 6 mg/24 hours must follow the dietary restrictions.
- Potentially fatal reactions may occur when any SSRI or TCA is coadministered with an MAOI. However, TCAs and MAOIs can be combined in refractory patients by experienced clinicians with careful monitoring.

Ketamine

- **Ketamine** is an older anesthetic agent, which modulates glutamate activity via extrasynaptic N-methyl-D-aspartate (NMDA) receptor antagonism resulting in increased BDNF activity and synaptogenesis.
- Ketamine has rapid antidepressant effects when used in intravenous doses of 0.5mg/kg for treatment refractory MDD.
- **Esketamine** is the single s-isomer of ketamine that has a higher affinity for the NMDA receptor than the r-isomer. Intranasal esketamine is FDA-approved and requires supervised, in-clinic self-administration (2–6 sprays per session) followed by 2 hours of in-clinic observation. In trials, patients received doses twice weekly for 4 weeks and variable dosing thereafter.
- Side effects include transient psychotomimetic/dissociative effects and blood pressure elevation (10–20 mm Hg) with both agents.

Brexanolone

- **Brexanolone** (exogenous allopregnanolone) is thought to exert antidepressant effect by allosteric modulation of $GABA_A$ receptors, which may increase 5HT and NE transmission and is FDA-approved for postpartum depression. Administration involves a 60-hour stepped dose, intravenous infusion.
- Common adverse effects are headache, dizziness, and somnolence. It has a mandatory Risk Evaluation and Mitigation Strategies (REMS) program with Elements to Ensure Safe Use (ETASU) due to the incidence of excessive sedation or loss of consciousness.

St. John's Wort

- **St. John's wort**, a herb containing hypericum, may be effective for mild-to-moderate depression. It is associated with several drug–drug interactions. All antidepressant regimens should be overseen by a trained healthcare professional.

TABLE 68-7 Dietary and Medication Restrictions for Patients Taking Monoamine Oxidase Inhibitors[a]

Foods to Avoid Completely	Approximate Tyramine Content (mg) Per Ounce
Aged cheeses (eg, cheddar, blue, Swiss, Camembert)	25–45
Chicken liver	60
Dry aged meats (eg, mortadella, salami, prosciutto)	2–45
Fava beans	Unknown
Kim chee	Unknown
Red wine	Variable
Sauerkraut	1–3
Smoked or pickled fish (eg, lox, caviar, pickled herring)	0–80
Soy sauce, fermented soy, miso	Varies
Tap beer	20–40
Yeast extract	2–60
Foods to Eat in Moderation	
American cheese, Parmesan cheese	<2
Canned, filtered beer	<2 per 12 oz (355 mL)
Havarti, brie	Thought to be low
Pepperoni	<2
Pizza (large commercial chains generally safe; avoid gourmet with aged cheeses and meats)	2 slices
White wine	<1 per 4 oz (120 mL)
Foods Without Restrictions	
Fresh dairy products (cottage cheese, cream cheese, fresh milk, ice cream, ricotta, sour cream, yogurt)	
Fresh meats (including fresh sausage)	
Processed meats (eg, lunch meat, hot dogs, ham)	
Spirits (eg, bourbon, gin, rum, vodka)	
Yeast bread products	

Medications to Avoid Completely

Antidepressants[a]	Dopamine	Methylphenidate
Amphetamines	Ephedrine	Reserpine
Appetite suppressants	Epinephrine	Sympathomimetics
Asthma inhalants	Guanethidine	Tryptophan
Buspirone	Levodopa	
Carbamazepine	Local anesthetics[b]	
Decongestants	Meperidine	
Dextromethorphan	Methyldopa	

[a]Tricyclic antidepressants may be used with caution by experienced clinicians in treatment-refractory populations.
[b]Those containing sympathomimetic vasoconstrictors.

SPECIAL POPULATIONS

Older Patients

- In older patients, depressed mood may be less prominent than other symptoms, such as loss of appetite, cognitive impairment, sleeplessness, fatigue, physical complaints, and loss of interest in usual activities.
- The SSRIs are often considered first-choice antidepressants for older patients. Bupropion, venlafaxine, and mirtazapine are also effective and well tolerated.
- Hyponatremia is more common in older patients.

Pediatric Patients

- Symptoms of depression in childhood include boredom, anxiety, failing adjustment, and sleep disturbance.
- Data supporting efficacy of antidepressants in children and adolescents are sparse. Fluoxetine and escitalopram are the only FDA-approved antidepressants for patients below 18 years of age.
- All antidepressants carry a black box warning for caution when using antidepressants in this population, and the FDA recommends specific monitoring parameters.
- Several cases of sudden death have been reported in children and adolescents taking desipramine and baseline electrocardiogram (ECG) is recommended.

Pregnancy

- Approximately 14% of pregnant women develop depression during pregnancy and women who discontinued antidepressant therapy were five times more likely to have a relapse during their pregnancy than were women who continued treatment.
- The absolute risk of antidepressant use in pregnancy is unknown.
- Risks reported with SSRIs use in pregnancy include low birth weight, respiratory distress, and congenital heart defects.
- The risks and benefits of drug therapy during pregnancy must be weighed, including concerns about untreated depression.
- Lack of current data exists regarding antidepressant exposure to infants during breastfeeding; however, sertraline may be preferred. The Motherisk program has the most up-to-date information.

Relative Resistance and Treatment-Resistant Depression

- Most "treatment-resistant" depressed patients have received inadequate therapy.
- The STAR*D study showed that one in three patients who did not achieve remission with an antidepressant became symptom-free when an additional medication (eg, bupropion SR or buspirone) was added, and one in four achieved remission after switching to a different antidepressant (eg, venlafaxine XR or bupropion, or sertraline).
- The current antidepressant may be stopped and a trial initiated with different agent (eg, mirtazapine or nortriptyline).
- Alternatively, the current antidepressant may be augmented by addition of another agent (eg, lithium or triiodothyronine [T_3]), or another antidepressant can be added. An atypical antipsychotic (eg, aripiprazole, quetiapine, brexpiprazole) can be used to augment antidepressant response.
- The practice guideline of the American Psychiatric Association recommends that after 6–8 weeks of antidepressant treatment, partial responders should consider changing the dose, augmenting the antidepressant, or adding psychotherapy or ECT. For patients with no response, options include changing to another antidepressant or the addition of psychotherapy or ECT. Figure 68-1 is an algorithm for treatment of depression including refractory patients.

EVALUATION OF THERAPEUTIC OUTCOMES

- Several monitoring parameters, in addition to plasma concentrations, are useful. Monitor regularly for adverse effects (Table 68-4), remission of target symptoms, and changes in social or occupational functioning. Assure regular monitoring for several months after discontinuation of antidepressants.
- Regularly monitor blood pressure of patients given serotonin–norepinephrine reuptake inhibitors.
- A pretreatment ECG is recommended before starting TCA therapy in children, adolescents, and patients over 40 years of age, and perform follow-up ECGs periodically.
- Monitor for suicidal ideation after initiation of any antidepressant, especially in the first few weeks of treatment and up to 30 days after treatment discontinuation.
- In addition to the clinical interview, use psychometric rating instruments to rapidly and reliably measure the nature and severity of depressive and associated symptoms.

See Chapter 85, Major Depressive Disorder, authored by Amy M. Vandenberg, for a more detailed discussion of this topic.

- *Opioid use disorder* (OUD) consists of intoxication and withdrawal from the substance for which there is no cure. Since 1999, the number of overdose deaths contributed to OUD has more than tripled. These deaths have involved opioid substances including prescription opioids (ie, natural opioids, semisynthetic opioids, and methadone), as well as heroin and synthetic opioids (ie, illicitly manufactured fentanyl).

PATHOPHYSIOLOGY

- The true etiology behind substance use disorders (SUD) is unknown. In general, it is felt that there needs to be a triad of the right patient, with the right genetic risk factors, being exposed to the right medication or substance in order for a SUD to occur.

CLINICAL PRESENTATION

- Signs and symptoms of opioid intoxication include euphoria, dysphoria, slurred speech, miosis, apathy, sedation, and attention impairment. Signs and symptoms of withdrawal include lacrimation, mydriasis, piloerection, diaphoresis, diarrhea, yawning, muscle aches, and insomnia. Pinpoint pupils, decreased breathing, pulmonary edema, loss of consciousness, and death may occur with opioid intoxication.
- The onset of withdrawal ranges from a few hours after stopping heroin to 3–5 days after stopping methadone. Duration of withdrawal ranges from 3–14 days. Occurrence of delirium suggests withdrawal from another drug (eg, alcohol).
- Symptoms can be scored on the Clinical Opiate Withdrawal Symptoms (COWS) assessment tool to assess severity of opioid withdrawal.
- Laboratory tests to obtain include a comprehensive metabolic panel to monitor serum electrolyte concentrations in the setting of significant vomiting or diarrhea; check liver function tests if using buprenorphine. Arterial blood gases, pulse oximetry, and capnography are useful to assess respiratory depression in opioid intoxication.

DIAGNOSIS

- The *Diagnostic and Statistical Manual of Mental Disorders*, 5th edition (*DSM-5*) defines SUD as "problematic pattern of substance use leading to clinically significant impairment or distress as manifested by at least two of eleven criteria occurring in the preceding 12-month period."
- These behaviors fall into the categories of: (1) impaired control, (2) social impairment, (3) risky use, and (4) pharmacological criteria, including tolerance and withdrawal, and are outlined in **Table 69-1**.
- SUDs occur in a broad range of severity from mild (2–3 symptoms) to moderate (4–5 symptoms) to severe (6 or more symptoms).
- *DSM-5* does not separate the diagnoses of substance abuse and substance dependence. Criteria are provided for SUD, accompanied by criteria for intoxication, withdrawal, substance-induced disorders, and unspecified substance-related disorders in some cases.
- *Addiction:* A primary chronic neurobiologic disease characterized by the inability to consistently abstain, impairment in behavioral control, craving, dysfunctional emotional response, and diminished recognition of significant problems with behaviors and interpersonal relationships.
- *Intoxication:* Development of a substance-specific syndrome after recent ingestion and presence in the body of a substance; it is associated with maladaptive behavior during the waking state caused by effects of the substance on the central nervous system (CNS).
- *Physical dependence:* A state of adaptation manifested by a drug-class–specific withdrawal syndrome that can be produced by abrupt cessation, rapid dose reduction, decreasing blood level of the drug, and/or administration of an antagonist.

801

TABLE 69-1	Eleven Criteria for Substance Use Disorder as Defined by *DSM-5*
Specific Category	**Specific Behavior**
Impaired Control	1. Substance is often taken in larger amounts or over a longer period of time than intended
Impaired Control	2. Persistent desire or continued unsuccessful efforts to cut down or control substance use
Impaired Control	3. Considerable amount of time is spent obtaining substance, using substance, or recovering from use of substance
Impaired Control	4. Craving or strong desire to use substance
Social Impairment	5. Recurrent use of substance is resulting in failure to fulfill major obligations at work, home, or school
Social Impairment	6. Continue to use substance despite persistent social or interpersonal problems
Social Impairment	7. Reducing or missing social, occupation, or recreational events due to substance use
Risky Use	8. Recurrent substance use in situations with increasing risk of physical harm
Risky Use	9. Continued use of substance despite knowledge of persistent or recurrent physical or psychological harm that was caused or worsened by the substance
Pharmacological Indicators	10. Tolerance as experienced by either: a. Need for increased amounts of the substance to achieve intoxication or desired result, or b. A noticeably decreased effect with continued use of the same amount of substance
Pharmacological Indicators	11. Withdrawal as experienced by either: a. Standard symptoms of withdrawal as defined by specific substance, or b. Use of a substance or a similar substance to relieve or avoid withdrawal symptoms

- *Substance dependence:* The continued use of the substance despite adverse substance-related problems.
- *Tolerance:* A state of adaptation in which exposure to a drug induces changes that result in a diminution of one or more of the drug's effects over time.
- *Withdrawal:* A substance-specific syndrome occurring after cessation of or reduction in intake of a substance that was used regularly.

OPIOIDS

- Deaths from prescription opioids have reached epidemic levels.
- **Heroin** can be snorted, smoked, and given IV. Complications of heroin use include overdoses, anaphylactic reactions to impurities, nephrotic syndrome, septicemia, endocarditis, and acquired immunodeficiency.
- **Hydrocodone** is the most widely abused pharmaceutical controlled substance in the United States.
- **Fentanyl** is a synthetic short-acting opioid which is 50–100 times more potent than morphine and approved for management of acute or chronic pain associated with advanced cancer. Most fentanyl-related morbidity and mortality have been linked to illicitly manufactured fentanyl and fentanyl analogs. It is often mixed with heroin or cocaine, with or without the user's knowledge. Several states have reported spikes in overdose deaths due to fentanyl and its analogs (eg, carfentanil).

- Opioids are commonly combined with stimulants (eg, cocaine [speedball]) or lcohol.
- **Methadone** has caused an increased number of deaths in recent years. Converting to methadone from other opioid agonists can be tricky, and lethal when done improperly. Peak respiratory depressant effects occur later and last longer than peak analgesic effects.
- **Dextromethorphan** and **loperamide** are over-the-counter drugs that cause depressant and mild hallucinogenic effects in high doses and significant hallucinations and CNS depression in excessive doses. Loperamide is sometimes taken with medications or foods that enhance its ability to cross the blood-brain barrier (ie, verapamil, methadone, cimetidine or grapefruit juice) to obtain CNS effects.
  - ✓ Loperamide side effects associated with supratherapeutic doses include possible cardiac arrhythmias including QTc interval prolongation, torsades de pointes, ventricular dysrhythmias, syncope, and cardiac arrest.
  - ✓ Acute overdoses of dextromethorphan can be treated with naloxone.

TREATMENT

- <u>Goals of Treatment</u>: Cessation of use of the drug, termination of drug-seeking behaviors, and return to normal functioning. The goals of treatment of withdrawal include prevention of progression to life-threatening severity, thus enabling comfort and functionality conducive to participation in a treatment program. OUD is a chronic disorder, and providing long-term medication decreases the risk of an accidental overdose or full relapse into opioid use.

NONPHARMACOLOGIC THERAPY

- The treatment of OUD may also include behavioral therapy, but participation in this should not be required for receiving medications. Behavioral therapy should be introduced if and when the patient is ready.

PHARMACOLOGIC THERAPY

- Naloxone is a key strategy in reducing opioid-related deaths because it may revive unconscious patients with respiratory depression. Naloxone is a competitive mu-opioid receptor antagonist that can be used in the reversal of an opioid overdose, but it may precipitate physical withdrawal in dependent patients. Table 69-2 outlines the naloxone delivery options.
- Patients and their caregivers should be educated on the availability of naloxone and the proper use of this agent. The World Health Organization (WHO) recommends that anyone who might witness an overdose should have access to naloxone and proper training. Many states have simplified the process to obtain naloxone to prevent opioid-related overdoses.

Withdrawal

- A variety of treatment regimens are used for patients during the acute opioid withdrawal phase and are summarized in Tables 69-3 and 69-4.
- Avoid unnecessary detoxification with drugs if possible (eg, if symptoms are tolerable), and provide patient-specific supportive care measures, such as fluids, until the patient stabilizes.
- The three FDA-approved medications used in OUD include **methadone, buprenorphine**, and **naltrexone**, all of which work by blocking the effects of the opioids and reducing or eliminating the cravings.

Methadone

- Methadone is a mu-opioid agonist that suppresses withdrawal symptoms and controls cravings for maintenance therapy.
- Once-daily dosing can range from 10 to 30 mg, depending on the patient's use pattern. This dose should be reduced to 10–20 mg for those over the age of 60, or if drug–drug interactions are identified.
- Dose adjustments of 5–10 mg should occur gradually, no sooner than every 4–7 days based on clinical response. Maintenance doses range between 60 and 120 mg/day.

TABLE 69-2	Naloxone Delivery Options			
	Intramuscular Injection	**Auto-Injector (Evzio)**	**Nasal Spray (Narcan)**	**Intranasal Spray (Atomizer)**
Description of device or what is provided to patient	Two single-use 0.4 mg/mL naloxone vials Two single-use 3-mL syringes, 23–25 gauge, 1–1.5 inch needles	One box of 2 mg/0.4 mL prefilled auto injectors that includes 2 devices and a trainer device	One box of two 4 mg/0.1 mL intranasal devices	2 mg/2 mL prefilled naloxone needleless syringe Two mucosal atomizer devices
Directions for use	Inject 1 mL intramuscularly in shoulder or thigh upon signs of opioid overdose. Call 911 immediately. May repeat once in 2–3 minutes if no response or patient is showing minimal response	Use one auto-injector by injecting in outer thigh by depressing and holding for 5 seconds. Voice automation will direct the patient. Call 911. May repeat ×1 in 2–3 minutes if no response or patient shows minimal response	Use full contents of spray in one nostril upon signs of opioid overdose. Call 911. May repeat ×1 in 2–3 minutes if no response or patient shows minimal response, using the other nostril	Spray one-half of contents of syringe into each nostril upon signs of opioid overdose. Call 911. May repeat ×1 in 2–3 minutes if no response or patient shows minimal response

Naloxone pearls

- Naloxone has not been shown to cause severe effects or side effects if administered to patients who are currently not taking opioids.
- Naloxone should be given if the patient is intoxicated by a combination of products since the naloxone will still work for the opioid but not for other products such as benzodiazepines or alcohol.

Naloxone counseling topics

- Overdose recognition, response, prevention
- Importance of seeking emergency medical care
- Proper device use and counseling of family members and caregivers
- Proper storage, shelf life. Periodically check expiration date
- Potential side effects associated with naloxone
- Availability of drug treatment program

General opioid safety counseling

- Take medication only prescribed for you, only take prescribed doses
- Do not mix opioids with alcohol or sleeping pills
- Always store all medications in a locked and secure place
- Dispose of unused medications appropriately
- Do not use opioids/drugs alone. Never buy opioids/drugs from unknown source
- Do not restart opioid at same dose if there is a period of abstinence. Overdose is possible due to lower tolerance

TABLE 69-3	Differences Between Medication-Assisted Therapy (MAT) Products		
	Methadone	**Extended-Release Injectable Naltrexone (XR-NTX)**	**Buprenorphine**
Pharmacology in OUD	Full opioid agonist at mu-opioid receptor with long half-life to allow for once-daily dosing for OUD	Antagonist at mu-opioid receptor (*note: does not provide analgesia and is not addictive*)	Partial agonist at mu-opioid receptor with long half-life (up to 36 hours via sublingual administration); blocks intoxicating effects of other opioids
Phase of treatment in OUD; effect	Medically supervised withdrawal, maintenance; reduces or eliminates withdrawal symptoms and cravings to use opioids, blocks or blunts the effects of illicit opioids	Prevention of relapse to opioid dependence following medically supervised withdrawal; reduces or eliminates cravings to use opioids and blunts or blocks the effects of illicit opioids	Medically supervised withdrawal, maintenance; reduces or eliminates withdrawal symptoms and cravings to use opioids and blocks or blunts the effects of illicit opioids
Route of administration used in MAT	Provided orally once daily: commonly given as liquid concentrate in OTPs but current guidelines also allow solid oral-dosage forms as well	IM extended-release (depot naltrexone) (*note: oral not as effective and use is not common in the treatment of OUD due to insufficient evidence of efficacy and poor medication adherence*)	Sublingual, buccal tablet, buccal film Other routes of administration available after meeting specific criteria: subdermal implant, subcutaneous extended-release injection
Restrictions for prescribing each product	CII; patient must meet Federal Opioid-Treatment Program standards; can be used in hospital settings for OUD treatment	Not a controlled substance but requires a prescription. All naltrexone products can be prescribed by general practitioners and in OUD treatment	CIII; requires waiver to prescribe outside of OTPs. Prescribers will receive separate DEA number with a "X" upon meeting requirements of DATA 2000. To confirm practitioner verification: https//www.samhsa.gov/bupe/lookup-form

(Continued)

TABLE 69-3	Differences Between Medication-Assisted Therapy (MAT) Products (*Continued*)		
	Methadone	**Extended-Release Injectable Naltrexone (XR-NTX)**	**Buprenorphine**
Restrictions for prescribing each product (continued)			Implant: prescribers must be certified in Probuphine REMS program to insert/remove implants
			Subcutaneous: healthcare settings and pharmacies must be certified in the Sublocade REMS program and only dispense the medication directly to a provider for administration
Patients that are commonly considered for this type of therapy	Patients with OUD; physiologically dependent on opioids and meet federal OTP admission criteria	Patients with OUD; patients who are abstinent from short-acting opioids for 7–10 days and long-acting opioids 10–14 days	Patients with OUD; physiologically dependent on opioids
Major side effects	Constipation, vomiting, dizziness, sedation, QTc prolongation, respiratory depression (risk is highest during initiation of methadone or dose titration and concurrent use of benzodiazepines or alcohol)	Injection site pain and tenderness, risk of injection site induration, toothache, LFT elevation, insomnia, nasopharyngitis	Constipation, vomiting, dizziness, sedation, insomnia, blurred vision, respiratory depression (highest risk with concurrent use of CNS depressants including benzodiazepines); sublingual buprenorphine/ naloxone sublingual and buccal film: oral hypoesthesia, oral mucosal erythema, glossodynia

CII, Schedule II prescription; CIII, Schedule III prescription; IM, intramuscular; LFT, liver function test; OTP, Opioid Treatment Program; OUD, opioid use disorder; REMS, Risk Evaluation and Mitigation Strategy.

TABLE 69-4 Extended-Release Products Approved by FDA for Opioid Use Disorder

Drug	Trade Name	Dose	Comments
Naltrexone tablets	Revia	Following a 7–10 day opioid-free period for short-acting opioids or a 10–14 day opioid-free period for long-acting opioids: begin with dose of 25 mg daily with food. If no signs of withdrawal, increase dose to 50 mg po daily	Should be part of a comprehensive treatment plan that includes psychosocial support Although specific dosage adjustments are not available for patient with hepatic dysfunction, reports of elevated LFTs have been reported; use with caution Use with caution in patients with renal impairment, although data are limited, naltrexone and active metabolite are renally excreted
Naltrexone XR injection	Vivitrol	Following a 7–10 day opioid-free period for short-acting opioids or a 10–14 day opioid-free period for long-acting opioids: 380 mg IM in gluteal area alternating buttocks; every 4 weeks or once a month	Must be administered by a healthcare provider Must use manufacturer provided needle and assess body size of patient at each visit so proper needle size is used Monitor injection site closely for any signs of abnormal pain and contact healthcare provider immediately if this occurs Dose adjustment is required in mild or moderate hepatic impairment. No data available in severe hepatic impairment No dose adjustments in mild renal impairment; use caution in patients with moderate-to-severe renal impairment, naltrexone and active metabolite are renally excreted
Buprenorphine	Probuphine	Four implants are inserted subdermally in the inner side of the upper arm and should remain in place for 6 months	Patients must meet specific criteria for use of Probuphine: a. Only indicated for patients who are opioid tolerant b. Demonstrates clinical stability on transmucosal buprenorphine with Subutex or Suboxone 8 mg/day or less (or transmucosal equivalent) for 3 months or longer without requiring supplemental dose adjustments *(Continued)*

TABLE 69-4 Extended-Release Products Approved by FDA for Opioid Use Disorder (Continued)

Drug	Trade Name	Dose	Comments
			Probuphine must be inserted or removed within a facility and by a certified provider who has completed the required live training
			It is recommended to not prescribe as-needed transmucosal buprenorphine products. If patient is requesting these products, reassessment is indicated
			Moderate-to-severe hepatic impairment: use not recommended
			Limited data in renal impairment, currently no dosage adjustments listed
Buprenorphine	Sublocade	For patients who have achieved clinical stability on equivalent of 8–24 mg of a transmucosal buprenorphine product daily	Must be administered by a healthcare provider
			Steady state occurs after 4–6 months; after discontinuation detectable buprenorphine levels could occur 12 months or longer; urine and plasma concentration correlations are not known
		Available in two extended-release solutions:	Injections must occur at least 26 days apart. Follow all manufacturer directions for preparation and injection
		a. 100 mg/0.5 mL	Do not give the injection at the belt or waistband area where pressure will occur
		b. 300 mg/1.5 mL	Counsel the patient that there will be a small bump at the injection site that will decrease in size over the next several weeks. Do not rub or massage this area
		Directions: inject 300 mg subcutaneously once a month in abdominal area for 2 months, then decrease dose to 100 mg once monthly in abdominal area	If needed, the most recently injected depot can be removed within the 14 days of injection under local anesthesia
			Doses can be adjusted back to 300 mg monthly for patients in whom benefits exceed risks
			Examine injection site each month for evidence of tampering
			Moderate-to-severe hepatic impairment: use not recommended
			Limited data in renal impairment, currently no dosage adjustments listed

IM, intramuscularly; LFTs, liver function tests; mg, milligram; mL, milliliters.

- Adverse effects seen with methadone use include sedation and respiratory depression.
- Methadone has many cytochrome P450 drug interactions, and concomitant use of alcohol or benzodiazepines can lead to overdose and use should be assessed.
- Methadone carries a risk of QT prolongation, which is increased when given with other drugs that also prolong the QT interval.
- The use of methadone for OUD treatment is only approved through the Opioid Treatment Program (OTP), controlled by the Drug Enforcement Agency (DEA) and Substance Abuse and Mental Health Services Administration (SAMHSA). Methadone for the treatment of OUD may be provided to patients during a hospital admission for treatment of other health conditions.

Buprenorphine

- Buprenorphine is a partial mu-receptor agonist that is available as buprenorphine alone or buprenorphine/naloxone formulations. **Table 69-5** outlines the products used in the treatment of OUD. Due to its partial agonist activity, buprenorphine does provide some intrinsic pain control and has a ceiling effect for respiratory depression. Buprenorphine can be abused.
- Initiation in the emergency room for patients who present with opioid withdrawal symptoms is a treatment option, and federal guidelines state that buprenorphine should be offered to patients with OUD who are appropriate candidates.
- Buprenorphine is a Schedule III controlled substance with specific prescribing restrictions. Refer to the DEA webpage for the most up-to-date regulations regarding buprenorphine prescribing. Sedation or intoxication is the main adverse effect seen with use.
- It is recommended that treatment starts with a COWS score of 12 or higher for the first dose, based on buprenorphine Risk Evaluation and Mitigation Strategy (REMS).
- Medically supervised withdrawal with buprenorphine consists of an induction phase and a dose reduction phase followed by maintenance. SAMHSA provides evidence-based recommendations for use of buprenorphine for opioid addiction through various Treatment Improvement Protocols (TIPs). The same buprenorphine preparation is commonly used for induction, stabilization, and maintenance for most patients.
- Induction helps patients switch from the opioid of abuse to buprenorphine, and the goal is to find the minimum dose of buprenorphine at which the patient discontinues or markedly diminishes use of the opioid of abuse and experiences no withdrawal symptoms, minimal or no side effects, and no craving. The initial induction doses should be administered as observed treatment.
- The stabilization phase starts when the patient is experiencing no withdrawal symptoms, is having minimal or no side effects, and no longer has uncontrollable cravings.
- The maintenance phase may be indefinite and should focus on psychosocial and family issues. Attention must be focused on psychosocial and family issues identified during the course of treatment that contribute to a patient's OUD.
- Patient education is important (**Table 69-6**).

Naltrexone

- Naltrexone is a mu-opioid antagonist that is available for OUD in both an oral tablet and an extended-release injectable formulation.
- After confirming patients have been opioid free for 7–10 days, the initial dose is 25 mg given once daily, which can be increased to 50 mg/daily. Extended-release injectable naltrexone (Vivitrol®) is FDA-approved for use following opioid detoxification to help prevent relapse.
- The main adverse effects include swelling, bruising, and pruritus at the injection site. Elevations in liver function tests may occur with oral use.

Alpha-2 Agonists

- **Clonidine** or **lofexidine** may be used to attenuate withdrawal symptoms such as anxiety, tachycardia, hypertension, chills, and piloerection.
- Adverse effects include hypotension, dizziness, and sedation.

TABLE 69-5 Oral Buprenorphine Products Used for Treating Opioid Use Disorder

	Buprenorphine SL Tablet	Suboxone SL Tablet	Zubsolv SL Tablet	Suboxone SL or Buccal Film	Bunavail Buccal Film
Strengths of products commercially available/Routes of administration	2 mg 8 mg	Buprenorphine/Naloxone 2 mg/0.5 mg 8 mg/2 mg	Buprenorphine/Naloxone 0.7 mg/0.18 mg 1.4 mg/0.36 mg 2.9 mg/0.71 mg 5.7 mg/1.4 mg 8.6 mg/2.1 mg 11.4 mg/2.9 mg	Buprenorphine/Naloxone 2 mg/0.5 mg 4 mg/1 mg 8 mg/2 mg 12 mg/3 mg	Buprenorphine/Naloxone 2.1 mg/0.3 mg 4.2 mg/0.7 mg 6.3 mg/1 mg
Recommended once-daily target maintenance dose and dosing ranges	Target maintenance dose 16 mg **Dosing range** 4–24 mg[a]	Target maintenance dose 16 mg/4 mg **Dosing range** 4 mg/1 mg to 24 mg/6 mg[b]	Target maintenance dose 11.4 mg/2.9 mg **Dosing range** 2.9 mg/0.71 mg to 17.2 mg/4.2 mg[a]	Target maintenance dose 16 mg/4 mg **Dosing range** 4 mg/1 mg to 24 mg/6 mg[a]	Target maintenance dose 8.4 mg/1.4 mg **Dosing range** 2.1 mg/0.3 mg to 12.6 mg/2.1 mg

[a]Doses higher than 24 mg/6 mg have not been shown to offer any further benefit.
[b]Doses higher than 17.2 mg/4.2 mg have not been shown to offer any added benefit.
SL, sublingual.
Note: Refer to individual product dosing information when switching formulations due to possible bioequivalence variability. Monitoring is recommended following a switch in products due to possible variation in response to different formulations.

| TABLE 69-6 | Patient Education Points for Buprenorphine Treatment |

Prior to Starting Buprenorphine Therapy and Repeat Education at Induction:

- **Communication with prescriber:** Tell your doctors all medications including over-the-counter, herbal, creams, injections, inhalants, street medications, etc. that you are currently taking. This is important so your doctor is aware of what is in your body and if there are any chances of a dangerous drug interaction. Additionally, tell all of your doctors you are taking buprenorphine. If you are being treated for pain, it is very important to tell your doctor you are taking buprenorphine.

- **Goals of therapy:** The goal of your first week of treatment is to improve the symptoms of withdrawal without causing any oversedation (making you too tired or feeling over medicated). Notify your doctor/prescriber if you are feeling overly tired/sedated or euphoric within 1–4 hours of your dose. Dose adjustments might occur initially and it will take a little time for the buprenorphine to become stable in your system. The goals of therapy include finding the right dose to eliminate withdrawal, decrease or even eliminate cravings for opioids, and block the effects of other opioids without severe side effects.

- **Product use:**
  - Buprenorphine products (tablets, sublingual film, and buccal film) are not equivalent. If you have to transition to a new buprenorphine product, a dose adjustment might be required.
  - Take your dose at regular intervals and only as prescribed.
  - If you miss a dose, take the dose as soon as possible. If it is almost time for the next dose, do not double your dose, take only the dose that is prescribed.
  - Leave medication in packaging until you are ready to use.
  - Do not swallow sublingual tablets or film. This can reduce the effect of buprenorphine and lead to withdrawal symptoms.
  - Sublingual tablets
    i. Place tablets under your tongue and allow the tablet to fully dissolve, which can take several minutes.
    ii. If your dose requires multiple tablets, all tablets can be placed under the tongue at one time. If this is uncomfortable, only place two tablets under the tongue at a time.
  - Sublingual film
    i. Drink water prior to placing the film to help the film dissolve easily.
    ii. Place film under the tongue, to the left or right of the center of the tongue, and allow to completely dissolve.
    iii. If you are prescribed 2 films at a time, place the second film on the opposite side of the tongue. Do not allow the films to touch.
    iv. If you are prescribed more than 2 films at a time, wait until previous films have dissolved and repeat the process.
  - Buccal film
    i. Wet the inside of your cheek with your tongue or rinse with water prior to placing film.
    ii. Hold the film by the edges with two fingers and place on inside of cheek until fully dissolved, which can take up to 30 minutes.
    iii. If you are prescribed 2 films, place the second film inside the opposite cheek.
    iv. Do not adjust the film placement or touch the film, do not chew or swallow the film
    v. Do not drink or eat until the film has completely dissolved.

- **Common side effects:** Some side effects can occur when taking buprenorphine. These do not happen all of the time and do not happen to everyone. If you are experiencing any of these side effects please tell your doctor immediately. Do not stop taking buprenorphine without first speaking to your doctor. The most common side effects include headache, nausea, constipation, abdominal pain, insomnia, sweating, and a possible feeling of weakness or lack of energy.

(Continued)

| TABLE 69-6 | Patient Education Points for Buprenorphine Treatment (*Continued*) |

- **Precautions and warnings**
  - Using alcohol while taking buprenorphine is very dangerous and can lead to increased risk of overdose and possibly death.
  - There is a risk of overdose and possibly death if taking buprenorphine with benzodiazepines or alcohol.
  - Using tobacco products prior to using buprenorphine decreases the absorption of buprenorphine, thereby decreasing its effectiveness.
  - Long-term buprenorphine maintenance is recommended in many cases. If you stop buprenorphine, there is a high risk of overdose if you return to illicit opioid use.
  - Buprenorphine is an opioid that can cause physical dependence. Do not stop taking buprenorphine without consulting your doctor. If you stop buprenorphine abruptly, you could experience withdrawal symptoms.
  - All medications, including buprenorphine, should be stored in a secure area, preferably in a locked cabinet or safe. It is important to keep medication away from children.
  - It is recommended that you do not drive, operate heavy machinery, or perform any dangerous activities until you are fully aware of how this medication affects you.
  - If you feel you have taken too much buprenorphine, you will need emergency medical attention immediately. Some possible signs include dizziness, confusion, unsteady or faint, slowed reflexes, or breathing slower.
  - Do not inject these products. Serious life-threatening infections could occur. Additionally, serious withdrawal reactions can also occur upon injecting many of these buprenorphine products.
- **Pregnancy:** It is very important to inform your doctors if you become pregnant.
- **Counseling options:** Recovery resources and counseling resources are available for you and your family. We can give you further information on this when you are ready.

Maintenance:

- **Adherence assessment:** If any discrepancies arise, initiate discussion to identify reasons for discrepancies
  - Complete pill/film count
  - Review PDMP
  - Confirm current buprenorphine dose
  - Review results of urine drug screen
- **Treatment assessment and counseling**
  - Review treatment goals and assess progress
  - Review and assess benefits and risks of continuing buprenorphine treatment
  - Discuss participation in counseling or encourage counseling if not receiving counseling

EVALUATION OF THERAPEUTIC OUTCOMES

- OUD is a chronic disorder that requires pharmacological treatment and psychosocial and educational support. Consistent monitoring for efficacy and appropriateness through treatment is critical.
- Monitoring for withdrawal reactions utilizing proper assessment scales (ie, COWS) can aid in evaluating the patient appropriately.
- Medication safety has to be considered based on unique side-effect profiles and drug-interaction concerns for the selected treatment regimen.
- Data from urine drug screens and profiles from the Prescription Drug Monitoring Program (PDMP) can provide critical information on the full clinical picture for each patient.
- Continual patient education must occur to ensure proper medication administration and safety as the therapy continues.

See Chapter 82, Substance-Related Disorders I: Overview and Depressants, Stimulants, and Hallucinogens, authored by Robin Moorman Li, Patrick Leffers, and Paul L. Doering, for a more detailed discussion of the topic.

CHAPTER 70

Schizophrenia

- *Schizophrenia* is characterized by positive symptoms (eg, delusions, disorganized speech [association disturbance], hallucinations, behavior disturbance [disorganized or catatonic], and illusions); negative symptoms (eg, alogia [poverty of speech], avolition, flat affect, anhedonia, and social isolation); and cognitive dysfunction (eg, impaired attention, working memory, and executive function) all leading to impaired psychosocial functioning.

PATHOPHYSIOLOGY

- Schizophrenia causation theories include genetic predisposition, obstetric complications with hypoxia, increased neuronal pruning, neurodevelopmental disorders, neurodegenerative theories, dopamine receptor defect, and regional brain abnormalities including hyper- or hypoactivity of dopaminergic processes in specific brain regions. Increased ventricular size and decreased gray matter have been reported.
- Alterations in glutamatergic neurotransmission resulting in increased neuronal pruning have also been implicated in schizophrenia pathogenesis. Genes controlling *N*-methyl-D-aspartate (NMDA) receptor activity are hypothesized to be part of this process.
- Studies have also shown increased susceptibility to immune/autoimmune disorders in schizophrenia, as well as abnormalities of autoantibodies and cytokine functioning.
- Positive symptoms may be closely associated with dopamine receptor hyperactivity in the mesocaudate, whereas negative and cognitive symptoms may be most closely related to dopamine receptor hypofunction in the prefrontal cortex.

CLINICAL PRESENTATION

- Symptoms of the acute episode may include being out of touch with reality; hallucinations (especially hearing voices); delusions (fixed false beliefs); ideas of influence (actions controlled by external influences); disconnected thought processes (loose associations); illogical conversation; ambivalence (contradictory thoughts); flat, inappropriate, or labile affect; autistic thinking (withdrawn and inwardly directed thinking); uncooperativeness, hostility, and verbal or physical aggression; impaired self-care skills; and disturbed sleep and appetite.
- After the acute psychotic episode has resolved, typically there are residual features (eg, anxiety, suspiciousness, lack of motivation, poor insight, impaired judgment, social withdrawal, difficulty in learning from experience, and poor self-care skills).
- Comorbid psychiatric and medical disorders (eg depression, anxiety disorders, substance abuse, and general medical disorders such as respiratory disorders, cardiovascular disorders, and metabolic disturbances) can also occur. Medication nonadherence is also common.

DIAGNOSIS

- The *Diagnostic and Statistical Manual of Mental Disorders*, 5th ed. (*DSM-5*), specifies the following diagnostic criteria:
  ✓ Continuous symptoms that persist for at least 6 months with at least 1 month of active phase symptoms (Criterion A) and may include prodromal or residual symptoms.
    o Criterion A: For at least 1 month, there must be at least two of the following present for a significant portion of time: delusions, hallucinations, disorganized speech, grossly disorganized or catatonic behavior, and negative symptoms. At least one symptom must be delusions, hallucinations, or disorganized speech.
    o Criterion B: Significantly impaired functioning.

- Before treatment, perform a mental status examination, physical (vitals including height and weight) and neurologic examination, complete family and social history, psychiatric diagnostic interview, and laboratory workup (complete blood count [CBC], electrolytes, hepatic function, renal function, electrocardiogram [ECG], fasting serum glucose, serum lipids, thyroid function, and urine drug screen).

TREATMENT

- <u>Goals of Treatment</u>: The goal is to alleviate target symptoms, avoid side effects, improve psychosocial functioning and productivity, achieve compliance with the prescribed regimen, integrate the patient back into the community, prevent relapse, and involve the patient in treatment planning.

NONPHARMACOLOGIC THERAPY

- Psychosocial rehabilitation programs to improve the patients' adaptive functioning are the mainstay of nondrug treatment for schizophrenia. Programs that involve the family aimed at supportive employment and housing are effective and considered "best practices" and decrease rehospitalization while improving functioning in the community.
- It is important to frame clinical decision making in the context of a mutual process involving patient and clinician.

PHARMACOLOGIC THERAPY

- Both first-generation antipsychotics (FGAs, also known as traditional) and second-generation antipsychotics (SGAs, also known as atypical) are used to treat schizophrenia. Available antipsychotics and dosage ranges are shown in **Table 70-1**.
- **Table 70-2** summarizes the long-acting injectable antipsychotics (LAIAs), including dosage range, conversion from oral to LAIA, and injection method/technique.
- The exact mechanism of action of antipsychotics is unknown. FGAs have been found to have high D_2 antagonism and low serotonin-2 receptor [5-HT$_{2A}$] antagonism. SGAs exhibit moderate-to-high D_2 antagonism and high 5-HT$_{2A}$ antagonism, and clozapine shows low D_2 antagonism and high 5-HT$_{2A}$ antagonism.
- Base antipsychotic selection on: (1) the need to avoid certain side effects, (2) concurrent medical or psychiatric disorders, and (3) patient or family history of response. **Figure 70-1** is an algorithm for management of schizophrenia. Clozapine has superior efficacy for suicidal behavior.
- In first-episode schizophrenia, initiate antipsychotic dosing at the lower end of the dosing range. Use of SGAs during the first acute episode results in greater treatment retention and relapse prevention compared to FGAs. **Aripiprazole, risperidone, or ziprasidone** may be preferred first line.
- Risperidone injection is more effective than oral risperidone in preventing relapse over a 1-year period for first episode schizophrenia. A long-acting antipsychotic should be considered during stages 1A, 1B, and 2.
- In Stage 3, **clozapine** monotherapy is recommended.
- For Stage 4, minimal evidence exists for any treatment option for patients who do not have adequate symptom improvement with clozapine. Use of antipsychotic combinations is controversial, as limited evidence supports increased efficacy, despite this practice being somewhat common.
- Predictors of antipsychotic response include prior response to the drug selected, absence of alcohol or drug abuse, acute onset and short duration of illness, later age of onset, affective symptoms, family history of affective illness, medication adherence employment, and good premorbid adjustment. Negative symptoms are generally less responsive to antipsychotic therapy.

TABLE 70-1	Available Antipsychotics and Dosage Ranges			
Generic Name	Trade Name	Starting Dose (mg/day)	Usual Dosage Range (mg/day)	Comments
First-generation antipsychotics				
Chlorpromazine	Thorazine	50–150	300–1000	Most weight gain among FGAs
Fluphenazine	Prolixin	5	5–20	
Haloperidol	Haldol	2–5	2–20	Higher dropout rate in first episode
Loxapine	Loxitane	20	50–150	
Loxapine inhaled	Adasuve	10	10; max 10 mg per 24 hrs	Approved REMS program only
Perphenazine	Trilafon	4–24	16–64	
Thioridazine	Mellaril	50–150	100–800	Significant QTc prolongation
Thiothixene	Navane	4–10	4–50	
Trifluoperazine	Stelazine	2–5	5–40	
Second-generation antipsychotics				
Aripiprazole	Abilify	5–15	15–30	
Asenapine	Saphris	5	10–20	Sublingual only, no food or drink for 10 minutes after administration
Brexpiprazole	Rexulti	1	2–4	
Cariprazine	Vraylar	1.5	1.5–6	Due to long half-life, steady state is not reached for several weeks
Clozapine	Clozaril	25	100–800	Check plasma level before exceeding 600 mg
Iloperidone	Fanapt	1–2	6–24	Care with dosing in CYP2D6 slow metabolizers
Lurasidone	Latuda	20–40	40–120	Take with food, $\geq$350 calories (1460 J)
Olanzapine	Zyprexa	5–10	10–20	Avoid in first episode because of weight gain
Paliperidone	Invega	3–6	3–12	Bioavailability increased when administered with food

(Continued)

			Usual	
		Starting	**Dosage**	
		Dose	**Range**	
Generic Name	**Trade Name**	**(mg/day)**	**(mg/day)**	**Comments**
Quetiapine	Seroquel	50	300–800	
Quetiapine XR	Seroquel XR	300	400–800	
Risperidone	Risperdal	1–2	2–8	
Ziprasidone	Geodon	40	80–160	Take with food, ≥500 calories (2100 J)

TABLE 70-1 Available Antipsychotics and Dosage Ranges (*Continued*)

Note: In first-episode patients, starting dose and target dose should generally be 50% of the usual dose range. See Long-Acting Injectable Antipsychotics in text for dosing of these agents.
REMS, Risk Evaluation and Mitigation Strategy; XR: extended release.

- An initial dysphoric response, (eg, dislike of the medication or feeling worse, combined with anxiety or akathisia) portends a poor drug response, adverse effects, and nonadherence.
- The importance of developing a therapeutic alliance between the patient and the clinician cannot be overemphasized.
- Table 70-3 outlines the relative adverse effect incidence of commonly used antipsychotics, which often follows their binding affinities.
- Anticholinergic side effects, most likely to occur with low-potency FGA, clozapine, and olanzapine, include impaired memory, dry mouth, constipation, tachycardia, blurred vision, inhibition of ejaculation, and urinary retention. Elderly patients are especially sensitive to these side effects.
- Sedation can be reduced if most or the entire antipsychotic daily dose is taken at bedtime.
- Antipsychotics are highly lipophilic, bind highly to membranes and plasma proteins, have large volumes of distribution, and are largely metabolized by cytochrome P450 (CYP) pathways (except ziprasidone). Pharmacogenetics may impact the pharmacokinetics of the antipsychotics.
- Most antipsychotics have elimination half-lives of 24 hours or more, except quetiapine and ziprasidone. Therefore, most can be dosed once daily.
- Antipsychotic pharmacokinetics can be significantly affected by concomitant enzyme inducers or inhibitors. Smoking is a potent inducer of hepatic enzymes and may increase antipsychotic clearance by as much as 50%. Asenapine, an inhibitor of CPY2D6, is the only antipsychotic that significantly affects the pharmacokinetics of other medications. Fluvoxamine, an inhibitor of CYP1A2, increases clozapine serum concentrations by two- to three-fold. Ketoconazole profoundly decreases lurasidone metabolism, and it is recommended that they not be used concomitantly. Carbamazepine reportedly decreases aripiprazole serum concentrations. Reduce the iloperidone dose by 50% when used with CYP2D6 inhibitors such as fluoxetine or paroxetine.

- **Initial Therapy**

- The goals during the first 7 days of treatment are decreased agitation, hostility, anxiety, and aggression and normalization of sleep and eating.
- Titrate the antipsychotic dose over the first few days to an average effective dose in (the middle of the ranges shown in Table 70-1), with the dose for first episode psychosis being half of that used for chronically ill patients. Rapid titration of dose is not recommended. If there is no improvement within 2 weeks at a therapeutic dose, then move to the next treatment stage in Figure 70-1.
- In partial responders who are tolerating the antipsychotic well, it may be reasonable to titrate above the usual dose range for 2–4 weeks with close monitoring.

Schizophrenia should be treated in the context of an interprofessional model that addresses the psychosocial needs of the patient, necessary psychiatric pharmacotherapy, psychiatric co-occurring mental disorders, treatment adherence, and any medical problems the patient may have.

FIGURE 70-1. Pharmacotherapy algorithm for treatment of schizophrenia.

TABLE 70-2 Summary of Available Long-Acting Injectable (LAI) Antipsychotics

Medication Name Parameter		Fluphenazine Decanoate	Haloperidol Decanoate	Risperidone (Risperdal Consta)	Risperidone (PERSERIS)
Dose range (mg)		12.5–100	20–450	12.5–50	90–120
PO Overlap		None	4 weeks (none if loading); use PO dose patient was taking prior to injection	3 weeks after first injection: use PO dose patient was taking prior to injection	None
Recommended maximum dose		100 mg every 2–3 weeks	450 mg every 4 weeks	50 mg every 2 weeks	120 mg
Initiation or loading dose		Can load	Can load	None	None
Time to peak		8–24 hours	4–11 days	4–5 weeks	4–6 hours
T_{ss}		2–3 months	2–3 months	6–8 weeks	60 days
Half-life		14.2 ± 2.2[a] days	21 days	3–6 days	9–11 days
Injection site	Gluteal	Yes	Yes	Yes	Abdominal only
	Deltoid	Yes	Yes	Yes	
Notes			Z-track	Subcutaneous injection	
				A starting dose of 12.5 mg is recommended in patients with hepatic or renal impairment	90 mg = 3 mg PO risperidone 120 mg = 4 mg PO risperidone

[a]Based on multiple-dose data. Single-dose data indicate a β-half-life of 6–10 days.
CrCl, creatine clearance; IM, intramuscular; LAIA, long-acting injectable; PO, oral; T_{ss}, time to steady state.

Paliperidone Palmitate (Invega Sustenna®)	Paliperidone Palmitate (Invega Trinza®) (1MPP)	Olanzapine Pamoate (Zyprexa Relprevv®) (3MPP)	Aripiprazole Monohydrate (Abilify Maintena®)	Aripiprazole (Lauroxil Aristada®)
39–234	273–819	150–405	160–400	441–882
None	None	None	2 weeks PO dose ranges from 10 to 20 mg/day	21 days PO overlap after first injection
234 mg every 4 weeks	819 mg every 3 months	300 mg every 2 weeks or 405 mg every 4 weeks	400 mg monthly	882 mg monthly
Initiation required	None required, dose used depends on last Invega Sustenna dose as follows: if 78 mg give 273 mg; if 117 mg give 410 mg; if 156 mg give 546 mg	Initiation required	None	None required, dose depends on PO dose as follows: If 10 mg/day PO give 441 mg/month IM; If 15 mg/day PO give 662 mg/month IM; If 20 mg PO give 882 mg/month IM
13 days	30–33 days	<1 week	5–7 days	5–6 days
7–11 months	Continues steady-state	3 months	3–4 months	4 months
25–49 days	84–89 days (deltoid) 118–139 days (gluteal)	30 days	29.9–46.5 days	29.2–34.9 days
Yes after 2nd dose	Yes	Yes	Yes	Yes for all dose strengths
Yes	Yes	No	No	Yes, but only 441 mg dose
Avoid use in patients with moderate-to-severe renal impairment (CrCl <50 mL/min [0.83 mL/sec])	Requires at least a 4-month trial with Invega Sustenna. Not recommended in patients with moderate or severe renal impairment (CrCl <50 mL/min [0.83 mL/sec])	Monitor for PDSS subject to REMS	Maintenance dose reduced to 300 mg if patient experiences adverse events. Dose adjustment needed in CYP2D6 slow metabolizers. Avoid use in patients taking CYP 3A4 inhibitors >14 days	May require up to 2 weeks of PO trial to establish tolerability to aripiprazole before initiating LAIA. Avoid use of strong CYP2D6 and 3A4 inhibitors on 662 and 882 mg dose, no adjustment needed for 441 mg dose

TABLE 70-3 Relative Side-Effect Incidence of Commonly Used Antipsychotics[a,b]

	Sedation	EPS	Anticholinergic	Orthostasis	Weight Gain	Prolactin
Aripiprazole	+	+/++[c]	+	+	+	+
Asenapine	+	+/++	±	+	++	+
Brexpiprazole	+	+/++[c]	+	+	+	+
Cariprazine	±	+/++[c]	+	+	+	+
Chlorpromazine	++++	+++	+++	++++	++	+++
Clozapine	+++	+	++++	++++	++++	+
Fluphenazine	+	++++	+	+	+	++++
Haloperidol	+	++++	+	+	+	++++
Iloperidone	+	±	+	+++	++	+
Lurasidone	++	++	+	+	+	+
Olanzapine	++	++	++	++	++++	+
Paliperidone	+	++++	+	++	++	++++
Perphenazine	++	++	++	+	+	++++
Quetiapine	++	+	++	++	++	+
Risperidone	+	++	+	++	++	++++
Thioridazine	+++	+++	+++	+++	+	+++
Thiothixene	+	++++	+	+	+	++++
Ziprasidone	++	++	+	+	+	+

[a]Side effects shown are relative risk based on doses within the recommended therapeutic range.
[b]Individual patient risk varies depending on patient-specific factors.
[c]Primarily akathisia.
EPS, extrapyramidal side effects—include dystonias, pseudoparkinsonism, akathisia, and tardive dyskinesia.
Relative side effect risk: ±, negligible; +, low; ++, moderate; +++, moderately high; ++++, high.

- Intramuscular (IM) antipsychotic administration (eg, aripiprazole 5.25–9.75 mg, ziprasidone 10–20 mg, olanzapine 2.5–10 mg, or haloperidol 2–5 mg) can be used to calm agitated patients. However, this approach does not improve the extent of response, time to remission, or length of hospitalization. IM **lorazepam**, 2 mg, as needed for agitation added to the maintenance antipsychotic is a rational alternative to an injectable antipsychotic. Combining IM lorazepam with olanzapine or clozapine is not recommended because of the risk of hypotension, central nervous system (CNS) depression, and respiratory depression.
- Inhaled **loxapine** powder, FDA-approved for acute agitation associated with schizophrenia or in adults, can be administered only in a healthcare facility and through the FDA-approved Risk Evaluation and Mitigation Strategy (REMS). Use is limited to one 10-mg inhaled dose per 24 hours. Patients with any lung disease associated with bronchospasm (eg, asthma, chronic obstructive pulmonary disease) are excluded. It may offer no advantage over IM and oral products.

Stabilization Therapy

- During weeks 2 and 3, the goal is to improve socialization, self-care, and mood. Dose titration may continue every 1–2 weeks as long as the patient has no side effects.
- If the patient begins to show an adequate response at a particular dose, then continue that dosage as long as symptoms continue to improve. Improvement in formal thought disorder may require an additional 6–8 weeks.

Maintenance Therapy

- The goal of maintenance therapy is relapse prevention; therefore, continue medication for at least 12 months after remission of the first psychotic episode. Many experts recommend treatment for at least 5 years, and lifetime pharmacotherapy at the lowest effective dose is necessary in most patients with schizophrenia.
- In general, when switching from one antipsychotic to another, the first should be tapered and discontinued over at least 1–2 weeks while the second antipsychotic is initiated and tapered upward. Slow titration of antipsychotics (especially FGAs and clozapine) can be done to avoid cholinergic rebound.

Management of Treatment-Resistant Schizophrenia

- Only clozapine has shown superiority over other antipsychotics; however, improvement occurs slowly, with 60% of patients improving if used for up to 6 months.
- Because of the risk of orthostatic hypotension, clozapine is usually titrated more slowly than other antipsychotics. If a 12.5-mg test dose does not produce hypotension, then 25 mg at bedtime is recommended, increased to 25 mg twice daily after 3 days, then increased in 25–50 mg/day increments every 3 days until a dose of at least 300 mg/day is reached.
- A 12-hour postdose clozapine serum concentration of at least 350 ng/mL (1.07 μmol/L) is associated with efficacy. Monitor serum concentrations of clozapine before exceeding 600 mg daily, in patients with unusual or severe adverse effects, in those concomitantly taking potentially interacting medications, in those with age or pathophysiologic changes suggesting altered kinetics, and in those suspected of medication nonadherence.
- Mood stabilizers (eg, **lithium, valproic acid**, and **carbamazepine**) may improve labile affect and agitation in patients with refectory schizophrenia. Selective serotonin reuptake inhibitors (SSRIs) may improve obsessive-compulsive symptoms that worsen or arise during clozapine treatment.
- Combining a FGA and SGA and combining different SGAs have been suggested, but no data support or refute these strategies. If tried, one of the drugs should be discontinued if there is no improvement within 6–12 weeks.

Extrapyramidal Side Effects

Dystonias

- Dystonias are prolonged tonic muscle contractions (occurring usually within 24–96 hours of dosage initiation or dosage increase); they may be life-threatening (eg, pharyngeal–laryngeal dystonias). Other dystonias are trismus, glossospasm, tongue protrusion, blepharospasm, oculogyric crisis, torticollis, and retrocollis. Risk factors include younger (male) patients and use of FGA, high-potency agents, and high dose.
- Treatment includes IM or IV anticholinergics (Table 70-4) or benzodiazepines. **Benztropine** 2 mg, or **diphenhydramine** 50 mg, may be given IM or IV, or **diazepam**, 5–10 mg by slow IV push, or **lorazepam**, 1–2 mg IM, may be given. Relief usually occurs within 15–20 minutes of IM injection or 5 minutes of IV administration.
- Prophylactic anticholinergic medications are reasonable when using high-potency FGAs (eg, haloperidol and fluphenazine) in young men or in patients with a prior dystonia. Risk can be minimized by using lower initial doses or by using an SGA.

Akathisia

- Akathisia occurs in 20%–40% of patients treated with high-potency FGA and consists of subjective complaints (feelings of inner restlessness) and/or objective symptoms (pacing, shifting, shuffling, or tapping feet).
- Reduction in antipsychotic dose is the best intervention but is not always feasible. Switching to an SGA is an option, although akathisia may occur with some SGAs. Aripiprazole, risperidone, quetiapine, and clozapine appear to have the lowest risk. Benzodiazepines should be avoided in patients with a history of substance abuse. **Propranolol** (up to 160 mg/day) is reported to be effective. Emerging literature suggests that agents with antagonist activity at the 5-HT$_2$ receptor (**cyproheptadine**, **mirtazapine**, and **trazodone**) may be protective against akathisia.

Pseudoparkinsonism

- There are four cardinal symptoms
  - ✓ Akinesia, bradykinesia, or decreased motor activity, including mask-like facial expression, micrographia
  - ✓ Tremor, predominantly at rest; decreasing with movement
  - ✓ Cogwheel rigidity; the patient's limbs yield in jerky, ratchet-like fashion when moved passively by the examiner
  - ✓ Stooped, unstable posture and slow, shuffling, or festinating gait
- Possible accessory symptoms include seborrhea, sialorrhea, hyperhidrosis, fatigue, weakness, dysphagia, and dysarthria.
- Risk factors include FGA use (especially in high dose), increasing age, and possibly female gender.
- Symptoms start 1–2 weeks after initiation of antipsychotic therapy or dose increase. Risk with SGAs is low except with risperidone in doses greater than 6 mg/day.
- **Benztropine** has a half-life that allows once- to twice-daily dosing. Typical dosing is 1–2 mg twice daily up to a maximum of 8 mg daily. **Diphenhydramine** produces more sedation (see Table 70-4). All of the anticholinergics have been abused for euphoriant effects. **Amantadine** is as effective as anticholinergics with less effect on memory.
- Attempt to taper and discontinue these agents 6 weeks to 3 months after symptoms resolve.

Tardive Dyskinesia

- Tardive dyskinesia (TD) is characterized by abnormal involuntary movements. The classic presentation is buccolingual-masticatory or orofacial movements that may interfere with chewing, wearing dentures, speech, respiration, or swallowing. Facial movements include frequent blinking, brow arching, grimacing, upward deviation of the eyes, and lip smacking. Restless choreiform and athetotic movements of the limbs

TABLE 70-4	Agents Used to Treat Extrapyramidal Side Effects	
Generic Name	Equivalent Dose (mg)	Daily Dosage Range (mg)
Antimuscarinics		
Benztropine[a]	1	1–8[b]
Biperiden[a]	2	2–8
Trihexyphenidyl	2	2–15
Antihistaminic		
Diphenhydramine[a]	50	50–400
Dopamine agonist		
Amantadine	NA	100–400
Benzodiazepines		
Lorazepam[a]	NA	1–8
Diazepam	NA	2–20
Clonazepam	NA	2–8
β-Blockers		
Propranolol	NA	20–160

[a]Injectable dosage form can be given intramuscularly for relief of acute dystonia.
[b]In treatment-refractory cases, dosage can be titrated to 12 mg/day with careful monitoring; nonlinear pharmacokinetics has been reported.
NA, not applicable.

occur in later stages. Movements may worsen with stress, decrease with sedation, and disappear with sleep.

- Screen at baseline and at least quarterly using the Abnormal Involuntary Movement Scale (AIMS) and the Dyskinesia Identification System Condensed User Scale (DIS-CUS) to detect TD.
- TD prevention includes: (1) use SGAs first-line; (2) biyearly TD screening; and (3) discontinue antipsychotics or switch to SGAs at the earliest symptoms of TD, if possible.
- Risk factors for TD include duration of antipsychotic therapy, higher dose, possibly cumulative dose, possibly female gender, increasing age, occurrence of acute extrapyramidal symptoms, poor antipsychotic response, diagnosis of organic mental disorder, diabetes mellitus, and mood disorders. With FGAs the prevalence of TD ranges from 20%–50%. With SGAs, the risk of TD is ~3.0% per year in nonelderly adults compared to 7.7% per year for FGAs.
- The American Academy of Neurology guideline recommends short-term treatment of TD with **clonazepam** or **ginkgo biloba**.
- **Deutetrabenazine** and **valbenazine** are vesicular monoamine transporter-2 (VMAT2) inhibitors approved for TD treatment in adults. Warnings associated with their use include suicidality, depression, and QT interval prolongation.

Other Antipsychotic Adverse Effects

Seizures

- The highest risk for antipsychotic-induced seizures is with chlorpromazine or clozapine. Seizures are more likely with initiation of treatment, higher doses, and rapid dose increases.

- Dosage reduction should occur for an isolated seizure, and anticonvulsant therapy is usually not recommended.
- If a change in antipsychotic therapy is required, risperidone, thioridazine, haloperidol, pimozide, trifluoperazine, and fluphenazine may be considered.

Thermoregulation

- Poikilothermia, the body temperature adjusting to the ambient temperature, can be a serious side effect of antipsychotic therapy in temperature extremes. Hyperpyrexia, leading to heat stroke, may be dangerous in hot weather or during exercise. Hypothermia is also a risk, especially in older individuals. These problems are more common with the use of low-potency FGAs and can occur with the more anticholinergic SGAs.

Neuroleptic Malignant Syndrome

- Neuroleptic malignant syndrome (NMS) occurs in 0.5%–1% of patients taking FGAs, and can occur with SGAs, including clozapine, but is less frequent.
- Symptoms develop rapidly over 24–72 hours (eg, body temperature exceeding 38°C [100.4°F]), altered level of consciousness, autonomic dysfunction (tachycardia, labile blood pressure, diaphoresis, and tachypnea), and rigidity.
- Myoglobinuria, leukocytosis, increases in creatine kinase (CK), aspartate aminotransferase (AST), alanine aminotransferase (ALT), and lactate dehydrogenase (LDH) are common.
- Discontinue antipsychotics and provide supportive care. Bromocriptine reduces rigidity, fever, and CK levels in up to 94% of patients. Amantadine has been used successfully in up to 63% of patients. **Dantrolene** has been used with favorable effects on temperature, heart rate, respiratory rate, and CK in up to 81% of patients.
- Antipsychotic rechallenge with the lowest effective dose of an SGA or low-potency FGA may be considered only after at least 2 weeks without antipsychotics. Monitor carefully and titrate the dose slowly.

Endocrine Effects

- Antipsychotic-induced prolactin elevations associated with galactorrhea, gynecomastia, decreased libido, and menstrual irregularities are common and are likely with FGAs, risperidone, and paliperidone. Possible management strategies include switching to an agent with lower risk (eg, aripiprazole, asenapine, iloperidone, lurasidone, brexpiprazole, and cariprazine). Dopamine agonists are not recommended due to potential psychosis exacerbation.
- Weight gain with antipsychotic therapy may be most likely with olanzapine, clozapine, risperidone, quetiapine, and iloperidone. Ziprasidone, aripiprazole, asenapine, lurasidone, brexpiprizole, and cariprazine appear to cause minimal weight gain.
- Patients with schizophrenia have a high prevalence of type 2 diabetes, which may be adversely affected by antipsychotics. Olanzapine and clozapine have the highest risk of causing new-onset diabetes, followed by risperidone and quetiapine. The risk with aripiprazole and ziprasidone is likely less than with other SGAs.

Cardiovascular Adverse Effects

- Orthostatic hypotension (defined as >20 mm Hg drop in systolic blood pressure upon standing) is greatest with low-potency FGAs, clozapine, iloperidone, quetiapine, and combination antipsychotics. Patients with diabetes and cardiovascular disease and older patients are predisposed. Dose reduction or changing to an antipsychotic with less α-adrenergic blockade may help, and tolerance may develop within 2–3 months.
- The low-potency piperidine phenothiazines (thioridazine), clozapine, iloperidone, and ziprasidone are the most likely to cause ECG changes, including increased heart rate, flattened T waves, ST-segment depression, and prolongation of QT and PR intervals. Thioridazine prolongs the QTc on average about 20 milliseconds longer

than haloperidol, risperidone, olanzapine, or quetiapine. For thioridazine, the effect is dose related, and the drug's labeling carries a boxed warning for torsades de pointes and sudden death.

- Iloperidone pharmacogenomic metabolism may increase the risk of QTc prolongation in CYP2D6 poor metabolizers. High IV doses of haloperidol also can prolong the QTc, and it also carries a boxed warning.

- Medication discontinuation should occur with QTc prolongation consistently exceeding 500 milliseconds. Torsades rarely happens in the absence of additional risk factors (eg, age greater than 60, female gender, preexisting cardiac or cerebrovascular disease, hepatic impairment, hypokalemia, hypomagnesemia, additional meds that prolong the QTc interval, metabolic inhibition by another medication, or preexisting QTc prolongation).

- In patients older than 50 years, pretreatment ECG and serum potassium and magnesium levels are recommended.

- Myocarditis is an infrequent and dose-independent adverse effect that is most likely to occur with clozapine but has been reported with quetiapine, and possibly with olanzapine. Recommended laboratory monitoring has been proposed with baseline and weekly monitoring of C-reactive protein (CRP) for the first 4 weeks, while troponin (I or T) and B-type natriuretic peptide monitoring has also been suggested. Cardiomyopathy, a potentially life-threatening adverse effect, can also be seen with clozapine, which typically presents later in the course of treatment than myocarditis, with an average time of onset of 14 months. Clozapine rechallenge after myocarditis is debated, and not recommended after cardiomyopathy.

- Those taking FGAs or SGAs have twice the risk of sudden cardiac death than nonusers. Use of antipsychotics was associated with a 1.53-fold increase in ventricular arrhythmia or sudden cardiac death.

- Compared to the general population, the risk of venous thromboembolism (VTE) is twofold higher in individuals with schizophrenia with both FGAs and SGAs associated with this risk. Although the mechanism of this risk is unknown, increased sedative side effects, metabolic side effects, antipsychotic effect on platelet aggregation, and hyperprolactinemia indirectly increasing venous stasis have been proposed.

Lipid Effects

- Some SGAs and phenothiazines cause elevations in serum triglycerides and cholesterol. Olanzapine, clozapine, and quetiapine have the highest risk for dyslipidemia.

- Weight gain, diabetes, and lipid abnormalities during antipsychotic therapy are consistent with development of metabolic syndrome (consisting of raised triglycerides, ≥ 150 mg/dL [1.70 mmol/L]), low high-density lipoprotein cholesterol (≤ 40 mg/dL [1.03 mmol/L] for males, ≤ 50 mg/dL [1.29 mmol/L] for females), elevated fasting glucose (≥ 100 mg/dL [5.6 mmol/L]), blood pressure elevation ($\geq 130/85$ mm Hg), and weight gain (abdominal circumference >102 cm [40 in.] for males, >89 cm [35 in.] for females).

Psychiatric Side Effects

- Aripiprazole has been associated with impulse control disorders such as pathological gambling, uncontrolled sexual urges, uncontrolled spending, binge or compulsive eating, and other intense urges.

Ophthalmologic Effects

- Exacerbation of narrow-angle glaucoma can occur with antipsychotics and/or anticholinergic use.

- Opaque deposits in the cornea and lens may occur with chronic phenothiazine treatment, especially chlorpromazine. Although visual acuity is not usually affected, periodic slit-lamp examinations are recommended with long-term phenothiazine use. Baseline and periodic slit-lamp examinations are also recommended for quetiapine-treated patients because of cataract development in animal studies.

- Thioridazine doses greater than 800 mg daily (the recommended maximum dose) can cause retinitis pigmentosa with permanent visual impairment or blindness.

Genitourinary System

- Urinary hesitancy and retention are common, especially with low-potency FGAs and clozapine, and in men with benign prostatic hyperplasia.
- Urinary incontinence may result from α-blockade, and among the SGAs, it is especially problematic with clozapine.
- Risperidone and paliperidone produce at least as much sexual dysfunction as FGAs, but other SGAs (which have a weaker effect of prolactin) pose less risk. Priapism, a sustained and painful erection that is unprovoked and persists for longer than an hour, is increasingly reported with antipsychotic medication use.

Hematologic System

- Antipsychotics can cause transient leukopenia, but it usually does not progress to clinical significance. Clozapine, chlorpromazine, and olanzapine have the highest risk for neutropenia.
- Agranulocytosis reportedly occurs in 0.01% of patients receiving FGAs, and it may occur more frequently with chlorpromazine and thioridazine. The onset is usually within the first 8 weeks of therapy.
- Agranulocytosis can manifest as sore throat, leukoplakia, erythema, and ulcerated pharynx. Patients with these symptoms taking antipsychotics should have an absolute neutrophil count (ANC). If the ANC is less than 500/μL (0.5×10^9/L), discontinue the antipsychotic with close monitoring for secondary infection.
- The risk of developing neutropenia or agranulocytosis with clozapine is approximately 3% and 0.8%, respectively. Increasing age and female gender increase risk. The greatest risk is between 1 and 6 months of initiating treatment. The baseline ANC must be at least 1500/μL (1.5×10^9/L) in order to start clozapine. Weekly ANC monitoring for the first 6 months is FDA mandated. After this time, if the ANC remains greater than 1500/μL (1.5×10^9/L), ANC monitoring can be decreased to every 2 weeks for the next 6 months. Subsequently, if all ANCs remain greater than 1500/μL (1.5×10^9/L) ANC monitoring can be decreased to monthly. If at any time the ANC drops to less than 500/μL (0.5×10^9/L), clozapine must be discontinued and the ANC monitored daily until it is greater than 1500/μL (1.5×10^9/L). Refer to the product labeling for more detailed information regarding ANC monitoring, including monitoring for mild and moderate leukopenia.

Dermatologic System

- Allergic reactions are rare and usually occur within 8 weeks of initiating therapy. They manifest as maculopapular, erythematous, or pruritic rashes.
- Contact dermatitis, on the skin or oral mucosa, may occur. Swallowing of the FGA oral concentrates quickly may decrease rashes on the oral mucosa.
- Ziprasidone can cause a rare but fatal skin reaction called Drug Reaction with Eosinophilia and Systemic Symptoms (DRESS).
- Both FGAs and SGAs can cause photosensitivity with severe sunburns. Patients should use maximal blocking sunscreens, hats, protective clothing, and sunglasses when in the sun.
- Blue-gray or purplish discoloration of skin exposed to sunlight may occur with higher doses of low-potency phenothiazines (especially chlorpromazine) given long term. This may occur with concurrent corneal or lens pigmentation.

Use in Pregnancy and Lactation

- Haloperidol is the best-studied FGA with approximately 400 reported exposures. A small study found a twofold elevated risk of preterm birth in women with schizophrenia taking FGAs as compared with mothers not taking antipsychotics. Risk of

TABLE 70-5	Antipsychotic Adverse Effects and Monitoring Parameters		
Adverse Reaction	**Monitoring Parameter**	**Frequency**	**Comments**
Adverse effect monitoring parameters for all antipsychotic medications			
Akathisia	Ask about restlessness or anxiety. Observe patient for restlessness. Barnes Akathisia Scale can also be used	Every visit	
Anticholinergic side effects	Ask patient about constipation, blurry vision, urinary retention, or unusual dry mouth	Every visit	
Glucose intolerance	FBS or HbA1c	At baseline, after 3 months, and if normal, then annually	
Hyperlipidemia	Lipid profile	At baseline, after 3 months, and if normal, then annually	
Orthostatic hypotension	Ask patient about dizziness on standing. If present, check BP and HR in sitting and standing positions	Every visit	The degree of orthostatic change in BP to produce symptoms varies. In general, a BP change of 20 mm Hg or more is significant
Hyperprolactinemia	In women, ask about expression of milk from the breast and menstrual irregularities. In men, ask about breast enlargement or expression of milk from nipples. If symptoms present, check serum prolactin level	Every visit	In the absence of symptoms, there is no need to monitor serum prolactin
Sedation	Ask patient about unusual sedation or sleepiness	Every visit	
Sexual dysfunction	Ask patient about decreased sexual desire, difficulty being aroused, or problems with orgasm	Every visit	Patients with schizophrenia have more sexual dysfunction than the normal population. Compare symptoms with medication-free state

(Continued)

TABLE 70-5	Antipsychotic Adverse Effects and Monitoring Parameters (*Continued*)		
Adverse Reaction	**Monitoring Parameter**	**Frequency**	**Comments**
Tardive dyskinesia	Standardized rating scale such as the AIMS or the DISCUS	At baseline, and then every 3 months for FGAs and every 6 months for SGAs	
Weight gain	Measure body weight, BMI, and waist circumference	At baseline, monthly for the first 3 months, and then quarterly	Waist circumference is the single best predictor of cardiac morbidity
Adverse effect monitoring parameters for specific antipsychotics			
Agranulocytosis	White blood cell (WBC) and absolute neutrophil counts (ANC)	At baseline, weekly for 6 months, then every 2 weeks for 6 months, and then monthly	Clozapine only
Sialorrhea or excess drooling	Ask patient about problems with excess drooling, waking in the morning with a wet ring on his or her pillow. Visual observation of the patient for drooling	Every visit	Clozapine only
Bronchospasm, respiratory distress, respiratory depression, respiratory arrest	Before administration, screen patients for a history of asthma, chronic obstructive pulmonary disease, or other lung disease associated with bronchospasm. Monitor patient every 15 minutes for a minimum of 1 hour after drug administration for signs and symptoms of bronchospasm (ie, vital signs and chest auscultation). Only one 10 mg dose can be given every 24 hours	Every dose administration	Inhaled loxapine only. Can only be administered in approved healthcare facilities registered in REMS program

(*Continued*)

TABLE 70-5	Antipsychotic Adverse Effects and Monitoring Parameters (*Continued*)		
Adverse Reaction	**Monitoring Parameter**	**Frequency**	**Comments**
Postinjection sedation/ delirium syndrome	Observe the patient for at least 3 hours after drug administration. Monitor for possible sedation, altered level of consciousness, coma, delirium, confusion, disorientation, agitation, anxiety, or other cognitive impairment	Every dose administration	Long-acting olanzapine pamoate monohydrate only. Can only be administered in approved healthcare facilities registered in REMS program

AIMS, abnormal involuntary movement scale; DISCUS, dyskinesia identification system condensed user scale, FBS, fasting blood sugar; FGA, first-generation antipsychotic; SGA, second-generation antipsychotic.

neonatal EPS is increased with in utero exposure to FGAs, with effects in the infant lasting for 3–12 months after birth.
- All SGAs cross the blood–placental barrier to varying degrees. A meta-analysis found a greater risk of birth defects and preterm births with first trimester exposure to SGA, but no specific abnormality was identified. Other larger studies also suggest that aripiprazole, olanzapine, quetiapine, risperidone, and ziprasidone collectively do not increase the risk of congenital malformations or cardiac malformation. Large, well-controlled studies are needed to clarify the safety of SGAs during pregnancy.
- For all of the FGAs, the overall relative infant doses (RID) obtained through breast-feeding is thought to be less than 10%, which is a common threshold indicating that these medications are safe for use. Olanzapine and quetiapine have reported RIDs of less than 4%. Risperidone and aripiprazole have higher RIDs up to approximately 9%. Breastfeeding while on clozapine is not recommended due to the risk of severe neutropenia and seizures in the infant.

EVALUATION OF THERAPEUTIC OUTCOMES

- Table 70-5 summarizes antipsychotic adverse effects, patient monitoring parameters, and frequency of monitoring parameters.
- The four-item Positive Symptom Rating Scale and the Brief Negative Symptom Assessment are brief enough to be useful in the outpatient setting to measure changes in symptomatology. Patient-rated self-assessments can also be useful, as they engage the patient in treatment and can open the door for patient education and addressing misconceptions. Clinicians should be assertive in attempting to achieve symptom remission.

See Chapter 84, Schizophrenia, authored by M. Lynn Crismon, Tawny Smith, and Peter F. Buckley, for a more detailed discussion of this topic.

- The *Diagnostic and Statistical Manual of Mental Disorders*, 5th ed., category of sleep–wake disorders encompasses insomnia, hypersomnolence, narcolepsy, breathing-related sleep disorders, circadian rhythm sleep–wake disorders, nonrapid eye movement (NREM) sleep arousal disorders, nightmare disorder, rapid eye movement (REM) sleep behavior disorder, restless legs syndrome, and substance/medication-induced sleep disorder.

SLEEP PHYSIOLOGY

- Humans typically have four to six cycles of NREM and REM sleep each night, each cycle lasting 70–120 minutes. Usually, there is progression through the four stages of NREM sleep before the first REM period.
- Stage 1 of NREM is the stage between wakefulness and sleep. Stages 3 and 4 sleep are called *delta sleep* (ie, slow-wave sleep).
- In REM sleep, there is a low-amplitude, mixed-frequency electroencephalogram, increased electrical and metabolic activity, increased cerebral blood flow, muscle atonia, poikilothermia, vivid dreaming, and fluctuations in respiratory and cardiac rate.
- Older individuals have lighter more fragmented sleep with more arousals and gradual reduction in slow-wave sleep.
- REM sleep is turned on by cholinergic cells. Dopamine has an alerting effect. Neurochemicals involved in wakefulness include norepinephrine and acetylcholine in the cortex and histamine and neuropeptides (eg, substance P and corticotropin-releasing factor) in the hypothalamus.
- Polysomnography (PSG) measures multiple electrophysiologic parameters simultaneously during sleep (eg, electroencephalogram, electrooculogram of each eye, electrocardiogram, electromyogram, air thermistors, abdominal and thoracic strain belts, and oxygen saturation) to characterize sleep and diagnose sleep disorders.

Insomnia

CLINICAL PRESENTATION

- Insomnia is subjectively characterized as trouble initiating or maintaining sleep associated with daytime consequences.
- Transient (two or three nights) and short-term (less than 3 months) insomnia is common. Chronic insomnia (more than 3 months duration) occurs in 9%–12% of adults and in up to 20% of older individuals.

DIAGNOSIS

- A complete diagnostic examination should include routine laboratory tests, physical and mental status examinations, as well as ruling out any medication- or substance-related causes.
- Causes of insomnia include stress; jet lag or shift work; pain or other medical problems; mood or anxiety disorders; substance withdrawal; stimulants, steroids, or other medications.

TREATMENT

- <u>Goals of Treatment</u>: Correct the underlying sleep complaint, improve daytime functioning, and avoid adverse drug effects.

TABLE 71-1	Nonpharmacologic Recommendations for Managing Insomnia

Stimulus control procedures

1. Establish regular time to wake up and to go to sleep (including weekends).

2. Sleep only as much as necessary to feel rested.

3. Go to bed only when sleepy. Avoid long periods of wakefulness in bed. Use the bed only for sleep or intimacy; do not read or watch television in bed.

4. Avoid trying to force sleep; if you do not fall asleep within 20–30 minutes, leave the bed and perform a relaxing activity (eg, read, listen to music) until drowsy. Repeat this as often as necessary.

5. Avoid blue spectrum light from television, smart phones, tablets, and other mobile devices.

6. Avoid daytime naps.

7. Schedule worry time during the day. Do not take your troubles to bed.

Sleep hygiene recommendations

1. Exercise routinely (three to four times weekly) but not close to bedtime because this can increase wakefulness.

2. Create a comfortable sleep environment by avoiding temperature extremes, loud noises, and illuminated clocks in the bedroom.

3. Discontinue or reduce the use of alcohol, caffeine, and nicotine.

4. Avoid drinking large quantities of liquids in the evening to prevent nighttime trips to the restroom.

5. Do something relaxing and enjoyable before bedtime.

NONPHARMACOLOGIC THERAPY

- Behavioral and educational interventions that may help include short-term cognitive behavioral therapy, relaxation therapy, stimulus control therapy, cognitive therapy, sleep restriction, paradoxical intention, and sleep hygiene education (**Table 71-1**).
- Management includes identifying the cause of insomnia, educating about sleep hygiene, managing stress, monitoring for mood symptoms, and eliminating unnecessary pharmacotherapy.
- In patients aged 55 years and older, cognitive behavioral therapy may be more effective than pharmacologic therapy at improving certain measures of insomnia.
- Transient and short-term insomnia should be treated with good sleep hygiene and careful use of sedative–hypnotics if necessary. Chronic insomnia calls for careful assessment for a medical cause, nonpharmacologic treatment, and careful use of sedative–hypnotics if necessary (**Figure 71-1**).

PHARMACOLOGIC THERAPY

- Antihistamines (eg, **diphenhydramine, doxylamine**, and **pyrilamine**) are less effective than benzodiazepines, but side effects are usually minimal. Their anticholinergic side effects may be problematic, especially in Older individuals.
- Antidepressants are good alternatives for patients who should not receive benzodiazepines, especially those with depression, pain, or a history of substance abuse.
  - ✓ **Amitriptyline, doxepin**, and **nortriptyline** are effective, but side effects include sedation, anticholinergic effects, adrenergic blockade effects, and cardiac conduction prolongation.
  - ✓ Low-dose doxepin is approved for sleep maintenance insomnia.
  - ✓ Mirtazapine may improve sleep, but may cause daytime sedation and weight gain.

831

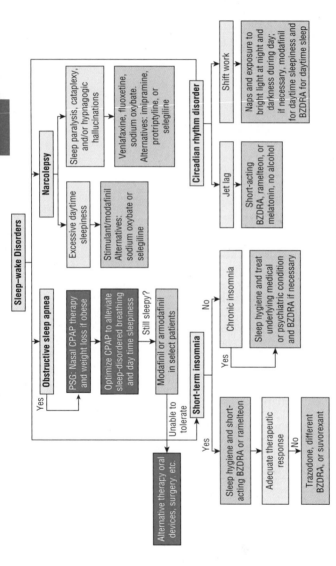

(BZDRA, benzodiazepine receptor agonist; CPAP, continuous positive airway pressure; PSG, Polysomnography.)

FIGURE 71-1. Algorithm for treatment of dyssomnias.

✓ **Trazodone**, 25–100 mg at bedtime, is often used for insomnia induced by selective serotonin reuptake inhibitors or bupropion and in patients prone to substance abuse. Side effects include serotonin syndrome (when used with other serotonergic drugs), oversedation, α-adrenergic blockade, dizziness, and rarely, priapism.

- **Suvorexant** (an orexinA and orexinB antagonist) turns off wake signaling. Doses of 10–20 mg at bedtime are indicated for difficulty initiating or maintaining sleep. Side effects include sedation and rarely narcolepsy-like symptoms. Use caution in patients with depression because suvorexant can worsen depression and trigger suicidal thinking in a dose-dependent manner.
- **Ramelteon** is a melatonin receptor agonist selective for the MT_1 and MT_2 receptors. The dose is 8 mg at bedtime. It is well tolerated, but side effects include headache, dizziness, and somnolence. It is not a controlled substance, and does not cause acute drowsiness similar to other insomnia agents. It is effective for patients with chronic obstructive pulmonary disease and sleep apnea.
- **Valerian**, an herbal product, is available without a prescription. The recommended dose is 300–600 mg. Purity and potency concerns are an issue. It may cause daytime sedation.
- The benzodiazepine receptor agonists (BZDRAs) are the most commonly used drugs for insomnia. They include the newer nonbenzodiazepine γ-aminobutyric acid$_A$ ($GABA_A$) agonists and the traditional benzodiazepines, which also bind to $GABA_A$. The FDA requires labeling regarding anaphylaxis, facial angioedema, complex sleep behaviors (eg, sleep driving, phone calls, and sleep eating).

Benzodiazepine Hypnotics

- The pharmacokinetics and dosing of BZDRAs are summarized in **Table 71-2**.
- Benzodiazepines have sedative, anxiolytic, muscle relaxant, and anticonvulsant properties. They increase stage 2 sleep and decrease REM and delta sleep.
- Overdose fatalities are rare unless benzodiazepines are taken with other central nervous system (CNS) depressants.
- **Triazolam** is distributed quickly because of its high lipophilicity, and it has a short duration of effect. Erythromycin, nefazodone, fluvoxamine, and ketoconazole reduce the clearance of triazolam and increase plasma concentrations.
- The effects of **flurazepam** and **quazepam** are long because of active metabolites and therefore they should not be used as first-line agents.
  - ✓ Side effects include drowsiness, psychomotor incoordination, decreased concentration, cognitive deficits, and anterograde amnesia, which are minimized by using the lowest dose possible.
  - ✓ Tolerance to daytime CNS effects (eg, drowsiness, decreased concentration) may develop in some individuals.
  - ✓ Rebound insomnia is minimized by using the lowest effective dose and tapering the dose upon discontinuation.
  - ✓ Long elimination half-life benzodiazepines are associated with falls and hip fractures; thus, **flurazepam** and **quazepam** should be avoided in older individuals.

Nonbenzodiazepine GABA$_A$ Agonists

- In general, the nonbenzodiazepine hypnotics do not have significant active metabolites, and they are associated with less withdrawal, tolerance, and rebound insomnia than the benzodiazepines.
- **Zolpidem** is comparable in effectiveness to benzodiazepine hypnotics, and it has little effect on sleep stages. Its duration is approximately 6–8 hours. Common side effects are drowsiness, amnesia, dizziness, headache, and gastrointestinal (GI) complaints. It appears to have minimal effects on next-day psychomotor performance. The usual dose is 5 mg in women, older persons, and those with liver impairment, and 5–10 mg in men. Sleep eating has been reported. It should be taken on an empty stomach.
- **Zaleplon** has a rapid onset, a half-life of ~1 hour, and no active metabolites. It decreases time to sleep onset, but does not reduce nighttime awakenings or increase

TABLE 71-2	Pharmacokinetics of Benzodiazepine Receptor Agonists				
Generic Name (Brand Name)	t_{max} (hours)[a]	Half-Life[b] (hours)	Daily Dose Range (mg)	Metabolic Pathway	Clinically Significant Metabolites
Estazolam (ProSom)	2	12–15	1–2	Oxidation	—
Eszopiclone (Lunesta)	1–1.5	6	2–3	Oxidation Demethylation	—
Flurazepam (Dalmane)	1	8	15–30	Oxidation N-dealkylation	Hydroxyethylflurazepam, flurazepam aldehyde N-desalkylflurazepam[c]
Quazepam (Doral)	2	39	7.5–15	Oxidation, N-dealkylation	2-Oxo-quazepam, N-desalkylflurazepam[c]
Temazepam (Restoril)	1.5	10–15	15–30	Conjugation	—
Triazolam (Halcion)	1	2	0.125–0.25	Oxidation	—
Zaleplon (Sonata)	1	1	5–10	Oxidation	—
Zolpidem (Ambien; Intermezzo)	1.6	2–2.6	1.75–10[d]	Oxidation	—

[a]Time to peak plasma concentration.
[b]Half-life of parent drug.
[c]N-desalkylflurazepam, mean half-life 47–100 hours.
[d]Oral and sublingual dosing 5–10 mg; sublingual tablets for middle-of-the night dosing 1.75–3.5 mg (1.75 mg for women, 3.5 mg for men).

the total sleep time. It does not appear to cause next-day psychomotor impairment. The most common side effects are dizziness, headache, and somnolence. The recommended dose is 10 mg (5 mg in older patients).

- **Eszopiclone** has a rapid onset and duration of action of up to 6 hours. The most common adverse effects are somnolence, unpleasant taste, headache, and dry mouth. It may be taken nightly for up to 6 months.

EVALUATION OF THERAPEUTIC OUTCOMES

- Assess patients with short-term or chronic insomnia after 1 week of therapy for drug effectiveness, adverse events, and adherence to nonpharmacologic recommendations. Patients should maintain a daily recording of awakenings, medications taken, naps, and an index of sleep quality.

Obstructive Sleep Apnea

PATHOPHYSIOLOGY

- Obstructive sleep apnea (OSA) is potentially life-threatening and characterized by repeated episodes of nocturnal breathing cessation followed by blood oxygen desaturation. It is caused by occlusion of the upper airway, and blood oxygen (O_2) desaturation can occur. Episodes may be caused by obesity or fixed upper airway lesions, enlarged tonsils, amyloidosis, and hypothyroidism. OSA is associated with motor vehicle accidents, depression, increased cancer risk, stroke, arrhythmias, hypertension, cor pulmonale, and sudden death.
- The apneic episode is terminated by a reflex action in response to the fall in blood O_2 saturation that causes an arousal with resumed breathing.

CLNICAL PRESENTATION AND DIAGNOSIS

- Heavy snoring, severe gas exchange disturbances, respiratory failure, and gasping occur in severe episodes. Patients with OSA usually complain of excessive daytime sleepiness (EDS). Other symptoms are morning headache, poor memory, and irritability.

TREATMENT

- <u>Goals of Treatment</u>: The goal is to alleviate sleep-disordered breathing and prevent complications (**Figure 71-1**).

NONPHARMACOLOGIC THERAPY

- Nonpharmacologic approaches are the treatments of choice (eg, weight loss [for all overweight patients], tonsillectomy, nasal septal repair, and nasal positive airway pressure [PAP], which may be continuous [CPAP] or bilevel). Other surgical therapies, such as uvulopalatopharyngoplasty and tracheostomy, may be necessary in severe cases.
- Management parameters are published by the American Academy of Sleep Medicine. Avoid all CNS depressants and drugs that promote weight gain. Angiotensin-converting enzyme (ACE) inhibitors can also worsen sleep-disordered breathing.

PHARMACOLOGIC THERAPY

- There is no drug therapy for OSA, and medications that worsen sleep should be avoided.
- **Modafinil** and **armodafinil** are approved by the FDA to improve wakefulness in those with residual daytime sleepiness. They should be used only in patients without cardiovascular disease who are using optimal PAP therapy.

EVALUATION OF THERAPEUTIC OUTCOMES

- Assess patients with OSA after 1–3 months of treatment for improvement in alertness, daytime symptoms, weight reduction, and compliance with PAP therapy. Bed partners can report on snoring and gasping.

Narcolepsy

PATHOPHSYIOLOGY

- Narcolepsy type 1 includes symptoms of cataplexy and occurs in 70%–80% of patients. Cataplexy is a sudden bilateral loss of muscle tone with collapse, which can be precipitated by high emotional situation. Narcolepsy type 2 does not include cataplexy.
- Dysfunction of the hypocretin/orexin neurotransmitter system may play a central role in narcolepsy. An autoimmune process may cause destruction of hypocretin-producing cells.

CLINICAL PRESENTATION AND DIAGNOSIS

- Narcolepsy can be diagnosed if the patient goes into REM sleep within 5 minutes of sleep. The narcolepsy tetrad includes EDS, cataplexy, hallucinations, and sleep paralysis. Patients complain of EDS, sleep attacks that last up to 30 minutes, fatigue, impaired performance, and disturbed nighttime sleep.

TREATMENT

- Goals of Treatment: The goal is to maximize alertness during waking hours and improve quality of life (**Figure 71-1**).

NONPHARMACOLOGIC THERAPY

- Provide patient and family education about misconceptions around the individual's behavior.
- Encourage good sleep hygiene and two or more daytime naps daily (as little as 15 minutes).

PHARMACOLOGIC THERAPY

- Pharmacotherapy (**Table 71-3**) focuses on EDS and REM sleep abnormalities.
- **Modafinil**, the standard for treatment of EDS, and **armodafinil** (the active R-isomer) are FDA-approved. They do not treat cataplexy. Evidence suggests no risk of tolerance, withdrawal, or risk of abuse. Side effects include headache, nausea, nervousness, and insomnia.
- **Amphetamines** and **methylphenidate** have a fast onset of effect and durations of 3–4 hours and 6–10 hours, respectively, for EDS. Amphetamines have more risk of abuse and tolerance. Side effects include insomnia, hypertension, palpitations, and irritability.
- Clinicians may prescribe sustained-release stimulants with scheduled administration times, and immediate-release stimulants to be taken as needed when the patient requires alertness (eg, driving, etc.).
- The most common treatments for cataplexy are the tricyclic antidepressants, serotonin norepinephrine reuptake inhibitors, and selective serotonin reuptake inhibitors. **Imipramine, protriptyline, clomipramine, fluoxetine,** and **nortriptyline** are effective in approximately 80% of patients. **Selegiline** improves hypersomnolence and cataplexy.
- **Atomoxetine** may improve cataplexy and sleepiness in children but appears to be less effective than other therapies in adults and older teenagers.
- **Sodium oxybate** (γ-hydroxybutyrate) improves EDS and decreases episodes of sleep paralysis, cataplexy, and hypnagogic hallucinations. Give at bedtime and repeat 2.5–4 hours later. Side effects include nausea, somnolence, confusion, dizziness, and incontinence.

TABLE 71-3 Dosing of Drugs Used to Treat Narcolepsy

Generic Name	Brand Name	Initial Dose (mg)	Usual Dose (mg)	Comments
Agents for excessive daytime somnolence				
Dextroamphetamine	Dexedrine	5–10	5–60	Concurrent use of amphetamines and acidic foods may reduce amphetamine absorption
Dextroamphetamine/ amphetamine salts[a]	Adderall	5–20	5–60	See above
Methamphetamine[b]	Desoxyn	5–15	5–15	See above
Lisdexamfetamine	Vyvanse	20–30	20–70	Prodrug of dextroamphetamine
Methylphenidate	Ritalin	10–40	30–80	May increase bleeding risk with warfarin therapy
Modafinil	Provigil	100–200	200–400	May reduce effectiveness of hormonal contraceptives
Armodafinil	Nuvigil	150	150–250	May reduce effectiveness of hormonal contraceptives
Sodium oxybate[c]	Xyrem	4.5 g/night	4.5–9 g/night	Do not use with other CNS depressants
Agents for cataplexy				
Atomoxetine	Strattera	18–100	40–100	Use lower doses in CYP2D6 poor metabolizers
Fluoxetine	Prozac	10–20	20–80	Cataplexy benefits occur sooner than antidepressant benefits
Imipramine	Tofranil	50–100	50–250	Anticholinergic side effects
Nortriptyline	Aventyl, Pamelor	50–100	50–200	Anticholinergic side effects
Protriptyline	Vivactil	5–10	5–30	
Venlafaxine	Effexor	37.5	37.5–225	May increase blood pressure
Selegiline	Eldepryl	5–10	20–40	Doses less than 10 mg/day do not require dietary tyramine restrictions

[a]Dextroamphetamine sulfate, dextroamphetamine saccharate, amphetamine aspartate, and amphetamine sulfate.
[b]Not available in some states.
[c]Also effective in treating cataplexy.

EVALUATION OF THERAPEUTIC OUTCOMES

- Patients with narcolepsy should keep a diary of frequency and severity of core symptoms. Monitoring parameters include reduction in daytime sleepiness, cataplexy, hypnagogic and hypnopompic hallucinations, and sleep paralysis.
- Assess patients regularly during medication titration, then every 6–12 months for side effects (eg, hypertension, sleep disturbances, and cardiovascular abnormalities).

See Chapter 89, Sleep–Wake Disorders, authored by John M. Dopp and Bradley G. Phillips, for a more detailed discussion of this topic.

CHAPTER 72

Substance Use Disorders: Alcohol, CNS Depressants, Stimulants, Nicotine

Substance use disorder (SUD) is a lifelong illness that consists of intoxication and withdrawal from the substance that may cause euphoria. Because this illness affects brain and behavior, it results in the inability to limit or control the use of legal and illegal substances.

PATHOPHYSIOLOGY

- The true etiology behind SUD is unknown. In general, it is felt that there needs to be a triad of the right patient, with the right genetic risk factors, being exposed to the right medication or substance in order for a SUD to occur.

Central Nervous System Depressants

CLINCAL PRESENTATION

ALCOHOL USE DISORDER

- Table 72-1 relates the effects of **alcohol** to the blood alcohol concentration (BAC).
- Alcohol withdrawal includes (1) a history of cessation or reduction in heavy and prolonged alcohol use and (2) the presence of two or more of the symptoms of alcohol withdrawal.
- There is 14 g of alcohol in 12 oz of beer, 5 oz of wine, or 1.5 oz (one shot) of 80-proof whiskey. This amount will increase the BAC by approximately 20–25 mg/dL (4.3–5.4 mmol/L) in a healthy 70-kg (154-lb) man. Deaths generally occur when BACs are greater than 400–500 mg/dL (87–109 mmol/L).
- Absorption of alcohol begins in the stomach within 5–10 minutes of ingestion. Peak concentrations are usually achieved 30–90 minutes after finishing the last drink.
- Alcohol is metabolized by alcohol dehydrogenase to acetaldehyde, which is metabolized to carbon dioxide and water by aldehyde dehydrogenase. Catalase and the microsomal alcohol oxidase system are also involved.
- Most clinical laboratories report BAC in milligrams per deciliter. In legal cases, results are reported in percentage (grams of alcohol per 100 mL of whole blood). Thus, a BAC of 150 mg/dL = 0.15% = 34 mmol/L.

BENZODIAZEPINES AND OTHER SEDATIVE–HYPNOTIC MISUSE

- Benzodiazepine intoxication is manifested as slurred speech, poor coordination, swaying, drowsiness, hypotension, nystagmus, and confusion.
- Likelihood and severity of withdrawal are a function of dose and duration of exposure. Gradual tapering of dosage is necessary to minimize withdrawal and rebound anxiety.
- Signs and symptoms of benzodiazepine withdrawal are similar to those of alcohol withdrawal, including dizziness, flu-like symptoms, impaired memory and concentration, nausea, vomiting, nightmares, visual disturbances, convulsions, muscle pain, anxiety, agitation, restlessness, confusion, irritability, hallucinations, delirium, seizures, and cardiovascular collapse. Withdrawal from short-acting benzodiazepines (eg, **oxazepam, lorazepam**, and **alprazolam**) has an onset within 12–24 hours of the last dose. **Diazepam, chlordiazepoxide**, and **clorazepate** have elimination half-lives (or active metabolites with elimination half-lives) of 24 to more than 100 hours. Thus, withdrawal may be delayed for up to 7 days after their discontinuation.

TABLE 72-1	Specific Effects of Alcohol Related to Blood Alcohol Concentration	
BAC (%)[a] (mmol/L)	Type of Impairment	Effect(s)
0.0–0.05 (0–12)	Mild	Mild speech/memory/attention/coordination/ balance impairment, relaxation, sleepiness
0.06–0.15 (13–34)	Increased	Impaired speech/memory/attention/ coordination/balance, risk of aggression, significantly impaired driving skills, increased risk of injury to self and others, moderate memory impairment
0.16–0.30 (35–65)	Severe	Impaired speech/memory/attention/ coordination/reaction time, balance significantly impaired, driving skills dangerously impaired, judgment and decision making dangerously impaired, blackouts, vomiting and signs of alcohol poisoning common, loss of consciousness
0.31–0.45 (66–98)	Life-threatening	Loss of consciousness, danger of life-threatening alcohol poisoning, significant risk of death

[a]Grams of ethyl alcohol per 100 mL of whole blood.
BAC, blood alcohol concentration.

- **Flunitrazepam** (Rohypnol) is most commonly ingested orally, frequently in conjunction with alcohol or other drugs. Often called a *date-rape drug*, it has been given to women (without their knowledge) to lower their inhibitions.
- **Zolpidem** is reported to have little liability for physical dependence, but tolerance and withdrawal have been reported.

CARISOPRODOL

- **Carisoprodol** is used for muscle spasms and back pain. **Meprobamate** is one of its metabolites.
- It can cause drowsiness, dizziness, vertigo, ataxia, tremor, irritability, headache, syncope, insomnia, tachycardia, postural hypotension, nausea, agitation, depression, weakness, and confusion.
- Overdose can cause stupor, coma, respiratory depression, and death.

DIAGNOSIS

- The *Diagnostic and Statistical Manual of Mental Disorders*, 5th ed. (*DSM-5*) defines SUD as "problematic pattern of substance use leading to clinically significant impairment or distress as manifested by at least two of eleven criteria occurring in the preceding 12-month period." See Diagnosis section in Chapter 69 for greater detail.
- The CAGE questionnaire or alcohol use disorders identification test (AUDIT) can be used to assess alcohol dependence/abuse.

TREATMENT

- <u>Goals of Treatment</u>: The goals include cessation of use of the drug, termination of drug-seeking behaviors, and return to normal functioning. The goals of treatment of withdrawal include prevention of progression to life-threatening severity, thus enabling comfort and functionality conducive to participation in a treatment program.

NONPHARMACOLOGIC THERAPY

- Treatment of drug dependence or addiction is primarily behavioral. The goal is complete abstinence, and treatment is a lifelong process. Most drug-dependence treatment programs embrace treatment based on the Alcoholics Anonymous approach (ie, a 12-step model).

PHARMACOLOGIC THERAPY

Alcohol Use Disorder

Intoxication

- In treating acute intoxications of central nervous system depressants, support of vital functions is critical.
- When toxicology screens are desired, blood or urine should be collected immediately upon arrival for treatment.

Withdrawal

- Treatment of withdrawal for alcohol is summarized in **Table 72-2**.
- Most clinicians agree that symptom-triggered treatment with benzodiazepines is the standard of care for alcohol detoxification.
- A common approach is the front-loading method using a long-acting benzodiazepine such as **diazepam** 10–20 mg or **chlordiazepoxide** 100 mg, repeated every 1–2 hours until the patient is sedated. The short-acting benzodiazepine lorazepam is also preferred because it can be administered IV, intramuscularly, or orally with predictable results (**Table 72-2**). Address fluid, electrolyte, and vitamin deficiencies as in **Table 72-2**.
- With symptom-triggered therapy, medication is given when the patient has symptoms and the Clinical Institute Withdrawal Assessment–Alcohol, Revised (CIWA-AR) score is ≥8. Various benzodiazepines may be used (**Table 72-2**) depending on patient-specific factors (ie, age and liver function). The patient should be reassessed hourly with continued doses given if the score is ≥8. The assessment timeframe can be extended to every 4–8 hours once the patient appears stable and their CIWA-AR score is <8.
- Alcohol withdrawal seizures do not require anticonvulsant drug treatment unless they progress to status epilepticus. Treat patients with seizures supportively. An increase in the dosage and slowing of the tapering schedule of the benzodiazepine used for detoxification or a single injection of a benzodiazepine may be necessary to prevent further seizure activity.

Dependence

- **Table 72-3** shows dosing and monitoring of drug therapy for alcohol dependence.
- **Disulfiram** deters a patient from drinking by producing an aversive reaction if the patient drinks. It inhibits aldehyde dehydrogenase in the pathway for alcohol metabolism, allowing acetaldehyde to accumulate, resulting in flushing, vomiting, headache, palpitations, tachycardia, fever, and hypotension.
  - ✓ Severe reactions include respiratory depression, arrhythmias, MI, seizures, and death. Inhibition of the enzyme continues for as long as 2 weeks after stopping disulfiram.
  - ✓ Prior to starting disulfiram, obtain baseline liver function tests (LFTs), and repeat at 2 weeks, 3 months, and 6 months, then twice yearly. Wait at least 24 hours after the last drink before starting disulfiram, usually at a dose of 250 mg/day.
- **Naltrexone** reduces craving and the number of drinking days. Do not prescribe it to patients currently dependent on opioids because it can precipitate severe withdrawal syndrome. A depot formulation allows monthly administration in a usual dose of 380 mg intramuscularly.
  - ✓ Naltrexone is hepatotoxic and contraindicated in patients with hepatitis, liver failure, or serum aminotransferase levels greater than five times normal. LFTs should

TABLE 72-2 Dosing and Monitoring of Pharmacologic Agents Used in the Treatment of Alcohol Withdrawal

Drug/Route	Dosage Range Per Day (Unless Otherwise Stated)	Indication	Monitoring	Duration of Dosing	Level of Evidence for Efficacy[a]
Multivitamin oral/IV	1 tablet	Malnutrition	Diet	At least until eating a balanced diet at caloric goal	B3
Thiamine oral/IV	100 mg	Deficiency	CBC, WBC, nystagmus	Empiric ×5 days. More if evidence of deficiency	B2
Crystalloid fluids IV (NS or D5–0.45 NS with 20 mEq [mmol] of KCl per liter)	50–100 mL/hr	Dehydration	Weight, electrolytes urine output, nystagmus if dextrose	Until intake and outputs stabilize and oral intake is adequate	A3
Clonidine oral (Catapres)	0.05–0.3 mg; Consider dose reduction in the elderly	Autonomic tone rebound and hyperactivity, hypertensive urgency	Shaking, tremor, sweating, blood pressure	3 days or less	B2
Clonidine transdermal (Catapres-TTS)	TTS-1 to TTS-3; Consider dose reduction in the elderly	Autonomic tone rebound and hyperactivity	Shaking, tremor, sweating, blood pressure	1 week or less. One patch only	B3
Antipsychotics oral/IV haloperidol (Haldol)	2.5–5 mg every 2–4 hours	Agitation unresponsive to benzodiazepines, hallucinations (tactile, visual, auditory, or otherwise), or delusions	Subjective response plus rating scale (CIWA-Ar or equivalent), ECG	Individual doses as needed	B1
Antipsychotics, atypical Quetiapine (Seroquel) oral	25–200 mg; dosage adjustment is necessary in hepatic impairment	Agitation unresponsive to benzodiazepines, hallucinations, or delusions in patients intolerant of conventional antipsychotics	Subjective response plus rating scale (CIWA-Ar or equivalent)	Individual doses as needed in addition to scheduled antipsychotic	C3
Aripiprazole (Abilify) oral/IV	5–15 mg				

Medication (route)	Dose	Use/Mechanism	Monitoring	Duration/Comments	Strength
Benzodiazepines (BZD)		Tremor, anxiety, diaphoresis, tachypnea, dysphoria, seizures	Subjective response plus CIWA-Ar rating scale or equivalent	Individual doses as needed. Underdosing is more common than overdosing	A2
Lorazepam (Ativan) oral/IV/IM	0.5–8 mg				
Chlordiazepoxide (Librium) oral	25–300 mg				
Diazepam (Valium) oral/IV/IM	5–40 mg				
Oxazepam (Serax) oral	15–30 mg				
Dexmedetomidine (Precedex) IV	0.2 mcg/kg/hr, titrate based on response	Adjunct to BZD for autonomic hyperactivity, sympathetic symptom control	Tremor, blood pressure, heart rate	5 days or less	B2
Phenobarbital (Luminal) oral/IV	30–260 mg	Adjunct to BZD, promotes BZD binding to GABA$_A$ receptor	Sedation, respiratory depression, blood pressure	5 days or less	B2
Alcohol oral		Prevent withdrawal	Subjective signs of withdrawal	Wide variation	C3
Alcohol IV		Prevent withdrawal	Subjective signs of withdrawal	Wide variation	C3

aStrength of recommendations, evidence to support recommendation: A, good; B, moderate; C, poor.

CBC, complete blood count; CIWA-Ar, Clinical Institute Withdrawal Assessment for Alcohol, revised; D5, dextrose 5%; ECG, echocardiogram; KCl, potassium chloride; NS, normal saline; WBC, white blood cell count.

Quality of evidence: (1) evidence from more than one properly randomized controlled trial; (2) evidence from more than one well-designed clinical trial with randomization, from cohort or case-control analytic studies or multiple time series, or dramatic results from uncontrolled experiments; and (3) evidence from opinions of respected authorities, based on clinical experience, descriptive studies, or reports of expert communities.

TABLE 72-3 Dosing and Monitoring of Pharmacologic Agents Used in the Treatment of Alcohol Dependence

Drug	Dosage Range Per Day	Indication	Monitoring	Duration of Dosing	Level of Evidence for Efficacy[a]
Disulfiram (Antabuse)	250–500 mg; use with caution in patients with hepatic disease or insufficiency	Deterrence	Facial flushing, liver enzymes	Indefinite	B2
Acamprosate (Campral)	999–1998 mg and higher (333 mg tablets) Dosage adjustment necessary in renal impairment	Craving	Patient-reported craving, renal function	Indefinite	A1
Naltrexone (ReVia)	50–100 mg; dosage adjustment may be needed in renal and liver impairment	Craving	Patient-reported craving	Indefinite	A1
Naltrexone (Vivitrol)	380 mg intramuscularly once every 4 weeks Risk of hepatotoxicity lower compared to oral formulation due to lack of first pass effect	Craving	Patient-reported craving	Indefinite	B2
Anticonvulsants (eg, lamotrigine [Lamictal], topiramate [Topamax], carbamazepine [Tegretol], valproic acid [Depakote], gabapentin [Neurontin])	Seizure disorder doses	Craving	Patient-reported craving, plasma drug levels	Indefinite	B2
Antidepressants (eg, clomipramine [Anafranil], bupropion [Wellbutrin], doxepin [Sinequan], fluoxetine [Prozac])	Depression doses	Craving, depression, anxiety	Patient-reported craving	Indefinite	B2

[a]Strength of recommendations: A, B, and C, good, moderate, and poor evidence to support recommendation, respectively.
Quality of evidence: (1) evidence from more than one properly randomized controlled trial; (2) evidence from more than one well-designed clinical trial with randomization, from cohort or case-control analytic studies or multiple time series, or dramatic results from uncontrolled experiments; and (3) evidence from opinions of respected authorities, based on clinical experience, descriptive studies, or reports of expert communities.

be done at baseline and 1–3 months after starting therapy, then annually. Use with caution in patients with moderate-to-severe renal impairment.

✓ Side effects include nausea, headache, dizziness, nervousness, insomnia, and somnolence.

- **Acamprosate** is a glutamate modulator that reduces alcohol craving.
  ✓ The most common acamprosate side effect is diarrhea.

Benzodiazepine Misuse and Dependence

Intoxication

- **Flumazenil** can be used for benzodiazepine overdoses and is contraindicated when cyclic antidepressant use is known or suspected because of seizure risk. Use with caution when benzodiazepine physical dependence is suspected, as it may precipitate withdrawal.

Withdrawal

- For benzodiazepine withdrawal, use the same drugs and dosages that are used for alcohol withdrawal (see **Table 72-3**).
- The onset of withdrawal from long-acting benzodiazepines may be up to 7 days after discontinuation of the drug. Initiate treatment at usual doses and maintain this dose for 5 days. Then taper over 5 days. Alprazolam withdrawal may require a more gradual taper of the benzodiazepine used for detoxification.

EVALUATION OF THERAPEUTIC OUTCOMES

ALCOHOL WITHDRAWAL AND DEPENDENCE

- Treating alcohol withdrawal takes precedence over the treatment of alcohol dependence.
- Close monitoring of withdrawal symptoms is essential to avoid progression to severe withdrawal.
- Patient counseling on potential adverse effects of medications used for alcohol dependence, followed by close monitoring and follow-up are necessary to assess therapeutic response and adherence.

BENZODIAZEPINE WITHDRAWAL

- Gradual taper of benzodiazepines should occur over 4–8 weeks and sometimes longer depending on the duration of use.
- Reduce the daily dose 10%–25% every 2 weeks to decrease the risk of severe withdrawal reactions and seizures.
- Minor abstinence symptoms (ie, anxiety, insomnia, irritability, sensitivity to light and sound, and muscle spasms) can remain for several weeks after the acute phase of withdrawal.

Central Nervous System Stimulants

PATHOPHYSIOLOGY

- **Nicotine** is a ganglionic cholinergic-receptor agonist with dose-dependent pharmacologic effects, including stimulation and depression in the central and peripheral nervous systems; respiratory stimulation; skeletal muscle relaxation; catecholamine release by the adrenal medulla; peripheral vasoconstriction; and increased blood pressure, heart rate, cardiac output, and oxygen consumption. Low doses produce increased alertness and improved cognitive functioning. Higher doses stimulate the "reward" center in the brain. Cigarette smoking is the leading cause of preventable morbidity and mortality in the United States. It increases the risks of cardiovascular diseases, lung cancer, other cancers, and nonmalignant respiratory diseases.

- **Cocaine** may be the most behaviorally reinforcing of all drugs. Ten percent of people who begin to use the drug "recreationally" go on to heavy use. Pharmacologically it blocks reuptake of catecholamine neurotransmitters.
  - ✓ The hydrochloride salt of cocaine is inhaled or injected. The high from snorting lasts 15–30 minutes. Smoking cocaine base (crack or rock) is almost instantly absorbed and causes intense euphoria. The high from smoking lasts 5–10 minutes. Tolerance to the "high" develops quickly. The elimination half-life of cocaine is 1 hour.
  - ✓ In the presence of alcohol, cocaine is metabolized to cocaethylene, a longer-acting compound than cocaine with a greater risk for causing death.
- **Methamphetamine** (known as speed, meth, and crank) can be taken orally, rectally, intranasally, by IV injection, and by smoking. Inhalation or IV injection results in an intense rush that lasts a few minutes. Methamphetamine has a longer duration of effect than cocaine. Ephedrine and pseudoephedrine can be extracted from cold and allergy tablets and converted to methamphetamine. In the United States, federal law requires that pseudoephedrine-containing products be kept behind a counter and that identification be shown at the time of purchase.
- **3,4-methylenedioxymethamphetamine (MDMA; Ecstasy or Molly)** is usually taken by mouth as a tablet, capsule, or powder, but it can also be smoked, snorted, or injected; if taken by mouth, effects last 4–6 hours.

CLINICAL PRESENTATION

NICOTINE WITHDRAWAL

- Abrupt cessation of nicotine results in withdrawal symptoms usually within 24 hours, including anxiety, cravings, difficulty concentrating, frustration, irritability, hostility, insomnia, and restlessness.

COCAINE INTOXICATION AND WITHDRAWAL

- Signs and symptoms of cocaine intoxication include agitation, euphoria, loquacity, sweating or chills, nausea, tachycardia, arrhythmias, respiratory depression, mydriasis, altered blood pressure, and seizures. Adverse effects seen with use include ulceration of nasal mucosa and nasal septal collapse.
- Withdrawal symptoms begin within hours of discontinuation and last up to several days. Signs and symptoms of withdrawal include fatigue, sleep disturbances, nightmares, depression, drug craving, changes in appetite, bradyarrhythmias, myocardial infarction (MI), and tremors.

METHAMPHETAMINE

- Intoxication may present as increased wakefulness, increased physical activity, decreased appetite, dental caries, increased respiration, hyperthermia, euphoria, irritability, insomnia, confusion, tremors, anxiety, paranoia, aggressiveness, convulsions, increased heart rate and blood pressure, stroke, and death.
- Individuals in withdrawal may exhibit depression, cognitive impairment, drug craving, dyssomnia, and fatigue, but they are usually not in acute distress. Duration of withdrawal ranges from 2 days to several months. Occurrence of delirium suggests withdrawal from another drug (eg, **alcohol**).

ECSTASY (MDMA) USE

- MDMA stimulates the CNS, causes euphoria and relaxation, and produces a mild hallucinogenic effect. It can cause muscle tension, nausea, impaired memory, impaired attention and reasoning, impaired incidental learning, chills, sweating, panic, anxiety, depression, hallucinations, convulsions, and paranoid thinking. It increases heart rate and blood pressure and destroys serotonin (5-HT)–producing neurons in animals. It is considered to be neurotoxic in humans.

DIAGNOSIS

- See Diagnosis section in Chapter 69 for greater detail.

TREATMENT

- <u>Goals of Treatment</u>: The goals include cessation of use of the drug, termination of drug-seeking behaviors, and return to normal functioning.

NONPHARMACOLOGIC THERAPY

Nicotine Use Disorder

- The Agency for Healthcare Research and Quality (AHRQ) and the United States Preventive Services Task Force (USPSTF) have developed treatment guidelines that use the 5 As (**A**sk about smoking, **A**dvise the person to quit through clear individualized messages, **A**ssess the patient's willingness to quit, **A**ssist in quitting, and **A**rrange follow-up and support).
- The USPSTF statement emphasized counseling sessions and highlighted the goal of reaching at least four in-person sessions.
- Minimal contacts, lasting <3 minutes that include the 5As, are more successful in increasing cessation rates than interventions involving no contact.
- Motivational interviewing with standard care or brief cessation advice improves quit rates modestly.
- Counseling alone can be effective but is further augmented by the addition of pharmacotherapy

Cocaine, Methamphetamine, and MDMA Use

- Active monitoring and management of vital organ function are required for a positive outcome.

PHARMACOLOGIC THERAPY

Nicotine Use Disorder

- First-line pharmacotherapies for smoking cessation include Nicotine Replacement Therapy (NRT), **bupropion sustained release**, and **varenicline**. Combinations of these should be considered if a single agent has failed. Second-line pharmacotherapies include **clonidine** and **nortriptyline** and should be considered if first-line therapy fails.

Nicotine Replacement Therapy

- Dosing and monitoring of pharmacotherapy for smoking cessation are shown in **Table 72-4**. Nicotine replacement therapy increases quit rates by 10%, with five products being available over the counter.
- The 2- and 4-mg gum and lozenge doses are recommended for those who experience time to first cigarette (TTFC) less than 30 minutes and greater than 30 minutes, respectively. The gum should be chewed slowly until a peppery or minty taste emerges and then parked between the cheek and gums to facilitate nicotine absorption. Generally, the gum should be used for up to 12 weeks at no more than 24 pieces per day and no more than 20 lozenges should be used in 1 day for up to 12 weeks. Patients should be given specific dosing and usage instructions for both the gum and lozenges to improve efficacy.
- The patch is available as nonprescription medication which has the highest rate of adherence. Patch use may be combined with as needed gum, lozenge, or nasal spray use. The initial patch dosage should be worn from 4 to 6 weeks, and then the dose should be tapered to the next strength every 2 weeks. A new patch should be placed on a relatively hairless location each morning.
- Nicotine nasal spray requires a prescription. It more than doubles long-term abstinence rates compared to placebo spray. Recommended duration of therapy is 3–6 months.

TABLE 72-4 First-Line Pharmacotherapy Treatment Options for Smoking Cessation

Drug	Dosing	Duration	Comments/Monitoring Parameters
Nicotine replacement therapies (NRTs)			
Nicotine patch	Based on cigarettes smoked per day: >10 cigs/day: Step 1: 21 mg/day: Weeks 1–6 Step 2: 14 mg/day: Weeks 7–8 Step 3: 7 mg/day: Weeks 9–10 <10 cigs/day: Step 2: 14 mg/day: 6 weeks Step 3: 7 mg/day: 2 weeks	10 weeks	Tapering dosing is considered optional after 6 weeks on a dose Patch can be worn for up to 24 hours per day If patient has sleep disturbances, remove patch at night and place one patch in morning (~16 hours per day) If waking up with cravings, patch should be worn for 24 hours Recommended to place patch on determined quit day Place a new patch on each day, hold patch on for 10 seconds to help adherence Rotate patches to avoid skin irritation
Nicotine gum	1st cigarette <30 minutes after waking: 4 mg 1st cigarette >30 minutes after waking: 2 mg Weeks 1–6: 1 piece of gum every 1–2 hours prn Weeks 7–9: 1 piece every 2–4 hours prn Weeks 10–12: 1 piece every 4–8 hours prn Then stop Do not exceed 24 pieces/day	12 weeks	Continuous use can lead to adverse effects (pyrosis, nausea, hiccups) 4 mg strength has shown to be more efficacious in heavy smokers over 6-week time period If patient uses with a cigarette, there is no major risk Counseling on proper use of gum: Repeat process until peppery sensation does not reoccur Use alternate sides of mouth when using chew and park method Park between cheek and gum after a peppery sensation becomes apparent Do not eat or drink 15 minutes before or during use of gum Chew each piece slowly

Lozenge available as Nicorette lozenge or Nicorette mini lozenge	1st cigarette <30 minutes after waking: 4 mg 1st cigarette >30 minutes after waking: 2 mg Weeks 1–6: 1 lozenge by mouth every 1–2 hours prn Weeks 7–9: 1 lozenge by mouth every 2–4 hours prn Weeks 10–12: 1 lozenge by mouth every 4–8 hours prn Then stop Do not exceed 20 lozenges/day	12 weeks	Counseling points: Do not eat or drink anything 15 minutes prior to or during lozenge use Allow the lozenge to dissolve slowly, approximately 20–30 minutes Nicotine release could create a tingling or warm sensation Do not chew or swallow the lozenge Periodically rotate the lozenge to different areas of the mouth
Nicotine oral inhaler + cartridge plus mouthpiece (Nicotrol*)	24–64 mg (6–16 cartridges) per day 1. Stop smoking completely before use 2. Use device by frequent continuous puffing (20 minutes) and use as needed (dosing is very individualized) based on nicotine needed 3. Recommended duration of treatment is 3 months 4. Gradual daily dose taper over 6–12 weeks	3–6 months	Patients should stop smoking prior to starting this product Most successful patients in trials; use ranged from 6 to 16 cartridges per day, 20 minutes continuous puffing Recommended duration of treatment: 3 months with subsequent weaning with gradual reduction over 6–12 weeks Treatment longer than 6 months has not been studied Precautions; patients with asthma, chronic pulmonary disease, history of recent myocardial infarction, serious arrhythmias, or worsening angina Pregnancy Category D
Nicotine metered nasal spray (Nicotrol NS*)	One spray (0.5 mg nicotine/spray) into each nostril one to two times each hour when craving cigarette Max. dose: 10 sprays per hour (max. of 80 sprays per day)	3 months	Two sprays is considered 1 dose Treatment duration is 3 months; safety beyond 6 months has not been studied Counseling: Breathe normally while administering spray, do not sniff or inhale deeply while administering spray For best results, use at least 16 sprays per day which has been found as the minimum effective dose

(Continued)

TABLE 72-4 First-Line Pharmacotherapy Treatment Options for Smoking Cessation (Continued)

Drug	Dosing	Duration	Comments/Monitoring Parameters
Non-nicotine replacement options			
Bupropion (Zyban)	150 mg by mouth daily × 3 days then 150 mg by mouth bid (dosing interval should be >8 hours)	3–6 months	Do not exceed 300 mg/day Recommend initiating therapy 1–2 weeks prior to set "quit" day Black box warning for neuropsychiatric warning and suicide warnings removed in 2016; downgraded to warning Pregnancy Category: C, excreted into breastmilk Monitor patients with renal/hepatic impairment Neuropsychiatric adverse events: black box warning removed in December 2016, warning remains Counseling points: might cause dry mouth, could cause insomnia
Varenicline (Chantix)	Start with dose titration: Days 1–3: 0.5 mg by mouth once daily Days 3–7: 0.5 mg by mouth twice daily Week 2 until end of treatment: 1 mg by mouth twice daily	3–6 months	Recommended to begin varenicline 1 week prior to quit day Maintenance up to 6 months of therapy is approved Renal impairment dosing for CrCl ≤30 mL/min (0.5 mL/sec) No dosing adjustment needed in hepatic impairment If patient has difficulty with cessation, recommend taper smoking by 50% each month with a goal of smoking abstinence in 12 weeks, continue varenicline for another 12 weeks for a full 24 week therapy Neuropsychiatric adverse events: black box warning removed in December 2016, warning remains Most common side effects: nausea, sleep problems, constipation, gas, vomiting Patients with intolerable insomnia might improve with lower doses

- Nicotine oral inhaler consists of a mouthpiece and plastic cartridge that is placed into the inhaler and delivers 4–10 mg of nicotine through vapor inhalation. Patients should actively puff on the inhaler for 5 minutes, adjusting use based on effect, as the cartridge can be used for up to 20 minutes of active puffing. The initial dosing is 6–16 cartridges/day for up to 12 weeks. A taper should be initiated after 6 weeks.
- NRT products have few side effects. Nausea and light-headedness may indicate nicotine overdose. Rotate the patch site to minimize skin irritation. Sleep disturbances are reported in 23% of patients using the patch. Eating or drinking anything except water should be avoided for 15 minutes before and during administration of the lozenge and gum. Long-term NRT may be needed in some patients.
- Electronic nicotine delivery systems (ENDS, or e-cigarettes) usage is controversial and continued research is needed to evaluate their efficacy and safety.

Bupropion and Varenicline

- Bupropion sustained release (SR) inhibits neuronal reuptake, and potentiates the effects of norepinephrine and dopamine. Its use is contraindicated in patients with current or past seizure disorder, current or prior diagnosis of bulimia or anorexia nervosa, and use of a monoamine oxidase inhibitor within the last 14 days. Concurrent use of medications that lower the seizure threshold is a concern.
  - ✓ Side effects of bupropion may include neuropsychiatric symptoms (in adults and pediatric patients), including depression, anxiety, agitation, hostility, suicidal thoughts/behavior, and attempted suicide.
- Varenicline is a partial agonist that binds selectively to nicotinic acetylcholine receptors with a greater affinity than nicotine, producing a lesser response than nicotine. It is also FDA-approved for 6 months of maintenance therapy. It may result in a higher rate of cessation than bupropion and single forms of NRT. It may be equally effective with combination NRT.
  - ✓ Side effects of varenicline may include suicidal thoughts and erratic and aggressive behavior. Screen patients for psychiatric illness or behavior change after starting varenicline. It may also be associated with a small increased risk of cardiovascular events.

Other Therapies

- **Clonidine** is an effective smoking-cessation treatment in doses varying from 0.15 to 0.75 mg/day orally and from 0.1 to 0.2 mg/day transdermally.
  - ✓ The most common clonidine side effects include dry mouth, dizziness, hypotension, sedation, and constipation. Monitor blood pressure. Abrupt discontinuation may result in nervousness, agitation, headache, tremor, and elevation in blood pressure.
- **Nortriptyline** is initiated 10–28 days before the quit date. The dose is initiated at 25 mg/day, gradually increasing to 75–100 mg/day. In trials, treatment duration was commonly 12 weeks.
  - ✓ Common side effects include sedation, dry mouth, blurred vision, urinary retention, tremor, and light-headedness.

Cocaine, Methamphetamine, and MDMA Use

Intoxication

- No antidotes or targeted therapies are available for these agents. When toxicology screens are desired, blood or urine should be collected immediately upon arrival for treatment.
- Treat pharmacologically only if the patient is agitated or psychotic. Injectable lorazepam 2–4 mg IM every 30 minutes to 6 hours can be used for agitation. Low-dose antipsychotics can be used short term for psychosis. Treat seizures supportively, but IV lorazepam or diazepam can be used for status epilepticus.

EVALUATION OF THERAPEUTIC OUTCOMES

NICOTINE USE DISORDER

- Tobacco cessation is a process that could take an extended period of time with extensive education and continual monitoring being vital to this process.
- The most effective treatment strategy for smoking cessation is a combination of behavioral and pharmacological treatment and frequent monitoring of both early on in the process is recommended.
- Patient counseling is vital to ensure maximum efficacy. Frequent reassessment should occur to evaluate breakthrough cravings, withdrawal symptoms, and relapses. Patients should be asked to immediately report any adverse effects to ensure adherence and prevent relapse.

COCAINE, METHAMPHETAMINE, AND MDMA USE

- When considering therapeutic outcomes, each treatment must be evaluated to determine efficacy and safety. Ongoing psychosocial and educational support is important to maximize outcomes.

Other Drugs of Abuse

PATHOPHYSIOLOGY

- **Catha edulis (Khat)** is a shrub native to the horn of Africa that when chewed produces stimulating effects. The psychoactive properties of this plant are due to several alkaloids including cathine and cathinone (thus the name cathinones). The pharmacology of the various cathinones and related drugs is not well studied. **Bath salts** (schedule I controlled substances) are synthetic, sympathomimetic, designer drugs that can cause intoxication, dependence, and death. **Flakka** is a new very potent cathinone that has become very popular in some counties in Florida.
- **Marijuana** (known as reefer, pot, grass, and weed) is a commonly used drug. Federally this drug continues to be illegal, although many states have passed laws allowing use. The active compounds within marijuana include the principal psychoactive component Δ^9-tetrahydrocannabinol **(THC)** and **cannabidiol** (CBD), which does not have psychoactive effects. Marijuana is most commonly smoked, but it can be orally ingested. After inhalation, the pharmacologic effects can be seen in about 10 minutes. Both THC and CBD are poorly bioavailable; therefore, peak concentrations occur in about 2 hours after ingestion. The single use terminal half-life of 24 hours is significantly elongated with chronic use due to accumulation and redistribution from fatty tissues. In chronic users, THC is detectable on toxicologic screening for up to 4–5 weeks after cessation of use
- Over 100 compounds are cannabinoid receptor agonists called **synthetic marijuana** (spice, K2, dream, red X dawn, and others). The product is inert dry plant material sprayed with these compounds.
- **Lysergic acid diethylamide (LSD)** can cause either agonist or antagonist effects on 5-HT activity. It is sold as tablets, capsules, a liquid, and on squares of decorated paper.
- Organic solvents inhaled by abusers include **gasoline, glue, aerosols, amyl nitrite, butyl nitrite, typewriter correction fluid, lighter fluid, cleaning fluids, paint products, nail polish remover, waxes,** and **varnishes.** Chemicals in these products include **nitrous oxide, toluene, benzene, methanol, methylene chloride, acetone, methylethyl ketone, methylbutyl ketone, trichloroethylene,** and **trichloroethane.**

CLINICAL PRESENTATION

SYNTHETIC CATHINONES (BATH SALTS) USE

- In addition to the stimulant effects of bath salts adverse effects include tachycardia, hypertension, diabetic ketoacidosis, paranoid psychosis, hyperthermia, agitation, headache, hyponatremia, and suicide.

MARIJUANA USE

- Initial effects of marijuana use include increased heart rate, dilated bronchial passages, and bloodshot eyes. Subsequent effects include euphoria, dry mouth, hunger, tremor, sleepiness, anxiety, fear, distrust, panic, incoordination, poor recall, amotivation, and toxic psychosis. Other physiologic effects include sedation, difficulty in performing complex tasks, and disinhibition. Endocrine effects include amenorrhea, decreased testosterone production, and inhibition of spermatogenesis. Recent findings suggest a neurotoxic effect on the adolescent brain.
- Cannabis use impairs driving performance, and is associated with increased risk of motor vehicle crashes.
- After abrupt discontinuation, heavy users may have a withdrawal syndrome characterized by irritability, anger, aggression, anxiety, depressed mood, restlessness, sleep difficulty, decreased appetite, or weight loss.
- Cannabinoid hyperemesis syndrome (CHS) is a syndrome of cyclical vomiting in habitual users that abates after discontinuation of cannabis.

SYNTHETIC CANNABINOID USE

- Toxic symptoms are similar to the effects of marijuana plus sympathomimetic effects, including agitation, anxiety, tachycardia, hypertension, nausea and vomiting, muscle spasms, seizures, tremors, paranoid behavior, nonresponsiveness, diaphoresis, hallucinations, and suicidal thoughts and behaviors.

LYSERGIC ACID DIETHYLAMIDE USE

- Signs and symptoms of LSD intoxication include mydriasis, tachycardia, diaphoresis, palpitations, blurred vision, tremor, incoordination, dizziness, weakness, and drowsiness; psychiatric signs and symptoms include perceptual intensification, depersonalization, derealization, illusions, psychosis, synesthesia, and flashbacks. It produces tolerance but is not addictive. There is no withdrawal syndrome.

INHALANT USE

- Physiologic effects include CNS depression, headache, nausea, anxiety, hallucinations, and delusions. With chronic use, the drugs are toxic to virtually all organ systems. Death may occur from arrhythmias or suffocation by plastic bags.

DIAGNOSIS

- See Diagnosis section in Chapter 69 for greater detail.

TREATMENT

- <u>Goals of Treatment</u>: The goals include cessation of use of the drug, termination of drug-seeking behaviors, and return to normal functioning.

NONPHARMACOLOGIC THERAPY

- Treatment for all most often centers on psychosocial interventions and supportive care.
- For marijuana use, nonpharmacologic therapy includes cognitive behavioral therapy (CBT), motivational enhancement therapy (MET), or a combination, which is synergistic.

PHARMACOLOGIC THERAPY

- Many patients with hallucinogen intoxication respond to reassurance.
- No antidotes or targeted therapies are available for these agents. When toxicology screens are desired, blood or urine should be collected immediately upon arrival for treatment.
- Treat pharmacologically only if the patient is agitated or psychotic. Injectable **lorazepam** 2–4 mg IM every 30 minutes to 6 hours can be used for agitation. Low-dose antipsychotics can be used short term for psychosis. Treat seizures supportively, but IV lorazepam or **diazepam** can be used for status epilepticus.

EVALUATION OF THERAPEUTIC OUTCOMES

- When considering therapeutic outcomes, each treatment must be evaluated to determine efficacy and safety. Ongoing psychosocial and educational support is important to maximize outcomes.

See Chapter 82, Substance-Related Disorders I: Overview and Depressants, Stimulants, and Hallucinogens and Chapter 83, Substance-Related Disorders II: Alcohol, Nicotine, and Caffeine, authored by Robin Moorman Li, Patrick Leffers, and Paul L. Doering, for a more detailed discussion of the topic.

CHAPTER

73 Acid–Base Disorders

- *Acid–base disorders* are caused by disturbances in hydrogen ion (H^+) homeostasis, which is ordinarily maintained by extracellular buffering, renal regulation of hydrogen ion and bicarbonate excretion, and ventilatory regulation of carbon dioxide (CO_2) elimination.

GENERAL PRINCIPLES

- Buffering refers to the ability of a solution to resist change in pH after the addition of a strong acid or base. The body's principal extracellular buffer system is the carbonic acid/bicarbonate (H_2CO_3/HCO_3^-) system.
- Most of the body's acid production is in the form of CO_2 and is produced from catabolism of carbohydrates, proteins, and lipids.
- There are four primary types of acid–base disturbances, which can occur independently or together as a compensatory response.
- Metabolic acid–base disorders are caused by changes in plasma bicarbonate concentration (HCO_3^-). Metabolic acidosis is characterized by decreased HCO_3^-, and metabolic alkalosis is characterized by increased HCO_3^-.
- Respiratory acid–base disorders are caused by altered alveolar ventilation, producing changes in arterial carbon dioxide tension ($PaCO_2$). Respiratory acidosis is characterized by increased $PaCO_2$, whereas respiratory alkalosis is characterized by decreased $PaCO_2$.

DIAGNOSIS

- Blood gases (**Table 73-1**), serum electrolytes, medical history, and clinical condition are the primary tools for determining the cause of acid–base disorders and for designing therapy.
- Arterial blood gases (ABGs) are measured to determine oxygenation and acid–base status (**Figure 73-1**). Low pH values (<7.35) indicate acidemia, whereas high values (>7.45) indicate alkalemia. The $PaCO_2$ value helps determine whether there is a primary respiratory abnormality, whereas the HCO_3^- concentration helps determine whether there is a primary metabolic abnormality. Steps in acid–base diagnosis and interpretation based on observed compensatory responses are described in **Tables 73-2** and **73-3**, respectively.

Metabolic Acidosis

PATHOPHYSIOLOGY

- Metabolic acidosis is characterized by a decrease in pH as a result of a primary decrease in serum HCO_3^- concentration, which can result from the buffering of an exogenous acid (consumption of HCO_3^-), accumulation of an organic acid because of a metabolic disturbance (eg, lactic acid and ketoacids), loss of bicarbonate-rich body fluids (eg, diarrhea, biliary drainage, or pancreatic fistula), or progressive accumulation of endogenous acids secondary to impaired kidney function (eg, phosphates and sulfates). Rapid administration of non–alkali-containing IV fluids can cause dilutional acidosis.

TABLE 73-1 Normal Blood Gas Values

	Arterial Blood	Mixed Venous Blood
pH	7.40 (7.35–7.45)	7.38 (7.33–7.43)
PO_2	80–100 mm Hg (10.6–13.3 kPa)	35–40 mm Hg (4.7–5.3 kPa)
SaO_2	95% (0.95)	70–75% (0.70–0.75)
PCO_2	35–45 mm Hg (4.7–6.0 kPa)	45–51 mm Hg (6.0–6.8 kPa)
HCO_3^-	22–26 mEq/L (mmol/L)	24–28 mEq/L (mmol/L)

HCO_3^-, bicarbonate; PCO_2, partial pressure of carbon dioxide; PO_2, partial pressure of oxygen; SaO_2, saturation of arterial oxygen.

TABLE 73-2 Steps in Acid–Base Diagnosis

1. Obtain ABGs and electrolytes simultaneously
2. Compare $[HCO_3^-]$ on ABG and electrolytes to verify accuracy
3. Calculate SAG
4. Is acidemia (pH <7.35) or alkalemia (pH >7.45) present?
5. Is the primary abnormality respiratory (alteration in $PaCO_2$) or metabolic (alteration in HCO_3^-)?
6. Estimate compensatory response (Table 73-3)
7. Compare change in $[Cl^-]$ with change in $[Na^+]$

ABG, arterial blood gases; $[Cl^-]$, chloride ion concentration; $[HCO_3^-]$, bicarbonate concentration; $[Na^+]$, sodium ion concentration; $PaCO_2$, partial pressure of carbon dioxide from arterial blood; SAG, serum anion gap.

- Serum anion gap (SAG) can be used to infer whether an organic or mineral acidosis is present. SAG is calculated as follows:

$$SAG = [Na^+] - [Cl^-] - [HCO_3^-]$$

The normal anion gap is approximately 9 mEq/L (mmol/L), with a range of 3–11 mEq/L (mmol/L). SAG is a relative rather than an absolute indication of the cause of metabolic acidosis.

CLINICAL PRESENTATION

- Chronic metabolic acidosis is relatively asymptomatic; major manifestations are bone demineralization with the development of rickets in children and osteomalacia and osteopenia in adults.
- Acute severe metabolic acidemia (pH <7.2) involves the cardiovascular, respiratory, and central nervous systems. Hyperventilation is often the first sign of metabolic acidosis. Respiratory compensation may occur as Kussmaul respirations (ie, deep, rapid respirations characteristic of diabetic ketoacidosis).
- The compensatory response for metabolic acidosis is to increase CO_2 excretion by increasing the respiratory rate.

TREATMENT

- The primary treatment is to correct the underlying disorder. Additional treatment depends on the severity and onset of acidosis.
- Manage asymptomatic patients with mild to moderate acidemia (HCO_3^- 12–20 mEq/L [mmol/L]; pH 7.2–7.4) with gradual correction of the acidemia over days to weeks using oral **sodium bicarbonate** or other alkali preparations (**Table 73-4**).

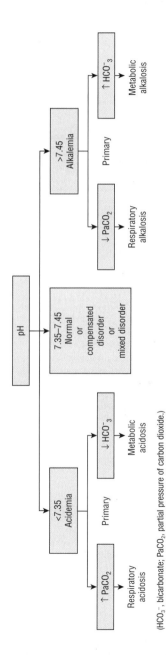

(HCO$_3^-$, bicarbonate; PaCO$_2$, partial pressure of carbon dioxide.)

FIGURE 73-1. Analysis of arterial blood gases.

TABLE 73-3	Guidelines for Interpretation of Acid–Base Disorders Based on Compensatory Responses
Acidosis	**Compensation**
Metabolic	$PaCO_2$ (in mm Hg) should decrease by 1.3 times the fall in plasma $[HCO_3^-]$ (in mEq/L or mmol/L)
Acute respiratory	The plasma $[HCO_3^-]$ should increase by 0.1 times the increase in $PaCO_2 \pm 3$ (in mm Hg)
Chronic respiratory	The plasma $[HCO_3^-]$ should increase by 0.35 times the increase in $PaCO_2 \pm 4$ (in mm Hg)
Alkalosis	**Compensation**
Metabolic	$PaCO_2$ (in mm Hg) should increase by 0.4–0.6 times the rise in plasma $[HCO_3^-]$ (in mEq/L or mmol/L)
Acute respiratory	The plasma $[HCO_3^-]$ should decrease by 0.2 times the decrease in $PaCO_2$ (in mm Hg), but usually not to <18 mEq/L (mmol/L)
Chronic respiratory	The plasma $[HCO_3^-]$ should fall by 0.35 times the decrease in $PaCO_2$ (in mm Hg), but usually not to <14 mEq/L (mmol/L)

$[HCO_3^-]$, bicarbonate concentration; $PaCO_2$, partial pressure of carbon dioxide from arterial blood; multiply values expressed in kPa by 7.519 to convert to mm Hg.

- The dose of bicarbonate can be calculated as follows:

$$\text{Loading dose (mEq or mmol/L)} = (V_d \ HCO_3^- \times \text{body weight}) \times$$
$$(\text{desired } [HCO_3^-] - \text{current } [HCO_3^-],$$

where $V_d \ HCO_3^-$ is the volume of distribution of HCO_3^- (0.5 L/kg).
- Intravenous alkali therapy can be used to treat patients with acute severe metabolic acidosis due to hyperchloremic acidosis, but its role is controversial in patients with lactic acidosis. Therapeutic options include **sodium bicarbonate** and historically, tromethamine, which is no longer available in the United States.
- Sodium bicarbonate is recommended to raise arterial pH to 7.2. However, an open-label, multicenter, controlled trial found that sodium bicarbonate administration did not reduce mortality at 28 days compared with no sodium bicarbonate administration. If IV sodium bicarbonate is administered, the goal is to increase, not normalize, pH to 7.2 and HCO_3^- to 8–10 mEq/L (mmol/L).

Metabolic Alkalosis

PATHOPHYSIOLOGY

- Metabolic alkalosis is *initiated* by increased pH and HCO_3^-, which can result from loss of hydrogen ions via the gastrointestinal (GI) tract (eg, nasogastric suctioning, vomiting) or kidneys (eg, diuretics, Cushing syndrome) or from gain of bicarbonate (eg, administration of bicarbonate, acetate, lactate, or citrate).
- Metabolic alkalosis is *maintained* by abnormal renal function that prevents the kidneys from excreting excess bicarbonate.

TABLE 73-4 Therapeutic Alternatives for Oral Alkali Replacement

Generic Name	Trade Name(s)	Milliequivalents of Alkali	Dosage Form(s)	Comment
Shohl's solution (sodium citrate/citric acid)	Bicitra (Willen)	1 mEq Na/mL; equivalent to 1 mEq bicarbonate	Solution (500 mg Na citrate, 334 mg citric acid/5 mL)	Citrate preparations increase absorption of aluminum
Sodium bicarbonate	Various (eg, Sodamint)	3.9 mEq bicarbonate/tablet (325 mg)	325 mg tablet	Bicarbonate preparations can cause bloating because of CO_2 production
		7.8 mEq bicarbonate/tablet (650 mg)	650 mg tablet	
	Baking soda (various)	60 mEq bicarbonate/tsp (5 g/tsp)	Powder	
Potassium citrate	Urocit-K (Mission)	5 mEq citrate/tablet	5 mEq tablet	Citrate preparations increase absorption of aluminum
Potassium bicarbonate/potassium citrate	K-Lyte (Bristol)	25 mEq bicarbonate/tablet	25 mEq tablet (effervescent)	Citrate preparations increase absorption of aluminum, while bicarbonate preparations can cause bloating
	K-Lyte DS (Bristol)	50 mEq bicarbonate/tablet (double strength)	50 mEq tablet (effervescent)	
Potassium citrate/citric acid	Polycitra-K (Willen)	2 mEq K/mL; equivalent to 2 mEq bicarbonate	Solution (1,100 mg K citrate, 334 mg citric acid/5 mL)	Citrate preparations increase absorption of aluminum
		30 mEq bicarbonate/unit dose packet	Crystals for reconstitution (3,300 mg K citrate, 1,002 mg citric acid/unit dose packet)	
Sodium citrate/potassium citrate/citric acid	Polycitra (Willen) Polycitra-LC (Willen)	1 mEq K, 1 mEq Na/mL; equivalent to 2 mEq bicarbonate	Syrup (Polycitra); solution (Polycitra-LC) (both contain 550 mg K citrate, 500 mg Na citrate, 334 mg citric acid/5 mL)	Citrate preparations increase absorption of aluminum

CLINICAL PRESENTATION

- No unique signs or symptoms are associated with mild to moderate metabolic alkalosis. Some patients complain of symptoms related to the underlying disorder (eg, muscle weakness with hypokalemia or postural dizziness with volume depletion) or have a history of vomiting, gastric drainage, or diuretic use.
- Severe alkalemia (pH >7.60) can be associated with cardiac arrhythmias and neuromuscular irritability.
- The compensatory response to metabolic alkalosis is respiratory, manifested as hypoventilation which increases $PaCO_2$.

TREATMENT

- Treatment is aimed at correcting the factor(s) responsible for maintaining the alkalosis and depends on whether the disorder is sodium chloride responsive or resistant (**Figure 73-2**).

Respiratory Alkalosis

PATHOPHYSIOLOGY

- Respiratory alkalosis is characterized by a decrease in $PaCO_2$ that leads to an increase in pH.
- $PaCO_2$ decreases when ventilatory CO_2 excretion exceeds metabolic CO_2 production, usually because of hyperventilation.
- Causes include increases in neurochemical stimulation via central or peripheral mechanisms, or physical increases in ventilation via voluntary or artificial means (eg, mechanical ventilation).

CLINICAL PRESENTATION

- Although usually asymptomatic, respiratory alkalosis can cause adverse neuromuscular, cardiovascular, and GI effects.
- Light-headedness, confusion, decreased intellectual functioning, syncope, and seizures can be caused by decreased cerebral blood flow.
- Nausea and vomiting can occur, probably due to cerebral hypoxia.
- Cardiac arrhythmias can occur in severe respiratory alkalosis.
- Serum electrolytes can be altered; serum chloride is usually increased; serum potassium, phosphorus, and ionized calcium are usually decreased.
- The initial compensatory response is to chemically buffer excess bicarbonate by releasing hydrogen ions from intracellular proteins, phosphates, and hemoglobin. If prolonged (>6 hours), the kidneys attempt to further compensate by increasing bicarbonate elimination.

TREATMENT

- Treatment is often unnecessary because most patients have few symptoms and only mild pH alterations (ie, pH not exceeding 7.50).
- Direct measures (eg, treatment of pain, hypovolemia, fever, infection, or salicylate overdose) can be effective. A rebreathing device (eg, paper bag) can help control hyperventilation in patients with anxiety/hyperventilation syndrome.
- Correct respiratory alkalosis associated with mechanical ventilation by decreasing the number of mechanical breaths per minute, using a capnograph and spirometer to adjust ventilator settings more precisely, or increasing dead space in the ventilator circuit.

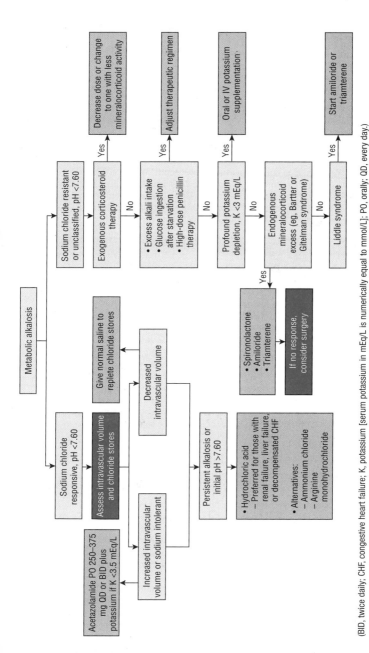

(BID, twice daily; CHF, congestive heart failure; K, potassium [serum potassium in mEq/L is numerically equal to mmol/L]; PO, orally; QD, every day.)

FIGURE 73-2. Treatment algorithm for patients with primary metabolic alkalosis.

Respiratory Acidosis

PATHOPHYSIOLOGY

- Respiratory acidosis is characterized by an increase in $PaCO_2$ and a decrease in pH.
- Respiratory acidosis results from disorders that restrict ventilation or increase CO_2 production, airway and pulmonary abnormalities, neuromuscular abnormalities, or mechanical ventilator problems.

CLINICAL PRESENTATION

- Neuromuscular symptoms include altered mental status, abnormal behavior, seizures, stupor, and coma. Hypercapnia can mimic a stroke or CNS tumor by producing headache, papilledema, focal paresis, and abnormal reflexes. CNS symptoms are caused by increased cerebral blood flow and are variable, depending in part on the acuity of onset.
- Initial compensatory response to acute respiratory acidosis is chemical buffering. If prolonged (>12–24 hours), proximal tubular HCO_3^- reabsorption, ammoniagenesis, and distal tubular H^+ secretion are enhanced, resulting in an increase in serum HCO_3^- concentration that raises pH to normal.

TREATMENT

- Provide adequate ventilation if CO_2 excretion is acutely and severely impaired ($PaCO_2$ >80 mm Hg [>10.6 kPa]) or if life-threatening hypoxia is present (arterial oxygen tension [PaO_2] <40 mm Hg [<5.3 kPa]). Ventilation can include maintaining a patent airway (eg, emergency tracheostomy, bronchoscopy, or intubation), clearing excessive secretions, administering oxygen, and providing mechanical ventilation.
- Treat underlying cause aggressively (eg, administration of bronchodilators for bronchospasm; narcotic or benzodiazepine antagonists to reverse effect of these agents on the respiratory center). Bicarbonate administration is rarely necessary and is potentially harmful.
- Chronic respiratory acidosis (eg, chronic obstructive pulmonary disease [COPD]) is treated essentially the same as acute respiratory acidosis with a few important exceptions. Oxygen therapy should be initiated carefully and only if the PaO_2 is less than 50 mm Hg (6.7 kPa) because the drive to breathe depends on hypoxemia rather than hypercarbia.
- For information on chronic respiratory acidosis, see Chapter 79.

Mixed Acid–Base Disorders

PATHOPHYSIOLOGY

- Failure of compensation is responsible for mixed acid–base disorders such as respiratory acidosis and metabolic acidosis, or respiratory alkalosis and metabolic alkalosis. In contrast, excess compensation is responsible for metabolic acidosis and respiratory alkalosis, or metabolic alkalosis and respiratory acidosis.
- Respiratory and metabolic acidosis can develop in patients with cardiorespiratory arrest, with chronic lung disease and shock, and with metabolic acidosis and respiratory failure.
- The most common mixed acid–base disorder is respiratory and metabolic alkalosis, which occurs in critically ill surgical patients with respiratory alkalosis caused by mechanical ventilation, hypoxia, sepsis, hypotension, neurologic damage, pain, or drugs; and with metabolic alkalosis caused by vomiting or nasogastric suctioning and massive blood transfusions.
- Mixed metabolic acidosis and respiratory alkalosis occur in patients with advanced liver disease, salicylate intoxication, and pulmonary–renal syndromes.

- Metabolic alkalosis and respiratory acidosis can occur in patients with COPD and respiratory acidosis who are treated with salt restriction, diuretics, and possibly glucocorticoids.

TREATMENT

- Treat mixed respiratory and metabolic acidosis by initiating oxygen delivery to improve hypercarbia and hypoxia. Mechanical ventilation can be needed to reduce $PaCO_2$. During initial therapy, give appropriate amounts of alkali to reverse the metabolic acidosis.
- Correct the metabolic component of mixed respiratory and metabolic alkalosis by administering **sodium and potassium chloride solutions**. Readjust the ventilator or treat the underlying disorder causing hyperventilation to treat the respiratory component.
- Treatment of mixed metabolic acidosis and respiratory alkalosis should be directed at the underlying cause.
- In metabolic alkalosis and respiratory acidosis, pH does not usually deviate significantly from normal, but treatment can be required to maintain PaO_2 and $PaCO_2$ at acceptable levels. Aim treatment at decreasing plasma bicarbonate with sodium and potassium chloride therapy, allowing renal excretion of retained bicarbonate from diuretic-induced metabolic alkalosis.

EVALUATION OF THERAPEUTIC OUTCOMES

- Monitor patients closely because acid–base disorders can be serious and even life-threatening.
- ABGs are the primary tools for evaluation of therapeutic outcome.

See Chapter 69, Acid–Base Disorders, authored by John W. Devlin and Thomas D. Nolin, for a more detailed discussion of this topic.

- *Acute kidney injury* (AKI) is a clinical syndrome generally defined by an abrupt reduction in kidney function as evidenced by changes in serum creatinine (Scr), blood urea nitrogen (BUN), and urine output.
- RIFLE (Risk, Injury, Failure, Loss of Kidney Function, and End-Stage Renal Disease), AKIN (Acute Kidney Injury Network), and the Kidney Disease: Improving Global Outcomes (KDIGO) clinical practice guidelines are three criteria-based classification systems developed to define and stage AKI in different patient populations (Table 74-1).
- All three staging systems have been validated across different patient populations, and their staging correlates closely with hospital mortality, cost, and length of stay.
- Scr and urine output are the main diagnostic criteria for each staging system.

PATHOPHYSIOLOGY

- AKI can be categorized as prerenal (resulting from decreased renal perfusion in the setting of undamaged parenchymal tissue), intrinsic (resulting from structural damage to the kidney, most commonly the tubule from an ischemic or toxic insult), and postrenal (resulting from obstruction of urine flow downstream from the kidney) (Figure 74-1).

CLINICAL PRESENTATION

- Patient presentation varies widely and depends on the underlying cause. Early recognition and cause identification are critical, as they directly affect the outcome of AKI. Outpatients often are not in acute distress; hospitalized patients may develop AKI after a catastrophic event.
- Symptoms in the outpatient setting include acute change in urinary habits, sudden weight gain, or severe abdominal or flank pain. Signs include edema, colored or foamy urine, and, in volume-depleted patients, postural hypotension, decreased jugular venous pressure, and dry mucous membranes.

DIAGNOSIS

- Thorough medical and medication histories, physical examination, assessment of laboratory values, and, if needed, imaging studies are important in the diagnosis of AKI.
- Scr cannot be used alone to diagnose AKI because it is insensitive to rapid changes in glomerular filtration rate (GFR). Scr lag behind the GFR's decline by 1-2 days, leading to a significant overestimation of GFR in the early stages of AKI and a potential delay in diagnosis of the syndrome. The use of BUN in AKI is very limited because urea production and renal clearance are heavily influenced by extrarenal factors such as critical illness, volume status, protein intake, and medications.
- Urine output measured over a specified period of time allows for short-term assessment of renal function, but its utility is limited to cases in which it is significantly decreased.
- In addition to BUN and Scr, selected blood and urine tests, and urinary sediment are used to differentiate the cause of AKI and guide patient management (Tables 74-2 and 74-3).
- Simultaneous measurement of urine and serum electrolytes and calculation of the fractional excretion of sodium (FE_{Na}) can help determine the etiology of AKI (see Table 74-2).

TABLE 74-1	RIFLE, AKIN, and KDIGO Classification Schemes for AKI[a]

RIFLE Category	Scr and GFR[b] Criteria	Urine Output Criteria
Risk	Scr increase to 1.5-fold or GFR decrease >25% from baseline	<0.5 mL/kg/hr for ≥6 hr
Injury	Scr increase to 2-fold or GFR decrease >50% from baseline	<0.5 mL/kg/hr for ≥12 hr
Failure	Scr increase to 3-fold or GFR decrease >75% from baseline, or Scr ≥4 mg/dL (354 μmol/L) with an acute increase of at least 0.5 mg/dL (44 μmol/L)	Anuria for ≥12 hr
Loss	Complete loss of function (RRT) for >4 weeks	
ESKD	RRT >3 months	

AKIN Criteria	Scr Criteria	Urine Output Criteria
Stage 1	Scr increase ≥0.3 mg/dL (27 μmol/L) or 1.5- to 2-fold from baseline	<0.5 mL/kg/hr for ≥6 hr
Stage 2	Scr increase >2- to 3-fold from baseline	<0.5 mL/kg/hr for ≥12 hr
Stage 3	Scr increase >3-fold from baseline, or Scr ≥4 mg/dL (354 μmol/L) with an acute increase of at least 0.5 mg/dL (44 μmol/L), or need for RRT	<0.3 mL/kg/hr for ≥24 hr or anuria for ≥12 hr

KDIGO Criteria	Scr Criteria	Urine Output Criteria
Stage 1	Scr increase ≥0.3 mg/dL (27 μmol/L) or 1.5–1.9 times from baseline	<0.5 mL/kg/hr for 6–12 hr
Stage 2	Scr increase 2–2.9 times from baseline	<0.5 mL/kg/hr for ≥12 hr
Stage 3	Scr increase three times from baseline, or Scr ≥4 mg/dL (354 μmol/L), or need for RRT, or eGFR[c] <35 mL/min/1.73 m^2 (0.34 mL/sec/m^2) in patients <18 years	Anuria for ≥12 hr

[a]For all staging systems, the criterion that leads to worst possible diagnosis should be used.
[b]GFR calculated using the Modification of Diet in Renal Disease (MDRD) equation.
[c]GFR calculated using the Schwartz formula.
AKI, acute kidney injury; AKIN, Acute Kidney Injury Network; ESKD, end-stage kidney disease; eGFR, estimated glomerular filtration rate; h, hours; KDIGO, Kidney Disease: Improving Global Outcomes; RIFLE, Risk, Injury, Failure, Loss of Kidney Function, and End-Stage Kidney Disease; RRT, renal replacement therapy; Scr, serum creatinine.

- The FE_{Na} is one of the better diagnostic parameters to differentiate the cause of AKI and is calculated as:

$$FE_{Na} = (U_{Na} \times Scr \times 100) / (U_{Cr} \times S_{Na})$$

where U_{Na} = urine sodium, Scr = serum creatinine, U_{Cr} = urine creatinine, and S_{Na} = serum sodium.

- A number of new serum and urinary biomarkers have been investigated to detect and predict the clinical outcomes of AKI, including tissue inhibitor of metalloproteinases 2 (TIMP-2) and insulin-like growth factor binding protein 7 (IGFBP7).

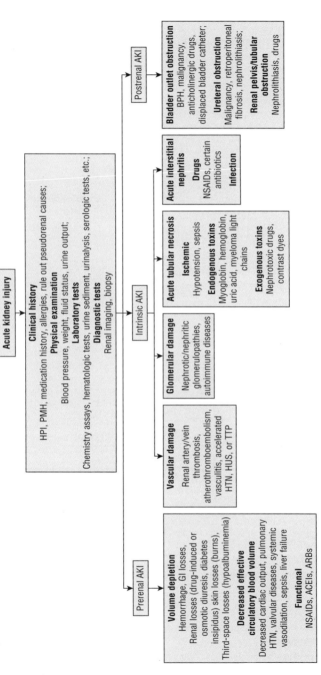

(ACEIs, angiotensin-converting enzyme inhibitors; ARBs, angiotensin receptor blockers; BPH, benign prostatic hyperplasia; GI, gastrointestinal; HPI, history of present illness; HTN, hypertension; HUS, hemolytic uremic syndrome; NSAIDs, nonsteroidal anti-inflammatory drugs; PMH, past medical history; TTP, thrombotic thrombocytopenic purpura.)

FIGURE 74-1. Classification of acute kidney injury (AKI) based on etiology.

TABLE 74-2	Diagnostic Parameters for Differentiating Causes of AKI[a]		
Laboratory Test	**Prerenal AKI**	**Intrinsic AKI**	**Postrenal AKI**
Urine sediment	Hyaline casts, may be normal	Granular casts, cellular debris	Cellular debris
Urinary RBC	None	2–4+	Variable
Urinary WBC	None	2–4+	1+
Urine Na (mEq/L or mmol/L)	<20	>40	>40
FE_{Na} (%)	<1	>2	Variable
Urine specific gravity	>1.018	<1.012	Variable

[a]Common laboratory tests are used to classify the cause of AKI. Functional AKI, which is not included in this table, would have laboratory values similar to those seen in prerenal AKI. The laboratory results listed under intrinsic AKI are those seen in acute tubular necrosis, the most common cause of intrinsic AKI.

AKI, acute kidney injury; FE_{Na}, fractional excretion of sodium; RBC, red blood cell; Scr, serum creatinine; WBC, white blood cell.

PREVENTION

- <u>Goals of Prevention</u>: The goals are to screen and identify patients at risk; monitor high-risk patients until the risk subsides; and implement prevention strategies when appropriate.

GENERAL APPROACH TO PREVENTION

Nonpharmacologic Therapy

- Intravenous fluids are routinely used in the prevention of AKI. KDIGO guidelines recommend isotonic crystalloids over colloids for intravascular volume expansion. Balanced solutions may offer some benefit compared to normal saline solutions.
- Fluids are the mainstay of therapy for prevention of contrast-induced acute kidney injury (CI-AKI), a common cause of acute tubular necrosis in the inpatient setting.
- KDIGO guidelines recommend either sodium bicarbonate or isotonic saline infusions in high-risk individuals receiving radiocontrast media. A common sodium bicarbonate regimen is 154 mEq/L (mmol/L) infused at 3 mL/kg/hr for 1 hour before the procedure and at 1 mL/kg/hr for 6 hours after the procedure. One frequently cited normal saline regimen is 1 mL/kg/hr for 12 hours pre- and post-procedure.
- Oral ingestion of a specific amount of water pre- and post-procedure is best reserved for outpatients with either normal or mildly impaired renal function undergoing elective procedures.

Pharmacologic Therapy

- Inadequate evidence exists to support use of ascorbic acid, an antioxidant, in the treatment or prevention of CI-AKI. The landmark PRESERVE trial demonstrated no benefit of *N*-acetylcysteine in the prevention of CI-AKI.
- Both hyper- and hypoglycemia are associated with adverse patient outcomes. Guidelines from the American Diabetes Association and Surviving Sepsis Campaign recommend a glycemic target range of 140–180 mg/dL (7.8–10 mmol/L) and less than 180 mg/dL (10 mmol/L), respectively, in critically ill patients.

TREATMENT OF ACUTE KIDNEY INJURY

- <u>Goals of Treatment</u>: Short-term goals include minimizing the degree of insult to the kidney, reducing extrarenal complications, and expediting recovery of renal function. Restoration of renal function to pre-AKI baseline is the ultimate goal.

TABLE 74-3	Urinary Findings as a Guide to the Etiology of Acute Kidney Injury	
Type of Urinary Evaluation	**Presence of**	**Suggestive of**
Urinalysis	Leukocyte esterases	Urinary tract infection
	Nitrites	Urinary tract infection
	Protein	
	Mild (<0.5 g/day)	Tubular damage
	Moderate (0.5–3 g/day)	Glomerulonephritis, pyelonephritis, tubular damage
	Large (>3 g/day)	Glomerulonephritis, nephrotic syndrome
	Hemoglobin	Glomerulonephritis, pyelonephritis, renal infarction, renal tumors, kidney stones
	Myoglobin	Rhabdomyolysis-associated tubular necrosis
	Urobilinogen	Hemolysis-associated tubular necrosis
Urine sediment	Microorganisms	Urinary tract infection
Cells	Red blood cells	Glomerulonephritis, urinary tract infection, renal infarction, papillary necrosis, renal tumors, kidney stones
	White blood cells	Urinary tract infection, interstitial nephritis
	Eosinophils	Drug-induced interstitial nephritis, renal transplant rejection
	Epithelial cells	Tubular necrosis
Casts	Granular casts	Tubular necrosis
	Hyaline casts	Prerenal azotemia
	White blood cell casts	Urinary tract infection, interstitial nephritis
	Red blood cell casts	Glomerulonephritis, renal infarct, lupus nephritis, vasculitis
Crystals	Urate	Postrenal obstruction
	Calcium phosphate	Postrenal obstruction

GENERAL APPROACH TO TREATMENT

- There is no specific treatment that can reverse AKI or hasten its recovery. Supportive measures that focus on hemodynamics, fluid balance, acid–base balance, and electrolyte homeostasis are the mainstays of therapy.

NONPHARMACOLOGIC THERAPY

- Fluid therapy is used to maintain or restore intravascular volume to assure adequate renal perfusion. Use IV fluids judiciously to prevent volume depletion and/or fluid overload which adversely affect kidney function and increase mortality.
- Serum electrolytes should be monitored daily. Hyperkalemia is the most common and serious electrolyte abnormality in AKI. Hypernatremia and fluid retention commonly occur, requiring calculation of daily sodium intake, including sodium contained in commonly administered antibiotics.
- Phosphorus and magnesium should be monitored, especially in patients with significant tissue destruction due to increased amounts of released phosphorus; neither is efficiently removed by dialysis.

TABLE 74-4	Common Indications for Renal Replacement Therapy
Indication for RRT	**Clinical Setting**
A: acid–base abnormalities	Metabolic acidosis (especially if pH <7.2)
E: electrolyte imbalance	Severe hyperkalemia and/or hypermagnesemia
I: intoxications	Salicylates, lithium, methanol, ethylene glycol, theophylline, phenobarbital
O: fluid overload	Fluid overload (especially pulmonary edema unresponsive to diuretics)
U: uremia	Uremia or associated complications (neuropathy, encephalopathy, pericarditis)

- Nutritional management of critically ill patients with AKI is complex due to multiple mechanisms for metabolic derangements. Nutritional requirements are altered by stress, inflammation, and injury that lead to hypermetabolic and hypercatabolic states.
- In severe AKI, renal replacement therapy (RRT), such as hemodialysis and peritoneal dialysis, is used to treat fluid overload, electrolyte disturbances (eg, hyperkalemia), acid–base imbalances, uremic complications, and pulmonary edema. See **Table 74-4** for indications for RRT in AKI. Intermittent and continuous (CRRT) options have different advantages (and disadvantages); the choice usually depends on physician preference and resources available. No difference in mortality or dialysis dependence has been shown; however, CRRT is generally preferred in hemodynamically unstable patients.
- Intermittent hemodialysis (IHD) is the most frequently used RRT and has the advantage of widespread availability and the convenience of lasting only 3–4 hours. Disadvantages include difficult venous dialysis access in hypotensive patients and hypotension due to rapid removal of large amounts of fluid.
- Several CRRT variants have been developed including continuous venovenous hemofiltration (CVVH), continuous venovenous hemodialysis (CVVHD), and continuous venovenous hemodiafiltration (CVVHDF) which differ in fluid clearance and solute removal. CRRT gradually removes solute, resulting in better tolerability by critically ill patients. Disadvantages include limited availability of equipment, need for intensive nursing care, and the need to individualize IV replacement, dialysate fluids, and drug therapy adjustments.
- Circuit clotting and filter patency limit CRRT performance requiring anticoagulation. The KDIGO Work Group recommends regional citrate as the preferred anticoagulant. This requires infusion of parenteral calcium which may limit feasibility of regional citrate when the supply of parenteral calcium is limited. The specific approach to anticoagulation is patient specific; if the patient requires systemic anticoagulation for an underlying comorbidity (eg, atrial fibrillation, artificial heart valve) no additional anticoagulation for RRT is needed.

PHARMACOLOGIC THERAPY

- Loop diuretics effectively reduce fluid overload but can worsen AKI. Equipotent doses of loop diuretics (**furosemide, bumetanide, torsemide**, and **ethacrynic acid**) have similar efficacy. KDIGO guidelines recommend limiting the use of loop diuretics to the management of fluid overload and avoiding their use for the sole purpose of prevention or treatment of AKI. Continuous infusions of loop diuretics appear to overcome diuretic resistance and to have fewer adverse effects than intermittent boluses but require more extensive and frequent monitoring.

TABLE 74-5 Common Causes of Diuretic Resistance in Patients with Acute Kidney Injury	
Causes of Diuretic Resistance	**Potential Therapeutic Solutions**
Excessive sodium intake (sources may be dietary, IV fluids, and drugs)	Remove sodium from nutritional sources and medications
Inadequate diuretic dose or inappropriate regimen	Increase dose, increase frequency, use continuous infusion, or add thiazide
Reduced oral bioavailability (usually furosemide)	Use parenteral therapy, switch to oral torsemide or bumetanide
Nephrotic syndrome (loop diuretic protein binding in tubule lumen)	Increase dose, add thiazide
Reduced renal blood flow	
Drugs (NSAIDs, ACEIs, vasodilators)	Discontinue these drugs if possible
Intravascular depletion	Intravascular volume expansion
Increased sodium resorption	
Distal nephron hypertrophy	Add thiazide, sodium restriction
Postdiuretic sodium retention	Dietary sodium restriction, use continuous infusion
Heart failure	Assess effective circulatory volume, increase dose, increase frequency, use continuous infusion
Cirrhosis	Assess effective circulatory volume, consider paracentesis
Acute tubular necrosis	Increase diuretic dose, diuretic combination therapy

ACEIs, angiotensin-converting enzyme inhibitors; NSAIDs, nonsteroidal anti-inflammatory drugs.

- Strategies are available to overcome diuretic resistance (Table 74-5). Combination therapy of loop diuretics plus a diuretic from a different pharmacologic class such as diuretics that work at the distal convoluted tubule (**thiazides**) or the collecting duct (**amiloride, triamterene**, and **spironolactone**) may have a synergistic effect. **Metolazone** is commonly used with a loop diuretic because, unlike other thiazides, it produces effective diuresis at GFR less than 20 mL/min (0.33 mL/sec).

Drug-Dosing Considerations

- Drug therapy optimization in AKI is a challenge. Confounding variables include residual drug clearance, fluid accumulation, and use of RRTs.
- Pharmacotherapy decisions should take into consideration the four distinct phases of AKI: initiation, extension, maintenance, and recovery phase. This requires frequent monitoring and adjustment of drug dosing to optimize therapy as kidney function stabilizes.
- Volume of distribution for water soluble drugs is significantly increased due to edema. Use of dosing guidelines for chronic kidney disease (CKD) does not reflect the clearance and volume of distribution in critically ill AKI patients.
- Patients with AKI may have a higher residual nonrenal clearance than those with CKD with similar creatinine clearances; this complicates drug therapy individualization, especially with RRTs.
- The mode of CRRT determines rate of drug removal, further complicating individualization of drug therapy. Rates of ultrafiltration, blood flow, and dialysate flow influence drug clearance during CRRT.

TABLE 74-6	Key Monitoring Parameters for Patients with Established Acute Kidney Injury
Parameter	**Frequency**
Fluid intake and output	Daily
Patient weight	Daily
Hemodynamics (eg, blood pressure, heart rate, mean arterial pressure.)	Hourly/Every shift
Blood chemistries	
Sodium, potassium, chloride, bicarbonate, calcium, phosphate, magnesium	Daily
Blood urea nitrogen/serum creatinine	Daily
Drugs and their dosing regimens	Daily
Nutritional regimen	Daily
Blood glucose	Daily (minimum)
Therapeutic drug monitoring of renally cleared drugs (eg, vancomycin aminoglycosides)	Highly variable, about three times weekly
Times of administered doses	Daily
Doses relative to administration of renal replacement therapy	Daily
Urinalysis, urinary output	
Calculate measured creatinine clearance	Every time measured urine collection performed
Calculate fractional excretion of sodium	Every time measured urine collection performed
Plans for renal replacement therapy	Daily

EVALUATION OF THERAPEUTIC OUTCOMES

- Vigilant monitoring of patient status is essential (Table 74-6).
- Perform therapeutic drug monitoring for drugs that have a narrow therapeutic index if results can be obtained in a timely manner.

See Chapter 60, Acute Kidney Injury, authored by Jenana Halilovic Maker, Lauren Roller, and William Dager, for a more detailed discussion of this topic.

- *Chronic kidney disease* (CKD) is defined as abnormalities in kidney structure or function, present for 3 months or longer.
- CKD is classified by glomerular filtration rate (GFR) and urinary albumin-to-creatinine ratio (uACR) based on the Kidney Disease: Improving Global Outcomes (KDIGO) guidelines for evaluation and management of CKD. The KDIGO classification system is referred to as CGA staging (*c*ause, *G*FR, *a*lbuminuria).
- A patient is classified with end-stage renal disease (ESRD) when their GFR is below $15 \, mL/min/1.73 \, m^2$ ($0.14 \, mL/sec/m^2$) and either chronic dialysis or kidney transplantation is needed to sustain life. KDIGO classification will be used in this chapter; the term CKD 5D indicates a patient with ESRD requiring dialysis as either hemodialysis (CKD 5HD) or peritoneal dialysis (CKD 5PD).
- Prognosis of CKD depends on cause of kidney disease, GFR at time of diagnosis, degree of albuminuria measured by uACR, and presence of other comorbid conditions. Please refer to *Pharmacotherapy: A Pathophysiologic Approach*, 11th ed., Chapter 61, Figure 61-1: KDIGO GFR and albuminuria categories and prognosis of CKD by category.

PATHOPHYSIOLOGY

- Clinical and sociodemographic risk factors for susceptibility to and initiation of CKD are useful for identifying individuals at risk of developing CKD. Clinical factors include, but aren't limited to, diabetes, hypertension, obesity, autoimmune diseases, systemic infections, family history of CKD, reduction in kidney mass, and low birth weight. Sociodemographic factors include older age, US ethnic minority status, low income or education, and exposure to certain chemical and environmental conditions.
- KDIGO recommends that prognosis be considered to help guide testing and treatment decisions. Validated estimating equations such as the kidney failure risk equation (KFRE) provide an accurate 2- and 5-year risk of progression to kidney failure for individuals with stage 3–5 CKD.
- Progression risk factors are associated with further decline in kidney function. Persistence of the underlying initiation factors (eg, diabetes mellitus, hypertension, glomerulonephritis) appears to be the most important predictor of progressive CKD.
- Most progressive nephropathies share a final common pathway to irreversible renal parenchymal damage and ESRD (**Figure 75-1**). Key elements of the pathway to ESRD include loss of nephron mass, glomerular capillary hypertension, and proteinuria.

CLINICAL PRESENTATION

- Progression of CKD from category 1 to 5 occurs over decades in the majority of people who are asymptomatic until they reach CKD 4 or 5. Signs and symptoms seen with stages 4–5 include fatigue, weakness, shortness of breath, mental confusion, nausea, vomiting, bleeding, anorexia, itching, cold intolerance, peripheral neuropathies, edema, weight gain, changes in urine output, and "foaming" of urine.

TREATMENT OF CKD

GENERAL APPROACH

- <u>Goals of Treatment</u>: The goal is to delay or prevent the progression of CKD while minimizing the development or severity of complications.
- Management should be based on KDIGO consensus guidelines to provide both evidence and opinion to optimize management of CKD.
- General nonpharmacologic recommendations for all CKD patients include exercise 30 minutes five times/week, weight loss if BMI >25 kg/m^2, smoking cessation, limit alcohol intake, and follow a low-sodium diet if hypertensive.

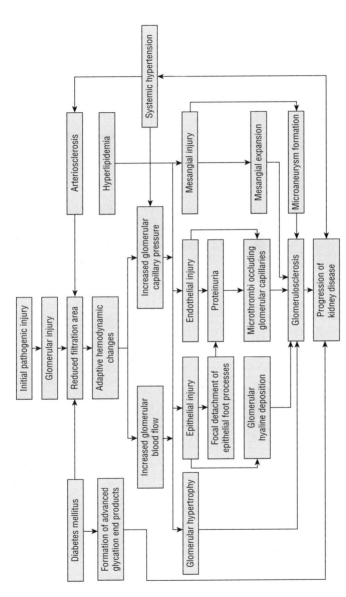

FIGURE 75-1. Proposed mechanisms for progression of kidney disease.

- General pharmacologic recommendations for all CKD patients include to adjust medication doses for kidney function, avoid herbal medicines, discuss over-the-counter medicines with pharmacist or other provider before self-medicating, discontinue potentially nephrotoxic/renally excreted drugs if estimated GFR (eGFR) <60 mL/min/1.73 m², adhere to vaccine recommendations, take aspirin as secondary prevention if indicated, and avoid oral phosphate-containing bowel preparations if GFR <60 mL/min/1.73 m².

PHARMACOLOGIC THERAPY

- Pharmacologic therapies to slow CKD progression include drugs with demonstrated benefits to reduce proteinuria and to manage the causal factors for CKD, primarily hypertension and diabetes.

Proteinuria

- First-line therapy for patients with diabetic CKD (DCKD) should include an **angiotensin-converting enzyme inhibitor (ACEI)** or an **angiotensin II receptor blocker (ARB)** if the patient's urine albumin excretion is in category A2 or greater (uACR between 30 and 300 mg/g [3–34 mg/mmol]). The antiproteinuric effect of ACEIs and ARBs is a class effect. Initiate therapy with the lowest recommended dose and increase dose until albuminuria is reduced by 30%–50% or side effects such as a greater than 30% decrease in eGFR or elevation in serum potassium occur (**Figure 75-2**).
- Achieving the target blood pressure is the primary goal for CKD patients with hypertension and a secondary goal is to control proteinuria.
- **Nondihydropyridine calcium channel blockers** are second- or third-line antiproteinuric drugs when an ACEI or ARB is contraindicated or not tolerated.
- Sodium glucose transport-2 inhibitors (SGLT-2) slow progression of DCKD by reducing glucose and sodium reabsorption in the proximal tubule of the kidney, resulting in a decrease in glomerular hyperfiltration and glomerular hypertension. In one trial **empagliflozin** reduced albuminuria, slowed eGFR decline, and reduced risk for progression to ESRD by 50% in patient with eGFR ≥30 mL/min/1.73 m².

Hypertension

- **Figure 75-2** provides an algorithm for recommended blood pressure goals based on the degree of albuminuria present and the choice of antihypertensive agent.
- For more information on hypertension, see Chapter 10.

Diabetes

- Screen patients with diabetes annually for CKD starting at the time of diagnosis of type 2 diabetes and 5 years after diagnosis of type 1 diabetes by ordering serum creatinine, eGFR, and uACR.
- Management of diabetes in patients with CKD includes reduction of proteinuria and achievement of target blood pressure and A1C.
- For more information on diabetes, see Chapter 19.

TREATMENT OF SECONDARY COMPLICATIONS

Anemia of CKD

- Desired outcomes of anemia management are to increase oxygen-carrying capacity, decrease signs and symptoms of anemia, and decrease the need for blood transfusions.
- Guide initiation of iron or erythropoiesis-stimulating agent (ESA) therapy by the patient's hemoglobin (Hb), transferrin saturation (TSat), and ferritin (**Table 75-1**). The risk of mortality and cardiovascular events is higher in CKD patients treated to higher Hb target values with an ESA. The target range for Hb in the CKD population is a topic of much debate.

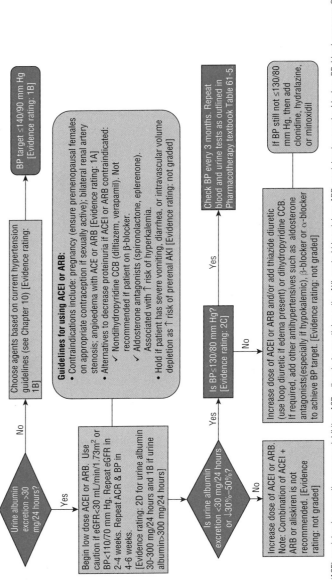

FIGURE 75-2. **Treatment of hypertension in chronic kidney disease.** (*Data from KDIGO Blood Pressure Work Group. KDIGO Clinical Practice Guideline for the Management of Blood Pressure in Chronic Kidney Disease. Kidney Int Suppl. 2012;2:337–414.*)

(ACEI, angiotensin-converting enzyme inhibitor; ACR, albumin-to-creatinine ratio; AKI, acute kidney injury; ARB, angiotensin receptor blocker; BP, blood pressure; CCB, calcium channel blocker; eGFR, estimated glomerular filtration rate.)

TABLE 75-1	KDIGO Recommendations for Initiation of Erythropoiesis-Stimulating Agents and Iron in Anemia of Chronic Kidney Disease		
	ND-CKD	**CKD 5HD and CKD 5PD**	**Pediatric CKD**
ESA initiation	If Hb <10 g/dL (100 g/L; 6.21 mmol/L). Consider rate of fall of Hb, prior response to iron, risk of needing a transfusion, risk of ESA therapy, and presence of anemia symptoms before initiating an ESA. [2C] Do not initiate if Hb ≥10 g/dL (100 g/L; 6.21 mmol/L). [2D]	Use ESAs to avoid drop in Hb to <9 g/dL (90 g/L; 5.59 mmol/L) by starting an ESA when Hb is between 9 and 10 g/dL (90 and 100 g/L; 5.59 and 6.21 mmol/L). [2B]	Selection of Hb concentration at which to initiate ESA therapy should include consideration of potential benefits (eg, improvement in QOL, school attendance, avoidance of blood transfusions) and potential harms. [2D]
Hb level	Do not use ESAs to *intentionally* increase Hb above 13 g/dL (130 g/L, 8.07 mmol/L). [1A] Do not use ESAs to maintain Hb above 11.5 g/dL (115 g/L; 7.14 mmol/L). [2C]	Do not use ESAs to *intentionally* increase Hb above 13 g/dL (130 g/L, 8.07 mmol/L). [1A] Do not use ESAs to maintain Hb above 11.5 g/dL (115 g/L; 7.14 mmol/L). [2C]	Suggest Hb range of 11–12 g/dL (110–120 g/L, 6.83–7.45 mmol/L). [2D]
Iron initiation[a]	If TSat is ≤30% (0.30) and ferritin is ≤500 ng/mL (mcg/L; 1120 pmol/L). [2C]	If TSat is ≤30% (0.30) and ferritin is ≤500 ng/mL (mcg/L; 1120 pmol/L). [2C]	If TSat is ≤20% (0.20) and ferritin is ≤100 ng/mL (mcg/L; 225 pmol/L). [1D]

[a]If TSat and serum ferritin are below suggested levels, consider iron supplementation if goal is to increase Hb and/or decrease ESA dose. *Note*: Serum ferritin is an acute-phase reactant—use clinical judgment when above 500 ng/mL (mcg/L; 1120 pmol/L).
CKD, chronic kidney disease; ESA, erythropoiesis-stimulating agent; Hb, hemoglobin; ND-CKD, nondialysis CKD patients; QOL, quality of life; TSat, transferrin saturation.
The strength of recommendation is indicated as Level 1, Level 2, or Not Graded. The quality of the supporting evidence is shown as A, B, C, or D.

- Kidney Disease Outcomes Quality Initiative (KDOQI) guidelines suggest a Hb range of 11–12 g/dL (110–120 g/L; 6.83–7.45 mmol/L) for all CKD patients, a target TSat of greater than 20% (>0.20), and a serum ferritin of greater than 100 ng/mL (mcg/L; >225 pmol/L) for CKD patients not requiring HD and greater than 200 ng/mL (mcg/L; >450 pmol/L) for CKD 5HD patients.
- Oral or IV **iron** supplementation is recommended in non-HD patients (eg, CKD category 3 or higher and PD patients). Supplementation with oral products (see Table 33-2) is more convenient but patients are likely to require IV iron supplementation to correct absolute iron deficiency, especially if they are receiving an ESA. Adverse effects of oral iron are primarily GI in nature and include constipation, nausea, and abdominal cramping which may negatively influence adherence.
- Soluble **ferric pyrophosphate citrate** is an iron compound added to the dialysate used for HD allowing for continuous iron administration during the procedure. Ferric pyrophosphate binds directly to transferrin, bypassing the reticuloendothelial system. The role of this agent in treating anemia of CKD is evolving.

- IV iron preparations have different pharmacokinetic profiles determined by the size of the iron-containing core and the composition of the surrounding carbohydrate shell (Table 75-2).
- Adverse effects of IV iron include allergic reactions, hypotension, dizziness, dyspnea, headaches, lower back pain, arthralgia, syncope, and arthritis. Some of these reactions can be minimized by decreasing the dose or rate of infusion. Non-dextran IV iron formulations have a better safety record than iron dextran. An analysis of anaphylaxis risk in patients newly exposed to IV iron products (including **dextran**, **gluconate**, **sucrose**, or **ferumoxytol**) reported the highest risk with iron dextran and the lowest risk with iron sucrose.
- Long-term IV iron administration introduces a risk of iron overload leading to hepatic, pancreatic, and cardiac dysfunction. Maintain target serum ferritin and TSat values to minimize risk.
- All available ESAs may be administered either IV or subcutaneously (SC) (Table 75-3). The biosimilar **epoetin-alfa epbx** is available in the United States with the same indications as the biological drug, **epoetin alfa**. SQ administration of epoetin results in a prolonged absorption phase leading to an extended half-life allowing target Hb to be maintained at doses 15%–30% lower than IV doses.
- The prolonged half-lives of **darbepoetin alfa** and **methoxy PEG-epoetin beta** allow for less frequent dosing.
- Causes of ESA resistance include iron deficiency, acute illness, inflammation, infection, chronic bleeding, aluminum toxicity, malnutrition, hyperparathyroidism, cancer, and chemotherapy.
- ESAs are well tolerated. Hypertension is the most common adverse event.
- **Figure 75-3** provides an approach to management of anemia in patients with CKD. For more information on anemia, see Chapter 33.

CKD-Related Mineral and Bone Disorder

- Desired outcomes for management of disorders of mineral and bone metabolism (CKD-MBD) are to "normalize" the biochemical parameters and prevent bone manifestations, cardiovascular and extravascular calcification, and the associated morbidity and mortality.
- The KDIGO-recommended targets for calcium, phosphorus, and PTH and frequency of monitoring based on the CKD category are given in **Table 75-4**.
- Recent guidelines emphasize avoiding hypercalcemia based on evidence linking higher calcium levels with mortality and nonfatal cardiovascular events. The change in the phosphorus recommendation from maintaining levels in the normal range to "toward the normal" is based on evidence linking both high- and low-phosphate concentrations with increased mortality.
- Calcium-phosphorus homeostasis is mediated through a complex interplay of hormones and their effects on bone, the gastrointestinal (GI) tract, kidneys, and the parathyroid gland. As kidney function declines, phosphate elimination decreases resulting in hyperphosphatemia and a decrease in serum calcium concentration. Hypocalcemia stimulates secretion of PTH. As kidney function declines, serum calcium balance can be maintained only at the expense of increased bone resorption, leading to alterations in structural integrity of bone and other consequences.

Treatment

- Dietary phosphorus restriction, dialysis, and parathyroidectomy are nonpharmacologic approaches to management of hyperphosphatemia and CKD-MBD.

Phosphate-Binding Agents

- Oral calcium compounds bind phosphate therefore decreasing phosphorus absorption from the gut and are first-line agents for controlling both serum phosphorus and calcium concentrations (Table 75-5). **Calcium carbonate** and **calcium acetate**

						Dose Ranges
TABLE 75-2	**IV Iron Preparations**					
Iron Compounds	**Brand Names**	**Half-Life (Hours)**	**Molecular Weight (Daltons)**	**FDA-Approved Indications**	**FDA-Approved Dosing**[a]	**Dose Ranges (mg)**[b,c]
Ferric carboxymaltose	Injectafer	7–12	150,000	Adult patients with intolerance to oral iron or who have had an unsatisfactory response to oral iron and in adult patients with CKD not on dialysis	Give 2 doses separated by at least 7 days of 750 mg per dose (if body weight is ≥50 kg) or 15 mg/kg per dose (if body weight is <50 kg) not to exceed 1500 mg per course. Give either IV push (100 mg/min) or diluted in not more than 250 mL of 0.9 NaCl as an infusion over at least 15 minutes	750
Ferumoxytol	Feraheme	15	750,000	Adult patients with intolerance to oral iron or who have had an unsatisfactory response to oral iron and in adult patients with CKD	510 mg (17 mL) as a single dose, followed by a second 510 mg dose 3–8 days after the initial dose. Dilute in 50–200 mL of 0.9% NaCl or 5% dextrose and administer as an IV infusion over 15 minutes	510
Iron dextran	INFeD	40–60	96,000	Patients with iron deficiency in whom oral iron is unsatisfactory or impossible	100 mg over 2 minutes (25 mg test dose required) Note: equation provided by manufacturer to calculate dose based on desired Hb	25–1000
Iron sucrose	Venofer	6	43,000	Adult and pediatric CKD 5HD patients aged 2 years and older	Adult: 100 mg over 2–5 minutes or 100 mg in maximum of 100 mL of 0.9% NaCl over 15 minutes per consecutive HD session Pediatric: 0.5 mg/kg not to exceed 100 mg per dose over 5 minutes or diluted in 25 mL of 0.9% NaCl administered over 5–60 minutes (give dose every 2 weeks for 12 weeks)	25–1000

					Indication	Dosing
					Adult and pediatric ND-CKD patients aged 2 years and older	Adult: 200 mg over 2–5 minutes on five different occasions within 14-day period. There is limited experience with administration of 500 mg diluted in a maximum of 250 mL of 0.9% NaCl over 3.5–4 hours on day 1 and day 14 Pediatric: see pediatric dosing for CKD 5HD (give dose every 4 weeks for 12 weeks)
					Adult and pediatric CKD 5PD patients aged 2 years and older	Adult: give 3 divided doses within 28 days as 2 infusions of 300 mg over 1.5 hours 14 days apart followed by one 400 mg infusion over 2.5 hours 14 days later. Dilute in a maximum of 250 mL of 0.9% NaCl Pediatric: see pediatric dosing for CKD 5HD (give dose every 4 weeks for 12 weeks)
Sodium ferric gluconate	Ferrlecit	1	350,000	62.5–1000	Adult and pediatric CKD 5HD patients aged 6 years and older receiving ESA therapy	Adult: 125 mg over 10 minutes or 125 mg in 100 mL of 0.9% NaCl over 60 minutes per HD session Pediatric: 1.5 mg/kg in 25 mL of 0.9% NaCl over 60 minutes per dialysis session; maximum dose 125 mg per dose

[a]Monitor for 30 minutes following an infusion; KDIGO guidelines recommend monitoring for 60 minutes (1B recommendation for iron dextran, 2C recommendation for non-dextran products).
[b]Dose ranges for iron deficiency in CKD. With the exception of ferric carboxymaltose and ferumoxytol, small doses (eg, 25–150 mg/week) are generally used for maintenance regimens.
[c]Larger doses (eg, 1 g) should be administered in divided doses.
Total dose for absolute iron deficiency is approximately 1 g in divided doses (1.5 g for ferric carboxymaltose).
CKD, chronic kidney disease; ESA, erythropoiesis-stimulating agent; ND-CKD, nondialysis CKD patients.

Diagnosis of Anemia of CKD^a (other causes ruled out)
Evaluate TSat and Ferritin

TSat <30% (<0.30), Ferritin <500 ng/mL (mcg/L; <1,120 pmol/L)

If goal is to ↑Hb without initiating an ESA or to ↓ESA dose, administer supplemental iron. [2C] IV: Give as single large dose or repeated smaller doses depending on formulation (see Table 75-2) [preferred route for CKD 5HD and CKD 5PD]

PO: 1-3 month course of 200 mg elemental iron per day [preferred route for ND-CKD]

Monitor Hb, TSat, and ferritin monthly.^c

If Hb increases too rapidly (see text) decrease ESA dose by 25% (if receiving an ESA). [2C]

If Hb does not increase appropriately (see text) and TSat <30% (<0.30), ferritin < 500 ng/mL (mcg/L;<1,120 pmol/L) give a course of IV iron.

If TSat and ferritin are above thresholds, see decision tree for ≥ 30%, Ferritin ≥500 ng/mL (mcg/L).

TSat ≥30% (≥0.30), Ferritin^b ≥ 500 ng/mL (mcg/L; ≥1,120 pmol/L)

If ESA naïve: Initiate ESA therapy (see Table 75-3). If receiving ESA therapy and Hb has not increased by 1 g/dL (10 g/L; 0.62 mmol/L) within 4 weeks, increase dose by 25%. Consider maintenance iron to avoid iron deficiency.

Monitor Hb and ferritin monthly.^c Monitor TSat and ferritin at least every 3 months (more frequent monitoring of iron indices may be warranted with initiation/increase in ESA).

If Hb increases too rapidly (see text) decrease ESA dose by 25%. [2C]

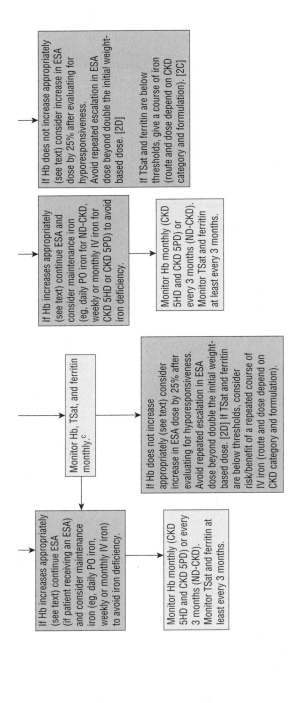

FIGURE 75-3 **Algorithm for management of anemia of CKD in adults.**

[a]See Table 75-1 and text for discussion of Hb levels.
[b]Clinical judgment should be used to determine if iron supplementation should be continued when ferritin >500 ng/mL (mcg/L; 1120 pmol/L).
[c]Weekly monitoring of Hb may be warranted. Wait at least 1 week after an IV dose of iron to measure TSat and ferritin.
(CKD, chronic kidney disease; ESA, erythropoiesis-stimulating agent; Hb, hemoglobin; ND-CKD, nondialysis CKD patients; TSat, transferrin saturation.)

TABLE 75-3	Erythropoiesis-Stimulating Agents in Chronic Kidney Disease			
Drug Name	Brand Name(s)	Starting Dose	Route of Administration	Half-Life (Hours)
Epoetin alfa	Epogen, Procrit	Adults: 50–100 units/kg three times per week Pediatrics: 50 units/kg three times per week	IV or SC	8.5 (IV) 24 (SC)
Epoetin alfa-epbx	Retacrit	See epoetin alfa information		
Darbepoetin alfa	Aranesp	Adults: ND-CKD: 0.45 mcg/kg once every 4 weeks CKD 5HD or CKD 5PD: 0.45 mcg/kg once per week or 0.75 mcg/kg every 2 weeks Pediatrics: 0.45 mcg/kg once weekly; may give 0.75 mcg/kg once every 2 weeks in ND-CKD patients	IV or SC	25 (IV) 48 (SC)
Methoxy PEG-epoetin beta	Mircera	All adult CKD patients: 0.6 mcg/kg every 2 weeks; once Hb stabilizes, double the dose and administer monthly (eg, if administering 0.6 mcg/kg every 2 weeks, give 1.2 mcg/kg every month)	IV or SC	134 (IV) 139 (SC)

CKD, chronic kidney disease; ND-CKD, nondialysis CKD patients; PEG, polyethylene glycol; SC, subcutaneous.

are the primary preparations used. **Sevelamer** is a nonabsorbable, nonelemental hydrogel that effectively lowers phosphorus and also lowers LDL and increases HDL.

- **Lanthanum carbonate** controls phosphorus and maintains PTH in the target range with less risk of hypercalcemia than calcium-containing binding agents. **Ferric citrate** and **sucroferric oxyhydroxide** are iron-based phosphate-binding agents.

- Adverse effects of all phosphate binders are generally limited to GI effects, including constipation, diarrhea, nausea, vomiting, and abdominal pain. Risk of hypercalcemia may necessitate restriction of calcium-containing binder use and/or reduction in dietary intake. Aluminum and magnesium binders are not recommended for regular use in CKD because aluminum binders have been associated with CNS toxicity and the worsening of anemia, whereas magnesium binders may lead to hypermagnesemia and hyperkalemia. The potential for iron overload should be considered with ferric citrate.

Vitamin D Therapy

- **Calcitriol**, 1,25-dihydroxyvitamin D_3, and vitamin D analogs directly inhibit or suppress PTH synthesis and also stimulate absorption of serum calcium by intestinal cells, which decreases PTH secretion by the parathyroid glands.

TABLE 75-4 KDIGO Monitoring and Goals for Calcium, Phosphorus, and Parathyroid Hormone

Parameter	Chronic Kidney Disease Stage			
	3	4	5	ESRD
Calcium[a]				
Monitoring frequency[b]	Every 6–12 months	Every 3–6 months	Every 1–3 months	Every 1–3 months
Goal	Avoid hypercalcemia [2C]	Avoid hypercalcemia [2C]	Avoid hypercalcemia [2C]	Avoid hypercalcemia [2C]
Phosphorus				
Monitoring frequency[b]	Every 6–12 months	Every 3–6 months	Every 1–3 months	Every 1–3 months
Goal	Toward the normal range [2C]	Toward the normal range [2C]	Toward the normal range [2C]	Toward the normal range [2C]
Intact PTH				
Monitoring frequency[b]	Based on baseline level and CKD progression	Every 6–12 months	Every 3–6 months	Every 3–6 months
Goal	Avoid progressively rising levels or levels persistently above the upper limit of normal [2C]	Avoid progressively rising levels or levels persistently above the upper limit of normal [2C]	Avoid progressively rising levels or levels persistently above the upper limit of normal [2C]	2–9 times the upper normal limit [2C]

[a]Usually corrected for albumin.
[b]Not graded.
See Table 75-1 for definitions of evidence grading in brackets.

TABLE 75-5 Phosphate-Binding Agents for Treatment of Hyperphosphatemia in Chronic Kidney Disease Patients

Category	Drug	Brand Name	Compound Content	Starting Doses	Dose Titration[a]	Comments[b]
Calcium-based binders	Calcium acetate (25% elemental calcium)	PhosLo Phoslyra	25% elemental calcium (169 mg elemental calcium per 667 mg capsule) 667 mg calcium acetate per 5 mL	1334 mg three times a day with meals	Increase or decrease by 667 mg per meal (169 mg elemental calcium)	Comparable efficacy to calcium carbonate with lower dose of elemental calcium Approximately 45 mg phosphorus bound per 1 g calcium acetate Evaluate for drug interactions with calcium
	Calcium carbonate[c]	Tums, Os-Cal, Caltrate	40% elemental calcium	0.5–1 g (elemental calcium) three times a day with meals	Increase or decrease by 500 mg per meal (200 mg elemental calcium)	Dissolution characteristics and phosphate binding may vary from product to product Approximately 39 mg phosphorus bound per 1 g calcium carbonate Evaluate for drug interactions with calcium
Iron-based binders	Ferric citrate	Auryxia	210 mg tablets (= 1 g ferric citrate)	420 mg ferric iron three times daily with meals	Increase or decrease dose by 1 or 2 tablets per meal	May increase serum iron, ferritin, and TSat May cause discolored (dark) stools Evaluate for drug interactions with iron
	Sucroferric oxyhydroxide	Velphoro	500 mg chewable tablets	500 mg three times daily with meals	Increase or decrease by 500 mg per day	May cause discolored (dark) stools Evaluate for drug interactions with iron

				Dose	Titration	Comments
Resin binders	Sevelamer carbonate	Renvela	800 mg tablet; 0.8 and 2.4 g powder for oral suspension	800–1600 mg three times a day with meals (once-daily dosing also effective)	Increase or decrease by 800 mg per meal	Also lowers low-density lipoprotein cholesterol; Consider in patients at risk for extraskeletal calcification; Risk of metabolic acidosis with sevelamer hydrochloride (less risk with carbonate formulation)
	Sevelamer hydrochloride	Renagel	400 and 800 mg tablets	800–1600 mg three times a day with meals	Increase or decrease by 800 mg per meal	May interact with cipro and mycophenolate mofetil
Other elemental binders	Lanthanum carbonate	Fosrenol	500, 750, and 1000 mg chewable tablets; 750 and 1000 mg oral powder	1500 mg daily in divided doses with meals	Increase or decrease by 750 mg/day	Potential for accumulation of lanthanum due to some GI absorption (long-term consequences unknown); Evaluate for drug interactions (eg, cationic antacids, quinolone antibiotics)
	Aluminum hydroxide	AlternaGel	Content varies (range 100–600 mg/unit)	300–600 mg three times a day with meals	Not for long-term use requiring titration	Not a first-line agent; risk of aluminum toxicity; do not use concurrently with citrate-containing products; Reserve for short-term use (4 weeks) in patients with hyperphosphatemia not responding to other binders; Evaluate for drug interactions

[a]Based on phosphorus levels, titrate every 2–3 weeks until phosphorus goal is reached.
[b]GI side effects are possible with all agents (eg, nausea, vomiting, abdominal pain, diarrhea, or constipation).
[c]Multiple preparations available that are not listed.
TSat, transferrin saturation.

TABLE 75-6 Vitamin D Agents

Nutritional Vitamin D

Generic Name	Brand Name	Form of Vitamin D	Dosage Forms	Initial Dose	Dosage Range	Frequency of Dosing or Dose Titration[a]
Ergocalciferol	Drisdol	D_2	PO	Varies based on 25(OH)D levels	400–50,000 international units	Daily (doses of 400–2000 international units)
Cholecalciferol[b]	Generic	D_3	PO			Weekly or monthly for higher doses (50,000 international units)
Calcifediol	Rayaldee	D_3	PO	30 mcg daily	30–60 mcg	Increase after 3 months if PTH above desired range

Vitamin D and Analogs

Generic Name	Brand Name	Form of Vitamin D	Dosage Forms	Initial Dose[c,d]	Dosage Range	Dose Titration[a]
Calcitriol	Rocaltrol	D_3	PO	0.25 mcg daily (varying doses administered three times per week are also used)	0.25–5 mcg	Increase by 0.25 mcg/day at 4–8 week intervals
	Calcijex		IV	1–2 mcg three times per week	0.5–5 mcg	Increase by 0.5–1 mcg at 2–4 week intervals
Doxercalciferol[e]	Hectorol	D_2	PO	ND-CKD: 1 mcg daily	5–20 mcg	Increase by 0.5 mcg at 2-week intervals for daily dosing or by 2.5 mcg at 8-week intervals for three times per week dosing

			ESRD: 10 mcg three times per week		Increase by 1–2 mcg at 8-week intervals
		IV	ESRD: 4 mcg three times per week	2–8 mcg	Increase by 1–2 mcg at 8-week intervals
Paricalcitol	Zemplar	D_2			
		PO	ND-CKD: 1 mcg daily or 2 mcg three times per week if PTH ≤500 pg/mL(ng/L; 54 pmol/L); 2 mcg daily or 4 mcg three times per week if PTH >500 pg/mL (ng/L; 54 pmol/L)	1–4 mcg	Increase by 1 mcg (for daily dosing) or 2 mcg (for three times per week dosing) at 2–4 week intervals
		IV	ESRD: 0.04–1 mcg three times per week	2.5–15 mcg	Increase by 2–4 mcg at 2–4 week intervals

aBased on PTH, calcium, and phosphorus levels. Decreases in dose are necessary if PTH is oversuppressed and/or if calcium and phosphorus are elevated.
bMultiple preparations are available that are not listed.
cDose ratios are as follows: 1:1 for IV paricalcitol to oral doxercalciferol, 1.5:1 for IV paricalcitol to IV doxercalciferol, and 1:1 for IV to oral calcitriol.
dDaily oral dosing most common for nonhemodialysis CKD patients, IV or PO dosing three times per week more often used in the hemodialysis population.
eProdrug that requires activation by the liver.
ESRD, end-stage renal disease; ND-CKD, nondialysis chronic kidney disease; PTH, parathyroid hormone.

- Serum calcium and phosphorus should be within the normal range before initiation and during continued vitamin D therapy. Adjust vitamin D dose every 2–4 weeks based on PTH concentrations and trends in calcium and phosphorus (Table 75-6).
- KDIGO does not advocate for routine use of calcitriol and vitamin D analogs in the nondialysis CKD population and suggests that they be reserved for patients with CKD stages 4–5.
- The newer vitamin D analogs **paricalcitol** and **doxercalciferol** may be associated with less hypercalcemia and hyperphosphatemia. Observational studies show all-cause and cardiovascular survival benefit with these agents.

Calcimimetics

- **Cinacalcet** and **etelcalcetide** reduce PTH secretion by increasing the sensitivity of the calcium-sensing receptor. The most common adverse events include nausea and vomiting.
- Since these agents lower serum calcium they should not be started if the serum calcium is less than the lower limit of normal. Start cinacalcet at 30 mg daily, which can be titrated to the desired PTH and calcium concentrations every 2–4 weeks to a maximum of 180 mg daily. Initiate etelcalcetide at 5 mg IV three times per week at the end of hemodialysis.

CARDIOVACULAR COMPLICATIONS OF CKD

CARDIOVASCULAR DISEASE

- CKD patients are at increased risk of CVD, independent of the etiology of their kidney disease and this is associated with much higher mortality rates. Traditional risk factors include diabetes, dyslipidemia, hypertension, smoking, and obesity. Nontraditional risk factors include proteinuria, hyperhomocysteinemia, anemia, inflammation, and abnormal calcium and phosphate metabolism, resulting in vascular calcification oxidative stress.
- CKD patients benefit from treatment of traditional risk factors. Aspirin is recommended for secondary prevention in all patients based on decreased mortality in observational studies.

HYPERLIPIDEMIA

- CKD with or without nephrotic syndrome is frequently accompanied by abnormalities in lipoprotein metabolism.
- KDIGO Lipid Guidelines recommend:
  1. Complete a fasting lipid profile in all adults with newly identified CKD.
  2. **Statin** treatment in adults ages 18–49 years with CKD but not treated with chronic dialysis or kidney transplantation, who have one or more of the following: known coronary disease; diabetes mellitus; prior ischemic stroke; estimated 10-year incidence of coronary death or nonfatal MI greater than 10%.
  3. Statin or statin/**ezetimibe** combination in adults >50 years with eGFR <60 mL/min/1.73 m^2 but not treated with chronic dialysis or kidney transplantation.
  4. Do not initiate statins or statin/ezetimibe combination therapy in adults with dialysis-dependent CKD. Continue these agents if patient is already taking them at the time of dialysis initiation.

See Chapter 61, Chronic Kidney Disease, authored by Joanna Q. Hudson, Lori D. Wazny, and Paul Komenda, for a more detailed discussion of this topic.

- *Fluid and electrolyte homeostasis* is maintained by feedback mechanisms, hormones, and many organ systems, and is necessary for the body's normal physiologic functions. Disorders of sodium and water, calcium, phosphorus, potassium, and magnesium homeostasis are addressed separately in this chapter.

DISORDERS OF SODIUM AND WATER HOMEOSTASIS

- Total body water (TBW) ranges from 45% to 60% of body weight depending on sex and age and is distributed primarily into two compartments: intracellularly (ICF; two-thirds [67%] of TBW), and one-third (33%) is contained in the extracellular space.
- *Effective osmoles* are solutes that cannot freely cross cell membranes, such as sodium and potassium. Addition of an isotonic solution to the extracellular fluid (ECF) does not change ICF volume because there is no change in effective ECF osmolality. Adding a hypertonic solution to the ECF decreases ICF volume, whereas adding a hypotonic solution increases it. **Table 76-1** summarizes the composition of commonly used IV solutions and their expected distribution into the ECF and ICF compartments.
- Hypernatremia and hyponatremia can be associated with conditions of high, low, or normal ECF sodium and volume. Both conditions are most commonly the result of abnormalities of water metabolism. It's important to understand the difference between *dehydration* (loss of TBW producing hypertonicity) and *hypovolemia* (volume depletion due to a symptomatic deficit in ECF volume).

HYPONATREMIA (SERUM SODIUM <135 mEq/L [mmol/L])
Pathophysiology

- Results from an excess of extracellular water relative to sodium because of impaired water excretion.
- Causes of nonosmotic release of arginine vasopressin (AVP), commonly known as *antidiuretic hormone*, include hypovolemia and decreased effective circulating volume as seen in patients with congestive heart failure (CHF), nephrotic syndrome, cirrhosis, and syndrome of inappropriate antidiuretic hormone (SIADH).
- Hyponatremia is classified as isotonic, hypertonic, or hypotonic depending on serum osmolity (**Figure 76-1**).
- Hypotonic hyponatremia, the most common form of hyponatremia, can be further classified as hypovolemic, euvolemic, or hypervolemic.
- Hypovolemic hypotonic hyponatremia is associated with a loss of ECF volume and sodium, with the loss of more sodium than water. It is seen in patients with diarrhea or in those taking thiazide diuretics.
- Euvolemic hyponatremia is associated with a normal or slightly decreased ECF sodium content and increased TBW and ECF volume. It is most commonly caused by SIADH.
- Hypervolemic hyponatremia is associated with an increase in ECF volume in conditions with impaired renal sodium and water excretion, such as cirrhosis, CHF, and kidney failure.

Clinical Presentation

- Most patients with hyponatremia are asymptomatic.
- Presence and severity of symptoms are related to the magnitude and rapidity of onset of hyponatremia. Hyponatremia that is severe or develops rapidly is associated with symptoms that progress from nausea and malaise to headache and lethargy and, eventually, to seizures, coma, and death.

TABLE 76-1 Composition of Common IV Solutions

Solution	Dextrose g/dL (kcal/L)	[Na$^+$] (mEq/L or mmol/L)	[K$^+$] (mEq/L or mmol/L)	[Cl$^-$] (mEq/L or mmol/L)	Other (mEq/L or mmol/L)	Osmolality (mOsm/kg or mmol/kg)	Tonicity	% ECF	% ICF	Free water (mL/L)
Dextrose 5% in water	5 (170)	0	0	0	—	253	Hypotonic	33	67	1000 mL
0.2% NaCl[a]	0	34	0	34	—	68	Hypotonic	50	50	750 mL
0.45% NaCl[b]	0	77	0	77	—	154	Hypotonic	67	33	500 mL
0.9% NaCl[c]	0	154	0	154	—	308	Isotonic	100	0	0 mL
Lactated Ringer's[d]	0	130	4	105	Lactate 28 Ca 4.8	273	Isotonic	97	3	0 mL
Plasma-Lyte A[e]	0.44 (21)	140	5	98	Acetate 27 Mg 3	294	Isotonic	100	0	0 mL
Plasma-Lyte 148[e]										
Normosol-R (pH 6.6)	0	140	5	98	Acetate 27 Mg 3	294	Isotonic	100	0	0 mL
Normosol-R (pH 7.4)										
3% NaCl[f]	0	513	0	513	—	1026	Hypertonic	100	0	−2331 mL

[a]Also referred to as *quarter normal saline.*
[b]Also referred to as *half normal saline.*
[c]Also referred to as *normal saline.*
[d]Also referred to as LR; also available commercially as Dextrose 5% LR.
[e]Plasma-Lyte A pH 7.4; Plasma-Lyte 148 pH 5.5.
[f]Hypertonic solution; results in osmotic removal of water from the ICF.
One g/dL is equivalent to 0.1 g/L; one kcal is equivalent to 4.18 kJ/L; Ca, calcium; Cl$^-$, chloride; ECF, extracellular fluid; ICF, intracellular fluid; IV, intravenous; K$^+$, potassium; Mg, magnesium; NA, not applicable; Na$^+$, sodium; NaCl, sodium chloride.

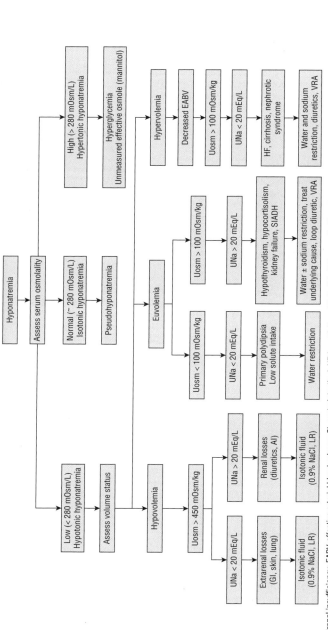

(AI, adrenal insufficiency; EABV, effective arterial blood volume; GI, gastrointestinal; HF, heart failure; LR, lactated Ringers; NaCl, sodium chloride; SIADH, syndrome of inappropriate antidiuretic hormone; UNa, urine sodium concentration [values in mEq/L are numerically equivalent to mmol/L]; Uosm, urine osmolality [values in mOsm/kg are numerically equivalent to mmol/kg]; VRA, vasopressin receptor antagonist.)

FIGURE 76-1. Algorithm for the assessment and treatment of hyponatremia.

- Patients with hypovolemic hyponatremia present with neurologic symptoms and also symptoms of hypovolemia, including decreased skin turgor, orthostatic hypotension, tachycardia, and dry mucous membranes.

Treatment

- Goals of Treatment: Resolve underlying cause of the sodium and ECF volume imbalance and safely correct the sodium and water derangements. Too rapid correction of serum sodium concentration can lead to an acute decrease in brain cell volume, contributing to the development of osmotic demyelination syndrome (ODS).

Acute or Severely Symptomatic Hypotonic Hyponatremia

- Symptomatic patients, regardless of fluid status, should initially be treated with 3% NaCl (513 mEq/L [mmol/L]) until symptoms resolve. Resolution of severe symptoms may require only a 5% increase in serum sodium; some clinicians suggest an initial target serum sodium of ~120 mEq/L (mmol/L).
- Treat SIADH with 3% saline plus, if the urine osmolality exceeds 300 mOsm/kg (mmol/kg), a loop diuretic (**furosemide**, 20–40 mg IV every 6 hours or **bumetanide**, 0.5–1 mg IV every 2–3 hours for several doses). Consider a continuous infusion if intermittent doses are not sufficient to manage edema.
- Treat hypovolemic hypotonic hyponatremia with 0.9% NaCl.
- Treat hypervolemic hypotonic hyponatremia with 3% NaCl and prompt initiation of fluid restriction. Loop diuretic therapy or **arginine vasopressin receptor antagonist (VRA)** is often required to facilitate urinary excretion of free water.

Nonemergent Hypotonic Hyponatremia

- Treatment of SIADH involves water restriction and correction of the underlying cause; discontinue drugs that could be a contributing factor. Restrict water intake to approximately 1000–1200 mL/day. Treat patients unable to restrict water sufficiently with NaCl tablets and a loop diuretic or **demeclocycline** (300 mg orally two to four times daily; onset of action in 3–6 days).
- VRAs or "vaptans" (eg, **conivaptan** [available IV only] and **tolvaptan** [15 mg orally daily]) can be used to treat SIADH as well as other causes of euvolemic and hypervolemic hypotonic hyponatremia that has been nonresponsive to other therapeutic interventions in patients with heart failure and SIADH. Fluid restriction should be avoided for the first 24–48 hours of starting VRA therapy when active sodium correction is occurring. Tolvaptan labeling currently includes a warning to NOT use it for more than 30 days and should not be used in patients with liver disease, including cirrhosis. The vaptans have dramatic effects on water excretion and represent a breakthrough in the therapy of hyponatremia and disorders of fluid homeostasis.
- Treatment of asymptomatic hypervolemic hypotonic hyponatremia involves correction of the underlying cause and restriction of water intake to less than 1000–1200 mL/day. Dietary intake of sodium chloride should be restricted to 1000–2000 mg/day.

HYPERNATREMIA (SERUM SODIUM >145 mEq/L [mmol/L])

Pathophysiology and Clinical Presentation

- Hypernatremia results from insensible water loss (evaporative water loss through skin and lungs), from hypotonic GI losses, or when patients are exposed to high temperatures. Diabetes insipidus (DI) causes a water diuresis. Hypernatremia may also result from hypertonic NaCl administration or from excess sodium intake from IV and enteral fluids and medications.
- Increase in serum sodium concentration and osmolality causes acute water movement from the ICF to the ECF. Symptoms are primarily caused by decreased brain cell volume and can include weakness, lethargy, restlessness, irritability, twitching, and confusion. Symptoms of a more rapidly developing hypernatremia include seizures, coma, and death.

Treatment

- <u>Goals of Treatment</u>: Correct serum sodium concentration at a rate that restores and maintains brain cell volume.
- Begin treatment of hypovolemic hypernatremia with 0.9% NaCl. After hemodynamic stability is restored and intravascular volume is replaced, replace free-water deficit with 5% dextrose or 0.45% NaCl.
- The correction rate should be approximately 1 mEq/L (1 mmol/L) per hour for hypernatremia that developed over a few hours and 0.5 mEq/L (0.5 mmol/L) per hour for hypernatremia that developed more slowly.
- Treat central DI with intranasal **desmopressin**, beginning with 10 mcg once daily. Titrate to 20 mcg twice daily based on serum sodium concentration. Oral tablets are available; poor bioavailability contributes to unpredictable response when transitioning between dosage forms.
- Treat nephrogenic DI by decreasing ECF volume with a thiazide diuretic and dietary sodium restriction (2000 mg/day), which can decrease urine volume by as much as 50%. Other treatment options include drugs with antidiuretic properties (Table 76-2).
- Treat sodium overload with loop diuretics (furosemide, 20–40 mg IV every 6 hours) and 5% dextrose at an appropriate rate.

EDEMA

Pathophysiology and Clinical Presentation

- Edema, defined as a clinically detectable increase in interstitial fluid volume, develops when excess sodium is retained either as a primary defect in renal sodium excretion or as a response to a decrease in the effective circulating volume despite an already expanded or normal ECF volume.
- Edema is usually due to heart, kidney, or liver failure, or a combination of these conditions.
- Edema is initially detected in the feet or pretibial area in ambulatory patients and in the presacral area in bed-bound individuals, and is described as "pitting" when a depression caused by briefly exerting pressure over a bony prominence does not rapidly refill.

Treatment

- Diuretics are the primary pharmacologic therapy for edema. Loop diuretics are the most potent, followed by thiazide diuretics and then potassium-sparing diuretics.

TABLE 76-2	Drugs Used in Central and Nephrogenic Diabetes Insipidus	
Drug	**Indication**	**Dose**
Desmopressin acetate	Central and nephrogenic	5–20 mcg intranasally q12–24 hr
Chlorpropamide	Central	125–250 mg orally daily
Carbamazepine	Central	100–300 mg orally twice daily
Clofibrate	Central	500 mg orally four times daily
Hydrochlorothiazide	Central and nephrogenic	25 mg orally q12–24 hr
Amiloride	Nephrogenic	5–10 mg orally daily
Indomethacin	Central and nephrogenic	50 mg orally q8–12 hr

DISORDERS OF CALCIUM HOMEOSTASIS

- ECF calcium is moderately bound to plasma proteins (40%), primarily albumin. Ionized or free calcium is the physiologically active form that is homeostatically regulated.
- Each 1 g/dL (10 g/L) drop in serum albumin concentration less than 4 g/dL (40 g/L) decreases total serum calcium concentration by 0.8 mg/dL (0.20 mmol/L).

HYPERCALCEMIA (TOTAL SERUM CALCIUM >10.2 mg/dL [>2.55 mmol/L])

Pathophysiology and Clinical Presentation

- Cancer and hyperparathyroidism are the most common causes of hypercalcemia. Primary mechanisms include increased bone resorption, increased GI absorption, and increased tubular reabsorption by the kidneys.
- Clinical presentation depends on the degree of hypercalcemia and rate of onset. Mild-to-moderate hypercalcemia (serum calcium concentration <13 mg/dL [<3.25 mmol/L] or ionized calcium concentration <6 mg/dL [<1.50 mmol/L]) can be asymptomatic.
- Hypercalcemia of malignancy develops quickly and is associated with anorexia, nausea and vomiting, constipation, polyuria, polydipsia, and nocturia. Hypercalcemic crisis is characterized by acute elevation of serum calcium to greater than 15 mg/dL (>3.75 mmol/L), acute kidney injury, and obtundation. Untreated hypercalcemic crisis can progress to oliguric acute kidney injury, coma, and life-threatening ventricular arrhythmias.
- Chronic hypercalcemia (ie, hyperparathyroidism) is associated with metastatic calcification, hypercalciuria, and chronic kidney disease secondary to interstitial nephrocalcinosis.
- Electrocardiographic (ECG) changes include shortening of the QT interval and coving of the ST-T wave.

Treatment

- Treatment approach depends on the degree of hypercalcemia, acuity of onset, and presence of symptoms requiring emergent treatment (**Figure 76-2**).
- Management of asymptomatic, mild-to-moderate hypercalcemia begins with attention to the underlying condition and correction of fluid and electrolyte abnormalities.
- Hypercalcemic crisis and acute symptomatic hypercalcemia are medical emergencies requiring immediate treatment. Rehydration with normal saline followed by loop diuretics (eg, furosemide, bumetanide) can be used in patients with normal to moderately impaired renal function. Normalization of total calcium may be seen within 24–48 hours.
- Initiate treatment with **calcitonin** in patients in whom saline hydration is contraindicated (**Table 76-3**). Onset of action is seen within 1–2 hours; however, the degree and extent of calcium reduction is often unpredictable.
- **Bisphosphonates** (eg, **pamidronate** and **zoledronic acid**) are indicated for hypercalcemia of malignancy. Total serum calcium decline begins within 2 days and nadirs in 7 days. Duration of normocalcemia varies but usually does not exceed 2–3 weeks, depending on treatment response of underlying malignancy.
- **Denosumab** is a monoclonal antibody approved for treatment of hypercalcemia of malignancy in patients refractory to bisphosphonate therapy.
- **Prednisone** or an equivalent agent is usually effective by reducing GI calcium absorption when hypercalcemia results from multiple myeloma, leukemia, lymphoma, sarcoidosis, and hypervitaminoses A and D. Onset of action is relatively slow.
- **Cinacalcet** is approved for management of parathyroid carcinoma, primary hyperthyroidism where parathyroidectomy is indicated but cannot be undertaken, and secondary hyperparathyroidism in patients with chronic kidney disease on dialysis.

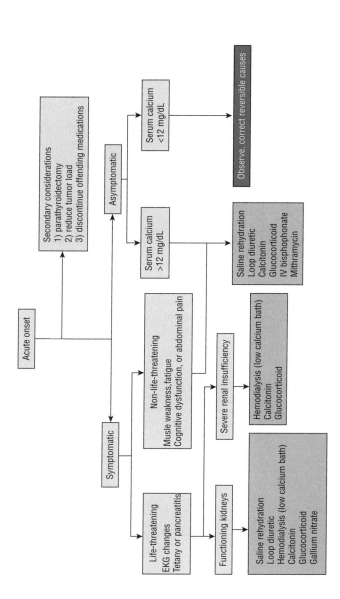

FIGURE 76-2. Pharmacotherapeutic options for the acutely hypercalcemic patient. Serum calcium of 12 mg/dL is equivalent to 3 mmol/L.

TABLE 76-3	Drug Dosing Table for Hypercalcemia		
Drug/ Brand Name	**Starting Dosage**	**Time Frame to Initial Response**	**Monitoring and Special Population Considerations**
0.9% saline ± electrolytes	200–300 mL/hr	24–48 hours	Electrolyte abnormalities, fluid overload, CI in advanced kidney disease, congestive heart failure
Loop diuretics Furosemide/ Lasix® Bumetandide/ Bumex® Torsemide/ Demadex®	40–80 mg IV q 1–4 hr of furosemide or equivalent	N/A	Electrolyte abnormalities (potassium and magnesium), CI in patients with allergy to sulfas (use ethacrynic acid)
Calcitonin/ Miacalcin®	4 units/kg q 12 hr SC/IM 10–12 units/hr IV	1–2 hours	Facial flushing, nausea/vomiting, allergic reaction, CI in patients with allergy to calcitonin
Pamidronate/ Aredia®	30–90 mg IV over 2–24 hours	2 days	Fever, fatigue, skeletal pain
Zoledronate/ Zometa®	4–8 mg IV over 15 minutes	1–2 days	Fever, fatigue, skeletal pain, CI in advanced kidney disease
Glucocorticoids	40–60 mg oral prednisone equivalents daily	3–5 days	Diabetes, osteoporosis, infection, CI in patients with serious infections, hypersensitivity

CI, contraindicated; SC, subcutaneous.

HYPOCALCEMIA (TOTAL SERUM CALCIUM <8.5 mg/dL [<2.13 mmol/L])

Pathophysiology

- Hypocalcemia results from altered effects of parathyroid hormone and vitamin D on the bone, gut, and kidney. Primary causes are postoperative hypoparathyroidism and vitamin D deficiency.
- Hypomagnesemia can be associated with severe symptomatic hypocalcemia that is unresponsive to calcium replacement therapy. Calcium normalization is dependent on magnesium replacement.

Clinical Presentation

- Clinical manifestations are variable and depend on the onset of hypocalcemia. Tetany is the hallmark sign of acute hypocalcemia, which manifests as paresthesias around the mouth and in the extremities; muscle spasms and cramps; carpopedal spasms; and, rarely, laryngospasm and bronchospasm.
- Cardiovascular manifestations result in ECG changes characterized by a prolonged QT interval and symptoms of decreased myocardial contractility often associated with CHF.

Treatment

- Acute, symptomatic hypocalcemia requires IV administration of soluble calcium salts (**Figure 76-3**). Initially, 100–300 mg of elemental calcium (eg, 1 g **calcium chloride**, 2–3 g **calcium gluconate**) should be given IV over 10–30 minutes (≤60 mg of elemental calcium per minute).

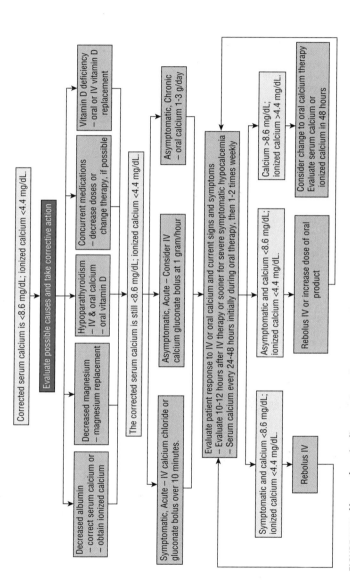

FIGURE 76-3. Hypocalcemia diagnostic and treatment algorithm. Serum calcium of 8.6 mg/dL is equivalent to 2.15 mmol/L. Ionized calcium of 4.4 mg/dL is equivalent to 1.1 mmol/L.

- The initial bolus dose is effective for only 1–2 hours; therefore, repeat doses should be given hourly as needed until severe, symptomatic patients are stabilized.
- Calcium gluconate is preferred over calcium chloride for peripheral administration because the latter is more irritating to veins.
- After acute hypocalcemia is corrected, the underlying cause and other electrolyte problems should be corrected. Magnesium supplementation is indicated for hypomagnesemia.
- Oral calcium supplementation (eg, 1–3 g/day of elemental calcium initially, then 2–8 g/day in divided doses) is indicated for chronic hypocalcemia due to hypoparathyroidism and vitamin D deficiency. If serum calcium does not normalize, add a vitamin D preparation.

DISORDERS OF PHOSPHORUS HOMEOSTASIS

HYPERPHOSPHATEMIA (SERUM PHOSPHORUS >4.5 mg/dL [>1.45 mmol/L])

Pathophysiology

- Most commonly caused by decreased phosphorus excretion, secondary to decreased glomerular filtration rate (GFR).
- Intracellular phosphate release can occur with rhabdomyolysis, hemolysis, and tumor lysis syndrome, a complication of chemotherapy associated with massive cell lysis with highest incidence in patients with acute leukemia and lymphoma.

Clinical Presentation

- Acute symptoms include nausea, vomiting, diarrhea, lethargy, obstruction of the urinary tract, and, rarely, seizures. Calcium phosphate crystals are likely to form when the product of the serum calcium and phosphate concentrations exceeds 50–60 mg^2/dL^2 (4–4.8 $mmol^2/L^2$).
- The major effect is related to the development of hypocalcemia and damage resulting from calcium phosphate crystal precipitation into soft tissues, intrarenal calcification, nephrolithiasis, or obstructive uropathy.
- For more information on hyperphosphatemia and renal failure, see Chapter 75.

Treatment

- The most effective way to treat nonemergent hyperphosphatemia is to decrease phosphate absorption from the GI tract with phosphate binders (see Chapter 75, Table 75-5).
- Severe symptomatic hyperphosphatemia manifesting as hypocalcemia and tetany is treated by the IV administration of calcium salts.

HYPOPHOSPHATEMIA (SERUM PHOSPHORUS <2.7 mg/dL [<0.9 mmol/L])

Pathophysiology

- Hypophosphatemia results from decreased GI absorption, reduced tubular reabsorption, or extracellular to intracellular redistribution.
- Hypophosphatemia is associated with chronic alcoholism, parenteral nutrition with inadequate phosphate supplementation, chronic ingestion of antacids, diabetic ketoacidosis, and prolonged hyperventilation.

Clinical Presentation

- Severe hypophosphatemia (serum phosphorus <1.5 mg/dL [<0.5 mmol/L]) has diverse clinical manifestations that affect many organ systems, including the following:
  - ✓ Neurologic manifestations: Progressive syndrome of irritability, apprehension, weakness, numbness, paresthesias, dysarthria, confusion, obtundation, seizures, and coma.

TABLE 76-4	Oral Phosphorus Replacement Therapy with Phosphate, Potassium, and Sodium Content Per Packet or Tablet		
Product	**Phosphate Content**	**Potassium Content**	**Sodium Content**
Packet			
Phos-NaK	250 mg (8 mmol)	280 mg (7.1 mEq)	160 mg (6.9 mEq)
Tablet			
Av-Phos 250 Neutral	250 mg (8 mmol)	45 mg (1.1 mEq)	298 mg (13 mEq)
K-Phos Neutral	250 mg (8 mmol)	45 mg (1.1 mEq)	298 mg (13 mEq)
K-Phos No. 2	250 mg (8 mmol)	88 mg (2.3 mEq)	134 mg (5.8 mEq)
Phospha 250 Neutral	250 mg (8 mmol)	45 mg (1.1 mEq)	298 mg (13 mEq)
Phospho-Trin 250 Neutral	250 mg (8 mmol)	45 mg (1.1 mEq)	298 mg (13 mEq)
Virt-Phos 250 Neutral	250 mg (8 mmol)	45 mg (1.1 mEq)	298 mg (13 mEq)

Phosphorus 31 mg = 1 mmol; potassium 39 mg = 1 mEq = 1 mmol; sodium 23 mg = 1 mEq = 1 mmol.

✓ Skeletal muscle dysfunction: Myalgia, bone pain, weakness, and potentially fatal rhabdomyolysis.
✓ Respiratory muscle weakness and diaphragmatic contractile dysfunction resulting in acute respiratory failure.
✓ Congestive cardiomyopathy, arrhythmias, hemolysis, and increased risk of infection can also occur.

- Chronic hypophosphatemia can cause osteopenia and osteomalacia because of enhanced osteoclastic resorption of bone.

Treatment

- Severe (<1.5 mg/dL; <0.5 mmol/L) or symptomatic hypophosphatemia should be treated with IV phosphorus replacement at a dose of 0.32–0.64 mmol/kg with normal kidney function. In critically ill trauma patients, doses up to 1 mmol/kg have been used.
- Asymptomatic patients or those who exhibit mild-to-moderate hypophosphatemia (1.5–2.7 mg/dL [0.5–0.9 mmol/L]) can be treated with oral phosphorus supplementation in doses of 1–2 g (32–64 mmol) daily in divided doses, with the goal of correcting serum phosphorus concentration in 7–10 days (Table 76-4).
- Monitor patients with frequent serum phosphorus and calcium determinations, especially if phosphorus is given IV or if renal dysfunction is present.

DISORDERS OF POTASSIUM HOMEOSTASIS

HYPOKALEMIA (SERUM POTASSIUM <3.5 mEq/L [mmol/L])

Pathophysiology

- Results from a total body potassium deficit or shifting of serum potassium into the intracellular compartment.
- Many drugs can cause hypokalemia (Table 76-5), and it is most commonly seen with use of loop and thiazide diuretics. Other causes of hypokalemia include diarrhea, vomiting, and hypomagnesemia.

TABLE 76-5	Mechanism of Drug-Induced Hypokalemia	
Transcellular Shift	**Enhanced Renal Excretion**	**Enhanced Fecal Elimination**
β_2-Receptor agonists	Diuretics	Laxatives
Epinephrine	Acetazolamide	Sodium polystyrene sulfonate
Albuterol	Thiazides	
Terbutaline	Indapamide	Phenolphthalein
Fomoterol	Metolazone	Sorbitol
Salmeterol	Furosemide	Patiromer
Isoproterenol	Torsemide	Sodium zirconium cyclosilicate
Ephedrine	Bumetanide	
Pseudoephedrine	Ethacrynic acid	
Tocolytic agents	High-dose penicillins	
Ritodrine	Nafcillin	
Nylidrin	Ampicillin	
Theophylline	Penicillin	
Levothyroxine	Mineralocorticoids	
Decongestants	Miscellaneous	
Caffeine	Aminoglycosides	
Insulin overdose	Amphotericin B	
Verapamil overdose	Cisplatin	
Barium overdose		

Clinical Presentation

- Signs and symptoms are nonspecific and variable and depend on the degree of hypo-kalemia and rapidity of onset. Mild hypokalemia is often asymptomatic.
- Cardiovascular manifestations include cardiac arrhythmias (eg, heart block, atrial flutter, paroxysmal atrial tachycardia, ventricular fibrillation, and digitalis-induced arrhythmias). In severe hypokalemia (serum concentration <2.5 mEq/L; mmol/L), ECG changes include ST-segment depression or flattening, T-wave inversion, and U-wave elevation.
- Moderate hypokalemia is associated with muscle weakness, cramping, malaise, and myalgias.

Treatment

- In general, every 1 mEq/L (mmol/L) decrease in potassium below 3.5 mEq/L (mmol/L) corresponds with a total body deficit of 100–400 mEq (mmol). To correct mild deficits, patients receiving chronic loop or thiazide diuretics generally need 40–100 mEq (mmol) of potassium.
- Whenever possible, potassium supplementation should be administered by mouth. Of the available salts, potassium chloride is most commonly used because it is the most effective for common causes of potassium depletion, use of diuretics, and with diarrhea.
- Limit IV administration to severe hypokalemia, patients exhibiting signs and symptoms such as ECG changes or muscle spasms, or inability to tolerate oral therapy. IV supplementation is more dangerous than oral therapy due to the potential for

hyperkalemia, phlebitis, and pain at the infusion site. Potassium should be administered in saline because dextrose can stimulate insulin secretion and worsen intracellular shifting of potassium. Generally, 10–20 mEq (mmol) of potassium is diluted in 100 mL of 0.9% NaCl and administered through a peripheral vein over 1 hour. ECG monitoring should be performed to detect cardiac changes.

HYPERKALEMIA (SERUM POTASSIUM >5 mEq/L [mmol/L])

Pathophysiology

- Hyperkalemia develops when potassium intake exceeds excretion or when the transcellular distribution of potassium is disturbed.
- Primary causes of true hyperkalemia include increased potassium intake, decreased potassium excretion, tubular unresponsiveness to aldosterone, and redistribution of potassium to the extracellular space.

Clinical Presentation

- Hyperkalemia is frequently asymptomatic; patients might complain of heart palpitations or skipped heartbeats.
- The earliest ECG change (serum potassium 5.5–6 mEq/L; mmol/L) is peaked T waves. The sequence of changes with further increases in serum potassium concentration is widening of the PR interval, loss of the P wave, widening of the QRS complex, and merging of the QRS complex with the T wave resulting in a sine-wave pattern.

Treatment

- Treatment depends on the desired rapidity and degree of lowering and the patient's clinical condition (**Figure 76-4, Table 76-6**).
- Calcium administration rapidly reverses ECG manifestations and arrhythmias, but it does not lower serum potassium concentrations. Calcium is short acting and therefore must be repeated if signs or symptoms recur.
- Rapid correction of hyperkalemia requires administration of drugs that shift potassium intracellularly (eg, insulin and dextrose, sodium bicarbonate, or albuterol).
- **Sodium polystyrene sulfonate** is a cation-exchange resin suitable for asymptomatic patients with mild-to-moderate hyperkalemia. Each gram of resin exchanges 1 mEq (1 mmol) of sodium for 1 mEq (1 mmol) of potassium. The sorbitol component promotes excretion of exchanged potassium by inducing diarrhea. The oral route is better tolerated and more effective than the rectal route.

DISORDERS OF MAGNESIUM HOMEOSTASIS

HYPOMAGNESEMIA (SERUM MAGNESIUM <1.4 mEq/L [<1.7 mg/dL; <0.70 mmol/L])

Pathophysiology

- Hypomagnesemia is usually associated with disorders of the intestinal tract or kidneys. Drugs (eg, aminoglycosides, amphotericin B, cyclosporine, diuretics, digitalis, and cisplatin) or conditions that interfere with intestinal absorption or increase renal excretion of magnesium can cause hypomagnesemia.
- Commonly associated with alcoholism.

Clinical Presentation

- Although typically asymptomatic, the dominant organ systems involved are the neuromuscular and cardiovascular systems. Symptoms include heart palpitations, tetany, twitching, and generalized convulsions.
- Ventricular arrhythmias are the most important and potentially life-threatening cardiovascular effect.

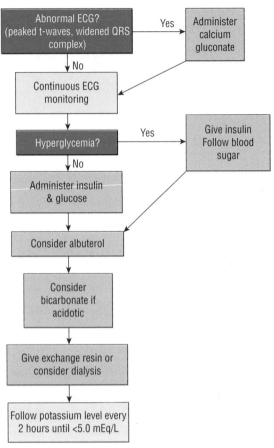

FIGURE 76-4. Treatment approach for hyperkalemia. Serum potassium of 5.0 mEq/L is equivalent to 5.0 mmol/L.

- ECG changes include widened QRS complexes and peaked T waves in mild deficiency. Prolonged PR intervals, progressive widening of the QRS complexes, and flattening of T waves occur in moderate-to-severe deficiency.
- Many electrolyte disturbances occur with hypomagnesemia, including hypokalemia and hypocalcemia.

Treatment

- The severity of magnesium depletion and the presence of symptoms dictate the route of magnesium supplementation. Intramuscular magnesium is painful and should be reserved for patients with severe hypomagnesemia and limited venous access. IV bolus injection is associated with flushing, sweating, and a sensation of warmth.
- The optimal oral magnesium regimen is unknown; 8–12 g of magnesium sulfate in divided doses over 24 hours followed by 4–6 g/day for 3–5 days is one widely accepted regimen when the serum magnesium concentration is greater than 1 mEq/L (1.2 mg/dL [0.5 mmol/L]). Sustained-release products are preferred due to improved patient compliance and less GI side effects (eg, diarrhea).

TABLE 76-6 Therapeutic Alternatives for the Management of Hyperkalemia

Medication	Dose	Route of Administration	Onset/Duration of Action	Acuity	Mechanism of Action	Expected Result
Calcium	1 g	IV over 5–10 minutes	1–2 minutes/10–30 minutes	Acute	Raises cardiac threshold potential	Reverses electrocardiographic effects
Furosemide	20–40 mg	IV	5–15 minutes/4–6 hours	Acute	Inhibits renal Na^+ reabsorption	Increased urinary K^+ loss
Regular insulin	5–10 units	IV or SC	30 minutes/2–6 hours	Acute	Stimulates intracellular K^+ uptake	Intracellular K^+ redistribution
Dextrose 10%	1000 mL (100 g)	IV over 1–2 hours	30 minutes/2–6 hours	Acute	Stimulates insulin release	Intracellular K^+ redistribution
Dextrose 50%	50 mL (25 g)	IV over 5 minutes	30 minutes/2–6 hours	Acute	Stimulates insulin release	Intracellular K^+ redistribution
Sodium bicarbonate	50–100 mEq (50–100 mmol)	IV over 2–5 minutes	30 minutes/2–6 hours	Acute	Raises serum pH	Intracellular K^+ redistribution
Albuterol	10–20 mg	Nebulized over 10 minutes	30 minutes/1–2 hours	Acute	Stimulates intracellular K^+ uptake	Intracellular K^+ redistribution
Hemodialysis	4 hours	N/A	Immediate/variable	Acute	Removal from serum	Increased K^+ elimination
Sodium polystyrene sulfonate	15–60 g	Oral or rectal	1 hour/variable	Nonacute	Resin exchanges Na^+ for K^+	Increased K^+ elimination
Patiromer	8.4–25.2 g	Oral	Hours/variable	Nonacute	Resin exchanges Ca^{++} for K^+	Increased K^+ elimination
Sodium zirconium cyclosilicate	5–15 g	Oral	1 hour/variable	Nonacute	Resin exchanges Na^+ for K^+	Increased K^+ elimination

- Administer IV magnesium if serum concentrations are less than 1 mEq/L (<1.2 mg/dL [<0.5 mmol/L]) or if signs and symptoms are present regardless of serum concentration. Infuse 4–6 g of magnesium over 12–24 hours and repeat as needed to maintain serum concentrations above 1 mEq/L (1.2 mg/dL [0.5 mmol/L]). Continue until signs and symptoms resolve. Reduce magnesium dose by 25%–50% with renal insufficiency.

HYPERMAGNESEMIA (SERUM MAGNESIUM >1.8 mEq/L [>2.3 mg/dL; >0.9 mmol/L])

Pathophysiology

- Magnesium concentrations steadily increase as the GFR decreases below 30 mL/min/1.73 m^2 and is generally associated with advanced CKD.
- Other causes include magnesium-containing antacids in patients with renal insufficiency, enteral or parenteral nutrition in patients with multiorgan system failure, magnesium for treatment of eclampsia, lithium therapy, hypothyroidism, and Addison disease.

Clinical Presentation

- Symptoms are rare when the serum magnesium concentration is less than 4 mEq/L (<4.9 mg/dL [<2 mmol/L]).
- The sequence of neuromuscular signs as serum magnesium increases from 5 to 12 mEq/L (6.1–14.7 mg/dL [2.5–6 mmol/L]) is sedation, hypotonia, hyporeflexia, somnolence, coma, muscular paralysis, and, ultimately, respiratory depression.
- The sequence of cardiovascular signs as serum magnesium increases from 3 to 15 mEq/L (3.7–18.4 mg/dL [1.5–7.5 mmol/L]) is hypotension, cutaneous vasodilation, QT-interval prolongation, bradycardia, primary heart block, nodal rhythms, bundle branch block, QRS- and then PR-interval prolongation, complete heart block, and asystole.

Treatment

- IV calcium (100–200 mg of elemental calcium; eg, calcium gluconate 2 g IV) is indicated to antagonize the neuromuscular and cardiovascular effects of magnesium. Doses should be repeated as often as hourly in life-threatening situations.
- Forced diuresis with 0.45% NaCl and loop diuretics (eg, furosemide, 40 mg IV) can promote magnesium elimination in patients with normal renal function or stage 1, 2, or 3 CKD. In dialysis patients, change to a magnesium-free dialysate.

EVALUATION OF THERAPEUTIC OUTCOMES

- The primary end point for monitoring treatment of fluid and electrolyte disorders is the correction of the abnormal serum electrolyte. In general, monitoring is initially performed at frequent intervals and, as homeostasis is restored, subsequently performed at less frequent intervals.
- Monitor all electrolytes as individual electrolyte abnormalities typically coexist with another abnormality (eg, hypomagnesemia with hypokalemia and hypocalcemia, or hyperphosphatemia with hypocalcemia).
- Monitor patients for resolution of clinical manifestations of electrolyte disturbances and for treatment-related complications.

See Chapter 66, Disorders of Sodium and Water Homeostasis, authored by Katherine H. Chessman and Jason Haney; Chapter 67, Disorders of Calcium and Phosphorus Homeostasis, authored by Amy Barton Pai and Angela L. Bingham; and Chapter 68, Disorders of Potassium and Magnesium Homeostasis, authored by Rachel W. Flurie, for a more detailed discussion of this topic.

CHAPTER 77

Allergic Rhinitis

- *Allergic rhinitis* involves inflammation of nasal mucous membranes in sensitized individuals when inhaled allergenic particles contact mucous membranes and elicit a response mediated by immunoglobulin E (IgE). There are two types: seasonal and persistent (formerly called "perennial") allergic rhinitis.

PATHOPHYSIOLOGY

- Airborne allergens enter the nose during inhalation and are processed by lymphocytes, which produce antigen-specific IgE, sensitizing genetically predisposed hosts to those agents. On nasal reexposure, IgE bound to mast cells interacts with airborne allergens, triggering release of inflammatory mediators.
- An immediate reaction occurs within seconds to minutes, resulting in rapid release of preformed and newly generated mediators from the arachidonic acid cascade. Mediators of immediate hypersensitivity include histamine, leukotrienes, prostaglandin, tryptase, and kinins. These mediators cause vasodilation, increased vascular permeability, and production of nasal secretions. Histamine produces rhinorrhea, itching, sneezing, and nasal obstruction.
- A late-phase reaction may occur 4–8 hours after initial allergen exposure due to cytokine release from mast cells and thymus-derived helper lymphocytes. This inflammatory response causes persistent chronic symptoms, including nasal congestion.

CLINICAL PRESENTATION

- Seasonal (hay fever) allergic rhinitis occurs in response to specific allergens (eg, pollen from trees, grasses, and weeds) present at predictable times of the year (spring and/or fall) and typically causes more acute symptoms.
- Persistent allergic rhinitis occurs year-round in response to nonseasonal allergens (eg, dust mites, animal dander, molds) and typically results in less variable, chronic symptoms.
- Many patients have a combination of both types, with symptoms year-round and seasonal exacerbations.
- Symptoms include clear rhinorrhea, sneezing, nasal congestion, postnasal drip, allergic conjunctivitis, and pruritic eyes, ears, or nose.
- In children, physical examination may reveal dark circles under the eyes (allergic shiners), a transverse nasal crease caused by repeated rubbing of the nose, adenoidal breathing, edematous nasal turbinates coated with clear secretions, tearing, and periorbital swelling.
- Patients may complain of loss of smell or taste, with sinusitis or polyps the underlying cause in many cases. Postnasal drip with cough or hoarseness can be bothersome.
- Untreated rhinitis symptoms may lead to disturbed sleep, malaise, fatigue, and poor work or school performance.
- Allergic rhinitis is associated with other conditions, including asthma, chronic rhinosinusitis, otitis media, nasal polyposis, respiratory infections, and dental malocclusions.
- Complications include recurrent and chronic sinusitis and epistaxis.

DIAGNOSIS

- Medical history includes careful description of symptoms, environmental factors and exposures, results of previous therapy, use of medications, previous nasal injury or surgery, and family history.
- Allergy testing can help determine whether rhinitis is caused by immune response to allergens. Immediate-type hypersensitivity skin tests are commonly used. Percutaneous testing is safer and more generally accepted than intradermal testing, which is usually reserved for patients requiring confirmation. The radioallergosorbent test (RAST) can detect IgE antibodies in the blood that are highly specific for a given antigen, but it may be slightly less sensitive than percutaneous tests.

TREATMENT

- <u>Goals of Treatment</u>: Minimize or prevent symptoms, prevent long-term complications, avoid or minimize medication side effects, provide economical therapy, and maintain normal lifestyle.
- **Figure 77-1** depicts a treatment algorithm for allergic rhinitis.

NONPHARMACOLOGIC THERAPY

- Avoiding offending allergens is important but difficult to accomplish, especially for perennial allergens. Mold growth can be reduced by keeping household humidity below 50% and removing obvious growth with bleach or disinfectant.
- Patients sensitive to animals benefit most by removing pets from the home, if feasible. Reducing exposure to dust mites by washing bedding on a hot cycle, replacing carpets with hard flooring, and using vacuum cleaners with HEPA filters has not been shown to provide a clinical benefit. Only encasing bedding in impermeable covers has some clinical benefit in children but not adults.
- Steps to prevent poor air quality in homes include avoiding wall-to-wall carpeting, using moisture control to prevent mold accumulation, and controlling sources of pollution such as cigarette smoke.
- Patients with seasonal allergic rhinitis should keep windows closed and minimize time spent outdoors during pollen seasons. Filter masks can be worn while gardening or mowing the lawn.
- Nasal saline irrigations may improve nasal symptoms and reduce medicine consumption. Adhesive nasal strips can facilitate breathing and reduce nasal obstruction.

PHARMACOLOGIC THERAPY

Antihistamines

- Histamine H_1-receptor antagonists bind to H_1 receptors without activating them, preventing histamine binding and action. They are effective in preventing the histamine response but not in reversing its effects after they have occurred. Antihistamines antagonize increased capillary permeability, wheal-and-flare formation, and itching.
- *Oral antihistamines* are divided into two categories: (1) nonselective (first-generation or sedating antihistamines) and (2) peripherally selective (second-generation or nonsedating antihistamines). However, individual agents should be judged on their specific sedating effects because variation exists among agents within these categories (**Table 77-1**).
- Antihistamines help control symptoms of sneezing, rhinorrhea, itching, and conjunctivitis. Symptom relief is caused in part by an anticholinergic drying effect that reduces nasal, salivary, and lacrimal gland hypersecretion.
- Antihistamines are only fully effective when taken 1–2 hours before anticipated exposure to the offending allergen. For seasonal allergic rhinitis, start treatment before the expected allergy season begins. Guidelines recommend that nonsedating agents be tried first, but tolerance to sedation from first-generation agents can develop after 4 days of treatment. If nonsedating agents are ineffective or too expensive,

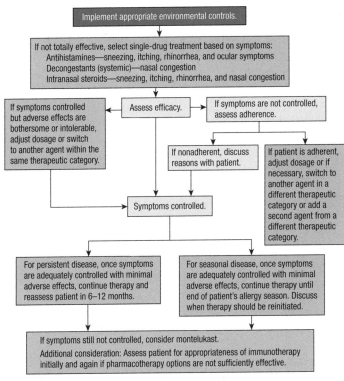

FIGURE 77-1. Treatment algorithm for allergic rhinitis.

first-generation agents may be used. For persistent allergic rhinitis, use an intranasal corticosteroid as an alternative to or in combination with systemic antihistamines.

- Drowsiness is the most frequent antihistamine side effect, and it can interfere with driving ability or adequate functioning. Sedative effects can be beneficial in patients who have difficulty sleeping because of rhinitis symptoms.
- Adverse anticholinergic such as dry mouth, difficulty in voiding urine, constipation, and cardiovascular effects may occur (Table 77-1). Antihistamines should be used with caution in patients predisposed to urinary retention and in those with increased intraocular pressure, hyperthyroidism, and cardiovascular disease.
- Other side effects include loss of appetite, nausea, vomiting, and epigastric distress. Taking medication with meals or a full glass of water may prevent gastrointestinal (GI) side effects.
- Table 77-2 lists recommended doses of oral agents.
- *Intranasal antihistamines*: **Azelastine** is a prescription-only intranasal antihistamine that relieves sneezing, rhinorrhea, and nasal pruritus of seasonal allergic rhinitis. The 0.1% product can be used in children for seasonal allergies, whereas the 0.15% product is labeled only for adults with either type of allergic rhinitis. However, guidelines favor use of intranasal antihistamines for seasonal but not persistent allergic rhinitis. Caution patients about the potential for drowsiness because systemic availability is ~40%. Patients may also experience drying effects, headache, and diminished effectiveness over time. **Olopatadine** is another intranasal antihistamine; it may cause less drowsiness because it is a selective H_1-receptor antagonist.

TABLE 77-1	Relative Adverse-Effect Profiles of Antihistamines	
Medications	**Relative Sedative Effects**	**Relative Anticholinergic Effects**
Alkylamine class, nonselective		
Brompheniramine maleate	Low	Moderate
Chlorpheniramine maleate	Low	Moderate
Dexchlorpheniramine maleate	Low	Moderate
Ethanolamine class, nonselective		
Carbinoxamine maleate	High	High
Clemastine fumarate	Moderate	High
Diphenhydramine hydrochloride	High	High
Phenothiazine class, nonselective		
Promethazine hydrochloride	High	High
Piperidine class, nonselective		
Cyproheptadine hydrochloride	Low	Moderate
Phthalazinone class, peripherally selective		
Azelastine (nasal only)	Low to none	Low to none
Bepotastine (ophthalmic only)	Low to none	Low to none
Piperazine class, peripherally selective		
Cetirizine	Low to moderate	Low to none
Levocetirizine	Low to moderate	Low to none
Piperidine class, peripherally selective		
Desloratadine	Low to none	Low to none
Fexofenadine	Low to none	Low to none
Loratadine	Low to none	Low to none
Olopatadine (nasal only)	Low to none	Low to none

- *Ophthalmic antihistamines*: **Levocabastine**, **olopatadine**, and **bepotastine** are ophthalmic antihistamines that can be used for conjunctivitis associated with allergic rhinitis. Systemic antihistamines are also usually effective for allergic conjunctivitis. Ophthalmic agents are a useful addition to nasal corticosteroids for ocular symptoms.

Decongestants

- Topical and systemic decongestants are sympathomimetic agents that act on adrenergic receptors in nasal mucosa to produce vasoconstriction, shrink swollen mucosa, and improve ventilation. They should only be used when nasal congestion is present. Decongestants work well in combination with antihistamines when nasal congestion is present.
- Topical decongestants are applied directly to swollen nasal mucosa via drops or sprays (Table 77-3). They result in little or no systemic absorption.
- Treatment should not exceed 3–5 days to avoid rhinitis medicamentosa (rebound vasodilation with congestion). Patients with this condition use more spray more often with less response. Abrupt cessation is an effective treatment, but rebound congestion may last for several days or weeks. Nasal corticosteroids have been used successfully

TABLE 77-2	Medication Dosing for Allergic Rhinitis		
Drugs	**Brand Names**	**Dosage for Adolescents[a] and Adults**	**Recommended Pediatric Doses**
Antihistamines			
Oral			
Nonselective			
Chlorpheniramine maleate	Various	Plain: 4 mg every 6 hours	6–11 years: 2 mg every 4–6 hours
		Extended release: 12 mg every 12 hours	2–5 years: 1 mg every 4–6 hours
Clemastine fumarate	Tavist	1.34 mg (1 mg base) twice daily, up to 2.68 mg 3 times daily; max. 8.04 mg/day (6 mg base/day)	6–11 years: syrup 0.67 mg (0.5 mg base) twice daily; max. 4.02 mg/day (3 mg base/day)
Diphenhydramine HCl	Benadryl, others	25–50 mg every 4–6 hours (max. 300 mg/day)	6–11 years: 12.5–25 mg every 4–6 hours; max. 150 mg/day
Peripherally selective			
Loratadine	Alavert, Claritin	10 mg once daily	6–12 years: 10 mg once daily or 5 mg twice daily
			2–5 years: 5 mg once daily
Fexofenadine	Allegra	60 mg every 12 hours or 180 mg once daily	2–11 years: 30 mg once daily
Cetirizine	Zyrtec	5–10 mg once daily	6–11 years: 5–10 mg once daily
			6 mo. to 5 years: 2.5 mg once daily
Levocetirizine	Xyzal	5 mg once daily (in the evening)	6–11 years: 2.5 mg once daily (in the evening)
			6 months–5 years: 1.25 mg once daily (in the evening)
Nasal			
Azelastine	Astelin, Astepro	1–2 sprays per nostril once or twice daily	2–11 years: 1 spray per nostril twice daily
Olopatadine	Patanase	Two sprays per nostril twice daily	6–11: 1 spray per nostril twice daily

(*Continued*)

TABLE 77-2	Medication Dosing for Allergic Rhinitis (Continued)		
Drugs	**Brand Names**	**Dosage for Adolescents[a] and Adults**	**Recommended Pediatric Doses**
Ophthalmic			
Bepotastine	Bepreve	1 drop into the affected eye(s) twice daily	2–11 years: 1 drop into the affected eye(s) twice daily
Levocabastine	Livostin	1 drop into the affected eye(s) 4 times daily	(Safety and efficacy not established)
Olopatadine	Patanol	1 drop into the affected eye(s) twice daily at intervals of 6–8 hours	3–11 years: 1 drop into the affected eye(s) twice daily at intervals of 6–8 hours
Decongestants			
Oral			
Pseudoephedrine	Various	60 mg every 4–6 hours Sustained release: 120 mg every 12 hours Controlled release: 240 mg once daily	6–11 years: 30 mg every 4–6 hours 2–5 years: 15 mg every 4–6 hours
Phenylephrine	Various	0–20 mg every 4 hours	6–11 years: 5 mg every 4 hours 2–5 years: 2.5 mg every 4 hours
Nasal			
Oxymetazoline	Various	2–3 sprays twice daily	6–11 years: 2–3 sprays twice daily
Phenylephrine	Various	2–3 sprays every 4 hours (0.25%–1%)	6–11 years: 2–3 sprays every 4 hours (0.25%) 2–5 years: 2–3 sprays every 4 hours (0.125%)
Nasal corticosteroids			
Beclomethasone	Beconase AQ	1–2 sprays in each nostril twice daily	6–11 years: 1 spray in each nostril twice daily
	Qnasl	2 sprays in each nostril once daily	4–11 years: 1 spray in each nostril once daily
Budesonide	Rhinocort Aqua	1 spray in each nostril once daily	6–11 years: 1 spray in each nostril once daily
Flunisolide	Various	Two sprays in each nostril twice daily	6–14 years: 2 sprays in each nostril twice daily

(Continued)

TABLE 77-2	Medication Dosing for Allergic Rhinitis (Continued)		
Drugs	Brand Names	Dosage for Adolescents[a] and Adults	Recommended Pediatric Doses
Fluticasone	Flonase	1–2 sprays in each nostril daily once daily	2–11 years: 1 spray in each nostril once daily
Mometasone	Veramyst, Nasonex, Nasacort	2 sprays in each nostril once daily	2–11 years: 1 spray in each nostril once daily
Triamcinolone	Nasacort AQ	2 sprays in each nostril once daily	2–11 years: 1 spray in each nostril once daily
Other nasal medications			
Cromolyn	Nasalcrom	1 spray in each nostril 3–4 times daily	2–11 years: 1 spray in each nostril 3–4 times daily
Ipratropium	Atrovent	2 sprays in each nostril 4 times daily	5–11 years: 2 sprays in each nostril 4 times daily
Leukotriene receptor antagonist			
Montelukast	Singulair	10 mg orally once daily	6–14 years: 5 mg chewable tablet once daily
			2–5 years: 4 mg chewable tablet or oral granules once daily
			6–23 months: 4 mg oral granules once daily

[a]Adolescent age is ≥12 years except for flunisolide and montelukast (≥15 years).

TABLE 77-3	Duration of Action of Topical Decongestants
Medications	**Durations of Action (hours)**
Short acting	
Phenylephrine hydrochloride	Up to 4
Intermediate acting	
Naphazoline hydrochloride	2–6
Tetrahydrozoline hydrochloride	
Long acting	
Oxymetazoline hydrochloride	Up to 12
Xylometazoline hydrochloride	

but take several days to work. Weaning off the topical decongestant can be accomplished by decreasing dosing frequency or concentration over several weeks. Combining the weaning process with nasal corticosteroids may be helpful.

- Other adverse effects of topical decongestants are burning, stinging, sneezing, and dryness of the nasal mucosa.
- These products should be used only when absolutely necessary (eg, at bedtime) and in doses that are as small and infrequent as possible. Duration of therapy should be limited to 3 days or less.
- **Pseudoephedrine** (Table 77-2) is an oral decongestant that has a slower onset of action than topical agents but may last longer and cause less local irritation. Rhinitis medicamentosa does not occur with oral decongestants. Doses up to 180 mg produce no measurable change in blood pressure or heart rate. However, higher doses (210–240 mg) may raise both blood pressure and heart rate. Systemic decongestants should be avoided in hypertensive patients unless absolutely necessary. Severe hypertensive reactions can occur when pseudoephedrine is given with monoamine oxidase inhibitors. Pseudoephedrine can cause mild CNS stimulation, even at therapeutic doses. Because of misuse as a component in the illegal manufacture of methamphetamine, pseudoephedrine is restricted to behind-the-counter sale with a limit on monthly purchases.
- **Phenylephrine** has replaced pseudoephedrine in many nonprescription antihistamine–decongestant combination products because of legal restrictions on pseudoephedrine sales.
- Combination oral products containing a decongestant and antihistamine are rational because of different mechanisms of action. However, antihistamines must be taken on a regular schedule, but decongestants should only be used when needed. Consumers should read product labels carefully to avoid therapeutic duplication and use combination products only for short courses.

Nasal Corticosteroids

- Intranasal corticosteroids reduce inflammation by reducing mediator release, suppressing neutrophil chemotaxis, reducing intracellular edema, causing mild vasoconstriction, and inhibiting mast cell–mediated, late-phase reactions.
- They relieve sneezing, rhinorrhea, itching, and nasal congestion (Table 77-2). Blocked nasal passages should be cleared with a decongestant or saline irrigation before administration to ensure adequate penetration of the spray. Advise patients to avoid sneezing or blowing their nose for at least 10 minutes after administration. Some patients improve within a few days, but peak response may require 2–3 weeks. The dosage may be reduced once a response is achieved.
- These agents are an excellent choice for persistent rhinitis and can also be excellent for seasonal rhinitis, especially if begun before exposure and the onset of symptoms. Recent guidelines suggest that nasal corticosteroids should be recommended as initial therapy for allergic rhinitis.
- Side effects are minimal and include sneezing, stinging, headache, epistaxis, and rare infections with *Candida albicans*.

Cromolyn Sodium

- **Cromolyn sodium**, a mast cell stabilizer, is available as a nonprescription nasal spray for symptomatic prevention and treatment of allergic rhinitis. It prevents antigen-triggered mast cell degranulation and release of mediators, including histamine. The most common side effect is local irritation (sneezing and nasal stinging).
- Nasal passages should be cleared before administration, and inhaling gently through the nose during administration enhances distribution to the entire nasal lining. Dosing must be repeated at 6-hour intervals to maintain the effect (Table 77-2).
- For seasonal rhinitis, treatment should be initiated just before the start of the offending allergen's season and continue throughout the season.

- In persistent rhinitis, improvement may not be seen for 2–4 weeks; antihistamines or decongestants may be needed during this initial phase of therapy.

Ipratropium Bromide

- **Ipratropium bromide** nasal spray is an anticholinergic agent that exhibits antisecretory properties when applied locally. It provides symptomatic relief of rhinorrhea associated with allergic and other forms of chronic rhinitis.
- It is not included in current treatment guidelines for allergic rhinitis and should be reserved for patients who fail or cannot tolerate other therapies. The optimal dose should be determined based on the specific patient's symptoms and response.
- Adverse effects are mild and include headache, epistaxis, and nasal dryness.

Montelukast

- **Montelukast** is a leukotriene receptor antagonist approved for treatment of persistent allergic rhinitis in children as young as 6 months and for seasonal allergic rhinitis in children as young as 2 years (Table 77-2).
- Montelukast is a third-line choice after antihistamines and nasal corticosteroids. Monotherapy is no more effective than peripherally selective antihistamines and is less effective than intranasal corticosteroids; however, the combination of montelukast and an antihistamine is more effective than an antihistamine alone. Montelukast monotherapy has been recommended for children with mild persistent asthma and coexisting allergic rhinitis.

Immunotherapy

- Immunotherapy is the process of administering doses of antigens responsible for eliciting allergic symptoms into a patient with the intent of inducing tolerance to the allergen when natural exposure occurs. Until recently, immunotherapy was only available for subcutaneous injection; sublingual dosage forms are now available for a limited number of allergens.
- Beneficial effects of immunotherapy may result from induction of IgG-blocking antibodies, reduction in specific IgE (long-term), reduced recruitment of effector cells, altered T-cell cytokine balance, T-cell anergy, and alteration of regulatory T cell activity.
- Good candidates for immunotherapy include patients with a strong history of severe symptoms unsuccessfully controlled by avoidance and pharmacotherapy and patients unable to tolerate adverse effects of drug therapy. Poor candidates include patients with medical conditions that compromise the ability to tolerate an anaphylactic-type reaction, patients with impaired immune systems, and patients with a history of nonadherence.
- For subcutaneous immunotherapy, very dilute solutions are given initially once or twice weekly. The concentration is increased until the maximum tolerated dose or highest planned dose is achieved. This maintenance dose is continued in slowly increasing intervals over several years, depending on clinical response. Better results are obtained with year-round rather than seasonal injections.
- Sublingual immunotherapy is available for ragweed, certain grasses, and house dust mite allergen. Ragweed and grass allergens are started 12 weeks before the allergen season and continued throughout the season. Because house dust mites cause persistent allergic rhinitis, this treatment is given year-round. The first dose is administered in the physician's office to allow observation of the patient for 30 minutes for hypersensitivity reactions. The patient places the tablet under the tongue where it dissolves; patients should not swallow for at least 1 minute. After the first dose is administered without incident, patients can take sublingual immunotherapy at home, but an auto-injectable epinephrine must be prescribed and available for immediate use.
- Adverse reactions with subcutaneous immunotherapy include mild induration and swelling at the injection site. More severe reactions (generalized urticaria, bronchospasm, laryngospasm, vascular collapse, and death from anaphylaxis) occur rarely.

Severe reactions are treated with epinephrine, antihistamines, and systemic corticosteroids. The most common reactions with sublingual immunotherapy are pruritus of the mouth, ears, and tongue; throat irritation; and mouth edema. Sublingual immunotherapy is only approved for persons age 18 year and older.

EVALUATION OF THERAPEUTIC OUTCOMES

- Monitor patients regularly for reduction in severity of identified target symptoms and presence of side effects.
- Ask patients about their satisfaction with the management of their allergic rhinitis. Management should result in minimal disruption to their normal lifestyle.
- The Medical Outcomes Study 36-Item Short Form Health Survey and the Rhinoconjunctivitis Quality of Life Questionnaire measure symptom improvement and parameters such as sleep quality, nonallergic symptoms (eg, fatigue and poor concentration), emotions, and participation in a variety of activities.

See Chapter e13, Allergic Rhinitis, authored by J. Russell May, for a more detailed discussion of this topic.

CHAPTER 78

Asthma

- *Asthma* is defined by the Global Initiative for Asthma (GINA) as a heterogeneous disease usually characterized by chronic airway inflammation. It is defined by a history of respiratory symptoms such as wheezing, shortness of breath, chest tightness, and cough that vary over time and in intensity, together with variable expiratory airflow limitation.

PATHOPHYSIOLOGY

- There is a variable degree of airflow obstruction (related to smooth muscle bronchospasm, edema, and mucus hypersecretion), bronchial hyperresponsiveness (BHR), and airway inflammation.
- In acute inflammation, inhaled allergens in allergic patients cause early-phase allergic reaction with activation of cells bearing allergen-specific immunoglobulin E (IgE) antibodies. After rapid activation, airway mast cells and macrophages release proinflammatory mediators such as histamine and eicosanoids that induce contraction of airway smooth muscle, mucus secretion, edema, and exudation of plasma in the airways. Plasma protein leakage induces a thickened, engorged, edematous airway wall and narrowing of lumen with reduced mucus clearance.
- Late-phase inflammatory reaction occurs 6–9 hours after allergen provocation and involves recruitment and activation of eosinophils, T lymphocytes, basophils, neutrophils, and macrophages. Eosinophils migrate to airways and release inflammatory mediators.
- T-lymphocyte activation leads to release of cytokines from type 2 T-helper (TH$_2$) cells that mediate allergic inflammation (interleukin [IL]-4, IL-5, and IL-13). Conversely, type 1 T-helper (TH$_1$) cells produce IL-2 and interferon-γ that are essential for cellular defense mechanisms. Allergic asthmatic inflammation may result from imbalance between TH$_1$ and TH$_2$ cells.
- Mast cell degranulation results in release of mediators such as histamine; eosinophil and neutrophil chemotactic factors; leukotrienes C$_4$, D$_4$, and E$_4$; prostaglandins; and platelet-activating factor (PAF). Histamine can induce smooth muscle constriction and bronchospasm and may contribute to mucosal edema and mucus secretion.
- Alveolar macrophages release inflammatory mediators, including proinflammatory and anti-inflammatory cytokines, reactive oxygen species, and eicosanoids. Production of neutrophil chemotactic factor and eosinophil chemotactic factor furthers the inflammatory process. Neutrophils also release mediators (PAFs, prostaglandins, thromboxanes, and leukotrienes) that contribute to BHR and airway inflammation. Leukotrienes C$_4$, D$_4$, and E$_4$ are released during inflammatory processes in the lung and produce bronchospasm, mucus secretion, microvascular permeability, and airway edema.
- Bronchial epithelial cells participate in inflammation by releasing eicosanoids, peptidases, matrix proteins, cytokines, and nitric oxide. Epithelial shedding results in heightened airway responsiveness, altered permeability of airway mucosa, depletion of epithelial-derived relaxant factors, and loss of enzymes responsible for degrading inflammatory neuropeptides. The exudative inflammatory process and sloughing of epithelial cells into the airway lumen impair mucociliary transport. Bronchial glands increase in size, and goblet cells increase in size and number.
- The airway is innervated by parasympathetic, sympathetic, and nonadrenergic inhibitory nerves. Normal resting tone of airway smooth muscle is maintained by vagal efferent activity, and bronchoconstriction can be mediated by vagal stimulation in small bronchi. Airway smooth muscle contains noninnervated β_2-adrenergic receptors that produce bronchodilation. The nonadrenergic, noncholinergic (NANC) nervous system in the trachea and bronchi may amplify inflammation by releasing nitric oxide.

CLINICAL PRESENTATION

CHRONIC ASTHMA

- Symptoms include episodes of shortness of breath, chest tightness, coughing (particularly at night), wheezing, or a whistling sound when breathing. These often occur with exercise but may occur spontaneously or in association with known allergens.
- Signs include expiratory wheezing (rhonchi) on auscultation; dry, hacking cough; and atopy (eg, allergic rhinitis or atopic dermatitis).
- Asthma can vary from chronic daily symptoms to only intermittent symptoms. Intervals between symptoms may be days, weeks, months, or years.
- Severity is determined by lung function, symptoms, nighttime awakenings, and interference with normal activity prior to therapy. Patients can present with mild intermittent symptoms that require no medications or only occasional short-acting inhaled β_2-agonists (SABAs) to severe chronic symptoms despite multiple medications.

ACUTE SEVERE ASTHMA

- Uncontrolled asthma can progress to an acute state in which inflammation, airway edema, mucus accumulation, and severe bronchospasm result in profound airway narrowing that is poorly responsive to bronchodilator therapy.
- Patients may be anxious in acute distress and complain of severe dyspnea, shortness of breath, chest tightness, or burning. They may be able to say only a few words with each breath. Symptoms are unresponsive to usual measures (ie, SABAs).
- Signs include expiratory and inspiratory wheezing on auscultation; dry, hacking cough; tachypnea; tachycardia; pallor or cyanosis; and hyperinflated chest with intercostal and supraclavicular retractions. Breath sounds may be diminished with severe obstruction.

DIAGNOSIS

CHRONIC ASTHMA

- Diagnosis is made primarily by history of recurrent episodes of coughing, wheezing, chest tightness, or shortness of breath and confirmatory spirometry.
- Patients may have family history of allergy or asthma or symptoms of allergic rhinitis or atopic dermatitis. History of exercise or cold air precipitating dyspnea or increased symptoms during specific allergen seasons suggests asthma. Patient may have excessive variability in twice-daily peak expiratory flows (PEF) over 2 weeks.
- Spirometry demonstrates obstruction (forced expiratory volume in 1 second [FEV_1]/forced vital capacity [FVC] <80%) with reversibility after inhaled β_2-agonist administration (at least 12% and 200 mL increase in FEV_1). If baseline spirometry is normal, challenge testing with exercise, methacholine, or mannitol can be used to elicit BHR.

ACUTE SEVERE ASTHMA

- PEF and FEV1 are <40% of normal predicted values. Pulse oximetry reveals decreased arterial oxygen and O_2 saturations.
- Arterial blood gases may reveal metabolic acidosis and low partial pressure of oxygen (PaO_2).
- Obtain the history and physical examination while initial therapy is provided, assessing for onset and causes of the exacerbation; severity of symptoms and if associated with anaphylaxis; medication use, adherence, and response to current therapy; and risk factors for asthma-related death (history of near-fatal asthma requiring intubation and mechanical ventilation, hospitalization or emergency care in the past year, recent use of oral corticosteroids, no current use of inhaled corticosteroids [ICS], overuse of SABA therapy [more than 1 canister/month], history of psychiatric disease

or psychosocial problems, poor medication adherence, lack of a written asthma action plan, and food allergy). During the physical exam, assess vital signs and identify any complicating factors (eg, pneumonia, anaphylaxis) and comorbid conditions that could be causing acute shortness of breath such as inhaled foreign body, heart failure, pulmonary infection, and pulmonary embolism.

- Measure lung function testing by PEF or FEV_1 before treatment if possible, 1 hour after start of treatment, and then periodically until response is achieved or no further improvement is evident. Monitor oxygen saturation closely, preferably by pulse oximetry.
- Arterial blood gases are typically reserved for patients who are poorly responsive to initial treatment or deteriorating.
- Obtain a complete blood count if there are signs of infection (fever and purulent sputum).

TREATMENT

- <u>Goals of Treatment</u>: The GINA long-term goals for asthma management include (1) achieve good control of symptoms and maintain normal activity levels, and (2) minimize future risk of exacerbations, fixed airflow limitation, and side effects. For acute severe asthma, the primary goal is prevention of life-threatening asthma by early recognition of signs of deterioration and early intervention.

NONPHARMACOLOGIC THERAPY

- Patient education is mandatory to improve medication adherence, self-management skills, and use of healthcare services.
- Short-term (approximately 2 weeks) home PEF monitoring can be used to assess treatment response. However, routine PEF monitoring is generally recommended only for patients with severe asthma or poor symptom perception.
- Avoidance of known allergenic triggers can improve symptoms, reduce medication use, and decrease BHR. Environmental triggers (eg, animals) should be avoided in sensitive patients, and smokers should be encouraged to quit.
- In acute asthma exacerbations, initiate oxygen therapy to achieve an arterial oxygen saturation of 93%–95% in adolescents and adults and 94%–98% in school-aged children and pregnant women or those with cardiac disease.
- Correct dehydration if present; urine specific gravity may help guide therapy in children when assessment of hydration status is difficult.

PHARMACOTHERAPY

General Approach

- Table 78-1 summarizes GINA recommendations for initial controller treatment in adults and adolescents with persistent asthma. Regardless of the long-term therapy, all patients must have an inhaled SABA available for quick relief of acute symptoms.
- Table 78-2 depicts the GINA stepwise approach for control-based management, which emphasizes three components: (1) ASSESS symptom control and risk factors, (2) ADJUST therapy and treat modifiable risk factors, and (3) REVIEW RESPONSE and optimize control about every 3 months. Step-down of controller treatment may be considered if symptoms have been well controlled and lung function has been stable for 3 months or longer. While engaging the patient in this effort, monitor symptoms and PEF and schedule follow-up. Stepping down ICS doses by 25%–50% at 3-month intervals is feasible and safe for most patients.
- The primary therapy of acute exacerbations includes inhaled SABAs and (depending on severity) systemic corticosteroids, inhaled ipratropium, intravenous (IV) magnesium sulfate, and oxygen. Treatments are typically administered concurrently to facilitate rapid improvement. Measure initial response 1 hour after the first three inhaled bronchodilator treatments.

TABLE 78-1	GINA Recommendations for Initial Controller Treatment in Adults and Adolescents
Symptom Presentation	**Preferred Treatment (Evidence Level)**
Symptoms or need for SABA less than 2×/mo; no waking due to asthma in last month; and no risk factors for exacerbations, including in prior year	No controller (D)
Infrequent symptoms, but patient has one or more risk factors for exacerbation (eg, low lung function, use of OCS in prior year, intensive care treatment for asthma ever)	Low-dose ICS (D)
Symptoms or need for SABA between 2×/mo and 2×/week, or patient wakes due to asthma more than once/mo	Low-dose ICS (D)
Symptoms or need for SABA >2×/week	Low-dose ICS[a] (A)
Troublesome symptoms most days or waking ≥1 ×/week, esp. if any risk factors exist	Medium/high-dose ICS or low-dose ICS/LABA[b] (A)
Symptoms consistent with severely uncontrolled asthma, or with an acute exacerbation	OCS short course AND start of high-dose ICS or moderate-dose ICS/LABA[b] (D)

[a]Less effective options are LTRA or theophylline.
[b]Not recommended for initial controller treatment in children ages 6–11 years.
(A), (B), (C), (D) = grade of evidence with A as the highest grade and D as the lowest grade.
ICS, inhaled corticosteroids; LABA, long-acting β_2-agonist; LTRA, leukotriene receptor antagonist; OCS, oral corticosteroids; SABA, short-acting β_2-agonist.

- **Figure 78-1** outlines strategies for self-management of worsening asthma.
- **Figure 78-2** is an algorithm for management of acute asthma exacerbations in acute care facilities (eg, emergency departments).

β_2-Agonists

- SABAs are the most effective bronchodilators. Aerosol administration enhances bronchoselectivity and provides more rapid response and greater protection against provocations (eg, exercise, allergen challenges) than systemic administration. In adults, administration as either continuous or intermittent (every 20 minutes for 3 doses) administration over 1 hour results in equivalent improvement. In acute severe asthma, continuous nebulization of a SABA (eg, albuterol) is recommended for patients having unsatisfactory response after three doses (every 20 minutes) of aerosolized β_2-agonists and potentially for patients presenting initially with PEF or FEV_1 values <30% of predicted normal.
- **Albuterol** and other inhaled SABAs are indicated for intermittent episodes of bronchospasm and are the treatment of choice for acute severe asthma and EIB. Regular treatment (four times daily) does not improve symptom control over as-needed use and is not indicated. Nonprescription inhaled **epinephrine** as Primatene Mist metered-dose inhaler is less effective than prescription SABAs and is only to be used for temporary relief of mild symptoms of intermittent asthma in patients ≥12 years old; patients should see a physician immediately if improvement is not seen within 20 minutes, symptoms become worse, or require more than 8 inhalations in a 24-hour period, or there are more than two episodes in a week.
- Two long-acting β_2-agonists (LABAs), **formoterol** (Foradil) and **salmeterol** (Serevent), provide bronchodilation for 12 hours or longer. The LABAs are preferred adjunctive therapy with ICS in adults and children ≥12 years old for step 3 and for children 6–11 years of age for steps 4 and 5. Combination treatment with ICS/LABA provides greater asthma control than increasing the dose of ICS alone while reducing

TABLE 78-2 GINA Stepwise Approach to Control Symptoms and Minimize Future Risk

Step	Preferred Option (Evidence Level)	Other Recommended Options (Evidence Level)
1	As-needed SABA (A)	Consider low-dose ICS, in addition to as-needed SABA, for patients at risk for exacerbations (B)
2	Low-dose ICS plus as-needed SABA (A)	LTRA (A)
		Low-dose ICS/LABA (A)
		ICS started with symptoms of allergic asthma, for seasonal treatment only (D)
3	Low-dose ICS/LABA, plus as-needed SABA for adults/adolescents	Medium-dose ICS for adults/adolescents (A)
	OR low-dose ICS/formoterol as both maintenance and reliever (A)	Low-dose ICS plus LTRA (A) or low-dose, sustained-release theophylline (B)
	For children 6–11 years of age, moderate-dose ICS, plus as-needed SABA	
4	Medium-dose ICS/LABA, plus as-needed SABA for adults/adolescents (B)	Add-on therapy with tiotropium for adults with exacerbation history (A)
	OR medium-dose ICS/formoterol as both maintenance and reliever (A)	Sublingual allergen immunotherapy in adults with allergic rhinitis and house dust mite sensitization if FEV_1 is >70% predicted
	For children 6–11 years of age, refer child to asthma specialist	
5	Referral to specialist and consideration of add-on treatment if asthma remains uncontrolled	Add-on anticholinergic (B): tiotropium if ≥12 years of age
		Add-on anti-IgE (A): omalizumab (subcutaneous) for moderate-to-severe allergic asthma if ≥6 years of age
		Add-on anti-interleukin-5 therapy (A): mepolizumab if ≥12 years (subcutaneous); reslizumab if ≥18 years) (intravenous)
		Add-on anti-interleukin 5 receptor (A): benralizumab if ≥12 years (subcutaneous)
		Sputum-guided treatment adjusted by eosinophilia >3% (0.03) (A)
		Bronchial thermoplasty in some adults with severe asthma (B)
		Add-on low-dose OCS (≤7.5 mg/day prednisone equivalent) (B)

ICS, inhaled corticosteroids; LABA, long-acting β_2-agonist; LTRA, leukotriene receptor antagonist; OCS, oral corticosteroids; SABA, short-acting β_2-agonist.

the frequency of mild and severe exacerbations. A SABA should be continued for acute exacerbations.

- Three ultra-LABAs (**indacaterol** [Arcapta Neohaler], **olodaterol** [Striverdi Respimat], and **vilanterol**) have a 24-hour bronchodilator duration of effect. Vilanterol is available only in combination with fluticasone furoate (Breo Ellipta) for once-daily

Effective asthma self-management education requires:

• Self-monitoring of symptoms and/or lung function

• Written asthma action plan

• Regular medical review

	All patients	**If PEF or FEV$_1$ <60% of best, or not improving after 48 hours**
	Increase reliever	Continue reliever
	Early increase in	Continue controller
	controller as below	Add prednisolone
	Review response	40-50 mg/day
		Contact doctor

EARLY or MILD   LATE OR SEVERE

Medication	Short-term change (1-2 weeks) for worsening asthma	Evidence Level
Increase usual reliever:		
Short-acting β$_2$-agonist (SABA)	Increase frequency of SABA use	A
	For pMDI, add spacer	A
Low dose ICS/formoterol[a]	Increase frequency of reliever use (maximum formoterol total 72 mcg/day	A
Increase usual controller:		
Maintenance and reliever ICS/formoterol[a]	Continue maintenance ICS/formoterol and increase reliever ICS/formoterol as needed[a] (maximum formoterol total 72 mcg/day)	A
Maintenance ICS with SABA as reliever	At least double ICS; consider increasing ICS to high dose (maximum 2000 mcg/day BDP equivalent)	B
Maintenance ICS/formoterol with SABA as reliever	Quadruple maintenance ICS/formoterol (maximum formoterol 72 mcg/day)	B
Maintenance ICS/other LABA with SABA as reliever	Step up to higher dose formulaion of ICS/other LABA, or consider adding a separate ICS inhaler (to maximum total 2000 mcg/day BDP equivalent)	D
Add oral corticosteroids (OCS) and contact doctor		
OCS (prednisone or prednisolone)	Add OCS for severe exacerbations (eg, PEF or FEV$_1$ <60% personal best or predicted), or patient not responding to treatment over 48 hours	A
	Adults: prednisolone 1 mg/kg/day (maximum 50 mg) usually for 5-7 days. *Children:* 1-2 mg/kg/day (maximum 40 mg) usually for 3-5 days	D
	Tapering is not needed if OCS are prescribed for < 2 weeks	B

BDP, beclomethasone dipropionate; FEV$_1$, forced expiratory volume in 1 second; ICS, inhaled corticosteroid; PEF, peak expiratory flow; SABA, short-acting β$_2$-agonist. Options are listed in order of evidence.

[a]ICS/formoterol maintenance and reliever regimen: lose dose budesonide or beclomethasone with formoterol. This regimen is not approved for children < 12 years in many countries.

FIGURE 78-1 Self-management of worsening asthma in adults and adolescents with a written asthma action plan. (*Adapted from Global initiative for Asthma. Global strategy for asthma management and prevention, 2018. Available from: www. ginasthma.org.*)

FIGURE 78-2 Management of asthma exacerbations in acute care facilities (eg, emergency departments).

dosing for asthma in adults ≥18 years old in the United States and for children and adults ≥12 years old in Europe. Products containing indacaterol and olodaterol are currently only indicated for COPD but are being evaluated for asthma.

• **Table 78-3** contains dosing guidelines for acute severe asthma exacerbations.

921

TABLE 78-3	Drug Doses for Treatment of Acute Severe Exacerbations of Asthma		
	Dosages		
Medications	**≥12 Years Old**	**<12 Years Old**	**Comments**
Inhaled β-agonists			
Albuterol nebulizer solution (5 mg/mL, 0.63 mg/3 mL, 1.25 mg/3 mL, 2.5 mg/3 mL)	2.5–5 mg every 20 minutes for three doses, and then 2.5–10 mg every 1–4 hours as needed, or 10–15 mg/hr continuously	0.15 mg/kg (minimum dose 2.5 mg) every 20 minutes for three doses, and then 0.15–0.3 mg/kg up to 10 mg every 1–4 hours as needed, or 0.5 mg/kg/hr by continuous nebulization	Only selective β$_2$-agonists are recommended. For optimal delivery, dilute aerosols to minimum of 4 mL at gas flow of 6–8 L/min. Use face mask if <4 years of age
Albuterol MDI (90 mcg/puff)	4–8 puffs every 30 minutes up to 4 hours, and then every 1–4 hours as needed	4–8 puffs every 20 minutes for three doses, and then every 1–4 hours as needed	In patients in severe distress, nebulization is preferred; use VHC-type spacer with face mask if <4 years old
Levalbuterol nebulizer solution (0.31 mg/3 mL, 0.63 mg/3 mL, 2.5 mg/1 mL, 1.25 mg/3 mL)	Give at one-half the milligram dose of albuterol above	Give at one-half the milligram dose of albuterol above	The single isomer of albuterol is twice as potent on a milligram basis Not recommended
Levalbuterol MDI (45 mcg/puff)	See albuterol MDI dose	See albuterol MDI dose above	See albuterol MDI dose; one-half as potent as albuterol on a microgram basis Not recommended
Anticholinergics			
Ipratropium bromide nebulizer solution (0.25 mg/mL)	500 mcg every 30 minutes for three doses, and then every 2–4 hours as needed	250 mcg every 20 minutes for three doses, and then 250 mcg every 2–4 hours	May mix in same nebulizer with albuterol; only add to β$_2$-agonist therapy
Ipratropium bromide MDI (18 mcg/puff)	8 puffs every 20 minutes as needed for up to 3 hours	4–8 puffs as needed every 2–4 hours	Not to be continued once hospitalized

(*Continued*)

TABLE 78-3	Drug Doses for Treatment of Acute Severe Exacerbations of Asthma (*Continued*)		
	Dosages		
Medications	**≥12 Years Old**	**<12 Years Old**	**Comments**
Corticosteroids			
Prednisone, methylprednisolone, prednisolone	50 mg in one or two divided doses (prednisone equivalent)	1 mg/kg (maximum 40 mg/day) in two divided doses (prednisone equivalent)	For outpatient "burst" use 1–2 mg/kg/day, maximum 60 mg, for 3–5 days in children and 40–60 mg/day in one or two divided doses for 5–7 days in adults

Note: No advantage has been found for very-high-dose corticosteroids in acute severe asthma, nor is there any advantage for IV administration over oral therapy. The usual regimen is to continue the oral corticosteroid for the duration of hospitalization. The final duration of therapy following a hospitalization or emergency department visit may be from 3 to 10 days. If patients are then started on an ICS, there is no need to taper the systemic corticosteroid dose. An ICS can be started at any time during the exacerbation.

Corticosteroids

- ICS are the preferred long-term control therapy for persistent asthma because of potency and consistent effectiveness; they are the only therapy shown to reduce risk of dying from asthma. See **Table 78-4** for comparative ICS doses; all agents are approved for once- or twice-daily dosing. Most patients with moderate disease can be controlled with twice-daily dosing of most ICS. In milder asthma, once-daily dosing is often sufficient to maintain control. More severe patients may require multiple daily dosing; after asthma is controlled, many patients can reduce the ICS dose and maintain control.
- Response to ICS is delayed; symptoms improve in most patients within the first 1–2 weeks and reach maximum improvement in 4–8 weeks. Maximum improvement in FEV_1 and PEF rates may require 3–6 weeks.
- Systemic toxicity of ICS is minimal with low-to-moderate doses, but risk of systemic effects increases with high doses (eg, growth suppression in children, osteoporosis, cataracts, dermal thinning, adrenal insufficiency). Local adverse effects include dose-dependent oropharyngeal candidiasis and dysphonia, which can be reduced by using a spacer device.
- Systemic corticosteroids (**Table 78-5**) are indicated in all patients with acute severe asthma not responding completely to initial inhaled β_2-agonist administration (every 20 minutes for 3 doses) and should be administered within 1 hour of presentation. IV therapy offers no advantage over oral administration except in patients unable to take oral medications. Adults are treated effectively with 5–7 days of oral prednisone (or equivalent), but children may require only 3–5 days. Dexamethasone for 1–2 days is an option for children and has the benefit of less vomiting. Continue full doses until the PEF reaches 70% of predicted normal or personal best. Tapering the dose after discharge is unnecessary if patients are prescribed an ICS for outpatient therapy.
- Because short-term (1–2 weeks), high-dose corticosteroids (1–2 mg/kg/day of oral prednisone) do not produce serious toxicities, the ideal strategy is to use systemic corticosteroids in a short "burst" and then maintain the patient on appropriate long-term control therapy with ICS.

Anticholinergics

- **Ipratropium bromide** (Atrovent HFA) and **tiotropium bromide** (Spiriva) produce bronchodilation only in cholinergic-mediated bronchoconstriction. Anticholinergics are effective bronchodilators but are not as effective as β_2-agonists. They attenuate but do not block allergen- or exercise-induced asthma in a dose-dependent fashion.

TABLE 78-4	Available Inhaled Corticosteroid Products, Lung Delivery, and Comparative Daily Dosages	
ICS	**Product**	**Lung Delivery[a]**
Beclomethasone dipropionate (BDP)	40 and 80 mcg/actuation HFA MDI	50%–60%
Budesonide (BUD)	90 or 180 mcg/dose DPI, Flexhaler	15%–30%
	200 and 500 mcg ampules, 1 mg	5%–8%
Ciclesonide (CIC)	80 or 160 mcg/actuation HFA MDI	50%
Flunisolide (FLU)	80 mcg/actuation HFA MDI	68%
Fluticasone furoate (FF)	100, 200 mcg/actuation DPI, Ellipta	80%–85%
Fluticasone propionate (FP)	44, 110, and 220 mcg/actuation HFA MDI	20%
	50, 100, and 250 mcg/dose DPI, Diskus	15%
Mometasone furoate (MF)	110 and 220 mcg/dose DPI, Twisthaler; 100 mcg and 200 mcg/actuation HFA MDI	11%

Comparative Daily Dosages (mcg) of Inhaled Corticosteroids

	Low Daily Dose Child[a]/Adult	Medium Daily Dose Child[a]/Adult	High Daily Dose Child[a]/Adult
BDP			
HFA MDI	80–160/80–240	>160–320/>240–480	>320/>480
BUD			
DPI	180–360/180–540	>360–720/>540–1080	>720/>1080
Nebules	500/UK	1000/UK	2000/UK
CIC HFA MDI	80–160/160–320	>160–320/>320–640	>320/>640
FLU			
HFA MDI	160/320	320/320–640	≥640/>640
FF DPI		UK/100	UK/200
FP			
HFA MDI	88–176/88–264	176–352/264–440	>352/>440
DPI	100–200/100–300	200–400/300–500	>400/>500
MF, DPI	110/110–220	220–440/>220–440	>440/>440

[a]5–11 years of age, except for BUD Nebules, which is 2–11 years of age. UK, unknown.

TABLE 78-5	Comparison of Systemic Corticosteroids			
Systemic	**Anti-Inflammatory Potency**	**Mineralocorticoid Potency**	**Duration of Biologic Activity (Hours)**	**Elimination Half-Life (Hours)**
Hydrocortisone	1	1	8–12	1.5–2
Prednisone	4	0.8	12–36	2.5–3.5
Methylprednisolone	5	0.5	12–36	3.3
Dexamethasone	25	0	36–72	3.4–4

Ipratropium bromide is approved by the US Food and Drug Administration (FDA) for maintenance treatment of bronchospasm associated with chronic obstructive pulmonary disease (COPD) but is not currently approved for treatment of asthma. Tiotropium bromide is also approved for once-daily maintenance treatment of COPD and is also indicated for the long-term, once-daily, maintenance treatment of asthma in patients $\geq$6 years of age.

- Time to reach maximum bronchodilation from aerosolized ipratropium is longer than from aerosolized SABAs (30–60 minutes vs. 5–10 minutes). However, some bronchodilation is seen within 30 seconds, and 50% of maximum response occurs within 3 minutes. Ipratropium bromide has a duration of action of 4–8 hours; tiotropium bromide has a duration of 24 hours.
- In acute asthma exacerbations, inhaled ipratropium bromide produces a further improvement in lung function of 10%–15% over inhaled β_2-agonists alone. When added to initial asthma therapy, ipratropium bromide reduces the hospitalization rate in patients with moderate-to-severe exacerbations.
- Inhaled ipratropium bromide should only be considered as adjunctive therapy in acute severe asthma not completely responsive to β_2-agonists alone.
- Tiotropium may be considered as add-on therapy in patients whose asthma is not well controlled with a medium-to-high dose of ICS and LABA combination therapy. Addition of tiotropium only modestly improves lung function, but it increases the time to severe exacerbation requiring oral corticosteroid treatment.

Leukotriene Modifiers

- **Zafirlukast** (Accolate) and **montelukast** (Singulair) are oral leukotriene receptor antagonists (LTRA) that reduce the proinflammatory and bronchoconstriction effects of leukotriene D_4. In persistent asthma, they improve pulmonary function tests, decrease nocturnal awakenings and β_2-agonist use, and improve symptoms. However, they are less effective than low-dose ICS, and they are less effective than LABAs when added to ICS for moderate persistent asthma. They are not used to treat acute exacerbations and must be taken on a regular basis, even during symptom-free periods. The adult zafirlukast dose is 20 mg twice daily, taken at least 1 hour before or 2 hours after meals; the dose for children ages 5–11 years is 10 mg twice daily. The adult montelukast dose is 10 mg once daily, taken in the evening without regard to food; the dose for children ages 6–14 years is one 5 mg chewable tablet daily in the evening.
- In general, the LTRA are well tolerated. An idiosyncratic syndrome similar to the Churg–Strauss syndrome, with marked circulating eosinophilia, heart failure, and associated eosinophilic vasculitis, has been reported rarely; a direct causal association has not been established. Because of reports of adverse neuropsychiatric events especially within a few weeks of starting therapy, monitor patients for signs of irritability, aggressiveness, and sleep disturbances; suicidality has also been reported rarely. There have been reports of fatal hepatic failure associated with zafirlukast.
- **Zileuton** (Zyflo) is a 5-lipoxygenase inhibitor; its use is limited due to potential for elevated hepatic enzymes, especially in the first 3 months of therapy, and inhibition of metabolism of drugs metabolized by CYP3A4 (eg, theophylline, warfarin). The dose of zileuton tablets is 600 mg four times daily with meals and at bedtime. The dose of zileuton extended-release tablets is two 600 mg tablets twice daily, within 1 hour after the morning and evening meals (total daily dose 2400 mg).

Biologic Agents

- These agents target the IgE pathway (relevant to allergic asthma) or IL-4, IL-13, and IL-5 pathways (relevant to the Th2 pathway and eosinophilic disorders) and are indicated for patients with moderate or severe asthma (depending upon the drug) along with other biomarkers or clinical indicators associated with treatment response. They are typically reserved for patients with moderate-to-severe persistent asthma who have been treated with dual therapy with ICS/LABA or triple therapy such as with ICS/LABA+ long-acting muscarinic antagonist (LAMA) and remain poorly controlled.

- **Omalizumab** (Xolair) is an anti-IgE antibody approved for treatment of allergic asthma not well controlled by oral or ICS. Dosage is determined by baseline total serum IgE (international units/mL [kIU/L]) and body weight (kg). Doses range from 150 to 375 mg subcutaneously (SC) at either 2- or 4-week intervals. Omalizumab is recommended for treating patients >6 years of age with moderate-to-severe asthma not adequately controlled by ICS, ICS/LABA, and in some cases, oral corticosteroids. Elevated levels of the fraction of exhaled nitric oxide (FeNO) at ≥19.5 ppb are predictive of an exacerbation rate reduction of ~50%. Because of a 0.2% incidence of anaphylaxis, observe patients for a reasonable period after injection because 70% of reactions occur within 2 hours. Some reactions have occurred up to 24 hours after injection.
- **Mepolizumab** (Nucala) and **reslizumab** (Cinqair) are monoclonal antibodies directed against IL-5 to block activation of the IL-5 receptor on eosinophils. **Benralizumab** (Fasenra) binds to the alpha subunit of the IL-5 receptor of eosinophils and prevents binding of IL-5, thus mitigating downstream eosinophilic inflammation. Mepolizumab and benralizumab are approved for patients ≥12 years old with severe asthma and are administered SC; reslizumab is approved for severe asthma in patients ≥18 years old and is administered IV. Mepolizumab and reslizumab are dosed every 4 weeks; benralizumab is dosed every 4 weeks for 3 months then every 8 weeks. Doses are to be administered in a healthcare setting by professionals who are prepared to manage anaphylaxis. Each of these drugs is indicated for patients with an "eosinophilic phenotype" (which has not been formally defined). However, a reduction in exacerbation rate of ~50% is observed when patients have a certain minimum peripheral blood eosinophil count that varies by drug.
- **Dupilumab** (Dupixent) targets the IL-4α receptor, thus blocking signaling of IL4 and IL-13, which are cytokines that promote IgE synthesis and inflammatory cell recruitment. Dupilumab is approved for patients with moderate-to-severe asthma age ≥12 years old with an eosinophilic phenotype and is administered SC every 2 weeks. Unlike mepolizumab, reslizumab, and benralizumab, FeNO levels >25 ppb in addition to blood eosinophil levels ≥150 cells/μL (0.15×10^9/L) is predictive of a response in reducing the asthma exacerbation rate by ~50%.

Magnesium Sulfate

- Magnesium sulfate is a moderately potent bronchodilator, producing relaxation of smooth muscle by blocking calcium ion influx into smooth muscles; it may also have anti-inflammatory effects.
- For patients with severe asthma exacerbations, a single 2 g IV infusion may reduce hospital admissions in adults who have an FEV_1 <25%–30% predicted upon arrival in the emergency department, children and adults who have persistent hypoxemia after standard treatment, and children whose FEV_1 remains <60% predicted after 1 hour of standard treatment. Adverse effects include hypotension, facial flushing, sweating, depressed deep tendon reflexes, hypothermia, and CNS and respiratory depression.

Methylxanthines

- Methylxanthines are rarely used today because of the high risk of severe life-threatening toxicity, numerous drug interactions, and decreased efficacy compared with ICS, LABAs, and biologics. **Theophylline** is a moderately potent bronchodilator with mild anti-inflammatory properties and is available for oral and IV administration. Theophylline dosing requires monitoring of serum concentrations for both efficacy and toxicity, including seizures and death. In addition, theophylline is eliminated primarily by metabolism via the hepatic CYP P450 microsomal enzymes (primarily CYP1A2 and CYP3A4), and drug interactions affecting metabolism significantly affect blood concentrations.

EVALUATION OF THERAPEUTIC OUTCOMES

- Focus the initial encounters on the patient's concerns, expectations, and goals of treatment. Basic education should include discussion of asthma as a chronic lung disease, the types of medications, and how they are to be used. Teach inhaler technique, advise the patient about when to seek medical advice, and provide written action plans. Both peak flow-based or symptom-based self-monitoring can be effective, if taught and followed correctly.
- At the first follow-up visit, reinforce the educational messages from the first visit and review of the patient's current medications, adherence, and any difficulties related to therapy.
- The two key components of effective asthma control are "symptom control" and "future risk of adverse outcomes." Assess symptom control by frequency of daytime and nighttime asthma symptoms, reliever medication use, and activity limitations; poor symptom control is also an indicator of future risk for exacerbations.
- Future risk of adverse outcomes includes assessment of risks for future exacerbations, fixed airflow limitation (and thus diminished response to therapy), and medication adverse effects. To assess the risk for future exacerbations, measure lung function before the start of treatment and then 2 months later when maximum response to controller medications is likely attained.
- During ongoing care, measure spirometry yearly but reserve long-term PEF monitoring for patients with severe asthma.
- Validated questionnaires can be administered regularly, such as the Asthma Control Test, Asthma Therapy Assessment Questionnaire, and Asthma Control Questionnaire.
- Ask patients about exercise tolerance because perceived good exercise tolerance may be biased by a sedentary lifestyle adapted to the frequency of bothersome symptoms.
- All patients on inhaled drugs should have their inhalation technique evaluated monthly initially and then every 3–6 months.
- After initiation of anti-inflammatory therapy or increase in dosage, most patients should experience decreased symptoms within 1–2 weeks and achieve maximum improvement within 4–8 weeks. Improvement in baseline FEV_1 or PEF should follow a similar time course, but decrease in BHR as measured by morning PEF, PEF variability, and exercise tolerance may take longer and improve over 1–3 months.

See Chapter 43, Asthma, authored by Kathryn V. Blake and Jason E. Lang, for a more detailed discussion of this topic.

Chronic Obstructive Pulmonary Disease

- Chronic obstructive pulmonary disease (COPD) is characterized by progressive airflow limitation that is not fully reversible. Two principal conditions (referred to as phenotypes) include:
  - ✓ *Chronic bronchitis*: Chronic or recurrent excess mucus secretion with cough that occurs on most days for at least 3 months of the year for at least 2 consecutive years.
  - ✓ *Emphysema*: Abnormal, permanent enlargement of the airspaces distal to the terminal bronchioles, accompanied by destruction of their walls, without fibrosis.

PATHOPHYSIOLOGY

- The most common cause of COPD is exposure to tobacco smoke. Inhalation of noxious particles and gases activates neutrophils, macrophages, and CD8$^+$ lymphocytes, which release chemical mediators, including tumor necrosis factor-α, interleukin-8, and leukotriene B$_4$. Inflammatory cells and mediators lead to widespread destructive changes in airways, pulmonary vasculature, and lung parenchyma, resulting in chronic airflow limitation.
- Oxidative stress and imbalance between aggressive and protective defense systems in the lungs (proteases and antiproteases) may also occur. Oxidants generated by cigarette smoke react with and damage proteins and lipids, contributing to cell and tissue damage. Oxidants also promote inflammation and exacerbate protease–antiprotease imbalance by inhibiting antiprotease activity.
- The protective antiprotease α_1-antitrypsin (AAT) inhibits protease enzymes, including neutrophil elastase. AAT deficiency increases risk for premature emphysema.
- Inflammatory exudate in airways leads to increased number and size of goblet cells and mucus glands. Mucus secretion increases and ciliary motility is impaired. There is thickening of the smooth muscle and connective tissue in airways. Chronic inflammation leads to scarring, fibrosis, and airflow obstruction.
- Arterial blood gas (ABG) abnormalities result from impaired gas transfer due to parenchymal damage and loss of alveolar-capillary networks. Significant ABG changes are usually not present until airflow limitation is very severe. In such patients, *hypoxemia* (low arterial oxygen tension—PaO$_2$ 45–60 mm Hg [6.0–8.0 kPa]) and *hypercapnia* (elevated arterial carbon dioxide tension—PaCO$_2$ 50–60 mm Hg [6.7–8.0 kPa]) can become chronic problems. Hypoxemia is initially associated with exertion but develops at rest as the disease progresses. Hypoxemia results from hypoventilation (V) of lung tissue relative to perfusion (Q) of the area. This low V/Q ratio progresses over several years, resulting in a consistent decline in PaO$_2$. As gas exchange worsens with disease progression, patients may exhibit chronic hypercapnia and are referred to as CO$_2$ retainers. In such patients, central respiratory response to chronically increased PaCO$_2$ is blunted. Serum pH is usually near normal because the kidneys compensate by retaining bicarbonate. If acute respiratory distress develops (eg, as with pneumonia or COPD exacerbation with respiratory failure) PaCO$_2$ may rise sharply, resulting in worsening respiratory acidosis.
- Chronic hypoxemia and changes in pulmonary vasculature lead to increases in pulmonary pressures, especially during exercise. Sustained elevated pulmonary pressures can lead to right-sided heart failure (cor pulmonale) characterized by right ventricle hypertrophy in response to increased pulmonary vascular resistance.
- Chronic airflow obstruction leads to air trapping, resulting in thoracic hyperinflation and flattening of diaphragmatic muscles, making them less efficient muscles of ventilation and predisposing patients to muscle fatigue, especially during exacerbations. Patients with thoracic hyperinflation have increased functional residual capacity

(FRC), which is the amount of air left in the lungs after exhalation. Increased FRC limits the amount of air the patient can inhale to fill the lungs and shortens the inhalation time, which may increase complaints of dyspnea.

- Loss of skeletal muscle mass and decline in overall health status can lead to ischemic cardiovascular events, cachexia, weight loss, osteoporosis, anemia, and muscle wasting.

CLINICAL PRESENTATION

- Initial symptoms include chronic cough and sputum production; patients may experience cough for several years before dyspnea develops. Dyspnea is worse with exercise and progressive over time, with decreased exercise tolerance or decline in physical activity. Chest tightness or wheezing may be present.
- Physical examination may be normal in milder stages. When airflow limitation progresses, patients may have shallow breathing, increased resting respiratory rate, "barrel chest" due to lung hyperinflation, pursed lips during expiration, use of accessory respiratory muscles, and cyanosis of mucosal membranes.

DIAGNOSIS

- Diagnosis is based on patient symptoms, history of exposure to risk factors such as tobacco smoke and occupational substances, and confirmation by pulmonary function testing, such as spirometry.
- Spirometry assesses lung volumes and capacities. Forced vital capacity (FVC) is the total volume of air exhaled after maximal inhalation, and FEV_1 is the total volume of air exhaled in 1 second. Postbronchodilator spirometry results should be used to assess lung function in patients with COPD. FEV_1 is measured 10–15 minutes after inhalation of a short-acting β_2-agonist or 30–45 minutes after a short-acting anticholinergic or a combination of the two agents. Airflow limitation is confirmed by a postbronchodilator FEV_1/FVC <70% (0.70).
- The Global Initiative for Chronic Obstructive Lung Disease (GOLD) guidelines suggest a four-grade classification of airflow limitation based on the FEV_1/FVC <70% (0.70), measured FEV_1 compared to predicted FEV_1 (%), and presence of symptoms: (1) mild, (2) moderate, (3), severe, or (4) very severe.
- Recommended patient assessment questionnaires to assess dyspnea and other measures of health status include the COPD Assessment Test (CAT), modified Medical Research Council (mMRC) Dyspnea Questionnaire, and the COPD Control Questionnaire (CCQ).

TREATMENT

- <u>Goals of Treatment</u>: Prevent or slow disease progression, relieve symptoms, improve exercise tolerance, improve overall health status, prevent and treat exacerbations, prevent and treat complications, and reduce morbidity and mortality.

NONPHARMACOLOGIC THERAPY

- Educate patients about their disease, treatment plans, and strategies to slow progression and prevent complications.
- Smoking cessation is the most important intervention to prevent development and progression of COPD. Reducing exposure to occupational dust and fumes as well as other environmental toxins is also important.
- Pulmonary rehabilitation programs include exercise training, breathing exercises, optimal medical treatment, psychosocial support, and health education.
- Administer the influenza vaccine annually during each influenza season. The CDC recommends giving the 23-valent pneumococcal polysaccharide vaccine (PPSV23) for people from ages 2 to 64 who have chronic lung disease, smokers over the age

of 18, and all people older than 65 years. The GOLD guidelines recommend the pneumococcal vaccine for COPD patients age $\geq$65 years of age and for patients <65 years old with comorbidities or FEV_1 <40% predicted.

- Once patients are stabilized as outpatients and pharmacotherapy is optimized, institute long-term oxygen therapy if either of the following conditions is documented twice in a 3-week period: (1) resting PaO_2 <5 mm Hg (7.3 kPa) or SaO_2 <88% (0.88) with or without hypercapnia, or (2) resting PaO_2 55–60 mm Hg (7.3–8.0 kPa) or SaO_2 <88% (0.88) with evidence of right-sided heart failure, polycythemia, or pulmonary hypertension. Oxygen can be delivered by nasal cannula at 1–2 L/min, providing 24%–28% (0.24–0.28) fraction of inspired oxygen (FiO_2) with a goal to raise PaO_2 above 60 mm Hg (8.0 kPa).

PHARMACOLOGIC THERAPY

- No COPD medication has been conclusively shown to slow lung function decline or prolong survival. The GOLD guidelines recommend that a combined "ABCD" classification system based on symptom severity and risk of future exacerbations be used as a stepwise approach to pharmacotherapy rather than FEV_1 measurements (Table 79-1). Symptom assessment should be measured at baseline and then during routine visits using CAT or mMRC. Defined cut points for patients exhibiting "more symptoms" and "less symptoms" have been established for CAT and mMRC. Frequency of exacerbations is assessed by reviewing exacerbation history for the past 12 months. Patients are assigned to an ABCD category based on these two assessments. Patients with at least two exacerbations in the last 12 months, or one exacerbation requiring hospitalization, are considered high risk for future

TABLE 79-1	Recommended Initial and Escalation Pharmacotherapy for Stable COPD	
Patient Category	**Initial Therapy**	**Escalation Therapy**
A (less symptoms, less exacerbation risk)	Offer either short- or long-acting bronchodilator, depending on symptoms	Continue therapy if beneficial or if re-education needed
		Stop therapy if intolerable adverse effects and switch to alternate class for symptom control
		Combine bronchodilator classes for additional symptom control
		If patient experiences exacerbations, reassess goals (ie, low vs. high risk for exacerbation) and follow escalation therapy as outlined in category C
B (more symptoms, less exacerbation risk)	Start LAMA or LABA for symptom control	Continue therapy if beneficial or if re-education needed
		Add long-acting bronchodilator if persistent symptoms on monotherapy (LAMA/LABA)
		If dual bronchodilators do not improve symptoms, consider stepping back to monotherapy AFTER assessing adherence and inhaler technique
		If patient experiences exacerbations, reassess goals (ie, low vs. high risk for exacerbation) and follow escalation therapy as outlined in category C

(Continued)

TABLE 79-1	Recommended Initial and Escalation Pharmacotherapy for Stable COPD (*Continued*)
Patient Category	**Initial Therapy**	**Escalation Therapy**
C (less symptoms, more exacerbation risk)	Start long-acting bronchodilator for exacerbation prevention; LAMA is preferred over LABA for initial therapy	Continue therapy if beneficial or if re-education needed
		Add long-acting bronchodilator if persistent symptoms on monotherapy (LAMA/LABA)
		If persistent exacerbations on long-acting bronchodilator monotherapy and eosinophil count <300/µL (0.3 × 10⁹/L), add additional long-acting bronchodilator (LAMA/LABA); dual bronchodilators are preferred due to better efficacy and lower risk of pneumonia
		If persistent exacerbations on long-acting bronchodilator monotherapy and eosinophil count ≥300/µL (0.3 × 10⁹/L), consider starting ICS/LABA instead of LAMA/LABA
		If persistent exacerbations on dual LAMA/LABA and eosinophil count ≥100/µL (0.1 × 10⁹/L), consider adding ICS
		If persistent exacerbations on dual LAMA/LABA and eosinophil count <100/µL (0.1 × 10⁹/L), consider roflumilast for patients with FEV_1 <50% (0.50) or azithromycin daily (nonsmokers or former smokers only)
		If persistent exacerbations on triple therapy (LAMA/LABA/ICS), consider roflumilast for patients with FEV_1 <50% (0.50) or azithromycin daily (nonsmokers or former smokers only)
		If recurrent exacerbations or pneumonia, consider withdrawal of ICS over 12 weeks
D (more symptoms, more exacerbation risk)	Start long-acting bronchodilator for exacerbation prevention; LAMA is preferred over LABA for initial therapy If highly symptomatic (ie, CAT >20), consider dual long-acting bronchodilators (LAMA/LABA) If blood eosinophil count ≥300/µL (0.3 × 10⁹/L), consider starting ICS/LABA instead of LAMA/LABA	Continue therapy if beneficial or if re-education needed If persistent exacerbations, follow escalation therapy as outlined in category C If recurrent exacerbations or pneumonia, consider withdrawal of ICS over 12 weeks

CAT, COPD Assessment Test; FEV_1, forced expiratory volume in 1 second; ICS, inhaled corticosteroid; LABA, long-acting β-agonist; LAMA, long-acting muscarinic antagonist; mMRC, modified Medical Research Council questionnaire; SABA, short-acting β-agonist; SAMA, short-acting muscarinic antagonist.

exacerbations (category C or D). Guidelines recommend that initial and escalation therapy be based on ABCD category classification.

• Bronchodilators are the mainstay of drug therapy; classes include short- and long-acting β_2-agonists, short- and long-acting muscarinic antagonists (anticholinergics), and methylxanthines. Short-acting inhaled bronchodilators relieve symptoms (eg, dyspnea) and increase exercise tolerance. Long-acting inhaled bronchodilators relieve symptoms, reduce exacerbation frequency, and improve quality of life and health status. Bronchodilators do not significantly improve measurements of expiratory airflow such as FEV_1.

Short-Acting Bronchodilators

• Either a short- or long-acting bronchodilator is recommended initially for patients with occasional symptoms (Table 79-1, category A). Short-acting bronchodilators are also recommended for all patients (categories A–D) as rescue or as-needed therapy to manage symptoms. Choices among short-acting bronchodilators include short-acting β_2-agonists (SABAs) or short-acting muscarinic antagonists (SAMAs). Both drug classes have a relatively rapid onset of action, relieve symptoms to a similar degree, and improve exercise tolerance and lung function. Short-acting bronchodilators do not reduce the frequency or severity of COPD exacerbations. If a patient does not achieve adequate symptom control with one agent, combining a SABA with a SAMA is reasonable.

• **Short-acting β_2-agonists (SABAs)** stimulate adenyl cyclase to increase formation of cyclic adenosine monophosphate (cAMP), which mediates relaxation of bronchial smooth muscle. They may also improve mucociliary clearance. SABAs have a rapid onset of effect; they cause only a small improvement in FEV_1 acutely but may still improve symptoms and exercise tolerance. The SABA choices include **albuterol** and **levalbuterol** (Table 79-2). Albuterol is most frequently used and is a racemic mixture

TABLE 79-2	Select Medications Used for Treatment of COPD[a]		
Generic (Brand) Name		**Dosage Form**	**Dosage Frequency[b]**
Short-acting β_2-agonists			
Albuterol sulfate (Proventil HFA, Ventolin HFA, Proair HFA)		MDI	Every 4–6 hrs PRN
Albuterol sulfate (Proair RespiClick)		DPI	Every 4–6 hrs PRN
Levalbuterol hydrochloride (Xopenex, generic)		NEB solution	Every 6–8 hrs PRN
Levalbuterol tartrate (Xopenex HFA)		MDI	Every 4–6 hrs PRN
Short-acting muscarinic antagonists (SAMAs)			
Ipratropium bromide (Atrovent HFA)		MDI	4 times/day PRN
Ipratropium bromide (generic)		NEB solution	3–4 times/day PRN
Long-acting β_2-agonists (LABAs)			
Arformoterol tartrate (Brovana)		NEB solution	Every 12 hrs
Formoterol fumarate (Perforomist)		NEB solution	Every 12 hrs
Indacaterol maleate (Arcapta Neohaler)		DPI	Once daily
Olodaterol hydrochloride (Striverdi Respimat)		SMI	Once daily
Salmeterol xinafoate (Serevent Diskus)		DPI	Twice daily
Long-acting muscarinic antagonists (LAMAs)			
Aclidinium bromide (Tudorza Pressair)		DPI	Twice daily
Tiotropium bromide (Spiriva Respimat)		SMI	Once daily
Tiotropium bromide (Spiriva Handihaler)		DPI	Once daily

(Continued)

TABLE 79-2	Select Medications Used for Treatment of COPDª (Continued)	
Generic (Brand) Name	Dosage Form	Dosage Frequencyᵇ
Glycopyrrolate (Lonhala Magnair)	NEB solution	Twice daily
Glycopyrrolate (Seebri Neohaler)	DPI	Twice daily
Umeclidinium bromide (Incruse Ellipta)	DPI	Once daily
Inhaled corticosteroids		
Beclomethasone dipropionate (Qvar 40, 80)	MDI	Twice daily
Budesonide (Pulmicort Flexhaler)	DPI	Twice daily
Flunisolide (Aerospan HFA)	MDI	Twice daily
Fluticasone propionate (Flovent HFA)	MDI	Twice daily
Mometasone furoate (Asmanex Twisthaler)	DPI	Twice daily
Combination inhalers		
SABA/SAMA: albuterol sulfate + ipratropium bromide (Duoneb, generic)	NEB solution	4–6 times/day PRN
SABA/SAMA: albuterol sulfate + ipratropium bromide (Combivent Respimat)	SMI	4–6 times/day PRN
LAMA/LABA: umeclidinium bromide + vilanterol trifenatate (Anoro Ellipta)	DPI	Once daily
LAMA/LABA: tiotropium bromide + olodaterol hydrochloride (Stiolto Respimat)	SMI	Once daily
LAMA/LABA: glycopyrrolate + indacaterol maleate (Utibron Neohaler)	DPI	Twice daily
LAMA/LABA: glycopyrrolate + formoterol fumarate (Bevespi Aerosphere)	MDI	Twice daily
ICS/LABA: budesonide + formoterol fumarate dehydrate (Symbicort)	MDI	Twice daily
ICS/LABA: fluticasone furoate + vilanterol trifenatate (Breo Ellipta)	DPI	Once daily
ICS/LABA: fluticasone propionate + salmeterol xinafoate (Advair Diskus, Airduo RespiClick)	DPI	Twice daily
ICS/LABA: fluticasone propionate + salmeterol xinafoate (Advair HFA)	MDI	Twice daily
ICS/LABA: mometasone furoate + formoterol fumarate (Dulera)	MDI	Twice daily
ICS/LAMA/LABA: fluticasone furoate + umeclidinium bromide +vilanterol trifenatate (Trelegy Ellipta)	DPI	Once daily
Oral medications		
Roflumilast (Daliresp)	Oral tablets	Once daily
Theophylline (Theo-24, generic)	Oral tablets, capsules	Once or twice daily (extended release)

ªNot all medications are FDA-approved for treatment of COPD.
ᵇConsult official product labeling or the medical literature for dosages used for COPD treatment.
DPI, dry power inhaler; hrs, hours; ICS, inhaled corticosteroid; inh, inhalations; LABA, long-acting β_2-agonist; LAMA, long-acting muscarinic antagonist; MDI, metered-dose inhaler; NEB, nebulized; PRN, as needed; SABA, short-acting β_2-agonist; SAMA, short-acting muscarinic antagonist; SMI, soft mist inhaler.

of (R)-albuterol (responsible for bronchodilation) and (S)-albuterol (which has no therapeutic effect). Levalbuterol is a single-isomer formulation of (R)-albuterol that offers no clear efficacy or safety advantages over albuterol, and it is more expensive. Inhalation is the preferred route for SABAs, and administration via metered-dose or dry powder inhalers (MDIs, DPIs) is at least as effective as nebulization therapy and is more convenient and less costly. Inhaled SABAs are generally well tolerated; they can cause sinus tachycardia and rhythm disturbances rarely in predisposed patients. Skeletal muscle tremors can occur initially but generally subside as tolerance develops. Older patients may be more sensitive and experience palpitations, tremors, and "jittery" feelings.

- **Short-acting muscarinic antagonists (SAMAs)** produce bronchodilation by inhibiting muscarinic receptor subtypes M_1, M_2, and M_3 in bronchial smooth muscle and mucus glands. This blocks acetylcholine, reducing cyclic guanosine monophosphate (cGMP), which normally acts to constrict bronchial smooth muscle, and decreasing mucus secretion. **Ipratropium bromide** is the most commonly prescribed SAMA in the United States (Table 79-2). Improvements in pulmonary function are similar to inhaled SABAs, although ipratropium has a slower onset of action (15–20 minutes vs. 5 minutes for albuterol) and more prolonged effect. Because of its slower onset, ipratropium may be less suitable for as-needed use but is often prescribed in this manner. In contrast to albuterol, patients may experience additional symptom improvement with a larger number of inhalations (eg, 6 puffs every 6 hours, maximum 24 puffs/day), whereas no additional improvement occurs with more frequent use than every 6 hours. The most frequent patient complaints are dry mouth, nausea, and occasionally metallic taste. Because it is poorly absorbed systemically, anticholinergic side effects are uncommon (eg, blurred vision, constipation, urinary retention, nausea, and tachycardia). Inhaled anticholinergics may rarely precipitate narrow-angle glaucoma symptoms.

Long-Acting Bronchodilators

- Long-acting bronchodilators are recommended for patients with persistent symptoms or in whom short-acting therapies do not provide adequate relief (Table 79-1, category B). Long-acting agents are also recommended for patients at high risk for exacerbation (categories C and D). Therapy can be administered as an inhaled long-acting β_2-agonist (LABA) or muscarinic antagonist (LAMA). Compared with short-acting agents, long-acting bronchodilators are more convenient for patients with persistent symptoms and are superior in improving lung function, relieving symptoms, reducing exacerbation frequency and need for hospitalization, and improving quality of life. LABAs and LAMAs are equally effective in managing symptoms, but LAMAs are more effective for preventing exacerbations and should be considered first-line monotherapy for patients at high risk for exacerbation. Treatment selection should consider individual patient response, tolerability, adherence, and economic factors.

- The available LABAs differ primarily by dosing frequency and device type (Table 79-2). **Arformoterol, formoterol, indacaterol,** and **olodaterol** have an onset of action similar to albuterol (<5 minutes), whereas **salmeterol** has a slower onset (15–20 minutes); however, none of these agents are recommended for acute relief of COPD symptoms. **Vilanterol** is available in the United States only in combination with an inhaled corticosteroid (fluticasone) or LAMA (umeclidinium). There is no dose titration for any of these agents; the starting dose is the effective and recommended dose for all patients.

- The available LAMAs differ in dosing frequency and device type (Table 79-2). They are more selective than ipratropium at blocking muscarinic receptors and dissociate slowly from M_3 receptors, resulting in prolonged bronchodilation. **Aclidinium, glycopyrrolate,** and **umeclidinium** have a faster onset of action (5–15 minutes) than **tiotropium** (80 minutes); however, none of these agents are recommended for acute relief of symptoms. There is no dose titration for any of these agents; the starting dose is the effective and recommended dose for all patients.

Combination Muscarinic Antagonists and β_2-Agonists

- Combination bronchodilator regimens are often used as symptoms worsen over time. Combining bronchodilators with different mechanisms of action allows use of the lowest possible effective doses and reduces potential adverse effects from individual agents. Short-acting bronchodilators may be combined for patients experiencing persistent symptoms, although step-up to long-acting bronchodilator monotherapy is usually preferred (Table 79-1).
- Guidelines recommend combining long-acting bronchodilators (LAMA/LABA) for patients who have persistent symptoms or recurrent exacerbations on bronchodilator monotherapy. The combination provides significant improvement in lung function, symptoms, and quality-of-life measures compared with LABA or LAMA monotherapy. In addition, dual long-acting bronchodilator therapy decreases the frequency of moderate-to-severe exacerbations compared to either LAMA or LABA monotherapy.

Methylxanthines

- **Theophylline** and **aminophylline** may produce bronchodilation by several mechanisms, including inhibition of phosphodiesterase, thereby increasing cAMP levels.
- Chronic theophylline use in COPD may improve lung function and gas exchange. Subjectively, theophylline reduces dyspnea, increases exercise tolerance, and improves respiratory drive.
- Methylxanthines have a limited role in COPD therapy because of the availability of LABAs and LAMAs as well as significant methylxanthine drug interactions and interpatient variability in dosage requirements. Theophylline may be considered in patients intolerant of or unable to use inhaled bronchodilators.
- Sustained-release theophylline preparations are most appropriate for long-term COPD management; they improve adherence and achieve more consistent serum concentrations than rapid-release products. Caution should be used in switching from one sustained-release preparation to another because of variability in sustained-release characteristics.
- Initiate theophylline therapy with 200 mg twice daily and titrate upward every 3–5 days to the target dose; most patients require 400–900 mg daily. Make dose adjustments based on trough serum concentrations. A therapeutic range of 8–15 mcg/mL (44–83 μmol/L) is targeted to minimize risk of toxicity. Once a dose is established, monitor concentrations once or twice a year unless the disease worsens, medications that interfere with theophylline metabolism are added, or toxicity is suspected.
- Common theophylline side effects include dyspepsia, nausea, vomiting, diarrhea, headache, dizziness, and tachycardia. Arrhythmias and seizures may occur, especially at toxic concentrations.
- Factors that decrease theophylline clearance and lead to reduced dosage requirements include advanced age, bacterial or viral pneumonia, heart failure, liver dysfunction, hypoxemia from acute decompensation, and drugs such as cimetidine, macrolides, and fluoroquinolone antibiotics.
- Factors that may enhance theophylline clearance and result in need for higher doses include tobacco and marijuana smoking, hyperthyroidism, and drugs such as phenytoin, phenobarbital, and rifampin.

Corticosteroids

- Anti-inflammatory mechanisms of corticosteroids in COPD include reducing capillary permeability to decrease mucus, inhibiting release of proteolytic enzymes from leukocytes, and inhibiting prostaglandins.
- The recommended role of inhaled corticosteroid (ICS) therapy is for patients at high risk of exacerbation (Table 79-1, categories C and D) who have recurrent exacerbations despite optimal therapy with inhaled bronchodilators. In order to best target therapy, consensus guidelines propose using blood eosinophil counts to identify patients with COPD who might benefit from chronic ICS treatment.

- The clinical benefits of ICS therapy (including decreased exacerbation frequency and improved lung function and health status) have been observed with combination therapy, primarily as an addition to LABA monotherapy. Given lack of supporting evidence, ICS monotherapy is not recommended for patients with COPD.
- For patients with recurrent exacerbations despite optimal long-acting bronchodilator monotherapy, combination therapy with dual long-acting bronchodilators (LAMA/LABA) is preferred over combination therapy with ICS/LABA (Table 79-1). Dual therapy with ICS/LABA may be considered instead of LAMA/LABA for patients with blood eosinophil counts ≥300 cells/μL (0.3 × 10^9/L).
- For patients with persistent symptoms and recurrent exacerbations on dual inhaled therapy, triple therapy with LAMA/LABA/ICS is recommended as initial escalation therapy (Table 79-1). Given the risk of adverse ICS effects, some clinicians avoid triple inhalation therapy for patients with persistent exacerbations and lower blood eosinophil counts (<100 cells/μL [0.1 × 10^9/L]) in favor of oral alternatives such as roflumilast or azithromycin.
- Short-term systemic corticosteroids may also be considered for acute exacerbations. Chronic systemic corticosteroids should be avoided in COPD because of questionable benefits and high risk of toxicity.
- The moderate-to-high ICS doses used in clinical trials of COPD have been associated with an increased risk of pneumonia and mycobacterial pulmonary infections. Other adverse effects include hoarseness, sore throat, oral candidiasis, and skin bruising. Severe side effects such as adrenal suppression, osteoporosis, and cataract formation occur less frequently than with systemic corticosteroids, but clinicians should monitor patients receiving high-dose chronic inhaled therapy. Treat patients with the lowest effective ICS dose to minimize risk of fracture.

Roflumilast

- **Roflumilast** is a phosphodiesterase 4 (PDE4) inhibitor that relaxes airway smooth muscle and decreases activity of inflammatory cells and mediators such as TNF-α and IL-8. Roflumilast is recommended for patients with recurrent exacerbations despite treatment with triple inhalation therapy (LAMA/LABA/ICS; Table 79-1). It may also be considered as escalation therapy for patients with recurrent exacerbations on dual long-acting bronchodilators (LAMA/LABA) who are not candidates for ICS, such as those with low blood eosinophil count (<100 cells/μL [0.1 × 10^9/L]) or who are at higher risk of adverse effects associated with ICS. Because theophylline and roflumilast have similar mechanisms of action, they should not be used together.
- Major adverse effects include diarrhea, nausea, decreased appetite, weight loss, headache and neuropsychiatric effects such as suicidal thoughts, insomnia, anxiety, and new or worsened depression. Although most symptoms usually resolve over time, a low starting dose (250 mcg orally once daily) is recommended for the first 4 weeks before increasing to the maintenance dose (500 mcg once daily). Caution is advised in patients with a history of depression or suicidality.
- Roflumilast is metabolized by CYP3A4 and 1A2; coadministration with strong CYP P450 inducers is not recommended due to potential for subtherapeutic plasma concentrations. Use caution when administering roflumilast with strong CYP P450 inhibitors due to potential for adverse effects.

Azithromycin

- Chronic **azithromycin** was associated with a lower rate of COPD exacerbation and improved quality-of-life scores in one study, but more patients in the azithromycin group reported hearing deficits (25% vs. 20% in the placebo group), and patients who continued to smoke did not achieve reduction in exacerbation frequency with azithromycin. Azithromycin was also associated with a higher rate of colonization with macrolide-resistant bacteria. In addition, the azithromycin product labeling includes a precaution about QT prolongation after a retrospective study reported increased cardiac events with short courses of azithromycin.

- Based on limited evidence supporting long-term treatment (beyond 1 year), current guidelines recommend to consider adding chronic azithromycin only for patients with recurrent exacerbations despite optimal therapy and who are not active smokers (Table 79-1). Clinicians may consider azithromycin for individual patients at high risk for exacerbations but must carefully weigh the risks and benefits of therapy.

α1-Antitrypsin Replacement Therapy

- For patients with inherited AAT deficiency-associated emphysema, treatment focuses on reduction of risk factors such as smoking, symptomatic treatment with bronchodilators, and augmentation therapy with replacement AAT.
- Several proprietary **alpha$_1$-proteinase inhibitors** are available: Glassia, Prolastin-C, Aralast, Aralast-NP, and Zemaira. Augmentation therapy is intended to maintain serum concentrations above the protective threshold of 10 μmol/L throughout the dosing interval. The recommended dosing regimen is 60 mg/kg IV given once weekly, usually at a rate of 0.08 mL/kg/min (consult individual product labeling), adjusted to patient tolerance. Augmentation therapy can cost over $50,000 annually.

COPD EXACERBATIONS

- A COPD exacerbation is defined as a change in the patient's baseline symptoms (dyspnea, cough, or sputum production) beyond day-to-day variability sufficient to warrant a change in management.
- The primary physiologic change is often a worsening of ABG values due to poor gas exchange and increased muscle fatigue. With severe exacerbations, profound hypoxemia and hypercapnia can be accompanied by respiratory acidosis and respiratory failure.
- Although criteria used to define acute exacerbations vary, most rely on a change in one or more of the following clinical findings: worsening dyspnea, increased sputum volume, or increased sputum purulence (Table 79-3).
- Additional symptoms may include chest tightness, increased need for bronchodilators, malaise, fatigue, and decreased exercise tolerance. Physical exam may reveal fever, wheezing, and decreased breath sounds. Obtain a sputum sample for Gram stain and culture and a chest x-ray to evaluate for new infiltrates.
- The diagnosis of acute respiratory failure is made based on an acute change in ABGs: an acute drop in PaO$_2$ of 10–15 mm Hg (1.3–2.0 kPa) or any acute increase in PaCO$_2$ that decreases the serum pH to 7.3 or less. Additional indications of respiratory failure include restlessness, confusion, tachycardia, diaphoresis, cyanosis, hypotension, irregular breathing, miosis, and unconsciousness.
- <u>Goals of Treatment</u>: (1) Minimize the negative consequences of the acute exacerbation (ie, reduce symptoms, prevent hospitalization, shorten hospital stay, prevent acute respiratory failure or death) and (2) prevent future exacerbations.

TABLE 79-3	Staging Acute Exacerbations of COPD
Mild (type 1)	One cardinal symptom^a plus at least one of the following: upper respiratory tract infection within 5 days, fever without other explanation, increased wheezing, increased cough, increase in respiratory or heart rate >20% above baseline
Moderate (type 2)	Two cardinal symptoms
Severe (type 3)	Three cardinal symptoms

^{a}Cardinal symptoms include worsening of dyspnea, increase in sputum volume, and increase in sputum purulence.

NONPHARMACOLOGIC THERAPY

- Provide oxygen therapy for patients with significant hypoxemia (eg, oxygen saturation <90% [0.90]). Use caution because many COPD patients rely on mild hypoxemia to trigger their drive to breathe. Overly aggressive oxygen administration to patients with chronic hypercapnia may result in respiratory depression and respiratory failure. Adjust oxygen to achieve PaO_2 >60 mm Hg (8.0 kPa) or oxygen saturation (SaO_2) >90% (0.90). Obtain ABG after oxygen initiation to monitor CO_2 retention resulting from hypoventilation.

- Noninvasive positive-pressure ventilation (NPPV) provides ventilatory support with oxygen and pressurized airflow using a face or nasal mask without endotracheal intubation. NPPV is not appropriate for patients with altered mental status, severe acidosis, respiratory arrest, or cardiovascular instability. Intubation and mechanical ventilation may be needed in patients failing NPPV or who are poor candidates for NPPV.

PHARMACOLOGIC THERAPY

Bronchodilators

- Dose and frequency of bronchodilators are increased during acute exacerbations to provide symptomatic relief. SABAs are preferred because of rapid onset of action. Muscarinic antagonists may be added if symptoms persist despite increased doses of β_2-agonists. LABAs or LAMAs should not be used for quick relief of symptoms or on an as-needed basis.

- Bronchodilators may be administered via MDI, DPI, or nebulization with equal efficacy. Nebulization may be considered for patients with severe dyspnea who are unable to hold their breath after actuation of an MDI.

- Theophylline should generally be avoided due to lack of evidence documenting benefit and the concern for adverse effects.

Corticosteroids

- Treatment with systemic corticosteroids in acute exacerbations improves oxygenation and recovery time, shortens hospitalization, and reduces risk of relapse.

- Although the optimal corticosteroid dose and duration are unknown, prednisone 40 mg orally daily (or equivalent) for 5 days is effective for many patients. If treatment is continued for longer than 2 weeks, employ a tapering oral schedule to avoid hypothalamic–pituitary–adrenal axis suppression.

Antimicrobial Therapy

- In order to limit unnecessary use, antibiotics should be initiated in any of these clinical situations: (1) patients presenting with three cardinal symptoms of acute exacerbation, (2) patients presenting with two cardinal symptoms as long as one is increased sputum purulence, and (3) patients requiring mechanical ventilation regardless of symptoms. Utility of sputum Gram stain and culture is questionable because some patients have chronic bacterial colonization of the bronchial tree between exacerbations. Use of C-reactive protein (CRP) as a biomarker to guide antimicrobial therapy decisions may be reasonable.

- Selection of empiric antimicrobial therapy should be based on the most likely organisms: Haemophilus influenzae, Moraxella catarrhalis, Streptococcus pneumoniae, and Haemophilus parainfluenzae. Drug-resistant pneumococci, β-lactamase–producing H. influenzae and M. catarrhalis, and enteric gram-negative organisms, including Pseudomonas aeruginosa, may be present in complicated acute exacerbations.

- Table 79-4 summarizes the most common organisms based on patient presentation and recommended antimicrobial therapy. Continue antimicrobial therapy for at least 5–7 days. If the patient deteriorates or does not improve as anticipated, hospitalization may be necessary, and more aggressive attempts should be made to identify potential pathogens responsible for the exacerbation.

TABLE 79-4	Recommended Antimicrobial Therapy for Acute Exacerbations of COPD	
Patient Characteristics	**Likely Pathogens**	**Recommended Therapy**
Uncomplicated exacerbations (<4 exacerbations per year, no comorbid illness)	*S. pneumoniae* *H. influenzae* *M. catarrhalis* *H. parainfluenzae* Resistance uncommon	Macrolide (azithromycin, clarithromycin) Second- or third-generation cephalosporin Doxycycline Therapies not recommended[a]: TMP/SMX, amoxicillin, first-generation cephalosporins, erythromycin
Complicated exacerbations (Age ≥65 and >4 exacerbations per year, presence of comorbid illness)	As above plus drug-resistant pneumococci, β-lactamase–producing *H. influenzae* and *M. catarrhalis*	Amoxicillin/Clavulanate Fluoroquinolone with enhanced pneumococcal activity (levofloxacin, gemifloxacin, moxifloxacin)
Presence of risk factors for colonization and infection with multi-drug resistant pathogens: ✓ Need for chronic corticosteroid therapy ✓ Recent hospitalization (90 days) ✓ Recent antibiotic therapy (90 days) ✓ Resident of long-term care facility	Some enteric gram-negatives As above plus *P. aeruginosa*	Fluoroquinolone with enhanced pneumococcal and *P. aeruginosa* activity (levofloxacin) IV therapy if required: β-lactamase–resistant penicillin with antipseudomonal activity, third- or fourth-generation cephalosporin with antipseudomonal activity

[a]TMP/SMX should not be used due to increasing pneumococcal resistance; amoxicillin and first-generation cephalosporins are not recommended due to β-lactamase susceptibility; and erythromycin is not recommended due to insufficient activity against *H. influenzae*.
TMP-SMX, trimethoprim-sulfamethoxazole.

EVALUATION OF THERAPEUTIC OUTCOMES

- In chronic stable COPD, assess pulmonary function tests annually and with any treatment additions or discontinuations. Other outcome measures are symptom scores, quality-of-life assessments, exacerbation rates, emergency department visits, and hospitalizations.
- In acute exacerbations of COPD, assess white blood cell count, vital signs, chest x-ray, and changes in frequency of dyspnea, sputum volume, and sputum purulence at the onset and throughout treatment of the exacerbation. In more severe exacerbations, ABG and SaO_2 should also be monitored.
- Evaluate patient medication adherence, side effects, and potential drug interactions at every encounter.

See Chapter 44, Chronic Obstructive Pulmonary Disease, authored by Sharya V. Bourdet and Dennis M. Williams, for a more detailed discussion of this topic.

CHAPTER

80 Benign Prostatic Hyperplasia

- *Benign prostatic hyperplasia* (BPH), is a non-cancerous condition in which an enlarged prostate compresses the urethra, blocking the outflow of urine.

PATHOPHYSIOLOGY

- Three types of prostate gland tissue are epithelial or glandular, stromal or smooth muscle, and capsule. Both stromal tissue and capsule are embedded with α_1-adrenergic receptors.
- The precise pathophysiologic mechanisms that cause BPH are not clear. Both intra-prostatic dihydrotestosterone (DHT) and type II 5α-reductase are thought to be involved.
- BPH commonly results from both static (gradual enlargement of the prostate) and dynamic (agents or situations that increase α-adrenergic tone and constrict the gland's smooth muscle) factors. Examples of drugs that can exacerbate symptoms include testosterone, α-adrenergic agonists (eg, decongestants), and those with significant anticholinergic effects (eg, antihistamines, phenothiazines, tricyclic antidepressants, antispasmodics, and antiparkinsonian agents).

CLINICAL PRESENTATION

- Patients present with a variety of signs and symptoms categorized as obstructive or irritative. Symptoms vary over time.
- Obstructive signs and symptoms result when dynamic and/or static factors reduce bladder emptying. Patients experience urinary hesitancy, urine dribbles out of the penis, and the bladder feels full even after voiding.
- Irritative signs and symptoms are common and result from long-standing obstruction at the bladder neck. Patients experience urinary frequency, urgency, and nocturia.
- Obstructive and irritative voiding symptoms are referred to as lower urinary tract symptoms (LUTS) which is not limited to BPH but may also be caused by neurogenic bladder or urinary tract infections.
- BPH progression may produce complications including chronic kidney disease, gross hematuria, urinary incontinence, recurrent urinary tract infection, bladder diverticula, and bladder stones.

DIAGNOSIS

- Includes careful medical history, physical examination, objective measures of bladder emptying (eg, peak and average urinary flow rate and postvoid residual [PVR] urine volume), and laboratory tests (eg, urinalysis and prostate-specific antigen [PSA]).
- On digital rectal examination, the prostate is usually but not always enlarged (>20 g), soft, smooth, and symmetric.

TREATMENT

- <u>Goals of Treatment</u>: The goals are to control symptoms, prevent progression of complications, and delay need for surgical intervention.

- Management options include watchful waiting, drug therapy, and surgical intervention. The choice depends on severity of signs and symptoms (Table 80-1).
- Watchful waiting is appropriate for patients with mild disease (Figure 80-1). Patients are reassessed at 6–12 month intervals and educated about behavior modification, such as fluid restriction before bedtime, minimizing caffeine and alcohol intake, frequent emptying of the bladder, and avoiding drugs that exacerbate voiding symptoms.

PHARMACOLOGIC THERAPY

- Pharmacologic therapy is appropriate for patients with moderate BPH symptoms and as an interim measure for patients with severe BPH.
- Pharmacologic therapy interferes with the stimulatory effect of testosterone on prostate gland enlargement (reduces the static factor), relaxes prostatic smooth muscle (reduces the dynamic factor), or relaxes bladder detrusor muscle (Table 80-2).
- Initiate therapy with an α_1-adrenergic antagonist for faster onset of symptom relief. Select a 5α-reductase inhibitor in patients with a prostate gland more than 40 g who cannot tolerate the cardiovascular adverse effects of α_1-adrenergic antagonists. Consider combination therapy for symptomatic patients with a prostate gland more than 40 g and PSA of 1.4 ng/mL (1.4 mcg/L) or more.
- Consider monotherapy with a phosphodiesterase inhibitor (PI) or use in combination with an α-adrenergic antagonist when erectile dysfunction and BPH are present.
- Combination therapy may reduce bothersome symptoms but may also result in increased risk of adverse effects and drug interactions, higher cost of treatment, and lower rates of adherence.

α-Adrenergic Antagonists

- α-Adrenergic antagonists relax smooth muscle in the prostate and bladder neck, increasing urinary flow rates by 2–3 mL/sec in 60%–70% of patients and reducing PVR urine volumes. These agents do not decrease prostate volume or PSA levels.
- **Prazosin, terazosin, doxazosin**, and **alfuzosin** are second-generation α_1-adrenergic antagonists. They antagonize peripheral vascular α_1-adrenergic receptors in addition to those in the prostate. Adverse effects include first-dose syncope, orthostatic hypotension, and dizziness. Current practice guidelines do not recommend prazosin due to multiple doses/day and significant cardiovascular adverse effects. Alfuzosin is less likely to cause cardiovascular adverse effects than other second-generation agents and is considered functionally and clinically uroselective.
- **Tamsulosin** and **silodosin**, third-generation α_1-adrenergic antagonists, are selective for prostatic α_{1A}-receptors. Therefore, they do not cause peripheral vascular smooth

TABLE 80-1	Categories of BPH Disease Severity Based on Symptoms and Signs	
Disease Severity	**AUA Symptom Score**	**Typical Symptoms and Signs**
Mild	≤7	Asymptomatic
		Peak urinary flow rate <10 mL/sec
		PVR urine volume >25–50 mL
Moderate	8–19	All of the above signs plus obstructive voiding symptoms and irritative voiding symptoms (signs of detrusor instability)
Severe	≥20	All of the above plus one or more complications of BPH

AUA, American Urological Association; BPH, benign prostatic hyperplasia; PVR, postvoid residual volume.

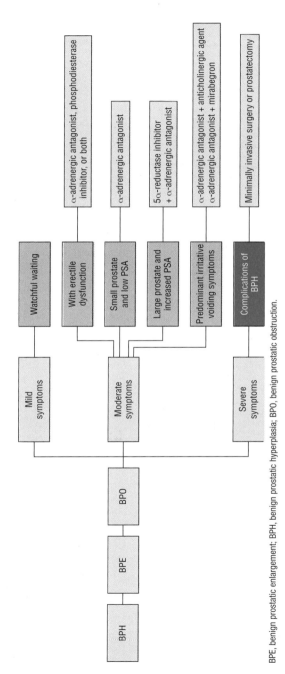

BPE, benign prostatic enlargement; BPH, benign prostatic hyperplasia; BPO, benign prostatic obstruction.

FIGURE 80-1. Management algorithm for benign prostatic hyperplasia (BPH).

TABLE 80-2	Dosing of Drugs Used in Treatment of Benign Prostatic Hyperplasia			
Drug	**Brand Name**	**Initial Dose**	**Usual Dose**	**Special Population Dose**
α-Adrenergic Antagonists				
Prazosin	Minipress	0.5 mg twice a day orally	1–5 mg twice a day orally	To uptitrate the dose, double the dose every 2 weeks.
Terazosin	Hytrin	1 mg at bedtime orally	10–20 mg daily orally	To uptitrate the dose, increase slowly to 2 mg, 5 mg, and then 10 mg daily in a stepwise fashion. Take extra care if the patient is taking other drugs that lower blood pressure.
Doxazosin	Cardura Cardura XL	1 mg daily orally 4 mg daily orally	8 mg daily orally 4–8 mg daily	For the immediate-release formulation, doses of 16 mg daily have been used for hypertension. For the XL formulation, increase from 4 to 8 mg daily after a 3- to 4-week interval. When switching from the immediate- to the extended-release formulation, start with 4 mg of the extended-release formulation no matter what maintenance dose of immediate-release doxazosin the patient is taking.
Alfuzosin	Uroxatral	10 mg daily orally	10 mg daily orally (no dose titration)	This extended-release formulation should not be chewed or crushed. It should be taken after meals and used cautiously in patients with creatinine clearance less than 30 mL/min (0.5 mL/sec).
Tamsulosin	Flomax	0.4 mg daily orally	0.4–0.8 mg daily orally	This extended-release formulation should not be chewed or crushed. It should be taken after meals. No dosage adjustment is needed in patients with renal or liver dysfunction. Allow several weeks before starting a dose before increasing to a higher dose.
Silodosin	Rapaflo	8 mg daily orally	8 mg daily orally (no dose titration)	This drug is contraindicated when creatinine clearance is less than 30 mL/min (0.5 mL/sec). If creatinine clearance is 30–50 mL/min (0.5–0.83 mL/sec), use 4 mg daily orally, preferably after the same meal each day. It should not be given to patients on potent CYP 3A4 inhibitors or with severe hepatic impairment.

5α-Reductase Inhibitors

Finasteride	Proscar	5 mg daily orally	No dosage adjustment in patients with renal impairment. Use cautiously in patients with hepatic impairment.
Dutasteride	Avodart	0.5 mg daily orally	No dosage adjustment in patients with renal impairment. Use cautiously in patients with hepatic impairment.
Dutasteride + tamsulosin	Jalyn	1 tablet (equivalent to 0.5 mg dutasteride + 0.4 mg tamsulosin) daily orally	No dosage adjustment needed in patients with renal or moderate hepatic impairment.

Phosphodiesterase Inhibitor

| Tadalafil | Cialis | 5 mg daily orally | If creatinine clearance is 30–50 mL/min (0.5–0.83 mL/sec), use 2.5 mg daily orally. Do not use if creatinine clearance is less than 30 mL/min (0.5 mL/sec). Use cautiously in patients with mild-to-moderate hepatic impairment. Avoid in patients with severe hepatic impairment. |

Anticholinergic Agents

| Darifenacin | Enablex | 7.5–15 mg daily orally | This extended-release formulation should not be chewed or crushed. To uptitrate the dose, double the dose after 2 weeks. If the patient is taking a potent CYP3A4 inhibitor (eg, ketoconazole, itraconazole, ritonavir, nelfinavir, and clarithromycin), do not exceed 7.5 mg daily orally. No dosage adjustment is needed for patients with renal impairment. Use a maximum dose of 7.5 mg daily for patients with moderate hepatic impairment. Do not use in patients with severe hepatic impairment. |

(Continued)

Drug	Brand Name	Initial Dose	Usual Dose	Special Population Dose
Fesoterodine	Toviaz	4 mg daily orally	4–8 mg daily orally	This extended-release formulation should not be chewed or crushed. If the patient is taking a potent CYP3A4 inhibitor (eg, ketoconazole, itraconazole, ritonavir, nelfinavir, and clarithromycin), do not exceed 4 mg daily orally. If the creatinine clearance is less than 30 mL/min (0.5 mL/sec), do not exceed 4 mg daily orally. Use is not recommended in patients with severe hepatic impairment.
Oxybutynin	Ditropan	5 mg two to three times a day orally	5–10 mg two to three times a day orally	Increase daily dose at 5 mg increments at weekly intervals. No specific dosing modifications available for patients with renal or hepatic impairment; use cautiously in these patients.
	Ditropan XL	5 mg daily orally	5–30 mg daily orally	This extended-release formulation should not be crushed or chewed. Increase daily dose at 5 mg increments at weekly intervals. No specific dosing modifications available for patients with renal impairment; use cautiously in these patients.
	Oxytrol TDS	1 patch (3.9 mg oxybutynin) twice weekly	1 patch (3.9 mg) twice weekly	Apply this transdermal patch to abdomen, hip, or buttock. Rotate application site. Do not expose patch to sunlight. No specific dosing modifications available for patients with renal or hepatic impairment; however, use cautiously in these patients.
	Gelnique 10% gel	1 g gel (100 mg oxybutynin) daily	1 g gel (100 mg oxybutynin) daily	This is available as premeasured dose packets. Apply to abdomen, thighs, upper arms, or shoulders. Wash hands after application. Do not bathe, shower, or swim for 1 hour after application. Cover application site with clothing until medication dries on skin. Rotate application site daily. No specific dosing modifications available for patients with renal or hepatic impairment; use cautiously in these patients.
Solifenacin	VESIcare	5 mg daily orally	5–10 mg daily orally	If the creatinine clearance is less than 30 mL/min (0.5 mL/sec) or the patient has moderate hepatic impairment, do not exceed 5 mg daily orally. Do not use if the patient has severe hepatic impairment. If the patient is taking a potent CYP3A4 inhibitor (eg, ketoconazole, itraconazole, ritonavir, nelfinavir, and clarithromycin), do not exceed 5 mg daily orally

TABLE 80-2 Dosing of Drugs Used in Treatment of Benign Prostatic Hyperplasia (*Continued*)

Tolterodine	Detrol	2 mg twice daily orally	1–2 mg twice daily orally	If the patient has significant renal impairment or severe hepatic impairment, limit dose to 1 mg twice a day.
	Detrol LA	4 mg daily orally	2–4 mg daily orally	This extended-release formulation should not be chewed or crushed. If the creatinine clearance is 10–30 mL/min (0.17–0.5 mL/sec) or the patient has mild/moderate hepatic impairment, do not exceed 2 mg daily orally. If the creatinine clearance is less than 10 mL/min (0.17 mL/sec), do not use Detrol LA. If the patient has severe hepatic impairment, use of the extended-release formulation is not recommended.
Trospium	Sanctura	20 mg twice daily orally	20 mg twice daily orally	Avoid alcohol ingestion for 2 hours after a dose. Use cautiously in patients with moderate or severe hepatic impairment. In patients older than 75 years, use the immediate-release formulation and start with 20 mg daily orally. If the creatinine clearance is less than 30 mL/min (0.5 mL/sec), use 20 mg immediate-release formulation.
	Sanctura XR	60 mg daily orally	60 mg daily orally	This extended-release formulation should not be chewed or crushed. This product is not recommended in patients with creatinine clearance less than 30 mL/min (0.5 mL/sec). It should be used cautiously in patients with severe hepatic impairment.
β₃-Adrenergic Agonist				
Mirabegron	Myrbetriq	25 mg daily orally	25–50 mg daily orally	This is an extended-release formulation. Do not chew, crush, or divide tablet. In patients with a creatinine clearance of 15–29 mL/min (0.25–0.48 mL/sec) or those with moderate hepatic impairment, the maximum daily dose is 25 mg daily. This drug is not recommended in patients with creatinine clearance less than 15 mL/min (0.25 mL/sec) or those with severe hepatic impairment.

muscle relaxation and associated hypotension. Dose titration is minimal and the onset of peak action is seen within a week.

- Potential drug interactions include decreased metabolism of α_1-adrenergic antagonists with CYP 3A4 inhibitors (eg, cimetidine and diltiazem) and increased catabolism of α_1-adrenergic antagonists with concurrent use of CYP 3A4 stimulators (eg, carbamazepine and phenytoin).
- Reduce the dose of silodosin in patients with moderate renal impairment or hepatic dysfunction.

5α-Reductase Inhibitors

- 5α-Reductase inhibitors interfere with the stimulatory effect of testosterone. These agents slow disease progression and decrease the risk of complications.
- Compared with α_1-adrenergic antagonists, disadvantages of 5α-reductase inhibitors include 6–12 months of use to maximally shrink the prostate, less likelihood of inducing objective improvement, and more sexual dysfunction. They are considered second-line therapy in sexually active males.
- **Dutasteride** inhibits types I and II 5α-reductase, whereas **finasteride** inhibits only type II.
- 5α-Reductase inhibitors may be preferred in patients with uncontrolled arrhythmias, poorly controlled angina, requirement for multiple antihypertensives, or intolerance to the hypotensive effects of α_1-adrenergic antagonists.
- Measure PSA at baseline and again after 6 months of therapy. If PSA does not decrease by 50% after 6 months of therapy in an adherent patient, evaluate the patient for prostate cancer.
- 5α-Reductase inhibitors are in FDA pregnancy category X and are therefore contraindicated in pregnant women. Women who are pregnant or seeking to become pregnant should not handle the tablets or have contact with semen from men taking 5α-reductase inhibitors.

Phosphodiesterase Inhibitors

- Increase in cyclic GMP by PIs relaxes smooth muscle in the prostate and bladder neck.
- **Tadalafil** 5 mg daily improves voiding symptoms but does not increase urinary flow rate or reduce PVR urine volume. Combination therapy with α-adrenergic antagonist results in significant improvement in LUTS, increased urinary flow rates, and decreased PVR volume.

Anticholinergic Agents

- Addition of **oxybutynin** and **tolterodine** to α-adrenergic antagonists relieves irritative voiding symptoms including urinary frequency, urgency, and nocturia. Start with lowest effective dose to determine tolerance of CNS adverse effects and dry mouth. Measure PVR urine volume before initiating treatment (should be less than 150 mL).
- Consider transdermal (eg, oxybutynin) or extended-release formulations (eg, tolterodine) or uroselective agents (eg, **darifenacin** or **solifenacin**) if systemic anticholinergic adverse effects are poorly tolerated.

B$_3$-Adrenergic Agonist

- **Mirabegron** is a β_3-adrenergic agonist that relaxes the detrusor muscle reducing irritative voiding systems, increases urinary bladder capacity, and increases the interval between voidings. It does not cause anticholinergic adverse effects and is an alternative to anticholinergic agents in patients with LUTS.

SURGICAL INTERVENTION

- Prostatectomy, performed transurethrally or suprapubically, is the gold standard for treatment of patients with moderate or severe symptoms of BPH and for all patients with complications.

- Retrograde ejaculation complicates up to 75% of transurethral prostatectomy procedures. Other complications seen in 2%–15% of patients are bleeding, urinary incontinence, and erectile dysfunction.

PHYTOTHERAPY

- Although widely used in Europe for BPH, phytotherapy with products such as saw palmetto berry (*Serenoa repens*), stinging nettle (*Urtica dioica*), and African plum (*Pygeum africanum*) should be avoided. Studies are inconclusive, and these agents are not regulated by the FDA.

EVALUATION OF THERAPEUTIC OUTCOMES

- The primary therapeutic outcome of BPH therapy is restoring adequate urinary flow with minimal treatment-related adverse effects. Assess efficacy 6–12 weeks after starting treatment.
- Outcome depends on the patient's perception of effectiveness and acceptability of therapy. The American Urological Association Symptom Score is a validated standardized instrument that can be used to assess patient quality of life.
- Objective measures of bladder emptying (eg, urinary flow rate and PVR urine volume) are useful measures in patients considering surgery.
- Monitor laboratory tests (eg, blood urea nitrogen, creatinine, and PSA) and urinalysis regularly. An annual digital rectal examination is recommended if life expectancy is at least 10 years.

See Chapter 100, Benign Prostatic Hyperplasia, authored by Mary Lee and Roohollah Sharifi, for a more detailed discussion of this topic.

CHAPTER 81

Erectile Dysfunction

- *Erectile dysfunction* (ED) is the persistent failure (minimum of 3 months) to achieve a penile erection suitable for sexual intercourse. Patients often refer to it as impotence.

PATHOPHYSIOLOGY

- ED can result from any single abnormality or combination of abnormalities of the four systems necessary for a normal penile erection. Vascular, neurologic, or hormonal etiologies of ED are referred to as *organic ED*. Patients who do not respond to psychogenic stimuli and have no organic cause for dysfunction have *psychogenic ED*.
- The penis has two corpora cavernosa and one corpus spongiosum, which contain interconnected sinuses that fill with blood to produce an erection that is sustained by occlusion of venous outflow from the corpora.
- Acetylcholine works with other neurotransmitters (ie, cyclic guanylate monophosphate [cGMP], cyclic adenosine monophosphate [cAMP], or vasoactive intestinal polypeptide) to produce penile arterial vasodilation and ultimately an erection.
- Organic ED is associated with diseases that compromise vascular flow to the corpora cavernosum (eg, peripheral vascular disease, arteriosclerosis, and essential hypertension), impair nerve conduction to the brain (eg, spinal cord injury and stroke), or impair peripheral nerve conduction (eg, diabetes mellitus). Secondary ED is associated with hypogonadism.
- Psychogenic ED is associated with malaise, reactive depression or performance anxiety, sedation, Alzheimer disease, hypothyroidism, and mental disorders. Patients with psychogenic ED generally have a higher response rate to interventions than those with organic ED.
- Social habits (eg, cigarette smoking and excessive ethanol intake) and medications (**Table 81-1**) can also cause ED.

CLINICAL PRESENTATION

- Signs and symptoms of ED can be difficult to detect. The patient's partner is often the first to report ED to the healthcare provider.
- Nonadherence to drugs thought to cause ED can be a sign of ED.

DIAGNOSIS

- Key diagnostic assessments include description of ED severity, medical, psychological, and surgical histories, review of concurrent medications, physical examination, assessment of cardiac reserve, and laboratory tests (ie, serum blood glucose, lipid profile, and testosterone level).
- Assess the severity of ED with a standardized questionnaire, such as the International Index of Erectile Function (IIEF).

TREATMENT

- <u>Goals of Treatment</u>: The goal is to improve the quantity and quality of penile erections suitable for intercourse.
- The first step in management of ED is to identify and, if possible, reverse underlying causes. Psychotherapy can be used as monotherapy for psychogenic ED or as an adjunct to specific treatments.
- Treatment options include vacuum erection devices (VEDs), drugs (**Table 81-2**), and surgery. Although no option is ideal, the least invasive options are chosen first (**Figure 81-1**).

TABLE 81-1 Medication Classes That Can Cause Erectile Dysfunction

Drug Class	Proposed Mechanism by Which Drug Causes Erectile Dysfunction	Special Notes
Anticholinergic agents (antihistamines, antiparkinsonian agents, tricyclic antidepressants, phenothiazines)	Anticholinergic activity	Second-generation nonsedating antihistamines (eg, loratadine, fexofenadine, or cetirizine) are associated with less erectile dysfunction than first-generation agents.
		Selective serotonin reuptake inhibitor (SSRI) and multiple receptor reuptake inhibitor antidepressants cause less erectile dysfunction than tricyclic antidepressants. Of the SSRIs, paroxetine, sertraline, fluvoxamine, and fluoxetine cause erectile dysfunction more commonly than venlafaxine, nefazodone, trazodone, bupropion, duloxetine, mirtazapine, escitalopram, or vilazodone.
		Phenothiazines with less anticholinergic effect (eg, chlorpromazine) can be substituted in some patients if erectile dysfunction is a problem.
Dopamine antagonists (eg, metoclopramide, phenothiazines)	Inhibit prolactin inhibitory factor, thereby increasing prolactin levels	Increased prolactin levels inhibit testicular testosterone production; depressed libido results.
Estrogens or drugs with antiandrogenic effects (eg, luteinizing hormone-releasing hormone superagonists, digoxin, spironolactone, ketoconazole, cimetidine)	Suppress testosterone-mediated stimulation of libido	In the face of a decreased libido, a secondary erectile dysfunction develops because of diminished sexual drive.
CNS depressants (eg, barbiturates, narcotics, benzodiazepines, short-term use of large doses of alcohol, anticonvulsants)	Suppress perception of psychogenic stimuli	

(Continued)

TABLE 81-1	Medication Classes That Can Cause Erectile Dysfunction (Continued)	
Drug Class	**Proposed Mechanism by Which Drug Causes Erectile Dysfunction**	**Special Notes**
Agents that decrease penile blood flow (eg, diuretics, peripheral β-adrenergic antagonists, or central sympatholytics [methyldopa, clonidine, guanethidine])	Reduce arteriolar flow to corpora	Any diuretic that produces a significant decrease in intravascular volume can decrease penile arteriolar flow.
		Safer antihypertensives include angiotensin-converting enzyme inhibitors, postsynaptic α₁-adrenergic antagonists (terazosin, doxazosin), calcium channel blockers, and angiotensin II receptor antagonists.
Miscellaneous	Unknown mechanism	
Finasteride, dutasteride		
Lithium carbonate		
Gemfibrozil		
Interferon		
Clofibrate		
Monoamine oxidase inhibitors (eg, phenelzine, isocarboxazid, tranylcypromine)		
Opioids		

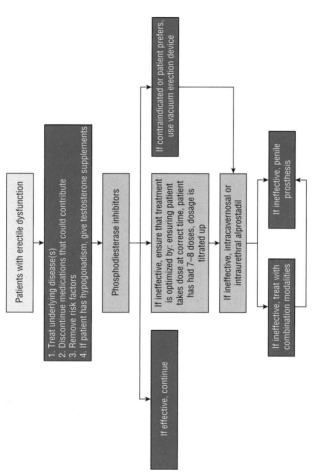

FIGURE 81-1. Algorithm for selecting treatment for erectile dysfunction.

TABLE 81-2 Dosing Regimens for Selected Drug Treatments for Erectile Dysfunction

Drug	Brand Name[a]	Initial Dose	Usual Range	Special Population Dose	Other
Phosphodiesterase Inhibitor					
Sildenafil	Viagra	50 mg orally 1 hour before intercourse	25–100 mg 1 hour before intercourse. Limit to one dose per day	In patients age 65 years and older, start with 25 mg dose. In patients with creatinine clearance less than 30 mL/min (0.5 mL/sec) or severe hepatic impairment, limit starting dose to 25 mg. In patients with mild-to-moderate hepatic impairment or those taking strong CYP3A4 inhibitors (eg, itraconazole, ketoconazole, or erythromycin), consider starting with 25 mg. In patients taking protease inhibitors, limit starting dose to 25 mg every 48 hours.	Generic formulations are available. Titrate dose so that erection lasts no more than 1 hour. High-fat foods decrease rate of absorption by 1 hour. Avoid taking dose with grapefruit juice. Contraindicated with nitrates by any route of administration.
Vardenafil	Levitra	5–10 mg orally 1 hour before intercourse	5–20 mg 1 hour before intercourse. Limit to one dose per day	In patients age 65 years and older, start with 5 mg Levitra. No dosage adjustment is required in patients with decreased creatinine clearance. In patients with moderate hepatic impairment, start with 5 mg Levitra. Use not recommended in patients with severe hepatic impairment. In patients taking strong P450 CYP3A4 inhibitors (eg, atazanavir, erythromycin, clarithromycin, ketoconazole, itraconazole), limit starting dose to 2.5 mg every 24 hours. In patients on ritonavir, limit dose to 2.5 mg every 72 hours. Not recommended in patients with congenital prolonged QT interval or in patients taking Type 1A or Type 3 antiarrhythmics.	Titrate dose so that erection lasts no more than 1 hour. High-fat foods decrease rate of absorption by 1 hour. Avoid taking dose with grapefruit juice. Contraindicated with nitrates by any route of administration.

Staxyn	10 mg tablet to dissolve on the tongue 1 hour before intercourse	10 mg tablet to dissolve on the tongue 1 hour before intercourse. Limit to one dose per day	Dose of Staxyn requires no adjustment in patients 65 years or older, patients with creatinine clearance less than 30 mL/min (0.5 mL/sec), or those with mild hepatic impairment. Do not use in patients with moderate or severe hepatic impairment or those taking moderately or highly potent P450 CYP3A4 inhibitors. Do not initiate Staxyn in patients taking α-adrenergic antagonists.	Staxyn should be taken without any liquid or food. The tablet should be placed on the tongue where it will dissolve. No uptitration of dose is recommended. Do not substitute Staxyn for Levitra, or vice versa.
Tadalafil	5–10 mg orally at least 30 minutes before intercourse OR 2.5–5 mg orally once daily	10–20 mg at least 30 minutes before intercourse. Limit to one dose per day 2.5–5 mg once daily. Limit to one dose per day	Dose of tadalafil requires no dosage adjustment in patients 65 years or older. In patients with creatinine clearance of 30–50 mL/min (0.5–0.83 mL/sec), limit starting dose to 10 mg every 48 hours; if less than 30 mL/min (0.5 mL/sec), limit starting dose to 5 mg every 72 hours. In patients with mild-to-moderate hepatic impairment, limit starting dose to 10 mg every 24 hours. Do not use in patients with severe hepatic impairment. In patients taking potent P450 CYP3A4 inhibitors, limit starting dose to 10 mg every 72 hours (if using it on demand) or 2.5 mg daily (if using a continuous daily regimen).	Generic formulations are available. Titrate dose so that erection lasts not more than 1 hour. Food does not affect rate or extent of drug absorption. Avoid taking dose with grapefruit juice. Contraindicated with nitrates by any route of administration. When taken with large amounts of ethanol, tadalafil may cause orthostatic hypotension.
	Cialis		

(Continued)

TABLE 81-2	Dosing Regimens for Selected Drug Treatments for Erectile Dysfunction (Continued)				
Drug	Brand Name[a]	Initial Dose	Usual Range	Special Population Dose	Other
Avanafil	Stendra	100 mg orally 15–30 minutes before intercourse	50–200 mg orally 15–30 minutes before intercourse. Limit to one dose per day.	In patients with creatinine clearance of 30–89 mL/min (0.5–1.49 mL/sec) or those with mild-to-moderate hepatic impairment, no dosage adjustment is needed. Not recommended if creatinine clearance is less than 30 mL/min (0.5 mL/sec), if the patient has severe hepatic disease, or if the patient is taking potent P450 CYP3A4 inhibitors. If the patient is taking moderate P450 CYP3A4 inhibitors (eg, erythromycin, fluconazole), the maximum recommended dose is 50 mg every 24 hours.	May be taken with or without food. Avoid taking dose with grapefruit juice. When taken with large amounts of ethanol, avanafil may cause orthostatic hypotension.
Prostaglandin E₁					
Alprostadil intracavernosal injection	Caverject, Edex	2.5 mcg intracavernosally 5–10 minutes before intercourse	10–20 mcg 5–10 minutes before intercourse. Maximum recommended dose is 60 mcg. Limit to not more than one injection per day and not more than three injections per week with a 24-hour interval between doses	In older adults, use the lowest effective dose. No specific dosage adjustment provided in labeling for patients with hepatic or renal impairment.	Titrate dose to achieve an erection that lasts 1 hour. Patient will require training on aseptic intracavernosal injection technique. Avoid intracavernosal injections in patients with sickle cell anemia, multiple myeloma, leukemia, severe coagulopathy, schizophrenia, poor manual dexterity, severe venous incompetence, severe cardiovascular disease, or Peyronie disease.

Drug	Brand	Dose	Dose	Considerations
Alprostadil intraurethral pellet	Muse	125–250 mcg intraurethrally 5–10 minutes before intercourse	250–1000 mcg just before intercourse. Limit to not more than two doses per day	In older adults, use the lowest effective dose. No specific dosage adjustment provided in labeling for patients with hepatic or renal impairment. Patient will require training on proper intraurethral administration techniques. Use applicator provided to administer medications to avoid urethral injury.
Testosterone Supplements				
Methyltestosterone	Android, Testred, Methitest	10 mg once daily	10–50 mg once daily	No dosage adjustment provided in labeling for patients with renal or hepatic impairment or older adults. Not recommended for use due to extensive first-pass hepatic catabolism and because it is associated with hepatotoxicity. May cause fluid retention in patients with renal or hepatic disease.
Testosterone buccal system	Striant	30 mg every 12 hours, morning and evening	30 mg every 12 hours, morning and evening	No dosage adjustment provided in labeling for patients with renal or hepatic impairment or older adults. Time the dose so that buccal system is removed before every morning and evening toothbrushing. Place buccal system just above incisor tooth in the mouth and hold in place for 30 seconds to adhere. To remove, slide buccal system down toward the tooth. With each dose, rotate site of administration to the alternate side of the mouth. Buccal tablet may become detached during eating. If this occurs, discard and replace with new buccal system. Do not chew or swallow buccal system.

(Continued)

957

TABLE 81-2 Dosing Regimens for Selected Drug Treatments for Erectile Dysfunction (*Continued*)

Drug	Brand Name[a]	Initial Dose	Usual Range	Special Population Dose	Other
Testosterone cypionate intramuscular injection	Depo-Testosterone	200–400 mg every 2–4 weeks	200–400 mg every 2–4 weeks (up to 6 weeks)	No dosage adjustment provided in labeling for patients with renal or hepatic impairment or older adults.	During the dosing interval, supraphysiologic serum concentrations of testosterone are produced during a portion of the dosing interval. This has been linked to mood swings.
Testosterone enanthate intramuscular injection	Delatestryl	200–400 mg every 2–4 weeks	200–400 mg every 2–4 weeks (up to 6 weeks)	No dosage adjustment provided in labeling for patients with renal or hepatic impairment or older adults.	During the dosing interval, supraphysiologic serum concentrations of testosterone are produced during a portion of the dosing interval. This has been linked to mood swings.
Testosterone undecanoate intramuscular injection	Aveed	750 mg as a single dose	750 mg as a single dose on Day 0, Week 4, and then 750 mg every 10 weeks	No dosage adjustment provided in labeling for patients with renal or hepatic impairment or older adults. Contraindicated in patients with serious hepatic or renal disease.	Only available in facilities certified through a Risk Evaluation and Mitigation Strategy Program. Administer by deep intramuscular injection into gluteal muscle. Avoid intravascular injection, which can lead to pulmonary oil embolism.
Testosterone transdermal patch	Androderm	4 mg as a single dose at bedtime	2–6 mg as a single dose at bedtime. Titrate dose 2 weeks after initiating a dose	No dosage adjustment is provided in labeling for patients with renal or hepatic impairment or older adults.	When administered at bedtime, serum concentrations of testosterone in the usual circadian pattern are produced. Apply to those sites recommended in the package labeling: upper arm, back, abdomen, and thigh. Rotate application sites every 7 days. May have to apply multiple patches at one time to achieve appropriate serum testosterone level. Avoid swimming, showering, or washing administration site for 3 hours after patch application.

| Testosterone gel | AndroGel 1% (25 mg/2.5 g), Testim 1% (25 mg/2.5 g) | 5–10 g of gel (equivalent to 50–100 mg testosterone, respectively) as a single dose in the morning | 5–10 g of gel (equivalent to 50–100 mg testosterone, respectively) as a single dose in the morning. Titrate dose up at 14-day intervals | No dosage adjustment provided in labeling for patients with renal or hepatic impairment or older adults. | Cover application site to avoid inadvertent transfer to others. Avoid swimming, showering, or washing administration site for 2 hours after gel application. Apply to those sites recommended in the product labeling. For AndroGel, apply to shoulders, upper arms, or abdomen. For Testim, apply to shoulders or upper arms only. Children and women should avoid contact with unclothed or unwashed application sites. Patients should wash hands with soap and water after administration of transdermal testosterone product. For patients who have difficulty measuring the appropriate dose using tubes of gel, it is also available in premeasured dose packets or from a pump dispenser. REMS assessments must be submitted to the FDA. |
| | AndroGel 1.6% (40.5 mg/2.5 g) | 2 pumps (equivalent to 40.5 mg testosterone) as a single dose in the morning | 2–4 pumps (equivalent to 40.5–81 mg) as a single dose in the morning. Titrate dose 14–28 days after starting treatment | No dosage adjustment provided in labeling for patients with renal or hepatic impairment or older adults. | Apply to shoulders and upper arms. Avoid swimming, showering, or washing administration site for 2 hours after application. Same precautions as listed above for 1% gel. REMS assessments must be submitted to the FDA. |

(Continued)

TABLE 81-2	Dosing Regimens for Selected Drug Treatments for Erectile Dysfunction (*Continued*)				
Drug	Brand Name[a]	Initial Dose	Usual Range	Special Population Dose	Other
Testosterone transdermal spray	Fortesta 2% (10 mg/actuation)	4 sprays (equivalent to 40 mg testosterone) every morning	4–7 sprays (equivalent to 40–70 mg testosterone) every morning. Titrate dose up at 14- to 35-day intervals	No dosage adjustment provided in labeling for patients with renal or hepatic impairment or older adults.	Must prime pump by pushing on pump three times. Apply to front or inner thighs only. Cover application site to avoid inadvertent transfer to others. Avoid swimming, showering, or washing administration site for 2 hours after spray application. Children and women should avoid contact with unclothed or unwashed application sites. Patients should wash hands with soap and water after administration of transdermal testosterone product. REMS assessments must be submitted to the FDA.
Testosterone transdermal solution	Axiron (30 mg/actuation)	One pump spray (equivalent to 30 mg testosterone) to left or right axilla daily	One to four pump sprays (equivalent to 30–120 mg testosterone, respectively) to left or right axilla daily. Titrate dose up at 14- to 35-day intervals	No dosage adjustment provided in labeling for patients with renal or hepatic impairment or older adults.	Limit application to axilla. Apply antiperspirant or deodorant before Axiron. If applying multiple spray doses, apply one spray, let dry, then apply second dose to each axilla. Avoid swimming, showering, or washing administration site for 2 hours after application. REMS assessments must be submitted to the FDA.
Testosterone subcutaneous implant pellet	Testopel	150–450 mg (equivalent to 2–6 pellets) as a single dose every 3–6 months	150–450 mg as a single dose every 3–6 months	No dosage adjustment recommended for renal or hepatic impairment or older adults.	Trained health professional is required to administer the dose. Should use sterile implanter kit. Administration of the dose requires a forearm incision and subcutaneous dose implant under local anesthesia. Clinical onset is delayed for 3–4 months after initial dose. Generic formulations are available in higher strengths: 100 or 200 mg per pellet.

[a]Common brand names are included in this table. Medications may be available with other brand names.

NONPHARMACOLOGIC TREATMENT

Vacuum Erection Device

- First-line therapy for older patients in stable relationships. Onset of action is slow (ie, 3–20 minutes). An erection can be prolonged through use of constriction bands or tension rings.
- Consider VEDs as second-line therapy after failure of oral or injectable drugs. Response rate improves with addition of **alprostadil** or a phosphodiesterase inhibitor (PI).
- VEDs are contraindicated in patients with sickle cell disease or a history of prolonged erections. Use cautiously in patients taking warfarin as the likelihood of penile bruising is increased.

Surgery

- Surgical insertion of a penile prosthesis, the most invasive treatment for ED, is used after failure of less invasive treatments and for patients who are not candidates for other treatments.

PHARMACOLOGIC TREATMENTS

Phosphodiesterase Type 5 Inhibitors

- Phosphodiesterase mediates catabolism of cGMP, a vasodilatory neurotransmitter in the corporal tissue.
- PIs are selective for isoenzyme type 5 in genital tissue. Inhibition of this isoenzyme in nongenital tissues (eg, peripheral vascular tissue, tracheal smooth muscle, and platelets) can produce adverse effects.
- Available agents (**avanafil, sildenafil, tadalafil,** and **vardenafil**) have different pharmacokinetic and pharmacodynamics profiles (**Table 81-3**). They are considered equally effective and comparable in safety despite no comparative clinical trial data.
- PIs are first-line therapy for younger patients. Effectiveness appears to be dose related; nonresponse rate is 30%–40%. Patient education is critical for clinical success.
- Hepatic metabolism of all four PIs can be inhibited by enzyme inhibitors of CYP 3A4. Use a lower starting dose to minimize dose-related adverse effects.
- Avoid exceeding prescribed doses due to increased frequency of adverse effects and inconsistent erectile responses.
- In usual doses, the most common adverse effects include headache, facial flushing, dyspepsia, nasal congestion, and dizziness that are all dose related.
- Sildenafil and vardenafil decrease systolic/diastolic blood pressure by 8–10/5–8 mm Hg for 1–4 hours after a dose. Although most patients are asymptomatic, multiple antihypertensives, nitrates, and baseline hypotension increase the risk of developing adverse effects. Avanafil is associated with similar decreases in blood pressure. Tadalafil is not associated with blood pressure decreases, but use with caution in patients with cardiovascular disease because of the inherent cardiac risk associated with sexual activity.
- Guidelines are available for stratifying patients on the basis of their cardiovascular risk (**Table 81-4**).
- Use PIs cautiously in patients at risk for retinitis pigmentosa and by pilots who rely on blue and green lights to land airplanes. Evaluate patients with sudden vision loss before continuing treatment.
- Tadalafil inhibits type 11 phosphodiesterase, which is thought to account for the dose-related back and muscle pain seen in 7%–30% of patients.
- PIs are contraindicated in patients taking nitrates. Use cautiously in patients taking α-adrenergic antagonists.

Testosterone-Replacement Regimens

- **Testosterone**-replacement regimens restore serum testosterone levels to the normal range (300–1100 ng/dL; 10.4–38.2 nmol/L). These regimens are indicated for

TABLE 81-3	Pharmacodynamics and Pharmacokinetics of Phosphodiesterase Inhibitors			
	Sildenafil (Viagra)	Vardenafil (Levitra/Staxyn)	Tadalafil (Cialis)	Avanafil (Stendra)
Inhibits PDE-5	Yes	Yes	Yes	Yes
Inhibits PDE-1	Yes	Yes	Minimally	Minimally
Inhibits PDE-6	Yes	Yes	No	Moderately
Inhibits PDE-11	No	No	Yes	No
Time to peak plasma level (hours)	0.5–1	0.7–0.9/1.5	2	0.5–0.8
Oral bioavailability (%)	40	15/21–44	36	15
Fatty meal decreases rate of oral absorption?	Yes	Yes/No[a]	No	No
Mean plasma half-life (hours)	3.7	4.4–4.8/4–6	18	4–5
Active metabolite	Yes	Yes/Yes	No	Yes
Is CYP 3A4 principally responsible for metabolism?	Yes	Yes	Yes	Yes
Other CYP enzymes responsible for metabolism	CYP 2C9, CYP 2C19, CYP 2D6	CYP 3A5, CYP 2C9	None	CYP 2C9
Percentage of dose excreted in feces	80	91–95/91–95	61	62
Percentage of dose excreted in urine	13	2–6/2–6	36	21
Clinical onset (minutes)	30	30/60	45	25–40
Duration (hours)	4–12	4–5/4–6	24–36	6+

[a]When Staxyn is taken with water, the area under the curve decreases by 29%.

TABLE 81-4	Recommendations of the Third Princeton Consensus Conference for Cardiovascular Risk Stratification of Patients Being Considered for Phosphodiesterase Inhibitor Therapy	
Risk Category	**Description of Patient's Condition**	**Management Approach**
Low risk	Has asymptomatic cardiovascular disease with <3 risk factors for cardiovascular disease	Patient can be started on phosphodiesterase inhibitor
	Has well-controlled hypertension	
	Has mild CHF (NYHA class I or II)	
	Has mild valvular heart disease	
	Has had a myocardial infarction >8 weeks ago	
Intermediate risk	Has ≥3 risk factors for cardiovascular disease	Patient should undergo complete cardiovascular workup and treadmill stress test to determine tolerance to increased myocardial energy consumption associated with increased sexual activity. Then, reclassify in low- or high-risk category
	Has mild or moderate, stable angina	
	Had a recent myocardial infarction or stroke within the past 2–8 weeks	
	Has moderate CHF (NYHA class III)	
	History of stroke, transient ischemic attack, or peripheral artery disease	
High risk	Has unstable or refractory angina, despite treatment	Phosphodiesterase inhibitor is contraindicated; sexual intercourse should be deferred
	Has uncontrolled hypertension	
	Has severe CHF (NYHA class IV)	
	Has had a recent myocardial infarction or stroke within past 2 weeks	
	Has moderate or severe valvular heart disease	
	Has high-risk cardiac arrhythmias	
	Has obstructive hypertrophic cardiomyopathy	

CHF, congestive heart failure; NYHA, New York Heart Association.

Reprinted with permission from Nehra A, Jackson G, Miner M, et al. The Princeton III Consensus Recommendations for the Management of Erectile Dysfunction and Cardiovascular Disease. Mayo Clin Proc. 2012;87(8):766–778.

symptomatic patients with hypogonadism as confirmed by both a decreased libido and low serum testosterone concentrations.

- Testosterone-replacement regimens correct secondary ED by improving libido. Improved muscle strength, sexual drive, and mood are observed within days or weeks of initiating treatment; however, improvements in ED or increased muscle mass may take months.

- Oral, buccal, parenteral, and transdermal products are available (see Table 81-2). Injectable regimens are preferred because they are effective, inexpensive, and do not have the bioavailability problems or adverse hepatotoxic effects of oral regimens. Testosterone patches, gels, and sprays are more expensive than other forms and should be reserved for patients who refuse injections.

- Screen patients 40 years and older for breast cancer, benign prostatic hyperplasia (BPH), and prostate cancer before starting therapy. Continue treatment for 3–6 months before an increase in dosage is considered.

- Testosterone replacement can cause sodium retention which can result in weight gain or exacerbate hypertension, congestive heart failure, and edema; gynecomastia; serum lipoprotein changes; and erythrocytosis.

- Oral testosterone-replacement regimens can cause hepatotoxicity, ranging from mildly elevated hepatic transaminases to serious liver diseases including peliosis hepatitis, hepatocellular and intrahepatic cholestasis, and benign or malignant tumors.

- Topical testosterone patches may cause contact dermatitis that responds to topical corticosteroids.

Alprostadil

- **Alprostadil**, or prostaglandin E_1, stimulates adenyl cyclase to increase production of cAMP, a neurotransmitter that ultimately enhances blood flow to and blood filling of the corpora.

- Alprostadil is approved as monotherapy for the management of ED. It is generally prescribed after failure of VEDs and PIs and for patients who cannot use these therapies. The intracavernosal route is more effective than the intraurethral route.

- *Intracavernosal* alprostadil is effective in 70%–90% of patients, but 30%–50% discontinue therapy during first 6–12 months. Perceived ineffectiveness, inconvenience of administration, unnatural, nonspontaneous erection, needle phobia, loss of interest, and cost of therapy are reasons given for discontinuation.

- *Intracavernosal* alprostadil is used successfully in combination with VEDs or vasoactive agents (eg, papaverine and phentolamine) that act by different mechanisms.

- *Intracavernosal* alprostadil acts rapidly, with an onset of 5–15 minutes. Duration of action is dose related and, within the usual dosage range, lasts less than 1 hour. To avoid adverse effects, the maximum number of injections is one daily and three weekly, with at least 24 hours between doses.

- Usual dose is 10–20 mcg up to a maximum of 60 mcg. The manufacturer recommends slow dose titration, but in clinical practice, most patients start with 10 mcg and titrate quickly.

- Local adverse effects occur during the first year of therapy, including cavernosal plaques or fibrosis at the injection site (2%–12% of patients), penile pain (10%–44%), and priapism (1%–15%). Penile pain is usually mild and self-limiting, but priapism (ie, painful, drug-induced erection lasting >1 hour) necessitates immediate medical attention.

- Use cautiously in patients at risk of priapism (eg, sickle cell disease, leukemia, or multiple myeloma) and bleeding complications secondary to injections.

- Instill *intraurethral* alprostadil, 125–1000 mcg 5–10 minutes before intercourse after emptying the bladder. No more than two doses daily are recommended.

- *Intraurethral* administration is associated with mild pain in 24%–32% of patients. Prolonged painful erections are rare.

- Female partners may experience vaginal burning, itching, or pain, which is probably related to transfer of alprostadil during intercourse.

Unapproved Agents

- A variety of commercially available and investigational agents have been used for management of ED. Examples include **yohimbine** (6–15 mg orally three times daily), **papaverine** (7.5–60 mg [single-agent therapy] or 0.5–20 mg [combination therapy] intracavernosal injection), and **phentolamine** (0.5–1 mg in combination with 30 mg papaverine; dose administered ranges from 0.1 to 1 mL of the mixture as an intracavernosal injection).

EVALUATION OF THERAPEUTIC OUTCOMES

- The primary therapeutic outcomes for ED are improving the quantity and quality of penile erections suitable for intercourse and avoiding adverse drug reactions and interactions.
- Assess the patient at baseline and after a treatment trial period of 1–3 weeks.
- Identify patients with unrealistic expectations and counsel accordingly to avoid adverse effects due to excessive use of erectogenic agents.

See Chapter 99, Erectile Dysfunction, authored by Mary Lee and Roohollah Sharifi, for a more detailed discussion of this topic.

- *Urinary incontinence* (UI) is loss of bladder control, leading to involuntary leakage of urine.

PATHOPHYSIOLOGY

- The urethral sphincter, a combination of smooth and striated muscles within and external to the urethra, maintains adequate resistance to the flow of urine from the bladder until voluntary voiding is initiated.
- Volitional and involuntary bladder contractions are mediated by activation of post-synaptic muscarinic receptors by acetylcholine. Bladder smooth muscle cholinergic receptors are mainly of the M_2 variety; however, M_3 receptors are responsible for both emptying contraction of normal micturition and involuntary bladder contractions, which can result in UI. Therefore, most pharmacologic antimuscarinic therapy is anti-M_3 based.
- Stimulation of beta-3 adrenergic receptors in the detrusor results in smooth muscle relaxation. β_3-agonists attenuate bladder contractility, which is useful for treatment of overactive bladder (OAB) and urgency incontinence.
- UI occurs as a result of overactivity or underactivity of the urethra, bladder, or both.
- Urethral underactivity is known as *stress UI* (SUI) and occurs during activities such as exercise, running, lifting, coughing, and sneezing. The urethral sphincter no longer resists the flow of urine from the bladder during periods of physical activity.
- Bladder overactivity is known as *urgency UI* (UUI) and is associated with increased urinary frequency and urgency, with or without urge incontinence. The detrusor muscle is overactive and contracts inappropriately during the filling phase.
- Urethral overactivity and/or bladder underactivity is known as *overflow* incontinence. The bladder is filled to capacity but is unable to empty, causing urine to leak from a distended bladder past a normal outlet and sphincter. Common causes of urethral overactivity include benign prostatic hyperplasia (see Chapter 80); prostate cancer (see Chapter 64); and, in women, cystocele formation or surgical overcorrection after SUI surgery.
- Mixed incontinence includes the combination of bladder overactivity and urethral underactivity.
- Functional incontinence is not caused by bladder- or urethra-specific factors but rather occurs in patients with conditions such as dementia or cognitive or mobility deficits.
- Many medications may precipitate or aggravate voiding dysfunction and UI (Table 82-1).

CINICAL PRESENTATION

- Signs and symptoms of UI depend on the underlying pathophysiology (Table 82-2). Patients with SUI generally complain of urine leakage with physical activity, whereas those with UUI complain of frequency, urgency, high-volume incontinence, and nocturia and nocturnal incontinence.
- Urethral overactivity and/or bladder underactivity is a rare but important cause of UI. Patients complain of lower abdominal fullness, hesitancy, straining to void, decreased force of stream, interrupted stream, and sense of incomplete bladder emptying. Patients can also have urinary frequency, urgency, and abdominal pain.

DIAGNOSIS

- A complete medical history, physical examination (ie, abdominal examination to exclude distended bladder, pelvic examination in women looking for evidence of

TABLE 82-1	Medications That Influence Lower Urinary Tract Function
Medications	**Effect**
Diuretics, acetylcholinesterase inhibitors	Polyuria resulting in urinary frequency, urgency
α-Receptor antagonists	Urethral muscle relaxation and stress urinary incontinence
α-Receptor agonists	Urethral muscle contraction (increased urethral closure forces) resulting in urinary retention (more common in men)
Calcium channel blockers	Urinary retention due to reduced bladder contractility
Opioid analgesics	Urinary retention due to reduced bladder contractility
Sedative hypnotics	Functional incontinence caused by delirium, immobility
Antipsychotic agents	Anticholinergic effects resulting in reduced bladder contractility and urinary retention
Anticholinergics	Urinary retention due to reduced bladder contractility
Antidepressants, tricyclic	Anticholinergic effects resulting in reduced bladder contractility (urinary retention), and α-antagonist effects resulting in reduced urethral smooth muscle contraction (stress incontinence)
Alcohol	Polyuria resulting in urinary frequency, urgency
ACEIs	Cough as a result of ACEIs may aggravate stress urinary incontinence

ACEIs, angiotensin-converting enzyme inhibitors.

prolapse or hormonal deficiency, and genital and prostate examination in men), and brief neurologic assessment of the perineum and lower extremities are recommended.
- For SUI, the preferred diagnostic test is observation of urethral meatus while the patient coughs or strains.
- For UUI, the preferred diagnostic tests are urodynamic studies. Perform urinalysis and urine culture to rule out urinary tract infection.
- For urethral overactivity and/or bladder underactivity, perform digital rectal examination or transrectal ultrasound to rule out prostate enlargement. Perform renal function tests to rule out renal failure.

TREATMENT

- Goals of Treatment: Restoration of continence, reduction in the number of UI episodes, and prevention of complications while minimizing adverse treatment consequences and cost.

NONPHARMACOLOGIC TREATMENT

- Nonpharmacologic, nonsurgical treatment options include behavioral interventions, external neuromodulation, anti-incontinence devices, and supportive interventions. Behavioral interventions (eg, lifestyle modifications, voiding schedule regimens, and pelvic floor muscle rehabilitation) are generally first-line treatment for SUI, UUI, and mixed UI.
- Surgery rarely plays a role in initial management of UI but can be required for secondary complications (eg, skin breakdown or infection). The decision to surgically treat symptomatic UI requires that lifestyle compromise warrant an elective operation and that nonsurgical therapy be proven undesirable or ineffective.

	Bladder	**Urethral**
Symptoms	**Overactivity (UUI)**	**Underactivity (SUI)**

TABLE 82-2 Differentiating Bladder Overactivity-Related UI (Urgency Urinary Incontinence) from Urethral Underactivity-Related UI (Stress Urinary Incontinence)

Symptoms	Bladder Overactivity (UUI)	Urethral Underactivity (SUI)
Urgency (strong, sudden desire to void)	Yes	Not common
Frequency with urgency	Yes	Rarely
Leaking during physical activity (eg, coughing, sneezing, lifting)	No	Yes
Amount of urinary leakage with each episode of incontinence	Large if present	Usually small
Ability to reach the toilet in time following an urge to void	No or just barely	Yes
Nocturnal incontinence (presence of wet pads or undergarments in bed)	Yes	Rare
Nocturia (waking to pass urine at night)	Usually	Seldom

PHARMACOLOGIC TREATMENT

Bladder Overactivity: Urgency Urinary Incontinence

- The pharmacotherapy of first choice for UUI includes antimuscarinic agents and β_3-adrenergic agonists drugs, which antagonize muscarinic cholinergic receptors (Table 82-3).

Oxybutynin

- **Oxybutynin immediate-release** (IR) is the oldest and least expensive treatment for UUI.
- Many patients discontinue oxybutynin IR because of adverse effects due to antimuscarinic effects (eg, dry mouth, constipation, vision impairment, confusion, cognitive dysfunction, and tachycardia), α-adrenergic inhibition (eg, orthostatic hypotension), and histamine H_1 inhibition (eg, sedation and weight gain).
- **Oxybutynin extended-release** (XL) is better tolerated than oxybutynin IR. Maximum benefits may take up to 4 weeks after dose initiation or escalation.
- **Oxybutynin transdermal system** (TDS) has similar efficacy but is better tolerated than oxybutynin IR presumably because this route avoids first-pass metabolism in the liver, which generates the metabolite thought to cause adverse events, especially dry mouth.
- **Oxybutynin gel** causes significantly less dry mouth than oxybutynin IR, but patients must be monitored for anticholinergic affects during long-term therapy, particularly frail patients.

Tolterodine

- **Tolterodine**, a competitive muscarinic receptor antagonist, is as effective as oxybutynin IR in efficacy outcomes with lower drug discontinuation rates.
- Tolterodine undergoes hepatic metabolism involving cytochrome (CYP) 2D6 and 3A4 isoenzymes. Therefore, elimination may be impaired by CYP 3A4 inhibitors, including fluoxetine, sertraline, fluvoxamine, macrolide antibiotics, azole antifungals, and grapefruit juice.

TABLE 82-3 Dosing of Medications Approved for OAB or UUI

Drug	Brand Name	Initial Dose	Usual Range	Special Population Dose	Comments
Anticholinergics/Antimuscarinics					
Oxybutynin IR	Ditropan	2.5 mg twice daily	2.5–5 mg two to four times daily		Titrate in increments of 2.5 mg/day every 1–2 months; available in oral solution
Oxybutynin XL	Ditropan XL	5–10 mg once daily	5–30 mg once daily		Adjust dose in 5-mg increments at weekly intervals; swallow whole
Oxybutynin TDS	Oxytrol Oxytrol for Women (OTC)		3.9 mg/day apply one patch twice weekly		Apply every 3–4 days; rotate application site
Oxybutynin gel 10%	Gelnique		One sachet (100 mg) topically daily		Apply to clean and dry, intact skin on abdomen, thighs, or upper arms/shoulders; contains alcohol
Oxybutynin gel 3%	Gelnique 3%		Three pumps (84 mg) topically daily		Same as above
Tolterodine IR	Detrol		1–2 mg twice daily	1 mg twice daily if patient is taking CYP3A4 inhibitors, or with renal/hepatic impairment	
Tolterodine LA	Detrol LA		2–4 mg once daily	2 mg once daily in patients taking CYP3A4 inhibitors or those with renal/hepatic impairment	Swallow whole; avoid in patients with creatinine clearance ≤10 mL/min (0.17 mL/sec)
Trospium chloride IR	Sanctura		20 mg twice daily	20 mg once daily in patients age ≥75 years or creatinine clearance ≤30 mL/min (0.5 mL/sec)	Take 1 hour before meals or on empty stomach; patients age ≥75 years should take at bedtime

(Continued)

TABLE 82-3	Dosing of Medications Approved for OAB or UUI (Continued)				
Drug	**Brand Name**	**Initial Dose**	**Usual Range**	**Special Population Dose**	**Comments**
Trospium chloride ER	Sanctura XR		60 mg once daily	Avoid in patients age ≥75 years or creatinine clearance ≤30 mL/min (0.5 mL/sec)	Take 1 hour before meals or on empty stomach; swallow whole
Solifenacin	VESIcare	5 mg daily	5–10 mg once daily	5 mg daily if patient is taking CYP3A4 inhibitors or with creatinine clearance ≤30 mL/min (0.5 mL/sec) or moderate hepatic impairment; avoid in severe hepatic impairment	Swallow whole
Darifenacin ER	Enablex	7.5 mg once daily	7.5–15 mg once daily	7.5 mg daily if patient is taking potent CYP3A4 inhibitors or with moderate hepatic impairment; avoid in severe hepatic impairment	Titrate dose after at least 2 weeks; swallow whole
Fesoterodine ER	Toviaz	4 mg once daily	4–8 mg once daily	4 mg daily if patient is taking potent CYP3A4 inhibitors or with creatinine clearance ≤30 mL/min (0.5 mL/sec); avoid in severe hepatic impairment	Prodrug (metabolized to 5-hydroxymethyl tolterodine); swallow whole
β₃-Adrenergic Agonist					
Mirabegron ER	Myrbetriq	25 mg once daily	25–50 mg once daily	25 mg once daily if creatinine clearance 15–29 mL/min (0.25–0.49 mL/sec) or moderate hepatic impairment; avoid in patients with ESRD or severe hepatic impairment	Swallow whole

CYP, cytochrome P450 enzyme; ER, extended-release; ESRD, end-stage renal disease; IR, immediate release; LA, long acting; OAB, overactive bladder; OTC, over-the-counter; TDS, transdermal system; UUI, urge urinary incontinence; XL, extended-release.

- Tolterodine's most common adverse effects include dry mouth, dyspepsia, headache, constipation, and dry eyes. The maximum benefit of tolterodine is not realized for up to 8 weeks after starting therapy or dose escalation.
- **Tolterodine long acting** (LA) offers once-daily dosing and may also take up to 8 weeks after starting therapy or dose escalation to see maximum benefit.
- **Fesoterodine fumarate** is a prodrug for tolterodine and is considered an alternative first-line therapy for UI in patients with urinary frequency, urgency, or urge incontinence.

Other Pharmacologic Therapies for Urgency Urinary Incontinence

- **Trospium chloride IR**, a quaternary ammonium anticholinergic, was shown to be noninferior to oxybutynin IR but was associated with less dry mouth. It causes the expected anticholinergic adverse effects with increased frequency in patients age 75 years or older. An extended-release product is also available.
- **Solifenacin succinate** and **darifenacin** are second-generation antimuscarinic agents. Both have been shown to improve urinary symptoms and quality-of-life. Drug interactions are possible if CYP 3A4 inhibitors are given with solifenacin succinate or CYP 2D6 or 3A4 inhibitors with darifenacin.
- **Mirabegron** is a β_3-adrenergic agonist alternative to anticholinergic/antimuscarinic drugs for managing UUI. It has modest efficacy as compared with placebo. Hypertension, nasopharyngitis, urinary tract infection, and headache are the most common adverse effects. It is a moderate inhibitor of CYP2D6.
- Use of other agents, including tricyclic antidepressants, **propantheline, flavoxate, hyoscyamine,** and **dicyclomine hydrochloride**, is not recommended. They are less effective, not safer, or have not been adequately studied.
- A systematic review of 94 randomized controlled trials with antimuscarinic drugs for UUI showed similar, small benefits for all drugs studied. Selection of initial drug therapy depends on side-effect profile, comorbidities, concurrent drug therapy, and patient preference in drug delivery methods (Table 82-4).
- **Botulinum toxin A** temporarily paralyzes smooth or striated muscle. It is indicated for the treatment of detrusor overactivity associated with neurologic conditions and OAB.
- Adverse effects of botulinum toxin A include dysuria, hematuria, urinary tract infection, and urinary retention (up to 20%). Therapeutic and adverse effects are seen 3–7 days after injection and subside after 6–8 months.

Urethral Underactivity: Stress Urinary Incontinence

- Treatment of SUI is aimed at improving urethral closure by stimulating α-adrenergic receptors in smooth muscle of the bladder neck and proximal urethra, enhancing supportive structures underlying the urethral epithelium, or enhancing serotonin and norepinephrine effects in the micturition reflex pathways.

Estrogens

- Historically, local and systemic **estrogens** have been the mainstays of pharmacologic management of SUI.
- A meta-analysis of 34 trials evaluating the use of local or systemic estrogen therapy on UI in postmenopausal women found that systemic administration of estrogen alone or in combination with progesterone resulted in UI worsening. There was some evidence that vaginal estrogen may improve UI, and reduce urgency and frequency.
- A meta-analysis of 17 trials of local estrogen compared to placebo or no treatment found beneficial effects on UI and OAB symptoms and some urodynamic parameters.
- Based on the results of these analyses, only topical estrogen products should be used for treatment of UI or OAB in postmenopausal women.

TABLE 82-4	Adverse Event Incidence Rates with Approved Drugs for Bladder Overactivity[a]			
Drug	**Dry Mouth**	**Constipation**	**Dizziness**	**Vision Disturbance**
Oxybutynin IR	71	15	17	10
Oxybutynin XL	61	13	6	14
Oxybutynin TDS	7	3	NR	3
Oxybutynin gel	10	1	3	3
Tolterodine	35	7	5	3
Tolterodine LA	23	6	2	4
Trospium chloride IR	20	10	NR	1
Trospium chloride XR	11	9	NR	2
Solifenacin	20	9	2	5
Darifenacin ER	24	18	2	2
Fesoterodine ER	27	5	NR	3
Mirabegron ER	3	3	3	NR

[a]All values constitute mean data, predominantly using product information from the manufacturers. IR, immediate release; LA, long acting; TDS, transdermal system; XL, extended-release; XR/ER, extended-release; NR, not reported.

α-Adrenergic Receptor Agonists

- Many open trials support the use of a variety of α-adrenergic receptor agonists in SUI. Combining an α-adrenergic receptor agonist with an estrogen yields somewhat superior clinical and urodynamic responses compared with monotherapy.
- Contraindications to these agents include hypertension, tachyarrhythmias, coronary artery disease, myocardial infarction, cor pulmonale, hyperthyroidism, renal failure, and narrow-angle glaucoma.

Duloxetine

- **Duloxetine**, a dual inhibitor of serotonin and norepinephrine reuptake indicated for depression and painful diabetic neuropathy, is approved in many countries for the treatment of SUI, but not in the United States. Duloxetine is thought to facilitate the bladder-to-sympathetic reflex pathway, increasing urethral and external urethral sphincter muscle tone during the storage phase.
- Six placebo-controlled studies showed that duloxetine reduces incontinent episode frequency and the number of daily micturitions, increases micturition interval, and improves quality-of-life scores. These benefits were statistically significant but clinically modest.
- Monitor patients taking concurrent CYP 2D6 and 1A2 substrates or inhibitors closely.
- The adverse event profile might make adherence problematic. Adverse events include nausea, headache, insomnia, dizziness, constipation, and dry mouth.

Overflow Incontinence

- Overflow incontinence secondary to benign or malignant prostatic hyperplasia may be amenable to pharmacotherapy (see Chapters 64 and 80).

EVALUATION OF THERAPEUTIC OUTCOMES

- Total elimination of UI signs and symptoms may not be possible. Therefore, realistic goals should be established for therapy.
- In the long-term management of UI, the clinical symptoms of most distress to the individual patient need to be monitored.
- Survey instruments used in UI research along with quantitating the use of ancillary supplies (eg, pads) can be used in clinical monitoring.
- Therapies for UI frequently have nuisance adverse effects, which need to be carefully elicited. Adverse effects can necessitate drug dosage adjustments, use of alternative strategies (eg, chewing sugarless gum, sucking on hard sugarless candy, or use of saliva substitutes for xerostomia), or even drug discontinuation.

See Chapter 101, Urinary Incontinence, authored by Eric S. Rovner, Jean Wyman, and Sum Lam, for a more detailed discussion of this topic.

APPENDIX

1

Pediatric Pharmacotherapy, Nutrition, and Neonatal Critical Care

TABLE A1-1	Opioid Administration for Acute and Severe Pain in Pediatrics
Intermittent IV or PO bolus administration (not as needed)	In 2018, the FDA announced limiting use of prescription opioid cough and cold medications containing codeine or hydrocodone in children <18 years old. Weak opioids (eg, codeine, hydrocodone, and oxycodone) often are combined with acetaminophen or an NSAID for moderate pain. With dose escalation of combination oral products, be aware that the dose does not exceed recommended daily amounts for acetaminophen or ibuprofen. One percent to 7% of the general population and up to 28% of some ethnic groups have a genetic variation in the enzyme cytochrome P450 2D6 that causes codeine to be converted to morphine faster and more completely. In 2012, the FDA issued a Drug Safety Communication stating that codeine use in certain children after tonsillectomy or adenoidectomy for obstructive sleep apnea syndrome led to deaths and life-threatening respiratory depression. Consider alternative analgesics for children undergoing tonsillectomy or adenoidectomy. If codeine or codeine-containing products are prescribed, then use the lowest effective dose for the shortest period of time on an as-needed basis. IV administration of codeine has been associated with allergic reactions related to histamine release. Parenteral administration of codeine is not recommended. Intermittent opioid administration is associated with wide fluctuation between peak and trough concentrations, so the patient may alternate between peak blood concentrations associated with untoward effects and trough concentrations associated with inadequate pain relief when being treated for severe pain. Oxycodone and morphine are available in a sustained-release formulation for use with chronic pain (not acute pain). The tablet must be swallowed whole and cannot be administered to patients through gastric tubes.
IV continuous infusion	Loading dose is administered to rapidly achieve a therapeutic blood concentration and pain relief (ie, morphine loading dose of 0.05–0.15 mg/kg in children; 0.1 mg/kg infused over 90 minutes in neonates). Loading dose is followed by a maintenance continuous infusion. Doses that are considered safe in children can cause respiratory depression and seizures in neonates because of decreased clearance, immature blood–brain barrier at birth that is more permeable to morphine, and an increased unbound fraction of morphine that increases CNS effects of the drug.
PCA	Gives patient some control over his or her pain therapy. PCA allows the patient to self-administer small opioid doses. The PCA-Plus (Abbott, Chicago, IL) pump allows the patient to receive a continuous infusion together with a set number of self-administered doses per hour. PCA helps to eliminate wide peak and trough fluctuations so that blood concentrations remain in a therapeutic range. Children as young as 5 or 6 years of age can master the use of PCA.

(Continued)

TABLE A1-1	Opioid Administration for Acute and Severe Pain in Pediatrics *(Continued)*
Epidural and intrathecal analgesia	Effective in the management of severe postoperative, chronic, or cancer pain. Spinal opioids can be administered by a single bolus injection into the epidural or subarachnoid space or by continuous infusion via an indwelling catheter. Dosage requirement by these routes is significantly less than with IV administration. Morphine, hydromorphone, fentanyl, and sufentanil are effective when administered intrathecally. Bupivacaine is the most commonly used local anesthetic in continuous epidural infusions. Fentanyl, morphine, or hydromorphone usually is combined with bupivacaine for epidural infusions.
Transdermal administration	Fentanyl and buprenorphine are available as a transdermal formulation. Multiple patches of an agent may be applied for patients who require higher doses. Disadvantage of transdermal administration is the requirement for an alternative short-acting opioid for break-through pain.
Transmucosal administration	Fentanyl lozenge is absorbed transmucosally. It is useful for providing analgesia during painful procedures. Advantages include rapid onset of action (within 15 minutes), short duration of action (60–90 minutes), and painless administration because no injection is needed. Common side effects are vomiting and mild-to-moderate oxygen desaturation. Doses of 10–15 mcg/kg provide blood concentrations equivalent to 3–5 mcg/kg IV.

FDA, Food and Drug Administration; IM, intramuscular; NSAID, nonsteroidal anti-inflammatory drug; PCA, patient-controlled analgesia; PO, by mouth.

TABLE A1-2	Frequency and Volume of Feedings in Infants	
Age	**Feedings Per Day**	**Volume Per Feeding, mL (ounces)**
Birth–1 week	6–10	30–90 (1–3)
1 week–1 month	7–8	60–120 (2–4)
1–3 months	5–7	120–180 (3–6)
3–6 months	4–5	180–210 (6–7)
6–9 months	3–4	210–240 (7–8)
9–12 months	3	210–240 (7–8)

TABLE A1-3	Composition of Human Milk Fortifiers[a] (Select Products and Nutrients)			
Nutrient	Similac HMF[b,c] Powder (Per Packet)	Enfamil HMF Powder (Per Packet)[b]	Similac HMF Hydrolyzed Protein Concentrated Liquid[b,c] (Per 5 mL)	Enfamil HMF Acidified Liquid[b,c] (Per 5 mL)
Calories, kcal	3.5	3.5	7	7.5
Protein, g	0.25	0.275	0.35	0.55
Fat, g	0.09	0.25	0.27	0.575
Sodium, mg	3.75	4	5	6.75
Potassium, mg	15.75	7.25	21	11.25
Calcium, mg	29.25	22.5	35	29
Magnesium, mg	1.75	0.25	2.2	0.46
Phosphorus, mg	16.75	12.5	20	15.75
Selenium, mcg	0.125	-	0.2	-
Iron, mg	0.08	0.36	0.11	0.44
Zinc, mg	0.25	0.18	0.3	0.24
Vitamin A, IU	155	237.5	197	290
Vitamin C, mg	6.25	3	7.7	3.8
Vitamin D, IU	30	37.5	35	47
Vitamin E, IU	0.8	1.15	1	1.4
Vitamin K, mcg	2	1.1	2.4	1.425

[a]Mix 1 packet (powder) or 5 mL (liquid) in 25 mL to make 24 kcal/oz (3.4 kJ/mL) concentration.
[b]Also contains linoleic acid, thiamin, riboflavin, pyridoxine, cyanocobalamin, niacin, folic acid, pantothenic acid, biotin, manganese, and copper.
[c]Also contains iodine, choline, and inositol.
HMF, human milk fortifier.
Source: Data from Abbott Nutrition, www.abbottnutrition.com; Mead Johnson, www.meadjohnson.com.

TABLE A1-4 Formulas for Premature Infants

Formula	Energy (kcal/oz) (kcal/dL)	Protein (g/dL)	Fat (g/dL)	Vitamin D (IU/mL)	Calcium (mg/dL)	Phosphorus (mg/dL)	Iron (mg/dL)
Mature human milk	65–70 (19.5–21)	1.03	3.5	Variable (based on mother's intake)	20–25	12–14	0.3–0.9
Premature infant formulas							
Similac Special Care 20	67.6 (20)	2.03	3.67	101.4	121.7	67.6	1.22
Similac Special Care 24	81.2 (24)	2.43	4.41	101.4	146.1	81.2	1.46
Similac Special Care 24 High Protein	81.2 (24)	2.68	4.41	121.7	146.1	81.2	1.46
Similac Special Care 30	101.4 (30)	3.04	6.71	182.6	152.2	101.4	1.83
Enfamil Premature 20	67.6 (20)	2.2	3.4	200	112	61	1.22
Enfamil Premature 24	81.2 (24)	2.7	4.1	240	134	73	1.46
Enfamil Premature 24 HP	81.2 (24)	2.9	4.1	240	134	73	1.46
Enfamil Premature 30	101.4 (30)	3.3	5.1	300	167	91	1.83
Postdischarge formulas							
Similac Neosure	74 (22)	2.1	4.1 MCT 25%	52	78	46	1.3
Enfamil EnfaCare/Enfamil NeuroPro EnfaCare	74 (22)	2.1	4 MCT 20%	53	90	50	1.3

MCT, medium–chain triglycerides. For results expressed in SI units: For energy expressed in kcal/dL multiply by 41.84 to convert to kJ/L; for energy expressed in kcal/oz multiply by 0.1415 to convert to kJ/mL; for fat or protein expressed in g/dL multiply by 10 to convert to g/L; for vitamin D expressed in IU/mL multiply by 1000 to convert to IU/L; and for calcium, phosphorus, or iron expressed in mg/dL multiply by 10 to convert to mg/L.

Source: Data from Abbott Nutrition, Abbott Laboratories, Columbus, Ohio; Mead Johnson Nutrition, Glenview, Illinois.

TABLE A1-5 World Health Organization (WHO) Guidelines for Oral Rehydration in Children

Recommended Volume of ORT to Correct Dehydration

Weight (kg)[a]	Age[a]	ORS, mL in First 4 Hr[b]
<5	<4 months	200–400
5–7.9	4–11 months	200–400
8–9.9	12–23 months	600–800
10–15.9	2–4 years	800–1200
16–29.9	5–14 years	1200–2200
≥30	≥15 years	2200–4000

Recommended Volume after Stooling to Prevent Dehydration

Age (y)	Recommended Volume (mL)	Maximum Daily Volume (mL)
<2	50–100	500
2–9	100–200	1000
≥10	At least 100–200, but as much as desired	2000

[a]Use age only if weight is not available.
[b]Volume for first 4 hr can also be calculated by multiplying the weight (kg) by 75.

TABLE A1-6 Oral/Enteral Hydration Solutions (Examples Only)

Product	Sodium (mEq/L)	Potassium (mEq/L)	Chloride (mEq/L)	Base (mEq/L)	CHO (g/L)	Osm (mOsm/L)	Other
Recommended Concentration	60–90	15–25	50–80	8–12	Equal to sodium; <111 mmol/L	200–310	
Rehydration solutions—replace fluid deficits							
WHO (UNICEF), original[a]	90	19.2	21	30	13.5	333	
WHO (UNICEF), modified	75	20	65	10	13.5	245	
Bana—Adult	68.6	10.3			2		
Ceralyte 70 (packets)	70	20	60	30	40 (rice)	<260	
Ceralyte 90 (packets)	90	20	80	30	40 (rice)	<275	
Drip Drop Solution	60	20	8	80	16	<200	
Pedialyte Advanced Care+[b]	60	20					Zinc
Maintenance solutions—prevent fluid deficits							
Pedialyte®, Pedialyte® Freezer Pops, Pedialyte Advanced Care[b]	45	20	35	30	25	388	Zinc
Ceralyte 50 (packets)	50	20	40	30	40 (rice)	<260	
Enfamil® Enfalyte®	50	20	40	30	20	251	
Clear liquids and sports drinks (for comparison only—not rehydration or maintenance solutions)							
Juice	2	30	–	0	69	730	
Soda	3	–	–	13	70	700	
Gatorade (G2)[c]	20	3.2	17	30	21	305	
Gatorade Prime[c]	40.5	7.6	17	30	195	305	

[a]Gold standard for rehydration solutions.
[b]Contains prebiotics.
[c]Other forms available; sugar-free Gatorade available; caution with sugar substitutes.
Source: Data from Manufacturers' websites; World Health Organization, apps.who.int/medicinedocs/en/d/Js4950e/2.4.html.

TABLE A1-7	Antimicrobial Dosage Regimens for Neonates for Early- and Late-Onset Sepsis[*]				
	Weight <1200 g	Weight 1200–2000 g		Weight >2000 g	
Drug	PNA 0–4 Weeks[a]	PNA 0–7 Days[a]	PNA 8–28 Days[a]	PNA 0–7 Days[a]	PNA 8–28 Days[a]
Antibacterials					
Ampicillin[b]	100 Q 12 hr	100 Q 12 hr	100 Q 8 hr	100 Q 8 hr	100 Q 6 hr
Cefazolin	25 Q 12 hr	25 Q 12 hr	25 Q 12 hr	25 Q 12 hr	25 Q 8 hr
Cefotaxime	50 Q 12 hr	50 Q 12 hr	50 Q 8 hr	50 Q 12 hr	50 Q 8 hr
Ceftazidime	50 Q 12 hr	50 Q 12 hr	50 Q 8 hr	50 Q 12 hr	50 Q 8 hr
Clindamycin	5 Q 12 hr	5 Q 12 hr	5 Q 8 hr	5 Q 8 hr	5 Q 6 hr
Imipenem	25 Q 12 hr	25 Q 12 hr	25 Q 8 hr	25 Q 12 hr	25 Q 8 hr
Meropenem[c]	20 Q 12 hr	20 Q 12 hr	20 Q 8 hr	20 Q 8 hr	20 Q 8 hr
Metronidazole	7.5 Q 24 hr	7.5 Q 24 hr	7.5 Q 12 hr	7.5 Q 12 hr	15 Q 12 hr
Nafcillin/Oxacillin	25 Q 12 hr[d]	25 Q 12 hr	25 Q 8 hr	25 Q 8 hr	25 Q 6 hr
Penicillin G (*GBS meningitis*)	100,000 Units Q 8 hr	100,000 Units Q 8 hr	112,500 Units Q 6 hr	100,000 Units Q 8 hr	112,500 Units Q 6 hr
Penicillin G (*Congenital syphilis*)	50,000 Units Q 12 hr	50,000 Units Q 12 hr	50,000 Units Q 8 hr	50,000 Units Q 12 hr	50,000 Units Q 8 hr
Piperacillin/ Tazobactam	75 Q 12 hr	75 Q 12 hr	75 Q 8 hr	75 Q 12 hr	75 Q 8 hr
Vancomycin	15 Q 18–24 hr	15 Q 12–18 hr	15 Q 8–12 hr	15 Q 8–12 hr	15 Q 6–8 hr
Antiviral					
Acyclovir	20 Q 12 hr[d]	20 Q 12 hr	20 Q 8 hr	20 Q 8 hr	20 Q 8 hr
Antifungals					
Amphotericin B Deoxycholate	1 Q 24 hr	1 Q 24 hr	1 Q 24 hr	1 Q 24 hr	1 Q 24 hr
Liposomal Amphotericin B	5 Q 24 hr	5 Q 24 hr	5 Q 24 hr	5 Q 24 hr	5 Q 24 hr
Fluconazole[e,f]	12 Q 24 hr	12 Q 24 hr	12 Q 24 hr	12 Q 24 hr	12 Q 24 hr

[a]PNA (postnatal age; chronologic age ≤28 days).
[b]For confirmed GBS meningitis, higher dosage may be required.
[c]Higher dosage may be required for meningitis.
[d]Changed to Q 8 hr dosing when patient is PNA ≥15 days.
[e]For treatment of candidemia/candidiasis, load with 25 mg/kg/dose; adjust for renal dosing if serum creatinine ≥1.3 mg/dL (115 μmol/L).
[f]Can be administered intravenously or orally.
[*]Dosage expressed in mg/kg/dose.

TABLE A1-8	Medications Used for Patient Ductus Arteriosus (PDA) Closure	
Medication	**Dosing Regimen**	**Monitoring Parameters**
Indomethacin	**Intravenous, intermittent:** PNA <48 hr: 0.1 mg/kg/dose Q 12–24 hr × 3 doses PNA 2–7 days: 0.2 mg/kg/dose Q 12–24 hr × 3 doses PNA >7 days: 0.25 mg/kg/dose Q 12–24 hr × 3 doses	Urine output (hold dose if <0.6 mL/kg/hr), serum creatinine (hold dose if >1.6 mg/dL [141 µmol/L]), platelets, signs of bleeding Blood pressure, murmur, respiratory status, echocardiogram
Ibuprofen	**Intravenous, intermittent:** "Standard-dose": 10 mg/kg/dose × 1 dose followed by 5 mg/kg/dose Q 24 hr × 2 doses "High-dose": 20 mg/kg/dose × 1 dose followed by 10 mg/kg/dose Q 24 hr × 2 doses High-dose regimen found to have higher closure rates compared to standard-dose without more frequent side effects	Urine output (hold dose if <0.6 mL/kg/hour), serum creatinine, platelets, signs of bleeding Blood pressure, murmur, respiratory status, echocardiogram
Acetaminophen	**Intravenous, intermittent:** 15 mg/kg/dose Q 6 hr × 3–7 days	Liver function tests Blood pressure, murmur, respiratory status, echocardiogram

PNA, postnatal age.

TABLE A1-9	Neonatal Dosing Recommendations for Commonly Used Analgesics and Sedatives		
Medication	**Uses**	**Dosing Regimen**	**Comments**
Sucrose 24% solution	Analgesia; mild procedural pain	<1 kg: 0.1 mL/dose 1–2 kg: 0.1–0.2 mL/dose >2 kg: 0.1–0.5 mL/dose	Administer 1–2 minutes prior to procedure May be applied to pacifier or directly to tongue Do not exceed 3 doses per procedure
Acetaminophen	Analgesia; mild-to-moderate postoperative or prolonged pain Analgesia; moderate-to-severe postoperative pain when used in combination with an opioid	**Oral:** GA 28–32 weeks: 10–12 mg/kg/dose Q 6–8 hr; max. dose 40 mg/kg/day GA 33–37 weeks: 10–15 mg/kg/dose Q 6 hr; max. dose 60 mg/kg/day Term, ≥10 days: 10–15 mg/kg/dose Q 4–6 hr; max. dose 75 mg/kg/day **Intravenous:** PMA 28–32 weeks: 10 mg/kg/dose Q 12 hr; max. dose 22.5 mg/kg/day	Not effective for acute procedural pain

(Continued)

TABLE A1-9	Neonatal Dosing Recommendations for Commonly Used Analgesics and Sedatives (*Continued*)		
Medication	**Uses**	**Dosing Regimen**	**Comments**
		PMA 33–36 weeks: 10 mg/kg/dose Q 8 hr; max. dose 40 mg/kg/day	
		PMA ≥37 weeks: 10 mg/kg/dose Q 6 hr; max. dose 40 mg/kg/day	
Morphine	Analgesia; moderate-to-severe prolonged or postoperative pain	**Intravenous, intermittent:** 0.05–0.1 mg/kg/dose Q 4–6 hr **Intravenous, continuous:** 0.01–0.03 mg/kg/hr	Preterm neonates may be more susceptible to hypotension, respiratory depression, apnea Titrate to effect Practitioners should be aware of potential adverse effects on neurodevelopment
Fentanyl	Analgesia; moderate-to-severe acute procedural pain, prolonged, or postoperative pain	**Intravenous, intermittent:** 0.5–3 mcg/kg/dose Q 2–4 hr **Intravenous, continuous:** 0.5–3 mcg/kg/hr	Administer bolus over 3–5 minutes, more rapid rates may cause chest wall rigidity Titrate to effect
Midazolam	Sedation; procedural or prolonged	**Intravenous, intermittent:** 0.05–0.1 mg/kg/dose **Intravenous, continuous:** GA 24–26 weeks: 0.02–0.03 mg/kg/hr GA 27–29 weeks: 0.03–0.04 mg/kg/hr GA ≥30 weeks: 0.03–0.06 mg/kg/hr	Myoclonus may occur especially in preterm neonates Titrate to effect Practitioners should be aware of potential adverse effects on neurodevelopment
Dexmedetomidine	Sedation, analgesia; prolonged	**Intravenous, continuous:** 0.1–0.3 mcg/kg/hr	Limited neonatal data

GA, gestational age; PMA, postmenstrual age.

(See the following chapters for more detailed discussions of these topics:

- *e/Chapter 19, Pediatrics: General Topics in Pediatric Pharmacotherapy, authored by Milap C. Nahata and Carol Taketomo*
- *e/Chapter 20, Pediatrics: Oral nutrition and Rehydration of Infants and Children, authored by Katherine H. Chessman*
- *e/Chapter 21, Pediatrics: Neonatal Critical Care, authored by Kirsten H. Ohler and Jennifer T. Pham)*

Geriatric Assessment and Pharmacotherapy

2

TABLE A2-1	Physiologic Changes with Aging
Organ System	**Manifestation**
Balance and gait	↓ Stride length and slower gait ↓ Arm swing ↑ Body sway when standing
Body composition	↓ Total body water ↓ Lean body mass ↑ Body fat ↔ or ↓ Serum albumin ↑ α_1-Acid glycoprotein (↔ or ↑ by several disease states)
Cardiovascular	↓ Cardiovascular response to stress ↓ Baroreceptor activity leading to ↑ orthostatic hypotension ↓ Cardiac output ↑ Systemic vascular resistance with loss of arterial elasticity and dysfunction of systems maintaining vascular tone ↑ Afterload ↓ Coronary perfusion
Central nervous system	↓ Size of the hippocampus and frontal and temporal lobes ↓ Number of receptors of all types and ↑ sensitivity of remaining receptors ↓ Short-term memory, coding and retrieval, and executive function Altered sleep patterns
Endocrine	↓ Estrogen, testosterone, thyroid-stimulating hormone, and DHEA-S levels Altered insulin signaling
Gastrointestinal	↓ Motility of the large intestine ↓ Vitamin absorption by active transport mechanisms ↓ Splanchnic blood flow ↓ Bowel surface area
Genitourinary	Atrophy of the vagina with decreased estrogen Prostatic hypertrophy with androgenic hormonal changes Detrusor hyperactivity may predispose to incontinence
Hepatic	↓ Hepatic size ↓ Hepatic blood flow ↓ Phase I (oxidation, reduction, hydrolysis) metabolism
Immune	↓ Antibody production in response to antigen ↑ Autoimmunity
Oral	Altered dentition ↓ Ability to taste salt, bitter, sweet, and sour
Pulmonary	↓ Respiratory muscle strength ↓ Chest wall compliance ↓ Arterial oxygenation and impaired carbon dioxide elimination ↓ Vital capacity ↓ Maximal breathing capacity ↑ Residual volume

(Continued)

TABLE A2-1	Physiologic Changes with Aging (*Continued*)
Renal	↓ Glomerular filtration rate ↓ Renal blood flow ↓ Filtration fraction ↓ Tubular secretory function ↓ Renal mass
Sensory	Presbyopia (diminished ability to focus on near objects) ↓ Night vision Presbycusis (high-pitch, high-frequency hearing loss) ↓ Sensation of smell and taste
Skeletal	↓ Skeletal bone mass (osteopenia) Joint stiffening due to reduced water content in tendons, ligaments, and cartilage
Skin/Hair	Thinning of stratum corneum ↓ Langerhans cells, melanocytes, and mast cells ↓ Depth and extent of the subcutaneous fat layer Thinning and graying of hair due to more hairs in the resting phase and shortening of the growth phase as well as changes in follicular melanocytes

Source: Data from Cefalu CA. Theories and mechanisms of aging. Clin Geriatr Med. 2011;27: 491–506; Alvis BD, Hughes CG. Physiology considerations in geriatric patients. Anesthesiol Clin. 2015;33:447–456.

TABLE A2-2	Age-Related Changes in Drug Pharmacokinetics
Pharmacokinetic Phase	**Pharmacokinetic Parameters**
Gastrointestinal absorption	Unchanged passive diffusion and no change in bioavailability for most drugs ↓ Active transport and ↓ bioavailability for some drugs ↓ First-pass metabolism, ↑ bioavailability for some drugs, and ↓ bioavailability for some prodrugs
Distribution	↓ Volume of distribution and ↑ plasma concentration of water-soluble drugs ↑ Volume of distribution and ↑ terminal disposition half-life ($t_{1/2}$) for lipid-soluble drugs
Hepatic metabolism	↓ Clearance and ↑ $t_{1/2}$ for some drugs with poor hepatic extraction (capacity-limited metabolism). Phase I metabolism may be affected more than Phase II ↓ Clearance and ↑ $t_{1/2}$ for drugs with high hepatic extraction ratios (flow-limited metabolism)
Renal excretion	↓ Clearance and ↑ $t_{1/2}$ for renally eliminated drugs and active metabolites

Source: Data from Reeve E, Wiese MD, Mangoni AA. Alterations in drug disposition in older adults. Expert Opin Drug Metab Toxicol. 2015;11:491–508; Shi S, Klotz U. Age-related changes in pharmacokinetics. Curr Drug Metab. 2011;12:601–610.

TABLE A2-3	Comparison of American Geriatrics Society Beers Criteria and STOPP Criteria
Criteria	**Organization**
Beers	Criteria are organized into five tables:
	1. PIMs for all older adults, organized according to organ system and therapeutic category
	2. PIMs for some older adults due to drug–disease or drug–syndrome interactions that might exacerbate disease/syndromes (eg, syncope, delirium, dementia, history of falls or fractures, history of gastrointestinal ulcers, urinary incontinence, benign prostatic hyperplasia, heart failure)
	3. PIMs to be used with caution (eg, aspirin for primary prevention, dabigatran/rivaroxaban—gastrointestinal bleeding in people >75 years)
	4. Potentially clinically important drug–drug interactions that should be avoided (eg, opioids, lithium, phenytoin, warfarin, avoid total of ≥3 CNS active drugs to reduce falls risk)
	5. Medications that should be avoided or have dosage reduced with varying levels of kidney function
STOPP	1. Organized according to physiological system (11 sections) and include drugs to avoid, drug–drug, dosing considerations for reduced renal function, and drug–disease interactions
	2. A section focused on general concepts that are not medication specific and include drug prescribed without evidence-based clinical indication, drug prescribed without recommended duration, and therapeutic duplication

Source: Data from O'Mahony D, O'Sullivan D, Byrne S, O'Connor MN, Ryan C, Gallagher P. STOPP/START criteria for potentially inappropriate prescribing in older people: Version 2. Age Ageing. 2015;44:213–218; 2019 American Geriatrics Society Beers Criteria Update Expert Panel. American Geriatrics Society 2019 updated Beers Criteria for potentially inappropriate medication use in older adults. J Am Geriatr Soc. 2019. doi:10.1111/jgs.15767.
PIM, potentially inappropriate medication.

TABLE A2-4	Medication Appropriateness Index

Questions to ask about each individual medication

1. Is there an indication for the medication?

2. Is the medication effective for the condition?

3. Is the dosage correct?

4. Are the directions correct?

5. Are the directions practical?

6. Are there clinically significant drug–drug interactions?

7. Are there clinically significant drug–disease interactions?

8. Is there unnecessary duplication with other medication(s)?

9. Is the duration of therapy acceptable?

10. Is this medication the least expensive alternative compared with others of equal utility?

Source: Reprinted from Hanlon JT, Schmader KE, Samsa GP, et al. A method for assessing drug therapy appropriateness. J Clin Epidemiol. 1992;45:1045–1051.

TABLE A2-5	Examples of Clinically Important Drug–Disease Interactions Determined by Expert Panel Consensus
Disease	**Drug or Drug Class**
Heart failure	NSAIDs, COX-2 inhibitors, thiazolidinediones, dronedarone
Heart failure with reduced ejection fraction	Nondihydropyridine calcium channel blockers
Syncope	Acetylcholinesterase inhibitors, peripheral nonselective α_1-blockers, tertiary tricyclic antidepressants, antipsychotics
Delirium	Anticholinergics, antipsychotics, benzodiazepines, corticosteroids, H_2-receptor antagonists, zolpidem and zoleplon ("z-hypnotics")
Cognitive impairment	Anticholinergics, antipsychotics, benzodiazepines, nonbenzodiazepine hypnotics, z-hypnotics
History of falls	Antiepileptics, antipsychotics, benzodiazepines, antidepressants, z-hypnotics, opioids
Parkinson disease	Antipsychotics (except quetiapine, clozapine, pimavanserin), metoclopramide, prochlorperazine, promethazine
Peptic ulcer disease	Aspirin in doses of 325 mg/day or more, NSAIDs
Chronic kidney disease stage IV and higher	NSAIDs
Urinary incontinence in women	Peripheral α_1-blockers

COX-2, cyclooxygenase 2; NSAIDs, nonsteroidal anti-inflammatory drugs.
Source: Data from 2019 American Geriatrics Society Beers Criteria Update Expert Panel. American Geriatrics Society 2019 updated Beers Criteria for potentially inappropriate medication use in older adults. J Am Geriatr Soc. 2019. doi:10.1111/jgs.15767.

TABLE A2-6	Atypical Disease Presentation in Older Adults
Disease	**Presentation**
Acute myocardial infarction	Only ~50% present with chest pain. In general, older adults present with weakness, confusion, syncope, and abdominal pain; however, electrocardiographic findings are similar to those in younger patients.
Congestive heart failure	Instead of dyspnea, older patients may present with hypoxic symptoms, lethargy, restlessness, and confusion.
Gastrointestinal bleed	Although the mortality rate is ~10%, presenting symptoms are nonspecific, ranging from altered mental status to syncope with hemodynamic collapse. Abdominal pain often is absent.
Upper respiratory infection	Older patients typically present with lethargy, confusion, anorexia, and decompensation of a preexisting medical condition. Fever, chills, and productive cough may or may not be present.
Urinary tract infection	Dysuria, fever, and flank pain may be absent. More commonly, older adults present with incontinence, confusion, abdominal pain, nausea or vomiting, and azotemia.

(See the following chapters for more detailed discussions of these topics:

- *e/Chapter 22, Geriatrics: The Aging Process in Humans and Its Effects on Physiology, authored by Krista L. Donohoe, Elvin T. Price, Tracey L. Gendron, and Patricia W. Slattum*
- *e/Chapter 23: Prescribing in the Older Adult, authored by Emily R. Hajjar, Lauren R. Hersh, and Shelly L. Gray*
- *e/Chapter 24: Assessing Health and Delivering HealthCare to Older Adults, authored by Leigh Ann Mike, Zachary A. Marcum, and Shelly L. Gray)*

TABLE A3-1	Pharmacokinetic Changes in Critical Illness		
Pharmacokinetic Parameter	**Changes in the Critically Ill**	**Etiologies**	**Example Drugs Affected**
Absorption	↓ Absorption	Perfusion abnormalities	Enteral, intramuscular, or subcutaneous drugs
		Decreased GI motility	*Itraconazole (capsules need an acidic medium for absorption), phenytoin (significant drug–nutrient interactions), subcutaneous enoxaparin (incompletely absorbed in the setting of vasopressors and edema)*
		Altered gastric pH	
		Bowel wall edema	
		Drug–nutrient interactions	
Distribution	↑ Vd	Large-volume resuscitation	Hydrophilic drugs
		Capillary leak syndrome	*Aminoglycosides, beta-lactams, daptomycin, hydromorphone, morphine, vancomycin*
		Ascites	
		Mechanical ventilation	
		Hypoalbuminemia	Albumin-bound drugs
			Amiodarone, ceftriaxone, midazolam, morphine, phenytoin, propofol, valproic acid, warfarin
		Extracorporeal circuits with expansive surface area (ECMO)	Lipophilic drugs
			Diazepam, fentanyl, fluoroquinolones, macrolides, midazolam, propofol
	↓ Vd	Decreased α1-acid glycoprotein	Drugs bound to α1-acid glycoprotein
			Azithromycin, carvedilol, fentanyl, lidocaine, olanzapine, phenobarbital
Metabolism	↑ Metabolism	Hepatic enzyme induction	Flow-dependent drugs (hepatic extraction ratio >0.7)
		Augmented hepatic blood flow	*Propofol, midazolam, morphine, metoprolol*
	↓ Metabolism	Hepatic enzyme inhibition	Flow-independent drugs (hepatic extraction ratio <0.3)
		Decreased hepatic blood flow	*Warfarin, diazepam, phenytoin*

(Continued)

TABLE A3-1	Pharmacokinetic Changes in Critical Illness (*Continued*)		
Pharmacokinetic Parameter	**Changes in the Critically Ill**	**Etiologies**	**Example Drugs Affected**
Excretion	↑ Clearance	Augmented renal clearance	Renally eliminated medications
		Extracorporeal removal	*Beta-lactam antibiotics, vancomycin, enoxaparin, gabapentin, levetiracetam*
	↓ Clearance	Acute kidney injury	Nephrotoxic medications
			Aminoglycosides, NSAIDs, antivirals, contrast

ECMO, extracorporeal membrane oxygenation; GI, gastrointestinal; NSAIDs, non-steroidal anti-inflammatory drugs; Vd, volume of distribution.

TABLE A3-2	Defining the Acronym: FAST HUGS BID	
Definition and Guidelines	**Purpose and Principles**	**Potential Pharmacologic Interventions**
Feeding	Replenish nutritional stores	Enteral nutrition formulas
American Society for Parenteral and Enteral Nutrition	Maintain gut function	Gastric motility agents
	Data suggest reductions in infectious complications (eg, pneumonia) and mortality with enteral nutrition	Parenteral nutrition
Analgesia	Maintain patient comfort due to interventions, procedures, or chronic pain	Acetaminophen
		Neuropathic-acting agents
	Analgesia-first approach (ie, analgosedation) to limit sedative agents	Nonsteroidal anti-inflammatory drugs
		Opioids
Sedation	Maintain patient comfort due to interventions or procedures	Benzodiazepines
		Dexmedetomidine
	Respiratory depression for mechanical ventilation and severe respiratory failure	Ketamine
		Propofol
	Lightest level of sedation possible preferred; daily sedation interruption	
Thromboembolic prophylaxis	Reduction in incidence of venous thromboembolism	Enoxaparin
		Heparin
	Balance with risk of bleeding	
Head-of-bed elevation (45°)	Reduces aspiration events and pneumonia	N/A

(*Continued*)

TABLE A3-2	Defining the Acronym: FAST HUGS BID (*Continued*)	
Stress **U**lcer prophylaxis	Reduction in stress-related mucosal damage (eg, gastrointestinal bleeding)	Histamine$_2$-receptor antagonists
	Risk based on risk factors related to bleeding (eg, coagulopathy)	Proton pump inhibitors
	Data inconsistent on benefits	
Glycemic control	Prevent hypoglycemia and hyperglycemia in setting of critical illness	Basal insulin
	Studies indicate improved mortality, length of stay, and reduced infections by prevention hyperglycemia	Insulin infusion
		Sliding scale insulin
	Hypoglycemia associated with increased mortality	
	Goal range dependent on population (eg, cardiac)	
Spontaneous breathing trial	Limits duration of mechanical ventilation	Decreasing analgesia/ Sedation
	Limits amount of sedatives a patient is exposed to	
Bowel regimen	Prevention of ileus with immobility or opiate therapy	Laxatives
		Stool softeners
Indwelling catheter removal	Removal of unnecessary lines and drains to prevent catheter-related infections	N/A
De-escalation of antibiotics	Constant evaluation of need/ Appropriateness for antibiotics	Antibiotics
	Reduction in multidrug-resistant organisms	

TABLE A3-3	Management of Pain, Agitation, and Delirium (PAD)
Assess for presence of PAD	
Pain	≥4 times per nursing shift and as needed with NRS, BPS, CPOT
Agitation/ Sedation	≥4 times per nursing shift and as needed with RASS and SAS
Delirium	Once per nursing shift and as needed with CAM-ICU and ICDSC
Identify and correct inciting factors when possible	
Establish patient-specific treatment goals	
Nonpharmacologic management	
Pain	Massage therapy, relaxation techniques, cold packs, manipulative medicine
Agitation	Manage pain and discomfort, provide reassurance, support, and empathetic explanations for procedures, diagnostic tests, and diagnoses, avoid excessive noise, immobility, constipation, and physical restraints
Delirium	Correct modifiable risk factors, promote diurnal sleep patterns, and orientation to person, place, circumstance, encourage family visitation, provide cognitive stimulation, mobility efforts, and limit sedation
Pharmacologic management	
Pain	Opioids and non-opioids for non-neuropathic, gabapentinoids for neuropathic pain, multimodal options for both
Agitation	Analgosedation, propofol, or dexmedetomidine for most patients. Reserve benzodiazepines for specific indications
Delirium	Dexmedetomidine for agitated delirium that interferes with weaning from mechanical ventilation. The role of antipsychotics is uncertain
Assess response to therapy; if not adequate, consider alternative approach	
Determine plan for withdrawal of pharmacotherapy and transition of care	

BPS, Behavioral Pain Scale; CAM-ICU, Confusion Assessment Method for the ICU; CPOT, Critical Care Pain Observational Tool; ICDSC, Intensive Care Delirium Screening Checklist; NRS, Numeric Rating Scale; RASS, Richmond Agitation Scale; SAS, Sedation Agitation Scale.

TABLE A3-4 Common ICU Medications Associated with Agitation and Delirium

Category	Medication or Class	Agitation	Delirium	With Use	With Withdrawal
Antibiotic	Cefepime	X	X	X	
	Macrolides	X		X	
	Fluoroquinolones	X	X	X	
	Voriconazole		X	X	
Anticholinergic	Diphenhydramine		X	X	
Anticonvulsant	Gabapentin	X			X
	Levetiracetam	X		X	
	Pregabalin	X			X
Antidepressant	Amitriptyline	X	X		X
	Selective serotonin reuptake inhibitors	X	X	X	X
	Serotonin norepinephrine reuptake inhibitors	X	X	X	X
Gabaminergic	Benzodiazepines	X	X	X	X
Miscellaneous	Corticosteroids	X	X	X	
	Digoxin	X	X	X	
	Ketamine	X	X	X	X
	Psychoactive medications	X	X	X	X

TABLE A3-5	Selected Pharmacotherapy Recommendations from the 2013 PAD and the 2018 PADIS Guidelines[a]	
Recommendation and Guideline Year		**Recommendation Grade[b]**
Pain		
Use opioids as first-line therapy for nonneuropathic pain (2013)		Strong
Use multimodal approach to decrease opioid exposure (2013 and 2018)		Conditional
Use enteral gabapentin, pregabalin, or carbamazepine with opioids for neuropathic pain (2013 and 2018)		Strong
Use enteral gabapentin, pregabalin, or carbamazepine with opioids for pain <u>after cardiovascular surgery</u> (2018)		Conditional
Use opioid (2013) or NSAID as an opioid alternative for procedural pain (2018) along with nonpharmacologic interventions		Conditional
Use an assessment-driven, protocol-based stepwise approach for pain management (2018)		Conditional
Use thoracic epidural anesthesia/analgesia for pain associated with abdominal aortic aneurysm surgery (2013)		Strong
Use thoracic epidural analgesia for pain associated with rib fractures (2013)		Conditional
Agitation/Sedation		
Use an analgesia-first sedation approach in mechanically ventilated patients (2013) in conjunction with an assessment-driven, protocol-base, stepwise approach for sedation management (2018)		Conditional
Titrate sedatives to light (vs. deep) sedation (2013 and 2018) or allow for daily sedative interruption		Strong (2013) and conditional (2018)
Propofol or dexmedetomidine are preferred over benzodiazepines for sedation (2013 and 2018)		Conditional
Delirium		
Do not use haloperidol or atypical antipsychotics to prevent delirium (2013 and 2018)		Conditional
Do not routinely use haloperidol or atypical antipsychotics to treat delirium (2018)		Conditional
Use dexmedetomidine for delirium in ventilated patients where agitation is precluding weaning or extubation (2018)		Conditional

[a]Barr J, Fraser GL, Puntillo K, et al. Clinical practice guidelines for the management of pain, agitation, and delirium in adult patients in the intensive care unit. *Crit Care Med*. 2013;41:263–306; Devlin JW, Skrobik Y, Gelinas C, et al. Clinical practice guidelines for the prevention and management of pain, agitation/sedation, delirium, immobility, and sleep disruption in adult patients in the intensive care unit. *Crit Care Med*. 2018;46:e825–e873.

[b]Strong recommendation that applies to almost all patients is based on moderate- to high-quality data where the benefits clearly outweigh the burdens; conditional recommendation that applies to most patients but with significant exceptions based on context using data that are conflicting, low quality, insufficient, or involve limited patient populations where there may be a close balance between benefits and burdens.

TABLE A3-6   Common ICU Analgesics and Sedatives Administered as Infusions

Drug	MOA	Dosing Range[a]	PK/PD Properties	ADR and Special Populations	Comments
Analgesics					
Fentanyl	μ agonist	25–200 mcg/hr LD = 50–100 mcg	1–2 min onset; 2–4 hr half-life; CYP3A metabolism; no active metabolites	Serotonin syndrome; caution with SSRI and SNRI	Rapid onset and offset Useful in kidney disease Less hypotension vs. morphine Interaction with CYP3A metabolized drugs (midazolam)
Hydromorphone	μ agonist	0.5–4 mg/hr LD = 0.5–2 mg	5–10 min onset; 2–3 hr half-life; glucuronidation; neurotoxic metabolite	Rare neurotoxicity due to metabolite accumulation in kidney disease	Slower onset than fentanyl, but longer duration No CYP interactions and no serotonin syndrome
Morphine	μ agonist	2–30 mg/hr LD = 2–5 mg	5–10 min onset; 3–4 hr half-life; demethylation and glucuronidation; active metabolites	Hypotension Accumulation of active metabolites in kidney disease	Venodilation from histamine release
Remifentanil	μ agonist	0.5–15 mcg/kg/hr LD = 1.5 mcg/kg	1–3 min onset; 3–4 min half-life; esterase metabolism; no active metabolites	Allows frequent evaluations of neurologic function Possible hypertension	Drug clearance unaffected by organ dysfunction Use IBW to dose obese patients Costly
Ketamine	NMDA receptor antagonist	0.05–0.4 mg/kg/hr	1 min onset; 2–3 hr half-life; demethylation; active metabolite	Psychological disturbances	Does not interfere with respiratory function Useful for opioid-tolerant patients
Sedatives					
Dexmedetomidine	Central α₂ agonist	0.2–1.4 mcg/kg/hr	5–10 min onset; 3 hr half-life; CYP2A6 metabolism and glucuronidation; no active metabolites	Bradycardia and hypotension	Does not interfere with respiratory function Allows "cooperative sedation" Opioid sparing properties Less delirium than midazolam

| Midazolam | GABA agonist | 1–5 mg/hr LD = 1–5 mg | 2–3 min onset; 3–11 hr half-life; CYP3A metabolism; active metabolites | Delirium Context-sensitive half-life | Less hypotension than propofol or dexmedetomidine Allows deep sedation and amnesia CYP3A interactions |
| Propofol | GABA agonist | 5–50 mcg/kg/min | 1–2 min onset; 3–12 hr half-life; CYP2B6 and CYP3A metabolism; no active metabolites | Hypotension PRIS Hypertriglyceridemia Pancreatitis | Allows easy goal titration and neurologic evaluations Can provide deep sedation with amnesia No analgesia Interacts with midazolam |

[a]Typical dosing range for adult ICU patients; analgesic dosing requirements for pain relief may exceed these recommendations as will sedative dosing requirements to produce deep sedation.

ADR, adverse drug reaction; cooperative sedation, ability to participate in care and follow commands; CYP, cytochrome P450; GABA, γ-aminobutyric acid; hr, hour; IBW, ideal body weight; LD, loading dose; min, minute; MOA, mechanism of action; NMDA, N-methyl-d-aspartate; PK/PD, pharmacokinetic/pharmacodynamic; PRIS, propofol-related infusion syndrome; SNRI, serotonin norepinephrine reuptake inhibitor; SSRI, selective serotonin reuptake inhibitor.

(See the following chapters for more detailed discussions of these topics:

- *e/Chapter 25, Critical Care: General Topics in Critical Care, authored by Adrian Wong and Sandra L. Kane-Gill*
- *e/Chapter 26, Critical Care: Pain, Agitation, and Delirium, authored by Gilles L. Fraser and Richard R. Riker*
- *e/Chapter 27, Critical Care: Considerations in Drug Selection, Dosing, Monitoring, and Safety, authored by Erin F. Barreto and Amy L. Dzierba)*

Drug Allergy

TABLE A4-1	Classification of Allergic Drug Reactions			
Type	Descriptor	Characteristics	Typical Onset	Drug Causes
I	Immediate (IgE mediated)	Allergen binds to IgE on basophils or mast cells, resulting in release of inflammatory mediators	Within 1 hour (may be within 1–6 hours)	Penicillin anaphylaxis, angioedema Blood products Polypeptide hormones Vaccines Dextran
II	Delayed; cytotoxic	Cell destruction occurs because of cell-associated antigen that initiates cytolysis by antigen-specific antibody (IgG) and complement. Most often involves blood elements	Typically >72 hours to weeks	Penicillin, quinidine, quinine, heparin, thiouracils, sulfonamides, methyldopa
III	Delayed; immune complex	Antigen–antibody (IgG or IgM) complexes form and deposit on blood vessel walls and activate complement. Result is a serum sickness-like syndrome or vasculitis	>72 hours to weeks	Penicillins, sulfonamides, minocycline, hydantoins
IV	Delayed; T cell–mediated	Antigens cause activation of T lymphocytes, which release cytokines and recruit effector cells	>72 hours	
	IVa	Th1 cells, interferon-γ, monocytes, and eosinophils respond to the antigen	1–21 days	Tuberculin reaction, contact dermatitis
	IVb	Th2 cells, interleukin-4, and interleukin-5 respond to the antigen	1–6 weeks	Maculopapular rashes with eosinophilia
	IVc	Cytotoxic T cells, perforin, granzyme B, FasL respond to the antigen	4–28 days	Bullous exanthems; fixed drug eruptions
	IVd	T cells and interleukin-8 respond to the antigen	>72 hours	Acute generalized exanthematous pustulosis

TABLE A4-2 Top 10 Drugs and Agents Reported to Cause Skin Reactions	
Drug Name	**Reactions per 1000 Recipients**
Amoxicillin	51.4
Trimethoprim–sulfamethoxazole	33.8
Ampicillin	33.2
Iopodate	27.8
Blood	21.6
Cephalosporins	21.1
Erythromycin	20.4
Penicillin G	18.5
Cyanocobalamin	17.9

Source: Data from Roujeau JC, Stern RS. Severe adverse cutaneous reactions to drugs. N Engl J Med. 1994;331:1272–1285.

TABLE A4-3 Treatment of Anaphylaxis

1. Remove the inciting allergen, if possible.
2. Assess airway, breathing, circulation, and orientation. Support the airway.
3. Cardiopulmonary resuscitation: Start chest compressions (100/min) if cardiovascular arrest occurs at any time.
4. Administer epinephrine 1:1000 (adults: 0.3–0.5 mg; children: 0.01 mg/kg) IM in the lateral aspect of the thigh.
5. Place the patient in a recumbent position.
6. Administer oxygen 8–10 L/min through facemask or up to 100% oxygen as needed; monitor by pulse oximetry, if available.
7. Repeat IM epinephrine every 5–15 minutes for up to 3 injections if the patient is not responding.
8. Establish IV line for venous access. Keep line open with 0.9% saline solution. For hypotension or failure to respond to epinephrine, administer 1–2 L at a rate of 5–10 mL/kg in the first 5–10 minutes. Children should receive up to 30 mL/kg in the first hour.
9. Consider nebulized albuterol 2.5–5 mg in 3 mL of saline for lower airway obstruction; repeat as necessary.
10. In cases of refractory bronchospasm or hypotension not responding to epinephrine because a β-adrenergic blocker is complicating management, glucagon 1d5 mg IV (20–30 mcg/kg; maximum, 1 mg in children) should be given IV over 5 minutes.
11. Give epinephrine by continuous IV infusion for patients with inadequate response to IM epinephrine and IV saline. Add 1 mg (1 mL of 1:1000) of epinephrine to 1000 mL of 0.9% saline solution; start infusion at 2 mcg/min and increase up to 10 mcg/min based on blood pressure, heart rate, and cardiac function.
12. Consider intraosseous access for either adults or children if attempts at IV access are unsuccessful.
13. Consider the antihistamine diphenhydramine (adults 25–50 mg; children 1 mg/kg, up to 50 mg) IM or by slow IV infusion.
14. Consider ranitidine 50 mg in adults and 12.5–50 mg (1 mg/kg) in children. The dose may be diluted in 5% dextrose in water to a volume of 20 mL and injected over 5 minutes.
15. Consider methylprednisolone 1–2 mg/kg/dose up to 125 mg (or an equivalent steroid) to reduce the risk of recurring or protracted anaphylaxis. Prednisone 20 mg orally can be given in mild cases. These doses can be repeated every 6 hours as required.

IM, intramuscular.
Source: Lieberman P, Nicklas RA, Randolph C, et al. Anaphylaxis: A practice parameter update 2015. Ann Allergy Asthma Immunol. 2015;115:341–384.

TABLE A4-4	Procedure for Performing Penicillin Skin Testing

Step 1: Prick Test

This will be performed first on the patient, before proceeding to intradermal testing.

a. Clean the volar surface of either forearm with an alcohol swab.

b. Using an ink pen, draw 3 vertical lines approximately 1 in. (2.5 cm) apart on the designated testing site of the arm.

c. Draw up 0.1 mL of the 4 solutions (Pre-pen, diluted Penicillin G, histamine positive control, and saline negative control) in 4 separate allergy syringes.

d. Apply a small drop of each solution to the separate pre-marked sites on the testing arm.

e. The histamine test site should be the most distal site from the elbow, followed up the arm by saline, Pre-Pen, and Pen G.

f. Puncture the epidermis using a twisting motion with a sterile 22–28 gauge needle at each drop site. Do not draw blood. Very little pressure is required.

g. Read the test in 15–20 minutes: (document test results below)

　1. Test is <u>negative:</u> change in diameter of the wheal is **less than** 3 mm than that observed with the negative control. <u>Proceed to intradermal test.</u>

　2. Test is <u>positive:</u> change in diameter of the wheal is **greater than** 3 mm than that observed with the negative control. As soon as a positive response is observed, the solution should be wiped off the skin. <u>Do not proceed to intradermal test.</u>

　3. The positive control (histamine skin test) should be positive to ensure the results are not falsely negative.

　4. The negative control (saline skin test) should be negative. If a wheal >2–3 mm develops after 20 minutes, repeat prick skin test. Upon retesting, if control still creates a wheal >2–3 mm after 20 minutes, discontinue test and notify the ID Physician and/or the ID Stewardship Pharmacist.

Step 2: Intradermal Test

Only conduct this test if the patient produced a negative result with the prick test in step 1.

a. Select 5 sites on the volar surface on the forearm. These sites should be on the opposite arm from the prick test if possible.

b. Using a 26–30 gauge, short bevel needle, intradermally inject 0.02 mL of Pre-Pen solution **twice** (separate at least 2 cm apart). Mark the margins of the initial blebs with an ink pen.

c. Using separate needles and syringes, intradermally inject diluted Pen G (0.02 mL = 200 units of penicillin) **twice** (separate at least 2 cm apart) and 0.02 mL of saline (separate at least 5 cm apart from other sites).

d. Read in 20 minutes: (document test results below)

　1. Test is <u>negative:</u> there is no increase in the original bleb and no greater reaction than the negative control site.

　2. Test is <u>positive:</u> bleb or wheal increases >2 mm from its original size or is >2 mm larger than the negative control. <u>Patient is NOT to receive penicillin.</u>

Step 3: (Optional) Oral Penicillin Challenge

a. If deemed necessary by ordering physician

　1. Oral penicillin (eg, amoxicillin 250 mg) challenge or graded challenge of target drug in a monitored setting for 30–45 minutes.

Source: Data from Jones BM, Bland CM. Penicillin skin testing as an antimicrobial stewardship initiative. Am J Health Syst Pharm. 2017;74:232–237.

TABLE A4-5 Characteristics of Drug Tolerance Protocols

Underlying Mechanism	Initial Dose	Duration of Protocol	Potential Outcome of Process	Duration of Induced Tolerance	Example
Immunologic IgE (desensitization)	Micrograms	Hours	Desensitization; render mast cells less responsive to degranulation	Temporary	β-Lactam antibiotics; taxanes
Immunologic non-IgE	Milligrams	Hours to days (eg, 6 hours–10 days)	Not known	Temporary	Delayed cutaneous reactions to trimethoprim–sulfamethoxazole in HIV-infected individuals
Pharmacologic	Milligrams	Hours to days (eg, 2 hours–5 days)	Cautious induction of a reaction followed by a shift in a metabolic process	Temporary	Aspirin
Undefined	Micrograms to milligrams	Prolonged; days to weeks	Not known	Temporary	Isolated cutaneous reactions to allopurinol

Source: Solensky R, Khan DA. Drug allergy: An updated practice parameter. Ann Allergy Clin Immunol. 2010;105:259–273.

TABLE A4-6	Induction of Drug Tolerance Protocol for IV Cephalosporin[a]

Preparation of Solutions

	Volume of Diluents (eg, 0.9% NSS)	Total to be Injected in Each Bottle	Final Concentration (mg/mL)
Solution 1	250 mL	10 mg	0.04
Solution 2	250 mL	100 mg	0.4
Solution 3	250 mL	1000 mg	4

Induction of Drug Tolerance Protocol

Step	Solution	Rate (mL/hr)	Time (min)	Administered Dose (mg)	Cumulative Dose (mg)
1	1	2	15	0.02	0.02
2	1	5	15	0.05	0.07
3	1	10	15	0.1	0.17
4	1	20	15	0.2	0.37
5	2	5	15	0.5	0.87
6	2	10	15	1	1.87
7	2	20	15	2	3.87
8	2	40	15	4	7.87
9	3	10	15	10	17.87
10	3	20	15	20	37.87
11	3	40	15	40	77.87
12	3	75	184.4	922.13	1000

[a]Full dose equals 1000 mg. Total time was 349.4 minutes.
NSS, normal saline solution.
Source: Solensky R, Khan DA. Drug allergy: An updated practice parameter. Ann Allergy Clin Immunol. 2010;105:259–273.

(See e/Chapter 104, Drug Allergy, authored by Christopher M. Bland and Bruce M. Jones, for a more detailed discussion of this topic.)

TABLE A5-1	Drugs Associated with Aplastic Anemia

Observational study evidence

Carbamazepine
Furosemide
Gold salts
Mebendazole
Methimazole
Nonsteroidal anti-inflammatory drugs
Oxyphenbutazone
Penicillamine
Phenobarbital
Phenothiazines
Phenytoin
Propylthiouracil
Sulfonamides
Thiazides

Case report evidence (*probable or definite* causality rating)

Acetazolamide
Aspirin
Captopril
Chloramphenicol
Chloroquine
Chlorothiazide
Chlorpromazine
Dapsone
Felbamate
Interferon alfa
Lisinopril
Lithium
Nizatidine
Pentoxifylline
Quinidine
Sulindac
Ticlopidine

MedWatch postmarketing reports 2009–2017

Adalimumab
Aliskiren
Amlodipine
Carvedilol
Dantrolene
Etanercept
Oxcarbazepine
Valsartan

TABLE A5-2	Drugs Associated with Agranulocytosis		
Observational Study Evidence	**Case Report Evidence (*Probable* or *Definite* Causality Rating)**		**MedWatch Postmarketing Reports 2009–2017**
β-Lactam antibiotics	Acetaminophen	Levodopa	Amlodipine
Carbamazepine	Acetazolamide	Meprobamate	Aripiprazole
Carbimazole	Ampicillin	Methazolamide	Benazapril
Clomipramine	Captopril	Methyldopa	Bocepravir
Digoxin	Carbenicillin	Metronidazole	Clozapine
Dipyridamole	Cefotaxime	Nafcillin	Defarasirox
Ganciclovir	Cefuroxime	NSAIDs	Fluoxetine
Glyburide	Chloramphenicol	Olanzapine	Haloperidol
Gold salts	Chlorpromazine	Oxacillin	Hydrochlorothiazide
Imipenem–cilastatin	Chlorpropamide	Penicillamine	Iacosamide
Indomethacin	Chlorpheniramine	Penicillin G	Leflunomide
Macrolide antibiotics	Clindamycin	Pentazocine	Levitiracetam
Methimazole	Clozapine	Phenytoin	Memantine
Mirtazapine	Colchicine	Primidone	Molindone
Phenobarbital	Doxepin	Procainamide	Olanzapine
Phenothiazines	Dapsone	Propylthiouracil	Oxcarbazepine
Prednisone	Desipramine	Pyrimethamine	Paliperidone
Propranolol	Ethacrynic acid	Quinidine	Pantoprazole
Spironolactone	Ethosuximide	Quinine	Pimozide
Sulfonamides	Flucytosine	Rifampin	Propafenone
Sulfonylureas	Gentamicin	Streptomycin	Quetiapine
Ticlopidine	Griseofulvin	Terbinafine	Rifabutin
Valproic acid	Hydralazine	Ticarcillin	Risperidone
Zidovudine	Hydroxychloroquine	Tolbutamide	Sulfasalazide
	Imipenem–cilastatin	Vancomycin	Thiothixene
	Imipramine		Trandolapril
	Lamotrigine		Ziprasidone

NSAID, nonsteroidal anti-inflammatory drug.

TABLE A5-3	Drugs Associated with Hemolytic Anemia

Observational study evidence

Phenobarbital

Phenytoin

Ribavirin

Case report evidence (*probable or definite* causality rating)

Acetaminophen

Angiotensin-converting enzyme inhibitors

β-Lactam antibiotics

Cephalosporins

Ciprofloxacin

Clavulanate

Erythromycin

Hydrochlorothiazide

Indinavir

Interferon alfa

Ketoconazole

Lansoprazole

Levodopa

Levofloxacin

Methyldopa

Minocycline

NSAIDs

Omeprazole

p-Aminosalicylic acid

Phenazopyridine

Probenecid

Procainamide

Quinidine

Rifabutin

Rifampin

Streptomycin

Sulbactam

Sulfonamides

Sulfonylureas

Tacrolimus

Tazobactam

Teicoplanin

Tolbutamide

Tolmetin

Triamterene

MedWatch postmarketing reports 2009–2017

Amlodipine

Bevacizumab

Chlorpropamide

Pegademase

Pioglitazone

Rosiglitazone

NSAID, nonsteroidal anti-inflammatory drug.

TABLE A5-4	Drugs Associated with Metabolic Hemolytic Anemia

Observational study evidence

Dapsone

Rasburicase

Case report evidence (*probable or definite* causality rating)

Ascorbic acid

Metformin

Methylene blue

Nalidixic acid

Nitrofurantoin

Phenazopyridine

Primaquine

Sulfacetamide

Sulfamethoxazole

Sulfanilamide

TABLE A5-5	Drugs Associated with Megaloblastic Anemia

Case report evidence (*probable or definite* causality rating)

Azathioprine

Chloramphenicol

Colchicine

Cotrimoxazole

Cyclophosphamide

Cytarabine

5-Fluorodeoxyuridine

5-Fluorouracil

Hydroxyurea

6-Mercaptopurine

Methotrexate

Oral contraceptives

p-Aminosalicylate

Phenobarbital

Phenytoin

Primidone

Pyrimethamine

Sulfasalazine

Tetracycline

Vinblastine

TABLE A5-6	Drugs Associated with Thrombocytopenia

Observational study evidence

Carbamazepine

Oxaliplatin

Phenobarbital

Phenytoin

Valproic acid

Case report evidence (*probable* or *definite* causality rating)

Abciximab

Acetaminophen

Acyclovir

Albendazole

Aminoglutethimide

Aminosalicylic acid

Amiodarone

Amphotericin B

Ampicillin

Aspirin

Atorvastatin

Bevacizumab

Bisoprolol

Capecitabine

Captopril

Chlorothiazide

Chlorpromazine

Chlorpropamide

Cimetidine

Ciprofloxacin

Clarithromycin

Clopidogrel

Dabigatran

Danazol

Deferoxamine

Diazepam

Diazoxide

Diclofenac

Diethylstilbestrol

Digoxin

Ethambutol

Isotretinoin

Itraconazole

Levamisole

Levofloxacin

Linezolid

Lithium

Low-molecular-weight heparins

Lurasidone

Measles, mumps, and rubella vaccine

Meclofenamate

Mesalamine

Methyldopa

Minoxidil

Morphine

Moxifloxacin

Nalidixic acid

Naphazoline

Naproxen

Nitroglycerin

Octreotide

Olmesartan

Oseltamivir

Oxacillin

p-Aminosalicylic acid

Pantoprazole

Penicillamine

Pentamidine

Pentoxifylline

Piperacillin

Primidone

Procainamide

Pyrazinamide

Quinidine

Quinine

Ranitidine

Recombinant hepatitis B vaccine

Red Bush Tea (Rooibos)

Medwatch postmarketing reports 2009–2017

Acarbose

Adalimumab

Ado-trastuzumab

Alfuzosin

Aliskirin

Amlodipine

Benazepril

Bocepravir

Bortezomib

Chlorambucil

Cladribine

Cotrimoxazole

Dalteparin

Dantrolene

Deferasirox

Didanosine

Drotecogin alfa

Efalizumab

Eltrombopag

Enoxaparin

Epirubicin

Epoprostenol

Eptifibatide

Ethionamid

Filgrastim

Fondaparinux

Glimepiride

Heparin

Hydrochlorothiazide

Indomethacin

Iloprost

Interferon beta 1a

Leflunomide

Losartan

Montelukast

Obinutuzumab

Octreotide

Oxcarbazepine

(Continued)

1005

TABLE A5-6	Drugs Associated with Thrombocytopenia (*Continued*)	
Enzalutamide	Rifampin	Palivizumab
Felbamate	Rivaroxaban	Pamidronate
Fenofibrate	Simvastatin	Pemetrexed
Fluconazole	Sirolimus	Pioglitazone
Gabapentin	Sulfasalazine	Pomalidomide
Gold salts	Sulfonamides	Propylthiouracil
Haloperidol	Sulindac	Quinine
Heparin	Tacrolimus	Raltegravir
Hydrochlorothiazide	Tamoxifen	Rosiglitazone
Ibuprofen	Tolmetin	Rosuvastatin
Inamrinone	Trastuzumab	Spironolactone
Indinavir	Trimethoprim	Sunitinib
Indomethacin	Vancomycin	Telmisartan
Interferon alfa-2b		Torsemide
Isoniazid		Trepostinil
		Ursodiol

(See e/Chapter 121, Drug-Induced Hematologic Disorders, authored by Elisa M. Greene and Tracy M. Hagemann, for a more detailed discussion of this topic.)

Drug-Induced Liver Disease

TABLE A6-1	An Approach to Evaluating a Suspected Hepatotoxic Reaction					
Points	−3	−1	0	+1	+2	+3
What is the temporal relationship? (days)						
From the start of therapy	–	–	??	<5	>90	5–90
From the end of therapy	>30	–	??	–	–	<30
Is there evidence of the concurrent use of a hepatotoxin[a]	Yes	Maybe	??	–	–	No
Is there an alternate cause, such as, viral hepatitis?	Yes	Most likely—Yes	??	Most likely—No		No
Are there extrahepatic signs or symptoms?						
Dermatologic: rash, palmar erythema, cutaneous vasculitis	–	–	No	Yes (+1 for each)	–	–
Dermatologic: spider nevi, white nails (aka Terry nails)	–	–	No	Yes (+1 for each)	–	–
Hematologic: coagulation disorders	–	–	No	Yes (+1 for each)	–	–
Endocrine disorders: insulin resistance, thyroid dysfunction	–	–	No	Yes (+1 for each)	–	–
Endocrine disorders: adrenal insufficiency, hypogonadism	–	–	No	Yes (+1 for each)	–	–
Skeletal muscular: arthralgias, arthritis	–	–	No	Yes (+1 for each)	–	–
Neurological: encephalopathy	–	–	No	Yes (+1 for each)	–	–
Portopulmonary hypertension	–	–	No	Yes (+1 for each)	–	–
Does the literature support a connection with this drug?						
Listed in the product labeling	–	–	–	–	–	Yes

(Continued)

1007

TABLE A6-1	An Approach to Evaluating a Suspected Hepatotoxic Reaction (*Continued*)					
Published reports in the literature	–	–		–	–	Yes	–
No information available, reaction is undocumented	–	–		Yes	–	–	–
	−3						**+4**
Results from a rechallenge with the drug.	Negative	–		–	–	–	Positive

[a]drug, herbal remedy, or other occupational exposure known to be potentially hepatotoxic.
A total score of <7 makes it unlikely that this is a hepatotoxic reaction. As the score approaches 14, the possibility that this is a hepatotoxic reaction increases toward certainty. ?? = uncertain.

TABLE A6-2	Environmental Hepatotoxins and Associated Occupations at Risk for Exposure
Hepatotoxin	Associated Occupations at Risk for Exposure
Arsenic	Chemical plant, agricultural workers
Carbon tetrachloride	Chemical plant workers, laboratory technicians
Copper	Plumbers, sculpture artists, foundry workers
Dimethylformamide	Chemical plant workers, laboratory technicians
2,4-Dichlorophenoxyacetic acid	Horticulturists
Fluorine	Chemical plant workers, laboratory technicians
Toluene	Chemical plant, agricultural workers, laboratory tech
Trichloroethylene	Printers, dye workers, cleaners, laboratory technicians
Vinyl chloride	Plastics plant workers; also found as a river pollutant

TABLE A6-3	Relative Patterns of Hepatic Enzyme Elevation versus Type of Hepatic Lesion			
Enzyme	**Abbreviations**	**Necrotic**	**Cholestatic**	**Chronic**
Alkaline phosphatase	Alk Phos, AP	↑	↑↑↑	↑
5′-Nucleotidase	5-NC, 5NC	↑	↑↑↑	↑
γ-Glutamyltransferase	GGT, GGTP	↑	↑↑↑	↑↑
Aspartate aminotransferase	AST, SGOT	↑↑↑	↑	↑↑
Alanine aminotransferase	ALT, SGPT	↑↑↑	↑	↑↑
Lactate dehydrogenase	LDH	↑↑↑	↑	↑

(*See e/Chapter 55, Drug-Induced Liver Disease, authored by William R. Kirchain and Rondall E. Allen, for a more detailed discussion of this topic.*)

TABLE A7-1	Drugs That Induce Apnea
Mechanism	**Relative Frequency of Reactions**
Central nervous system depression	
Narcotic analgesics	F
Barbiturates	F
Benzodiazepines	F
Other sedatives and hypnotics	I
Tricyclic antidepressants	R
Phenothiazines	R
Ketamine	R
Promazine	R
Anesthetics	R
Antihistamines	R
Alcohol	R
Levodopa	R
Oxygen	R
Respiratory muscle dysfunction	
Aminoglycoside antibiotics	I
Polymyxin antibiotics	I
Neuromuscular blockers	I
Quinine	R
Digitalis	R
Myopathy	
Corticosteroids	F
Diuretics	I
Aminocaproic acid	R
Clofibrate	R

F, frequent; I, infrequent; R, rare.

TABLE A7-2	Drugs That Induce Bronchospasm
Mechanism	**Relative Frequency of Reactions**
Anaphylaxis (IgE-mediated)	
Penicillins	F
Sulfonamides	F
Serum	F
Cephalosporins	F
L-Asparaginase	F
Papain	F
Pancreatic extract	I
Psyllium	I
Subtilase	I
Tetracyclines	I
Allergen extracts	I
Cimetidine	R
Direct airway irritation	
N-acetylcysteine	F
Bisulfite	F
Smoke	F
Smoke inhaled steroids	I
Acetate	R
Crromolyn	R
Precipitating IgG antibodies	
β-Methyldopa	R
Carbamazepine	R
Spiramycin	R
Cyclooxygenase inhibition	
Aspirin/NSAIDs	F
Phenylbutazone	I
Acetaminophen	R
Anaphylactoid mast-cell degranulation	
Iodinated-radiocontrast media	I
Benzalkonium chloride	I
Opioid analgesics	I
Iron-dextran complex	I
Local anesthetics	I
Steroidal anesthetics	I
Platinum	R
Pancuronium bromide	R
Ethylenediamine	R
Pharmacologic effects	
β-Adrenergic agonists	I-F

(Continued)

TABLE A7-2	Drugs That Induce Bronchospasm (*Continued*)
Cholinergic stimulants	I
Anticholinesterases	R
α-Adrenergic receptor blockers	R
Ethylenediamine tetraacetic acid	R
Unknown mechanisms	
ACE inhibitors	I
Monosodium glutamate	I
Anticholinergics	R
Hydrocortisone	R
Isoproterenol	R
Piperazine	R
Tartrazine	R
Sulfinpyrazone	R
Zinostatin	R
Losartan	R

ACE, angiotensin-converting enzyme; F, frequent; I, infrequent; Ig, immunoglobulin; NSAIDs, nonsteroidal anti-inflammatory drugs; R, rare.

TABLE A7-3	Tolerance of Anti-Inflammatory and Analgesic Drugs in Aspirin-Induced Asthma
Cross-Reactive Drugs	**Drugs with No Cross-Reactivity**
Diclofenac	Acetaminophen[a]
Diflunisal	Benzydamine
Fenoprofen	Chloroquine
Flufenamic acid	Choline salicylate
Flurbiprofen	Corticosteroids
Hydrocortisone hemisuccinate	Dextropropoxyphene
Ibuprofen	Phenacetin[a]
Indomethacin	Salicylamide
Ketoprofen	Sodium salicylate
Mefenamic acid	
Naproxen	
Noramidopyrine	
Oxyphenbutazone	
Phenylbutazone	
Piroxicam	
Sulindac	
Sulfinpyrazone	
Tartrazine	
Tolmetin	

[a]A very small percentage (5%) of patients with aspirin-hypersensitivity react to acetaminophen and phenacetin.

TABLE A7-4	Drugs That Induce Pulmonary Edema
Mechanism	**Relative Frequency of Reactions**
Cardiogenic pulmonary edema	
Excessive intravenous fluids	F
Blood and plasma transfusions	F
Corticosteroids	F
β_2-Adrenergic agonists	I
Sodium diatrizoate	R
Hypertonic intrathecal saline	R
Phenylbutazone	R
Noncardiogenic pulmonary edema	
Heroin	F
Methadone	I
Morphine	I
Oxygen	I
Propoxyphene	R
Ethchlorvynol	R
Chlordiazepoxide	R
Salicylate	R
Hydrochlorothiazide	R
Triamterene + hydrochlorothiazide	R
Leukoagglutinin reactions	R
Iron–dextran complex	R
Methotrexate	R
Cytosine arabinoside	R
Nitrofurantoin	R
Dextran 40	R
Fluorescein	R
Amitriptyline	R
Colchicine	R
Nitrogen mustard	R
Epinephrine	R
Metaraminol	R
Bleomycin	R
Iodide	R
Cyclophosphamide	R
VM-26	R

F, frequent; I, infrequent; R, rare.

TABLE A7-5	Drugs That Induce Pulmonary Infiltrates with Eosinophilia (Löffler Syndrome)
Drug	**Relative Frequency of Reactions**
Nitrofurantoin	F
para-Aminosalicylic acid	F
Amiodarone	F
Iodine	F
Captopril	F
Bleomycin	F
L-tryptophan	F
Methotrexate	F
Phenytoin	F
Gold salts	F
Sulfonamides	I
Penicillins	I
Carbamazepine	I
Granulocyte-macrophage colony-stimulating factor	I
Imipramine	I
Minocycline	I
Nilutamide	I
Propylthiouracil	I
Sulfasalazine	I
Tetracycline	R
Procarbazine	R
Cromolyn	R
Niridazole	R
Chlorpromazine	R
Naproxen	R
Sulindac	R
Ibuprofen	R
Chlorpropamide	R
Mephenesin	R

F, frequent; I, infrequent; R, rare.

TABLE A7-6	Drugs That Induce Pneumonitis and/or Fibrosis
Drug	**Relative Frequency of Reactions**
Oxygen	F
Radiation	F
Bleomycin	F
Busulfan	F
Carmustine	F
Hexamethonium	F
Paraquat	F
Amiodarone	F
Mecamylamine	I
Pentolinium	I
Cyclophosphamide	I
Practolol	I
Methotrexate	I
Mitomycin	I
Nitrofurantoin	I
Methysergide	I
Sirolimus	I
Azathioprine, 6-mercaptopurine	R
Chlorambucil	R
Melphalan	R
Lomustine and semustine	R
Zinostatin	R
Procarbazine	R
Teniposide	R
Sulfasalazine	R
Phenytoin	R
Gold salts	R
Pindolol	R
Imipramine	R
Penicillamine	R
Phenylbutazone	R
Chlorphentermine	R
Fenfluramine	R
Leflunomide	R
Mefloquine	R
Pergolide	R

F, frequent; I, infrequent; R, rare.

TABLE A7-7	Possible Causes of Pulmonary Fibrosis

Idiopathic pulmonary fibrosis (fibrosing alveolitis)

Pneumoconiosis (asbestosis, silicosis, coal dust, talc berylliosis)

Hypersensitivity pneumonitis (molds, bacteria, animal proteins, toluene diisocyanate, epoxy resins)

Smoking

Sarcoidosis

Tuberculosis

Lipoid pneumonia

Systemic lupus erythematosus

Rheumatoid arthritis

Systemic sclerosis

Polymyositis/dermatomyositis

Sjögren syndrome

Polyarteritis nodosa

Wegener granuloma

Byssinosis (cotton workers)

Siderosis (arc welders' lung)

Radiation

Oxygen

Chemicals (thioureas, trialkylphosphorothioates, furans)

Drugs (see Tables A7-5, A7-6, and A7-8)

TABLE A7-8	Drugs That May Induce Pleural Effusions and Fibrosis	
Mechanism	**Relative Frequency of Reactions**	
Idiopathic		
Methysergide	F	
Practolol	F	
Pindolol	R	
Methotrexate	R	
Nitrofurantoin	R	
Drug-induced lupus syndrome		
Procainamide	F	
Hydralazine	F	
Isoniazid	R	
Phenytoin	R	
Mephenytoin	R	
Griseofulvin	R	
Trimethadione	R	
Sulfonamides	R	
Phenylbutazone	R	
Streptomycin	R	
Ethosuximide	R	
Tetracycline	R	
Pseudolymphoma syndrome		
Cyclosporine	R	
Phenytoin	R	

F, frequent; I, infrequent; R, rare.

(See e/Chapter 47, Drug-Induced Pulmonary Diseases, authored by Hengameh H. Raissy and Michelle Harkins, for a more detailed discussion of this topic.)

TABLE A8-1	Drug-Induced Kidney Structural–Functional Alterations

Tubular epithelial cell damage

Acute tubular injury/necrosis
  Aminoglycoside antibiotics
  Radiographic contrast media
  Cisplatin, carboplatin
  Ifosfamide
  Amphotericin B
  Cyclosporine, tacrolimus
  Adefovir, cidofovir, tenofovir
  Pentamidine
  Foscarnet
  Zoledronate

Osmotic nephropathy
  Mannitol
  Dextran
  IV immunoglobulin (sucrose)
  Hydroxyethyl starch

Hemodynamically mediated kidney injury

Angiotensin-converting enzyme inhibitors
Angiotensin II receptor blockers
SGLT-2 inhibitors

NSAIDs
Cyclosporine, tacrolimus
OKT3

Obstructive nephropathy

Crystal nephropathy
  Acyclovir
  Sulfonamides
  Indinavir, atazanavir
  Foscarnet
  Methotrexate
  Ascorbic acid, ethylene glycol, orlistat

Nephrolithiasis
  Sulfonamides
  Triamterene
  Indinavir, atazanavir
Nephrocalcinosis
  Oral sodium phosphate solution

Glomerular disease

Minimal change disease
  NSAIDs, COX-2 inhibitors
  Lithium
  Pamidronate
  Interferon-α and β
Membranous disease
  NSAIDs
  Penicillamine
  Captopril

Focal segmental glomerulosclerosis
  Pamidronate
  Interferon-α and β
  Lithium
  Sirolimus
  Anabolic steroids
  Tyrosine kinase inhibitors

(Continued)

TABLE A8-1	Drug-Induced Kidney Structural–Functional Alterations (*Continued*)

Tubulointerstitial disease

Acute allergic interstitial nephritis	Chronic interstitial nephritis
Penicillins	Cyclosporine
Ciprofloxacin	Lithium
NSAIDs, cyclooxygenase-2 inhibitors	Aristolochic acid
Proton pump inhibitors	Papillary necrosis
Loop diuretics	NSAIDs, combined phenacetin, aspirin, and caffeine analgesics

Renal vasculitis, thrombotic microangiopathy, thrombosis, and cholesterol emboli

Vasculitis and thrombosis	Methamphetamines
Hydralazine	Cyclosporine, tacrolimus
Propylthiouracil	Adalimumab
Allopurinol	Bevacizumab
Penicillamine	Cholesterol emboli
Gemcitabine	Warfarin
Mitomycin C	Thrombolytic agents

TABLE A8-2	Potential Risk Factors for Aminoglycoside Nephrotoxicity

(A) Related to aminoglycoside dosing

Large total cumulative dose

Prolonged therapy

Trough concentration exceeding 2 mg/L[a]

Recent previous aminoglycoside therapy

(B) Related to synergistic nephrotoxicity. Aminoglycosides in combination with

Cyclosporine

Amphotericin B

Vancomycin

Diuretics

Iodinated radiographic contrast agents

Cisplatin

NSAIDs

(*Continued*)

| TABLE A8-2 | Potential Risk Factors for Aminoglycoside Nephrotoxicity (*Continued*) |

(C) Related to predisposing conditions in the patient

Preexisting kidney disease

Diabetes

Increased age

Poor nutrition

Shock

Gram-negative bacteremia

Liver disease

Hypoalbuminemia

Obstructive jaundice

Dehydration

Hypotension

Potassium or magnesium deficiencies

[a]The equivalent concentration in SI molar units is 4.3 μmol/L for tobramycin and 4.2 μmol/L for gentamicin.

| TABLE A8-3 | Recommended Interventions for Prevention of Contrast Nephrotoxicity |

Intervention	Recommendation	Recommendation Grade[a]
Contrast	Minimize contrast volume/dose	A-1
	Use noniodinated contrast studies	A-2
	Use low- or iso-osmolar contrast agents	A-2
Medications	Avoid concurrent use of potentially nephrotoxic drugs (eg, NSAIDs, aminoglycosides)	A-2
Isotonic sodium chloride (0.9%)	Initiate infusion 3–12 hours prior to contrast exposure and continue 6–24 hours postexposure	A-1
	Infuse at 1–1.5 mL/kg/hr adjusting postexposure as needed to maintain a urine flow rate of 150 mL/hr	
	Alternatively, in urgent cases, initiate infusion at 3 mL/kg/hr, beginning 1 hour prior to contrast exposure, then continue at 1 mL/kg/hr for 6 hours postexposure	

[a]*Strength of recommendations*: A, B, and C are good, moderate, and poor evidence to support recommendation, respectively. *Quality of evidence*: (1) evidence from more than one properly randomized, controlled trial; (2) evidence from more than one well-designed clinical trial with randomization, from cohort or case-controlled analytic studies or multiple time series, or dramatic results from uncontrolled experiments; and (3) evidence from opinions of respected authorities, based on clinical experience, descriptive studies, or reports of expert communities.

TABLE A8-4	Drugs Associated with Allergic Interstitial Nephritis

Antimicrobials

Acyclovir	Indinavir
Aminoglycosides	Rifampin
Amphotericin B	Sulfonamides
β-Lactams	Tetracyclines
Erythromycin	Trimethoprim–sulfamethoxazole
Ethambutol	Vancomycin

Diuretics

Acetazolamide	Loop diuretics
Amiloride	Triamterene
Chlorthalidone	Thiazide diuretics

Neuropsychiatric drugs

Carbamazepine	Phenytoin
Lithium	Valproic acid
Phenobarbital	

Nonsteroidal anti-inflammatory drugs

Aspirin	Ketoprofen
Indomethacin	Phenylbutazone
Naproxen	Diclofenac
Ibuprofen	Cyclooxygenase-2 inhibitors
Diflunisal	
Piroxicam	

Miscellaneous

Acetaminophen	Immune checkpoint inhibitors
Allopurinol	Lansoprazole
Interferon-α	Methyldopa
Aspirin	Omeprazole
Azathioprine	p-aminosalicylic acid
Captopril	Phenylpropanolamine
Cimetidine	Propylthiouracil
Clofibrate	Radiographic contrast media
Cyclosporine	Ranitidine
Glyburide	Sulfinpyrazone
Gold	Warfarin sodium

(See Chapter 63, Drug-Induced Kidney Disease, authored by Thomas D. Nolin and Mark A. Perazella, for a more detailed discussion of this topic.)

Drug-Induced Ophthalmic Disorders

TABLE A9-1	Common Drug-Induced Ophthalmic Disorders, Causative Agents, and Treatment Recommendations	
Reactions	**Causative Agents**	**Treatment Recommendations**
Cataracts	Alkylating agents (busulfan)	Surgical removal of cataract
	Antiestrogens (tamoxifen)	
	Corticosteroids	
	Statins	
Dry eye	Alpha-1 antagonists (alfuzosin, tamsulosin, terazosin)	Nonpharmacologic therapy: (1) warm compresses, (2) increase fluid intake, (3) use humidifier
	Alpha-2 agonists (apraclonidine, brimonidine)	Increase tear volume: (1) consider artificial tears or other topical lubricants, (2) punctal occlusion
	Anticholinergics (atropine, homatropine, hyoscine, ipratropium, tolterodine)	
	Anticonvulsants (valproic acid)	Decrease inflammation: (1) 0.05% cyclosporine ophthalmic drugs, (2) LFA-1 antagonist ophthalmic drops, (3) short-term ophthalmic glucocorticoids
	Antihistamines (cetirizine, chlorpheniramine, diphenhydramine, doxylamine)	
	Antimalarials (chloroquine, hydroxychloroquine)	Medication changes: (1) discontinue medication, (2) use preservative-free ophthalmic drops
	Antineoplastics (busulfan, cyclophosphamide)	
	Antipsychotics (thioridazine)	
	Anxiolytics (lorazepam)	
	Beta agonists (acebutolol)	
	Beta blockers (atenolol, propranolol)	
	Benzalkonium chloride	
	Bisphosphonates	
	Cannabinoids (dronabinol)	
	Systemic decongestants (pseudoephedrine)	
	Diuretics (furosemide, indapamide, metolazone)	
	Oral contraceptives	
	Retinoids (isotretinoin)	
	Topical decongestants (naphazoline)	
	Tricyclic antidepressants (amitriptyline)	

(Continued)

APPENDICES

TABLE A9-1	Common Drug-Induced Ophthalmic Disorders, Causative Agents, and Treatment Recommendations	
Floppy iris syndrome	Alpha-1 antagonists Benzodiazepines Chlorpromazine Donepezil Duloxetine Finasteride Quetiapine	Preoperative screening for previous and/or current use of causative agents Consider cataract surgery before initiation of alpha-1 antagonist therapy Intracameral alpha-adrenergic agonists (epinephrine, phenylephrine) Intraoperative devices: (1) iris retractors, (2) OVDs, (3) pupil expanders
Optic neuropathy	Amiodarone Ethambutol Linezolid PDE-5 inhibitors (avanafil, sildenafil, tadalafil, vardenafil)	Discontinuation of causative drug as medically appropriate Regular ophthalmic examinations
Retinopathy	Aminoquinolines (hydroxychloroquine, chloroquine) Antiestrogens (tamoxifen) Phenothiazines (chlorpromazine, thioridazine) Retinoids (isotretinoin)	Monitor via regular ophthalmic examinations, patient-reported signs and symptoms Vision loss is irreversible

LFA-1, lymphocyte function-associated antigen 1; OVDs, ophthalmic viscosurgical devices; PDE-5, phosphodiesterase 5.

(See Chapter e112, Drug-Induced Ophthalmic Disorders, authored by Rena Gosser, for a more detailed discussion of this topic.)

Index

Note: Page numbers followed by "*f*" and "*t*" denote figures and tables, respectively.

Index

Index

Index

Index

Index

Index

Index

Index

Index